Accident & Emergency

For Elsevier

Content Strategist: Mairi McCubbin
Content Specialist: Alison McMurdo
Project Manager: Srividhya Vidhyashankar
Designer/Design Direction: Hitchen Miles
Illustration Manager: Jennifer Rose
Illustrator: Antbits Ltd

Accident & Emergency

Theory into Practice

THIRD EDITION

Edited by

Brian Dolan BSc(Hons), MSc(Oxon), MSc(Nurs), RMN, RGN, CHSM
Director of Service Improvement, Canterbury District Health Board, Christchurch, New Zealand;
Director, Dolan & Holt Consultancy Ltd., UK; Formerly Vice Chair, Royal College of Nursing
Emergency Care Association, UK

Lynda Holt MA, DipHS RGN, EN(G), FInstLM
Managing Director, Health Service 360; Founder, Lynda Holt Academy, UK; Formerly Chair, Royal
College of Nursing Emergency Care Association, UK

BAILLIÈRE TINDALL

ELSEVIER

Edinburgh London New York Oxford Philadelphia St Louis Sydney Toronto 2013

BAILLIÈRE
TINDALL
ELSEVIER

First edition 2000
Second edition 2008
Third edition 2013
Reprinted 2016

ISBN 978-0-7020-4315-4

British Library Cataloguing in Publication Data
A catalogue record for this book is available from the British Library

Library of Congress Cataloging in Publication Data
A catalog record for this book is available from the Library of Congress

Notices
Knowledge and best practice in this field are constantly changing. As new research and experience broaden our understanding, changes in research methods, professional practices, or medical treatment may become necessary.

Practitioners and researchers must always rely on their own experience and knowledge in evaluating and using any information, methods, compounds, or experiments described herein. In using such information or methods they should be mindful of their own safety and the safety of others, including parties for whom they have a professional responsibility.

With respect to any drug or pharmaceutical products identified, readers are advised to check the most current information provided (i) on procedures featured or (ii) by the manufacturer of each product to be administered, to verify the recommended dose or formula, the method and duration of administration, and contraindications. It is the responsibility of practitioners, relying on their own experience and knowledge of their patients, to make diagnoses, to determine dosages and the best treatment for each individual patient, and to take all appropriate safety precautions.

To the fullest extent of the law, neither the Publisher nor the authors, contributors, or editors, assume any liability for any injury and/or damage to persons or property as a matter of products liability, negligence or otherwise, or from any use or operation of any methods, products, instructions, or ideas contained in the material herein.

Printed in Great Britain

Contents

PART 8 Professional issues in the ED

    Lynda Holt

37. Clinical decision-making 537
    Emma Tippins

38. Ethical issues 545
    Karen Sanders

39. Law 553
    Nicola Meeres

40. Health and safety 561
    Kim Sunley

41. Managing issues of culture and power in the ED 571
    Sandra Richardson & Tracey Williams

42. Creating patient flow 577
    Richard Hamilton, Brian Dolan & Michael Ardagh

    Appendix: Normal values 587

    Index 589

Contributors

Prof Michael Ardagh MBChB, DCH, FACEM, PhD
Emergency Physician, Professor of Emergency Medicine, Christchurch School of Medicine and Health Sciences, New Zealand

Tamsin Attenburrow, PGDip (HealSci), RN
Clinical Coach, Emergency Department, Christchurch Hospital, Canterbury District Health Board, New Zealand

Brian Boag BSc (Critical Care), PGDE, PGCHE, RN(A), RN(M), RNT
Senior Lecturer, Faculty of Education, Health and Science, University of Derby, UK

Gerry Bolger MHM, RN
Former Chair of the Royal College of Nursing In-flight Nurses Association and Recent Programme Director for Quality in Nursing Care at the Department of Health (England)

Dr Michael Brown BSc (Hons), MSc, PhD, PGCE, RGN, RNLD, RNT, FHEA
Senior Lecturer, Edinburgh Napier University and Nurse Consultant, NHS Lothian, UK

David Corkill BN, MEmergN, MAdvPrac (Health Prof Edu), Grad Dip App Sc
Emergency Nurse Educator, Emergency Department, Gold Coast Hospital, Queensland, Australia

Caroline Delaforce RGN, RMN
Clinical Nurse, Bayside Mental Health Service Cleveland, Queensland, Australia

Orla Devereux DipMgt, RGN, RM
Clinical Nurse Manager, Emergency Department, Mayo General Hospital, Castlebar, Ireland

Brian Dolan BSc(Hons), MSc(Oxon), MSc(Nurs), RMN, RGN, CHSM
Director of Service Improvement, Canterbury District Health Board, Christchurch, New Zealand; Director, Dolan & Holt Consultancy Ltd., UK; Vice Chair, RCN Emergency Care Association, UK

Kate Gilmour MEmergN, RN
Current Nurse Practitioner Candidate
Early Discharge Emergency Nurse (EDDI nurse), Gold Coast Emergency Department, Queensland, Australia

Paula Grainger MN (Clin), PhD Candidate, RN
Nurse Coordinator, Clinical Projects, Emergency Department, Christchurch Hospital, Christchurch, New Zealand

Richard Hamilton BSc
Business Development Manager, Canterbury District Health Board, New Zealand

Lynda Holt MA, DipHS RGN, EN(G), FInstLM
Managing Director, Health Service 360; Founder, Lynda Holt Academy, UK; Formerly Chair, Royal College of Nursing Emergency Care Association, UK

Heather Josland MHlthSc, PG Cert (Tchg), RN
School of Nursing, Christchurch Polytechnic Institute of Technology (CPIT), New Zealand

Dr Tim Kilner PhD, PGCE, DipIMC RCSEd, RN, BN
Principal Lecturer, Paramedic Sciences, Coventry University, Coventry, UK

Amy Lamb BSc, MSc
Senior Sister, Paediatric Accident and Emergency, Central Manchester University Hospitals NHS Foundation Trust, UK

Prof Janet Marsden BSc, MSc, PhD, RGN, OND, FRCN, FRSM, FFEN
Professor of Ophthalmology and Emergency Care, Manchester Metropolitan University, Manchester, UK

Barry McCarthy RCpN, DipN (NZ), GradCertClinEd
Nursing Director, Emergency Services, Sunshine Coast Health Service District, Queensland, Australia

Nicola Meeres Barrister BA (Hons), DipHE
Associate, Dolan & Holt Consultancy Ltd, Stratford upon Avon, Warwickshire, UK

Samantha Minett BSc (Hons), RN (Adult), RN (Child)
Paediatric Sister, Emergency Department, Colchester Hospital University Foundation Trust, Colchester, UK

Chris Morrow-Frost BA (Hons), DipN
Clinical Site Manager, Chelsea and Westminster Hospital, London, UK

Tim Morse BSc (Hons), MSc, PGCHE, DPSN, RGN
Senior Lecturer in Emergency Care, Coventry University, Coventry, UK

Dr Barbara Neades DipN, BN, PhD, CertA&E, PGCertEd (FE), RNT, ALS (I), TNCC (P), M Phil Law & Ethics Med, RMN, RGN, FFEN
Senior Lecturer, Edinburgh Napier University, Edinburgh, UK

Cormac Norton BSc (Hons), MSc (Health Studies), PGCert, DipPSN (Critical Care), RGN
Senior Lecturer, Emergency Care, De Montfort University, Leicester, UK

Mike Paynter PGDip, CertA&E, RGN, RN, REMT, FFEN
Consultant Nurse, Somerset NHS Foundation Trust, Bridgwater Community Hospital, Somerset, UK

Dr Stewart Piper MSc, PhD, PGDE, RGN
Senior Lecturer, Faculty of Health, Social Care and Education, Anglia Ruskin University, UK

Dr Sandra Richardson BA, PhD, DipSocSci, DipHealSci, DipTertTeach, RGON
Senior Lecturer, Centre for Postgraduate Nursing Studies, University of Otago, New Zealand; Nurse Researcher, Emergency Department, Christchurch Hospital, Canterbury District Health Board, New Zealand

Tina Roche BN, MNSci
(Nurse Practitioner)
Emergency Nurse Practitioner, Queensland Health Forensic and Scientific Services, Queensland, Australia

Karen Sanders MA, RGN, RNT
Senior Lecturer, Faculty of Health and Social Care, London South Bank University, UK

Valerie Small MSc, PG Dip CHSE, A&E Cert, RGN, RNT, RNP, RANP
Advanced Nurse Practitioner (Emergency),
St James's Hospital, Dublin; Associate Lecturer, Trinity College Dublin, Ireland

Richard Smith Grad Cert EN, RN, TNCC (Ins)
Director of Nursing, Marie Rose Centre, Metro South Health Service, Queensland, Australia

Margaret Sowney BSc (Hons), MSc, RNT, RGN, RNLD
Lecturer, School of Nursing, University of Ulster, Londonderry, Northern Ireland

Matthew Stuart DipHE, RN (Child)
Children's Nurse Practitioner, Colchester Hospital University NHS Foundation Trust, UK

Catherine Sumsky GradCertPaediatricCritCare, GradDipChild and Family Health, Grad Dip Clinical Teaching, MNursing, APLS Instructor, RN, CM
Nurse Educator, Emergency, Sydney Children's Hospital, Randwick, Australia

Kim Sunley CMIOSH
Senior Employment Relations Adviser, Royal College of Nursing, London, UK

Jo-Anne Timms Grad Dip Emerg N, MEmergN, MNursing, Nurse Practitioner, Dip Bus, RN
Assistant Director Nursing, Emergency Department Gold Coast Hospital, Adjunct Lecturer, Griffith University, Gold Coast, District Disaster Representative, Queensland, Australia

Emma Tippins MSc, RN
Lead Nurse Emergency Care, Heatherwood and Wexham Park NHS Foundation Trust, UK

Jenni Ward DipAppSc, BAppSc, MHs (Nsg), RN, FRCNA
Education Coordinator, Trauma Service, Princess Alexandra Hospital, Brisbane, Queensland, Australia

Tracey Williams PGCert (HealSci), RGON
Associate Clinical Nurse Manager
Emergency Department, Christchurch Hospital, Canterbury District Health Board, New Zealand

It's a source of mild wonder to reflect how quickly the years have passed since the first edition of *Accident & Emergency: Theory into Practice* was published in 2000. Back then, we proclaimed part of the *raison d'être* for the book was that we did not believe the existing books on the market met the comprehensive and changing professional and educational needs of UK emergency nurses.

Hopefully, the third edition in your hands now and the 15 reprints of the previous editions are testament to doing something right in meeting those needs. That we now have authors from New Zealand, Australia and the Republic of Ireland is also indicative of the broad international reach and appeal this textbook has achieved, something that is a great credit to all the authors, and readers, who have gone before and continue with us in this edition.

Since 2000, the landscape of emergency care has continued to shift and change. The introduction of emergency care access targets in different countries over the last decade to ensure patients are seen, treated and admitted or discharged in a timely fashion may have had its detractors, however, these targets have been instrumental in fostering the kind of whole health system reform that is needed to ensure the patient's journey has as little time wasted as is clinically appropriate.

To all those who think targets are, to paraphrase Irish writer George Bernard Shaw, some kind of 'conspiracy against the professions', it was emergency nurses in particular who led the way for many years in calling for a whole health systems response to crowding in emergency departments (EDs). While one can hit a target and miss the point of it, on balance, for the vast majority of patients they have been a blessing, saving them time that had usually been spent waiting, whether it was for assessment, diagnostics, referrals, treatment and too often, admission. This new edition introduces a chapter dedicated to Creating Patient Flow which both illustrates and underlines why improving emergency care must be a whole-systems rather than just an ED response by underlining that it is flow not volumes of patients that determine the effectiveness of any health system.

The eight-part core structure that has proved so successful from previous editions is also retained, so, we have Trauma Management; Trauma Care; Psychological Dimensions; Life Continuum; Physiology for ED Practice; Emergency Care; Practice Issues in Emergency Care and Professional Issues in Emergency Care.

We appreciate the feedback you have given us about this approach and it has always been especially satisfying to visit emergency departments and minor injuries units, and many other settings besides, where a battered and much-thumbed copy of our book lies readily available to staff to dip into as required. We are particularly excited that, for the first time, this edition of *Accident & Emergency: Theory into Practice* will also be available electronically enabling it to reach emergency nurses in the most remote enclaves of practice.

Emergency nursing and its development are a never-ending journey and those who practice it can inhabit a world where the youngest young and the oldest old, as well as the most and least ill or injured may be seen in just a few hours, or even minutes. Exhilarating at times, frustrating occasionally but never dull. Even for those who do other things in their careers it remains a truism that 'once an emergency nurse, always an emergency nurse'! So, welcome to the third edition of *Accident & Emergency: Theory into Practice*, about which all of us in the family of emergency nursing can say 'this is our guide to make ourselves even better emergency nurses to further improve the patient care we are proud to deliver – wherever we may be'.

Stratford upon Avon, 2013

Brian Dolan
Lynda Holt

PART 1

Trauma management

Pre-hospital care

Tim Kilner and Tim Morse

1

CHAPTER CONTENTS

Introduction

Pre-hospital care is defined as care and treatment provided at the scene of an accident or acute and sudden illness in an ambulance, emergency vehicle or helicopter (Advanced Life Support Group 2011a, Ahl & Nystrom 2012). Historically, nurses have played an important role in the shaping of pre-hospital emergency care in the UK. The contribution of the hospital flying squad and the cardiac ambulance and the nurses working on them should not be underestimated. Not only did these teams provide a service that filled a therapeutic vacuum in patient care, but they were also instrumental in the development and evolution of these services. The work of both the flying squad and the cardiac ambulance significantly influenced the development of ambulance service and ultimately the birth of the paramedic.

The demise of the hospital flying squad has resulted from a reduced need, partly because of the increasing sophistication of ambulance service provision, enabling ambulance staff to manage increasingly complex clinical situations, complemented by the role played by immediate care doctors responding to incidents in partnership with the ambulance service. Perhaps more influential in the demise of the mobile hospital team has been the increasing workloads of Emergency Departments (ED) and their limited resources to release staff to attend incident scenes on a regular basis.

The role for nurses in responding to the scene of emergency incidents has substantially contracted; however, the potential for nursing input at the scene of a major incident remains a possibility. There are developing areas of pre-hospital practice in which the role of nurses remains, firstly the role in inter-hospital transfer of the critically ill and injured, and secondly working as Emergency Care Practitioners (ECPs).

Whatever role nurses play in their contribution to pre-hospital emergency care, they must be able to do so safely and competently. The professional requirements, set down by the Nursing and Midwifery Council (2008), to provide high standards of practice at all times, to use the best available evidence, to keep skills and knowledge up to date and to recognize and work within the limits of personal competence remain valid when working in the pre-hospital environment just as they do in the ED.

Major incidents

It is neither essential nor desirable for all acute hospitals to be able to provide a mobile team in the event of a major incident. The responsibilities for ensuring mobile teams are available rests with the relevant regional or national health commissioning body. They may nominate those hospitals who will be responsible for deploying a Medical Emergency Response Incident Team (MERIT) to the scene of the incident, if requested to do so (DoH Emergency Preparedness Division 2005). In areas where active immediate care or British Association for Immediate Care (BASICS) schemes are operating, the relevant health board may nominate them to provide the on scene response rather than the acute hospitals. It is, however, essential that the emergency department staff are familiar with the local arrangements in their area.

http://dx.doi.org/10.1016/B978-0-7020-4315-4.00001-2

Those hospitals that are identified as being able to provide a MERIT must ensure staff identified to deploy, the staff must understand the role they are to fulfil in the event of an incident, have the necessary competencies to fulfil that role and have received training to fulfil those competencies (DoH Emergency Preparedness Division 2005, 2007, Bland 2011).

However, there are circumstances, although infrequent, when an ED may be requested to provide medical and nursing support at the scene of a major incident to support their ambulance service colleagues. Given that such incidents are likely to be complex and high profile there is a risk that staff agree to respond without carefully considering if they and their fellow healthcare providers can bring additional expertise that will be of clear benefit to patient care and, in addition, to those services already provided.

Use and function of mobile teams

It is essential that guidelines for the call-out of the team and its intended role are clearly defined in the major incident procedures of all interested parties, predominantly, but not exclusively, the acute hospital, the ambulance trust, and the health authority. There is, unfortunately, a long history of hospital teams being called to the scene of an incident where their role has not been clearly defined beforehand, resulting in the team, at best, contributing little to patient outcome and, at worst, putting themselves and others at risk.

In addition to the clarity of purpose, any proposed team activity must be supported with education, training, rehearsal and operational experience. Failure to do so will result in an ill-equipped, poorly trained, undisciplined team working in an environment in which there is no place for them. The need for regular update training and rehearsal is evermore important because requests for assistance are relatively rare, team members are unlikely to have much experience in this aspect of practice.

Unfortunately there is little guidance available to help organizations identify the best use of the mobile team, the criteria for deployment, the equipment the team should have access to and the training team members require. Although arguing for a medical specialty of pre-hospital and retrieval medicine, the Faculty of Pre-hospital Care, Royal College of Surgeons of Edinburgh, give an insight into what competencies may be required of team members in executing their role (Faculty Pre-hospital Care, Royal College of Surgeons of Edinburgh, 2008). They suggest that the specialist role include:

- supporting complex decision making – balancing the risks and benefits associated with at-scene clinical interventions
- supporting complex transport decisions – balancing the risks and benefits associated with pre-hospital triage, mode of transport and level of clinical escort
- provision of alternative forms of analgesic drugs and techniques
- provision of pre-hospital procedural sedation
- provision of pre-hospital emergency anaesthesia
- provision of organ support

- supporting the clinical use of critical care drugs and infusions, such as anaesthesia, vasoactive drugs and blood products
- use of complex monitoring and near patient investigation techniques, such as invasive haemodynamic monitoring and ultrasound.

In addition to the clinical skills required to provide added value to patient care, it is essential that team members have the skills that allow them to operate safely in the pre-hospital environment. They must be both safe and competent to work in environments that are inherently dangerous and where clinical conditions are suboptimal, such as poor lighting, confined spaces, and inclement weather. Additional specialist skills may also be necessary when working at incidents that involve potential hazardous materials.

The problem of an armed perpetrator on scene preventing access to victims is a relatively common problem in so-called 'spree killing' incidents. The perpetrators often commit suicide, but even if this happens confirmation of scene safety often takes time. A comprehensive armed police response is almost always more rapid in urban areas, since this is where most incidents occur. A slower response in more rural locations is almost inevitable. In 2010 twelve people were killed by a gunman in Cumbria, a rural county in the UK. The gunman was mobile and was able to operate at multiple locations for more than two hours before shooting himself. In July 2011, where a lone gunman killed 77 people in Norway, the scene at Utøya Island was additionally complicated by the presence of a powerful long-range weapon and separation of the scene from the mainland by water (Lockey 2012).

Training and rehearsal with colleagues from other disciplines is essential in order to understand on scene command and control procedures and the roles adopted by others. The team should provide something in addition to that of other members of the multidisciplinary team. There is little point in a team arriving on scene and replicating the care that could easily be provided by the ambulance service, and who are more familiar with the operating environment from their day-to-day work.

Potential team members must be familiar with their local plan, to be aware of any requirements for them to provide a MERIT, and their role in the team if requested to participate. Plans should provide outline guidance on the role of the MERIT; however, it is incumbent upon the Ambulance Incident Commander (AIC) and the Medical Incident Commander (MIC) to clearly define the role and purpose of deploying a MERIT and giving advice on the best way of executing their role (DoH Emergency Preparedness Division 2005). This guidance provides examples of the specific skills the team may bring to the scene, such as provision of analgesia or the specialist support of children. There is, however, a clear expectation that the team has received appropriate training for this role.

Resourcing the team often results in the hospital being depleted of key, experienced personnel at a time when their expertise is in greatest demand. Plans must take this into account, ensuring that those required by the regional health board to provide a MERIT response are able to take action

Box 1.1

Essential equipment for mobile teams

- Carbon fibre helmet with chin strap and visor. Helmet should be green in colour with 'nurse' or 'doctor' in white lettering on each side
- Ear defenders — for team members and the patient
- Fire-retardant suit — designed to offer some protection to the wearer should a fire occur, but not designed to allow the wearer to enter a fire
- Warm underclothing — essential during cold weather, especially if the incident is likely to be protracted
- High-visibility jacket — with designation clearly marked front and back. Jacket to have green shoulder and fluorescent lower section with reflective bands
- Heavy duty gloves
- Latex gloves
- Oil- and acid-resistant boots. Wellington boots are not appropriate for the demands of pre-hospital care; they are cold, limit movement and are prone to having liquids poured into them

Additional essential equipment

- Personal identification and money
- Notebook — ideally plasticized with water-resistant pen
- Action card

(After Hodgetts T, McNeill I, Cooke M (2000) The Pre-Hospital Emergency Management Master. London: BMJ Publishing Group.)

to ensure that a team can be assembled with appropriately skilled staff, when required to do so. The plan should not require action that would knowingly deplete essential services and expose the organization and patients to unacceptable risk.

The plan should also identify the equipment that is available to the MERIT, ensuring that it is appropriately packaged for clinical needs, operation and manual handling. The team must also have access to appropriate personal protective equipment, primarily for their safety but with due consideration to the identification of team members and key roles. Staff must therefore be familiar with the clinical and safety equipment they require and the safe and appropriate use of that equipment in the pre-hospital environment. Equipment should, as far as possible, be both compatible and interchangeable with the local ambulance service (Box 1.1).

Deployment of the team

Deployment of the team is often delayed, principally for logistical reasons, such as assembly of the team, collection of the equipment, and availability of transport for the team. Transport is a particular problem as most ambulances and their staff will be committed to patient care and transport and it may be some time before a vehicle is made available to transport the team. In the case of natural disasters, such as flooding or earthquakes, transport may be particularly badly affected due to road damage and loss of infrastructure (Dolan 2011a,b, Dolan et al. 2011).

The AIC is responsible for coordinating ambulance resources at the scene of the incident and, in conjunction with the MIC, coordinating the activity of other NHS resources at the scene of the incident. On arrival at the scene the MERIT must report to the MIC, or the AIC if the MIC has not yet arrived on scene. Under no circumstances should the MERIT self-task at the scene.

The MERIT is likely to deploy close to the incident site, but outside the inner cordon surrounding the actual incident site, a casualty clearing point will be established. This is the interface between the incident site and the chain of evacuation. It is at this point that the MERIT may be of most use.

Triage for transport

Patients will initially be treated by ambulance personnel prior to evacuation to the casualty clearing point. At the casualty clearing station the mobile team will reassess patients prior to making further treatment and transport decisions, identifying those patients who should be dispatched to hospital immediately and those who may wait a short time. The team may also become involved in the care of the critically injured and those patients with less severe injuries prior to their transportation to the receiving hospital. The team should be able to provide complex clinical interventions such as anaesthesia, sedation, and complex pain management. The team may be also able to provide interventions that currently fall outside the remit of ambulance paramedics, such as tube thoracotomy.

Clinical prioritization and decision making may be assisted by the use of major incident triage algorithms. These algorithms vary from the conventional triage operated on a daily basis in the emergency department as they give a low priority for both treatment and transportation of those with critical injury, who will require large amounts of resource to care for them and are unlikely to survive. Where resources are plentiful these patients would be of a high priority, but in a major incident their priority is low, given that providing the required resources may deprive many others, with potentially survivable injuries, of care. This form of triage is often difficult for nurses and doctors to accept, but the aim is to do the greatest good for the greatest number (Barnes 2006).

Triage for treatment usually follows the triage sieve approach (Life Support Group 2011a). This is a physiologically based system that considers the ability to walk, the patency of the airway, the respiratory rate and the capillary refill rate of pulse rate. The physiological parameters are appropriate for adults (Fig. 1.1). For children, the paediatric triage tape provides a suitable alternative with age-appropriate physiological parameters, whilst retaining the algorithm structure of the triage sieve (Wallis & Carley 2006).

After initial treatment in situ and in the casualty clearing station, patients must be prioritized for transport to hospital. Triage for transport employs the triage sort system (Life Support Group 2011a), which is somewhat less crude than the triage sieve. The triage sort requires the measurement of the Glasgow Coma Scale, respiratory rate and systolic blood

This is carried out to rapidly determine priorities for treatment and is initially carried out at the incident site

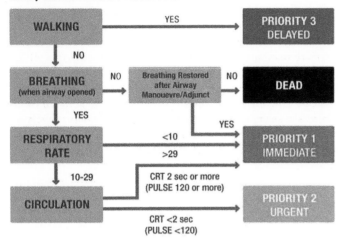

Figure 1.1 ● Triage sieve. ● (After Hodgetts T, Cooke M, McNeill I (2002). The Pre-Hospital Emergency Management Master. London: BMJ Books.)

pressure (Fig. 1.1). Again this relates specifically to adult patients. For children the Paediatric Early Warning Score (PEWS) (Duncan et al. 2006) or Paediatric Advanced Warning Score (PAWS) (Advanced Life Support Group 2011b, Egdell et al. 2008) systems may be more appropriate.

Inter-hospital transfer

There is an increased awareness within the ambulance service that patients need not be taken to the closest emergency department, but to a hospital most likely to be able to meet their needs. For example, it may be permissible to take a patient with a serious head injury directly to a hospital with neurosurgical facilities and bypass the local emergency department. This principle is well established in patients with confirmed acute myocardial infarctions being taken directly to hospitals providing emergency primary angioplasty services. The practice of bypassing local emergency departments has become increasingly viable with the proliferation of air ambulance services.

There are, however, still occasions where the critically ill or injured patient must be transferred from one hospital to another. This work may be undertaken by air ambulance services, some operating 24 hours per day, but others restricted to flying during daylight hours. A number of patients continue to be transported between facilities with the need for a nurse or nurse and doctor escort. There remains the debate whether this role should be undertaken by emergency nurses or by critical care nurses.

The fact remains that from whatever discipline the nurse comes from they must have the requisite skills to be able to care for the patient in transit. The professional requirements remain in that the nurse must recognize and work within the limits of personal competence (NMC 2008). One might argue that the requisite skills mirror those identified by the Faculty of Pre-hospital Care, Royal College of Surgeons of Edinburgh (2008):

- supporting the clinical use of critical care drugs and infusions
- use of complex monitoring and near patient investigation techniques.

One would also expect that nurses intending to adopt this role had developed the skills and competencies through training and rehearsal. In particular they should be familiar with the specific issues that result from the environment. They must be able to work in a confined space and in a moving vehicle. They must also be aware of the difficulties that occur, including not having limitless supplies of electricity or oxygen. For example, will infusion pumps have sufficient battery power to last the journey, even if the journey is delayed or the infusion rate is increased? Is there sufficient oxygen to ventilate the patient for the entire journey, again including unexpected delays or an increase in the required inspired oxygen?

Equipment used for inter-hospital transfers must be fit for purpose and, where possible, interchangeable with the ambulance service. Equipment must also be adequately package for the environment, given the limited space, lack of surfaces for equipment, and appropriate means for securing in the vehicle. It is not appropriate to take unsecured and loose pieces of equipment on a transfer. It is equally unacceptable for a handful of drugs to be taken in a vomit bowl or in the nurse's pocket. Transfers must be conducted in a safe and professional manner.

Emergency care practitioner

In 2000 the Joint Royal Colleges Ambulance Liaison Committee proposed the development of the role of the Practitioner in Emergency Care (PEC). This work introduced the concept that some patients could be adequately assessed and treated at home or the scene of incident without the need for transportation to hospital. Up until this point the vast majority of patients attended by the ambulance service would be transported to the local emergency department.

Over the past decade the role has evolved into that of the Emergency Care Practitioner (ECP); however, the title PEC was never really adopted. Despite a promising start the role of the ECP has not developed as quickly as many would have liked and the numbers of trained ECPs working in ambulance trusts is variable. However, despite some reservations and operational difficulties one interesting development appears to have endured, the employment of emergency nurses as ECPs alongside their paramedic-qualified ECP colleagues. Perhaps this should not be entirely surprising as the skills required in the assessment, treatment and discharge of patients with mainly minor injuries and illness is well established in the role of the Emergency Nurse Practitioner. There are, of course, new skills for emergency nurses working as ECPs to develop, some more obvious than others. For example, emergency nurses used to working in teams need to adapt to be comfortable working as a solo responder, without the range of equipment and patient testing available in the emergency department. Wound care including suturing, for example, has some added complexity in the patient's home when compared with a treatment room in the emergency department.

ECPs may be tasked to a range of emergency calls, such as cardiac arrests or road traffic collisions. This often presents nurse ECPs with a steep learning curve; learning advanced driving skills, scene assessment and management, and resuscitation as a solo responder. Many skills are transferable, but the emergency nurse should not assume that because they are, for example, an Advanced Life Support (ALS) provider they would be able to manage a cardiac arrest single handed in the community. Emergency nurses have much to learn from their paramedic colleagues as paramedics have much to learn from their emergency nurse colleagues.

Conclusion

Nurses can make a valuable contribution to the delivery of pre-hospital patient care and outcome as part of a multidisciplinary team in a major incident, provided their role is clear and that they are properly trained and equipped for the role. The same is true for emergency nurses involved in the inter-hospital transfer of critically ill and injured patients. Emergency nurses with additional training and experience can and do make a valuable contribution to patient care in the pre-hospital environment as ECPs. It will be interesting to see how this role evolves in the next decade.

References

Advanced Life Support Group, 2011a. Major Incident Medical Management and Support: The Practical Approach at the Scene, third ed. BMJ Books, London.

Advanced Life Support Group, 2011b. Advanced Paediatric Life Support: The Practical Approach, fifth ed. BMJ Books, London.

Ahl, C., Nystrom, M., 2012. To handle the unexpected: The meaning of caring in pre-hospital emergency care. International Emergency Nursing 20 (1), 33–41.

Barnes, J., 2006. Mobile medical teams: Do A&E nurses have the appropriate experience? Emergency Nurse 13 (9), 18–23.

Bland, S., 2011. Pre-hospital emergency care. In: Smith, J., Greaves, I., Porter, K. (Eds.), Oxford Desk Reference: Major Trauma, Oxford Medical Publications, Oxford.

Dolan, B., 2011a. Rising from the ruins. Nursing Standard 25 (28), 22–23.

Dolan, B., 2011b. Emergency nursing in an earthquake zone. Emergency Nurse 19 (1), 12–15.

Dolan, B., Esson, A., Grainger, P., et al., 2011. Earthquake disaster response in Christchurch, New Zealand. Journal of Emergency Nursing 37 (5), 506–509.

Duncan, H., Hutchison, J., Parshuram, C.S., 2006. The Pediatric Early Warning System score: A severity of illness score to predict urgent medical need in hospitalized children. Journal of Critical Care 09; 21 (3), 271–278.

Egdell, P., Finlay, L., Pedley, D.K., 2008. The PAWS score: Validation of an early warning scoring system for the initial assessment of children in the emergency department. Emergency Medicine Journal 25 (11), 745–749.

Hodgetts, T., Cooke, M., McNeil, T., 2002. The Pre-Hospital Emergency Management Master. BMJ Books, London.

Wallis, L.A., Carley, S., 2006. Validation of the paediatric triage tape. Emergency Medicine Journal 23, 47–50.

Trauma life support

2

Cormac Norton

CHAPTER CONTENTS

Introduction

Trauma remains the leading cause of death among those under 40 years of age and it is suggested that after cardiovascular disease and cancer, traumatic injury is the leading cause of death across all ages in the developed world (O' Reilly 2003 Span et al. 2007, Greaves et al. 2009). Injuries kill some 5 million people each year, equating to 9 % of worldwide deaths, and young people between the ages of 15 and 44 account for approximately 50 % of global mortality due to trauma (Middleton 2011). There are an estimated 20 000 cases of serious/multiple injuries in England annually (National Audit Office 2010) resulting in approximately 5400 deaths and a significant proportion of victims suffer permanent disability. It is important to acknowledge that these serious injuries, commonly referred to as 'major' trauma, represent a small proportion of workload annually for most Emergency Departments (EDs) – approximated at 0.2 % of normal activity (National Audit Office 2010). In the current economic climate some may question why such an emphasis is placed upon this area of emergency care. The rationale for this may be explained by considering the age group most affected by this epidemic. People under 40 years who may be in gainful employment could work until 65 or more years of age. This employment reflects tax revenue and personal expenditure. This in effect supports the national economy. The loss of those individuals from society from a purely financial perspective is significant. Effective care and treatment may prevent death or disability. It is crucial that quality of care and resources reflect the needs of this demographic. As Cole (2004) notes, the human cost of trauma on society is incalculable.

Reflecting a concept described by the Resuscitation Council (UK) (2010) the 'chain of survival' in trauma care is important when attempting to reduce mortality/morbidity from serious injury (Lott et al. 2009). The continuum of care from scene of accident to definitive care should remain intact. Put simply, communication and standards of care are crucial. The Advanced Trauma Life Support (ATLS®) programme (American College of Surgeons 2008), which follows a sequence of priorities of care, with the objective of minimizing mortality and morbidity, has been widely adopted for trauma patients throughout the world. The adoption of this international system offers many benefits for both the practitioner and patient. ATLS is utilized throughout the UK; a practitioner working in London, for example, should expect to be able to operate the same principles of trauma care in Aberdeen. The system in effect is a language – improving communication between professionals.

The initial assessment component of the system comprises:

- preparation
- primary survey
- resuscitation
- secondary survey
- continuous monitoring and evaluation
- definitive care.

The application of these components and maintenance of the chain of survival is reliant upon excellent teamwork. The composition of the team will vary from hospital to hospital. The principles however remain unchanged:

- strong leadership
- competent team members
- good organization and communication
- excellent cooperation between all medical specialists involved (Lott et al. 2009).

Much of the emphasis on trauma care is on medical assessment and intervention, and defining the role of the nurse within the trauma team can be difficult (Table 2.1).

Table 2.1 Nursing roles within the trauma team

Assessment	Observation of respiratory rate, pulse, BP, capillary refill time, GCS
Intervention	Basic airway management, insertion of vascular access, phlebotomy, i.v. fluid/blood product administration, application of splinting
Monitoring	ECG/cardiac monitoring, arterial lines, capnography, repetition of observations and documentation
Communication	Reassurance and information for the conscious patient, liaison between team members/specialist involvement, communication with tertiary/specialist centres
Leadership	Activating trauma team, coordinating nursing care (including care of relatives/significant others)

This chapter will follow through the sequence of events; in reality, however, many activities occur in parallel or simultaneously and involve a number of team members. For the multiply injured patient, resuscitation of physical condition takes immediate priority, but psychological needs must not be overlooked. For the conscious patient this role is crucial as many patients will have a vivid recollection of the immediate care following their injury. This is an area that nurses may influence greatly through effective communication.

Preparation

High-quality care is important in the pre-hospital phase of trauma care and time spent on scene with the patient should be kept to the minimum (Pre-Hospital Trauma Life Support

Committee 2002). Much debate remains regarding the extent to which pre-hospital practitioners should instigate advanced trauma interventions – the so-called 'scoop and run' versus 'stay and play'. Smith & Conn (2009) contend that there has been no proven benefit to the patient of advanced interventions, e.g., chest drain insertion or rapid sequence induction and endotracheal intubation. This evidence, however, was specific to urban environments, and its validity to more remote incidents may be questionable. The focus of pre-hospital care should be on airway management, control of haemorrhage, immobilization and transfer of the patient to the nearest and most appropriate facility. In many instances, the ambulance service alerts the ED to the impending arrival of a multiply injured patient. This allows time for appropriate preparation of personnel and environment. Irrespective of the level of staffing, a systematic approach to care should apply on every occasion and it should be constantly monitored to maintain optimum effectiveness and efficiency (Sexton 1997). Equally, safety measures are imperative for both staff and patients to ensure no needless harm is caused (see Table 2.2).

Table 2.2 Safety measures during trauma care*

Minimum safety requirements for team members	Gloves Aprons Goggles Lead aprons, where appropriate
Patient safety	Effective infection control measures Maintenance of temperature e.g., blankets or provision of Bair Hugger©

*It is assumed that all staff have been immunized against hepatitis B

Primary survey

The ATLS approach requires a two-stage approach to the management of the patient. The first stage, or primary survey, follows an adapted ABCDE format similar to the initial assessment applied in medical emergencies (Resuscitation Council (UK) 2010). The adaptation introduces cervical spine control, control of haemorrhage and, importantly, environmental control (American College Surgeons 2008). Environmental control should be interpreted as the prevention of hypothermia. The importance of this will be discussed later in this chapter. It may help to remember the adapted approach as AcBDE. The addition of the letter 'F' as Fahrenheit may help some remember the need for temperature control (Table 2.3).

The primary survey is a rapid assessment aiming to detect life-threatening problems and dealing with them as they are discovered. Although the survey would appear to occur sequentially, i.e., Ac, B then C etc., in fact in the team context each component may be assessed simultaneously. In many cases in the UK an anaesthetist may assess and manage the airway while another member assesses breathing, another controls haemorrhage, and so on.

Table 2.3 Sequence of primary survey

	Activity
Ac	Airway with cervical spine control
B	Breathing
C	Circulation and control of haemorrhage
D	Disability
E	Exposure
F	**Fahrenheit** – control of environment

Airway with cervical spine control

The management of a patient's airway takes precedence over all other aspects of patient care. Cervical spine control should be instigated simultaneously. The ability of the patient to answer simple questions confirms that the airway is patent and that sufficient oxygen is perfusing the brain to elicit a reply. A physical examination of the airway should still be undertaken (American College of Surgeons 2008).

If the patient does not respond to a simple question, airway obstruction should be assumed and measures should be taken to relieve this immediately. The most common reason for obstruction in the unconscious patient is partial or complete occlusion of the oropharynx by the tongue. Saliva, vomit and blood may exacerbate the problem. Interventions should begin with the simplest, progressing to the more complex if necessary. A chin lift or jaw thrust should pull collapsed soft tissues out of the airway. Any debris or foreign bodies must be physically removed. Suction can be very effective, using a tonsil tip/rigid (Yankeur) suction catheter. Cole (2004) recommends the tip of the Yankeur suction catheter be kept in sight to ensure it is not inserted too deeply causing the patient's gag reflex to be stimulated. Equally, blind finger sweeps should not be used as this may further push foreign objects into the airway.

More active measures may be required for those who are unable to maintain their own airway. A nasopharyngeal airway will ensure patency in the conscious patient, without causing a gag reflex. This may be particularly useful for those with a fluctuating conscious level. Caution should be exercised, however, in patients with a head injury. The presence of a fracture of the base of skull precludes the use of this device, as accidental placement of the airway in the cranial vault is a possibility (Greaves et al. 2009). For the unconscious patient, an oropharyngeal (Guedel) airway may be helpful; however, its use increases the risk of vomiting.

Many multiply injured patients need emergency endotracheal (ET) intubation early on in their management. This procedure carries with it certain risks, particularly in the trauma patient. Cervical spine immobilization must be maintained throughout intubation, making the procedure more complex. The patient is often shocked, can have a damaged airway, and frequently has a full stomach. ET intubation in inexperienced hands can be fraught with danger. Ideally, it should be performed by someone with appropriate trauma and anaesthetic skills.

If oral or nasal intubation fails to secure an airway in the patient with obstruction within 60 seconds, and the patient cannot be ventilated with a bag-valve-mask (BVM) system for reasons such as facial fractures, the nurse should prepare for an emergency cricothyroidotomy. Several periods of apnoea caused by repeated attempts at intubation can result in dangerous levels of hypoxia. A needle cricothyroidotomy can establish a temporary airway swiftly, but will need to be followed by a surgical cricothyroidotomy or a tracheostomy within 30–45 minutes.

A definitive airway should be established if there is any doubt about the patient's ability to maintain airway integrity (American College of Surgeons 2008). After any intervention the patency of the airway should be re-checked. A cuffed tube placed in the trachea is the gold standard for securing and protecting the airway. However, the laryngeal tube airway and the intubating laryngeal mask airway (LMA) are recent advances in airway management that can facilitate intubation in the patient with a difficult airway (American College of Surgeons 2008, Stoneham et al. 2001).

Patients suffering significant blunt force trauma or having a mechanism of injury that would lead the practitioner to suspect an injury above the clavicles should be considered to have a cervical spine injury unless proven otherwise. The same principles should be applied where the patient has an altered level of consciousness. This is commonly the case in the patient whose mechanism of injury is complicated by the ingestion of alcohol. To prevent secondary injury to the spinal cord the neck must be immobilized. This is achieved using a rigid cervical collar and head blocks with tape.

It should be noted that immobilizing a patient in a supine position increases the risk to an unsecured airway from aspiration of stomach contents. It is imperative therefore that the patient is never left unsupervised, and that functioning suction equipment is readily available. Communication with the conscious patient will need to be adapted. The practitioner should approach the patient from an angle that removes temptation for the patient to try to move their head.

For those patients who are unable to remain still and might be thrashing around on the trolley, a semi-rigid collar can be applied until the patient is calm enough to tolerate more confining measures. Neurological examination alone does not exclude a cervical spine injury. Remember also that a patient who is agitated should be considered hypoxic until proven otherwise.

Breathing

A patent airway does not automatically mean that the patient is able to breathe properly. The patient's chest should be watched carefully, for the rise and fall of the chest wall, on both sides. The assessor should listen for breath sounds and feel for exhaled breath. If the patient is not breathing or is breathing inadequately, mechanical ventilation using a BVM system with high-flow oxygen should be instituted. This is usually more effective when performed by two people, one to seal the airway and one to squeeze the self-inflating bag.

Efficiency of breathing should be established by applying the acronym RIPPA: *R*espiratory rate, *I*nspection, *P*alpation, *P*ercussion and *A*uscultation (Table 2.4).

Breathing that is unequal or asymmetrical may indicate bony injury or an underlying pneumothorax. Pulse oximetry is a valuable monitor, as peripheral oxygen saturation is a good measure of breathing efficiency; however, it must be remembered that the reading may not be accurate in a shocked, hypothermic, or burned trauma patient (Casey 2001). Where the patient is intubated, the use of colorimetric carbon-dioxide-measuring devices is regarded as essential to ensure correct tube placement. All trauma patients should receive high-flow oxygen (American College of Surgeons 2008). Metabolic demand following serious injury increases significantly. Inadequate oxygen delivery to cells can result in cell damage. In some cases this can result in an inflammatory response known as systemic inflammatory response syndrome (SIRS) similar to that seen in the septic patient (Adams & Osborne 2009). This can further complicate the condition of a seriously injured patient. A concentration of approximately 95% arterial saturation can be achieved by administering oxygen at 15 L/min through a non-rebreather oxygen mask.

Any life-threatening condition encountered during the assessment of breathing should be corrected immediately. These include:

- airway obstruction
- tension pneumothorax
- open pneumothorax (sucking chest wound)
- massive haemothorax
- flail chest
- cardiac tamponade.

Sucking chest wounds should be covered. Chest decompression will be required immediately in the event of a tension pneumothorax, as this dramatically compromises ventilation and circulation. Equipment for inserting a chest drain should be prepared following a needle thoracentesis. A large flail segment with pulmonary contusion or a massive haemothorax should be treated straight away. If the patient is unable to maintain adequate ventilation unassisted, endotracheal intubation may be required, with mechanical ventilation. After any

manoeuvre is used to correct inadequate ventilation, breathing should always be rechecked.

Circulation with haemorrhage control

The most significant contributions to developments in trauma care in recent years have emanated from military medical/nursing care (Champion & Leitch 2012). Conflicts in Afghanistan and Iraq in particular have forced military surgeons to adapt and improve interventions to improve outcomes in the most extreme injuries (Duncan & Moran 2009, Greaves et al. 2009). Many of these developments have made their way into civilian trauma care. Despite improvements in trauma care, uncontrolled bleeding contributes to 30–40% of trauma-related deaths and is the leading cause of potentially preventable early in-hospital deaths (Kauver et al. 2006, Span et al. 2007). Hypotension in the injured patient should be assumed to be due to haemorrhage until proven otherwise (Duncan & Moran 2009). Although assessment of circulation and control of bleeding would usually follow assessment of airway and breathing where assessment is sequential, there are occasions where control of haemorrhage may take precedence. Catastrophic haemorrhaging, i.e., rapid bleeding likely to result in imminent death, for example, following stab injury, should be dealt with immediately. The military adapt the ATLS protocol to <C>AcBCDE, where <C> represents control of catastrophic haemorrhage (Greaves et al. 2009, Sapsford 2008). This may take the form of direct pressure and elevation where possible. In specific circumstances, however, particular measures may need to be taken that were previously unavailable or avoided in civilian trauma care. Two specific interventions include the judicious use a tourniquet, and the use of haemostatic agents, e.g., Celox®.

Determination of the patient's circulatory status should be made by assessing:

- skin colour and general appearance – check for the presence of pallor, diaphoresis (sweating) and temperature of extremities
- pulse – rate, depth and volume. Tachycardia in the presence of a normal blood pressure (normotension) may be the only indication of hypovolaemia in the injured patient. The absence of a pulse following serious injury is a very poor prognostic indicator. Very few patients recover from a cardiac arrest in this situation. The most recent ATLS guidelines recommend that where a patient suffering penetrating trauma has no cardiac output that no resuscitation effort should be made (American College of Surgeons 2008)
- conscious level – the reduction in cellular perfusion in hypovolaemia results in anxiety in the early stages or confusion/agitation in later stages. These are important signs, and the nurse communicating with the patient may be in the ideal position to observe any alteration in this.

Fluid resuscitation (the replacement of fluid in the presence of hypovolaemia) is the subject of much debate and research in recent years. To facilitate fluid administration at least two short, wide-bore cannulae are inserted (14–16 gauge) into

Table 2.4 Assessment of breathing (RIPPA)	
Respiratory rate	Observing rate and peripheral oxygen saturation
Inspection	Symmetry of chest expansion, cyanosis, use of accessory muscles, tracheal shift from the midline, engorged neck veins, any sucking chest wounds
Palpation	Crepitus, surgical emphysema, sites of tenderness
Percussion	This may help determine the presence of haemothorax or pneumothorax
Auscultation	Bilateral air entry, presence of abnormal or absence of sounds

large veins as proximal in peripheries as possible, e.g., antecubital fossa. Lines should not be placed in injured extremities if they can be avoided. It is important to remember that the rate of intravenous (i.v.) infusion is not determined by the size of the vein, but by the internal diameter of the cannula, and is inversely affected by its length. Where venous access proves difficult or impossible alternatives include venous cut down or intraosseous cannulation (Hunt & Hunt 2011).

The ATLS system currently advocates the principle of fluid challenge. According to this protocol an initial fluid bolus of two litres of warmed Hartmann's solution is administered through a blood-giving set (American College of Surgeons 2008). The patient's response to this 'fluid challenge' is then determined to decide whether further fluid/blood product is required. Patients will either respond:

- rapidly – patients return to a normal cardiovascular state and remain normal
- transiently – patients return to a normal cardiovascular state for a brief period, but begin to deteriorate thereafter
- minimal or no response – patients fail to respond or respond to a minimal extent.

There is evidence to suggest that in some circumstances fluid resuscitation should be related to pulse pressures, e.g., the presence of a radial pulse. This equates to a systolic blood pressure of at least 70 mmHg (Duncan & Moran 2009; Geeraedts et al. 2009; Greaves et al. 2009). This approach is known as permissive hypotension. The rationale behind this approach is that the systolic blood pressure of >70 mmHg would be sufficient to perfuse vital organs, but importantly would not be a pressure high enough to disrupt a newly formed clot at the site of bleeding. Fluid is given in 250 mL boluses to maintain a palpable radial pulse. This is particularly important in so-called 'incompressible' bleeding, e.g., intra-abdominal or pelvic bleeding. The exception to this approach would be the presence of a significant head injury. In this situation higher minimum pressures are required to maintain cerebral perfusion pressure (Greaves et al. 2009).

A blood sample should be taken for full blood count, urea and electrolyte analysis, grouping and cross-matching of at least six units at the time of cannula insertion. Where a blood sample is taken following cannula insertion it should be taken at a point distal to the site of fluid administration to prevent errors in analysis of the sample. Women of child-bearing years should have a pregnancy test. These can be performed on a urine sample if possible or from blood where facilities exist.

It is an obvious statement that the best replacement for lost blood is blood itself, however, blood is a valuable and scarce commodity that takes time to cross match and prepare. O-negative blood can be used and should be stored in small quantities in the ED for such cases. Patient blood samples should be taken early, as infusion of large quantities of O-negative blood can cause difficulties with grouping and cross-matching later. In the interim, intravenous fluids in the form of crystalloids or colloids can be administered. There has been debate in the past regarding which fluid was optimal. Crystalloids are cheaper than colloids, and are more effective in restoring intravascular volume (Schierhout & Roberts 1998). Hartmann's solution is a good

option; however 0.9% sodium chloride ('normal' saline) is an acceptable alternative (American College of Surgeons 2008). It is important to remember that for every millilitre of estimated blood volume lost, three millilitres of crystalloid should replace it. Neither fluid can enhance oxygen-carrying capacity or enable coagulation. The volume of fluid should therefore be cautious to avoid haemodilution and subsequent coagulopathies.

Occult bleeding, for example, from fractured long bones, can be the cause of hypovolaemia. Haemorrhage control therefore should take into account the need for interventions such as traction of long bones or pelvic splinting (Geeraedts et al. 2009).

Cardiac monitoring provides circulatory information from the heart rate and rhythm. It also provides an indicator of hypoxia, hypoperfusion, myocardial contusion, or hypothermia in the form of arrhythmias or ectopic beats. Pulseless electrical activity (PEA) is suggestive of profound hypovolaemia, cardiac tamponade, or tension pneumothorax (Resuscitation Council (UK) 2010) and has a poor prognosis unless the cause can be found and treated immediately.

Monitoring the patient's fluid intake and output is a vital part of the ED nurse's role. Knowing precisely how much and what kind of fluid the patient has received are essential in determining subsequent fluid management.

Urinary catheters and nasogastric tubes should be considered part of the resuscitation of the patient. Urine output is a sensitive measure of renal perfusion and an invaluable way to assess success of the resuscitation. A urinary catheter attached to a urometer should be inserted, providing no contraindications exist, such as blood at the urinary meatus, scrotal haematoma or a high-riding prostate, which would indicate urethral damage (American College of Surgeons 2008, Greaves et al. 2009). A urometer will ensure that accurate hourly measurements of urine output can be taken. If urethral catheterization is contraindicated due to urethral damage, a suprapubic catheter should be inserted by a suitably skilled team member. A urinary output of more than 50 mL/h in an adult is a good indicator of satisfactory tissue perfusion. The urine that is voided initially should be tested for blood and saved for microscopy and subsequent possible drug analysis.

A nasogastric tube should be inserted to decompress the stomach, thereby helping to avoid regurgitation. This can be caused by a paralytic ileus or air in the stomach as the result of assisted manual ventilation. A gastric tube may also identify blood in the gastric contents. A nasogastric tube should not be inserted if a cribriform plate fracture is suspected, in case it is inadvertently passed into the cranial vault. In this event, the tube can be inserted orally.

Disability: neurological status

A simple and rapid assessment of neurological status should take place during the primary survey. The evaluation should establish level of consciousness, pupil size and reaction. The Glasgow Coma Scale (GCS) is the commonest method used for the assessment of level of consciousness and a sequence of readings will tend to show fairly subtle changes quickly.

Continuity in measurement is important and measurements should be made by the same person.

As part of the GCS, painful stimulus is sometimes required. There is much variation in the nature of the stimulus. Some areas advocate the use of a sternal rub, while others suggest pressure over the supraorbital ridge or pinching of the trapezius muscle (Waterhouse 2009). Whatever the stimulus method used, the level should not be so excessive as to cause damage to the skin or underlying soft tissues. Be aware of patients with spinal cord injury and upper limb fractures as they may feel painful stimulus but be unable to respond with limb movement. In all cases painful stimuli should be kept to a minimum.

Normal pupil size ranges from 2–5 mm, with a difference of 1 mm being acceptable. As the light is shone in each eye, both eyes should be tested for responsiveness. A decreased level of consciousness should alert the assessor to four possibilities:

- decreased cerebral oxygenation (hypoxia and hypoperfusion)
- central nervous system injury (traumatic brain injury, intracranial haemorrhage)
- drug or alcohol intoxication
- metabolic derangement (hypoglycaemia, sepsis, SIRS).

Exposure/environmental control

At the end of the primary survey, every item of clothing must be removed, without risking any further damage to the patient (American College of Surgeons 2008). It is prudent at this point to log-roll the patient so that the back, which comprises 50% of the body, can be fully examined and the rescue board can be removed, along with any debris or retained clothing. Failure to assess the back of the patient can mean that the assessor misses a life-threatening injury. However, rolling a patient with an unstable pelvic fracture can result in further pelvic haemorrhage, so minimal movement and gentle handling are crucial (Little et al. 2001).

Hypothermia in trauma

Trauma patients are at risk from hypothermia (<35°C). Many have been exposed to cold, wet conditions, and blood loss can contribute further to a drop in core temperature. Hypothermia increases morbidity and mortality by a factor of up to three and must be prevented or reversed (Ireland et al. 2011). Secondary hypothermia should be prevented from occurring in the resuscitation room. This is an important aspect of nursing care that should not be neglected in what can be a busy and distracting environment. Various measures can be used, including:

- warm blankets over the patient from a warming cabinet
- i.v., blood and lavage fluids warmed to 39°C
- adequate environmental temperature in resuscitation area
- specifically designed warming plate suspended over patient trolley
- controlled exposure of the patient
- external warming device, e.g., Bair Hugger®.

Full history

A comprehensive history surrounding the patient and event will ensure a quicker idea of the status of the patient. Ambulance crews, paramedics, witnesses and relatives are an invaluable source of information. If the patient is conscious, they may possibly hold the most relevant information.

An AMPLE history helps plan patient care:

A – allergies

M – medication currently used

P – past illness/pregnancy

L – last ate or drank

E – events/environment related to the injury.

Details regarding the mechanism of injury can indicate the site and seriousness of many potential injuries. This information can help target specific treatment strategies, e.g., a fall of 30 cm is less likely to have significance than a fall of 2 m. In this situation the incidence of spinal injury increases and appropriate measures can be taken (Dickinson 2004).

Any pre-existing disease in a trauma patient increases their chances of dying, so clinicians need as much information as possible about medical history.

X-rays should be used carefully and should not delay resuscitation. Following primary survey the most appropriate X-rays taken are of the chest and pelvis. These X-rays provide information that may help lead the initial resuscitation of the patient. Evidence of a pneumothorax or fractured pelvis, for example, will help focus interventions. If clinically indicated, cervical X-rays may also be taken. These are:

- unconscious/intoxicated patients
- neck pain/tenderness
- abnormal neurological signs or symptoms (Hoffman et al. 2000).

A clear cervical spine X-ray may provide valuable information about serious injury. However, when appropriate, these and any other X-rays required can be deferred to the secondary survey. A major pitfall in the immediate assessment of cervical spine integrity is a failure to recognize that early imaging on its own is inadequate to safely clear the spine (Little et al. 2001).

Pain relief can be overlooked during the activity of resuscitation, but it is an essential part of good patient care. Intravenous opiates work well, but intramuscular routes are not appropriate in acute situations. Entonox can provide useful pain relief during the early stages, but should be avoided if there is the possibility of a pneumothorax. Any drug administered should be carefully recorded in the appropriate place. It is easy to lose track of what drugs have been given during a busy resuscitation.

Good communication, explanation and gentle handling are important preliminaries to analgesia. Correct immobilization of fractures will also relieve a great deal of pain. Other sources of discomfort should be excluded, e.g., full bladder. Analgesia should not be avoided just because the patient has a head injury, but it should be carefully administered and the patient must be monitored afterwards.

Secondary survey

The primary survey and resuscitation must be completed before the secondary survey begins (Robertson & Al-Haddad 2013). If, at the end of the primary survey, the patient's condition remains unstable, each step should be repeated until stability is achieved. During the secondary (head-to-toe) survey, less obvious injuries, which may pose a latent threat to life, should be detected.

At this stage assessment of vital signs every five minutes should be initiated:

- temperature – rectal or tympanic membrane
- pulse (radial, femoral or carotid) – rate, rhythm and volume
- respiration and peripheral oxygen saturation
- blood pressure
- GCS.

Vital signs should be monitored by the same person to avoid assessor variability.

Trauma patients are vulnerable to the effects of pressure on their skin, and every effort should be made to prevent any unnecessary risk (Swartz 2000). Patients who arrive in the ED on a spine board should be transferred from it as soon as is safe (Cooke 1998). Wet and soiled linen must be removed as soon as possible.

Head and face

The patient should be asked about any pain he may be experiencing and examined for evidence of injury to the bones or soft tissue, mouth or eyes. Otorrhoea or rhinorrhoea should be noted.

Swelling may prevent adequate examination of the eyes, later, so assess:

- visual acuity – this may be modified to suit the situation using either a specifically designed hand-held Snellen chart, or asking the patient to read printed text at a set distance
- pupil size and movement
- penetrating injury
- bleeding into the anterior chamber (hyphaema)
- contact lenses (remove before swelling occurs)
- eye movement–this may provide evidence of orbital floor fracture.

Neck

Patients with facial or head trauma must be presumed to have cervical spine injury until this has been excluded by an expert. Cervical spine immobilization should be maintained at all times. If immobilizing devices must be removed, manual in-line immobilization should be substituted. While maintaining careful cervical spine immobilization, the neck should be examined for any obvious injury to the bones or soft tissues. Any evidence of damage should lead the assessor to be concerned about potential airway obstruction. The assessor should check for tracheal deviation or distended neck veins, which may indicate a missed tension pneumothorax or cardiac tamponade.

Chest

The patient should be asked about pain or dyspnoea. Any sign of obvious injury should be noted, e.g., sucking chest wounds, bruising, paradoxical movements, subcutaneous emphysema, bruising or crepitus over the ribs. Life-saving interventions should already have been performed for open chest wounds or tension pneumothorax.

It is important to remember that every patient has a posterior chest, which should already have been examined during the log-roll at the end of the primary survey. A 12-lead ECG will determine dysrhythmias and may indicate cardiac contusion. This is demonstrated by elevation of the ST-segment of the affected area, atrial fibrillation, or an unexplained tachycardia.

Abdomen

An assessment of pain should be made, providing the patient is conscious. The abdomen should be examined for any obvious injury, distension, rigidity, guarding, contusions, scars, and bowel sounds. Such an examination should be careful and thorough, as bleeding into the abdomen from damaged organs is frequently the cause of life-threatening hypovolaemia. The most important aspect of the abdominal assessment is to determine whether the patient requires surgery or not.

A naso- or orogastric tube and a urinary catheter should have been inserted during the primary survey and is always inserted before diagnostic peritoneal lavage (DPL) is performed. Such measures will ensure that abdominal and pelvic organs are less likely to be damaged during the procedure. DPL and focused abdominal ultrasonography (FAST) are quick diagnostic procedures to determine intra-abdominal bleeding. They are indicated when results of physical examination are equivocal or the patient is unable to participate in the assessment. They should always be performed by, or in the presence of, the surgeon who will be acting upon any positive findings. Remember that DPL in an unstable patient is looking only for frank blood. If the DPL does not reveal gross blood, then the search must be continued for another site of blood loss.

Pelvis and genitalia

Patients should be asked about pain and whether they have an urge to pass urine. Male patients should be examined for bruising, blood at the urinary meatus, priapism, and scrotal bruising/oedema. The presence of femoral pulses should be ascertained. If a digital rectal examination was not performed when the patient was log-rolled at the end of the primary survey, it should be carried out now. The assessor should look for blood

Table 2.5 Considerations required for primary survey in children

Airway/cervical spine control	Children's airways are more susceptible to obstruction. Cartilage in the larynx and trachea will be more pliable than in an adult, and the tongue is proportionally larger within the mouth Cervical spine control and assessment is particularly difficult in children, as they may be unable to communicate the presence or absence of any neck tenderness. Immobilization may also cause distress in the conscious child
Breathing	As with adults, 100% oxygen is required via a non-rebreather mask. Signs of respiratory distress may be different, e.g., nasal flaring, intercostals recession, or grunting Tension pneumothorax in children is more common. It is crucial that these are detected and managed rapidly (Greaves et al. 2009)
Circulation	A stethoscope should be used to determine pulse rate in children less than 2 years old (RCN 2007) Early close monitoring is essential, as children may compensate for hypovolaemia better than adults, thus potentially hiding early clues of shock Vascular access may need to be via intraosseous routes (Resuscitation Council (UK) 2006)
Disability	A modified GCS is available for children under 5 years of age. This modifies the verbal response section, e.g., able to smile/interacts well to irritable or unresponsive
Exposure/control of environment	Children are at a higher risk of hypothermia due to their larger body surface area. Exposure for examination/intervention should be therefore kept to a minimum

in the rectum, which may indicate damage to the gut or pelvis. A high-riding prostate may be indicative of urethral injury, and loss of sphincter tone is often associated with spinal injury. Bony fragments may also be felt, indicating pelvic damage.

A vaginal examination should be performed in women, to look for blood and lacerations resulting from either direct damage or pelvic fractures. The pelvic ring should not be 'rocked' by applying heavy manual pressure to the iliac crests, but should be carefully examined to investigate for lack of continuity. 'Rocking' can be extremely painful and causes further damage and bleeding.

Extremities

Both arms and legs should be examined for contusion or deformity. Each should be assessed for:

- pain
- pallor
- pulse
- paraesthesia
- paralysis
- cold
- perspiration
- instability
- crepitus.

Any injuries should be realigned and splinted. Every time this is done, the limb must be reassessed. Any open wounds should be covered with a sterile dressing. If at any time during the secondary survey a patient's condition deteriorates, returning to the primary survey with institution or reinstitution of resuscitative measures is essential. The primary and secondary surveys should be repeated to ascertain any deterioration in the patient's condition.

Special care should be taken to examine body regions where injuries are easily missed or underestimated:

- back of head and scalp
- neck beneath semi-rigid collar
- back, buttocks and flanks
- groin creases, perineum and genitalia.

Trauma in children

Injury following an accident is the second leading cause of death in children (Greaves et al. 2009). The number of childhood deaths has declined over the past 30 years. This has been attributed to effective injury prevention strategies. Nurses may play a key role in this regard with effective advice and health promotion advice. Encouraging parents to provide children with cycle helmets being one such example.

Whilst many of the principles for managing children are the same as for adults, it is essential that team members with paediatric experience are available. The priorities for assessment and management are identical. Some of the approaches to the care of the injured child will need to be modified, due to key differences in managing the seriously injured child (Table 2.5). The differences lie in children's anatomy, physiology (Table 2.6) and emotional development. It can be difficult for the inexperienced to recognize early problems.

Greaves et al. (2009) recommend thorough preparation where the arrival of the injured child can be anticipated. Knowledge of the age of the child allows for a calculation of weight, drug dosages, fluid volumes and endotracheal tube sizes where appropriate. Children can sustain significant injury to the intrathoracic structures without evidence of any skeletal trauma. Children have not had the experience

Table 2.6 Normal parameters for vital signs in children (Resuscitation Council 2006)

Age	Respiratory rate	Heart rate	Systolic BP (mmHg)
Neonatal (up to 4 weeks)	40–60	120–160	>60
Infant < 1 year	30–40	110–160	70–90
Toddler 1–2 years	25–35	100–150	75–95
Pre-school 3–4 years	25–30	95–140	85–100
School 5–11 years	20–25	80–120	90–100
> 12 years	14–20	60–100	100–120

Table 2.7 Considerations required for primary survey in the older person

Airway/cervical spine control	Degenerative changes make cervical spine injury more likely X-rays may be more difficult to interpret due to co-morbidities, e.g., osteoarthritic changes
Breathing	Decreased lung volume and compliance Co-existing respiratory conditions, e.g., COPD will exacerbate any increased requirement for oxygen following injury The thorax becomes less compliant making it more vulnerable to fracture
Circulation	Pre-existing cardiac conditions or vascular disease will compromise the body's ability to compensate for hypovo-laemic shock Vasoconstrictor response becomes slower with age. Medication, e.g., beta-blocker, may mask tachycardias or affect compensatory mechanisms to shock
Disability	Older patients are more likely to suffer with dementia or mental health problems making assessment of mental status very difficult
Exposure/control of environment	Delayed and decreased shivering response, decreased ability to produce heat and a slower metabolic rate will make the older patient more vulnerable to hypothermia. A structural and functional change in the skin increases the risk of the older patient developing pressure ulcers. This is a particularly important aspect of care that falls well within the sphere of nursing responsibility

to develop the emotional coping strategies of adults. Particular attention should be paid to psychological considerations. This is particularly important where the child's has been immobilized to protect their cervical spine. This may be terrifying for a child. If at all possible, someone known to the child is almost always a helpful support in the trauma room and should be given the opportunity to stay throughout the resuscitation.

Trauma in the older person

There are an increasing number of elderly trauma patients, not least because of demographic changes in the population (Greaves et al. 2009) (Table 2.7).

The elderly are more at risk of developing irreversible shock than younger people. They are more likely to be chronically dehydrated, which, in addition to shock, can move the process very quickly to irreversibility.

Definitive care

Once the trauma patient has been assessed using the ABCDE approach, has been successfully resuscitated and has undergone a head-to-toe assessment to find all injuries, they can be moved on to the next stage of care. Definitive care may be provided in the operating theatre, intensive care unit or a specialist treatment unit (e.g., burns care). Serious injuries are treated and definitive plans for the comprehensive care of the patient are made. It is essential the patient is in the best condition possible to undergo transfer either within the hospital or to another care facility. It is this aspect of trauma care that has seen the most significant recommendation in government policy and approach to major trauma in England. Following the development of a successful trauma network in London, a report from the National Audit Office (2010) has recommended extending the approach nationwide. The report indicates that the creation of trauma networks could improve patient outcome following serious injury.

The system draws on experience from the military and the US where seriously injured patients are met by highly trained specialists and managed in specialist care facilities where their injuries are definitively managed (Miller 2010). The most apt example of this may be the patient with a serious head injury, who is transported by helicopter from the scene of their injury, directly to a facility with a neurosurgical unit. Delay is minimized, optimizing potential recovery. A 20% reduction in mortality from serious head injury has been demonstrated between the US and UK using this approach (Davenport et al. 2010).

Current recommendations (National Audit Office 2010) divide the UK into geographical regions, and within those regions will be a trauma network. The hospitals providing care are awarded a 'level' that determines the ability to manage the various specialities and facilities the seriously injured patient will require. Level 1 trauma centres, for example, will have an ED consultant doctor available 24 hours a day, have a helipad and have all surgical specialities that may be required. Level 2 centres may have 24-hour ED facilities but may lack the specialities required. Level 3 centres may lack the specialities required and the ability to provide 24-hour CT scanning, for example (Miller 2010). Each regional trauma network would have one level 1 centre and several level 2 and 3 centres.

Copies of the comprehensive records and reports, which must be kept up to date, should accompany patients wherever they are transferred. While a resuscitation is in progress, it is tempting to leave documentation until afterwards. Pre-printed trauma sheets can be useful, both to save time and to act as an aide memoire. Fully comprehensive notes, regarding all details of the patient, contribute significantly to high standards of communication supporting the patient, and are vital to good care, not to mention medico-legal and audit purposes.

Family members and loved ones should be kept fully informed of the proceedings. The distress experienced by this group of people during resuscitation can be far longer lasting than that experienced by the patient. If possible, someone should be allocated to liaise between the resuscitation room and relatives. Although the nurse may be the ideal person, chaplains, social workers, or staff from other areas of the hospital can often assume this role. Relatives can provide important information, and they should be included in patient care planning. Inviting relatives into the trauma room is appropriate in some instances (Royal College of Nursing & British Association for Accident and Emergency Medicine 1995, Barratt & Wallis 1998, Nykiel et al. 2011, Barratt & Wallis 1998). (See also Chapter 14: Care of the Bereaved.)

Psychological aspects

Over recent years trauma management has continued to develop alongside technical advances and evidence-based practices. As this has grown, so has the deeper understanding of the effects of trauma at a psychological level. Where trauma care has expanded from the ED setting to definitive and specialist care, so the psychological needs and the long-term social effects of events must be considered.

Most of the resources associated with trauma management in terms of funding, education, and research are directed towards physiological and life-threatening aspects. However, some of the more lasting effects are from the emotional damage trauma has inflicted on patients and their relatives (Larner 2005).

Psychological aspects of care must be addressed early if long-term damage is to be avoided. There is strong belief that immediate intervention assists with the healing of any psychological trauma. Basic interventions, including clear explanations, addressing patient's fears and considering physical comfort, will make a difference during the acute phase of resuscitation. As members of the trauma team everyone takes a role assisting with the psychological support of the patient, although practically this role is often considered to be the remit of the nurse, who can make a significant contribution by combining nursing skills with the increasingly sophisticated methods of managing trauma.

The psychological impact of managing the seriously injured patient on staff should not be underestimated. Simple measures such as peer support, reflection, or simply allowing the same team to work together soon after the event can help minimize the impact of distressing events. In some cases more formal approaches including formal debriefing or counselling may be required. It is important to note, however, that involvement in this process should be voluntary rather than mandatory as it may not be suitable for all staff.

Conclusion

Good trauma care relies heavily on a multidisciplinary approach. Not all trauma team members give 'hands-on' care, but each department and speciality has a valuable part to play. Successful initial assessment using a systematic approach every time, by every team member, will ensure that injuries are not missed. This gives the trauma patient the best possible chance of a complete and speedy recovery.

A great deal of progress has been made over the last two decades, but there still remains a great deal to do. In the past, trauma patients have died as the result of relatively simple problems such as hypovolaemia and hypoxia. Many of us are now aware of ways to prevent such deaths. However, it is essential that all those who come into contact with trauma patients have the necessary skills and knowledge. Investment in training of this nature is a small price to pay for a reduction in trauma deaths.

References

Adam, S., Osborne, S., 2009. The systemic inflammatory response, sepsis and multiple organ dysfunction. Critical Care Nursing – Science and practice. Oxford University Press, Oxford.

American College of Surgeons, 2008. Advanced Trauma Life Support, eighth ed. American College of Surgeons, Chicago.

Barratt, F., Wallis, D.N., 1998. Relatives in the resuscitation room: their point of view. Journal of Accident and Emergency Medicine 15, 109.

Casey, G., 2001. Oxygen transport and the use of pulse oximetry. Nursing Standard 15 (47), 46–53.

Champion, H.R., Leitch, R.A., 2012. Combat casualty management. In: Lenquist, S. (Ed.), Medical Incident Response to Major Incidents and Disasters. Springer-Verlag, Berlin.

Cole, E., 2004. Assessment and management of the trauma patient. Nursing Standard 18 (41), 45–51.

Cooke, M.W., 1998. Use of the spinal board within the accident and emergency department. Journal of Accident and Emergency Medicine 15, 108–109.

Davenport, R., Tai, N., West, A., et al., 2010. A major trauma centre is a speciality hospital not a hospital of specialities. British Journal of Surgery 97 (1), 109–117.

Dickinson, M., 2004. Understanding the mechanism of injury and kinetic forces involved in traumatic injuries. Emergency Nurse 12 (6), 30–35.

Duncan, N., Moran, C., 2009. Initial resuscitation of the trauma victim. Orthopaedics and Trauma 21 (1), 1–8.

Geeraedts, L., Kaasjager, H., van Vugt, A., et al., 2009. Exsanguination in trauma; A review of diagnostics and treatment options. Injury: International Journal Care of the Injured 40, 11–20.

Greaves, I., Porter, K., Garner, J., 2009. Trauma Care Manual, second ed. Hodder Arnold, London.

Hoffman, J., Mower, W., Wolfson, A., et al., 2000. Validity of a set of clinical criteria to rule out injury to the cervical spine in patients with blunt trauma. National Emergency X-radiography Utilisation Study Group. New England Journal of Medicine 343, 94–99.

Hunt, P., Hunt, F., 2011. Fluid resuscitation therapy. In: Smith, J., Greaves, I., Porter, K. (Eds.), Oxford Desk Reference: Major Trauma. Oxford Medical Publications, Oxford.

Ireland, S., Endacott, R., Cameron, P., et al., 2011. The incidence and significance of accidental hypothermia in major trauma: A prospective observational study. Resuscitation 82 (3), 300–306.

Larner, S., 2005. Common psychological challenges for patients with newly acquired disability. Nursing Standard 19 (28), 33–39.

Little, G., Kelly, M., Glucksman, E., 2001. Critical pitfalls in the immediate assessment of the trauma patient. Trauma 3, 43–51.

Lott, C., Araujo, R., Cassar, M., et al., 2009. The European Trauma Course (ETC) and the team approach: Past, present and future. Resuscitation 80, 1192–1196.

Middleton, P., 2011. The Trauma Epidemic. In: Smith, J., Greaves, I., Porter, K. (Eds.), Oxford Desk Reference: Major Trauma. Oxford Medical Publications, Oxford.

Miller, S., 2010. How trauma networks can improve patient care. Emergency Nurse 18 (6), 14–18.

National Audit Office, 2010. Major Trauma Care in England. The Stationery Office, London.

Nykiel, L., Denicke, R., Schneider, R., et al., 2011. Evidence-based practice and family presence: paving the path for bedside nurse scientists. Journal of Emergency Nursing 37 (1), 9–16.

Resuscitation Council (UK), 2006. European Paediatric Life Support. Resuscitation Council (UK), London.

Resuscitation Council (UK), 2010. Resuscitation Guidelines 2010. Resuscitation Council, London.

Robertson, LC., Al-Haddad, M., 2013. Recognizing the critically ill patient. Anaesthesia and Intensive Care Medicine 14 (1), 11–14.

Sapsford, W., 2008. Should the 'C' in 'ABCDE' be altered to reflect the trend towards hypotensive resuscitation. Scandinavian Journal of Surgery 97, 4–11.

Schierhout, G., Roberts, I., 1998. Fluid resuscitation with colloid or crystalloid solutions in critically ill patients. British Medical Journal 316 (7136), 961–964.

Sexton, J., 1997. Trauma epidemiology and team management. Emergency Nurse 5 (1), 14–16.

Smith, R.M., Conn, A., 2009. Pre-hospital care: Scoop and run or stay and play? Injury, International Care of the Injured 4054, S23–S26.

Span, D.R., Cerny, V., Coats, T.J., et al., 2007. Management of trauma following major trauma: A European guideline. Critical Care 11, R17.

Stoneham, J., Riley, B., Brooks, A., et al., 2001. Recent advances in trauma management. Trauma 3, 143–150.

Swartz, C., 2000. Resuscitation considerations to prevent pressure ulcers in trauma patients. International Journal of Trauma Nursing 6, 16–18.

Waterhouse, C., 2009. The use of painful stimulus in relation to Glasgow Coma Scale observations. British Journal of Neuroscience Nursing 5 (5), 209–214.

Major incidents

3

Tim Morse and Tim Kilner

Introduction

Incidents involving large numbers of injured individuals are not as uncommon as people may like to believe, although over the years the profiles of these incidents have changed. Incidents are often associated with industry, transportation, mass gatherings, and terrorism. Carley & Mackway-Jones (2005) found on average, 3–4 major incidents occurred in the UK every year from 1966 to 1996 (range 0–11). Table 3.1 lists a few examples of incidents occurring over the last 20 years in the UK.

At a local level the threat of a major incident occurring in the UK has often been viewed as remote; however, the terrorist events in New York and Washington on September 11th 2001 that killed 2996 people, the Madrid bombing that killed 191 people and injured over 1700 and on the London Underground attack on 7th July 2005, which killed 52 and injured over 700 people certainly heightened awareness and the increasing terrorist risk. Consequently, major incident planning has assumed a greater priority than previously, although there may still be an element of denial by assuming that such events will happen elsewhere (Lennquist 2012).

By their very nature, major incidents are unpredictable, the only certainty being that at some time, somewhere, the unexpected will happen. But when it does, the health services must be able to respond rapidly, mobilizing additional human and material resources. Procedures must also be in place to make the most efficient use of those resources in the given circumstances. Achieving this requires the health services to be proactive in the planning of emergency management measures, thus reducing the need for reactive management in an extremely stressful situation. The Emergency Department (ED) provides the focus for the hospital's patient-care activity during the response to an incident.

This chapter discusses the role of the health services in contingency planning and service provision for major incidents. Consideration will be given to hospital-based activity, both in general terms and specifically in relation to in-hospital emergency services. The on-scene response to a major incident is considered in Chapter 1.

In England the primary source of guidance to assist the NHS in planning a response to a major incident is contained in the Department of Health Emergency Preparedness Division (2007) *Mass Casualties Incidents: A Framework for Planning*, which is influenced by the requirements of the Civil Contingencies Act 2004 (Home Office 2004). Guidance for Scotland, Wales and Northern Ireland is issued by the Health Departments of each of the Administrations.

Definition

Guidance from the Department of Health (HSE 1996a,b) defines a major incident as: 'any occurrence that presents serious threat to the health of the community, disruption

http://dx.doi.org/10.1016/B978-0-7020-4315-4.00003-6

Table 3.1 Examples of major incidents in the UK since 1996			
1996	Terrorist bomb Canary Wharf	2 dead	100 injured
1996	Shooting Dunblane	17 dead	13 injured
1996	Rail collision Watford South Junction	1 dead	69 injured
1997	100-vehicle collision A12 Essex		50 injured
1997	26-vehicle collision A19 north Yorkshire	1 dead	4 injured
1997	110-vehicle collision M42 Worcestershire	3 dead	62 injured
1997	Rail collision Southall	7 dead	160+ injured
1997	Hot-air balloon crash into cables Yorkshire	1 dead	13 injured
1997	Gas explosion south London		8 injured
1998	Gas leak in factory York		31 injured
1998	Terrorist bomb Omagh	29 dead	200+ injured
1999	Rail collision Cheshire		27 injured
2000	Rail collision Hatfield	4 dead	35 injured
2001	Explosion in steelworks Port Talbot	2 dead	13 injured
2001	Rail/road vehicle collision Selby	10 dead	76+ injured
2002	Coach collision Cumbria		43 injured
2002	Coach collision Berkshire	7 dead	35 injured
2002	100-vehicle collision Oxford	2 dead	20+ injured
2002	30–50-vehicle collision north Yorkshire		24 injured
2002	Coach collision Heathrow	5 dead	40 injured
2003	Rail collision Chancery Lane		32 injured
2003	Minibus collision Manchester	7 dead	7 injured
2004	Fire at care home Glasgow	10 dead	6 injured
2004	Factory explosion Glasgow	9 dead	40+ injured
2004	Rail collision Upton Nevet	7 dead	150 injured
2005	Multiple terrorist explosion London	52 dead	700+ injured
2005	Birmingham tornado		30 injured
2007	Coach crash M4/M25	2 dead	67 injured
2009	Ottery St Mary event - explosion		12 injured
2009	Coach collision Penzance	2 dead	47 injured
2010	Car bomb Northern Ireland		No-one injured
2010	Shooting Cumbria	12 dead	11 injured

to service, or causes (or is likely to cause) such numbers or types of casualties as to require special arrangements to be implemented by hospitals, ambulance trusts or primary care organizations'.

This definition reflects the departure from the view that major incidents only result from the 'big bang' scenario such as a rail collision or a building collapse. Guidance now recognizes that major incidents can also occur in a variety of different ways (NHS Management Executive 1998, National Audit Office 2002), such as

- rising tide – such as a developing infectious disease epidemic or an outbreak of Legionnaires' disease (Smith et al. 2005)
- cloud on the horizon – a serious incident elsewhere that may develop and need preparatory action such as a cloud of toxic gas from a fire at an industrial plant
- headline news – public alarm about a personal threat
- internal incident – such as a fire in the hospital or power failure
- deliberate – such as the release of chemical, biological, radiation or nuclear material
- pre-planned major events – such as sporting or entertainment mass gatherings.

Planning

Each NHS organization must have a major incident plan based upon risk assessment, cooperation with partners, communicating with the public, and information sharing. It is the Chief Executive's responsibility to ensure such a plan is in place and to keep the Trust Board up to date with the plan (Department of Health Emergency Preparedness Division 2005, 2011).

The plan should outline actions for the acute Trust to discharge its responsibilities, namely:

- provide a safe and secure environment for the assessment and treatment of patients
- provide a safe and secure environment for staff that will ensure the health, safety and welfare of staff, including appropriate arrangements for the professional and personal indemnification of staff
- provide a clinical response, including provision of general support and specific/specialist healthcare to all casualties, victims and responders
- liaise with the ambulance service, local Primary Care Organizations (PCOs) including GPs, out-of-hours services, Minor Injuries Units (MIUs) and other primary care providers, other hospitals, independent sector providers, and other agencies in order to manage the impact of the incident
- ensure there is an operational response to provide at-scene medical cover using, for example, BASICS and other immediate-care teams where they exist; members of these teams will be trained to an appropriate standard; the Medical Incident Commander should not routinely be taken from the receiving hospital so as not to deplete resources
- ensure that the hospital reviews all its essential functions throughout the incident

- provide appropriate support to any designated receiving hospital or other neighbouring service that is substantially affected
- provide limited decontamination facilities and personal protective equipment to manage contaminated self-presenting casualties
- acute Trusts will be expected to establish a Memorandum of Understanding (MOU) with their local Fire and Rescue Service on decontamination
- acute Trusts will need to make arrangements to reflect national guidance from the Home Office for dealing with the bodies of contaminated patients who die at the hospital
- liaise with activated health emergency control centres and/or on call PCO Officers as appropriate
- maintain communications with relatives and friends of existing patients and those from the incident, the Casualty Bureau, the local community, the media and VIPs.

The very nature of major incidents brings together diverse groups of professionals in large numbers, each group having distinct roles and responsibilities. When faced with the complexities of a major incident, it is unrealistic to expect such a large multidisciplinary team to function in an effective and coordinated manner without detailed prior planning. It is therefore essential that planning assumes an appropriately high priority.

Training

There is an expectation that staff understand the role they would adopt in a major incident, have the competencies to fulfil that role and have received training to fulfil those competencies. There is some evidence to suggest that staff are not entirely familiar with the action they should take in a major incident (Carr et al. 2006, Milkhu et al. 2008, Linney et al. 2011). It is suggested that acute Trusts should consider providing annual training and development for staff to enable them to meet these expectations. There is also a requirement for all NHS organizations to undertake a live exercise every three years, a table-top exercise each year and a test of communication cascades every six months (Department of Health Emergency Preparedness Division 2005). However, despite these exercises their must be a recognition for acute hospital trusts to coordinate their role with the surrounding primary healthcare organizations, as they may also lack in preparedness (Day et al. 2010).

Large-scale exercises serve a number of purposes:

- enabling major incident plans to be tested
- allowing the rehearsal of practical skills in realistic environments
- working alongside other services, establishing working relationships with individuals and organizations likely to be involved in a true response.

However, large exercises do not allow detailed scrutiny of any one aspect of the plan; rather, there is a superficial overview of the plan as a whole. Large-scale exercises should be as realistic as possible in all respects and be based upon the more

likely incidents that may occur locally, to gain full benefit from testing the emergency response and making the experience as meaningful as possible.

The timing of an exercise is also of importance. If possible, it is preferable not to advise personnel exactly when the exercise will take place, as forewarning will inevitably create a false state of preparation and readiness that will not truly reflect the response to a 'real' incident. However, there is a need to ensure that exercises do not unduly disrupt the normal functioning of the service, so an acceptable compromise must be reached when planning and informing staff of exercises. The organization and enactment of full or 'live' exercises are expensive in terms of time, personnel and resources, and these factors make exercises of considerable financial cost. Combining exercises with other services and agencies, many of which also have statutory requirements to exercise, can keep costs to a minimum. It may be that in some circumstances other forms of exercise, which may be more cost-effective and appropriate in meeting response and training needs, should also be considered.

Small-scale exercises allow part of the plan to be examined in detail, utilizing skill and task-specific activities, but do not always highlight problems that may occur when influenced by the activity of other departments or organizations. Table-top exercises allow a greater range of activities to be scrutinized in detail, but are largely theoretical and may not highlight logistical problems or poor skill levels resulting from inadequate training.

In addition to table-top exercises, using computer video serious gaming technology, can create a near reality likeness to an actual event. Knight et al. (2010) developed serious gaming technology to support the decision making involved in triaging patients. The benefit of this technology compared with large exercises is that it is cheaper in terms of resources, and the student can revisit the situation again.

Given that each method has limitations, perhaps there is a case for exercise and training to make use of a combination of these techniques and not to be reliant upon one method.

The hospital should carry out an internal communications/call-in exercise at least every six months and exercise communications systems between themselves and the ambulance service at regular intervals. Exercising of plans also provides an opportunity to review procedures and make amendments in the light of lessons learned from testing implementation. Lack of practice in implementing the plan allows deficits, inconsistencies, and errors to go undetected until a major incident occurs.

While selection, training, and motivation can be expected to create greater resilience in staff involved in major incidents than among the rest of the population, there is also evidence that staff are not completely immune to adverse effects of trauma work (Alexander 2005). Staff may be exposed to:

- gruesome sights, sounds and smells and other materials
- on-site dangers and interpersonal violence
- distressing survivor stories
- powerlessness – being unable to help at the level they wish.

It is important, therefore, to ensure staff have sufficient rest, exercise and opportunity to talk, when they feel able to do so, to those whom they trust (Alexander & Klein 2011).

Major incident alerting procedures

In the event of a 'big bang' major incident it is likely the ambulance service will be the first to become aware of the incident. In this case they will be responsible, on confirmation of the incident, for alerting all appropriate partners within the health community. That noted, there are plenty of examples of major incidents, such as the Omagh bombing in Northern Ireland in 1998 (Lavery & Horan 2005) and the Canterbury earthquake in New Zealand in 2011 (Dolan 2011a,b, Dolan et al 2011) where patients presented to the ED some minutes before the first ambulances.

The acute trust should be alerted by one of two messages: either 'major incident standby' indicating a major incident may need to be declared, or 'major incident declared – activate plan', indicating that the major incident plan should be implemented and all appropriate action should commence.

The alert will be terminated with either 'major incident – cancelled', indicating a stand down from the alert and a halt to the implementation of the plan, or 'major incident stand down', indicating that all live casualties have left scene, but some may still be en route to hospital.

In the event of a 'rising tide' incident the alert is most likely to come from either the Strategic or Regional Health Authority or from one of the Primary Care Organizations. Acute Trusts may declare a major incident, initiated by the most senior person available in the Trust at that time, and this may result from an incident where casualties self-present prior to the ambulance service being aware. In such cases it is essential that the ambulance service are immediately alerted and updated as a matter of urgency.

The hospital's response to a major incident alert

The emergency department

The primary responsibility of the ED is the reception and treatment of patients. This will include the establishment of reception areas and treatment areas with appropriate access and egress to control patient flow, and decontamination facilities where necessary. Systems should be implemented to provide clinical records for each patient and for the management of patients' possessions.

During this stage of the incident, relevant nursing and medical staff will be contacted and deployed to activity predetermined by individual action cards. If additional nursing staff are required by the ED, then an appropriately designated person should initiate a 'call-in' procedure. Other involved areas in the hospital will also activate similar procedures, which may also involve the use of personnel from voluntary organizations. It is often advisable to call in staff rostered for the next shift but one in the department, as this allows for an already rostered fresh shift to come in relieving those involved in the initial response and allows the present and called-in shifts an opportunity to rest. This is not always possible as the bulk of the current shift may be rostered for the shift after next, e.g., today's late shift staff are tomorrow's early shift staff.

It may also be advisable to distinguish ED nurses and doctors from other staff deployed to the department from elsewhere by the use of identifying tabards. If possible, additional staff deployed into ED should have ED or critical-care experience and should not be utilized in treatment teams without the presence of at least one experienced ED nurse. Nurses from other areas can play useful roles in dealing with minor injuries and in transferring casualties from the treatment areas to admission wards.

Receipt of casualties

Within the ED, all of the patients in the department at the time of the major incident alert should have the situation explained to them and their conditions reassessed. Those awaiting treatment or with minor injuries should be given any appropriate first aid treatment and advised to go home, attend their local community hospital, or see their GP. More seriously injured or ill patients should be rapidly stabilized and transferred to a ward.

It should be borne in mind that during a major incident the ED may still receive casualties who have not been involved in the incident, especially if they make their own way to the department. Moreover, patients involved in an incident may make their own way to the department and these should be included within the documentation used during the incident. In either case, the department should provide facilities to treat them but not confusing them with the casualties involved in the major incident. The department should prepare facilities for the reception and treatment of casualties according to their priority for treatment. This commonly involves the utilization of appropriately identified areas, adjacent to the ED if possible, for the collection and treatment of those with a lower clinical priority. Within the ED and other areas identified for casualty reception and treatment, appropriate types and amounts of equipment should be prepared. To enable this essential equipment to be rapidly available for use, stocks should be held in an easily accessible place within the department, and planning with the central sterile supply department, pharmacy and other departments should enable additional supplies to be quickly procured to replenish the stocks held in ED, such as chest drain packs and controlled analgesic drugs.

Each patient should receive a uniquely numbered identification bracelet and set of records, different to those used by the rest of the hospital. As immediate identification of the casualty may be difficult and time consuming, this unique number will accompany the patient throughout the hospital system. The triage labels used at the incident scene should also be uniquely numbered and, if it is practical to use this number within the hospital as well, tracking of the casualty will be assisted.

In the ED, arrangements should be made to receive and treat casualties with appropriate priority. On arrival at the hospital all patients should be re-triaged, documented and directed to an appropriate treatment area. However, in a mass casualty situation, managing a large number of casualties means that the view of 'doing the greatest good for the greatest number' (Jenkins et al. 2008) should be applied; a philosophy which is different in normal everyday ED work.

Triage should be carried out by a triage team consisting of an experienced ED doctor and nurse. If separate entrances have been designated for minor and other categories, due to the geography of the hospital, two triage teams may be needed. Each patient will be assigned a triage category and a unique identification number – preferably the same as on the triage label from the scene. Further identification and documentation of patients will take place as their condition allows, and will be carried out by members of the police documentation team and hospital administrative staff. Information regarding the numbers and identities of patients will be compiled by the police documentation team and relayed at regular intervals to the police's casualty bureau, where it will be combined with information from the scene, rest centres, mortuary and other sources, such as transport companies' passenger lists.

Patient care

Treatment may be facilitated by organizing available staff into 'treatment teams'. A treatment team can consist of two doctors and two nurses. At least one of the nurses should be an ED nurse. Each 'immediate priority' patient will require one treatment team for their care in the department. However, one team should be able to manage the care of two or three urgent priority patients, and the area designated for delayed priority ('minor') patients should be manageable using two teams. The medical and nursing staff in ED should aim to treat, stabilize and transfer immediate and urgent casualties out of the initial treatment areas as rapidly as possible, to allow treatment of the maximum number of casualties. However, in reality, the number of immediate and urgent patients that a hospital will be able to accept will be limited by the number of intensive care, high-dependency care and operating theatre spaces available.

While casualties in the minor area may be initially regarded as having a low priority, their conditions may change. It is therefore important that at least some of the nurses allocated to this area are suitably experienced and are able to re-triage casualties into higher categories when required and arrange for their transfer to a more appropriate treatment area as necessary, especially as areas designated for the treatment of minor injuries may be geographically separated from the main ED treatment areas, such as an outpatients department.

Transfer teams will also be required to transfer critically ill patients from the treatment area to critical care areas or to the operating theatres. These teams may consist of a doctor and a nurse, preferably both with critical care experience, and preferably two porters, as medical and nursing staff are needed for patient care and should not be pushing trolleys. The transfer of non-critical casualties to their admission destination can be facilitated by a nurse and a porter. In order that there is continuity of care for casualties and of record keeping and handover, it may prove useful for one nurse to remain with the patients in immediate and urgent categories during their stay in the ED. However, the practicality of this arrangement will depend upon the number of casualties involved and the number of nurses available. It may be that this role should be fulfilled by a nurse drafted into the department from elsewhere in the hospital. During a major incident the knowledge and skills of the emergency nurse are at a premium, and if their numbers are limited then they are probably best utilized in the care of critical casualties and in a resource and organization of care role, making use of other hospital nurses drafted into the department.

Hospital response

The hospital will establish a Hospital Coordinating Team (HCT) typically made up of a senior clinician, a senior nurse and a senior manager. The primary function of the HCT is to manage the hospital's response and ensure effective deployment of staff.

If the hospital is to receive patients, it is also likely that routine operating lists will be suspended and as many intensive care and high dependency spaces as possible made free. In addition, it may be thought necessary to clear as many beds as possible in other wards by means of early discharges and by transferring patients to other, unaffected hospitals – the use of the voluntary aid societies and their vehicles may be indicated for this task as the ambulance service is unlikely to be able to support this activity. The Civil Contingencies Home Office Act (2004) now places statutory responsibilities on primary care organizations to cooperate with other responders to an incident and to have a plan in place. It should be possible, in theory at least, for beds to be made available in a major incident but there is a reliance on primary care organizations having plans for some surge capacity in the event of such an emergency.

Restriction of access

Maintaining security, controlling access to the hospital and the containment of casualties, relatives and the media in specified areas of the hospital are vital tasks essential to the effectiveness of the hospital's response. Full security and containment arrangements must be in place as soon as possible after the hospital has received notification to activate its plan.

If possible, access to all involved areas should be limited to one entrance and egress to one exit. All other entrances should be locked or closed by security personnel. Only those staff with appropriate identification should be allowed into the hospital, the ED and associated treatment and collection points. Major incidents cause a convergence of individuals and groups on the hospital, focusing upon the ED. Well-meaning and interested hospital and non-hospital nursing and medical staff, various volunteers and voluntary groups will cause a disrupted and confused response and their access must be prevented.

It is advisable that hospital staff do not leave their own departments or come to the hospital until they are requested to do so via the recognized communication channels. A decision will also have to be made whether or not to use non-requested, non-hospital medical, nursing and other volunteers who offer their services. The potential legal ramifications of using possibly unqualified impostors and/or the possibility of negligence claims resulting from their practices may well outweigh any useful function that they may be able to perform.

The media

The media, which will no doubt have gathered at the hospital, should be provided with regular and accurate press releases. The media are under pressure during a major incident to meet deadlines and if they do not receive adequate and appropriate information they may set about seeking it out for themselves. It is not uncommon for members of the media to attempt to gain access to patients/relatives in ED and other clinical settings such as ITU and wards by pretending to be members of staff. Walter (2011) notes, however, that news reporting, particularly live from the scene, may give vital information to the more remote commanders and to the wider health response before the normal communication channels can generate a properly informed report. The needs of the media should be addressed in ways that will not compromise the emergency response of the hospital and its staff or the confidentiality of casualties and relatives. Only designated members of staff, who preferably have been prepared for this role, should address the media and only statements prepared in consultation with the appropriate emergency services and approved by the hospital's major incident coordination team should be released. Any access to casualties and staff should be very carefully controlled, with ground rules being agreed and consent obtained before any interviews take place.

Medico-legal issues

During the response to a major incident in the hospital or at the scene, nurses must consider a number of legal and professional issues. Major incident scenes are considered to be 'scenes of crime' until proven otherwise and consideration must be given to the preservation of forensic evidence. Such evidence, e.g., clothing, debris, etc., may leave the scene with casualties and, as a result, be present in the ED and other areas of the hospital. Every effort should be made to collect and preserve this evidence in collaboration with the police. Of course, in all circumstances, preservation of life takes priority over the preservation of evidence.

Criminal investigations and prosecutions, civil actions, official inquiries and inquests are all possible following a major incident. Some of the staff involved in the management of the incident is likely to be required to provide statements and/or give evidence. It should also be remembered that all documentation completed during the incident can be used not only as a source of evidence to explain what happened, but possibly also to suggest negligence.

Although staff are working under considerable pressure at the time of an incident, all documentation should be adequate, clear and accurate (Carvalho et al. 2011). Nurses should consider that the pressures of a major incident do not remove their professional accountability for practice, and they may well be asked to justify the actions that they took, both inside and outside the ED, at a later date. Staff should also be aware that the plan, including any action cards, is a written document and, as such, essentially becomes an approved policy document of the organization and provides standards and descriptions of expected activities against which the actions of staff may be judged by any investigation, whether internal or external.

Aftermath

During and in the aftermath of a major incident, it is important to recognize that both casualties and staff may be psychologically and/or spiritually affected by events that are outside the normal range of experience. As a consequence they may be at risk of developing post-trauma stress reactions and doubting long-held beliefs (Firth-Cozens et al. 2000).

Hospital major incident plans must include arrangements to provide patients, relatives, and staff with appropriate psychological and spiritual support during and after the event. Psychological support may be provided by appropriately trained personnel from the mental health professions or other statutory or voluntary bodies. Religious representatives from the major groupings should also be available, as well as a contact list of representatives from a broad range of spiritual beliefs so that individual needs may be met as far as is possible. Both psychological and spiritual support should be available from the outset and throughout the incident. Follow-up services such as psychological debriefing should also be made available to all of those involved as part of the plan.

Conclusion

Major incidents are rare, but they do happen. It is essential that organizations' plans are based on risk assessment and take into account other major incident plans within the health community and the work of Local Resilience Fora. For the plans to be successful individuals need to be familiar with their role within the plans and the actions they need to take and to be appropriately skilled, trained and rehearsed for that role.

References

Alexander, D., 2005. Early mental health intervention after disasters. Advances in Psychiatric Treatment 11 (1), 12–18.

Alexander, D., Klein, S., 2011. Major incidents. In: Smith, J., Greaves, I., Porter, K. (Eds.), Oxford Desk Reference: Major Trauma. Oxford Medical Publications, Oxford.

Carley, S., Mackway-Jones, 2005. Major Incident Medical Management and Support: The Practical Approach in the Hospital. Blackwell Publishing, Advanced Life Support Group, Oxford.

Carr, E.R.M., Chatrath, P., Palan, P., 2006. Audit of doctors' knowledge of major incident policies. Annals of the Royal College of Surgeons of England 88 (3), 313–315.

Carvalho, S., Reeves, M., Orford, J., 2011. Fundamental Aspects of Legal, Ethical and Professional Issues in Nursing, second ed. Quay Books, London.

Day, T., Challen, K., Walter, D., 2010. Major incident planning in primary care trusts in north-west England. Health Services Management Research 23, 25–29.

Department of Health Emergency Preparedness Division, 2005. The NHS Emergency Planning Guidance. Department of Health, London.

Department of Health Emergency Preparedness Division, 2011. The NHS Emergency Planning Guidance: Planning for the management of burn-injured patients in the event of a major incident: interim strategic national guidance. Department of Health, London.

Dolan, B., 2011a. Rising from the ruins. Nursing Standard 25 (28), 22–23.

Dolan, B., 2011b. Emergency nursing in an earthquake zone. Emergency Nurse 19 (1), 12–15.

Dolan, B., Esson, A., Grainger, P., et al., 2011. Earthquake disaster response in Christchurch, New Zealand. Journal of Emergency Nursing 37 (5), 506–509.

Firth-Cozens, J., Midgley, S.J., Burgess, C., 2000. Questionnaire survey of post-traumatic stress disorder in doctors involved in the Omagh bombing. British Medical Journal 319, 1609.

Home Office, 2004. Civil Contingencies Act. Home Office, London.

HSE, 1996a. Emergency Planning in the NHS: Health Services Arrangements for Dealing with Major Incidents, vol. 1. Department of Health, London.

HSE, 1996b. Emergency Planning in the NHS: Health Services Arrangements for Dealing with Major Incidents, vol. 2. Department of Health, London.

Knight, J.F., Carley, S., Tregunna, B., et al., 2010. Serious gaming technology in major incident training: A pragmatic controlled trial. Resuscitation 81, 1175–1179.

Lavery, G.G., Horan, E., 2005. Clinical review: Communication and logistics in the response to the 1998 terrorist bombing in Omagh, Northern Ireland, Critical Care 9, 401–408.

Linney, A.C.S., Kernohan, W.G., Higgins, R., 2011. The identification of competencies for an NHS response to chemical, biological, nuclear and explosive (CBRNe) emergencies. International Emergency Nursing 19, 96–105.

Milkhu, C.S., Howell, D.C.J., Glynne, P.A., et al., 2008. Mass casualty incidents: Are NHS staff prepared? An audit of one NHS foundation trust. Emergency Medicine Journal 25 (10), 562–564.

National Audit Office, 2002. Facing the Challenge: NHS Emergency Planning in England. National Audit Office, London.

Smith, A.F., Wild, C., Law, J., 2005. The Barrow-in-Furness legionnaires' outbreak: qualitative study of the hospital response and the role of the major incident plan. Emergency Medicine Journal 22 (4), 251–255.

Walter, D., 2011. Communication. In: Smith, J., Greaves, I., Porter, K. (Eds.), Oxford Desk Reference: Major Trauma. Oxford Medical Publications, Oxford.

Transportation of the acutely ill patient

4

Gerry Bolger

CHAPTER CONTENTS

Introduction

This chapter outlines the nursing care and operational considerations in regard to transportation of the acutely ill person. It will build upon areas elsewhere in this book and will identify the pre-, peri- and post-transportation issues and the care needs of people in transportation. The focus of this chapter will primarily be on secondary rather than primary transportation, as other chapters such as Chapters 1 and 3 make reference to pre-hospital care and the assessment prior to transportation. It links the social trends on movement of people with the need to provide rapid transportation.

Travel trends

With the onset of travel, especially aviation, more people travel year on year. Since the middle of the last century there has been a significant increase in travel:

- between 1950 and 2005, international tourism arrivals expanded at an annual rate of 6.5%, growing from 25 million to 806 million travellers
- the income generated by these arrivals grew at an even stronger rate reaching 11.2% during the same period, outgrowing the world economy to reach around US$680 billion in 2005
- while in 1950 the top 15 destinations absorbed 88% of international arrivals, in 1970 the proportion was 75% and decreased to 57% in 2005, reflecting the emergence of new destinations, many of them in developing countries (United Nations World Tourism Organization 2010, European Travel Commission 2011).

The United Nations World Tourism Organization (UNWTO) stated that of the 922 million international tourist arrivals in 2008, air transport accounted for about 52% of arrivals and marine transport 6%.

- since 1984, trends in UK travel abroad have risen from 22 million residents to 58.6m in 2009; equally travel to the UK from abroad has also increased since 1984 with 13.6 million overseas residents rising to 28.9m in 2009 (Office of National Statistics 2010)
- the US had 56 million international visitors from 213 countries during 2007, up 10% from 2006; total arrivals were also up 9% from 2000, the former record year for

total non-resident visitation to the country (International Trade Administration 2008).

Travel, and specifically tourism, is a significant economic factor for both the UK and the world global economy at large. According to the Office of National Statistics (ONS 2010), spending by overseas residents within the UK has increased from £4.6 billion in 1984 to £16.6bn in 2009.

With mass movement of people there is also the corresponding movement of organisms and disease, which presents many health challenges. Firstly, as the human body can be a host for a number of organisms, mobilization of diseases across countries and continents is far easier when compared to 50 or 60 years ago. Secondly, as some parts of the world become more affluent, travelling is no longer seen as a luxury, and ease of travel means that more people have access to and the means to travel to different destinations.

Thirdly, as people live longer and many long-term conditions become the norm, the potential for illness, relapse, injury or deterioration requires the need for transportation of chronic and acutely ill patients often across long distances using modes of transport not originally intended for the care of the ill person. As such, this creates challenges in the environment of care and the associated assessment and operational factors required to provide this care. This chapter will discuss these in more detail.

Trends in admissions to critical care settings

Critical care admissions data collected by the NHS in England provide some insight into the patterns and reasons for admission to critical care units. Data from the first publication from Hospital Episodes Statistics (HES) in England show that 82 % of critical care records in the period April 2008–March 2009 were available, with 50 % of admissions showing detailed sources (Health and Social Care Information Centre 2009). While 45 % of data does not identify the reason for admission, of the remaining data just over 1 in 4 or 28 % are unplanned admissions with the majority being local admissions resulting in over 36 000 critical care transfers. While tertiary transfers are just fewer than 2900 cases, repatriations from neighbouring hospitals or overseas are recorded in over 3000 transfers. The dataset goes on to show that approximately 1 in 6 patients being admitted into a critical care bed will require a transfer and transportation.

Types of transportation

There are broadly three types of transportation:

- *primary* transportation refers to the initial response of the acutely ill or injured from the scene of accident or incident to a care facility
- *secondary* transportation is any onward movements following the primary transportation; also sometimes called *tertiary* transportation to specialist care or repatriation

when it refers to moving someone back to their country of domicile after they become ill or injured abroad
- *patient transport* refers to general movement; patient transport service (PTS) is used for routine transportation of patients to and from hospital care, such as outpatients appointments or discharge to their place of residence.

In the UK, the development of regional trauma centres and specialist centres, e.g., burn units, neurosurgical units (if not contained within trauma centres), specialist neonatal units (level 1), will mean secondary transfer will probably be necessary. The role of the nurse in the preparation, both pre-transfer and co-ordination of care by communicating with the receiving hospital/centre is key in the safe and effective transfer of the acutely ill or injured person.

Primary transfers

This is the transfer of the acutely ill or injured person to a care setting that offers care for the injuries or illness. This is following the immediate stabilization of the casualty or person, which allows for transportation. The primary purpose is to get the victim to a place of care as quickly and as safely as possibly without exacerbating the situation, injury or presenting complaint. This may be to a trauma centre for immediate life-saving intervention, or to a general accident and emergency service for ongoing care after stabilization, assessment of other conditions, or other potential factors that may require intervention. This will only happen following stabilization prior to transport.

Because of the need for rapid intervention, transportation and support, time is a critical factor in insuring a fast transfer to the appropriate care setting. This will often mean only one or two modes which may be considered: road or air. In the majority of cases, because of limited aircraft availability the transport will usually be a road transfer. This is discussed further in the chapter.

The mode of transport will influence what care is needed pre-transportation. For example, it may be necessary to intubate in advance rather than attempt to intubate in transit because of space, movement and other external factors. The steps required for the pre-hospital care environment are discussed in Chapter 1.

Secondary transfers

As the name suggests, this is the transfer of the acutely ill or injured person needing transfer to another care setting for further or specialist care. This occurs after the initial primary transfer to a care setting for stabilization or management of injuries, and is sometimes referred to as 'inter-hospital transfers' if between local hospitals. If the clinical condition of the ill or injured person warrants it and there is a need to transfer to a speciality unit for on-going care, this is referred to as *tertiary* transfers.

Transfers back to the care setting responsible for the person's on-going condition (including back to their country of domicile), or where rehabilitation is appropriate, are classed as *repatriation* transfers. Because of the distances involved, the patient's clinical condition and resources will influence the appropriate mode of transportation. The Association of Anaesthetists of Great Britain and Ireland has developed recommendations that are summarized in Box 4.1.

Box 4.1

Factors affecting transfers

- The clinical condition of the acutely ill or injured person
- The distance to the secondary care (or tertiary care) facility
- The availability of specialist services and support
- The availability and cost of the transfer resources

Association of Anaesthetists of Great Britain and Ireland (2009).

Patient transport services

A third type of transportation is patient transport services, which are provided for patients requiring routine transportation to and from hospital for appointments and to transport them from hospital to home when clinically appropriate. This type of transportation is planned in advance, sometimes requires clinical warrants to be provided and is by road in most, if not all, cases. As this service is aimed at non-acutely ill patients, this chapter will not discuss the issues of patient transport services.

Factors affecting transfers

Several factors need to be balanced and risk assessed to ensure a successful transfer. The decision to make the transfer needs to be a multi-professional decision as each profession will bring their unique and valid perspectives ensures adequate preparation to such care. While the responsibility rests with the lead clinician, it is good practice to have a multi-professional input into secondary transfer to ensure appropriate risk assessment and planning takes place.

In some cases it is worth considering what, if any, alternatives to secondary transfers may be available, especially if the patient's clinical condition is of concern. One such option is a visiting clinical team or service, especially for some surgical procedures. For example, cardiothoracic teams operate over a regional or geographic area rather than transferring acutely ill patients.

A key operational issue that is often overlooked is that unless a local policy dictates otherwise, secondary transfers, i.e., tertiary and repatriations transfers, should not route via the Emergency Department (ED) unless there has been deterioration in the patient's condition or a new event requiring immediate intervention. Being sent to the ED for registration purposes is poor practice (Box 4.2).

Modes of transportation

With the advent of emergency call centres, coupled with evidence-based decision-making algorithms, there is now a

Box 4.2

Key principles of transfer

1. Transfer can be safely accomplished even in extremely ill patients. Those involved in transfers have the responsibility for ensuring that everything necessary is done to achieve this
2. The need for transfers between hospitals is likely to increase. Transfers for non-clinical reasons should only take place in exceptional circumstances, and ideally only during daylight hours
3. The decision to transfer must involve a senior and experienced clinician
4. Hospitals should form transfer networks to coordinate and manage clinically indicated transfers
5. Networks should take responsibility for ensuring that arrangements can be made for accepting transfers to an agreed protocol with minimal administrative delays
6. Protocols, documentation and equipment for transfers should be standardized within networks
7. All doctors and other personnel undertaking transfers should have the appropriate competencies, qualifications and experience. It is highly desirable that this should include attendance at a suitable transfer course
8. A professional, dedicated transfer service has many advantages and is the preferred method of transferring suitable patients
9. Hospitals must ensure that suitable transfer equipment is provided
10. Hospitals must ensure that they have robust arrangements to ensure that sending personnel on a transfer does not jeopardize other work within the hospital
11. Hospitals must ensure that employees sent on transfers have adequate insurance cover and are made aware of the terms and limitations of this cover
12. Arrangements must be in place to ensure that personnel and equipment can safely and promptly return to base after the transfer
13. Details of every transfer must be recorded and subject to regular audit and review

(Data from Association of Anaesthetists of Great Britain and Ireland (2009) *AAGBI Safety Guidelines: Inter-hospital Transfer.* London: Association of Anaesthetists of Great Britain and Ireland.)

move away from dispatching two-person road ambulances, especially in cities and urban areas in parts of the UK. The initial response in some parts of England is now a single paramedic responder on a motorbike. Their role is to provide an initial response, provide care and call in for supportive back up based on that initial assessment or triage. While triage was historically developed for battlefield prioritization, it is now used routinely by emergency response services.

While progress in transportation over the last 100 years has increased the mode of transport options, the majority of both primary and secondary transfers have been by road transportation. Historically, ambulances provided a basic collection and removal of the ill or injured person. They now provide a mobile primary response service by providing the initial assessment, stabilization prior to transportation to ongoing care at a hospital base. Aircraft and helicopters provide a means of rapid movement of people over long distances, offering significant advances to the survival of injured or ill patients. While each mode of transport has benefits they also have risks, and the choice of mode is as important as the response itself.

Considerations on appropriate transportation

The mode of transport may have already been determined in some situations. In most cases the primary response will be a ground response due to resource availability. Not all ambulance response services will have air support, which is either provided at a regional or country level and then against strict criteria. Ground response will be appropriate in most cases, however there are some options and variances that should be considered. The mode of transport is a key factor in the management of the acutely ill person.

Where any of these factors are compromised then alternatives need to be considered, assuming such supportive resources exist or can be accessed. Holleran & Rhoades (2005) discuss these and similar factors in their work. In some parts of the UK air support may be provided by special request from neighbouring authorities, especially when road transportation in isolated areas or the victim's condition is serious, rapid transportation to a facility may warrant the use of a primary helicopter. The Intensive Care Society (2002) suggests that for long journeys where road access is difficult, air transport may be quicker; however the perceived speed of air transport must be balanced against organizational delays and inter-vehicle transfers.

Ground transportation

Ground response is the most common. It is used for both primary and secondary transportation widely across the UK as well as internationally. The accepted form is the dedicated road ambulance vehicle.

Internationally, ambulance vehicles are specially adapted to provide a primary response as well as supportive care in transportation of the acutely ill adult. In the UK specialist retrieval teams and ambulances are developed, such as the CATS – the Children's Acute Ambulance Service – specialist retrieval teams that support the acutely ill child by sending, stabilizing, and preparing a child for transfer to a tertiary service.

Modern vehicles all have life-saving equipment with automatic external defibrillators, suction, and a wide range of medication to support critical care to obstetric care. These will have 240 volt AC power, a secure critical care trolley and carry a ventilator and syringe drivers. It is more usual to request an ambulance from the local ambulance service to perform the transfer (Box 4.3).

Air transportation

Used to move injured soldiers in World War I in Italy (Bellini 2008), and in common use by World War II, aircraft have advanced over time since then to be pressurized, comfortable and a common mode of general transportation. However,

Box 4.3

The European Committee for Standardization specifications for ambulances

Patient transport ambulances (Types A1, A2)

Generally only used for the non-emergency transportation of patients, either between facilities or between a facility and a residence. The emphasis is on transportation; such ambulances have limited treatment or equipment space. Smaller communities may also use such ambulances because of cost, particularly if there is no Advanced Life Support (ALS) service, or if another vehicle or pre-hospital response crew provides ALS.

Emergency ambulances (Type B)

This is the most commonly seen type of emergency ambulance. This vehicle type permits increased treatment space and also the ability to store significantly larger amounts of medical equipment. Such vehicles will typically respond independently to emergency calls, providing some level of treatment. For high-priority emergency calls, these will often be supplemented by the response of a pre-hospital response or British Association of Immediate Care (BASICS) support response crew.

Mobile intensive care unit (Type C)

This type of ambulance is commonly seen in the movement of high-acuity (ICU) patients between hospitals. It provides adequate space for not only the medical equipment commonly seen in ambulances, but also to accommodate hospital equipment such as ventilators, during transport. In some locations, vehicles of this design may be used to provide mobile resuscitation services, either supplemented by a pre-hospital response or Notarzt response, equivalent to the BASICS support response crew.

movement by air has limitations and the response will be determined by key factors. Response by air is influenced by whether it is a primary or secondary response. The major advantages of an air response are both speed by the reduction in journey time and the ability to get the acutely ill or injured person from point A to B with minimal changes or delays.

However, aircraft were never developed or intended as ambulances or designed for the acutely ill or injured. Aircraft are in effect long tubes flying at great speed at reduced internal air pressure. The higher the aircraft flies the greater the need for pressurization at an altitude that normal healthy people can breathe normally. Normal jet aircraft cruise between 11 000–12 200 metres (36 000–40 000 feet) and are pressurized to be between 1 800–2 400 metres (6000–8000 feet), which supports normal respiration in normally healthy people. Above 3 048 meters (10 000 feet) hypoxia becomes a major issue and consciousness is not sustainable without supplemental oxygen.

Effect of air pressure on acutely ill

Impact of available oxygen

In the last 100 years there has been a growing understanding of the impact of air travel and the changes in pressure to human physiology. Martin (2001), Rainford & Grandwell (2006) and Holleran (2009) outline in detail how changes in air pressure affect the human body.

Figure 4.1 • Relationship between atmospheric pressure (mmHg) and altitude (ft) • (British Thoracic Society (2004) *Managing Passengers with Respiratory Disease Planning Air Travel Summary for Primary Care*. London, British Thoracic Society. Adapted by permission from BMJ Publishing Group Limited.)

Although the percentage of oxygen in inspired air is constant at different altitudes, the fall in atmospheric pressure at higher altitude decreases the partial pressure of inspired oxygen and hence the driving pressure for gas exchange in the lungs. An ocean of air is present up to 9 000–10 000 m, where the troposphere ends and the stratosphere begins. The weight of air above us is responsible for the atmospheric pressure, which is normally about 100 kPa at sea level. This atmospheric pressure is the sum of the partial pressures of the constituent gases, oxygen and nitrogen, and also the partial pressure of water vapour (6.3 kPa at 37°C). As oxygen is 21 % of dry air, the inspired oxygen pressure at sea level (Peacock 1998) (Fig 4.1) is calculated as follows:

$$0.21 \times (100 - 6.3) = 19.68 \text{ kPa}$$

Because of the effect of falling barometric pressure, even while pressurized to 2 438 metres (8 000 feet), for the majority of people there are no adverse effects despite the partial pressure of oxygen being at 120 mmHg (16.0 kPa), which corresponds to 75 % of the sea-level value of oxygen at 160 mmHg (21.3 kPa). This means a reduction in arterial oxygen tension from 95 mmHg (12.7 kPa) to between 53–64 mmHg (7.0–8.5 kPa), so oxygen saturation reduces from 97 % saturation on the ground (at sea level) to between 80–92 % at cruising altitude 2 438 metres (8 000 feet) (British Medical Association 2004). This is known as the oxygen disassociation curve and is covered in more detail in Chapter 23.

For healthy individuals there are usually no adverse effects; however, individuals with health problems that can affect the transportation, delivery or uptake of oxygen will need careful planning, management, monitoring and support during transport by air. These conditions include, but are not limited to, pulmonary disease, cardiac failure, anaemia, infection, or any organ susceptible to a reduction in oxygen, e.g., cerebral disease (trans-ischaemic attacks or cerebrovascular accidents).

Impact of pressure on main organs

Boyle's gas law, where *Pressure × Volume = Constant*, means that as an aircraft ascends and pressure drops, gas expands. The expansion will be affected by the reduction in air pressure, and at 2 438 metres (8 000 feet) this means an increase in expanded gas of approximately 30 %. Where gas can pass freely there is no problem; however, there can be problems where there is trapped or limited free gas movement, including in any organ which has had surgery in the proceeding 14 days.

This means that any object which has air in an enclosed space will expand. For patients, this affects drains, intravenous giving sets and infusion bags, colostomy bags and even the surface they are lying on if it has enclosed air. It also affects the human body including the gastrointestinal tract, sinuses, teeth, and the ear canal. As such, any person who has had recent surgery where air will have entered the body should not fly without prior medical clearance, and this is usually not less than 10 days for the air to be naturally absorbed.

There are particular consequences for those who have circulatory problems or inability to carry oxygen, e.g., anaemia or hypovolaemia, with haemoglobin less than 7.5 gm/dL, as these travelers are at risk of hypoxia and require supplemental oxygen or transfusion to correct the anaemia. This would also include any patient where hypoxia could exacerbate an underlying problem, e.g., the cerebral or cardiac condition, those with trans-ischaemic attacks, or a cerebral vascular accident, because the reduced partial pressure of O_2 can increase the CO_2 in the cerebral tissue and potentially put them at risk of a further attack or worse an extension. Likewise, this includes any patient with myocardial blockages or a recent cardiac event.

Second are those patients with an underlying respiratory problem, chronic obstructive airways disease or left ventricular failure. Because of the oxygen disassociation curve principles, at sea level these patients are already compromised and a partial reduction due to the gas laws in an aircraft could mean a rapid de-saturation. It is imperative that ongoing monitoring of the patient oxygen saturation is maintained, and should their saturated O_2 rate fall below that on the ground, or below 85 %, that they are given supplemental oxygen. This includes those patients with COPD as the drop in O_2 is significant and will expose them to hypoxia. Supplemental oxygen is usually available in 2 and 4 litres flow rate per minute. It is essential to ensure an adequate amount of oxygen for the whole journey plus a reserve in case of a delay.

To ensure safe and uneventful transportation by air, the person travelling should be assessed for travel thoroughly by a suitably qualified aero-medical doctor. If it is deemed necessary that the person needs a clinical escort, it should be by a suitably qualified and trained aero-medical repatriation nurse or doctor.

At lower flying levels, aircraft cabins, including helicopters, are usually not pressurized. However, they are susceptible to the effects of turbulence, vibration, can be cold, and with helicopters noise. As a result, some equipment, e.g., stethoscopes, is unusable in the air. Sphygmomanometers containing mercury are restricted, so digital sphygmomanometers must be used. Furthermore, temperature affects the ability to record oxygen saturation and a low saturation due to cold peripheral extremities rather than hypoxia should be considered.

On commercial aircraft each airline is responsible for providing medical clearance for its patients prior to flight. The International Air Transport Association (2010) issued medical clearance guidance to airlines and their governing bodies to support suitability to fly. Box 4.4 summarizes the main impact of changes in air pressure on key organs.

 Box 4.4

Effect of gas on main organs

- *Ear* (minimal impact) – gas is released from the Eustachian tubes by yawning; however where otitis media is present travel by air should not occur due to the significant risk of ruptured ear drum
- *Sinuses* – while normally not a problem, due to mucus build up there is a low risk of barosinusitis
- *Lungs* – normally no problem; however, where there has been history of pneumothorax the British Thoracic Society (2004) has issued guidance on a wide range of respiratory conditions and assessment, especially those with oxygen saturation levels below 95 %. When transferring a patient with a pneumothorax a one-way flutter valve (or Heimlich valve) should be connected to the draining tube to prevent the effect of gas expansion affect the thoracic tissue
- *Abdomen* – Normal gas releasing happens over time; however those with colostomies or urostomies need to be alerted to the effect of flying and the need to have a bag empty of air prior to flying otherwise risk of bursting will occur. It is possible for the abdomen to contain up to 1 000 mL of gas at altitude

Contraindications to air travel

While for most patients in most situations travel by air is acceptable, there are a number of conditions where air travel is contraindicated (World Health Organization 2010). However, while some commercial airlines will accept a number of these conditions, a specialized air ambulance would be an alternative approach with appropriate medical and nursing support (Box 4.5).

Primary response by air

A primary response by air usually uses helicopters because they can land and take off from places inaccessible by ground and other vehicles. Most trauma centres now have a helipad facilitating point-to-point transfers and rapid interventions; it is used primarily as air transfer as it may reduce transportation by a quarter of normal road response time. They also operate in lower altitudes, thus reducing any impact of changes of altitude on the body especially below 610 metres (2 000 feet). Specific primary response/transportation helicopters will be set up with key clinical equipment to support the retrieval and transportation of the acutely ill or injured person.

Box 4.5

Contraindications to air travel

Travel by air is normally contraindicated in the following cases:
- Infants less than 48 hours old
- Women after the 36th week of pregnancy (32nd week for multiple pregnancies)
- Those suffering from:
  - angina pectoris or chest pain at rest
  - any active communicable disease
  - decompression sickness after diving
  - increased intracranial pressure due to haemorrhage, trauma or infection
  - infections of the sinuses or of the ear and nose, particularly if the Eustachian tube is blocked
  - recent myocardial infarction and stroke–elapsed time since the event depending on severity of illness and duration of travel
  - recent surgery or injury where trapped air or gas may be present, especially abdominal trauma and gastrointestinal surgery, craniofacial and ocular injuries, brain operations, and eye operations involving penetration of the eyeball
  - severe chronic respiratory disease, breathlessness at rest, or unresolved pneumothorax
  - sickle-cell anaemia
  - psychotic illness, except when fully controlled

The above list is not comprehensive, and fitness for travel should be decided on a case-by-case basis (World Health Organization 2010).

The adverse factors that can affect the patient's physiological response as well as impact the ability of the medical personnel to perform certain functions and procedures are:
- noise
- vibration
- motion sickness
- and reduced or inability to maintain temperature management (Martin 2001).

The latter issue of temperature management is usually not an overarching factor as the transfer duration is relatively short time-wise. The majority of journeys are usually less than 30 minutes' duration and rarely exceed one hour.

Unless these issues adversely affect the movement of the injured or acutely ill patient, air transportation may be the mode of choice, especially in ensuring rapid supportive care. Undoubtedly helicopter primary transfers have saved thousands of lives worldwide since their introduction, especially among the most critically ill (Nicholl et al. 1995, Chipp et al. 2010).

The initial preparation and nursing considerations for a primary transfer will be the same as for a road ambulance transfer. The patient will need to have had a primary survey, most if not all cases will require c-spine immobilization and have adequate airway with venous access should there be a need to rapidly infuse. The level of consciousness and mechanism of injury, or underlying condition may require further preparation of intubation to ensure a patent airway. It is possible to provide infusions in these types of transfers.

A key risk time is the loading and unloading of the patient, and vigilance in ensuring that the patient's limbs do not get caught in stretchers. It is key that all members follow the lead of the clinical/medical lead especially with monitoring and clinical tubing. Only approved monitoring equipment authorized by the appropriate aviation authorities should be used (Box 4.6).

Secondary repatriation by air

Pressurized twin or jet engine aircraft usually do air transfers, although for some secondary responses helicopters may be an option, especially for the acutely ill and medium-length transfers.

Aircraft in the UK are not usually dedicated to air responses unlike in other parts of Europe, the US and Australasia, although some companies that specialize in air repatriation have adapted and dedicated aircraft. In the UK, the majority of secondary air transfers will be from the Islands and from remote parts of the UK to tertiary services. The Intensive Care Society (2002) recommends that air transportation in a fixed wing aircraft should be considered for distances greater than 150 miles, and helicopter in place of long road journeys or where roads are inaccessible.

Search and rescue

A final service in transportation of people is 'search and rescue'. In the UK, the Coast Guard manages this with Royal Air Force support for helicopter rescue. Its primary purpose is to retrieve the person from the situation, whether it is at sea, mountainous terrain, or on the side of a cliff, and then transport them to land or a place where care can take place. As well as possible trauma injuries, these people are prone to hypothermia.

Special considerations for transportation by air

Regardless of aircraft type, space is a major issue. In the majority of cases, where a patient is placed on a stretcher the patient will be positioned feet forward against the side of the aircraft, meaning access from either the left or right is not possible. This has major implications for access and also positioning, so care must be taken to note the skin integrity before, during and after the flight and secondary transport, with all corresponding actions to prevent pressure ulceration.

The patient is positioned in an aircraft on Joint Aviation Authorities (JAA)/Civil Aviation Authority (UK) CAA approved stretchers, with four-point (over shoulder and abdomen) safety belts. In commercial aircraft and smaller

Box 4.6

The transfer process

As secondary transfers either relocate a primary injured patient from one hospital or facility to another, there is usually sufficient time to plan and prepare both the patient and agree a time with the accepting hospital or facility when they can expect or receive the patient. The steps in this process will vary slightly by region and hospital but principally are:

1. Before any transfer, the patient is accepted by a named consultant or clinician at the receiving hospital or faculty on a specified date.

2. The patient will be transported by the mode appropriate to their clinical condition taking into account accepted best practice, and any national or regional transfer guidance as well as economic and logistical factors. This will usually be decided by the dispatching hospital and where more than one mode is used, will have ensured the onward transfer by road ambulance and return of the transfer staff.

3. The transferred patient is clinically assessed immediately prior to transfer to ensure they are suitable for transfer, this assessment should include key nursing assessments including assessment for potential complications of pressure ulcers, and should this be a potential risk, action taken and interventions are duly documented.

4. The dispatching hospital or unit will ensure that the patient's next-of-kin and any significant other(s) are informed of the transfer, the location, time and provide a contact name/number for them to liaise with.

5. The patient will be accompanied by appropriately trained clinical staff being trained to transfer in the mode, and able to work and respond to deterioration in that environment who will ensure that the patient's dignity is maintained; monitoring the patient throughout the progress, documenting all monitoring and actions.

6. Clinical information will have been provided to the accepting clinical team in advance and should the accepting individual or team not be on duty when the patient arrives, that this information will have been passed to a named individual who will be able to accept and will be responsible for assessing the patient on arrival.

7. Because this is a secondary transfer, the patient will go straight to the clinical area, unless there has been deterioration in the patient's condition or a new event warranting immediate assessment in an emergency unit. The transportation team, or named transfer nurse/doctor will remain with the patient until the assessing clinical staff have accepted the patient. If there is a likely delay this may be omitted subject to the nursing staff being comfortable with accepting the patient (and subject to local policy).

8. All clinical information will be provided, including radiological investigation, diagnostic investigations and clinical notes to reduce unnecessary duplication, delay in treatment and exposure to unnecessary procedures. The patient's property should also accompany them unless there is good reason that this is not practical. The patient's medication should be administered in line with recommended best practice (Royal College of Nursing 2006), especially in nurse-led transfers, and the medication are both prescribed and dispensed to the named patient.

9. Infection prevention is a key issue for all healthcare providers, as such the dispatching hospital will provide a report on the infectious status of the patient being admitted, and unless this is available or unclear, the receiving unit may choose to isolate the patient, unless clinically contraindicated, while maintaining their care.

10. The transferring clinical team will maintain confidentiality and apply universal precautions, follow infection prevention and control procedures including decontamination following the transfer.

jets, the space above the person is usually restricted. Lastly, because of the gas laws of physics, any equipment that has air in it will expand.

Commercial airlines require any patient to be screened by their own staff, they require either an Incapacitated Passengers Handling Advice (INCAD) form and/or a Medical Information Form (MEDIF). If they are frequent travelers they are likely to have a Frequent Travelers medical card; however, these are only relevant to those individuals requiring mobility and clearance assistance rather than for transfer in an acute phase.

These forms help the airlines assess the level of risk of an interrupted journey, as the cost of a diversion is hugely expensive financially, operationally and adversely affects their reputation. They also ensure that all the appropriate support of supplemental oxygen, transfer arrangement and assistance on board and disembarking are in place.

More recently, many commercial airlines do not carry stretchers and require the patient to walk or to be wheeled to their seat, and should they need to lie down during the flight, airline now offer club seats or first class alternatives. Some airlines, e.g., Lufthansa, provide dedicated units for stretcher patients to support privacy and dignity. Where an airline cannot carry a person, such as risk to the person, infectious risk, or they are unsuitable candidates, the only alternative is a privately hired aircraft.

Venous Thromboembolisms

In the 1990s awareness of deep vein thrombosis (DVT), now considered part of venous thromboembolism (VTE), as part of long-haul flying came under scrutiny. The UK House of Lords Science and Technology Committee investigated and produced *Air Travel and Health* that identified those who are at low, medium and higher risk of developing DVT/VTEs in flight (UK Parliament 2000). A subsequent report (UK Parliament 2007) further looked at DVT/VTEs and other issues raised in the first report. The issues around DVT/VTEs were considered as part of a wider World Health Organization Research Into Global Hazards of Travel (WRIGHT) project that was developed to confirm that the risk of VTE is increased by air travel. The study also determined the magnitude of risk, the effect of other factors on the risk, and the effect of preventive measures on risk (Box 4.7).

While there is still a lack of clarity on how to prevent air-related DVTs, the use of aspirin is yet to be clearly identified as a reputable source. However, the use of low-molecular-weight heparin in the prevention of DVT in higher-risk groups, including those who have previously had a DVT, is well established but it is not clear how it should be used in the prevention of travel-related DVT (British Medical Association 2004, Katsumata et al. 2012).

Special considerations

In all cases patient safety must be paramount in the transportation of patients or acutely ill persons. When dealing with specialist cases, e.g., intensive care patients, patients with traumatic brain or neurological injury, paediatric patients and neonates, specialist attention is required.

Box 4.7

Venous thromboembolism and air travel

- Travelling for more than four hours in any form of transport approximately doubled the risk of VTE
- The absolute risk of VTE for a flight of more than four hours was 1 in 6000 passengers, rising to about 1 in 1000 passengers for longer journeys and multiple flights
- The longer the flight, including multiple trips, the greater the risk of developing VTE
- There is no difference in the relative risk of VTE if the cabin pressure was reduced
- Those who were very short, very tall or overweight were at slightly greater risk
- Travelling by air accentuated other pre-existing VTE risk factors, e.g., use of oral contraceptives and the presence of prothrombotic blood abnormalities
- 'Hyper-responders' seemed to react to unspecified flight-related factors. If an individual had a risk factor the likelihood of him developing VTE increased dramatically after an 8-hour flight

(UK Parliament (2007) *House of Lords Science and Technology Committee Air Travel and Health: An Update*. London, The Stationery Office.)

When preparing all transfers, it is paramount that specialist teams are considered, possibly using retrieval/collection teams if they exist. The suitably qualified (in the relevant specialty) and experienced clinical staff should follow the nationally agreed or professionally developed transfer guidelines (Middleton 2011). This should also include any specific documentation required as recommended.

Transfer of adult intensive care patients

In 1997 there were an estimated 11 000 tranfers (Association of Anaesthetists of Great Britain and Ireland 2009), however figures for the number of such transfers carried out currently are difficult to obtain as there is no national reporting (Intensive Care Society 2011). There are a number of international and national guidance documents (Association of Anaesthetists of Great Britain and Ireland 2009, Clinical Resource Efficiency and Resource Team 2006), which outline the key priorities. While these discuss the operational and skills level of the practitioner (Holleran 2002), there is also a need for nurses to have a suitable level of training to provide effective transfer and transportation support.

The Intensive Care Society (2002) issued guidance that covers an array of core service provision at EDs, consultant cover, transportation guidance on the number of staff and skills set, equipment and preparation, including competence of transport personnel, the role of nursing staff, the role of critical care networks, and the need for dedicated equipment.

While the rate of adverse events by clinically specialized teams is low (Kue et al. 2011), this requires adequate preparation of the team and the equipment. To support practitioners there is a need for adequate preparation (Bambi & Day 2010) and transportation checklists (Intensive Care Society 2002,

Nocera 2002) have emerged that support practice around key areas. The Intensive Care Society guidelines include a number of checklists, for example: 'Is the patient stable for transport' covering airway, ventilation, circulation, metabolic, neurology, trauma, and monitoring and 'Are you ready for departure'. These checklists are further supported by detailed guidance in the document.

Transfer of patients with neurological injuries

Patients who have developed brain or neurological injuries following trauma require special attention. The mechanism of injury will determine what care is required and the resulting injury may require treatment after initial resuscitation of other life-threatening injuries.

These types of injuries require rapid discussion, usually consultant-to-consultant prior to transfer. The Association of Anaesthetists of Great Britain and Ireland (2006) developed recommendations for the transfer of patients with brain injuries (Box 4.8).

Box 4.8

Safe transfer of patients with brain injury guidance

1. High-quality transfer of patients with brain injury improves outcome.
2. There should be designated consultants in the referring hospitals and the neuroscience units with overall responsibility for the transfer of patients with brain injuries.
3. Local guidelines on the transfer of patients with brain injuries should be drawn up between the referring hospital trusts, the neurosciences unit and the local ambulance service. These should be consistent with established national guidelines. Details of the transfer of responsibility for patient care should also be agreed.
4. While it is understood that transfer is often urgent, thorough resuscitation and stabilization of the patient must be completed before transfer to avoid complications during the journey.
5. All patients should be intubated and ventilated if they meet any of the following criteria:
   - Glasgow coma score of 8 or less
   - Significantly deteriorating conscious level, i.e., fall in motor score of two or more of the following factors: loss of protective laryngeal reflexes; hypoxaemia (PaO_2 <13 kPa on oxygen); hypercarbia ($PaCO_2$ >6 kPa); spontaneous hyperventilation causing $PaCO_2$ <4.0 kPa; bilateral fractured mandible; or copious bleeding into the mouth (e.g., from skull base fracture).
6. Patients with brain injuries should be accompanied by a doctor with appropriate training and experience in the transfer of patients with acute brain injury. They must have a dedicated and adequately trained assistant. Arrangements for medical indemnity and personal accident insurance should be in place.
7. The standard of monitoring during transport should adhere to previously published standards.

(Association of Anaesthetists of Great Britain and Ireland (2006) Recommendations for the Safe Transfer of Patients with Brain Injury. London: Association of Anaesthetists of Great Britain and Ireland.)

Transfer of children

Acutely ill paediatric transfers require the same attention to preparation and management as critical care transfers. The Royal College of Anaesthetists (2001) made the following recommendation on the transfer of paediatric patients; a transfer is normally undertaken by the paediatric emergency transfer team and where this is not feasible the following:

- there should be a designated consultant with the responsibility for transfers
- functional mobile equipment and relevant guidelines should be available
- all patient transfers should be accompanied by a trained doctor with a minimum of two years' experience who has the ability to perform tracheal intubation and is accompanied by a trained assistant, either an ICU nurse or Operating Department Practitioner.

There will be times when a transfer to another care centre is appropriate, and guidelines for the transfer of ambulatory paediatric patients are recommended in these cases (Clinical Resource Efficiency and Resource Team 2001) (Box 4.9). While speedy intervention into paediatric care is important, Killion & Stein (2009) argue that air versus road ambulance transfers have no impact on patient outcome. Further studies in Australia suggest that different approaches can influence transfer time (Soundappan et al. 2007).

Consideration of infection

Infection prevention and control are as applicable within hospital care as well as external to hospital care. A significant amount of meticillin-resistant *Staphylococcus aureus* and other organisms are transferred into and between care settings from

Box 4.9

Ambulatory paediatrics: guidelines for referrals and transfer

- An experienced paediatrician is needed when the unit is open, together with experienced nursing, clerical and other staff
- The service needs close association with, or inclusion of, a paediatric community nursing service
- Appropriate referrals are children considered by a general practitioner or ED staff to need further assessment, observation or investigation but likely to return home after a short period in the ambulatory unit
- The GP or ED must contact ambulatory unit staff to arrange the referral, especially if the child is acutely ill and needs paediatric expertise immediately
- Transfer arrangements must be carefully worked out with the local ambulance service
- Attendance will also be appropriate for some children who require follow up after discharge from hospital or initial attendance at the ambulatory unit, but this should not be used as a substitute for referral to a paediatric outpatient clinic

(Clinical Resource Efficiency and Resource Team (2001) Ambulatory Paediatrics Guidelines for referrals and transfer. Belfast, CREST.)

outside of hospital care. Transferring patients between hospitals poses significant risks to established infection control procedures, and each hospital will have localized policies in how patients are accepted and managed on arrival.

Some organizations will want confirmation of the status of a patient's infectious status with regard to specific or a range of organisms. While it is unlikely that someone will be denied treatment because of their infectious status, operationally this can delay when someone is accepted, especially with regards isolation facilities.

The transferring crew must follow universal precautions. The Department of Health in England have issued some guidance on 'Reducing infection through effective practice in the pre-hospital environment' (Department of Health 2008a). The document covers a range of topics from hand hygiene, personal protective equipment, aseptic technique and environmental cleanliness, through to the decontamination of ambulance stretcher beds. The nurse and medical escorts must ensure appropriate disposal of infectious clinical equipment.

Conclusion

Health systems, commissioners and providers of health need to be aware of the emerging forces around the movement of people in general to both predict and manage increasing numbers who need care and will require transportation. Nurses, especially those in EDs, critical care areas and those involved in transportation of patients are well placed to assess, plan the pathway of transportation, implement that care and evaluate it. Evaluation needs to be against the three outcome domains for quality (Department of Health 2008b):

1. the anticipated and expected experience: was the experience for the patient as anticipated, was all done to improve that experience?
2. the effectiveness of the need to transport: was the outcome after the transfer anticipated and could only have resulted from the transfer? Was the mode of transport the appropriate one, both for outcome and cost?
3. the safety: was a risk assessment in place to identify potential problems or harms? Did any occur? And what did the nursing intervention in place do to reduce harm?

With a growing body of evidence on the trends, outcomes, experiences and not just data, nurses and healthcare practitioners will be increasingly better placed to influence and improve the effects of care.

References

Association of Anaesthetists of Great Britain and Ireland, 2006. Recommendations for the Safe Transfer of Patients with Brain Injury. Association of Anaesthetists of Great Britain and Ireland, London.

Association of Anaesthetists of Great Britain and Ireland, 2009. AAGBI safety guideline - Inter-hospital Transfer. Association of Anaesthetists of Great Britain and Ireland, London.

Bambi, S., Day, D., 2010. The risk of intrahospital transport to patients. 'Keeping patients safe during intrahospital transport'. Critical Care Nurse 30 (6), 14–16.

Bellini, C., 2008. An historical perspective of early Italian air medical transport. Air Medical Journal 27 (6), 286–292.

British Medical Association, 2004. The Impact of Flying on Passenger Health: A Guide oor Healthcare Professionals. British Medical Association, London.

British Thoracic Society, 2004. Managing Passengers with Respiratory Disease Planning Air Travel Summary for Primary Care. British Thoracic Society, London.

Chipp, E., Warner, R.M., McGill, D.J., et al., 2010. Air ambulance transfers of adult patients to a UK regional burn centre: Who needs to fly? Burns 36 (8), 1201–1207.

Clinical Resource Efficiency and Resource Team, 2001. Ambulatory Paediatrics Guidelines for referrals and transfer. CREST, Belfast.

Clinical Resource Efficiency and Resource Team, 2006. Protocol for the Inter Hospital Transfer of Patients and their Records. CREST, Belfast.

Department of Health (England), 2008a. Ambulance Guidelines: Reducing Infection Through Effective Practice in the Pre-hospital Environment. Department of Health, London.

Department of Health (England), 2008b. High Quality Care for All: NHS Next Stage Review Final Report. Department of Health, London.

European Travel Commission, 2011. European Tourism in 2010: Trends & Prospects. European Travel Commission, Brussels.

Health and Social Care Information Centre, 2009. Hospital Episode Statistics 2008–2009. HSCIC, London.

Holleran, R., 2002. Challenges in transport nursing. Australian Emergency Nursing Journal 5 (1), 7–11.

Holleran, R., 2009. ASTNA Patient Transport: Principles and Practice, fourth ed. Mosby, St Louis.

Holleran, R., Rhoades, C., 2005. Ask the experts. Critical Care Nurse 25 (1), 58–59.

Intensive Care Society, 2002. Guidelines for the Transport of the Critically Care Adult. Intensive Care Society, London.

Intensive Care Society, 2011. Guidelines for the Transport of the Critically Ill Adult, third ed. ICS, London.

International Air Transport Association (IATA), 2010. Medical Manual, third ed. International Air Transport Association, Geneva.

International Trade Administration (USA), 2008. 2007 International Arrivals into the United States. Department of Commerce, Washington.

Katsumata, Y., Kimura, K., Sano, M., et al., 2012. Frequent long-distance flyer's undesirable mileage: an organized thrombus stuck in PFO. Journal of Thrombolysis 33 (3), 296–298.

Killion, C., Stein, H.M., 2009. The impact of air transport on neonatal outcomes. Newborn & Infant Nursing Reviews 9 (4), 207–211.

Kue, R., Brown, P., Ness, C., et al., 2011. Adverse clinical events during intrahospital transport by a specialized team: a preliminary report. American Journal of Critical Care 20 (2), 153–164.

Martin, T., 2001. Handbook of Patient Transportation. Greenwich Medical Media Ltd, London.

Middleton, P., 2011. Trauma retrieval. In: Smith, J., Greaves, I., Porter, K.M. (Eds.), Oxford Desk Reference: Major Trauma. Oxford University Press, Oxford.

Nicholl, J.P., Brazier, J.E., Snooks, H.A., 1995. Effects of London helicopter emergency medical service on survival after trauma. British Medical Journal 311 (6999), 217–222.

Nocera, N., 2002. The N.E.W.S. Checklist: Enhancing interhospital transfer of trauma patients. Australian Emergency Nursing Journal 5 (1), 12–14.

Office of National Statistics, 2010. Travel Trends, 2009 edition. Office of National Statistics, London.

Parliament, U.K., 2000. House of Lords Science and Technology Committee Air Travel and Health. The Stationery Office, London.

Parliament, U.K., 2007. House of Lords Science and Technology Committee Air Travel and Health: An Update. The Stationery Office, London.

Peacock, A.J., 1998. Oxygen at high altitude. British Medical Journal 317 (7165), 1063–1066.

Rainford, D.P., Grandwell, D.G., 2006. Ernsting's Aviation Medicine, fourth ed. Hodder, London.

Royal College of Nursing, 2006. Royal College of Nursing In-flight Nurses Association Clarification and Guidance on the Management and Administration of Medicines in the In-Flight Setting. Royal College of Nursing, London.

Soundappan, S.V., Holland, A.J., Fahy, F., et al., 2007. To study the appropriateness of, and time taken, to transfer pediatric trauma patients in New South Wales to The Children's Hospital at Westmead (CHW), a pediatric trauma center. The Journal of Trauma 62 (5), 1229–1233.

United Nations World Tourism Organization, 2010. World Tourism Barometer. UNWTO, Madrid.

World Health Organization, 2010. Mode of travel: Health considerations. In International Travel and Health, 2010 edition. World Health Organization, Geneva.

PART 2

Trauma care

Head injuries

5

Karen Sanders

Introduction

There are no reliable up-to-date figures for the total denominator of attendees who attend Emergency Departments (EDs) with a head injury (National Institute for Health and Clinical Excellence 2007). The role of ED staff is to diagnose and appropriately treat a large number of patients presenting following a head injury. Neurological damage occurs both at the time of the injury (primary insult) and evolves over the following minutes, hours and days (secondary insult). Patient outcomes improve where secondary insults are treated early, and where successful responses result in limiting and preventing further injury caused by secondary insult. Wyatt et al. (2008) argue that emergency nurses are 'fundamental to keeping morbidity to a minimum by being vigilant and prevent secondary brain injury.'

While 90% of traumatic brain injuries (TBIs) are considered mild (Vos et al. 2012), it is the world's leading cause of morbidity and mortality in individuals under the age of 45 years old (Wilson 2011). It is estimated that the ED attendance rate in the UK for patients with head injuries is close to 700 000 patients (National Institute for Clinical Excellence 2007) and that 20 % of these are admitted to hospital. Half of those who die from TBI do so within the two hours of the injury. Approximately 30 % of admitted patients with a Glasgow Coma Score (GCS) of <13 will die, and if the GCS is <8, this increases to 50% (Wilson 2011).

The most common causes of a minor head injury are falls (22–43 % of injuries), assaults (30–50 % of injuries), and road traffic accidents (25 % of injuries) (Department of Health 2001, National Institute for Health and Clinical Excellence 2007). In the UK, 70–88 % of individuals that sustain a head injury are male, 10–19 % are aged 65 years or greater, and 40–50 % are children. Alcohol may be involved in up to 65 % of adult head injuries and road traffic accidents account for a large proportion of moderate to severe head injuries. Traumatic injury in which severe head injury plays a major role in over 50 % of cases, is a leading cause of death in those aged 25 years or less (Maartens & Lethbridge 2005); 5–10 % of patients who suffer a severe head injury also suffer a cervical spine injury.

It is vital that the emergency department staff caring for patients with head injuries has a good knowledge and understanding of the anatomy and physiology of the skull, the brain and its related structures along with the physiological processes that maintain homeostasis. Such knowledge and understanding allows the nurse to relate the mechanisms of injury to the brain injuries suffered and thus assess, plan, evaluate, and implement the care and management needed by the patient at any particular stage following the injury.

A structured approach to the care of head-injured patients should be initiated based on current valid evidence. The Brain Trauma Foundation has developed recommendations for the management of moderate and severe head injuries (Bratton et al. 2007) in collaboration with the Advanced Trauma Life Support (ATLS) system (American College of Surgeons 2008), providing a mechanism for assessment and immediate management and minimizes the risk of secondary brain injury in adults. For children the Advanced Paediatric Life Support (APLS) system (Advanced Life Support Group 2011) should be employed (National Institute for Health and Clinical Excellence 2007). These guidelines are based on class II (studies based on prospectively collected data and the retrospective analysis of reliable data) and III (studies based on retrospectively collected data) evidence. There is a lack of class I (prospective randomized controlled trials) evidence to support practice.

Anatomy and physiology

The skull

The skull is a rigid bony cavity composed of 29 individual bones: the 8 bones of the cranium, 14 facial bones, the 6 ossicles of the ear, and the hyoid bone. To ensure maximum protection, strength and support, bony capsules surround the brain, the eyes, the nasal passages, and the inner ear; bony buttresses extend upwards from the teeth through the facial bones. To relieve the potential weight, the skull is made lighter by the paranasal sinuses, which also give resonance to the voice.

The cranium is one of the strongest structures in the body and provides the bony protection for the brain. It is composed of the parietal (2), occipital, frontal, temporal (2), sphenoid, and ethmoid bones. Figure 5.1 shows an exploded view of the cranial skull; however, the bones are fused along main sutures, the sagittal, coronal, lambdoidal, and squamosal. The facial bones form the framework for the nasal and oral cavities and include the zygomatic bones (2), palatine bones

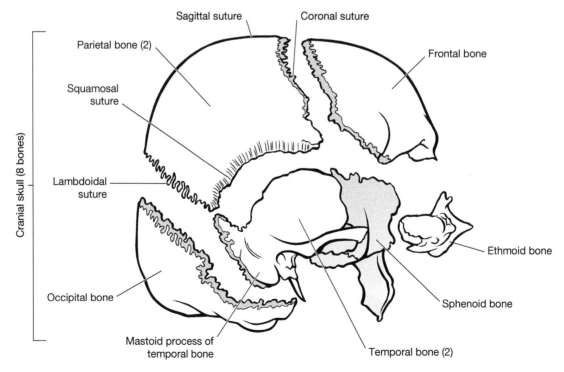

Figure 5.1 • Exploded view of the cranial skull.

(2), mandible, maxilla (2), lacrimal bones (2), nasal bones (2), vomer and the inferior nasal concha (2) (Fig. 5.2).

Figure 5.3 shows the irregular internal surfaces of the skull. These irregular surfaces/bony protrusions account for injury to the brain as it moves within the skull under acceleration/deceleration forces.

The meninges

The brain and the spinal cord are encased by three layers of membrane – the dura mater, the arachnoid mater, and the pia mater, known collectively as the meninges (Fig. 5.4).

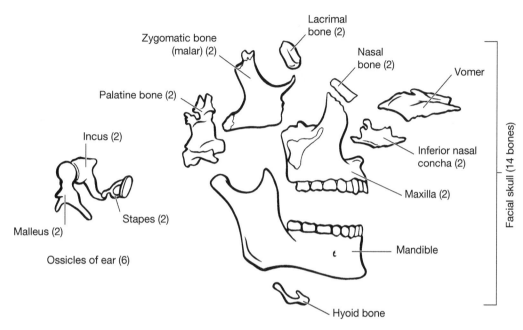

Figure 5.2 • Exploded view of the facial skull.

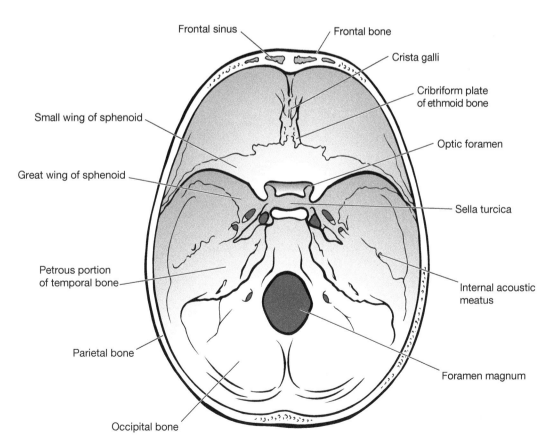

Figure 5.3 • View of the base of the skull from above.

Dura mater

The dura mater consists of two layers: the outer layer is the periosteal layer of the skull, which terminates at the foramen magnum, and the inner layer is a strong, thick membrane that is continuous with the spinal dura mater. There is a potential space between the two dura, except at the falx cerebri, which divides the left and right hemispheres of the cerebrum; the tentorium cerebelli, which divides the cerebrum and cerebellum; the falx cerebelli, which divides the lateral lobes of the cerebellum; and the diaphragm sellae. The dura creates a roof for the sella turcica (which houses the pituitary gland). These compartments provide support and protection for the brain and form the sinuses, which drain venous blood from the brain (Crossman & Neary 2000, Lindsey et al. 2004).

Arachnoid mater

The arachnoid mater is a fine serous membrane that loosely covers the brain. There is a potential space between this and the inner dura mater, known as the subdural space. Between the arachnoid mater and the pia mater is an actual space, known as the subarachnoid space, which contains the arachnoid villi, cerebrospinal fluid (CSF), and small blood vessels.

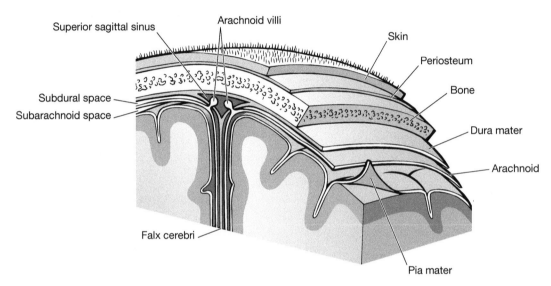

Figure 5.4 • The cranial meninges.

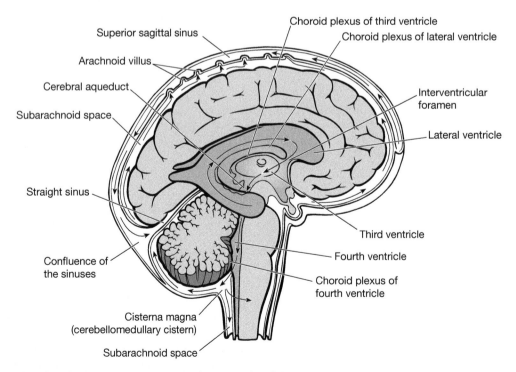

Figure 5.5 • Ventricles of the brain and circulatory path of cerebrospinal fluid through the cranial pathways.

Pia mater

The pia mater follows the convolutions and is attached to the surface of the brain. It consists of fine connective tissue, housing the majority of the blood supply to the brain.

The ventricles and cerebrospinal fluid

Within the brain there are four connected cavities called ventricles, which contain CSF. These are the left and right lateral ventricles, the third ventricle and the fourth ventricle. The lateral ventricles lie in the cerebral hemispheres, the third in the diencephalon, and the fourth in the brain stem. The lateral ventricles are connected to the third ventricle by the interventricular foramen, sometimes known as the foramen of Munro, and the third ventricle is connected to the fourth by the cerebral aqueduct, sometimes known as the aqueduct of Sylvius (Fig. 5.5).

CSF is a clear, colourless fluid composed of water, some protein, oxygen, carbon dioxide, sodium, potassium, chloride and glucose. Its purpose is to protect the brain from injury by providing a cushioning effect. The major source of CSF is from the secretions of the choroid plexus, found in the ventricles. The choroid plexus produces approximately 500 mL of CSF daily; however, the average adult brain only holds between 125 and 150 mL. CSF is renewed and replaced approximately three times daily, being reabsorbed through the arachnoid villi, which drain into the superior sagittal sinus, when the CSF pressure exceeds the venous pressure. Normal CSF pressure is 60–180 mmH$_2$O in the lumbar puncture position (lateral recumbent) and 200–350 mmH$_2$O in the sitting position.

The brain

The brain consists of three main areas:

- cerebrum
- cerebellum
- brain stem.

The major structures within the brain are summarized in Box 5.1.

Cerebrum

The cerebrum consists of two cerebral hemispheres, which are partially separated by the longitudinal fissure and connected at the bottom by the corpus callosum. It is generally accepted that one hemisphere (usually the left) is more highly developed than the other. The left side of the brain has been shown to control the right side of the body, spoken and written language, scientific reasoning and numerical skills, whereas the right side is more concerned with emotion and artistic and creative skills. However, at birth, the hemispheres are of equal ability and very early injury to one side or another usually results in skills being acquired by the opposite side of the brain. Each cerebral hemisphere has an area of grey matter called the basal ganglia, which assists in the motor control of fine body movements.

The surface area of the cerebral cortex (grey matter) on the surface of the brain is much increased by the presence of gyri and sulci (Fig. 5.6), resulting in a 3:1 proportion of grey to white matter. Below the cortex lies the white matter. The cerebral hemispheres are composed of four lobes, the frontal, parietal, temporal and occipital lobes. Box 5.2 summarizes the main functions of these lobes.

The diencephalon is located deep into the cerebrum and consists of the thalamus, hypothalamus, subthalamus and epithalamus. It connects the midbrain to the cerebral hemispheres. The hypothalamus includes several important structures, such as the optic chiasma, the point at which the two optic tracts cross, and the stalk of the pituitary gland (hypophysis).

Cerebellum

The cerebellum is situated behind the pons and attached to the midbrain, pons and medulla by three paired cerebellar peduncles. It consists of three main parts:

- the cortex
- the white matter, which forms the connecting pathways for impulses joining the cerebellum with other parts of the central nervous system
- four pairs of deep cerebellar nuclei.

The cerebellum is the processing centre for coordination of muscular movements, balance, precision, timing, and body positions. It does not initiate any movements and is not involved with the conscious perception of sensations.

Brain stem

The brain stem is the connection between the brain and the spinal cord and is continuous with the diencephalon above and the spinal cord below. Within the brain stem are ascending and descending pathways between the spinal cord and parts of the brain. All cranial nerves except the olfactory (1) and the optic (2) nerves emerge from the brain stem (Fig. 5.7). The brain stem is formed from three main structures:

- midbrain
- pons
- medulla.

The midbrain connects the pons and the cerebellum to the cerebrum. It is involved with visual reflexes, the movement of the eyes, focusing and the dilatation of the pupils. Contained within the midbrain and upper pons is the reticular activating system, which is responsible for the 'awake' state.

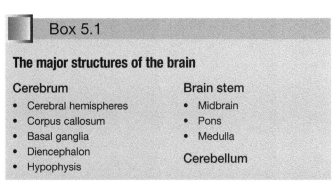

Box 5.1

The major structures of the brain

Cerebrum
- Cerebral hemispheres
- Corpus callosum
- Basal ganglia
- Diencephalon
- Hypophysis

Brain stem
- Midbrain
- Pons
- Medulla

Cerebellum

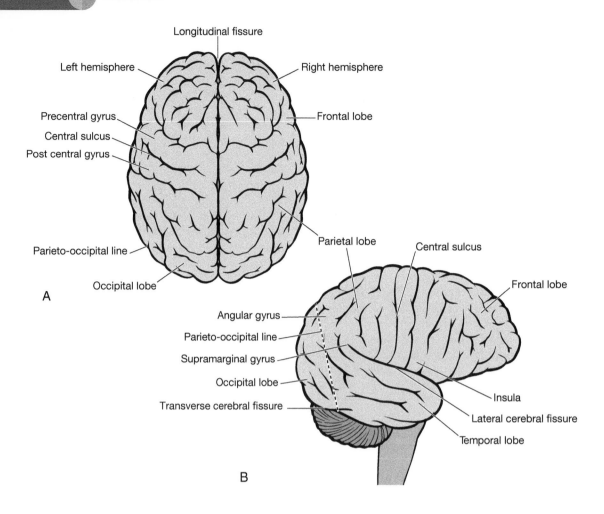

Figure 5.6 • Gyri, sulci and fissures of the cerebral hemispheres. (A) Superior view. (B) Right lateral view.

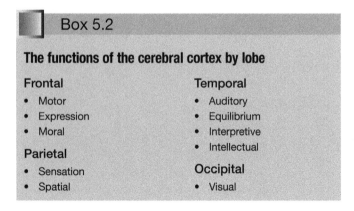

Box 5.2

The functions of the cerebral cortex by lobe

Frontal
- Motor
- Expression
- Moral

Parietal
- Sensation
- Spatial

Temporal
- Auditory
- Equilibrium
- Interpretive
- Intellectual

Occipital
- Visual

The pons is located between the midbrain and the medulla and serves as a relay station from the medulla to higher structures in the brain. It is involved with the control of respiratory function.

The medulla connects the pons and the spinal cord. The point of decussation of the pyramidal tract occurs within the medulla. The vital centres associated with autonomic reflex activity are present in its deeper structure. These are the cardiac, respiratory and vasomotor centres and the reflex centres of coughing, swallowing, vomiting and sneezing.

Cerebral circulation

The brain is supplied with blood by four major arteries: two internal carotid arteries, which supply most of the cerebrum and both eyes; and two vertebral arteries, which supply the cerebellum, brain stem and the posterior part of the cerebrum. Before the blood enters the cerebrum it passes through the circle of Willis, which is a circular shunt at the base of the brain consisting of the posterior cerebral, the posterior communicating, the internal carotids, the anterior cerebral and the anterior communicating arteries (Figs 5.8 and 5.9). These vessels are frequently anomalous; however, they allow for an adequate blood supply to all the brain, even if one or more is ineffective.

The venous drainage from the brain does not follow a similar pathway (Fig. 5.10). Cerebral veins empty into large venous sinuses located in the folds of the dura mater. Bridging veins connect the brain and the dural sinuses and are often the cause of subdural haematomas. These sinuses empty into the internal jugular veins, which sit on either side of the neck

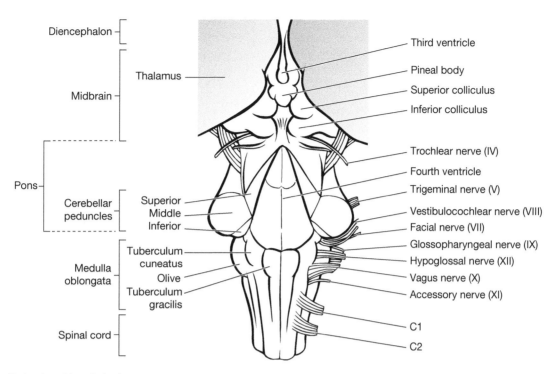

Figure 5.7 • Brain stem (dorsal view).

Figure 5.8 • Major arteries of the head and neck.

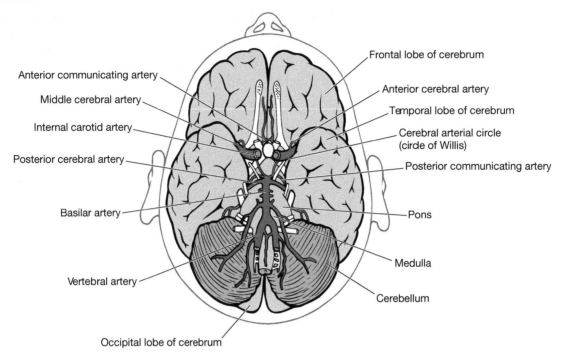

Figure 5.9 • Cerebral circulation.

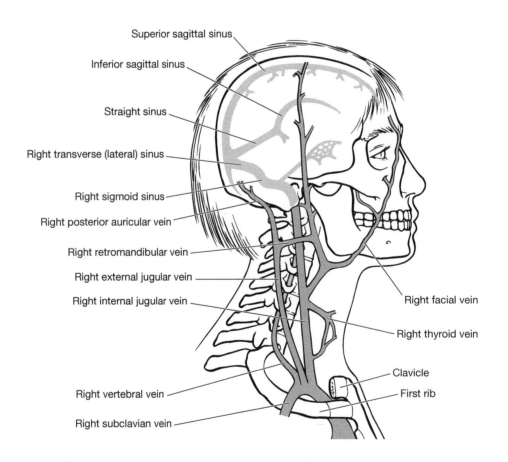

Figure 5.10 • Major veins of the head and neck.

and return the blood to the heart via the brachiocephalic veins.

The brain, especially the grey matter, has an extensive capillary bed, requiring approximately 15–20 % of the total resting cardiac output, about 750 mL/min. Glucose, required for metabolism in the brain, requires about 20 % of the total oxygen consumed in the body for its oxidation. Blood flow to specific areas of the brain correlates directly with the metabolism of the cerebral tissue.

Physiology of raised intracranial pressure

Intracranial pressure (ICP) represents the pressure exerted by the CSF within the ventricles of the brain (Hickey 2009). The exact pressure varies in different areas of the brain. The normal range is 0–15 mmHg in adults, 3–7 mmHg in children, and 1.5–6 mmHg in term babies when measured from the foramen of Munro.

ICP is fundamental in maintaining adequate brain function. The brain lies in the skull, a rigid compartment. The contents of the skull are non-compressible, i.e., brain tissue (80 %), intravascular blood (10 %) and cerebrospinal fluid (10 %). Normally these components maintain a fairly constant volume, therefore creating dynamic equilibrium therein. Should one or more components increase for whatever reason, the Monro-Kellie hypothesis states that another component must decrease in quantity in order to maintain the dynamic equilibrium and thus maintain adequate cerebral blood flow (CBF). If this does not occur, ICP rises, leading to brain injury (Hickey 2009). Dynamic equilibrium is maintained by a number of compensatory mechanisms, these include:

- increasing CSF absorption
- decreasing CSF production
- shunting of CSF to the spinal subarachnoid space
- vasoconstriction – reducing cerebral blood flow.

In severe traumatic brain injury the compensatory mechanisms are rapidly exhausted (Deitch & Dayal 2006). They fail in the healthy adult brain when the ICP reaches 20 mmHg. Once exhausted, small increases in brain mass, blood, or CSF volume have a profound effect on ICP. Chestnut et al. (1993) demonstrated a clear correlation between the length of time patient's ICP remains greater than 20 mmHg and an increased mortality and morbidity rate.

Maintenance of the dynamic equilibrium in the brain is further aided by autoregulation. Pressure autoregulation is the ability of the brain to maintain a relatively constant CBF over a wide range of cerebral perfusion pressures (50–150 mmHg). Pressure autoregulation is initiated by cerebral perfusion pressure (CPP), which is defined as the blood pressure gradient across the brain and is calculated by subtracting ICP from the systemic mean arterial pressure (MAP):

$$CPP = MAP - ICP$$

CPP is used as an indicator of CBF, and therefore oxygen delivery to the brain. Current recommendations suggest that in adults the CPP should lie between 50–70 mmHg, although adults with intact pressure autoregulation may tolerate higher CPP values (Bratton et al. 2007). When the patient's MAP falls and/or the patient's ICP increases, there is a risk that the cerebral perfusion pressure will fall to too low a value to maintain adequate CBF. This results in cerebral hypoxia and secondary brain injury in the form of cerebral ischaemia and potentially infarction. Autoregulation fails when CPP falls below 50 mmHg or rises above 150 mmHg, resulting in CPP and CBF become dependent on the systemic blood pressure alone.

Chemo autoregulation is triggered by changes in extracellular pH and metabolic by-products. Changes in PCO_2 or a dramatic reduction in PO_2 (Fig. 5.11) may trigger this. Hypercapnia >45 mmHg (or 6 kPa) (Albano 2005) is a potent vasodilator that induces hyperaemia and cerebral blood volume increases, without an adequate decrease in CSF; as a result of the compensatory response the ICP will rise. Hypocapnia <45–>30 mmHg (or 6–4 kPa) considered a critical low value (Garner & Amin 2007) is a potent vasoconstrictor that reduces brain mass and induces hypoaemia; as a result cerebral blood flow and volume decrease leading to a risk of secondary ischaemia and potentially an infarction if not treated (Albano 2005).

Classification of head injuries

Head injuries can be classified under three anatomical sites:

- the scalp
- the skull
- the brain.

Figure 5.11 • Autoregulation of the brain.

Patients often present with a combination of injuries. The pathophysiology of brain injury is multivariate, complex, and evolutionary. Neurological damage occurs both at the time of the injury (primary insult) and evolves over the following minutes, hours and days (secondary insult). Patient outcomes improve where secondary insults are treated early, and where successful responses result in limiting and preventing further injury.

Scalp injuries

There are four types of injury to the scalp:

- *abrasion* – minor injury that may cause a small amount of bleeding. Treatment may not be required, but ice applied to the area may reduce any haematoma formation (Hickey 2009)
- *contusion* – no break in the skin, but bruising to the scalp may cause blood to leak into the subcutaneous layer
- *laceration* – a cut or tear of the skin and subcutaneous fascia that tends to bleed profusely. Bleeding from the scalp alone is unlikely to cause shock in the adult. In small children, a scalp laceration may be sufficient to cause hypovolaemia. Scalp lesions should be explored under local anaesthetic for foreign bodies and/or skull fracture with a skull X-ray if there is any doubt about the diagnosis. Lesion(s) should be sutured or glued according to their depth and position
- *subgaleal haematoma* – a haematoma below the galea, a tough layer of tissue under the subcutaneous fascia and before the skull. The veins here empty into the venous sinus, and thus any infection can spread easily to the brain, despite the skull remaining intact. There is controversy surrounding the treatment of subgaleal haematomas, due to the risks of infection; therefore some doctors argue that it is best to evacuate the haematoma, while others suggest that it is best to let it reabsorb.

If the scalp injuries are only part of other injuries, it is important they are documented to allow further investigation at a more appropriate time. They may need to be cleaned and dressed or temporarily sutured.

Skull injuries

Skull fractures indicate that the head has suffered a major impact. Patients who suffer skull fractures have a high incidence of intracranial haematoma. Skull fractures are classified into five groups:

- *linear* – these are the most common types of injury. They usually result from low-velocity direct force. They are usually diagnosed from skull X-ray and need no specific treatment
- *depressed* – usually evident clinically, but a skull X-ray to discover the full extent of the potential brain damage

is usually necessary. Management is dependent on the severity of the fracture and whether there are any accompanying injuries. If there are no other injuries requiring surgical management, they may not be surgically elevated, due to the risks of infection. However, surgical intervention will normally be necessary if there are bone fragments embedded in the brain so as to elevate the bone fragments and manage the brain trauma
- *open* – usually evident clinically. Usually managed according to the severity of the injury. If debris is dispersed in the brain tissue then surgery will be required and there is a heightened risk of infection
- *comminuted* – these are detected on skull X-ray. These patients should be closely observed and any neurological deficits managed appropriately. Surgical intervention is usually required. If there are bone fragments imbedded in the brain tissue then surgery will be required to elevate the bone fragments and manage the brain trauma
- *basal* – these are diagnosed clinically as they are difficult to detect on X-ray. Signs include CSF leakage from the nose (rhinorrhoea) or the ear(s) (otorrhoea). Rhinorrhoea or otorrhoea indicates that a skull base fracture has breached the dura and formed a communication between the intracranial contents and an air sinus. This places the patient at risk of meningitis while the CSF leak continues. If CSF leakage is suspected, the fluid should be tested for glucose and the 'halo test' performed, where a small amount of fluid is placed on blotting paper; if CSF is present it will separate from blood and form a yellow ring around the outside of the blood. Patients with a base of skull fracture may also have retroauricular bruising (Battle's signs) and periorbital bruising ('panda eyes' or 'raccoon eyes'): 80–90 % of cases seal within two weeks and neurosurgical intervention is usually not considered until this time has elapsed. An exception is a fracture of the posterior wall of the frontal sinus, visualized on CT scan, where anterior fossa repair may be undertaken early.

Brain injuries

Severe brain injury is uncommon because the skull and scalp absorb the majority of the impact of the assault. The amount of brain damage suffered is relative to the force/energy of the assault. A high-energy head injury results when: a pedestrian is struck by a motor vehicle, an occupant is ejected from a motor vehicle, a person falls from a height of greater than 1 metre or more than five stairs (a lower threshold for the height of falls should be used when dealing with infants and young children under 5 years old), following a diving accident, following a high-speed motor vehicle collision, following a rollover motor accident, or a bicycle collision (National Institute for Health and Clinical Excellence 2007).

Damage to the brain as a result of trauma includes both the immediate (primary) injury caused at the moment of the impact and the secondary injury that develops during the first few minutes, hours or days after the impact (Box 5.3).

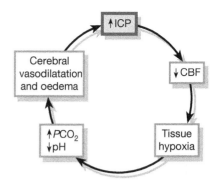

Figure 5.12 • Cycle of progressive brain swelling.

 Box 5.3

Types of brain injury

Primary brain injury
- Disruption of brain vessels
- Haemorrhagic contusion
- Diffuse axonal injury

Secondary brain injury

Extracranial insults
- Systemic hypotension
- Hypoxaemia
- Hypercarbia
- Disturbances of blood coagulation

Intracranial insults
- Haematoma (extradural, subdural, intracerebral)
- Cerebral oedema (see Fig. 5.12)
- Infection

These secondary injuries may have extracranial or intracranial causes.

There are no interventions that can prevent the primary brain injury. Secondary brain injuries, which further exacerbate the primary neuronal injury and lead to a worsening outcome depending upon their duration and severity, are largely preventable. The two main causes of secondary injury are delayed diagnosis and treatment of intracranial haematomas, and failure to correct systemic hypoxaemia and hypotension (Fig. 5.12). Brain injuries are usually categorized as either focal or diffuse injuries.

Focal injuries

Focal injuries occur in a specific area of the brain. The mechanism of injury is usually blunt injury and acceleration/deceleration injury.

Cerebral contusion (bruising of the surface of the brain) is sustained as the brain hits the bony protuberances of the skull at the site of the impact (coup injury) and at the opposite side of the brain during deceleration (contrecoup injury). Cerebral contusion is a common type of brain injury, which is diagnosed by CT scan, and is most commonly seen at the frontal and temporal lobes as a result of the irregular surfaces/bony protrusions of the skull. The term contusion is used when the pia mater has not been breached. The brain swells around the site(s) of the contusion(s). Bleeding may occur into the contusion(s). If the contusion(s) is (are) large and/or widespread, the swelling may cause the ICP to rise. Nausea, vomiting and visual disturbances are common clinical signs.

Cerebral lacerations of the cortical surface commonly occur in similar locations to contusions, and are most commonly seen at the frontal and temporal lobes as a result of irregular surfaces/bony protrusions of the skull. The term laceration is used when the pia mater is torn.

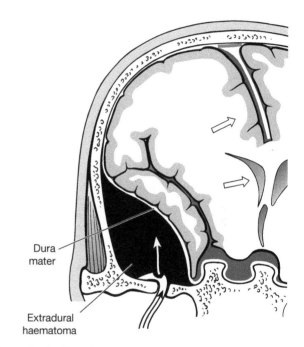

Dura mater

Extradural haematoma

Figure 5.13 • Extradural haematoma.

Haematoma

Extradural haematoma (EDH) is an accumulation of blood in the extradural space between the periosteum on the inner side of the skull and the dura mater (Fig. 5.13). Most are associated with skull fracture and are commonly caused by a laceration to the middle meningeal artery or vein, or less commonly to the dural venous sinus, following an insult to the temporal-parietal region. Consequentially, the parietal and parieto-temporal areas of the brain are affected. In 85% of patients the EDH will be accompanied by a skull fracture (Hudak & Gallo 1994).

Patients with skull fractures may be neurologically intact on admission and later deteriorate as the EDH develops. Most often the primary brain injury causes some disturbance of consciousness and the developing haematoma results in rapid neurological deterioration (Kwiatkowski 1996). Patients with EDHs most commonly present with a history of transient loss of consciousness, followed by lucidity for a period (hours to days) dependent on the rate of the bleed, irritation and headache. Patients then rapidly lose consciousness and deteriorate

Figure 5.14 ● Subdural haematoma.

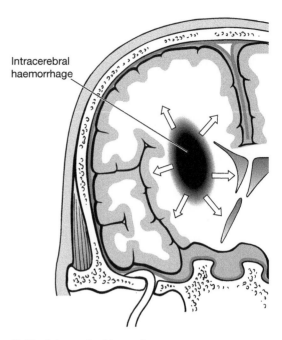

Figure 5.15 ● Intracerebral haematoma.

very quickly. Late signs are seizures, ipsilateral pupil dilatation, unconsciousness, and contralateral hemiplegia. Surgical treatment is required to evacuate the haematoma and ligate the damaged blood vessel.

Relatives, friends and/or carers often require a great deal of reassurance, as they often feel responsible for not bringing the patient to hospital earlier.

Subdural haematoma (SDH) is an accumulation of blood between the dura mater and arachnoid mater. SDHs are caused by the rupture of bridging veins from the cortical surfaces to the venous sinuses (cortical veins) (Fig. 5.14).

SDHs can be seen in isolation, but more commonly are associated with accompanying brain injury, i.e., cerebral contusions and/or intracerebral haematomas. They are the most common intracranial mass result from head trauma (Maartens & Lethbridge 2005). In most cases a large contusion is found at the frontal or temporal surface of the brain. SDHs are predisposed with increasing age and alcoholism. Both groups can suffer regular falls and have a degree of cerebral atrophy, which puts strain on the bridging veins and coagulopathy. Subdural haematomas are classified as acute, subacute and chronic:

- *acute* (ASDH) refers to symptoms which manifest before 72 hours post-injury. Most patients harbouring an acute SDH are unconscious immediately following major cerebral trauma. The expanding haematoma then causes additional deterioration (Duffy 2001)
- *subacute* refers to symptoms which manifest between 72 hours and 3 weeks post-injury
- *chronic* refers to symptoms which manifest after 3 weeks post-injury. The injury may have been considered as minor and the patient often does not remember a particular predisposing injury.

The most common symptom of a SDH is a headache, which progressively intensifies and is eventually accompanied by vomiting, cognitive impairment(s), a depressed level of consciousness, and a focal deficit, which will vary depending on severity of the injury. Even in the absence of focal deficit, increasing ICP may lead to cognitive impairment and eventually a depressed level of consciousness (Watkins 2000). SDHs are often associated with other injuries, and therefore the symptoms can become confused within a general head injury picture. Small SDHs may be treated conservatively, as they will reabsorb over time. Larger SDHs will require evacuation, due to the secondary damage they cause.

A poor outcome is likely if the SDH is bilateral, it accumulates rapidly or there is a greater than 4-hour delay in the surgical management of an ASDH. Increased patient age and underlying accompanying brain injury also lead to a poor outcome.

Intracerebral haematoma (ICH) is caused by bleeding within the substance of the brain (Fig. 5.15). ICH usually affects the white matter and the basal ganglia found deep within the brain parenchyma. ICHs are related to contusions as a result of a major impact, and are usually found in the frontal, temporal, and parietal lobes. Other causes include penetrating and missile injuries and shearing of blood vessels deep within the brain following an acceleration/deceleration injury. Symptoms include headache, contralateral hemiplegia, ipsilateral dilated/fixed pupil and deteriorating level of consciousness, progressing to deep coma (GCS < 8). Treatment tends to be conservative, due to the difficulties of evacuating haematomas situated so deeply within the brain. Mortality is high within this group of patients.

Subarachnoid haemorrhage (SAH) is seen in 30–40% of patients following severe traumatic brain injury. The mortality and morbidity rates are double in these patients compared with those with similar injury without the SAH component

Box 5.4

Grading concussion

Grade I – no loss of consciousness, transient confusion and rapid return to normal function

Grade II – confusion and mild amnesia

Grade III – profound confusion with pre- and post-traumatic amnesia

Grade IV – loss of consciousness, variable confusion, amnesia

Box 5.5

Symptoms of mild diffuse axonal injury

- Headache
- Fatigue
- Irritability
- Poor concentration
- Dizziness
- Poor balance
- Depression

(Dearden 1998). The patient either suffered the SAH prior to the insult and thus the SAH is possibly the cause of the incident (Sakas et al. 1995), or the vessels in the subarachnoid space are damaged by the shearing forces at the time of the insult.

Diffuse injuries

Diffuse injuries occur throughout the brain rather than in a specific area of the brain. They result in generalized dysfunction. Diffuse injuries range from concussion with no residual damage, to diffuse axonal injury and persistent vegetative state. Diffuse injury occurs in 50–60% of patients with severe head trauma and is the commonest cause of unconsciousness, the vegetative state and subsequent disability (Graham et al 1995).

Concussion is a transient form of diffuse injury that occurs following blunt trauma. It causes a temporary neuronal dysfunction because of transient ischaemia or neuronal depolarization. This manifests as a headache, dizziness, inability to concentrate, disorientation, irritability, and nausea. Concussion can occur with or without memory loss. Concussion is graded in line with the severity of symptoms (Box 5.4).

Recovery is usually rapid, but if neurological symptoms persist, a CT scan should be performed to rule out more severe injuries. Skull X-ray should only be performed if the mechanisms of injury or existing clinical findings are suggestive of a skull fracture. Most patients with concussion can be discharged with an accompanying adult. If there has been a loss of consciousness greater than ten minutes the patient should be admitted for observation even if he appears fully recovered.

Approximately one-third of patients with head injuries who are discharged from emergency departments have persistent post-concussion-type symptoms, such as headache, fatigue, inability to concentrate, irritability, and anxiety, persisting for several months due to mild diffuse axonal injury (Jackson 1995). The majority of these patients will have been knocked out for a short time and may have other mild neurological signs. As there is no treatment for mild diffuse axonal injury, and recovery is usually spontaneous, reassurance and psychological support are vital to the patient's recovery (Box 5.5).

Acute axonal injury is usually the result of an acute rotation/deceleration injury, typically following a road traffic accident (Fig. 5.16). The patient usually becomes unconscious rapidly after injury, due to the shearing injury to the brain.

Mortality is high in this patient group, and those who do survive usually suffer severe neurological dysfunction.

Initially a CT scan may show little abnormality, but gradually with repeated scans, many small diffuse haemorrhagic areas will begin to appear, commonly in the corpus callosum, often associated with traumatic intraventricular haemorrhage and the brain stem. As a result of these injuries the patient may also develop autonomic dysfunction and exhibit symptoms such as excessive sweating, hyperpyrexia, and hypertension. Severe generalized cerebral oedema usually accompanies such injuries. Management and treatment involve maximizing cerebral perfusion and the prevention of secondary brain injury.

Cerebral oedema – This is a consistent reaction of the brain to an insult and it usually develops during the first 3–5 days following the insult causing an increase in ICP. Cerebral oedema following severe traumatic brain injury affects almost all patients to a greater or lesser degree. The opening of the blood–brain barrier is a central prerequisite to the development of cerebral oedema (Fernandes & Landolt 1996). Four pathophysiological mechanisms of cerebral oedema have been proposed (Table 5.1).

Table 5.1 Types and causes of cerebral oedema

Types of oedema	Cause
Vasogenic	
Blood vessel damage Extends slowly over a period of 72 hours	Contusion
Cytotoxic	
Cell membrane pump failure	Hypoxaemia/ischaemia
Hydrostatic	
High vascular transmural pressure	Loss of autoregulation Post brain decompression
Hypo-osmotic	
Low plasma osmotic pressure (serum sodium < 120 mEq/L)	Hyponatraemia (dilutional/ mannitol)

Cerebral ischaemia occurs whenever the delivery of oxygen and substrates to the brain falls below its metabolic needs, as a result of hypoxia (cardiac arrest, obstructive airway, cervical

Figure 5.16 • Diffuse axonal injury.

spinal injury and prolonged epileptic-type seizures), hypotension and/or intracranial hypertension (raised ICP).

Blood flow in and around areas of brain tissue damaged by trauma may be abnormal. Vasomotor paralysis also occurs in and around areas of brain tissue damaged by trauma. Blood vessels lose the ability to control their own resistance actively with subsequent loss of blood pressure autoregulation and reactivity to CO_2. Cerebral blood flow thus becomes pressure dependent, rendering these areas of brain more susceptible to ischaemia at lower blood pressures and more likely to sustain injury at higher pressures.

Cerebral ischaemia may be global or focal, complete or incomplete. Incomplete ischaemia differs from complete ischaemia in that there is a continuing supply of glucose to the brain tissue despite tissue hypoxia. The glucose sustains anaerobic metabolism, which increases the brain lactic acid level. Neuronal damage occurs above a certain threshold. This effect is the basis for concern that increased peri-ischaemia glucose levels may increase and/or hasten the ischaemia tissue damage. Ischaemia leads instantly to cerebral oedema, which in turn worsens ischaemia (Farnsworth & Sperry 1996).

As the $PaCO_2$ increases, unaffected normal blood vessels dilate, however blood is shunted away from the abnormal areas of the brain that do not respond to CO_2 and is known as the 'steal phenomenon'. An inverse steal (Robin Hood phenomenon) occurs when the $PaCO_2$ is reduced and the unaffected, normal blood vessels vasocontrict, shunting blood to the abnormal areas of the brain that do not constrict (Darby et al. 1988).

The concept of *ischaemia penumbra* states that the area of the brain around an ischaemic brain, where blood flow provides sufficient oxygenation for the cells to survive but insufficient oxygenation for the cells to maintain normal neuronal function, can re-establish normal function if blood flow and oxygenation to this area is rapidly improved. Cerebral ischaemia is the single most important factor in determining the outcome in severe traumatic brain injury: ischaemia lesions are found in 90% of patients at post-mortem (Dearden 1998).

Management

Patients who have sustained a head injury should be assessed and managed according to clear principles and standard practice as embodied in the ATLS system (American College of Surgeons 2008) and for children the APLS system (Advanced Life Support Group 2011) should be employed (Bavetta & Benjamin 2002, National Institute for Health and Clinical Excellence 2007). The main focus of the assessment should be the risk of clinically important brain and cervical spine injuries. Due attention should also be paid to co-existing injuries and other concerns the healthcare team may have, e.g., non-accidental injury.

External referrals

Community health services, e.g., general practice, paramedics, NHS walk-in centres, dental practitioners and NHS minor injury clinics, and telephone advice services, e.g., NHS Direct, should refer people who have sustained a head injury to the ambulance services for emergency transport to the ED if they have experienced any of the following:

- GCS less than 15 at any time since the injury
- any loss of consciousness as a result of the injury
- any focal neurological deficit since the injury, e.g., problems understanding, speaking, reading or writing, loss of sensation in a part of the body, problems balancing, general weakness, problems walking, and any changes in eyesight
- any seizure since the injury
- any suspicion of a skull fracture or penetrating head injury, e.g., CSF leakage from the nose (rhinorrhoea) or the ear(s) (otorrhoea), black eye(s) with no associated damage around the eye(s), bleeding from one or both ears, new deafness in one or both ears, bruising behind one or both ears, penetrating injury signs, or visible trauma to the scalp or skull
- a high-energy head injury

• the injured person or their carer is incapable of transporting the injured person safely to the hospital emergency department without the use of ambulance services, providing any other risk factors indicating emergency department referral are present (National Institute for Health and Clinical Excellence 2007).

Telephone advice services e.g., NHS Direct should refer people who have sustained a head injury to a hospital emergency department if the related history indicates any of the following risk factors:

• amnesia for events before or after the injury: the assessment of amnesia will not be possible in preverbal children and is unlikely to be possible in any child under 5 years old
• persistent headache since the injury
• any loss of consciousness as a result of the injury from which the injured person has now recovered
• any vomiting episode since the injury: clinical judgement should be used regarding the cause of vomiting in those aged less than or equal to 12 years and whether referral is necessary
• any previous cranial neurosurgical intervention
• history of bleeding or clotting disorders
• current anticoagulant therapy such as warfarin
• current drug or alcohol intoxication
• age greater than or equal to 65 years
• suspicion of non-accidental injury
• irritability or altered behaviour particularly in infants and young children
• continuing concern by the Helpline's personnel about the diagnosis (National Institute for Health and Clinical Excellence 2007).

In the absence of the factors listed above the telephone advice services should advise the injured person to seek medical advice from community health services, e.g., general practice and NHS walk-in centres if any of the following factors are present:

• adverse social factors, e.g., no one able to supervise the injured person at home
• continuing concern by the injured person or their carer about the diagnosis (National Institute for Health and Clinical Excellence 2007).

History

Accurate history-taking gives vital clues to the type and potential severity of the head injury (Shah 1999) (Box 5.6). This may have to be obtained from a witness or paramedic. If the history is obtained from the patient, it should be corroborated by a witness/relative if possible.

Assessment

Management of head injury in the emergency department revolves largely around the assessment of the risks of, and the prevention or limiting of, secondary brain injury (the

Box 5.6

History-taking in head injury
• Mechanism of injury
• Time elapsed
• Period of loss of consciousness
• Any pre/post-traumatic amnesia
• Condition since injury, such as nausea, vomiting, confusion, visual disturbance, lethargy or dizziness

Box 5.7

Causes of secondary brain injury
• Hyperpyrexia
• Cerebral ischaemia
• Cerebral oedema
• Raised intracranial pressure
• Infection
• Metabolic disorder
• Evolving intracranial bleed
• Hypotension

causation of secondary brain injury is shown in Box 5.7) and of injury to the cervical spine, whilst the patient awaits definitive treatment such as surgery to evacuate haematoma. Due attention should also be paid to co-existing injuries.

Patients presenting to the emergency department with a GCS less than or equal to 8 should be assessed early by an anaesthetist or critical-care physician to provide appropriate airway management and to assist with resuscitation (National Institute for Health and Clinical Excellence 2007). The recommended primary investigation of choice for the detection of acute clinically important brain injuries is CT imaging (National Institute for Health and Clinical Excellence 2007). CT scanning was generally reserved for patients with moderate or severe head injuries (GCS less than 13) and should be undertaken within 30 minutes of admission to the ED (National Institute for Health and Clinical Excellence 2007). MRI for safety, logistic and resource reasons is not currently indicated as the primary investigation, although additional information of importance to the patient's prognosis can sometimes be detected using MRI, care must be taken to ensure that the patient does not harbour an incompatible device, implant, or foreign body. Skull X-ray(s) are the recommended primary investigation of choice for skull fractures (Box 5.8). If CT scanning is not available, then skull X-rays along with high-quality patient observations have a vital role. Early imaging, rather than admission and observation for neurological deterioration, reduces the time needed to detect life-threatening complications and is associated with a better outcome (National Institute for Health and Clinical Excellence 2007). Indications for CT scanning are listed in Box 5.9.

Box 5.8

Indications for skull X-ray
- Suspected penetrating injury
- Decreased consciousness (if GCS below 8/15, CT is indicated)
- Altered neurology
- CSF from nose or ear
- Significant scalp bruising or swelling
- Difficulty in clinical examination, where mechanism of injury is suggestive of fracture

Box 5.9

Indications for urgent CT scanning following a head injury
- GCS less than 13 at any point since the injury
- GCS 13–14, two hours after the injury
- Suspected open or depressed skull fracture
- Clinical symptoms of basal skull fracture
- Post-traumatic seizure
- Focal neurological deficit(s)
- More than one episode of vomiting (clinical judgement should be used regarding the cause of vomiting in those children 12 years or younger, and whether imaging is necessary)
- Amnesia for greater than 30 minutes of events prior to the assault. This assessment is not possible in children 5 years or younger

CT should be immediately requested in patients with any of the following risk factors, providing they have experienced some loss of consciousness or amnesia since the assault:
- Age 65 years or older
- Coagulopathy (clotting disorder or current treatment with warfarin)
- A high-energy head injury

CT scanning and the results should be analysed within one hour of the request having been received by the radiology department in patients with the following risk factors:
- GCS less than 13 at any point since the injury
- GCS 13–14, two hours after the injury
- Suspected open or depressed skull fracture
- Any signs of basal skull fracture
- Post-traumatic seizure
- Focal neurological deficit(s)
- More than 1 episode of vomiting (clinical judgement should be used regarding the cause of vomiting in those children 12 years or younger, and whether imaging is necessary)
- Amnesia for greater than 30 minutes of events prior to the assault. This assessment is not possible in children 5 years or younger
- Age 65 years or older providing that loss of consciousness or amnesia has been experienced
- Coagulopathy (history of bleeding, clotting disorder or current treatment with warfarin) providing that loss of consciousness or amnesia has been experienced
- A high-energy head injury (National Institute for Health and Clinical Excellence 2007)

Neurological assessment

Full neurological assessment forms part of the secondary survey, as should a thorough examination of the scalp for lacerations, haematoma, or evidence of a depressed skull fracture. The assessment and classification of patients who have suffered a head injury should be guided primarily by the adult (16 years or older) and paediatric versions of the GCS and its derivative the Glasgow Coma Score (National Institute for Health and Clinical Excellence 2007). The paediatric version should include a 'grimace' alternative to the verbal score to facilitate assessment in the pre-verbal or intubated patients.

The GCS, developed by Teasdale & Jennett (1974) continues to be the gold standard for assessing consciousness (Addison & Crawford 1999, Stern 2011) (Table 5.2 and Fig. 5.17). The GCS measures arousal, awareness, and activity by assessing eye opening (E), verbal response (V), and motor response (M). Each activity is allocated a score, therefore enabling objectivity, ease of recording, and comparison between recordings. It also provides useful information for patient outcome prediction. The score should be based on the sum of 15 and to avoid confusion this denominator should be specified, e.g., 13/15. When recording the GCS it is important to record the three separate response scores as well as the total GCS score, i.e., E2, V3, and M4, GCS = 9 (National Institute for Health and Clinical Excellence 2007).

When applying verbal stimulus, it is good practice to commence with normal voice and then increase volume to elicit a response. It is important to ascertain whether the patient is deaf, wears a hearing aid, and whether English is the patient's spoken language. When applying a painful stimulus, it is good practice to commence with light pressure and then increase to elicit a response. When assessing motor function, always record the response from the best arm. There is no need to record left and right differences, as the GCS does not aim to measure focal deficit. It is not appropriate to measure leg response unless unavoidable, i.e., injury to both arms, as a spinal reflex rather than a brain-initiated response might be initiated (Teasdale & Jennett 1974).

The GCS may be misleading in patients who have a high cervical injury or brain stem lesion, and in those who are hypoxic, suffering haemodynamic shock, or suffer from epileptic seizures. These patients may be unable to move their limbs or show no responses to stimuli. It is important to attempt to assess the spinal patient using facial movements, being aware of the possibility of a combined head and neck injury. Patients who show no response should be re-evaluated following correction of any shock or hypoxia (National Institute for Health and Clinical Excellence 2007). Post-resuscitation, the GCS with specific emphasis on the motor response score is a powerful predictor of outcome (Hunningher & Smith 2006).

The GCS assessment should be accompanied by an assessment of pupil size and reactivity, limb movement and vital signs observations:

- blood pressure
- respiration rate
- heart rate

Table 5.2 Adult and paediatric Glasgow Coma Scale

Eye opening		Motor response		Verbal response	
Adult (16 years and older)					
Spontaneous	4	Obeys	6	Orientated	5
To speech	3	Localizes	5	Confused	4
To pain	2	Normal flexion	4	Inappropriate	3
None	1	Abnormal flexion	3	Incomprehensible	2
		Extensor response	2	None	1
		None	1		
Child					
Spontaneous	4	Obeys commands or performs normal spontaneous movements	6	Alert, babbles, coos, words or sentences to usual ability	5
To speech	3	Localizes to painful stimuli or withdraws to touch	5	Less than usual ability and/or spontaneous irritable cry	4
To pain	2	Withdrawal to painful stimuli	4	Cries inappropriately	3
None	1	Abnormal flexion	3	Occasionally whimpers and/or moans	2
		Abnormal extension	2	None	1
		None	1		
Pre-verbal child or intubated patient					
Spontaneous	4	Obeys commands or performs normal spontaneous movements	6	Spontaneous normal facial/oro-motor activity	5
To speech	3	Localizes to painful stimuli or withdraws to touch	5	Less than usual	
To pain	2	Withdrawal to painful stimuli	4	Spontaneous ability or only response to touch stimuli	4
None	1	Abnormal flexion	3	Vigorous grimace to pain	3
		Abnormal extension	2	Mild grimace to pain	2
		None	1	None	1

- temperature
- blood oxygen saturation (National Institute for Health and Clinical Excellence 2007).

As well as providing a baseline for assessing the patient's progress, vital signs give important information about potential secondary brain injury, e.g., respiration rate and cerebral hypoxia. When assessing vital signs in conjunction with GCS, it is important to remember the following:

- hypotension is only of neurological origin in end-stage brain injury or spinal shock; other causes of hypotension, such as hypovolaemia, should be investigated
- Cushing's triad (hypertension, bradycardia and bradypnoea) indicates a life-threatening rise in ICP
- pyrexia with hypertension may indicate autonomic dysfunction.

Limb movement is useful to assess for focal damage. However, although it is usual for a hemiparesis or hemiplegia to occur on the contralateral side to the lesion, it may occur on the ipsilateral side. This is due to indentation of the contralateral cerebral peduncle and is known as a false localizing. Spontaneous movements are observed for equality. If there is little or no spontaneous movement, then painful stimuli must be applied to each limb in turn, comparing the result. As already stated it is most appropriate to complete this while assessing the motor component of the GCS.

Pupils are assessed for their reaction to light, size and shape, i.e., cranial nerves II (optic) and III (oculomotor) activity. Each pupil needs to be assessed and recorded individually. Pupils are measured in millimetres, the normal range being 2–6 mm in diameter. They are normally round in shape and abnormalities are described as ovoid, keyhole, or irregular (Hickey 2009). A bright light is shone into the side of each eye to assess the pupils' reaction to light. This should produce a brisk constriction in both pupils, the consensual light reaction. Herniation of the medial temporal lobe through the tentorium directly damages the oculomotor (CNIII) nerve, resulting in dilation of the pupil and an

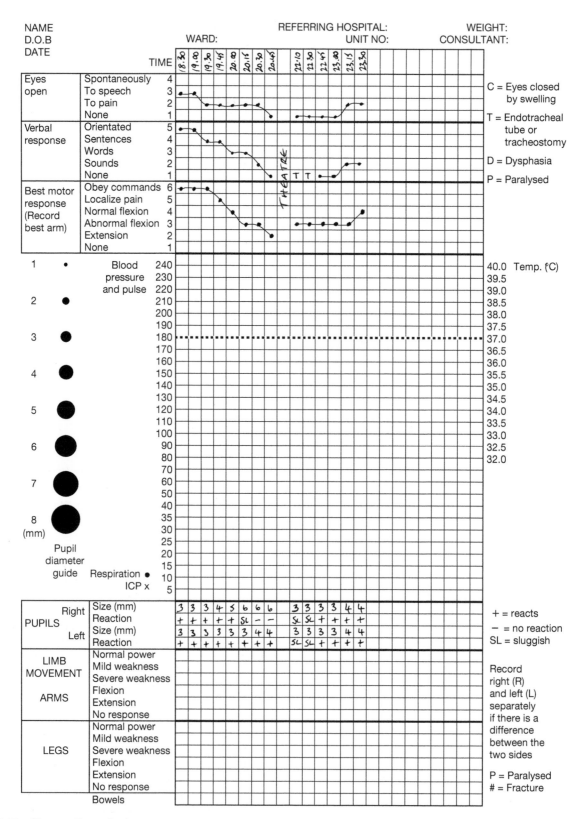

Figure 5.17 • Glasgow Coma Scale.

impaired reaction to light. The pupil dilates on the side of the lesion.

Patients with head injuries can be classified into three groups depending on their GCS:

- a score of 13–15 is indicative of a minor head injury. In some patients, a one-point drop in their GCS can be alcohol- or drug-induced. This necessitates extra vigilance from nursing staff as alcohol and/or drugs may mask subtle changes in the patient's cognition or conscious level
- a GCS of 9–12 suggests a moderate head injury, or a more serious injury evolving. Any changes in the patient's condition should be closely monitored
- a severe head injury is classed by a GCS of 8 or less. These patients are potentially at risk of secondary brain injury, and their GCS and vital signs should be monitored at frequent intervals.

Admission to hospital

Patients should be admitted if:

- they have suffered a new surgically significant abnormality on imaging
- the patient has not returned to a GCS equal to 15 after imaging, regardless of the imaging results
- they fulfil the criteria for CT scanning but this cannot be done within the appropriate period, either because CT is not available or because the patient is not sufficiently co-operative to allow scanning
- the patient has continuing worrying signs of concern to the clinicians, e.g., persistent vomiting and severe headache
- the patient has received sedation or general anaesthetic during CT imaging
- the patient has other sources of concern to the clinicians, e.g., drug and/or alcohol intoxication, other injuries, shock, suspected non-accidental injury, and cerebrospinal fluid leak (National Institute for Health and Clinical Excellence 2007).

Patients should undergo urgent reassessment by the clinician in charge of the case if any of the following responses occur:

- development of agitation or abnormal behaviour
- a sustained (at least 30 minutes) drop of one point in GCS level (greater weight should be given to a drop of one point in the motor score of the GCS)
- any drop of greater than two points in GCS level regardless of duration or GCS sub-scale
- development of severe or increasing headache or persisting vomiting
- new or evolving neurological symptoms or signs such as pupil inequality or asymmetry of limb or facial movement (National Institute for Health and Clinical Excellence 2007).

Box 5.10

Typical head injury advice sheet

- General advice about observing a patient every two hours; ensure he wakes easily and is orientated when awake. Ensure the patient is able to move all limbs
- You should return to hospital if any of the following occur:
  - Persistent vomiting
  - Confusion
  - Excessive sleeping; difficulty in rousing patient
  - Severe headache
  - Double vision
  - Limb weakness
  - Convulsions or 'passing out'
  - Discharge of blood/fluid from nose/ears
- You should not drink alcohol until all symptoms have subsided
- The name and telephone of the hospital should be included

Management of minor traumatic head injury

The majority of patients treated in emergency departments with head injury will have a 'minor' head injury and the majority will be discharged home. A thorough assessment of the patient's condition should be performed, which should include pulse, respiration, blood pressure, pupil size and reaction, and the patient's GCS (Caton-Richards 2010). Although only 1% of head-injured patients have skull fractures (Ramrakha & Moore 1997), there are certain circumstances where a skull X-ray is appropriate (Box 5.8).

The key to managing minor head injury is giving adequate information and advice to the patient and his carer. The patient should be advised to rest quietly, avoid stressful situations, should be discouraged from taking part in strenuous activities and from undertaking long periods of visual display unit work or watching television which will exacerbate any headache. The patient should not stay at home alone for the first 48 hours after leaving hospital. Simple analgesia, such as paracetamol, that should be sufficient to alleviate headaches without masking other signs of deterioration should be suggested. The patient should be discouraged from taking alcohol or non-prescribed drugs until symptoms have subsided. The patient should not play any contact sport for at least three weeks after the injury without talking to their doctor or other appropriately qualified clinician first. Written advice should always be given to the patient/carer to reinforce any verbal information (Box 5.10). (See also Chapter 34 – Health Promotion.)

When discussing the outcomes of a minor head injury, it is important that the emergency nurse explains post-concussion-type symptoms to the patient. Head-injured patients should be discharged into the care of a responsible adult. Not all patients with a minor head injury are appropriate for discharge (Box 5.11). Particular care is needed with patients who are intoxicated and/or have taken drugs where neurological assessment is unreliable.

Box 5.11

Indications for hospital admission

- Decreased consciousness
- Neurological deficit
- Severe headache and persistent vomiting
- Confusion
- Intoxication rendering clinical assessment unreliable
- Coexisting conditions such as clotting disorders
- Social circumstances making discharge unwise

Management of severe traumatic head injury

Despite the fact that patients who have suffered severe injury to the brain may recover completely if they are treated quickly and appropriately, it is also possible that the patient may suffer serious disability or even death (National Institute for Health and Clinical Excellence 2007). Indeed, head injury accounts for the majority of trauma deaths in young adults in Europe (Tagliaferri et al. 2006). Age is a significant factor in determining outcome, especially in patients who become deeply unconscious. The mortality rate is 19% in patients aged 20, but 71% in those aged 60 and over (Hickey 2009).

The management of patients with severe traumatic head injury is multi-dimensional and complex. The aim of management of the head-injured patient is to prevent and treat secondary physiological insults. Monitoring of ECG, direct arterial blood pressure, central venous pressure, and pulse oximetry is mandatory in all patients who have suffered from a severe traumatic brain injury. Regular arterial blood gas analysis, measurement of blood glucose and sodium and core temperature monitoring are also required to optimize treatment strategies.

There is a developing base of evidence to guide the management of patients with traumatic brain injury. A study by Patel et al. (2002) looked at the effect of neurocritical care, delivered by specialist staff and based on protocol-driven therapy, they found improved outcomes. It is universally accepted that initial management of severe traumatic brain injury requires urgent cardiopulmonary resuscitation, emergency CT scan, transfer to a neurosurgical centre, and appropriate surgical intervention, and guidelines covering this initial care are generally well established in practice (Intensive Care Society 1997, McNaughton & Harwood 2002,). In the US, the practice of ensuring that pre-hospital care, triage, and admission to designated trauma centres are coordinated within regional trauma systems has been seen to improve the outcomes for individuals with traumatic brain injury (Ghajar 2000). There is little evidence in the UK as to whether patients transported directly to a neurosciences centre compared to those who are taken to their nearest district hospital experience a better outcome (National Institute for Health and Clinical Excellence 2007). Level III evidence from Patel et al. (2002) concluded that specialist neurocritical care is associated with a significant improvement in outcome for patients with TBI.

Trauma services in the UK are presently being organized into a formal system similar to that in the US. In London four trauma networks have been established (Healthcare for London 2009). Extracranial complications occur frequently in severe traumatic brain injury and studies suggest that some complications are highly influential in determining patient outcome. Management should follow the sequence laid down by ATLS (National Institute for Health and Clinical Excellence 2007, American College of Surgeons 2008).

Assessment and management

Airway and cervical spine

Airway management is paramount in preventing hypoxia (PO_2 <60 mmHg or 8 kPa). Hypoxia is the second most influential cause of secondary brain injury after hypotension and leads to a worse outcome (Chesnut et al. 1993). Prevention of such insults during initial resuscitation at the scene of the injury, during transfer and during hospitalization may have a major impact on outcome (Royal College of Paediatrics and Child Health 2001). Oedema and/or debris following injury, loss of the gag reflex and/or vomiting may threaten airway patency. If a clear airway cannot be maintained with simple aids, such as a Guedel or oropharyngeal airway, then intubation should be performed. Cervical spine immobilization should be maintained until a full risk assessment and imaging (if deemed necessary) has been undertaken and the possibility of a neck injury has been excluded. If urgent intubation is indicated, it should be assumed that the patient has a full stomach, and cricoid pressure should be applied to prevent vomiting or gastric regurgitation. In adults, this should be maintained until the cuff of the endotracheal tube is inflated, creating a secure airway. Short-acting sedatives and muscle relaxants should always be used for intubation, to minimize the risk of raised ICP due to noxious stimulation and coughing. Suctioning should be kept to a minimum as it also raises ICP.

Breathing

In patients with isolated head injury, acute lung injury (ALI) is common. Studies show ALI occurrence in 20% of patients with a post-resuscitative GCS of 8 or less. ALI is an additional marker of the severity of brain injury and is associated with an increased risk of morbidity and mortality (Bratton & Davis 1997). Neurogenic pulmonary oedema (NPE) represents the most severe form of ALI and is typically reported in cases of fatal or near-fatal head injuries (Bratton & Davis 1997). The development of neurogenic pulmonary oedema may be remarkably rapid and is usually associated with an acute and significant rise in ICP. The exact mechanism responsible for this acute condition seen after severe traumatic brain injury and after abrupt elevations in ICP is unclear. It is generally accepted that there is a neurological pathway following central nervous system injury and that it is the result of massive sympathetic outflow, possibly mediated by the hypothalamus. The classic form appears early, within minutes to a few hours after injury, while the delayed form progresses slowly over a period of 12 to 72 hours (Durieux 1996).

Some studies have shown a link between CPP management and acute respiratory distress syndrome (ARDS) (Contant et al. 2001, Robertson 2001). Induced hypertension to raise CPP can cause increased pulmonary hydrostatic pressures and thereby increase the amount of water accumulating within the lungs. The results of a randomized trial comparing two head injury management strategies, one ICP targeted and the other CPP targeted, showed a fivefold increase in the incidence of ARDS in the CPP targeted group where CPP was maintained >70 mmHg (Robertson 2001).

The pathophysiological changes result in the rapid development of interstitial oedema and subsequent increased pulmonary shunt, decreased compliance, and loss of alveoli surface area. Signs and symptoms include dyspnoea, cyanosis, pallor, sweating, a weak rapid pulse, and the production of pink frothy sputum. Primary treatment consists of employing therapeutic interventions aimed at reducing ICP and to normal limits providing appropriate ventilation support and management, controlling carbon dioxide levels, and maximizing oxygenation with minimal effect on cardiac output. This complicates the management of severe traumatic brain injury, many of the therapies used to protect the lungs e.g., reduced tidal volume, permissive hypoxia and hypercarbia, increased levels of positive tracheal end pressure, and prone lying, causes a rise in ICP or decreased CPP (Robertson et al. 1999).

The neurophysiology of breathing is complex and involves several areas of the brain. Following head injury the normal pattern of breathing is easily disrupted, leading to hypoxia. Hypoxia is a major cause of cerebral ischaemia. Approximately 60% of patients with severe traumatic brain injury become hypoxaemic without ventilatory support or added oxygen and require advanced ventilatory support within a short period of time.

In patients with traumatic brain injury the effects of hypotension and hypoxia appear to be more profound than those that result when hypoxic and/or hypotensive episodes of similar magnitude occur in trauma patients without neurological involvement (Bratton et al. 2007). It is important to maintain adequate oxygenation, as a rising PCO_2 level initiates autoregulation, causing cerebral vasodilatation and a rise in ICP. If unchecked, this may lead to secondary brain injury.

Patients with head injuries should be given oxygen via a facemask and reservoir bag. Respiratory function must be monitored closely with regular arterial blood gases (ABGs) and continuous O_2 saturation measurement. If bradypnoeic, the patient's respiratory function should be assisted as soon as possible following the severe traumatic brain injury.

Intubation and ventilation should be implemented immediately in the following circumstances:

- GCS <8
- loss of protective laryngeal reflexes
- ventilatory insufficiency as judged by arterial blood gases:
- hypoxaemia (PaO_2 <13 kPa on oxygen) or hypercarbia ($PaCO_2$ >6 kPa)
- spontaneous hyperventilation (causing $PaCO_2$ >4 kPa)
- irregular respirations (National Institute for Health and Clinical Excellence 2007).

Intubation and ventilation should be implemented before the start of a transfer in the following circumstances in addition to the above:

- significantly deteriorating conscious level (one or more points on the motor score), even if not coma
- unstable fractures of the facial skeleton
- copious bleeding into the mouth, e.g., base of skull fracture
- seizures (National Institute for Health and Clinical Excellence 2007).

The goal is to achieve and maintain normocapnia, a PaO_2 greater than 13 kPa, $PaCO_2$ 4.5–5.0 kPa, unless there is clinical or radiological evidence of raised intracranial pressure, in which case more aggressive hyperventilation is justified (National Institute for Health and Clinical Excellence 2007). Hypoxemia, hypercapnia, hypocapnia and acidosis that result from either inadequate ventilation or hypermetabolism following traumatic brain injury are all associated with poor outcomes. Induced hyperventilation should be used to reduce PCO_2 levels, but this should be discussed with a neurosurgeon first (Bullock & Teasdale 1996). Hyperventilation is only recommended as a temporary measure in order to reduce elevated ICP. It should not be used in the first 24 hours after injury when CBF is reduced (Bratton et al. 2007). If hyperventilation is used, the inspired oxygen concentration should be increased (National Institute for Health and Clinical Excellence 2007).

Cardiac

High levels of sympathetic activity and of circulating catecholamines after severe traumatic brain injury can have an adverse effect on cardiac function, basal metabolic rate, and vascular and neuronal function in the central nervous system (Clifton et al. 1983). The magnitude of this hyperdynamic cardiovascular state occurring after severe head injury does not necessarily correlate with ICP, GCS or CT findings (Clifton et al. 1981). There is both clinical and experimental evidence to suggest that cerebral neurogenic factors cause arrhythmias in normal hearts, with fatal arrhythmias being reported in otherwise healthy brain-injured patients (McLeod 1982, Oppenheimer et al. 1990). A wide variety of atrial and ventricular arrhythmias, abnormalities of the QRS complex, T-wave and ST segment and QT prolongation have been documented and occur most commonly in patients with diffuse injury, oedema, and contusions. In two seminal studies, 31% of patients admitted with head injury exhibited some form of cardiac arrhythmia (Hersch 1961) and cardiac arrhythmias were observed in 41 out of 100 patients admitted with acute subdural haematoma, with more than half of these showing ventricular arrhythmias ranging in severity from premature ventricular contractions to ventricular tachycardia and ventricular fibrillation (Van der Ark 1975). Elevations of pulse greater than 120 beats per minute have been found in one-third of patients with severe traumatic brain injury.

It is generally accepted that hypotension related to trauma is not caused by head injury, although it can be related to head injury per se in children. However, there is some evidence that episodes of hypotension following severe traumatic brain injury may be of neurogenic origin in a small proportion of patients, and that this is not simply attributable to devastating, non-survivable brain injury (Chesnut et al 1998).

Hypotension is usually a result of systemic hypovolaemia following multiple traumas. According to the Brain Trauma Foundation, hypotension is a systolic blood pressure of <90 mmHg (Bratton et al. 2007). The diagnosis and treatment of life-threatening extracranial injuries take priority over intracranial injuries according to ATLS protocols. The causes of hypotension should be identified rapidly as the provision of appropriate treatment and fluid resuscitation is imperative to prevent a drop in mean BP, CBF and CPP leading to cerebral ischaemia and secondary brain injury. Hypotension is a predominant contributing factor in secondary brain injury and has the highest correlation with morbidity and mortality (Schreiber et al. 2002). Chesnut et al. (1993) report that a single episode of hypotension during the pre-hospital phase in patients with a severe traumatic brain injury is associated with increasing morbidity and doubling mortality. Until ICP monitoring is established the aim should be to achieve a target mean arterial pressure of 90 mmHg or more or a systolic BP >120 mmHg by infusion of fluid and vasopressors as indicated. In children, blood pressure should be maintained at a level appropriate for the child's age (Brain Trauma Foundation 2007, Maas et al. 1997, National Institute for Health and Clinical Excellence 2007). Children aged > 10 years have the same hypotension threshold definition as adults (Badjatia et al. 2007).

Several factors need to be considered in the fluid management of patients following severe traumatic brain injury:

- clinical and laboratory assessment of volume status
- the effects of different fluids on CPP and cerebral oedema
- osmotic therapy
- water and electrolyte disturbances.

Following traumatic brain injury the blood–brain barrier is likely to be disrupted, and different solutions have differing effects on cerebral oedema. If the serum osmolarity falls, water moves across the blood–brain barrier along the altered osmotic gradient, causing cerebral oedema, increased ICP and decreased CPP. The use of hypotonic fluids should, therefore, be avoided.

Since 0.9% saline is isotonic, it has a negligible effect on brain water and has become the crystalloid of choice in the management of traumatic brain injury. Resuscitation with 0.9% saline requires four times the volume of blood lost to restore haemodynamic parameters; therefore, blood loss from other injuries should be replaced with blood products (Spiekermann & Thompson 1996).

The use of hypertonic saline solutions has become the crystalloid of choice for volume resuscitation in the management of traumatic brain injury. The evidence base for its use in adults is weak; however there is some evidence of its beneficial effects in children and paediatric guidelines recommend the use of hypertonic saline as a continuous infusion (Adelson et al. 2003). Hypertonic saline is an osmotherapeutic agent that induces a shift of fluid from the intracellular to the extracellular space across the osmotic gradient it generates. It therefore reduces brain water (cerebral oedema) and potentially decreases ICP, increases blood volume, and increases plasma sodium, making it suitable for patients who are fluid depleted, e.g., following acute trauma. (Deem 2006). Studies in the human traumatic brain injury population demonstrate that hypotonic saline is not associated with the rebound intracranial hypertension often seen with mannitol (Bratton et al. 2007).

Based on data from various studies, it is widely accepted that glucose-containing solutions should not be used in the fluid management of patients following severe traumatic brain injury unless specifically indicated to correct hypoglycaemia. The mechanism by which glucose worsens neurological injury is not fully understood; however, it is believed that, in the presence of ischaemia, glucose is metabolized anaerobically leading to an accumulation of lactic acid. Increased lactic acid is thought to decrease intracellular pH, leading to vasodilatation, compromise cellular function, ischaemia and ultimately cause infarction. An alternative explanation proposes that hyperglycaemia worsens ischaemia by decreasing CBF. Other studies suggest that hyperglycaemia decreases cerebral adenosine levels, and adenosine is an inhibitor of the release of excitatory amino acids that are thought to play a major role in ischaemic cell death (Spiekermann & Thompson 1996).

Accurate fluid balance (input and output) observations are essential. The patients should have a urinary catheter and hourly urine output recordings.

Once a normal circulating volume has been established, noradrenaline (norepinephrine) is often the drug of choice for extrinsic support of blood pressure due to its vasoconstricting properties and superior augmentation of CPP (Steiner et al. 2004).

In the late stages of head injury, hypertension occurs with bradycardia and bradypnoea. Hypertension is a late sign of pending brain injury. Arterial blood pressure increases in an attempt to maintain the cerebral perfusion pressure in the brain. The decrease in respiration and heart rates are due to pressure on the medullary reflex areas. These signs often precede brain stem death. This is referred to as Cushing's triad.

Severe traumatic brain injury can be complicated by the development of a coagulopathy that can worsen blood loss and delay invasive neurosurgical treatment. Studies have reported a positive correlation between the presence and severity of disseminated intravascular coagulation (DIC) and the degree of brain injury, assessed by plasma fibrinogen degradation product levels. Although most of the acute coagulopathies associated with brain injury are not preventable, prompt treatment can be effective in reducing morbidity. Clotting studies at the time of admission to the ED can be valuable in predicting the occurrence of delayed injury, and early follow-up CT scanning is advocated in the patient with coagulopathy (Piek et al. 1992, May et al. 1997).

Disability

Uncontrolled elevation in ICP is the most common cause of mortality, morbidity and secondary brain injury after severe TBI, since it alters tissue perfusion causing cerebral ischaemia and potential infarction. It is imperative that signs of raised ICP are recognized, documented and treated promptly. Disorientation, irritation, headache, seizures, nausea and vomiting are all possible indicators of raised ICP, and later signs include deterioration in the GCS, deteriorating limb function and pupillary changes and finally alteration in the vital signs (Cushing's triad).

Mannitol has been considered the most effective agent to reduce cerebral oedema and ICP in patients with intracranial hypertension (Bullock 1995). The Brain Trauma Foundation (2007) suggests that hypertonic saline as a bolus infusion may be used as an effective alternative to mannitol however it states that the limitations of the research conducted so far does not allow for a conclusion to be reached (Bratton et al. 2007). Mannitol reduces ICP as a result of its osmotic effects; mannitol may also reduce ICP by improving cerebral microcirculatory flow and oxygen delivery. However, mannitol opens the blood–brain barrier and this effect may become harmful after multiple doses and can exacerbate ICP by increasing brain swelling. Repetitive administration can potentially increase ICP, since mannitol accumulates within brain tissue, reversing osmotic shift and increasing cerebral oedema. The peak effect of mannitol on ICP occurs within 15 minutes of administration, but its effects on serum osmolarity last 2 to 6 hours, depending on the dose and clinical condition of the patient. Mannitol increased serum sodium levels and is excreted entirely by the kidneys, therefore there is increased risk of acute renal failure (acute tubular necrosis) if administered in large doses, particularly if serum osmolarity is >320 mOsm/L. Mannitol raises urine osmolarity and specific gravity, therefore these variables cannot be used to diagnose diabetes insipidus.

The ICP-lowering effect of bolus administration of mannitol appears to be equal over the range 0.25–1.0 g/kg, although the duration of activity may be somewhat shorter with the lower dose. Under most circumstances, the lower dose should be used in order to minimize the risk of hyperosmolality and avoid a negative fluid balance. Guidelines recommend mannitol 20 % be given as an intravenous infusion over 15 to 20 minutes, and repeated as necessary. Blood osmotic pressure must be monitored and serum osmolarity kept below 315 mOsm/L. They also recommend that if mannitol has insufficient effect then frusemide can be given additionally (Maas et al. 1997, Brain Trauma Foundation 2007).

Blood viscosity

Cerebral blood flow can be influenced by blood viscosity, of which haematocrit is the single most important determinant. Blood viscosity increases logarithmically with increasing haematocrit and the optimal level is probably about 35 %. Cerebral blood flow is reduced by haematocrit levels over 50 % and increased with haematocrit levels below 30 %. This compensatory mechanism allows sufficient oxygen delivery in healthy individuals even with haematocrit levels of 20 %.

Studies suggest that a haematocrit of 30–34 % may result in optimal oxygen delivery to brain tissue. However, if maximum vasodilatation already exists, haemodilution may decrease oxygen delivery and lead to increases in cerebral blood volume (CBV) and therefore ICP (Cesarini 1996).

Drugs

It is common practice for severe traumatic brain injury patients to be empirically managed with a protocol that includes the routine use of sedatives, analgesics, and neuromuscular blocking agents to facilitate mechanical ventilation and to treat intracranial hypertension.

Intravenous sedation agents cause a dose-dependent reduction in cerebral metabolism, CBF and ICP while maintaining pressure autoregulation and CO_2 reactivity. The use of barbiturates in traumatic brain injury is controversial and has largely been replaced by propofol, which has similar cerebrovascular effects but a more favourable pharmacological profile. Propofol has become the sedative of choice but care must be taken to avoid hypotension (Kelly 2000, Kelly et al. 1999).

Fentanyl and morphine are frequently administered to manage pain, facilitate mechanical ventilation, and potentiate the effect of sedation.

Neuromuscular blocking drugs have no direct effect on ICP but may prevent rises produced by coughing and straining on the endotracheal tube. However, such agents are not associated with improved outcome and their use is the subject of much debate (Prielipp & Coursin 1995); their use should only be employed when sedation alone proves inadequate.

Patients with CSF leakage are usually prescribed prophylactic antibiotics, because of the high risk of bacterial meningitis. The available evidence, however, does not support the use of prophylactic antibiotics (Watkins 2000).

Corticosteroids have been used in the treatment of certain neurological conditions since the 1950s. There is no doubt about their value in producing rapid improvement in patients with brain tumours associated with oedema, and there is evidence of benefit in the early administration of high-dose methylprednisolone in spinal cord injury but no evidence to support their use in the management of patients with traumatic brain injury. CRASH Trial Collaborators (2004, 2005) state, after a major study involving over 10 000 adults, that patients with traumatic brain injuries should *not* be given corticosteroids, as they increase the risk of death or severe disability.

Temperature control

Following traumatic brain injury, temperature regulation may be disrupted as a result of damage to the hypothalamus. Fever can make an existing neurological dysfunction more apparent and may worsen an ongoing insult. The brain's metabolic rate for oxygen increases by 6–9 % for every degree Celsius rise in temperature. In the acute phase of head injury, therefore, hyperthermia should be treated since it will exacerbate cerebral ischaemia and adversely affect outcome.

Hypothermia as a treatment in severe traumatic brain injury has been a major area of research during the last decade. Brain Trauma Foundation guidelines cautiously support prophylactic hypothermia as being associated with significantly higher GCS outcomes, but this is based on limited research (Bratton et al. 2007).

The interim results of a large multi-centre study showed that cooling to 32–33°C within 10 hours of injury improved neurological recovery in patients presenting with head injury and a GCS of 5–7 but not those with a lower GCS. However, this study was terminated early with no clear benefit established (Marion et al. 1997).

Some studies suggest that hypothermia provides protection against secondary injury, specifically hypotension and hypoxia, and that there may be a therapeutic window for neuroprotection in the early stages following the primary injury (Yamamoto et al. 1999). Whether this protection can be sustained over longer periods remains to be determined.

A randomized trial evaluating the use of mild hypothermia during intracranial aneurysm surgery found that, compared with normothermic patients, more patients in the hypothermic group had good outcomes and fewer of these patients had neurological deficits at the time of discharge (Hindman et al. 1999). In a further study on CBF and oxygen metabolism during mild hypothermia (33–34°C) in elective aneurysmal surgery, positron emission tomography (PET) showed luxury perfusion in almost all cases, providing the first PET evidence of decreased CBF and metabolic rate of O_2 during hypothermia in humans (Kawamura et al. 2000).

There is some evidence of increased mortality in the general trauma population for patients admitted with hypothermia, and at least one study demonstrated an increased incidence of infection in head injured patients subjected to hypothermia (Sutcliffe 2001, Brain Trauma Foundation 2007).

Seizure activity

Seizure activity reflects disordered electrical discharges in the damaged brain and results in local loss of autoregulation, increased metabolic activity in the brain with concomitant increases in cerebral blood flow and tissue lactic acidosis, which may aggravate ICP. Seizures are seen in 5–15% of patients after traumatic brain injury, especially those who have suffered a haematoma, penetrating injury, including depressed skull fracture with dural penetration, and focal neurological signs or intracranial sepsis (Dunn 1996, Watkins 2000).

In the conscious patient a single seizure requires only supportive treatment, but in the comatose patient every seizure can threaten life or neurological function and should be treated promptly. Patients having seizures should be protected from harm, if they are not in any danger they should not be handled. Extra vigilance is required, frequent GCS observations should be performed until the pre-seizure state is regained. The seizure should be observed for origin, sequence of events and time of start/finish. This information should be clearly documented in the patient's notes. No generally accepted classification of seizures exists, but it is useful to distinguish between non-focal seizures, where loss of consciousness is the primary event, followed by convulsions affecting all four limbs, and focal or partial seizures, where activity is confined to one area of the cerebral cortex. The continuous neuronal firing that occurs during non-focal seizure activity causes a massive increase in the brain's requirement for oxygen. If a corresponding increase in the supply of oxygen is not provided then hypoxia, ischaemia, and potential infarction will result. Anticonvulsant drugs should be used if two or more seizures occur (Watkins 2000). If seizure activity is continuous, i.e., status epilepticus or serial fitting, severe cerebral oedema may occur.

Positioning

Many studies have been undertaken to determine the influence of body position on ICP and CPP and establish the best practices for positioning of severe traumatic brain injury patients (Sullivan 2000). It has been demonstrated that head elevation decreases ICP and that head rotation and neck flexion are associated with increased ICP, decreased jugular venous return, and localized changes in cerebral blood flow. In the light of these findings, it is common practice to position head-injured patients in bed with their head elevated above the heart to varying degrees (0–30°) provided they have an adequate blood pressure and there are no contraindications, in neutral alignment with the trunk, in order to reduce ICP.

Gastric decompression

If gastric decompression is indicated, the orogastric route should be used as the nasogastric route carries the risks of trauma to the brain and the introduction of infection.

Transfer to a specialist neurosurgical unit

In an attempt to improve outcome for patients with traumatic brain injury the National Institute for Health and Clinical Excellence (2007) recommends an improvement in the rate at which such patients are transferred to the specialist neurosciences unit. Patients who have suffered an isolated severe head injury should ideally receive their treatment in a specialist neurosciences unit, regardless of the need for neurosurgery (National Institute for Health and Clinical Excellence 2007). Patients should be referred to a neurosurgeon where:

- a new surgically significant abnormality is seen on imaging
- a persisting coma (GCS less than or equal to 8) is seen after initial resuscitation
- an unexplained confusion, which persists for more than four hours is seen
- deterioration in GCS score after admission is seen. (Greatest attention should be paid to motor response deterioration)
- progressive focal neurological signs are seen
- an epileptic seizure without full recovery is seen
- a definite or a suspected penetrating injury is seen
- a cerebrospinal fluid leak is seen (National Institute for Health and Clinical Excellence 2007).

Once the decision to transfer has been made, it is imperative that the patient is thoroughly resuscitated and stabilized prior to transfer to avoid complications during the journey.

The neck should be fully examined to identify or exclude cervical injury (see also Chapter 7). Chest or abdominal injuries (Chapters 8 and 9) should be treated if potentially life-threatening and fractures splinted where appropriate (see Chapter 6). Airway management is a major cause for concern during transfer. Unconscious patients, those who are vomiting or those whose condition appears to be deteriorating (GCS less than 8) should be intubated and ventilated prior to transfer (National Institute for Health and Clinical Excellence 2007).

Any patient being transferred should be accompanied by a clinician with at least two years' experience in an appropriate specialism, e.g., anaesthesia or a paediatrician, and one who has received supervised training in the transfer of patients with a severe head injury, along with a competent nurse escort (National Institute for Health and Clinical Excellence 2007). During transfer, the patient should be carefully observed and ECG, oxygen saturation levels, and blood pressure should be monitored continuously (Parkins 1998). If the patient is not sedated, pupil size and reaction and GCS should be recorded. All documentation and results of clinical investigations, such as CT, should accompany the patient (Jones 1993).

Sedation and neuromuscular blocking drugs are essential to optimizing the transport of patients with a traumatic head injury. In the absence of outcome-based studies the choice of sedative is left to the physician, and neuromuscular blocking agents should only be employed when sedation alone proves inadequate (Maas et al. 1997, Brain Trauma Foundation 2007).

Surgical treatment

Delay in surgical treatment of TBI has been shown to be a major preventable cause of morbidity and mortality. In a typical series of patients who had surgery for Acute Sub-Dural Haematoma (ASDH), more than 70% had a functional recovery, i.e., good recovery or moderate disability, if the delay from injury to operation was less than two hours. Where the delay was 2–4 hours, just over 60% made a functional recovery. Where the delay was more than four hours after the injury, fewer than 10% made a functional recovery (Watkins 2000). The Royal College of Surgeons of England recommends that, in all circumstances, life-saving decompressive surgery must be available to all patients who require it, within four hours of the injury (Royal College of Surgeons 1999, Flannery & Buxton 2001).

Some lesions may be inaccessible to the neurosurgeon or be in such sensitive areas of the brain that the risks of surgery are too great. Alternatively, brain injury may be diffuse and surgical intervention inappropriate. Whether all haematomas must be removed remains controversial and this is particularly so in the management of intracerebral haematomas and haemorrhagic contusions. While some surgeons advocate early surgery in such cases, experience has shown that despite surgical treatment, post-operative intracranial hypertension continues to occur in virtually all patients. Guidelines outlining the specific indications for surgery are based on biological and pathophysiological principles, published evidence, and practical experience (Maas et al. 1997, Brain Trauma Foundation 2007).

Indications for decompressive surgery:

- intracranial mass lesions with >5 mm midline shift or basal cistern compression on CT scan

- a surgically significant (1 cm thick) extradural haematoma and acute subdural haematoma needs evacuation within 2–4 hours of injury to achieve optimal chance of recovery

- a conservative approach is generally adopted for small haemorrhagic contusions or other small intracerebral lesions, but operation should be considered urgent for a large intracranial haematoma (>20–30 ml) based on position, clinical condition, and ICP

- skull fracture depressed greater than the thickness of the skull or compound fractures with a torn dura (Maas et al. 1997, Brain Trauma Foundation 2007).

Decompressive craniotomy

The practice of wide bone removal for the treatment of intracranial hypertension due to cerebral oedema, refractory to medical management, has a long history and remains controversial. Polin et al. (1997) concluded that provided surgery was performed before ICP exceeded 40 mmHg for a sustained period and within 48 hours of injury, decompressive craniectomy showed a statistical advantage over medical treatment. Decompressive craniectomy, which can also increase oedema formation, is usually reserved as a last resort (Maas et al. 1997).

Brain stem death testing

The diagnosis of brainstem death is usually made in the intensive care unit.

Preconditions

- diagnosis compatible with brainstem death

- presence of irreversible structural brain damage

- presence of apnoeic coma preconditions.

Exclusions

- o therapeutic drug effects (sedatives, hypnotics, muscle relaxants)
- o hypothermia (temp >35°C)
- o metabolic abnormalities
- o endocrine abnormalities
- o intoxication.

Clinical tests

1. Confirmation of absent brain stem reflexes
   - o no pupillary response to light
   - o absent corneal reflex
   - o no motor response within cranial nerve distribution
   - o absent gag reflex
   - o absent cough reflex
   - o absent vestibulo-ocular reflex

2. Confirmation of persistent apnoea
   - o pre-oxygenation with 100% oxygen for 10 minutes
   - o allow $PaCO_2$ to rise above 5.0 kPa before test
   - o disconnect from ventilator
   - o maintain adequate oxygenation during test

- allow $PaCO_2$ to climb above 6.65 kPa
- confirm no spontaneous respiration
- reconnect ventilator

3. Two experienced practitioners should perform clinical tests
- at least one should be a consultant: both must be competent to perform the tests, i.e., intensivists/neurologists/neurosurgeons
- neither should be part of the transplant team
- the tests should be performed on two separate occasions
- there is no necessary prescribed time interval between the tests.

These conditions limit the probability of the full testing occurring in the emergency department; however, some or all of the tests may be performed, either to complete a clinical picture or to reach an endpoint in an inevitable situation.

Conclusion

Head trauma can have a devastating effect on a person's life and some mortality and morbidity are inevitable. McMillan et al. (2011) noted that head injury is associated with increased vulnerability to death for at least 13 years after hospital admission. The emergency nurse who is equipped with the evidence-based knowledge and skills to manage patients with traumatic brain injury is fundamental to keeping morbidity and mortality to a minimum.

References

Adelson, P.D., Bratton, S.L., Carney, N.A., et al., 2003. Guidelines for the acute medical management of severe traumatic brain injury in infants, children and adolescents. Paediatric Critical Care Medicine 4 (3), S1–S75.

Addison, C., Crawford, B., 1999. Not bad, just misunderstood. Nursing Times 95, 52–53.

Advanced Life Support Group, 2011. Advanced Paediatric Life Support: The Practical Approach. West Sussex, Wiley-Blackwell.

Albano, C., 2005. Innovations in the management of cerebral injury. Critical Care Nurse Quarterly 28 (2), 135–149.

American College of Surgeons, 2008. Advanced Trauma Life Support, seventh ed. American College of Surgeons, Chicago.

Badjatia, N., Carney, N., Crocco, T.J., et al., 2007. Guidelines for prehospital management of traumatic brain injury, second ed. Prehospital Emergency Care 12 (1), S1–S52.

Brain Trauma Foundation, 2007. American Association of Neurological Surgeons' Joint section on neurotrauma and critical care guidelines for the management of severe head injury, third ed. Journal of Neurotrauma 13, 641–734.

Bratton, S.I., Davis, R.L., 1997. Acute lung injury in isolated traumatic brain injury. Neurosurgery 40 (4), 707–712.

Bratton, S.L., Chesnut, R.M., Ghajar, J., et al., 2007. Guidelines for management of severe traumatic brain injury, third ed. Journal of Neurotrauma 24 (Suppl. 1), S1–S106.

Bullock, R., 1995. Mannitol and other diuretics in severe neurotrauma. New Horizons 3 (3), 443–452.

Bullock, R., Teasdale, G., 1996. Head injuries. In: Skinner, D., Driscoll, R., Earlam, R. (Eds.), ABC of Trauma. BMJ Publishing Group, London.

Caton-Richards, M., 2010. Assessing the neurological status of patients with head injuries. Emergency Nurse 17 (10), 28–31.

Cesarini, K.G., 1996. Pathophysiology of cerebral ischaemia. In: Palmer, J.D. (Ed.), Manual of Neurosurgery. Churchill Livingstone, London.

Chesnut, R.M., Gautille, T., Blunt, B.A., et al., 1998. Neurogenic hypotension in patients with severe head injuries. Journal of Trauma 44 (6), 958–963.

Chesnut, R.M., Marshall, L.F., et al., 1993. The role of secondary brain injury in determining outcome from severe head injury. Journal of Trauma Injury: Infection and Critical care 34 (2), 216–222.

Clifton, G.L., Ziegler, M.G., Grossman, A., 1981. Circulating catecholamines and sympathetic activity after head injury. Neurosurgery 8, 10–14.

Clifton, G.L., Robertson, C.S., Kyper, K., et al., 1983. Cardiovascular response to severe head injury. Journal of Neurosurgery 3, 447–454.

Contant, C.F., Valadka, A.B., Shankar, M.D., et al., 2001. Adult respiratory distress syndrome: a complication of induced hypertension after severe head injury. Journal of Neurosurgery 95, 560–568.

Crossman, A.R., Neary, D., 2000. Neuroanatomy – An Illustrated Colour Text, second ed. Churchill Livingstone, Edinburgh.

Darby, J., Yonas, H., Marion, D.W., et al., 1998. Local 'inverse steal' induced by hyperventilation in head injury. Neurosurgery 23, 84.

Dearden, N.M., 1998. Mechanism and prevention of secondary brain damage during intensive care. Clinical Neuropathology. 17 (47), 221–228.

Deem, S., 2006. Management of acute brain injury and associated respiratory issues. Respiratory Care 51 (4), 357–367.

Deitch, E.A., Dayal, S.D., 2006. Intensive care unit management of the trauma patient. Critical Care Medicine 34 (9), 2294–2301.

Department of Health, 2001. Hospital episode statistics 2000–2001. Department of Health, London.

Duffy, C., 2001. Anaesthesia for head injury. In: Gupta, A.K., Summors, A. (Eds.), Notes in Neuroanaesthesia and Critical Care. Greenwich Medical Media, London.

Dunn, L.T., 1996. Post-traumatic epilepsy. In: Palmer, J.D. (Ed.), Manual of Neurosurgery. Churchill Livingstone, London.

Durieux, M.E., 1996. Anaesthesia for head trauma. In: Stone, D.J., Sperry, R.J. (Eds.), The Neuroanaesthesia Handbook. Mosby, St. Louis.

Farnsworth, S.T., Sperry, R.J., 1996. Neurophysiology. In: Stone, J.D., Sperry, R.J. et al., (Eds.), The Neuroanaesthesia Handbook. Mosby, St Louis.

Flannery, T., Buxton, N., 2001. Modern management of head injuries. Journal of the Royal College of Surgeons (Edinburgh) 46, 150–153.

Garner, A., Amin, Y., 2007. The management of raised intracranial pressure: a multidisciplinary approach. British Journal of Neurosciences Nursing 3 (11), 516–521.

Ghajar, J., 2000. Traumatic brain injury. Lancet 356, 923–929.

Graham, D.I., Hume Adams, J., Nicoll, J.A.R., et al., 1995. The nature, distribution and causes of traumatic brain injury. Brain Pathology 5, 397–406.

Healthcare for London, 2009. The shape of things to come: Developing New High-quality Major Trauma and Stroke Services for London: Compact Consultation Document. Healthcare for London, London.

Hersch, C., 1961. Electrocardiographic changes in head injuries. Circulation 23, 853–860.

Hickey, J.V., 2009. The Clinical Practice of Neurological and Neurosurgical Nursing, sixth ed. Lippincott Williams & Wilkins, Philadelphia.

Hindman, B.J., Todd, M.M., Gelb, A.W., et al., 1999. Mild hypothermia as a protective therapy during intracranial aneurysm surgery: a randomized prospective pilot trial. Neurosurgery 44, 23–33.

Hudak, C.M., Gallo, B.M., 1994. Critical Care Nursing, sixth ed. JB Lippincott, Philadelphia.

Hunningher, A., Smith, M., 2006. Update on the management of severe head injury in adults. Care of the Critically ill 22 (5), 124–129.

Intensive Care Society, 1997. Guidelines for the Transport of the Critically Ill Adult. Intensive Care Society, London.

Jackson, S., 1995. Not so minor head injuries? Emergency Nurse 3 (1), 19–22.

Jones, H., 1993. Safe transfer. Nursing Times 89 (41), 31–33.

Kawamura, S., Suzuki, A., Hadeishi, H., et al., 2000. Cerebral blood flow and oxygen metabolism during mild hypothermia in patients with subarachnoid haemorrhage. Acta Neurochir (Wein) 142 (10), 1117–1121.

Kelly, D.F., 2000. Sedation after severe head injury: beneficial to final outcome? European Journal of Anaesthesiology 17 (Suppl. 18), 43–54.

Kelly, D.F., Goodale, D.B., Williams, J., et al., 1999. Propofol in the treatment of moderate and severe head injury: a randomized prospective double-blind trial. Journal of Neurosurgery 90 (6), 1042–1052.

Kwiatkowski, S., 1996. Traumatic acute intracranial haematoma. In: Palmer, J.D. (Ed.), Manual of Neurosurgery, Churchill Livingstone, London.

Lindsey, K.W., Bone, I., Callander, R., 2004. Neurology and Neurosurgery Illustrated, fourth ed. Churchill Livingstone, Edinburgh.

Maartens, N., Lethbridge, G., 2005. Head and neck trauma. In: O'Shea, R.A. (Ed.), Principles and Practice of Trauma Nursing, Elsevier Churchill Livingstone, Edinburgh.

Maas, A.I.R., Dearden, M., Teasdale, G.M., et al., 1997. European Brain Injury Consortium Guidelines for management of severe head injury in adults. Acta Neurochir (Wien) 139, 286–294.

Marion, D.W., Penrod, L.E., Kelsey, S.F., et al., 1997. Treatment of traumatic brain injury with moderate hypothermia. New England Journal of Medicine 336 (8), 560–566.

McLeod, A.A., Neil-Dwyer, G., Meyer, C.H.A., et al., 1982. Cardiac sequelae of acute head injury. British Heart Journal 47, 221–226.

McMillan, T.M., Teasdale, G.M., Weir, C.J., et al., 2011. Death after head injury: the 13 year outcome of a case control study. Journal and Neurology and Neurosurgical Psychiatry.

McNaughton, H., Harwood, M., 2002. Traumatic brain injury: assessment and management. Hospital Medicine 63, 8–12.

National Institute for Health and Clinical Excellence, 2007. Head Injury Triage, Assessment, Investigation and Early Management of Head Injury in Infants, Children and Adults. NICE, London.

Oppenheimer, S.M., Cochetto, D.F., Hachinski, V.C., 1990. Cerebrogenic cardiac arrhythmias. Acta Neurology 47, 513–519.

Parkins, D.R., 1998. Transportation of the injured: head injuries. Pre-hospital Immediate Care 2, 25–26.

Patel, H.C., Menon, D.K., Tebbs, S., et al., 2002. Specialist neurocritical care and outcome from head injury. Intensive Care Medicine 28, 547–553.

Piek, J., Chesnut, R.M., Marshall, L.F., et al., 1992. Extracranial complications of severe head injury. Journal of Neurosurgery 77, 901–907.

Polin, S., Shaffrey, M.E., Bogaev, C.A., et al., 1997. Decompressive craniectomy in the treatment of severe refractory post-traumatic cerebral oedema. Neurosurgery 41, 84–94.

Prielipp, R.C., Coursin, D.B., 1995. Sedative and neuromuscular blocking drug use in critically ill patients with head injuries. New Horizons 3 (3), 456–468.

Ramrakha, P., Moore, K., 1997. Oxford Handbook of Acute Medicine. Oxford University Press, Oxford.

Robertson, C.S., 2001. Management of cerebral perfusion pressure after traumatic brain injury. Anaesthesiology 95(6) 15, 13–17.

Robertson, C.S., Valadka, A.B., Hannay, H.J., et al., 1999. Prevention of secondary insults after severe head injury. Critical Care Medicine 27, 2086–2095.

Royal College of Paediatrics and Child Health, 2001. Guidelines for Good Practice: Early Management of Patients with a Head Injury. Royal College of Paediatrics and Child Health, London.

Royal College of Surgeons, 1999. Report of the Working Party on the Management of Patients with Head Injury. Royal College of Surgeons, London.

Sakas, D.E., Dias, L.S., Beale, D., 1995. Subarachnoid haemorrhage presenting as a head injury. British Medical Journal 310, 1186–1187.

Schreiber, M., Aoki, N., Scott, B.G., Beck, J.R., 2002. Determinants of mortality in patients with severe blunt head injury. Archives of Surgery 137, 285–290.

Shah, S., 1999. Neurological assessment. Nursing Standard 13 (22), 49–56.

Spiekermann, B.F., Thompson, S.A., 1996. Fluid management. In: Stone, D., Sperry, R.J. et al., (Eds.), The Handbook of Neuroanaesthesia. Mosby, St Louis.

Sullivan, J., 2000. Positioning of patients with severe traumatic brain injury: research based practice. Journal of Neuroscientific Nursing 32 (4), 204–209.

Stern, S., 2011. Observing and recording neurological dysfunction. Emergency Nurse 18 (10), 28–31.

Sutcliffe, A., 2001. Hypothermia (or not) for the management of head injury. Care of the Critically Ill 17 (5), 162–165.

Tagliaferri, F., Compagnone, C., Korsic, M., et al., 2006. A systematic review of brain injury epidemiology in Europe. Acta Neurochir (Wien) 148, 255–268.

Teasdale, G., Jennett, B., 1974. Assessment of coma and impaired consciousness: a practical scale. The Lancet 2 (7872), 81–84.

Van der Ark, G.D., 1975. Cardiovascular changes with acute subdural haematoma. Surgical Neurology 5 (3), 305–308.

Vos, P.E., Alekseenko, Y., Battistin, L., et al., 2012. Mild traumatic brain injury. European Journal of Neurology 19 (2), 191–198.

Watkins, L.D., 2000. Head injuries: general principles and management. Surgery 18 (7), 219–224.

Wilson, M., 2011. Major incidents. In: Smith, J., Greaves, I., Porter, K. (Eds.), Oxford Desk Reference: Major Trauma. Oxford Medical Publications, Oxford.

Wyatt, J.P., Illingworth, R.N., Graham, C.A., et al., 2008. Oxford Handbook of Emergency Medicine, third ed. Oxford University Press, Oxford.

Yamamoto, M., Marmarou, C.R., Stiefel, M.F., et al., 1999. Neuroprotective effect of hypothermia on neuronal injury in diffuse traumatic brain injury coupled with hypoxia and hypotension. Journal of Neurotrauma 16 (6), 487–499.

Skeletal injuries

6

Lynda Holt

CHAPTER CONTENTS

http://dx.doi.org/10.1016/B978-0-7020-4315-4.00006-1

Introduction

Skeletal and soft tissue injuries range in severity from life- or limb-threatening to self-limiting minor injuries. International research has demonstrated that patients with musculoskeletal injuries represent approximately 25% of the Emergency Department (ED) workload. It is imperative for emergency nurses to be able to assess musculoskeletal injury and identify life- or limb-threatening trauma, some of which may not seem devastating at first glance.

This chapter will provide the underpinning anatomy and physiology of the musculoskeletal system, before looking at areas such as pelvis, neck of femur and limb injuries. Each of these will be examined in detail, principles of assessment and management will be discussed, and particular problems related to specific injuries will be identified.

Anatomy and physiology

In order to appreciate the impact of injury, it is necessary for the emergency nurse to have a thorough understanding of the make-up and purpose of the human skeleton (Fig. 6.1) and skeletal muscle. The skeleton comprises two parts with specific functions:

- *the axial skeleton*, consisting of the skull, vertebral column, ribs and sternum – supports and protects vital organs
- *the appendicular skeleton*, consisting of the shoulder girdle, pelvic girdle and limbs – provides shape and facilitates movement.

Bone is a form of connective tissue comprising three major components:

- organic matrix of collagen – creates tensile strength
- mineral matrix of calcium and phosphate – creates rigidity and strength
- bone cells, including osteoblasts, osteoclasts, osteocytes and fibroblasts.

Compact cortical bone is found on outer parts of all bone; it forms the shaft of long bones and encloses marrow cavities (Fig. 6.2). Compact bone contains Haversian systems consisting of Haversian canals, blood vessels, connective tissues, nerve fibers and lymphatic vessels with osteocytes that facilitate the exchange of nutrients and waste. Cancellous bone is found at the ends of the long bone and in the vertebrae and flat bones. Cancellous bone is organized in a lattice system known as trabeculae and contains fewer Haversian canals. Red and fatty bone marrow fills the cavities in this lattice.

The periosteum is a fibrous tissue layer covering bone, but not cartilage or synovial joints. It transmits blood vessels and nerve fibres. The periosteum also provides attachments for ligaments and muscles. Beneath this layer are osteoblasts which aid bone growth, as a result, the periosteum does not attach to the bone surface until adulthood when growth is complete. Because of the abundant nerve supply, the periosteum is responsible for bone pain. Damage to periosteum or pressure on it from tumours or trauma can cause severe pain.

Bone cells

Osteoblasts are present on all bone surfaces and form a uniform layer. Their purpose is the synthesis and secretion of collagen and protein, and they promote calcification during rapid phases of this process, e.g., fracture repair. Osteoblasts create the trabeculae of cancellous bone.

Osteocytes form from osteoblasts trapped in matrix. The exact function of these cells is not known, but they appear to act as a pump, controlling calcium release in response to hormones.

Osteoclasts are found near the bone surface. They destroy dead bone and are responsible for reabsorption of bone. They are very mobile and are found in great numbers where bone is undergoing erosion. Their activity is controlled by a number of hormones including parathyroid and thyroxin.

Joints

Joints are the area of contact between bone and bone, or bone and cartilage. They are classified by the type of movement they permit.

Fibrous joints permit no movement at all, e.g., skull joints. Fibrous connective tissue merges into the periosteum of each bone.

Cartilaginous joints permit limited movement because of flexible cartilage between bones. The symphyses have cartilage pads, or discs, between bones, e.g., symphysis pubis or intervertebral joints. Complex ligament arrangements stabilize these cartilage pads to limit movement and facilitate recoil. Synchondroses are cartilage joints that ossify into bone in adulthood preventing movement, e.g., epiphysis of long bone.

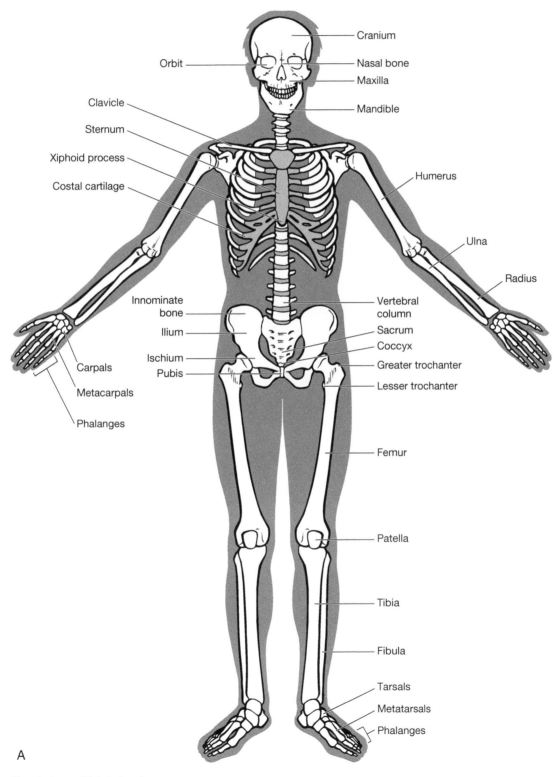

A

Figure 6.1 • The skeleton. (A) Anterior view.

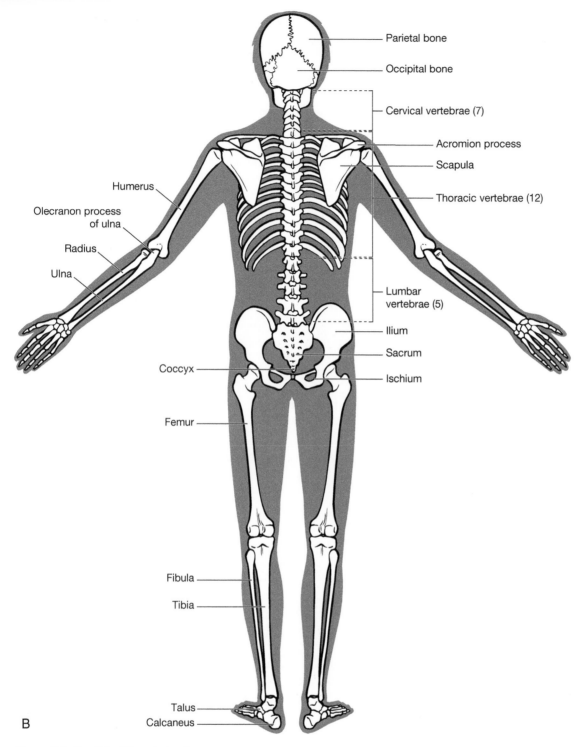

Parietal bone

Occipital bone

Cervical vertebrae (7)

Acromion process

Scapula

Thoracic vertebrae (12)

Humerus

Olecranon process
of ulna

Radius

Ulna

Lumbar
vertebrae (5)

Ilium

Sacrum

Coccyx

Ischium

Femur

Fibula

Tibia

Talus

Calcaneus

B

Figure 6.1, Cont'd • (B) posterior view.

Synovial joints form most of the body's joints. They are further classified by the type and range of movement they allow (see Table 6.1). All synovial joints have a number of similar structured features. They are enclosed in a capsule that is lined with a synovial membrane, which secretes synovial fluid. Bone ends are not in direct contact and are covered by hyaline cartilage. The fibrous capsule is held in place by a number of ligaments.

Muscular system

Muscle tissue is formed to convert chemical energy into mechanical contraction, creating movement. Movements are generated both at joints and in soft tissue. Muscles also assist in maintaining body posture and muscular activity is associated with maintaining body heat.

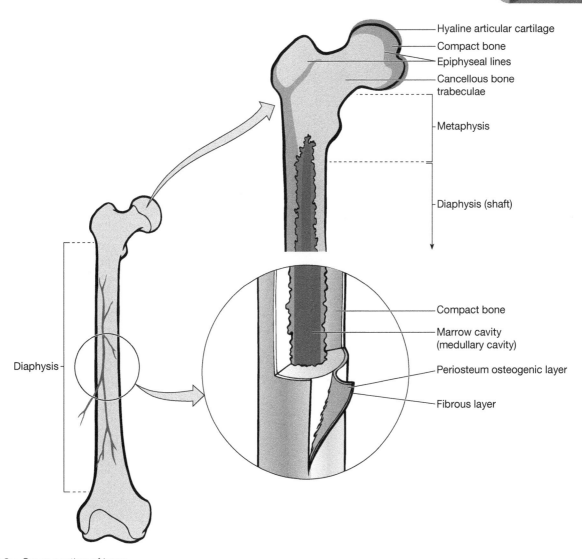

Figure 6.2 • Cross-section of bone.

Muscles are made up of bundles of fibres (fasciculi). The length of these fibres relates to the range of movement the muscle performs; that is, the longer the fibre, the greater is the range of movement. The number of fibres relates to the strength of the muscle. Muscles are attached to the periosteum by tendons. There are two points of attachment, the origin of which remains fixed during contraction while the insertion moves. Skeletal muscles have a rich blood supply which increases dramatically during exercise.

Tendons

Tendons are made up of fibrous connective tissue carrying parallel bundles of collagen fibres. This gives greater flexibility but prevents stretching when under pressure, such as in muscle contraction. They act like a spring, allowing the transition of movement from muscle to bone. Tendons have a sparse blood supply that inhibits healing if damaged.

Ligaments

Ligaments are made up of bundles of collagen that are not designed to stretch. They are attached to bone and are responsible for maintaining joint stability. Undue force may tear some fibres, resulting in them being painful, swollen and in severe cases can result in unstable joints.

Pelvic injury

Anatomy and physiology

The pelvis is designed to provide structure, strength for weight-bearing and protection of internal organs. It houses the rectum, bladder and, in women, the reproductive organs. The pelvis forms a ring, comprising the sacrum and two innominate bones, each made up of an ilium, pubic bone and ischium (Fig. 6.3).

These bones are supported by strong ligaments at the sacroiliac joint and a cartilaginous joint at the symphysis pubis. In children the innominate bones are supported by cartilage until they fuse around 16–18 years of age. The pelvis has a rich blood supply from the internal and external iliac arteries. The stability of the pelvic ring is dependent on the strong posterior sacroiliac, sacrotuberous and sacrospinous ligaments. Disruption of the pelvic ring can result in significant trauma to the neurovascular and soft tissue structures it protects.

Mechanism of injury

Major trauma to the pelvic girdle is relatively uncommon and accounts for approximately 3–6% of all skeletal injuries and 20% of polytrauma cases (Smith 2005); however, the mortality associated with major pelvic fractures may reach 57% where shock is present on the patient's arrival (Starr et al. 2002). Most pelvic fractures are caused by motorcycle accidents, accidents involving pedestrians, direct crush injuries, or falls from a height (American College of Surgeons 2008). Falls are also the second highest cause of unintentional death after motor vehicles (Middleton 2011).

Fracture patterns

In adults, isolated pelvic fractures rarely occur. This is because of the strength and ligamentous stretch of the pelvic ring. If significant force is applied, two or more breaks in the pelvic ring are likely to occur. The pelvis has predictable areas of strength and weakness, and therefore, in adults, potential patterns of fractures are easy to predict. In children, the increased elasticity of the pelvis prior to fusion of the innominate bones makes isolated fractures far more likely.

Lateral compression (LC) fractures (graded I, II, III) are caused by a side impact, usually to motorcyclists or pedestrians in collision with vehicles. A compression fracture of the pubic bone or rami is combined with compression fracture on the side of impact (Fig. 6.4A). With greater force of impact, the iliac wing on the side of the impact will also

Table 6.1 Classification of synovial joints

Type of joint	Site	Range of movement
Hinge	Elbow Fingers Ankle Toes	Flexion Extension
Pivot	Vertebral column	Rotation
Gliding	Shoulder girdle Vertebral column	Limited motion in several directions
Ball and socket	Hip Shoulder	Extensive range ofmovement: flexion, extension, rotation
Saddle	Hand Base of thumb	Flexion Extension Abduction Adduction Opposition
Ellipson	Wrist Hand Foot	Flexion Extension Abduction Adduction Opposition

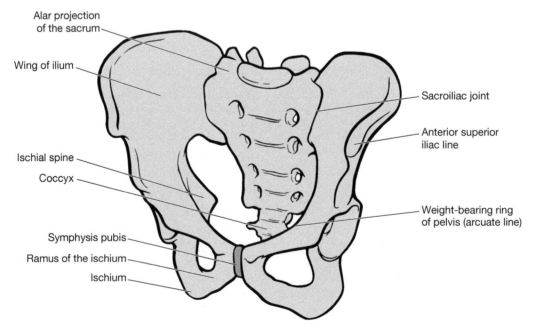

Figure 6.3 • The pelvis.

Alar projection of the sacrum
Wing of ilium
Ischial spine
Coccyx
Symphysis pubis
Ramus of the ischium
Ischium
Sacroiliac joint
Anterior superior iliac line
Weight-bearing ring of pelvis (arcuate line)

break; this is a grade II injury (Fig. 6.4B). A grade III injury involves an additional fracture on the opposite side to the impact (Fig. 6.4C).

Anteroposterior compression (APC) fractures (graded I, II, III) are caused by direct pressure or crushing and result in the pelvis opening outwards from wings rather like a book. The result is the fracturing of the pubis or rami together with sacroiliac distribution. In grade I injuries, the symphysis is separated by less than 2 cm (Fig. 6.5A); in grade II injuries the sacrospinous and sacrotuberous ligaments rupture (Fig. 6.5B); and in grade III injuries the iliolumbar ligament can rupture (Fig. 6.5C). This type of pelvic fracture has double the mortality rate of the lateral compression injuries.

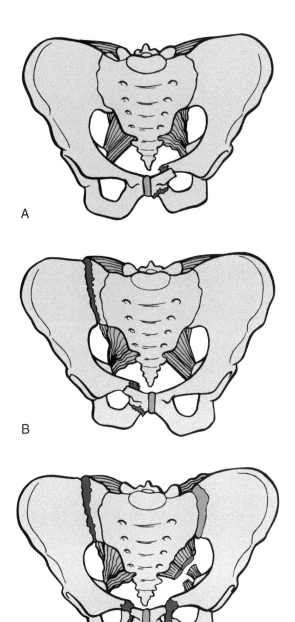

Figure 6.4 • Lateral compression fractures of the pelvis. (A) Grade I, (B) grade II, (C) grade III.

Vertical shearing force fractures result from falls or from knees hitting a car dashboard with great speed. The pattern of injury is similar to anteroposterior compression, but with vertical displacement (Fig. 6.6). With combined mechanical forces, such as being run over by a motor vehicle, a combination of the above fracture patterns may occur simultaneously.

Patterns of single fracture injury to the pelvis include:

- *acetabulum* – these are not common in isolation, but can occur with direct force to the leg, driving the head of the femur into the acetabulum
- *sacrum* – again these are uncommon in isolation, but can result from a backward fall or falls from a height
- *coccyx* – this is often fractured by falls onto the buttocks, particularly in women where the coccyx is more prominent
- *single pubic ramus* – these appear to be common in elderly patients following falls; however, evidence suggests that they usually occur with other pelvic injuries that are not initially detected
- *avulsion fractures* – these occur in young athletes, where excessive muscle strain can avulse growth cartilage on the apophyseal plates
- *iliac wing fractures* – these injuries commonly result from direct trauma and should always be considered in conjunction with intra-abdominal injury.

Assessment of pelvic ring injury

Fractures involving the pelvic ring carry potentially life-threatening complications if not rapidly identified and treated. Because of the force exerted to cause such fractures, attendant injury to underlying organs and haemorrhage is common and associated with high morbidity and mortality rates. Injuries can include among others: neurological, 26 %; rectal/gastrointestinal tract, 7 %; renal, 7 %; and bladder, 10 % (Scalea & Burgess 2004); urethral, up to 24 % (Ingram et al. 2008); ureteral, 7 % (penetrating trauma) to 18 % (blunt trauma) (Lynch et al. 2005) as well as genitalia; haematuria and haemodynamic instability due to hypovolaemic shock (Routt et al. 2002).

Mechanisms of injury should give some clues as to a potential pelvic fracture. The assessing nurse should carry out a primary assessment following the ABCDE approach laid out in Advanced Trauma Life Support (ATLS) guidelines (American College of Surgeons 2008). A patient with a pelvic ring fracture will have severe pelvic pain and progressive flank, perianal or scrotal swelling and bruising. Disruption of the pelvic ring can also be identified by differences in leg length and external rotation of a leg without an associated limb fracture.

Mechanical instability of the pelvis can be tested by manual manipulation or compression of the pelvis. This should be carried out only once by an experienced clinician and only when X-rays have excluded unstable pelvic fractures. It is a very painful procedure for the patient and undue force carries the risk of exacerbating haemorrhage. When the clinician manipulates the pelvis, pressure should be applied gently to the

Figure 6.5 • Anteroposterior compression fractures of the pelvis. (A) Grade I, (B) grade II, (C) grade III.

Figure 6.6 • Pelvic ring fracture.

iliac crest. If the pelvis has rotated, the clinician will be able to close the ring by gently pushing the iliac crests together. Most patients with a pelvic ring fracture will have moderate to severe hypotension.

Assessment should also include examination of the groin, perineal area and genitalia. Femoral pulses should be checked on both sides. Absent pulses are indicative of damage to the external iliac artery and emergency surgery is required to preserve the limb of the affected side. Decreased pulse pressure should be closely monitored, as it may be indicative of a worsening systemic condition or damage to the iliac artery. The perineum should be inspected for laceration and bleeding. Prophylactic antibiotics should be prescribed for wounds because of the high infection risk from faecal flora (Ruiz 1995).

In men, the testicles should be examined as a swollen testicle is indicative of testicular rupture requiring surgical decompression. The penis should be examined for blood at the meatus, suggestive of urethral damage. In women, the vulva should be examined and the vagina and urethral meatus inspected for blood. In male and female patients where there is no evidence of urethral injury, a urinary catheter should be inserted. If urethral injury is likely then suprapubic catheterization should be considered for bladder decompression. A rectal examination should be performed to test sphincter tone; a reduction in tone is suggestive of a sacral fracture. Frank blood is usually indicative of a rectal tear and surgical intervention is necessary. In men, the position of the prostate should be established as a high, boggy prostate indicates a urethral transection.

Management of pelvic ring fractures

Pelvic fracture can be a life-threatening injury often accompanied by significant haemorrhage and injury to the genitourinary system (Hauschild et al. 2008). Arterial injuries occur in 20 % of patients and posterior fractures are more likely than anterior fractures to cause bleeding. Initial management focuses on volume replacement, stabilization of fractures and, therefore, the rate of haemorrhage and pain control. Fluid replacement should follow ATLS guidelines with a rapid infusion of warmed crystalloid fluid, ideally Ringer's lactate or Hartmann's solution (American College of Surgeons 2008). Ringer's solution closely resembles the electrolyte content of plasma and therefore provides transient intravascular expansion followed by interstitial and intracellular replacement. Normal saline can be used, but large amounts are not recommended because it can induce hypercholaemic acidosis. After an initial 2 L, or 20 mL/kg in children, blood or colloid solutions should be commenced. The patient's haemodynamic condition should be continuously monitored during this period.

Haemorrhage control relies on fracture stabilization. Early external fixation provides definitive haemorrhage control. As an interim measure, longitudinal skin traction can be used (American College of Surgeons 2008). The use of a pneumatic anti-shock garment (PASG) also known as military anti-shock trousers (MAST) serves a dual purpose of haemorrhage and pain control. It provides mechanical stabilization of the fractures and external counter-pressure. When used, circulation to extremities should be regularly checked as compartment syndrome is a known risk. Decompression should take place in a controlled environment, at a pace that does not exacerbate haemodynamic instability, generally in the operating theatre. The use of PASG in no longer emphasized in ATLS as Dickinson & Roberts (2004) found that there was no benefit from their use, while Mattox et al. (1989) demonstrated PASG increased morbidity and mortality. Pain control is initiated by fracture immobilization with intravenous opiates; inhaled analgesia, such as entonox in the conscious patient may be used where not contraindicated by other potential injuries.

Uncomplicated, isolated pelvic fractures not involving the pelvic ring should be assessed in a similar manner. The management of these injuries is usually conservative. Patients usually require hospital admission for initial bed rest, pain control and rehabilitation support. Most of these fracture injuries have an uncomplicated recovery pattern. Acetabular fractures, however, have a high morbidity rate. They are caused by extreme force, commonly road traffic accidents (RTAs), where the knees hit the dashboard at speed. Long-term prognosis is improved by surgical intervention (Snyder 2002).

Hip injury

Anatomy and physiology

The femoral head and neck lie within the joint capsule of the hip joint. The head of the femur moves within the acetabulum. This is supported by three ligaments: iliofemoral, ischiofemoral and pubofemoral. Blood supply to the head of the femur is largely from the profunda femoris artery, which has circumflex branches around the neck of femur, off which smaller branches supply the head. This pattern of blood supply is particularly vulnerable to disruption from impacted fractures, hence the high risk of vascular necrosis with neck of femur fractures. The periosteum is very thin or non-existent around the neck of femur, therefore making it very susceptible to fractures. This susceptibility increases with age, particularly for women where osteoporosis has further weakened bone strength.

Classification of fractures

Neck of femur

Garden's classification of neck of femur (NOF) fractures has been used for almost 50 years (Garden 1964). He highlighted four stages of fracture (Fig. 6.7):

- *Stage I* represents impacted fractures. The trabeculae and cortex are pushed into the femoral head. This is considered a stable fracture as the inferior cortex usually remains intact. This type of fracture is not very susceptible to avascular necrosis and therefore operative treatment usually entails pinning rather than prosthetic replacement of the femoral head. Union rates are good and morbidity is low following this treatment (Ruiz 1995).
- *Stage II* is a non-displaced fracture across the entire femoral neck. Because there is no impaction, the fracture is unstable, but as there is no displacement the risk of avascular necrosis is low. These injuries are therefore fixed with screws.
- *Stage III* is a displaced fracture, with the femoral head abducted in relation to the pelvis. Fragments of the fracture are in contact with each other. Disruption of the blood supply is common and for this reason operative repair usually involves the insertion of a prosthesis to replace the femoral head.
- *Stage IV* are similar to stage III fractures in that they are displaced, but the femoral head is adducted in relation to the pelvis, fracture fragments are completely separated and avascular necrosis is likely. In most cases, prosthetic replacement of the femoral head is the treatment of choice in younger patients; however, attempts may be made to reduce and internally fixate the fracture. This prevents degeneration of the acetabulum caused over time by a prosthesis.

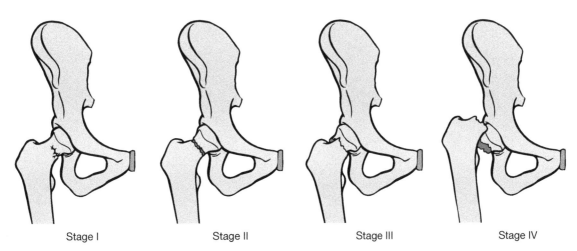

Stage I   Stage II   Stage III   Stage IV

Figure 6.7 • Garden's classification of femoral neck fractures: stages I–IV.

Intertrochanteric fractures

Although these have specific differences from NOF fractures, the assessment of injury and initial emergency management is similar. In terms of anatomy, the main difference is in bone density, as periosteum is present over the trochanters, although osteoporosis has a detrimental effect in women. In younger people and older men these fractures are far less common than NOF fractures. These injuries are not affected by avascular necrosis as the circumflex arterial branches of the NOF are not damaged. Because of the periosteum, the risk of non-union is also lower.

Several fracture classifications are used and all have slight variations from each other. To provide a general idea of fracture classification, Kyle et al. (1979) described four types of injury (Fig. 6.8):

- *Type I* – stable, undisplaced intertrochanteric fracture, requiring simple internal fixation.
- *Type II* – stable but displaced with fragmentation of the lesser trochanter; these are internally fixed.
- *Type III* – unstable fractures of the greater trochanter with posteromedial comminuted bone and deformity. These are fixed, but if a stable reduction cannot be achieved because of the amount of comminuted bone, osteotomy to the base of greater trochanter may be performed.
- *Type IV* – these have the components of type III fractures, but also have subtrochanteric fractures. Internal fixation is attempted using screws and sliding plates.

In children, NOF or intertrochanteric fractures are uncommon and are caused by severe force. Internal fixation is not the treatment of choice because of growth patterns. Children are treated with bed rest and traction.

Assessment of patients with hip injury

These patients are usually elderly, predominantly women, and commonly attend the ED following a fall. The average age of a person with a hip fracture is 84 years for men and 83 years for women; 76% of fractures occur in women. Mortality is high; about 10% of people with a hip fracture die within one month of injury and one-third within 12 months (National Clinical Guideline Centre 2011).

The patient usually complains of groin pain and pain through the thigh to the knee. Pain is worsened by any movement and the majority of patients will have been unable to weight-bear since injury. In most NOF and intertrochanteric fractures, the injured limb will be externally rotated and is shortened if displacement exists at the fracture site. Neurovascular integrity should be checked distally to the fracture, although damage of this type is extremely uncommon. The patient's haemodynamic status should be regularly observed, particularly with intertrochanteric fractures where blood loss from surrounding tissues is higher than NOF fractures. The patient's general health should be discussed and pre-existing medical

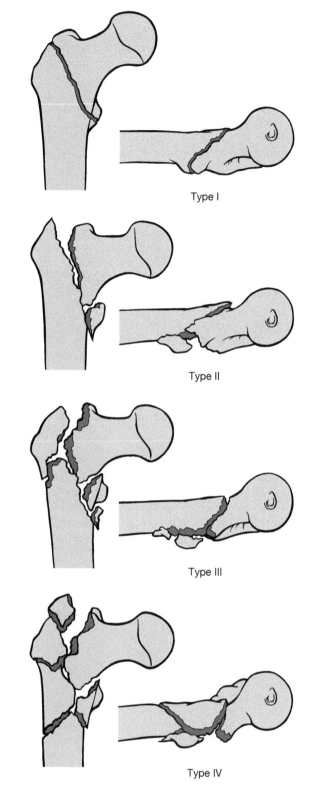

Type I

Type II

Type III

Type IV

Figure 6.8 ● Kyle's classification of intertrochanteric fractures.

conditions and medication established. It is also necessary to establish the cause of the fall to rule out medical reasons. The patient's hydration and nutritional status should be assessed, as should skin integrity and risk level for pressure sores (Lisk et al. 2011).

Initial management

In most instances, these fractures can be broadly diagnosed clinically. X-rays provide supplementary information necessary for ongoing management. As a result, patients with clinically diagnosed fractures should receive appropriate analgesia, such as morphine sulphate, prior to X-ray. Hydration at an early stage reduces mortality, and therefore intravenous fluids should be commenced, particularly for patients with intertrochanteric fractures where blood loss is greater. Regular observations should be undertaken to ensure haemodynamic stability is maintained, and to ensure the patient is neither dehydrated nor becomes overloaded by fluid replacements. Early oxygen therapy has been demonstrated to be beneficial as hypoxaemia is evident in elderly patients with a fractured NOF. Most hospitals now have fast-track policies to get patients into a ward bed and off hard emergency trolleys (Audit Commission 2000). If tissue viability is to be maintained, this together with regular pressure area care is vital (Wickham 1997). If the patient's general condition prohibits internal repair of the fracture, skin traction is advised at the earliest opportunity.

Hip dislocation

The majority of hip dislocations occur in people with total hip replacements or femoral head replacements. Hip dislocations in patients who have not had previous hip surgery are uncommon and demand a great deal of force. Posterior dislocation is commonly caused by high-impact RTAs where the patient's knee hits the dashboard and account for about 90 % of non-prosthetic dislocations. The patient will present in severe pain, with an internally rotated, flexed leg. Neurological examination is important, particularly in those with marked internal rotation, as the dislocation may compress the sciatic nerve and its branches, resulting in deficits especially in the perineal nerve region. Anterior dislocation is much less frequent and results from a fall from a height where the patient lands on an extended leg. This type of injury can be confused with a fractured NOF in elderly patients, and therefore careful history-taking and limb assessment are vital.

In both anterior and posterior dislocations, early limb relocation is essential. Closed reduction should be performed, provided associated fractures of the femoral head have been excluded. Management priorities in ED involve pain relief, X-ray and relocation of the hip joint under sedation. Once the hip is relocated, the patient should be admitted for traction. If relocation attempts are unsuccessful with conscious sedation in the ED, then urgent transfer to theatre for closed or open reduction under general anaesthetic is appropriate.

Limb injury

Anatomy and physiology

Limbs form part of the appendicular skeleton and are vital for movement. Both arms and legs comprise long bones, with complex joints and bone systems in the hands and feet. Limb

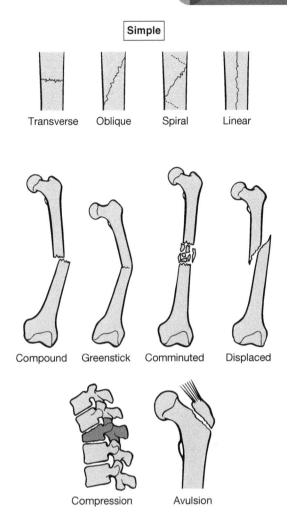

Figure 6.9 • Fracture classification.

injuries treated in the ED fall into two categories: fractures and soft tissue injury.

Classification of fractures

A break or fracture of the bone occurs when it is no longer able to absorb the mechanical energy placed on it. This usually results from trauma (Bickley & Szilagyi 2008). Fractures are classified into the following groups (Fig. 6.9):

- *simple* – this is deemed a closed fracture because the skin is intact and the fracture is undisplaced. These can be further categorized by the direction in which the fracture travels:
  - ○ – transverse: across the bone
  - ○ – oblique: at an angle to the length of the bone
  - ○ – spiral: encircle the bone in a spiral around its diameter
  - ○ – linear: runs parallel with the axis of the bone
- *compound* – this is an open fracture where the skin has been punctured either internally by the bone or externally from the surface the skin came in contact with during the trauma. These can exist with any of the above types of fracture. It is also possible for fracture fragments

to puncture blood vessels, nerves and organs. All compound fractures warrant prophylactic antibiotics and tetanus prophylaxis if not covered (Clasper & Ramasamy 2011)

- *greenstick* – these occur in children and are incomplete fractures, they are like a bent twig that disrupts the bone cortex but does not pass right through
- *comminuted* – fragmented fracture with two or more pieces
- *displaced* – bone ends are completely separated at the fracture site
- *compression* – adjacent bones are compacted
- *avulsion* – bone ends or condyles pulled off when the ligaments remain intact under extreme force.

Fracture healing follows a specific pattern. It has three main phases: inflammatory, reparative and remodelling.

The inflammatory phase lasts approximately 72 hours. Initially a homeostatic response to the physiological damage to bone, tissue and blood vessels occurs. A clot is formed in which the fibrin networks collect debris, blood and marrow cells. Capillary network increases over 24 hours and neutrophils invade the area. In the following 48 hours, phagocytosis takes place. In the reparative stage chondroblasts and osteoblasts proliferate. The chondroblasts unite fracture ends in a fibrous tissue called callus which begins to calcify after 14 days. During this phase osteoblasts create the trabeculae of cancellous bone while osteoclasts destroy dead bone. Remodelling takes several months: osteoblasts and osteoclasts restore bone shape, replacing cancellous with compact bone (Fig. 6.10).

Assessment of limb injury

Following ATLS principles, assessment of extremity injury should take place after only the primary survey is completed and more serious injuries are dealt with. The assessment has three stages:

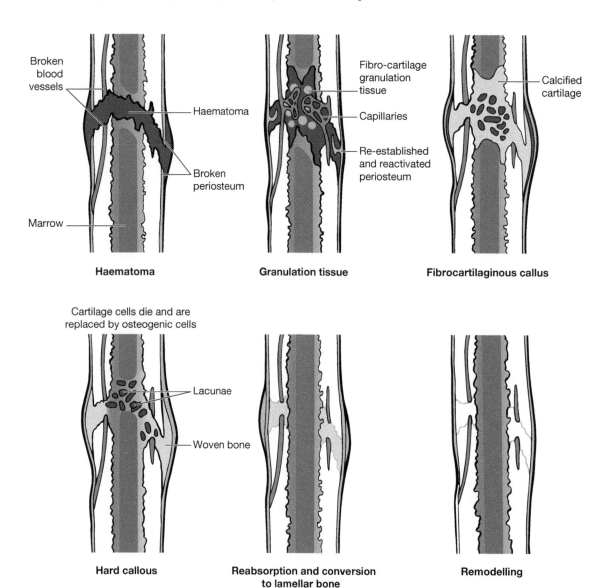

Figure 6.10 • Bone healing process.

- *identification* and intervention in life-threatening haemorrhage (primary survey)
- *identification* and intervention in limb-threatening haemorrhage (secondary survey)
- *identification* and management of other limb injuries.

Assessment should follow a set pattern regardless of how severe or trivial an injury may appear. The assessing nurse should establish the history, perform an examination and, if appropriate, refer the patient for X-ray. When assessing the history, the nurse should establish a number of factors (Box 6.1). Mechanism of injury should include what happened, the direction and magnitude of force, and how long the patient was exposed to the force. When determining symptoms, the nurse should establish pain, loss of function and perceived swelling. The nurse should also enquire about the duration of symptoms and whether they are worsening or improving. Past history should include pre-existing injuries to that limb, medical conditions that affect the musculoskeletal system or bone density, and factors which would influence recovery.

Box 6.1

Establishing history of musculoskeletal injury

- Mechanism of injury
- Symptoms
- Duration
- Pain
- Previous relevant injury, illness, medication

Examination

Examination should follow a specific pattern, starting from the joint above, moving through the site of the injury, and finally checking neurovascular function distal to the injury. Principles of examination are shown in Box 6.2. Examination starts from the joint above the injury site to assess both function and limits of injury and to gain the patient's cooperation and confidence. It should be systematic and considering of both the bony and soft tissue structures involved. The examination should also include assessment of pain, and factors influencing it, such as movement, pressure and guarding (Bickley & Szilagyi 2009).

If a patient presents with a mechanism of injury or the clinical examination is suggestive of a fracture then X-ray should be requested. X-rays should not, however, be performed for purely medico-legal reasons (Ward 1999).

Femoral fractures

The femur is the longest, strongest human bone. It is surrounded by muscles and is fed by the profunda femoris artery. The shaft of femur also has a good collateral blood

Box 6.2

Principles of examination

Look

- Colour
- Perfusion
- Deformity
- Swelling
- Wounds
- Bruising
- Symmetry with opposite limb

Feel

- Palpate from joint above injury
- Identify tender spots
- Note areas of reduced sensation
- Note obvious crepitus – *never* test for crepitus because of the pain it causes
- Assess distal pulses and capillary refill
- Test temperature of the limb
- Test sensation distal to wound

Move

- Assess active movement
- Assess passive movement
- Test resistance to establish muscle injury

Function

- Observe how patient uses limb
- Observe for either reduced or increased range of movement
- Observe walking/weight-bearing for lower limbs

supply in the periosteum. Most of the bleeding associated with femoral fracture is due to rupture of small branches of the profunda femoris artery. The femur only fractures under great force and the most common causes of injury are RTAs, particularly motorcycle accidents, pedestrian vs motor-vehicle accidents and falls (Nowotarski et al. 2000); particularly where bone density is compromised or the fall is from a significant height.

Assessment

Fractures of the femur fall into three anatomical categories: proximal, mid-shaft and distal. Examination findings are shown in Box 6.3. The patient should be carefully assessed for signs of hypovolaemic shock as blood loss from a closed shaft of femur fracture averages 1200 mL (Cadogan 2004). Although isolated femoral fractures rarely cause significant shock, fractures occurring with other traumatic injury do contribute to significant hypovolaemia. Observation should therefore be vigilant and X-ray will confirm diagnosis. Severe muscle spasms cause significant pain following femoral fracture and also cause the limb to shorten. Crepitus occurs over the fracture site as bone pieces move (O'Steen 2003).

> ### Box 6.3
>
> **Assessment of femoral fracture**
> - Severe pain in thigh
> - Reduced leg movement – unable to weight-bear
> - Deformity – shortening because of muscle spasm and external rotation in proximal fractures
> - Swelling in surrounding tissue due to soft tissue damage and bleeding
> - Crepitus – possibility of damage to popliteal nerves and blood vessels. Check distal circulation and sensation

Management priorities

Management priorities in the ED are twofold: preventing secondary damage and pain control. Preventing secondary damage includes managing blood loss by initiating intravenous fluid replacement. Reduction in blood loss and significant pain reduction can be achieved by correct application of an appropriate traction splint, such as a pneumatic Donway traction splint or a traditional Thomas half-ring splint or its modified version Hare traction splint may be used. These stabilize the fracture until definitive repair can take place. In doing this, the extent of the trauma to surrounding soft tissue is minimized. Pain is reduced because bone ends are immobilized. Distal and proximal pulses, capillary refill and sensation should be rechecked after splint application. If the fracture is open, broad-spectrum antibiotics should be given and the patient's tetanus status checked. The wound should be covered with a damp dressing; care should be taken to avoid wound maceration if a delay to surgery is possible. Povidone-iodine soaks are commonly used because of the devastating effects of infection (see also Chapter 24). Intravenous analgesia should also be given. Fractured femurs take about 8–16 weeks to heal in an adult and 6–12 weeks in a child. Definitive treatment is usually internal fixation for an adult, which means they can usually be walking within two weeks post-surgery. Surgery is not recommended for children because of growth and speed of repair; therefore traction is recommended for older children, and plastering with hip spica for toddlers and small children.

Supracondylar fractures of the femur are assessed in the same way as shaft fractures. The mechanisms of injury are similar, with pain usually localized to the knee. Fractures involving the femoral condyles usually involve the knee joint and there may be associated knee joint injuries, particularly osteochondral fractures of the patella (Rowley & Dent 1997). These fractures do not cause the same extent of blood loss as shaft fractures and are repaired by either long leg casting or surgery.

Lower leg injury

The principles of assessment are common to all limb injuries and have been highlighted earlier in the chapter. This section describes specific advice, identifying common mechanisms of injury, assessment findings and initial management.

Patellar fractures and dislocations

Patellar fractures occur following a direct blow or fall onto the knee. Indirect twisting injury can also result in a fracture as the patella is ripped apart by the quadriceps muscles. The patient presents with pain, swelling and a knee effusion. As a result, range of movement is restricted, particularly full extension. Usually, patellar fractures can be repaired by long leg cylindrical casting for 4–6 weeks. Surgical intervention is necessary for open fractures, those fractures where fragmentation of the patella leaves gaps greater than 4 mm and longitudinal fractures.

Patellar dislocation results from a direct blow to the medial aspect of the knee, common in football or similar contact sports. The knee locks and remains in a flexed position. On examination, obvious lateral deformity is present with medial tenderness and pain on attempted movement. Acute swelling between 2 and 12 hours of injury is likely to indicate haemarthrosis (Rourke 2003, Adams 2004). Treatment seeks to relocate the patella. This is usually straightforward and achieved by extension of the knee. It is painful because of muscle spasm and therefore analgesia and muscle relaxants should be used. A supportive long leg bandage should then be applied, or a long leg cast.

Tibial plateau fractures

Tibial plateau injury commonly occurs from pedestrian/car accidents, usually at lower speeds where the car bumper hits the standing pedestrian. Fractures also occur as a result of a fall from a height, causing compression of the plateau, or they may occur in elderly patients with osteoporotic bones. Patients usually present with pain and swelling over the fracture site and inability to weight-bear. Swelling varies considerably, with haemarthrosis sometimes present. Diagnosis of tibial plateau fractures is usually by X-ray and is classified using the Schatzker classification system (Schatzker et al. 1979) which records six levels of injury:

- I: split lateral condyle without displacement
- II: split fragmented lateral condyle with depression of the fragment
- III: compression of the lateral (IIIA) or central (IIIB) condyle with depressed displacement
- IV: medial condyle
- V: bicondylar
- VI: bicondylar with complete dissociation of metaphysis from diaphysis – extending into the tibial shaft.

Choice of treatment is dictated by the classification of the injury, displacement of fragments, and the condition of skin, tissue and muscles. Conservative treatment includes long leg plaster casting, traction and functional cast bracing and is reserved for classes I–IV where surgery is not otherwise indicated. Internal fixation is more common because of the morbidity risk of prolonged immobilization, particularly in older patients (Harris & Haller 1995).

Tibial shaft fractures

Mechanisms of injury are varied. The tibia has little muscular protection, so fractures from direct blows are the commonest long bone fracture. They are also the most common open fracture. As the tibia is vulnerable to torsional injuries, for example in sporting injuries, and force transmitted through the feet is high, the incidence of injury is high (Smith 2005), particularly in children. Similar mechanisms cause tibial and fibular fracture, although much more force is needed to break both bones. Direct trauma tends to cause transverse or comminuted fractures, and indirect trauma causes oblique and spiral fractures. The patient presents with localized pain and is usually unable to weight-bear. Surrounding soft tissue damage varies from a haematoma, causing swelling, to an open wound caused by fracture ends. Treatment for tibial fractures varies: children with greenstick fractures need casting for 6 weeks; in adults, displaced fractures may need internal fixation. ED documentation of the neurovascular status is vital as the risk of compartment syndrome is high. Therefore admission for 24 hours, observation and limb elevation should be considered in very swollen proximal tibial fractures. Pain is managed with intravenous opiates and the lower leg should be plastered as soon as possible. Circumferential casts must *never* be applied in the acute phase because of the inherent risk of compartment syndrome.

Fibular fractures

Isolated fibular fractures are not common and usually occur in conjunction with tibial fractures. Isolated fibular fractures usually occur as a result of direct trauma to the lateral aspect of the calf. Distal fibular/malleolar fractures occur with excessive rotational forces. They are discussed in more detail under ankle injury below. The patient will complain of pain over the fracture site, with radiation along the length of the fibula on palpation. Because the fibula is not a weight-bearing bone, the patient may be walking with discomfort. Swelling is usually minimal. Depending on the degree of pain, isolated fractures are treated by either plaster cast or compression bandage.

Tibial and fibular fractures

Combined tibial and fibular fractures are fairly common in contact sports, such as football. In injuries where indirect force causes the fracture, the tibia and fibula may be fractured in different places. Commonly, the tibial shaft fractures at the distal third, and because of a twisting mechanism the fibula fractures at the proximal end. This reinforces the need to assess from the joint above to the joint below the injury. If injury is caused by direct force and both bones are fractured at the same level, the leg will appear unstable and flexible at the fracture site. It is important that temporary immobilization occurs as soon as possible, both to reduce pain and to prevent further soft tissue damage. These fractures will need surgical fixation (Gordon et al. 2012).

Ankle fractures

Most ankle injuries seen in the ED are soft-tissue injuries (Eisenhart et al. 2003). Patients with fractures risk significant morbidity if these are not identified and treated early. The ankle is a complex hinge joint made up of three bones: the tibia, fibula and talus, and three collateral ligaments: the lateral, medial and interosseous. These ligaments stabilize the ankle joint; the lateral ligament allows for some inversion of the joint, whereas the medial and interosseous have less stretch (Fig. 6.11). Injury patterns can be classified by the mechanism of injury (Box 6.4 and Fig. 6.12).

Isolated lateral malleolar fractures can occur following inversion injury. Patients present with pain, swelling, ecchymosis and bony tenderness on the lateral aspect of the ankle and are usually unable to weight-bear (Hopkins 2010). Most isolated fractures are either a chip or avulsion fracture with ligament injury. These can be treated by a below-knee weight-bearing cast. Some fractures above the joint line or comminuted fractures may warrant surgical intervention. Isolated medial malleolar fractures are less common and usually result from a direct blow or eversion and, occasionally, inversion injury. The patient presents with pain over the medial aspect,

Figure 6.11 • Bony anatomy of the ankle.

Box 6.4

Lauge-Hansen classification of ankle injury

Supination – adduction (inversion injury)

- Stage I – fracture of lateral malleolus at joint level or below, or tear of lateral collateral ligament
- Stage II – as above with fracture of medial malleolus

Supination – lateral rotation

- Stage I – rupture of anterior tibiofibular ligament
- Stage II – as above with spiral fracture of distal fibula
- Stage III – as above with posterior tibiofibular ligament disruption with/without avulsion fracture of posterior malleolus
- Stage IV – as above with medial malleolar fracture

Pronation – abduction

- Stage I – transverse fracture of medial malleolus or deltoid ligament tear
- Stage II – as above with posterior and anterior tibiofibular ligament disruption with/without avulsion fracture of posterior malleolus
- Stage III – as above with fracture of distal fibula at ankle joint level

Pronation – lateral rotation

- Stage I – transverse fracture of medial malleolus or tear or deltoid ligament
- Stage II – as above with disruption of anterior tibiofibular ligament and interosseous membrane
- Stage III – as above with fracture of distal bone 6 cm or greater above joint
- Stage IV – as above with posterior tibiofibular ligament disruption with/without avulsion fracture of posterior malleolus

(Mayeda DV (2009) Ankle and foot. In: Marx J, Hockberger R, Walls R, eds. Rosen's Emergency Medicine: Concepts and Clinical Practice, 7th edn. St Louis: Mosby Year Book.)

swelling and limited range of movement. Usually, the patient will be non-weight-bearing (Wyatt et al. 1999). Simple avulsion fractures can be managed by below-knee casting. Fractures into the joint space should be referred for specialist opinion as internal fixation may be necessary.

Bi-malleolar fractures involve two of the lateral, medial and posterior malleoli, usually the lateral and medial. The patient presents with a history of inversion or eversion injury and will have bilateral bony tenderness and swelling, with or without deformity, and will be non-weight-bearing. These are unstable fractures with a significant risk of ankle dislocation. The ankle should be temporarily immobilized, adequate pain relief should be given and hospital admission facilitated. Restoration of function requires accurate medial malleolus reduction and joint space alignment (Mayeda 2009). Good outcomes are also dependent on skilled plastering and surveillance for weeks. Increasingly surgeons prefer to avoid these uncertainties by routine accurate internal fixation (McRae 2006). Lateral malleolar reduction is desirable but less crucial. This is usually achieved by open reduction and fixation in theatre, but can be achieved by closed methods if surgery is contraindicated.

Tri-malleolar fractures involve the posterior malleolus as well and are usually combined with ankle dislocation. They are caused by falls or, most commonly, tripping, e.g., off a kerb. Management priorities are limb realignment (see discussion of dislocations below) and subsequent internal fixation, using the same principles as for bi-malleolar fractures.

The standard X-ray evaluation for the acutely injured ankle includes lateral, anteroposterior and mortice views. The requirement for X-ray of the adult ankle or foot may be determined using the Ottawa Ankle Rules (Stiell et al. 1992). These have shown that X-rays are only required for the ankle if there is any pain in the malleolar region and:

- bone tenderness over the posterior aspect of the distal 6 cm of the lateral malleolus or
- bone tenderness over the posterior aspect of the distal 6 cm of the medial malleolus or
- inability to weight-bear for at least four steps both immediately after the injury and at the time of assessment in ED.

Foot X-ray is required if there is pain in the midfoot region and:

- bone tenderness at the navicular or
- bone tenderness at the base of the fifth metatarsal or
- inability to weight-bear for at least four steps both immediately after the injury and at the time of assessment in ED.

The Ottawa ankle rules (Fig. 6.13) apply to adults (>18 years) and have a >98% sensitivity for detecting clinically significant malleolar ankle injuries. They also reduce the number of ankle X-rays by up to 40% (Bachmann et al. 2003).

Ankle dislocation

Ankle dislocation occurs when significant force applied to the joint results in loss of opposition of the articular surfaces.

Dislocation occurs in one of four directions: anterior, lateral, superior and posterior. Posterior is the most common (Fig. 6.14). Stability of the ankle is normally maintained by tight articulation of the talus with the tibia and fibula. Isolated ankle dislocation is extremely rare (Georgilas & Mouzopoulos 2008) and may well be due to the amount of force required. It is usually associated with malleolar fractures and ligament rupture. Common causes of dislocation are sports injuries, direct force or RTAs (Harris 1995). Complicated dislocations associated with multiple ankle fractures are most common in osteoporotic women.

On examination the ankle will be oedematous, the joint locked, with the distal tibia prominent under stretched skin. Management priorities in the ED are to preserve neurovascular integrity. Early reduction is crucial, since delay may increase risk of neurovascular compromise or damage to articular cartilage. If there appears to be neurovascular compromise, the ankle dislocation should be reduced urgently, without waiting for X-rays. If neurovascular integrity appears intact, X-rays can be obtained, but the foot should remain supported to prevent further injury. Reduction should be carried out swiftly after X-ray. Nitrous oxide is a useful initial

Supination
Adduction injury

Stage I

Stage 2

Supination
Lateral rotation injury

Stage IV

Pronation
Abduction injury

Stage I

Stage II

Pronation
Lateral rotation injury

Stage IV

Figure 6.12 • Ankle fracture (based on Lauge-Hansen classification). • (After Mayeda DV (2009) Ankle and foot. In: Marx J, Hockberger R, Walls R, eds. Rosen's Emergency Medicine: Concepts and Clinical Practice, 7th edn. St Louis: Mosby Year Book.)

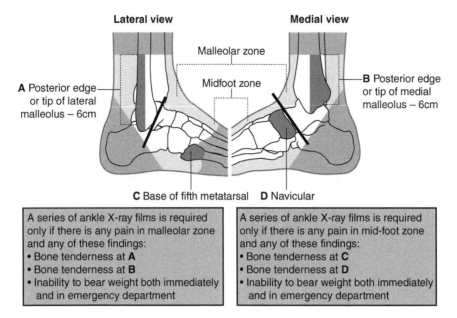

Figure 6.13 ● Ottawa ankle rules assessment.

The labels in the figure read:

Lateral view | Medial view

Malleolar zone

Midfoot zone

A Posterior edge or tip of lateral malleolus – 6cm

B Posterior edge or tip of medial malleolus – 6cm

C Base of fifth metatarsal | **D** Navicular

A series of ankle X-ray films is required only if there is any pain in malleolar zone and any of these findings:
• Bone tenderness at **A**
• Bone tenderness at **B**
• Inability to bear weight both immediately and in emergency department

A series of ankle X-ray films is required only if there is any pain in mid-foot zone and any of these findings:
• Bone tenderness at **C**
• Bone tenderness at **D**
• Inability to bear weight both immediately and in emergency department

Figure 6.14 ● Ankle dislocations. (A) Posterior; (B) anterior; and (C) lateral.

pain relief, for its therapeutic effects of analgesia, increasing oxygen intake and for its distraction potential, i.e., by getting the patient to concentrate on breathing (Bowie 2011). While the dislocation is being reduced, the patient should have adequate intravenous analgesia and muscle relaxant. The patient's cardiac and respiratory function should be monitored during this procedure.

Ankle reduction is at least a two-person job. It is achieved by flexing the patient's knee to reduce tension on the Achilles tendon. One carer supports the lower leg while the other applies downward traction to the foot and force is applied in the opposite direction to that of the original injury. An additional clinician should be present whenever intravenous analgesia and muscle relaxant are given to monitor and protect the patient's cardiorespiratory state. When reduction is completed, neurovascular integrity should be rechecked, by checking for pedal pulse, capillary refill and sensation. The ankle should then be immobilized in an above-knee plaster that is either bivalved or guttered, because of the degree of

swelling associated with fracture manipulation. Most patients need internal fixation of associated fractures.

Foot fractures

The foot has 28 bones with 57 articulating surfaces and is divided into three anatomical areas (Fig. 6.15). It is considered vital for balance, movement and as a shock absorber for movement.

The hindfoot

The talus supports the body weight and forces above by allowing movement at the ankle joint and between the calcaneus and midfoot. It is well secured by ligaments surrounding the ankle joint and therefore fracture is uncommon (Harris 1995). In the event of injury to the talus, the risk of

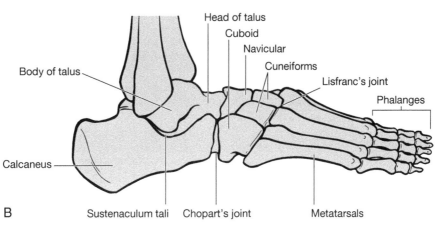

Figure 6.15 • The right foot (A) Dorsal view and (B) lateral view.

complication is high because 60% of the surface is covered by articular cartilage and vascular supply is low, creating a significant threat of avascular necrosis. It is usually injured as a result of falls, landing on the heel or forefoot, causing fractures through the body or neck of the talus. Fractures to the neck of the talus also result from head-on RTAs, where the driver's foot is pressed against compressed floors or pedals, causing extreme dorsiflexion.

The patient will present with ankle pain, there may be visible disruption to normal ankle anatomy and swelling is common. Fractures to the talar neck are usually treated by below-knee casting, but if any displacement cannot be reduced, open reduction is necessary. Fractures to the talar

body frequently require internal fixation. Fractures of the talar head are extremely uncommon and management varies with the extent of the injury and associated injuries. Specialist orthopaedic advice should be sought for specific management.

The calcaneus

This is the largest bone of the foot and it absorbs the body's weight when standing or moving. The calcaneus is a relatively hollow bone consisting of an outer thin cortical shell filled with cancellous bone. As a result, it fractures when subjected to vertical forces such as falling from a height.

There is an associated crush fracture of the lumbar spine in about 10 % of cases resulting from a fall. The Achilles tendon attaches to the tuberosity and can cause an avulsion fracture when damaged. Fractures resulting from a fall are most common in men between 30 and 50 years old, whereas avulsion fractures are more common in women showing signs of osteoporosis.

The patient presents with pain over the rear of the foot and both sides of the heel. Swelling is usually present and patients are usually unable to weight-bear on their heel. If the presentation to ED is a few hours post-injury, a horseshoe-shaped bruise may be present. Calcaneal fractures are categorized into two groups: those involving the subtalar joint and those which do not, i.e., extra-articular fractures. The outcome for patients with extra-articular fractures is considerably better than those involving the subtalar joint. Extra-articular fractures are managed conservatively with compression and elevation in the first instance. After swelling has subsided, the injury is immobilized in a cast. The majority of fractures will involve the subtalar joint and the prognosis for these patients is poor. About 50 % have some long-term problems from the injury (Mayeda 2009), including restricted movement, pain and subtalar arthritis. Most are treated with internal fixation. Fractures to other bones of the foot are not uncommon, and patients with suspected calcaneum fractures, or those who have fallen over six feet, must have a full examination of the spine and lower leg (Larsen 2002).

The midfoot

This region includes the navicular, cuboid, cuneiform and metatarsal bones. The midfoot provides foot flexibility. Fractures to this area are uncommon and result from direct force, such as crush injuries. Transverse dislocation of the forefoot results from direct force. Patients present with localized tenderness and swelling. These injuries heal well and can usually be treated with below-knee non-weight-bearing casts. There are two exceptions to this: the first relates to avulsion fractures of the navicular, which occur as a result of eversion injury. If 20 % or more of the articular surface is avulsed, the fracture should be internally fixed, if less than 20 % is avulsed, a below-knee cast should be adequate. The second exception is the Lisfranc dislocation, which occurs when the forefoot is dislocated across the metatarsal joints. This is an extremely rare condition, occurring in one in 55 000 cases (Mayeda 2009). Neurovascular compromise is common, partly because the force necessary to cause dislocation also causes extensive soft tissue damage, resulting in oedema and vascular compromise. The patient presents with moderate to severe midfoot pain and large amounts of swelling which can hinder diagnosis. There is usually a shortening of the foot length, compared with the uninjured foot, and the injured foot will have transverse broadening.

Patients with Lisfranc dislocation will not be able to stand on their toes. Treatment of this injury revolves around rapid reduction of the dislocation and cast immobilization, because the risk of circulation compromise and subsequent necrosis is so high. If a base of second metatarsal fracture coexists, an accurate reduction may not be possible, or will prove unstable. In such cases, internal fixation should be considered. Hospital admission is usually necessary during the initial days post-injury, whatever the method of reduction.

The forefoot

The forefoot consists of the five metatarsal bones and the phalanges.

Metatarsal fractures

The metatarsals are susceptible to fractures because of their length. The mechanisms of fracture vary; the second and third metatarsals are relatively fixed and therefore susceptible to stress fractures. The first, fourth and fifth metatarsals are more mobile. Fractures are caused by direct blows to the foot, e.g., a heavy object falling across the foot.

Twisting injury can also result in fractures, particularly of the second to fourth metatarsals. The patient presents with swelling over the foot, localized pain and inability to weight-bear. Reduction of swelling is imperative as skin necrosis and neurovascular compromise can occur. Elevation of the foot is essential. Most fractures can be managed by immobilization in a short leg cast.

Fifth metatarsal fracture, also known as a Jones fracture is one of the most common foot injuries (Herrera-Soto et al. 2007). It usually results from an inversion injury causing sudden contraction of the peroneus brevis muscle. The tendons joining this muscle with the base of the fifth metatarsal can cause an avulsion fracture. The management of fifth metatarsal fractures is either neighbour (or buddy) strapping and crutches or a below-knee cast, depending on the patient's pain. Occasionally, displaced fractures require internal fixation.

First metatarsal fractures warrant special consideration because of the weight-bearing capacity of the first metatarsal and its contribution to balance and stability. If the metatarsal head has been displaced in plantar rotation, the patient will have trouble with weight-bearing and with the 'push-off' mechanism in walking. Many of these fractures can be reduced in ED with adequate analgesia, and then immobilized in a cast. If reduction cannot be achieved in this manner, internal fixation should be considered.

Phalangeal fractures

These result from stubbing injury or from dropping heavy objects on toes. The patient presents with pain, swelling and often bruising or a subungal haematoma. The clinical symptoms can make fracture diagnosis difficult and often X-rays do not offer much assistance (Mayeda 2009). If angulation or deformity of the toe exists, then X-rays are more helpful. Most fractures can be managed by neighbour strapping and elevation. Obviously angulated fractures should be reduced using a digital block, then the toe neighbour strapped. Big toe fractures needing reduction may warrant immobilization in a cast with toe support.

Shoulder injury

The shoulder girdle consists of three bones: the scapula, the clavicle and the humerus (Fig. 6.16). The shoulder attaches the arms to the axial skeleton. These are interconnected at the acromioclavicular, glenohumeral, coracoclavicular and sternoclavicular articulations and muscles from the rib cage and cervical spine. The glenohumeral joint (GHJ) is where the head of the humerus articulates with the glenoid fossa of the scapula providing the majority of the shoulder girdle movement. The sternoclavicular joint (SCJ) links the arm to the axial skeleton, via the clavicles, the upper and lateral manubrium sterni and the cartilage of the first rib. The SCJ deltoid, pectorals and trapezius muscles maintain the normal position of the shoulder. The acromioclavicular joint (ACJ) permits the 'gliding' motion of the articular end of the lateral clavicle on the medial aspect of the anterior acromion and rotation of the scapula on the clavicle during abduction of the arm (Knapton 1999). The clavicle is attached to the scapula by acromioclavicular and coracoclavicular ligaments, the latter incorporating both the conoid and trapezoid ligaments and is the stronger of the two. If any of the ligaments weaken or tear, the shoulder has a greater tendency to dislocate.

Scapular fractures

The scapula is situated above and lateral to the posterior thorax. It is well protected from injury by thick muscle and extreme force is necessary to fracture it. Injuries commonly result from high-speed road traffic accidents, crushing or falls. Occasionally, a scapular fracture occurs as a result of electric shock, when one or both scapulae are fractured (Rana & Banerjee 2006). Fractured scapulae most frequently occur in young men (O'Steen 2003) because of the force needed to cause fractures and associated injuries such as pneumothorax, chest wall injury or related shoulder girdle injuries.

Anatomically, scapular fractures fall into three categories (Fig. 6.17):

- *Type I fractures* are difficult to palpate because of thick muscle and pain. An adducted shoulder and the mechanism of injury should suggest possible fracture, which can be confirmed on X-ray (Knapton 1999). Treatment is usually conservative and involves pain relief and simple immobilization using a broad arm sling on the injured side. Controversy exists over the benefits versus risks of plating scapular body fractures. It has been suggested that scapular fractures have a better outcome when treated operatively (Cole 2002) despite reluctance by clinicians after historically choosing conservative therapy because of high post-operative complication rates as argued by Schmidt et al. (1992).

- *Type II fractures* involve the acromion and coracoid process. They occur from direct trauma and are similar in that patients have pain over the site of injury and adduction of the shoulder. They differ in that acromion fractures cause pain on elbow flexing, while in coracoid fractures the patient actively flexes the elbow as a form of pain relief. Both types are usually managed conservatively unless concurrent shoulder girdle injury exists, such as dislocation or clavicular fracture.

- *Type III fractures* involve the scapula neck or glenoid fossa. They result from lateral to medial rotation of the humeral head. The patient presents with pain around the humeral head and on shoulder adduction, and is

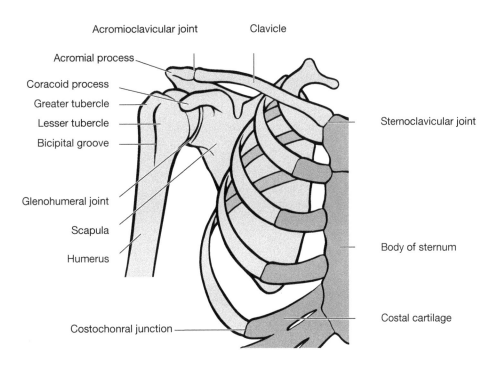

Acromioclavicular joint   Clavicle

Acromial process

Coracoid process

Greater tubercle

Lesser tubercle

Bicipital groove

Sternoclavicular joint

Glenohumeral joint

Scapula

Humerus

Body of sternum

Costal cartilage

Costochondral junction

Figure 6.16 • The shoulder girdle.

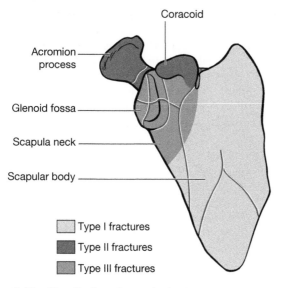

Coracoid

Acromion process

Glenoid fossa

Scapula neck

Scapular body

☐ Type I fractures
■ Type II fractures
☐ Type III fractures

Figure 6.17 • Classification of scapular fractures.

Table 6.2 Classification of clavicular fractures		
Type	**Mechanism of injury**	**Frequency (% of all clavicular fractures)**
Proximal third	Direct blow to anterior chest	5
Mid-third	Indirect force to lateral aspect of shoulder	80
Distal third	Direct blow to top of shoulder	15

of non-union. Complications frequently include malunion, regardless of the support mechanism used. While malunion is of little functional or cosmetic consequence, a persistent sharp clavicular spike may cause discomfort against clothes and require excision (Kelly 2004). Patients should be advised that a residual palpable or visible deformity may be present after healing has occurred (Smith 2005).

usually supporting an injured arm. Treatment involves immobilization of the arm on the injured side; however, difficulty in regaining full range of movement following this injury is high.

Clavicular fractures

The clavicle provides anterior support for the shoulder. It is a slightly S-shaped bone that articulates laterally with the acromion process and medially with the sternum. The clavicle gives definition to body shape as well as providing protection for the subclavian neurovascular bundle. Clavicle fractures make up 5% of all fractures, so are not uncommon and in children and adolescents it is a particularly common fracture (O'Steen 2003). Fracture of the clavicle is most commonly due to a violent upwards and backwards force such as a fall on the outstretched hand. Less commonly, the clavicle may be fractured by blows or falls on the point of the shoulder.

Clavicular fractures are divided into three groups: proximal third fracture, mid-clavicular fracture and distal fractures (Table 6.2).

Common presenting symptoms include pain over the fracture site, crepitus and sometimes a palpable deformity. The patient is usually supporting the arm of the injured side. In mid-clavicular fractures, deformity is common. The patient presents with a downward shoulder stump, sometimes rotated inward and forward. This is due to gravitational forces and contraction of the pectoralis major. The proximal fragment is displaced upward. Because of the location of the neurovascular bundles and the great blood vessels, a careful assessment of neurovascular function of the arm on the injured side must be carried out. Management of clavicular fracture is usually conservative. Immobilization with a simple sling is as effective as other less comfortable methods and is therefore the treatment of choice. Displaced fractures of the distal third often require surgical repair because of the risk

Shoulder dislocation

The glenohumeral joint of the shoulder girdle is a shallow synovial ball and socket joint that comprises five joints and three bones. The wide range of movement carried out at the shoulder, and its lack of bony stability, predisposes the joint to dislocation. Two main patient groups can be identified: men between the ages of 20 and 30 years (Zacchilli & Owens 2010), and women over 60 years, and approximately 55–60% of shoulder dislocations are recurrent (Proehl 2009). Glenohumeral joint dislocation can be categorized into four groups: anterior (>90% of dislocations), posterior (<5%), inferior (<1%) and superior (<1%).

Anterior dislocation

Anterior dislocations occur following a fall onto an outstretched hand where the arm is extended and externally rotated. They can also be caused by direct trauma to the posterolateral aspect of the shoulder.

The patient presents in extreme pain, usually holding the injured arm in abduction and external rotation (Genge Jagmin 1995). On examination, the shoulder will be obviously deformed when compared with the uninjured side. It will have a square appearance over the lateral aspect and the acromial process will be prominent (Fig. 6.18). Assessment should include a detailed examination of neurovascular function (Box 6.5).

Box 6.5

Assessment of neurovascular function following shoulder injury

- Posterior cord of brachial plexus – test for wrist extension
- Axillary nerve damage – test for sensation over lateral aspect of upper arm
- Axillary artery damage – test for brachial pulse

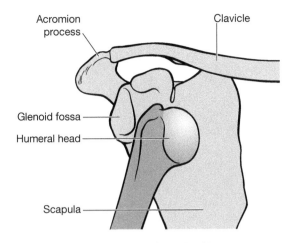

Figure 6.18 • Anterior dislocation of the shoulder.

Before shoulder dislocation is treated, humeral fracture should be excluded on X-ray. Fractures of the humeral head or neck prohibit early reduction of dislocation in the ED and orthopaedic opinion should always be sought. If no fracture exists, reduction of shoulder dislocation should be carried out as soon as possible. Prompt reduction is always necessary as the procedure becomes more difficult as time passes and the dislocation may prove irreducible (Mills et al. 1995), partly because muscle spasm increases with the length of time the joint is dislocated. Early relocation is also vital in maintaining the integrity of the humeral head. Because the scapular neck is harder than the humeral head, a compression fracture occurs, causing long-term deformity to the humeral head (Hill-Sachs deformity), which leads to recurrent dislocation. This is thought to occur in between 11 and 50 % of patients with anterior dislocation.

Four types of anterior dislocation exist, classified by the exact position of the humeral head. Management is broadly the same. Successful reduction of shoulder dislocation depends on overcoming muscle spasm. This is achieved by intravenous administration of muscle relaxant, such as midazolam, together with appropriate analgesia, usually opiates. The mechanics of shoulder reduction are achieved by traction or leverage, or a combination of both.

Traction methods include laying the patient prone with the injured arm over the side of the trolley and hanging a 5–7 kg weight, depending on the patient's muscularity, on the affected arm. Over 20–30 minutes this reduces muscle spasm by gently elongating muscles, pulling the humeral head off the scapular and allowing the rotator cuff muscles to relocate it in the glenoid fossa. This method is thought to be less painful than some more aggressive relocations and the risk of complication is low (Quaday 1995). There are several approaches to reduction available: two-person traction/counter-traction using a sheet, two-person traction/counter-traction using foot in the patient's armpit, external rotation leverage, Kocher's leverage technique and Spaso Miljesic leverage method.

The most commonly used and safest traction method of reduction is a two-person traction/counter-traction approach.

One person applies longitudinal traction to the injured arm, reducing muscle spasm, while the other person applies counter-traction by wrapping a sheet around the patient's chest and under the axilla of the injured side and then pulling towards the patient's ear on the unaffected side. This helps to disengage the humeral head from the scapula. Traditional traction/counter-traction methods of putting a foot in the patient's armpit and then pulling on the arm are not recommended because of their high association with neurovascular injury and lower success rate than other methods (Quaday 1995).

Leverage techniques involve some traction to lift the humeral head off the scapula, but then lever it back into place. These methods are fast, but increase the risk of injury to the glenoid rim or humeral shaft. The external rotation method of reduction is the least traumatic. It works by slowly adducting the injured arm and then flexing the elbow to 90°. The elbow is then held in place while the forearm is externally rotated by its own weight and gravity, not by force. This allows the smallest profile of the humeral head to be relocated into the glenoid fossa. The traditional method of leverage is Kocher's technique. This involves a three-step external/internal rotation manoeuvre which is both painful for the patient and dangerous because of the high risk of vascular tearing, rotator cuff injury and humeral fracture. A third technique is the Spaso Miljesic method: with the patient supine grasp the arm around the wrist or distal forearm. Gradually lift the arm vertically, applying gentle traction. Slightly externally rotate while maintaining vertical traction. Pauses may be required when muscular spasm occurs in which case the traction is maintained while movement is halted until the spasm passes (Yuen et al. 2001). If reduction cannot be achieved, orthopaedic referral should be made for manipulation under general anaesthetic.

Whatever method of reduction is used, it is important that neurovascular integrity is rechecked, and an X-ray taken to check position. The affected arm is often immobilized to prevent re-dislocation, however Hovelius et al. (2008) found that there were no long-term differences between patients who were immobilized compared with those who were allowed immediate mobilization. Where immobilization is chosen, the arm should be adducted and internally rotated. To prevent shoulder stiffness, the patient should be advised to extend the elbow and rotate the arm to a neutral position several times a day. In older patients, the risk of joint stiffness is greater, and therefore it is usual to remobilize the arm sooner than in younger people. Patients over 40 years should not be immobilized for longer than three weeks. The rate of re-dislocation is higher in younger people but settles over time (Hovelius et al. 2008).

Posterior dislocation

The anatomy of the shoulder girdle makes posterior dislocation difficult because the glenoid fossa is positioned posteriorly to the humeral head. The angle of the scapula helps to buttress this structure. When dislocation occurs, the humeral head sits behind the glenoid and usually below the acromion (Fig. 6.19).

Posterior dislocation is caused by a fall onto an outstretched hand where the arm is flexed and internally rotated.

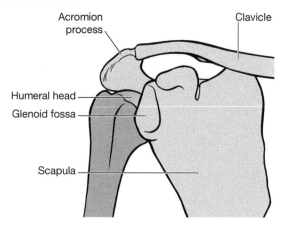

Figure 6.19 • Posterior dislocation of the shoulder.

Posterior dislocation also occurs following significant electric shock, epileptic seizures and, occasionally, from direct force to the anterior aspect of the shoulder. The patient will have severe pain and will present holding the arm in internal rotation, supported in a sling-type position. There is usually a loss of definition of the anterior shoulder and a prominent acromial and coracoid process, with the humeral head sometimes palpable posteriorly. The patient is unable to lift the arm above 90° and cannot externally rotate.

Diagnosis should be made from the mechanism of injury and patient presentation as anteroposterior X-rays are inconclusive and up to 50% of posterior dislocations are missed initially (Quadray 1995). Lateral and axillary X-ray views will confirm diagnosis. Neurovascular injury is less common with posterior dislocation because the major structures lie anterior to the joint and are thus protected. Although closed reduction with muscle relaxant and analgesia may be attempted, orthopaedic consultation should determine this.

Because of the strong anterior muscle mass, reduction in ED is usually only recommended for elderly or frail patients and reduction under general anaesthetic is generally required. If attempts at reduction are made in ED, the process involves slow in-line traction, while maintaining internal rotation, with gentle pressure on the humeral head to lift it off the glenoid. If reduction is attempted, neurovascular integrity should be checked afterwards and X-rays performed. The affected arm should be immobilized but not internally rotated. For this reason, shoulder spicas are often used to create slight external rotation. Immobilization should not exceed four weeks.

Upper arm injury

The humerus is surrounded by strong muscle compartments: anteriorly the biceps and posteriorly the triceps. The neurovascular bundle lies on the medial border of the biceps and contains the brachial artery, the brachial vein and the medial and ulnar nerves. The radial nerve runs posteriorly until it reaches the distal humerus, where it travels laterally until it is anterior to the humerus. The muscle design of the upper arm is appropriate for pulling or hanging activities.

Humeral fractures are common in two main patient groups:

- women aged between 56 and 65 years, usually with osteoporosis – fractures occur as a result of a fall and occasionally direct force; injury is usually to the proximal humerus, neck or shaft
- young men aged between 16 and 24 years – mechanisms of injury include RTAs (transverse humeral fractures), falls from a significant height (oblique or spiral fractures) and stress fractures from throwing actions.

The patient will present holding their arm close to their chest, with localized pain, extensive bruising or shoulder pain in fractures of the humeral neck. The upper arm is usually swollen and may have obvious shortening with normal movement at the point of fracture. Very careful neurovascular assessment is necessary, especially with distal third fractures as both the brachial plexus and axillary nerve may be damaged. Circulation should be assessed at the brachial pulse, radial pulse and along the ulnar and brachial arteries. The axillary artery is the most common to sustain vessel injury and may be present with any combination of limb pain, paraesthesia, pallor, no pulse, a cool limb and paralysis. Capillary refill of the fingertips and hand should also be assessed. Sensory and motor function should be checked in line with radial, ulnar and median nerve activity.

The muscle masses help to splint humeral fractures, and gravity helps with lengthening and aligning the bone. However, this is a very painful option for the patient, and nonunion is common. Although exact alignment is not vital because the shoulder's mobility can compensate, four basic steps to fracture management should be followed:

- traction to restore length and align fragment
- any angulation should be reduced
- initial immobilization for pain control and healing
- encourage mobilization of shoulder and elbow to prevent loss of function.

A number of immobilization methods exist. Hanging casts and U-slabs have been used for many years as a method of immobilizing the upper arm. As well as being extremely uncomfortable and restrictive for patients, these casts can cause posterior angulation of the fracture (Ciernick et al. 1991); and since they are not adjustable they cannot ensure that the soft tissues are compressed as swelling decreases and atrophy ensues or enable the patient to move the arm several times a day to passively flex and extend the elbow, emphasizing extension of the joint. Slings are commonly used, but these offer little immobilization or pain control. The treatment of choice appears to be an interlocking upper arm functional brace with forearm support. These have 95% excellent functional rotation and 85% minimal shortening of the limb (Zagorski et al. 1988). Functional bracing is contraindicated in: fractures with axial distraction between the fragments due to higher risk of delayed or nonunion; open fractures with major soft-tissue damage or with vascular injuries that require surgical repair; bilateral humeral fractures; and polytrauma who are unable to walk are best treated by surgical stabilization. Open reduction with internal fixation is usually performed for open or severely comminuted

Figure 6.20 • The elbow joint. (A) Anterior view; (B) posterior view; and (C) lateral view.

fractures and in patients with multiple fractures where conservative management would delay overall recovery and mobility.

Elbow injury

The elbow joint is a hinge-like articulation and consists of the distal humerus, radius, ulna and olecranon (Fig. 6.20). The distal humerus forms two columns; the lateral and medial epicondyles form the proximal part of these columns and are significant for their muscle attachment facilitating wrist movement. The wrist extensors originate from the lateral epicondyle, and flexors from the medial epicondyle. The trochlea articulates with the olecranon to allow flexion/extension at the elbow, and the capitellum allows pronation and supination of the forearm by articulation with the radial head. The radial nerve travels around the humerus to the anterior of the lateral epicondyle, and supplies the wrist and finger extensors. Because of its proximity to the distal humerus, it is very susceptible to injury. The medial nerve travels anterior to the humerus with the brachial artery. It provides sensation to the thumb and index finger and coarse hand movement, such as grip. If the nerve is damaged above the elbow, the index finger cannot be flexed (Ochsner's test). If damaged in the forearm, the interphalangeal thumb joint cannot be flexed if the base of the thumb is held to immobilize it.

The ulnar nerve crosses behind the medial epicondyle and is therefore susceptible to damage when elbow injury occurs. It supplies the flexor muscles and intrinsic hand nerves. Sensation to the ulnar side of the hand is also provided by the ulnar nerve. The brachial artery travels down the anterior aspect of the humerus and crosses the elbow with the median nerve. This is the major blood supply to the hand and forearm and compromise of this supply following injury can result in

Volkmann's ischaemia. This is muscle wasting of the hand and forearm which leads to contracture.

Supracondylar fractures

These are distal humerus fractures, proximal to the epicondyles. They are the most common fracture in children and adolescents, accounting for 50–70% of elbow fractures (El-Adl et al. 2008) and 30% of all limb fractures in under-7-year-olds (Babal et al. 2010). Supracondylar fractures are categorized into two groups depending on the mechanism of injury: extension and flexion fractures.

Extension fractures

This type of fracture is caused by a fall onto an outstretched hand with the elbow locked in extension (Fig. 6.21). This results in posterior displacement of the distal fragment of the humerus, and puts neurovascular structures at risk because of the jagged proximal humerus which becomes anteriorly angulated. This injury is most common in those under 15 years of age, because the tensile strength of the ligaments and joint capsule is greater than that of bone, and therefore fracture occurs. In adults, the reverse is true and dislocation of the elbow joint is more common (Magnusson 2009).

The patient will present holding the arm partially flexed. There is usually severe pain and swelling above the elbow. A thorough assessment should be made of neurovascular and motor function, as injury to the radial nerve occurs in about 8% of patients (Tsai & Ruiz 1995) (Table 6.3).

Management depends on clinical findings. If circulatory compromise exists then immediate reduction should be considered in the ED. This carries significant risk of neurovascular damage and should only be carried out in limb-threatening situations. In most cases prompt reduction of the fracture should be carried out in theatre. In undisplaced fractures, a plaster backslab can be applied, and provided neurovascular integrity is maintained the patient can be discharged with limb care advice and fracture clinic follow-up.

Flexion fractures

These are less common than extension fractures and comprise approximately 2–4% of the total number of supracondylar fractures (Babal et al. 2010). They are caused by direct force to a flexed elbow, from a fall or a blow (Fig. 6.22). The patient will have significant pain around

Figure 6.21 ● Supracondylar extension fracture.

Figure 6.22 ● Supracondylar flexion fracture.

Table 6.3 Assessing neurological function following elbow injury			
Nerve	**Position**	**Motor function**	**Sensory function**
Radial	Spirals humerus to anterior of lateral epicondyle	Wrist and finger extensor muscles – test for wrist drop on elbow flexion and forearm pronation	Snuff box area and dorsal aspect of thumb – test for sensation
Median	Anterior to humerus	Coarse hand movement, e.g., grip	Thumb and index finger – test for sensation
		Test location of injury – above elbow there will be inability to flex index finger: below elbow there will be inability to flex thumb	
Ulna	Posterior to medial epicondyle	Flexor muscles of wrist and fingers and intrinsic muscles of the hand – damage can present as claw-like hand	Palmar and dorsal aspects of ulnar half of hand

the site and will be supporting the injured arm in a flexed position, but the olecranon prominence will be decreased. There may be a prominent proximal fragment of the humerus anteriorly, and these injuries are commonly seen in open fractures. Although nerve damage is less likely with flexion fractures, the ulnar nerve is at risk because of fracture displacement. Vascular injury is uncommon. If only minimal displacement exists, the fracture can be treated by closed reduction and an above-elbow back-slab in flexion. Fractures with significant displacement or open injuries should have open reduction and internal fixation of the fracture.

Elbow dislocation

Although elbow dislocation is not uncommon in adults, considerable force is needed to cause dislocation. As a result, a 1 in 3 likelihood of an associated fracture exists. The most common type of dislocation is posterior, where the coronoid process slips back and lies in the olecranon fossa, or impacts into the distal humerus. The joint capsule is damaged and collateral ligaments are torn.

The patient will have pain, the arm will be supported in mid-flexion and the limb will appear shortened. The olecranon is prominent. Careful neurovascular examination is essential, especially of the nerve and brachial artery. The median nerve may be assessed by feeling the muscle while the patient attempts to resist the thumb being pressed from a vertical position against the plane of the hand (Smith 2005). The brachial artery can be assessed by checking the radial pulse.

Management involves urgent relocation for both pain control and neurovascular integrity. This is achieved with muscle relaxants and adequate analgesia followed by a traction/counter-traction approach where one carer applies sustained traction distally from the wrist followed by flexion with posterior pressure. When the reduction is completed, range of movement should be checked to rule out a mechanical blockage, neurovascular integrity should be rechecked, and then the arm should be immobilized in at least 90% flexion. Medial, lateral and anterior dislocations can also occur, but these are less common and should be managed by the orthopaedic team.

Radial head fractures

In this type of fracture the radial head becomes compressed upwards against the capitellum following a fall onto an outstretched hand. It is an important feature in elbow flexion/extension and forearm rotation. The patient will present with localized pain, which is worse with passive rotation of the forearm and an inability to fully extend the forearm. The presence of a fat pad elevation on X-ray is recognized as associated with an underlying radial head fracture in recent trauma (O'Dwyer et al. 2004). For management purposes, fractures are classified into three types (Table 6.4).

Table 6.4 Classification and management of radial head fractures

Type	Description	Management
I	Undisplaced	Sling with early mobilization
II	Marginal fracture with displacement	Joint aspiration if necessary Sling and early mobilization
III	Comminuted fracture	Treatment options vary from internal fixation to partial or total extension of the radial head

Forearm injury

The forearm consists of two long bones: the radius and ulna. They run essentially parallel, although the ulna is straight and the radius bows laterally to allow supination and pronation. The radius and ulna articulate with each other at both ends and are held together by the elbow and wrist joints and their ligaments. The radiocarpal joint connects the radius and the articular disc of the ulna with the carpal bones. This allows palmar and dorsiflexion of the wrist and abduction of the ulna. The union and alignment of the radius and ulna are vital to the function of the forearm and wrist.

Fracture of both radius and ulna

This occurs following a direct blow, fall or road traffic accident involving significant force or longitudinal compression. These fractures are commonly open and nearly always displaced because of the force needed to break both bones. Injury commonly occurs where the mid- and distal thirds merge because there is less muscle protection. These fractures are easy to diagnose as the patient presents with severe pain and marked deformity, sometimes with abnormal movement of the forearm, which mainly depends on the degree of deformity. If there is no angulation or displacement, a long arm plaster of Paris (POP) slab with 90° flexion of the elbow is applied. Usually open reduction with internal fixation is required because displacement is common. If good reduction is not achieved and maintained, non-union of the bones or union with loss of function will occur.

Ulnar fractures

Ulnar shaft fractures sometimes known as nightstick fractures are caused by direct force to the arm, commonly when it is raised to protect the face from injury. The patient presents with pain over the area, and swelling and deformity if the fracture is displaced. Management depends on the degree of displacement. Fractures with more than 50% displacement or 10% of angulation should be internally fixed as they carry a significant risk of non-union. Fractures with less displacement/angulation can be treated in a long arm POP cast with the elbow in 90° flexion and the forearm in a neutral position. Non-displaced fractures initially treated by immobilization respond well to early remobilization at about ten days post-injury.

Proximal ulnar fractures rarely occur independently and are associated with radial head dislocation. This is called a Monteggia fracture and four major classifications of these exist (Wilkins 2002), these are defined by the position of the radial head. Monteggia fractures have a better outcome in children compared with adults (Wilkins 2002). In adults, these fractures are associated with increased morbidity including the complications of reduced function, non-union, infection and the need for revisionary surgery (Fayaz & Jupiter 2010). Radial nerve paralysis can also occur as a result of compression from the displaced radial head. This causes weak wrist and hand extensors. It has been argued that the implications of distal ulnar fractures are often insufficiently appreciated and may result in ineffective treatment, especially compared to distal radius fractures (Logan & Lindau 2008). Greenstick fractures of the ulna are often difficult to detect, which in part accounts for the reason that Monteggia fractures are frequently overlooked in children.

The patient presents with localized pain and, depending on the position of the radial head, it may be palpable, and shortening of the forearm may also be noted. The patient will resist any movement of the elbow. Management involves open reduction and internal fixation in adults, as non-union and persistent dislocation of the radial head is common. A closed reduction under general anaesthetic can usually be achieved in children, as slight radial angulation of the ulna will not restrict movement.

Fractures of the radius

Proximal third fractures are rare because of the muscular support attached to the forearm. When they do occur, these fractures are usually caused by direct force to the forearm. The patient usually has pain around the fracture site and pain on longitudinal compression of the radius. Deformity is not as easy to detect as in other forearm fractures because of the amount of soft tissue surrounding the proximal radius. Associated ulnar injury is common because of the force needed to fracture the radius at this level.

The shape of the radius must be maintained to restore function. In proximal third fractures this is complicated by the force exerted by the supinator and biceps brachii muscles, creating supination and displacement of the proximal fragment. The pronator teres muscle causes pronation of the distal fragment which compounds deformity. This deforming process can occur within a POP cast, and therefore if fractures occur proximal to the point of pronator teres insertion in the mid-third of the radius, internal fixation of the fracture is recommended. Fractures in the proximal fifth of the radius are unsuitable for internal fixation because orthopaedic metalwork/hardware cannot be accommodated. These fractures should be treated in a long arm cast with 90° elbow flexion and forearm supination to minimize muscle forces and maintain reduction. The outcome of closed reduction is better in children than in adults.

Distal third shaft fractures also occur because of direct force, but are more common because of the lack of soft tissue protection. Isolated fractures are less common than more complicated injury (Goldberg et al. 1992). Dislocation of the radio-ulnar joint is usually concomitant with fractures around the mid-shaft and distal shaft junction. This is called a Galeazzi fracture. These fractures have a high incidence of long-term functional disability and chronic pain when untreated (Perron et al. 2001). Pain is the primary diagnostic feature. Tissue swelling may obscure deformity, but shortening is sometimes apparent. The deforming forces, shown in Table 6.5, make closed reduction less successful than open reduction with internal fixation.

Table 6.5 Deforming forces in Galeazzi fractures

Mechanism	Deformity
Gravity	Subluxation or dislocation of radio-ulnar joint Angulation of radial fracture
Pronator quadratus	Rotation of distal fragment in a proximal and volar direction
Brachioradialis	Shortening because of distal fragment rotation
Thumb abductors and extensors	Compounds shortening

Wrist injury

Anatomically, the wrist is an area that contains multiple joints connected by ligaments. It extends from the distal radius and ulna to the distal carpal bones (Fig. 6.23). Injury to the wrist usually results from a fall onto an outstretched hand, which causes hyperextension of the hand and force to be exerted on the volar aspect of the radius causing fracture. Injury pattern varies with age, gender and the amount of force involved. The distal radius is a common site of injury in adults. Fractures of this area are broadly grouped into three categories depending on the displacement of the distal radius and ulna. They are known as Colles', Smith's and Barton's fractures.

Colles' fracture

The most common of these fractures is the Colles' fracture (Fig. 6.24). This describes a distal radius fracture with dorsal displacement of the distal fragment. This causes a loss of the usual volar tilt and pronation of the distal fragment over the proximal fragment. An associated ulnar styloid fracture is present in 60% of cases (Cooney et al. 1991). The injury is most prevalent in women over 50 years, particularly those with signs of osteoporosis. Colles' fractures are easy to identify at initial assessment as the patient presents with classic dinner-fork deformity of the wrist because of dorsal displacement and loss of volar angulation (Harness et al. 2004).

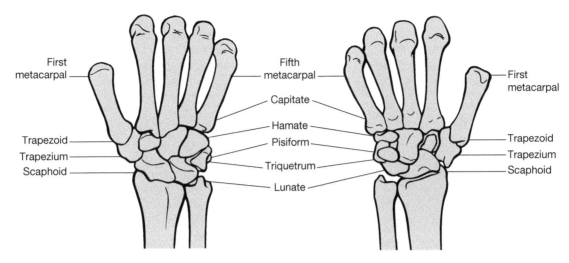

Figure 6.23 • The wrist injury.

Figure 6.24 • Colles' fracture.

The patient usually has significant swelling around the fracture site and localized pain. Nerve involvement is not uncommon and paraesthesia may be present in areas served by the median or ulnar nerve. Severe swelling can cause vascular compromise and compartment syndrome. Neurovascular function should therefore be carefully checked on assessment. All the digits should be touched to ensure there is feeling and therefore neurological deficit is present, and capillary refill should also be checked. Patients need adequate analgesia and a full explanation of what is going to happen before any examination of the wrist is undertaken (Summers 2005). Management priorities involve restoration of anatomical alignment, in particular the degree of volar tilt, and the exact restoration of a neutral radio-ulnar joint if good function of the wrist is to be restored. Fractures with minimal displacement with no shortening and maintenance of volar tilt are managed in a forearm POP back-slab or split cast with the hand pronated and ulnar deviation, and flexion at the wrist (Brown 1996).

Most displaced fractures can be managed by closed reduction in the ED. To facilitate this, adequate analgesia is required. Debate persists as to which method of anaesthesia is most appropriate, and various methods are discussed in Chapter 26. Bier's block is often favoured by orthopaedic staff, but

demands skilled operators. Haematoma block requires less skill but carries the risk of subsequent tissue toxicity from the lidocaine used, and has been criticized for providing inadequate anaesthesia to complete the reduction (Cooney et al. 1991). Despite this, haematoma block is commonly used and is successful in the treatment of elderly women. As a general rule, haematoma block is not suitable for Colles' fracture reduction in younger patients, particularly men with greater muscle spasm creating resistance to reduction. An accurate reduction is vital for restoration of full function in younger patients, and therefore multiple attempts at manipulation are sometimes needed. This is more easily facilitated under Bier's block.

The reduction involves a traction/counter-traction approach, with the first person applying longitudinal traction through the hand to lengthen the radius, while the second applies counter-traction through the forearm until disimpaction of the distal fragment can be felt. Then the first person applies pressure to the top of the distal fragment to reduce it. Again, volar movement will be felt and visible deformity should be resolved. The wrist should be immediately immobilized in a POP slab with ulnar deviation and wrist flexion. Post-reduction X-rays should be obtained to establish the degree of volar tilt, length and neutral radio-ulnar joint position (Greaves & Jones 2002). If this cannot be achieved by closed manipulation, open reduction and internal fixation should be considered. In complicated or severely comminuted injuries, open reduction and internal fixation should be considered and closed manipulation not attempted in ED.

Compartment syndrome, which is the compression of nerves and blood vessels in an enclosed space, can lead to permanent damage of these structures. Summers (2005) recommends the following symptoms of compartment syndrome – the 'five Ps' – should be discussed with patients, stressing that, if any of these symptoms manifest themselves, patients should contact their ED for advice.

The five Ps are:

- persistent pain
- pallor, when fingers lose their healthy colour

- pulselessness: instruction needs to have been given on how to perform capillary refill testing and interpret results
- paraesthesia
- paralysis.

As patients with Colles' type fracture are often older, their social circumstances should be established before discharge to make sure they can cope at home.

Smith's fractures

In both anatomical presentation and mechanism of injury, a Smith's fracture represents the opposite of a Colles' fracture. The distal radius is displaced proximally and the distal fragment is volar to the radial shaft. There are three classifications depending on the direction of the fracture (Fig. 6.25).

The mechanism of injury is an impact on the distal aspect of the hand. Because significant force is needed to cause this fracture, the cause is usually an RTA or cyclist going over the handlebars. Smith's fractures are most common in young men. The patient presents with severe pain, obvious volar

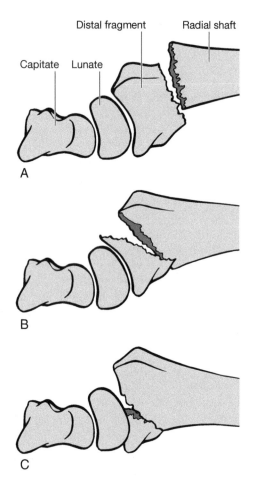

Figure 6.25 • Smith's fracture: classification of anterior displacement. (A) Type I–transverse fracture; (B) type II–oblique fracture from proximal volar surface through dorsal particular surface; (C) type III–oblique fracture with joint space involvement (same as Barton fracture-dislocation).

deformity of the wrist, making the hand appear anteriorly displaced, and often swelling to the dorsal aspect of the wrist. Neurological compromise to median and ulnar nerves is possible with significant deformity, as is vascular compromise. Careful triage will highlight these complications.

Type I fractures can usually be treated in the ED. Closed manipulation involves restoring length and dorsal alignment of the radius. This can be achieved using Bier's block anaesthesia and manual traction. Once deformity is corrected, the arm should be immobilized in an above-arm split POP cast with the forearm in a supinated position.

Type II and type III fractures are unstable injuries and, to ensure maximum functional recovery, orthopaedic advice should also be sought. Open reduction with internal fixation is usually required.

Barton's fractures

These are distal radius fractures with volar or dorsal dislocation of radiocarpal joint. Volar fractures are more common than dorsal (Harness et al. 2004). It differs from Colles' or Smith's fracture in that there is always intra-articular dislocation present. Barton's fractures are often associated with high-velocity trauma (Aggarwal & Nagi 2004) although they can result from a fall upon an outstretched, pronated arm.

Treatment is usually by surgery as conservative care has an elevated risk of complications, including 'early osteoarthrosis, deformity, subluxation, and instability' (Aggarwal & Nagi 2004).

Carpal fractures

The carpal bones form two rows (see Fig. 6.23). The proximal row consists of the scaphoid, lunate, triquetrum and pisiform bones. The scaphoid has a bridging position with the distal row which consists of the trapezium, capitate and hamate bones. These bones are supported by three strands of ligaments stemming from the radial styloid. The radial and ulnar arteries provide vascular supply, and the radial, ulnar and median nerves provide neurological function.

Fractures of the carpal bones are less common than other wrist injuries averaging at 8% compared to phalanges (59%) and metacarpals (33%) (Van Onselen et al. 2003, Dennis et al. 2011). These fractures are often associated with ligament injury, creating an unstable wrist joint. Long-term disability is not uncommon in missed fractures. Assessment of wrist injury should focus on the mechanism of injury, force involved, and exact site of impact as well as the age of the patient, wrist anatomy and relative strengths change with age.

Scaphoid fracture

Because of its unique position in relation to the radius and both rows of carpal bones, the scaphoid is the most commonly fractured carpal bone and accounts for between 2 and 7% of all orthopaedic fractures (McNally & Gillespie 2004). It occurs in both adults and children, most often between early teens and mid-life. The oblong-shaped scaphoid bone derives its name from the Greek word '*skaphos*' meaning 'boat' and is divided into four anatomical areas (Fig. 6.26).

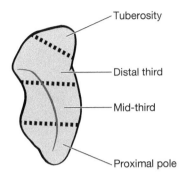

Figure 6.26 • The scaphoid bone.

The scaphoid has a good vascular supply to the middle and distal areas, but the proximal pole has no dedicated blood supply. This results in a high incidence of vascular necrosis if fracture union is not rapidly achieved. Scaphoid fractures are usually classified as stable or unstable and time taken to union differs with the fracture location (Box 6.6). Stable fractures that are incomplete or completely undisplaced, heal rapidly and are treated with immobilization. An unstable fracture has been defined as displacement of the fracture by 1 mm or more on X-ray.

Box 6.6

Herbert's classification of scaphoid fractures

Type A (stable)
- A1 Crack fractures
- A2 Tubercle fractures

Type B (unstable)
- B1 Distal third
- B2 Waist
- B3 Proximal pole
- B4 Carpal dislocation
- B5 Comminuted

The most common mechanism of injury is a fall onto an outstretched hand. Externally, there is little visible evidence of a fracture, although swelling can sometimes be present. The patient will have generalized pain, which is worse on wrist movement, particularly gripping actions. On examination, patients will have specific tenderness in the anatomical snuffbox. The anatomical snuffbox is on the radial aspect of the dorsum of the wrist. They may also have pain when longitudinal pressure is applied to the thumb and index finger, and pain on dorsiflexion of the wrist. To assess the snuffbox, ask the patient to hyperextend the thumb with the wrist slightly deviated in the radial aspect. In this position the snuffbox becomes visible. The scaphoid can be palpated proximally in the floor of the snuffbox. The trapezium can be palpated distally. This test is sensitive but not specific (Phillips et al. 2004). Tenderness of the scaphoid tubercle is also a sensitive test

but is more specific. To examine this with one hand extend the patient's wrist while applying pressure on the scaphoid tuberosity at the proximal wrist crease with the other. If there is no tenderness with these two tests, a scaphoid fracture is unlikely.

Because of the location of pain and lack of external signs, patients often delay attending the ED as they do not automatically relate symptoms with a broken bone.

X-ray findings can be misleading as up to 20 % of patients with scaphoid fracture have normal initial X-rays (McNally & Gillespie 2004). Fractures not initially visible on X-ray will be apparent between 10–14 days post-injury (Hunter 2005). For this reason diagnosis should be based on clinical findings, specifically, mechanism of injury and localized tenderness in the anatomical snuffbox. Management of scaphoid fractures can be controversial (Hunter 2005). At present most non-complex fractures are treated conservatively with an excellent healing rate, however where the facilities and skill exist surgical treatment is increasing in popularity with a 100 % union rate and reduced immobilization time required (Vinnars et al. 2008). A general consensus exists that all fractures, whether clinical or radiological, should be immobilized as failure to do this can result in delayed or non-union healing or avascular necrosis. A POP cast or splint that incorporates the forearm and thumb, with the wrist in slight volar flexion, should be used. Complicated fractures should be referred to the orthopaedic team because of the risk of avascular necrosis. Some fractures are internally fixed at an early stage to prevent non-union and to ensure good functional recovery (Chin et al. 2009).

Lunate fracture

The lunate is in the middle of the proximal carpal row and rests in the lunate fossa of the radius. Injury of the lunate bone is relatively uncommon because it is protected by the lunate fossa. When fracture does occur it is usually due to a fall onto an outstretched hand, where force is taken through the heel of the hand. The patient presents with mid-dorsal pain and wrist weakness; however, swelling is uncommon. As a result, attendance in the ED is sometimes days or weeks after the initial injury.

Radiological evidence of fracture is not always obvious, therefore clinical diagnosis is necessary based on location of pain and mechanism of injury. Non-displaced fractures should be treated in a forearm POP cast, with orthopaedic follow-up. Displaced fractures are prone to avascular necrosis and non-union, with a potential for secondary osteoarthritis. For this reason, patients should be referred to the orthopaedic team for possible internal fixation.

Triquetrum fractures

The triquetrum is the second most commonly fractured carpal bone. Such fractures often occur with other carpal fractures or perilunate dislocation. Isolated injury is less common and usually minor. Triquetrum fractures are usually caused by hyperextension injury of significant force. The patient usually complains of pain over the dorso-ulnar area of the wrist. Management involves a short arm POP cast or splint for

3–6 weeks in the case of isolated injury or referral to the orthopaedic team where the fracture is associated with other wrist injuries. Other carpal fractures generally occur as part of a more complicated hand or wrist injury, and demand specialist orthopaedic input after initial diagnosis in the ED.

Perilunate and lunate dislocation

These dislocations occur as a result of disruption to the lesser arc of ligaments. They can be graded into four groups depending on the degree of disruption (Box 6.7). They are caused by extreme hyperextension, which might occur due to a motorcycle accident or fall from a height. Because of the force needed to cause perilunate and/or lunate dislocation, concurrent injury is common. The patient presents with extreme pain and a fork-type deformity, and is usually unable to hold the fingers in a flexed position. Nerve disruption is not uncommon, so paraesthesia may also be present. Fractures and severe ligament disruption are usual with these injuries, which should always be managed by the orthopaedic team and often require open reduction when associated with fractures.

Hand injury

The hand is a complex structure whose skeletal outline is shown in Fig. 6.27. The back of the hand is referred to as the dorsal aspect and the palm of the hand the volar aspect. The

> ### Box 6.7
>
> ### Stages of perilunate disruption and midcarpal dislocation
>
> - Stage 1: scapholunate instability – due to torn radioscaphoid and scapholunate interosseous ligaments with/without scaphoid fracture
> - Stage 2: dorsal perilunate dislocation – capitate dislocates dorsally from lunate at the midcarpal joint
> - State 3: disruption of lunate and triquetrum — occurs with avulsion fracture of triquetrum with/without scaphoid or capitate fracture
> - Stage 4: volar dislocation of lunate
>
> (After Mayfield JK et al. (1980) Carpal dislocations: pathomechanics and progressive perilunar instability. Journal of Hand Surgery 5(3), 226-241.)

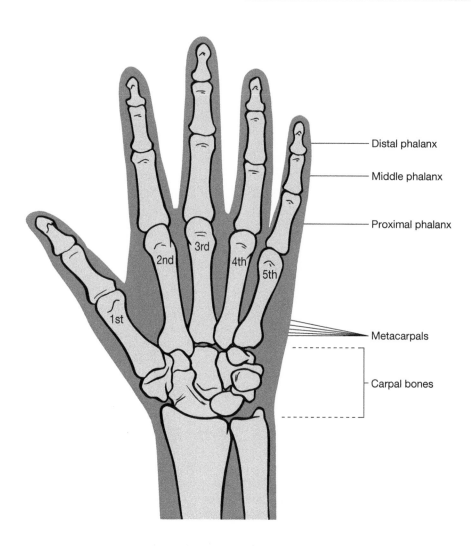

Figure 6.27 • Anatomy of the hand.

intricate mechanisms of hand movement are particularly vulnerable to injury because of its environmental exposure and functional purpose. Hand function relies on intact muscle and tendon structures and sensory motor connection to the central nervous system, as well as adequate circulation. The treatment of any hand injury revolves firstly around restoring function and secondly around appearance. Anatomy will be considered in greater detail where relevant to specific injuries.

Thumb injury

The flexor surface of the thumb is perpendicular to that of the fingers and has a saddle joint which allows 45° of rotation. The range of thumb movements includes flexion/extension, adduction/abduction and opposition. It provides both strength and grip. Thumb fractures are treated differently from other metacarpal fractures because of the degree of functional restoration needed.

First metacarpal shaft fractures

These usually occur in the proximal half of the bone and are often associated with adduction of the distal segment. Management usually involves longitudinal traction and POP cast incorporating the thumb. Early orthopaedic follow-up is advisable.

Base of first metacarpal fractures

These are usually more complicated and result from flexion injuries, commonly from clenched fists. They can be classified as intra-articular fractures, such as Bennett's fractures, or extra-articular transverse or oblique fractures.

Extra-articular fractures occur within the joint capsule, but do not involve the articular surface of the joint (Fig. 6.28) and are the most common fracture type. These injuries are usually managed by closed reduction and POP cast incorporating the thumb. In order to retain good function, it is important not to hyperextend the thumb at the metacarpophalangeal joint. Some oblique fractures may remain unstable with closed reduction and plaster immobilization alone, and therefore orthopaedic referral for percutaneous pinning is necessary.

Intra-articular fractures can be divided into two groups: the more common Bennett's fracture and Rolando's fracture. The Bennett's fracture is categorized by the displacement of the metacarpal shaft while the palmar articular fragment retains its correct anatomical location as shown in Fig. 6.29. The mechanism of injury is similar to that of an extra-articular fracture, with interpersonal fracas being a common cause of injury. The patient has limited movement of the base of the thumb with pain and swelling around the area. Effective emergency management is essential to prevent degenerative post-traumatic arthritis and to restore adequate range of movement. This injury is considered unstable because of the adductor pollicis longus tendon, which is attached to the base of the first metacarpal. Its tensile strength prevents union of

fracture without the aid of percutaneous pins or orthopaedic reduction and internal fixation.

Rolando's fracture is similar to a Bennett's fracture, but in addition to the palmar articular fragment remaining in place, the dorsal fragment displaces from the base, creating a Y-shaped or more severely comminuted base of metacarpal fracture. Mechanism of injury and patient presentation are similar to those of a Bennett's fracture, but the prognosis is poor

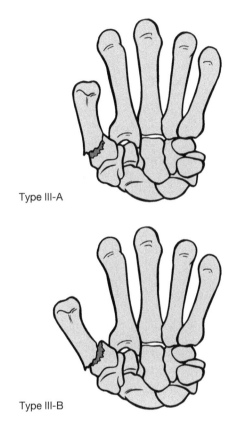

Type III-A

Type III-B

Figure 6.28 • Extra-articular fracture to the base of the first metacarpal.

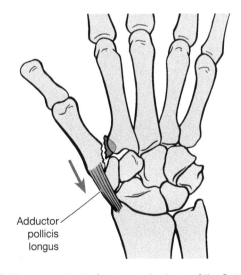

Adductor pollicis longus

Figure 6.29 • Intra-articular fracture to the base of the first metacarpal (Bennett's fracture).

as functional integrity is difficult to restore with orthopaedic reduction and internal fixation or closed reduction and immobilization. Persistent pain and degenerative arthritis are common.

Phalangeal fractures of the thumb are generally managed in the same manner as fingers.

Second to fifth metacarpal fractures

The metacarpals are anatomically sectioned into base, shaft, neck and head. Unlike other long bones, the base is at the proximal point and the head at the distal end.

Base of metacarpal fractures (II–IV)

The patient presents with a history of a fall onto an outstretched hand or punch injury. The fractures are often associated with carpal fractures and second and third metacarpal base fractures often have intra-articular involvement, but this causes little or no disability because of the relative immobility of the second and third carpo-metacarpal (CMC) joint. As a result, treatment focuses on maintaining patient comfort. A removable splint is the treatment of choice. Fractures of the fourth and fifth metacarpal bases are usually associated with CMC dislocation. Fourth metacarpal base fractures can usually be managed in the ED with closed reduction and splinting followed up by the orthopaedic team. Fifth metacarpal base fractures will usually require pinning because of displacement.

Good fracture alignment is necessary to retain normal mobility of the CMC joint. When splinting hand injuries, it is vital that metacarpo-phalangeal joints are immobilized in at least 70° of flexion to prevent shortening of the collateral ligaments. If these ligaments contract during immobilization, the patient is left with considerable disability because of joint stiffness.

Shaft of metacarpal fracture

These are caused by a number of mechanisms of injury (Table 6.6). Principles of management revolve around correction of any rotation, angulation and shortening of the finger to ensure functional recovery. Even a small degree of rotation can cause problems with flexion of the metacarpo-phalangeal joint. Effective closed reduction and immobilization are usually achievable in ED unless severe swelling or open fractures exist. If rotation cannot be corrected with manipulation, the patient should be referred for percutaneous pinning or orthopaedic reduction and internal fixation.

Metacarpal neck fractures

Second and third metacarpal neck fractures often need wiring to correct angulation in order to restore functional mobility, and therefore orthopaedic opinion should be sought. The fourth metacarpal is more mobile and neck fractures will heal without functional deficit even if volar angulation at the

Table 6.6 Metacarpal shaft fractures

Type	Cause
Transverse	Direct blow
Oblique	Torque force
Comminuted	Crush injury/gunshot wound

metacarpal neck exists. However, any rotation in these fractures must be corrected to prevent functional deficit.

Fifth metacarpal neck fracture, known as Boxer's fracture, is one of the most common hand injuries treated in the ED and usually results from a punch injury. Management of these fractures is controversial (Winter et al. 2007), but there is a consensus that any rotational injury needs manipulation and either splinting or wiring. Volar angulation can, however, be treated in a number of ways, ranging from orthopaedic reduction and internal fixation to no treatment and early mobilization (Winter et al. 2007).

Clinical trials (Rusnak 1995) have found that no treatment at all or supportive splinting which facilitates mobilization has quicker functional repair, with minimal cosmetic deformity in the majority of cases. Where closed reduction is carried out, maintaining that reduction is difficult without causing further damage to the function of the hand. This is because 70° of flexion at the metacarpo-phalangeal joint is necessary to prevent contractures, but this position will not provide the three-point fixation needed to stabilize the metacarpal neck.

If the patient is exceptionally concerned about the cosmetic result and the possible loss of knuckle definition, then surgical fixation should be considered; however, recovery is significantly slower with this method. Whatever method is used, the patient should have adequate follow-up from a hand surgeon to ensure the fullest functional potential is achieved. Metacarpal head fractures should be managed conservatively unless they are displaced or comminuted, when an orthopaedic opinion should be sought.

Fracture of phalanges

As with other hand fractures, the key management priority is to maintain good function by correcting rotation. Neighbour-strapping is usually the treatment of choice for uncomplicated fractures.

Soft tissue injury

Soft tissue injuries are commonly treated in ED and are usually considered 'minor' in nature by emergency staff. The impact on the patient, however, is far from minor; loss of normal function in the short term is common, usually because of pain. If soft tissue injuries are not detected and treated properly, long-term or recurrent problems can occur. Soft tissue injury (STI) is the all-encompassing term given to injury to muscles, ligaments, tendons and skin. As a result, the diagnosis of a STI has a number of possible causative factors. The common ones are described below.

A treatment common to all STIs is that of non-steroidal anti-inflammatory drugs (NSAIDs). This treatment is becoming increasingly questioned. NSAIDs can reduce pain and swelling enabling earlier mobilization and therefore recovery. However, the argument is that swelling is a recognized part of the healing process and this treatment should not routinely be used on acute injuries (Stovitz & Johnson 2003).

Sprains

These are injuries to the fibres of ligaments supporting a joint. This results from abnormal movement of the joint causing stretching and tearing of the ligament. The degree of this varies from partial tearing to total disruption of the ligament complex supporting a joint (Table 6.7).

Table 6.7 Classification of sprains

	Physiology	Clinical signs
First degree	Minor tearing of ligament fibres with mild haemorrhage	Minimal swelling Tenderness over ligaments – worse with motion, stressing the ligaments
Second degree	Partial tear with moderate haemorrhage and reduced active motion	Significant pain – worse with passive movement and swelling Injuries prone to recurrence and can cause joint instability
Third degree	Complete rupture of ligament Moderate haemorrhage with significant loss of function	Less painful with significant swelling and abnormal motion of joint on active/passive movement Usually need surgical repair if joint instability exists

The patient will present with mechanisms of injury and symptoms similar to those with fractures. The joint has often been subjected to forces in opposite or abnormal directions, creating joint stress. The patient will usually describe a sudden onset of acute pain, and often describe hearing a 'snap' at the time of injury. Many patients are convinced this means they have broken their limb and the nurse must therefore be careful to assess the injury thoroughly and provide the appropriate reassurance (Loveridge 2002, Smith 2003) without offending by implying the injury should not be seen in ED. Although specific injury management can vary, common RICE principles of sprain management apply:

- *Rest* – most acute sprains benefit from a 48-hour period of rest, with minimal use.
- *Ice* – used as a first aid measure either as an ice pack, or wrapped crushed ice. The intention is to help decrease both pain and swelling although there is little evidence to confirm improved clinical outcomes result in its use (Collins 2008).

The patient should be advised to apply the ice for 10–15 minutes every 2–3 hours for the first 12 hours post-injury.

- *Compression* – elastic tubular bandages or strapping are utilized to provide support for the injury and help to reduce swelling although there is debate about the efficacy of elasticated tubular bandages (Beynnon et al. 2006). Where a tubular bandage is applied, the patient should remove it at night to prevent oedema distal to the injury. In severe sprains, POP casts or braces may be more appropriate for specific injuries.
- *Elevation* – together with ice packs and rest, elevation of the injured part helps to reduce the accumulation of blood and lymph in tissues surrounding the injury, which in turn reduces both pain and healing time (Safran et al. 1999). This is particularly important for distal limb injuries, such as those of the hand, foot or ankle.

Strains

These are injuries to muscles and tendons. They occur after forced stretching or sudden violent contraction. As with sprains, the severity of strain injury is classified by the extent of damage (Table 6.8).

Table 6.8 Classification of strains

	Physiology	Clinical signs
First degree	Minor tearing of muscle/tendon unit	Spasm, swelling and localized pain
Second degree	More severe pain but incomplete tearing of fibres	Muscle spasm, swelling, localized pain and loss of strength
Third degree	The muscle or tendon is completely disrupted with separation of muscle from tendon, tendon from muscle or tendon from bone	Palpable defect is often present Muscle spasm, pain, swelling and loss of function

Treatment of strains is similar to that of sprains. Management of first-degree strains involves rest, ice, compression and elevation as described under 'sprains' above. Second-degree injuries may require immobilization, depending on the site affected, and usually take longer to heal. Third-degree injuries should be immobilized and the patient referred for early orthopaedic consultation at the fracture/STI clinic. Some injuries benefit from surgical repair, but many require simple immobilization. Many factors influence this decision: the site of injury, as well as the age, activity level and occupation of the patient (Loveridge 2002).

Tendinitis

This is an inflammatory condition usually caused by overuse. Less commonly it is caused by direct trauma. The patient complains of pain at the point where the tendon attaches to bone. Pain is worse on movement and function is sometimes restricted. Occasionally, palpable crepitus exists. Common sites include the rotator cuff of the shoulder (supraspinatus tendonitis), the insertion of hand extensors to the humeral lateral epicondyle (tennis elbow), the medial epicondyle (golfer's elbow), the radial aspect of the wrist (De Quervain's tenosynovitis) and the Achilles tendon. Management principally involves rest. NSAIDs are often used but their efficacy is currently debated particularly where overuse and degeneration are present (Khan et al. 2000).

Bursitis

This is inflammation of the bursa. The bursa is a sac of synovial fluid situated between muscle, tendon and bony prominences to facilitate movement. Bursitis can result from friction between the bursa and musculoskeletal tissue, direct trauma or infection. It results in inflammation and oedema, which causes sac engorgement, and the area becomes painful.

This condition is most common in middle age (Genge Jagmin 1995). The patient usually presents to the ED with a swelling at 2–3 days post-injury or strain. Pain can increase gradually over this time or may be of sudden onset. It is usually worse on movement and radiates distally from the site of bursitis. The area will appear classically inflamed with erythema and swelling and will be hot to the touch. Areas commonly affected include the knee (Adams 2004), elbow and big toe (gout bursitis).

If infection is suspected, e.g., following a puncture wound, or if the patient has pyrexia, the bursa should be aspirated and the aspirate sent to the laboratory for culture. Otherwise, the injured area should be managed conservatively with rest and analgesia with or without NSAIDs.

Haematoma

This is a collection of blood resulting from vascular injury within the soft tissues, bone or muscle. It is a result of direct or blunt trauma. Large haematomas not only threaten homeostasis, due to loss of circulatory volume, but are also a potential host for infection. As a result, surgical drainage and antibiotic therapy may be necessary. Smaller haematomas can be treated with compression bandages, ice as described above, and elevation.

Contusions

These usually result from direct trauma, which results in localized pain, swelling and bruising. Most are self-limiting and symptoms are relieved by ice treatment, analgesia and early mobilization.

Specific soft tissue injuries

There are a number of soft tissue injuries that are so commonly treated in EDs that they warrant individual discussion within this chapter.

Knee injury

The knee gives support and flexibility to body movement. Ligaments and musculotendinous structures maintain its stability. The knee joint is the most complicated joint in the body (Snell 2000, Adams 2004) and because of its load-bearing task it is very susceptible to injury, particularly during sporting activities such as rugby and football. Medial injuries tend to be the most common; lateral injuries, however, are often more disabling. A history of an audible snap at time of injury is suggestive of anterior cruciate rupture. The mechanism of injury gives a strong indication of the likely structural damage, so accurate history-taking is vital (Table 6.9).

Table 6.9 Mechanisms of knee injury

Force	Cause	Injury
Hyperextension Forced flexion	Running/sudden deceleration, e.g., from rugby tackles	Tearing of anterior cruciate ligament
Twisting or flexed knee injury	Direct or blunt trauma	Meniscal injury
Valgus stress with external rotation	Skiing	Medial collateral ligament injury
Varus stress internal rotation	Skiing in snow plough position	Lateral collateral ligament
Direct force	Fall, hitting dashboard in RTA	Posterior cruciate ligament

Examination of the knee should be carried out with the patient undressed and lying on a trolley. The nurse should look at both knees to detect subtle differences. Bruising, swelling or redness are all signs of soft tissue injury. A rapid onset of swelling is indicative of haemarthrosis, which could be the result of ligament/meniscus tear or a fracture of the tibial plateau and is therefore an indication for X-ray. Aspiration may be carried out in strict aseptic conditions, both for symptom relief and for diagnostic purposes. If the aspirate contains fat globules then a fracture is present. All patients with a rapid-onset haemarthrosis have significant knee trauma and should be referred for orthopaedic follow-up. Swelling which has a gradual onset usually represents a reactionary effusion. These may also be aspirated for symptom relief if large or restrictive.

The nurse should carefully assess knee movement, as this will give clues as to what ligamentous damage exists. Most ligament injuries can be healed with the treatment described above for sprains. Because of the load-bearing nature of the knee tendon, ruptures are often associated with fractures and frequently need surgical repair. For this reason, patients with total ruptures should be referred to the orthopaedic team.

Patients may also present to the ED with knee pain but no history of trauma. In such presentations other diagnoses such as Baker's cyst, osteoarthritis or in rare cases septic arthritis should be considered.

Achilles tendon rupture

The Achilles tendon is the largest, thickest and strongest tendon in the body and after the quadriceps is the second most ruptured supporting tissue (Kerr 2005). Achilles tendon rupture is a common tennis and badminton injury, associated with sudden jumping movements with a heavy landing. The patient complains of a sudden sharp pain at the back of the ankle, not dissimilar to a direct blow. Swelling is present in some cases, as is bruising, but often it is simply pain and the mechanism of injury which initially indicate Achilles tendon rupture. The calf squeeze test (Simmonds' test) is useful in confirming diagnosis. The patient kneels backwards over a chair or lies face down on a trolley with the ankles over the end. When the calf is squeezed, plantar flexion of the ankle should occur unless the Achilles tendon is ruptured (Bickley & Szilagyi 2008). All of these patients should be referred for orthopaedic follow-up.

Most are initially managed in long leg equinous plaster, with the ankle in plantar flexion. Some patients benefit from surgical repair, particularly young athletic people. Patient outcomes appear similar whether or not open repair is performed (Mayeda 2009). Achilles tendinitis should not be confused with partial rupture. Tendinitis is caused by overuse or sudden change in activity such as dancing or running. The patient will have localized pain, swelling and crepitus over the tendon. The range of movement will be normal but painful. The patient should be treated with rest and analgesia with or without NSAIDs.

Ankle sprain

Large numbers of patients with ankle injuries are treated in ED, and one of the priorities for ED nurses lies with identifying serious or potentially limb-threatening injury (Loveridge 2002). Assessment for all ankle injuries should be systematic and thorough, although the majority will turn out to be straightforward sprains. Assessment should include mechanism of injury, the most common being an inversion injury causing damage to the anterior talofibular ligaments. This results from slipping off kerbs or twisting the ankle in a manner where the sole of the foot turns inwards.

Eversion injury is less common, but is more likely to be associated with an avulsion fracture and causes damage to the deltoid ligament; it is characterized by an injury where the sole of the foot turns outwards. Patients will often have heard a 'snap' or 'crack' at the time of injury which they will probably associate with a broken bone. The nurse needs to provide reassurance as well as a thorough assessment, particularly when an X-ray is not clinically indicated (see Ottawa ankle rules, Fig 6.13). The patient with an ankle sprain usually has pain at the site of injury, swelling over that area, and reduced mobility because of pain. Examination usually identifies the area immediately below the respective malleolus to be the most severe point of pain, as opposed to a fracture where pain is worse over the bony prominence.

Management involves initial rest with compression bandaging, intermittent ice therapy and support. Recovery usually takes 2–4 weeks; however, most long-term problems stem from prolonged immobilization. For this reason, patients

Table 6.10 The rotator cuff muscles

Muscle	Action
Infraspinatus	External rotation
Teres minor	External rotation
Subscapularis	Internal rotation
Supraspinatus	Internal rotation

should be encouraged to exercise the ankle gently and resume activity after 1–2 weeks as pain and swelling permit.

Rotator cuff injury

The varied mobility of the shoulder joint makes it susceptible to injury (Ryan 2004). Shoulder stability is maintained by the rotator cuff. It comprises a sheath of muscles listed in Table 6.10. Degenerative conditions such as rheumatoid arthritis are not uncommon and increase the likelihood of injury. Acute injury includes tearing or tendinitis. The supraspinatus is the most commonly injured area; this results from falls with hyperextension or hyperabduction of the shoulder. Rest and analgesia comprise the management of choice, and most patients benefit from orthopaedic follow-up, as recurrent injury is not uncommon.

Rotator cuff tendinitis is usually a chronic condition, but a patient may present to the ED following an acute exacerbation. Unlike a rotator cuff tear, the patient will describe a gradually worsening discomfort, inability to sleep and decreased range of movement. Analgesia with or without NSAIDs and rest are the treatment of choice.

Thumb sprain

Stability and function of the thumb rely on the ulnar collateral ligament (UCL). Injury to the UCL is caused by hyperextension of the thumb from ball games or a fall, or by hyperabduction, usually from falling while moving, such as during skiing and are known as 'Greenkeeper's thumb'. If the history is suggestive of a UCL injury and the patient has pain in that area, then an X-ray should be performed to exclude a fracture before joint stability is formally tested. If no fracture is present, the joint should be examined with the thumb in flexion and extension to determine stability. If UCL rupture is suspected, the patient should be referred to the orthopaedic team, as open surgical repair is often beneficial. If an uncomplicated sprain exists then adhesive tape strapping in the form of a thumb spica will provide the compression and rest the joint to enable the sprain to heal.

Mallet finger

This occurs as a result of forced flexion of the distal interphalangeal (DIP) joint or by a direct blow to the end of the finger, and is an injury commonly sustained by netball players. It is caused by rupture or avulsion of the extensor tendon. If an avulsion fracture of the distal phalanx is present, healing is usually more rapid than a tendon rupture. The patient presents in the ED with pain and a deformed finger and is unable to actively extend the fingertip distal to the DIP joint, causing drooping of the distal phalanges which may be slight or severe (Wang & Johnston 2001). Management involves splinting the finger to below the DIP joint in slight hyperextension. Patient education and cooperation are vital to the success of this treatment. The splint is usually plastic and needs to be removed frequently to clean the finger and prevent skin damage. It is important, however, that hyperextension of the DIP joint is maintained during this time. The patient should therefore be taught to apply and remove the splint while supporting the fingertip on a firm surface.

Compartment syndrome

Compartment syndrome is a common but potentially life-threatening condition that requires prompt treatment and recognition. Caused by high pressure in a closed fascial space so that capillary perfusion is too low for tissue viability, it is well recognized as a potentially devastating complication of fractures (Edwards 2004, Kashuk et al. 2009). If this pressure is allowed to rise and stay high, it causes permanent damage to the soft tissue structures and nerves within that compartment. The limbs contain compartments, so injuries where swelling occurs have the potential to cause compartment syndrome. The forearm contains dorsal and volar compartments, and the lower leg is divided into four compartments: lateral, anterior, superficial posterior and deep posterior. In addition to internal tissue swelling, constricting dressings or POP which is too tight can cause compartment syndrome. This is one reason why casts on new injuries tend to be either split or bivalved or back-slabs are applied.

Tissue pressure rises for a number of reasons, and often the primary injury is not in itself devastating. Any injury with the potential for haemorrhage or tissue swelling can result in compartment syndrome. There is no correlation between fractures and severity and tissue pressure. If pressure rises there is an increased volume in that area. There are two main causes:

- bleeding into the compartment, perhaps following a fracture or rupture of small vessels, will result in clot formation and increased compartmental pressure
- muscle swelling – this usually occurs after a period of ischaemia, e.g., following vascular damage.

During the ischaemic period, fluid leaks into tissues through damaged capillaries and membranes. When blood supply is restored, however, this situation continues because of capillary damage. This results in muscle oedema. This is why compartment syndrome is so common after major burn injury or as a follow-up to major crush injuries. Increased tissue pressure leads to hypoperfusion of the structure within the affected compartment. Tissue perfusion rises, restricting

venous return and causing reduced blood flow in major vessels; therefore the patient will have no tangible change in systemic blood pressure and pulses in the affected compartment will remain palpable. Tissue ischaemia can cause irreversible muscle and nerve damage unless nurses are familiar with the physiology of compartment syndrome and do not rely solely on traditional determinants, such as major pulses, to assume all is well.

The patient will complain of severe pain that is incompatible with the severity of the injury and paraesthesia. Pain may also occur away from the site of the primary injury. Symptoms are usually worse on movement or manual compression of the compartment. The patient often complains of numbness of the extremities distal to the compartment because of neurological compression. Motor function may also be impaired.

If any restrictive splints or dressings are in place these should be removed and the limb elevated in an attempt to reduce swelling. Initial treatment with mannitol can decompress compartment syndrome and avoid the need for surgery (Porter & Greaves 2003); however, if conservative treatment fails to restore sensation and relieve pain, fasciotomy will be necessary to prevent long-term damage. Fasciotomy has a high complication rate, however, as it transforms a closed lesion into an open wound (Fitzgerald et al. 2000). In all patients susceptible to compartment syndrome, early involvement of the orthopaedic and/or vascular team is essential. Specialist tissue-pressure monitoring gives an accurate portrait of how the patient is responding to conservative management and an indication of how quickly to intervene with fasciotomies. If left unchecked, the cycle of oedema and ischaemia results in muscle infarction, nerve injury and permanent loss of function in the extremity (Edwards 2004).

Conclusion

Musculoskeletal injury is one of the most common types of presentation to EDs. As this chapter has highlighted, it is imperative for emergency nurses to be able to assess musculoskeletal injury and identify life- or limb-threatening trauma, some of which may not seem devastating at first glance. An understanding of the underpinning anatomy and physiology of the musculoskeletal system has been provided in order to inform clinical decision-making and meet the needs of the individual patient and avoid long-term, preventable disability. As most of these patients will be discharged from the ED, the nurse has a crucial role as health educator in ensuring the patient looks after their injury, and prevents or minimizes long-term sequelae. In doing so, the emergency nurse may be assured of delivering quality care to this vulnerable group of patients.

References

Adams, N., 2004. Knee injuries. Emergency Nurse 11 (10), 19–27.

Aggarwal, A.K., Nagi, O.N., 2004. Open reduction and internal fixation of volar Barton's fractures: A prospective study. Journal of Orthopaedic Surgery 12 (2), 230–234.

American College of Surgeons, 2008. Advanced Trauma Life Support, eighth ed. American College of Surgeons, Chicago.

Audit Commission, 2000. United they Stand: Coordinating Care for Elderly People with Hip Fractures. The Stationary Office, London.

Babal, J.C., Mehlman, C.T., Klein, G., 2010. Nerve injuries associated with pediatric supracondylar humeral fractures: A meta-analysis. Journal of Pediatric Orthopedics 30 (3), 253–263.

Bachmann, L.M., Kolb, E., Koller, M.T., et al., 2003. Accuracy of Ottawa ankle rules to exclude fractures of the ankle and mid-foot: a systemic review. British Medical Journal 326 (7386), 405–406.

Beynnon, B.D., Renström, P.A., Haugh, L., et al., 2006. A prospective, randomized clinical investigation of the treatment of first-time ankle sprains. American Journal of Sports Medicine. 34 (9), 1401–1412.

Bickley, L.S., Szilagyi, P.G., 2008. Bates' Guide to Physical Examination and History Taking, tenth ed. Lippincott, Williams & Wilkins, Philadelphia.

Bickley, L.S., Szilagyi, P.G., 2009. Bates' Pocket Guide To Physical Examination And History Taking, sixth ed. Lippincott, Williams & Wilkins, Philadelphia.

Bowie, D., 2011. Choosing the right pain relief for patients with soft-tissue injuries. Emergency Nurse 19 (2), 28–30.

Brown, A.F.T., 1996. Accident & Emergency Diagnosis and Management. Butterworth-Heinemann, Oxford.

Cadogan, M., 2004. Femur injuries. In: Cameron, P., Jelinek, G., Kelly, A.M., Murray, L., Brown, A.F.T., Heyworth, J. (Eds.), Textbook of Emergency Medicine, second ed. Churchill Livingstone, Edinburgh.

Chin, H.W., Propp, P.A., Orban, D.J., 2009. Forearm and wrist. In: Marx, J., Hockberger, R., Walls, R. (Eds.), Rosen's Emergency Medicine: Concepts and Clinical Practice, seventh ed. Mosby Year Book, St Louis.

Ciernick, I.F., Meier, L., Hollinger, A., 1991. Humeral mobility after treatment with a hanging cast. Journal of Trauma 31 (2), 230–233.

Clasper, J., Ramasamy, A., 2011. Open fractures. In: Smith, J., Greaves, I., Porter, K. (Eds.), Oxford Desk Reference: Major Trauma. Oxford Medical Publications, Oxford.

Cole, P.A., 2002. Scapula fractures. Orthopedic Clinics of North America 33 (1), 1–18.

Collins, N.C., 2008. Is ice right? Does cryotherapy improve outcome for acute soft tissue injury? Emergency Medicine Journal 25 (2), 65–68.

Cooney, W.P., Linscheid, R.L., Dobyns, J.H., 1991. Fractures and dislocations of the wrist. In: Rockward, C.A., et al. (Eds.), Fractures in Adults, vol. 1. JB Lippincott, Philadelphia.

Dennis, H.H., Sze, A.C., Murphy, D., 2011. Prevalence of carpal fracture in Singapore. Journal of Hand Surgery 36 (2), 278–283.

Dickinson, K., Roberts, I., 2004. Medical antishock trousers (pneumatic antishock garments) for circulatory support in patients with trauma [Cochrane review]. Cochrane Database Systematic Review 4, 2–CD001856.

Edwards, S., 2004. Acute compartment syndrome. Emergency Nurse 12 (3), 32–38.

Eisenhart, A.W., Gaeta, T.J., Yens, D.P., 2003. Osteopathic Manipulative Treatment in the Emergency Department for Patients With Acute Ankle Injuries. Journal of the American Osteopathic Association 103 (9), 417.

El-Adl, W.A., El-Said, M.A., Boghdady, G.W., et al., 2008. Results of treatment of displaced supracondylar humeral fractures in children by percutaneous lateral cross-wiring technique. Strategies in Trauma and Limb Reconstruction 3 (1), 1–7.

Fayaz, H.C., Jupiter, J.B., 2010. Monteggia fractures in adults. Acta Chirurgiae Orthopaedicae et Traumatologiae Cechoslovaca 77 (6), 457–462.

Fitzgerald, A.M., Wilson, Y., Quaba, A., et al., 2000. Long-term sequelae of fasciotomy wounds. British Journal of Plastic Surgery 53 (8), 690–693.

Garden, R.S., 1964. Stability and union in subcapital fractures of the femur. Journal of Bone and Joint Surgery 46-B, 630.

Genge Jagmin, M., 1995. Musculoskeletal injuries. In: Kitt, S., Selfridge-Thomas, J., Proehl, J.A., Kaiser, J. (Eds.), Emergency Nursing: A Physiologic and Clinical Perspective, second ed. Saunders, Philadelphia.

Georgilas, I., Mouzopoulos, G., 2008. Anterior ankle dislocation without associated fracture: a case with an 11 year follow-up. Acta Orthopaedica Belgica 74 (2), 266–269.

Goldberg, H.D., Young, J.W.R., Reiner, B.I., 1992. Double injuries of the forearm: a common occurrence. Radiology 185 (1), 223–227.

Gordon, W.T., Grijalva, S., Potter, B.K., 2012. Damage control and austere environment external fixation: Techniques for the civilian provider. Journal of Orthopaedic Advances 21 (1), 22–31.

Greaves, L., Jones, J., 2002. Practical Emergency Medicine. Arnold, London.

Harness, N., Ring, D., Jupiter, J.B., 2004. Volar Barton's fractures with concomitant dorsal fracture in older patients. The Journal of Hand Surgery 29A (3), 439–445.

Harris, C.R., 1995. Ankle injuries. In: Ruiz, E., Cicero, J.J. (Eds.), Emergency Management of Skeletal Fractures. Mosby, St Louis.

Harris, C.R., Haller, P.R., 1995. The tibia and tibula. In: Ruiz, E., Cicero, J.J. (Eds.), Emergency Management of Skeletal Fractures. Mosby, St Louis.

Hauschild, O., Strohm, P.C., Culemann, U., et al., 2008. Mortality in patients with pelvic fractures: results from the German pelvic injury register. The Journal of Trauma Injury, Infection and Critical Care 64 (2), 449–455.

Herrera-Soto, J.A., Scherb, M., Duffy, M.F., et al., 2007. Fractures of the fifth metatarsal in children and adolescents. Journal of Pediatric Orthopedics 27 (4), 427–431.

Hopkins, M., 2010. A comparative analysis of the application of the Ottawa ankle rule. International Emergency Nursing 18 (4), 188–195.

Hovelius, L., Olofsson, A., Sandström, B., et al., 2008. Nonoperative treatment of primary anterior shoulder dislocation in patients forty years of age and younger: A prospective twenty-five year follow-up. The Journal of Bone & Joint Surgery 90 (5), 945–952.

Hunter, D., 2005. Diagnosis and management of scaphoid fractures: a literature review. Emergency Nurse 13 (7), 22–26.

Ingram, M.D., Watson, S.G., Skippage, P.L., et al., 2008. Urethral injuries after pelvic trauma: Evaluation with urethrography. RadioGraphics 28 (6), 1631–1643.

Kashuk, J.L., Moore, E.E., Pinski, S., et al., 2009. Lower extremity compartment syndrome in acute care surgery paradigm: safety lessons learned. Patient Safety in Surgery 3 (11), 11–16.

Khan, K.M., Cook, J.L., Taunton, J.E., et al., 2000. Overuse tendinosis, not tendonitis part 1: a new paradigm for a difficult clinical problem. The Physician and Sports Medicine 28 (5), 38–48.

Kelly, A.M., 2004. Injuries of the shoulder girdle. In: Cameron, P., Jelinek, G., Kelly, A.M., Murray, L., Brown, A.F.T., Heyworth, J. (Eds.), Textbook of Emergency Medicine, second ed. Churchill Livingstone, Edinburgh.

Kerr, J., 2005. Achilles tendon injury: assessment and management in the ED. Emergency Nurse 13 (2), 32–38.

Knapton, P., 1999. Shoulder injury: A case study. Emergency Nurse 6 (10), 25–28.

Kyle, R.F., Gustilo, R.B., Premer, R.F., 1979. Analysis of 622 intertrochanteric hip fractures: a retrospective and prospective study. Journal of Bone and Joint Surgery 61 (2), 216.

Larsen, D., 2002. Assessment and management of foot and ankle fractures. Nursing Standard 17 (6), 37–46.

Lisk, R., Raison, N., Lawton, K., et al., 2011. Improving the management of pressure ulcer care in fracture neck of femur patients Communications to the Spring Meeting of the British Geriatrics Society. p32. 4–6_May_2011 BT Convention Centre Liverpool.

Logan, A.J., Lindau, T.R., 2008. The management of distal ulnar fractures in adults: a review of the literature and recommendations. Strategies in Trauma and Limb Reconstruction 3 (2), 49–56.

Loveridge, N., 2002. Lateral ankle sprains. Emergency Nurse 10 (2), 29–33.

Lynch, T.H., Martínez-Piñeiro, L., Plas, E., et al., 2005. EAU guidelines on urological trauma. European Urology 47 (1), 1–15.

Magnusson, A.R., 2009. Humerus and Elbow. In: Marx, J., Hockberger, R., Walls, R. (Eds.), Rosen's Emergency Medicine: Concepts and Clinical Practice, seventh ed. Mosby Year Book, St Louis.

Mattox, K.L., Bickell, W., Pepe, P.E., et al., 1989. Prospective MAST study in 911 patients. Journal of Trauma 29 (8), 1104–1111.

Mayeda, D.V., 2009. Ankle and foot. In: Marx, J., Hockberger, R., Walls, R. (Eds.), Rosen's Emergency Medicine: Concepts and Clinical Practice, seventh ed. Mosby Year Book, St Louis.

Mayfield, J.K., Johnson, R.P., Kilcoyne, R.F., 1980. Carpal dislocations: pathomechanics and progressive perilunar instability. Journal of Hand Surgery 5 (3), 226–241.

McNally, C., Gillespie, M., 2004. Scaphoid fractures. Emergency Nurse 12 (1), 21–25.

McRae, R., 2006. Pocketbook of Orthopaedics and Fractures. Churchill Livingstone, Edinburgh.

Middleton, P., 2011. Trauma retrieval. In: Smith, J., Greaves, I., Porter, K.M. (Eds.), Oxford Desk Reference: Major Trauma. Oxford University Press, Oxford.

Mills, K., Morton, R., Page, G., 1995. Color Atlas and Text of Emergencies, second ed. Mosby-Wolfe, London.

National Clinical Guideline Centre, 2011. The management of hip fracture in adults. Royal College of Physicians, London.

Nowotarski, P.J., Turen, C.H., Brumback, R.J., et al., 2000. The Journal of Bone and Joint Surgery America 82 (6), 781.

O'Dwyer, H., O'Sullivan, P., Fitzgerald, D., et al., 2004. The fat pad sign following elbow trauma in adults: its usefulness and reliability in suspecting occult fracture. Journal of Computer Assisted Tomography 28 (4), 562–565.

O'Steen, D., 2003. Orthopaedic and neurovascular trauma. In: Newbery, L. (Ed.), Sheehy's Emergency Nursing: Principles and Practice, fifth ed. Mosby, St Louis.

Perron, A.D., Hersh, R.E., Brady, W.J., et al., 2001. Orthopedic pitfalls in the ED: Galeazzi and Monteggia fracture-dislocation. American Journal of Emergency Medicine 19 (3), 225–228.

Phillips, T.G., Reibach, A.M., Slomiany, W.P., 2004. Diagnosis and management of scaphoid fractures. American Family Physician 70 (5), 879–884.

Porter, K., Greaves, I., 2003. Crush injury and crush syndrome: a consensus statement. Emergency Nurse 11 (6), 26–30.

Proehl, J., 2009. Emergency Nursing Procedures, fourth ed. WB Saunders, Philadelphia.

Quday, K., 1995. Shoulder injuries. In: Ruiz, E., Cicero, J.J. (Eds.), Emergency Management of Skeletal Fractures, Mosby, St Louis.

Rana, M., Banerjee, R., 2006. Scapular Fracture After Electric Shock. Annals of the Royal College of Surgeons England 88 (2), 143.

Rourke, K., 2003. An orthopaedic nurse practitioner's practical guide to evaluating knee injuries. Journal of Emergency Nursing 29 (4), 366–372.

Routt Jr., M.L., Nork, S.E., Mills, W.J., 2002. High energy pelvic ring disruptions. Orthopedic Clinics of North America 33, 59–72.

Rowley, D.I., Dent, J.A., 1997. The Musculoskeletal System: Core Topics in the New Curriculum. Arnold, London.

Ruiz, E., 1995. Pelvic, sacral and acetabular fractures. In: Ruiz, E., Cicero, J.J. (Eds.), Emergency Management of Skeletal Fractures. Mosby, St Louis.

Rusnak, R.A., 1995. Examination of the hand and management of finger-tip injuries. In: Ruiz, E., Cicero, J.J. (Eds.), Emergency Management of Skeletal Fractures. Mosby, St Louis.

Ryan, A., 2004. Rotator cuff tears. Emergency Nurse 12 (4), 27–37.

Safran, M.R., Achazewski, J.E., Benedetti, R.S., et al., 1999. Lateral ankle sprains: a comprehensive review. Part 2: treatment and rehabilitation with an emphasis on the athlete. Medicine and Science in Sports and Exercise 31 (7), S438–S447.

Scalea, T.M., Burgess, A.R., 2004. Pelvic fractures. In: Moore, E.E., Feliciano, D.V., Mattox, K.L. (Eds.), Trauma, fifth ed. McGraw-Hill, New York.

Schatzker, J., McBroom, R., Bruce, D., 1979. The tibial plateau fracture: the Toronto experience, 1968–1975. Clinical Orthopeadics and Related Research 138, 94–104.

Schmidt, M., Armbrect, A., Havermann, D., 1992. Results of surgical management of scapula fractures. 78th annual meeting of the Swiss Society of Accident Surgery and Occupational Diseases. Z-Unfallchir Versicherungsmed 85, 186–188.

Smith, M., 2003. Ankle sprain: A literature search. Emergency Nurse 11 (3), 12–16.

Smith, M., 2005. Orthopaedic trauma. In: O'Shea, R.A. (Ed.), Principles and Practice of Trauma Nursing. Elsevier Churchill Livingstone, Edinburgh.

Snell, R.S., 2000. Clinical Anatomy for Medical Students, sixth ed. Lippincott Williams, Wilkins, Philadelphia.

Snyder, P.E., 2002. Fractures. In: Maher, A.B., Salmond, S.W., Pellino, T.A. (Eds.), Orthopaedic Nursing, second ed. WB Saunders, Philadelphia.

Starr, A.J., Griffin, D.R., Reinert, C.M., et al., 2002. Pelvic ring disruptions: Prediction of associated injuries, transfusion requirement, pelvic arteriography, complications, and mortality. Journal of Orthopaedic Trauma 16 (8), 553–561.

Stiell, I.G., Greenberg, G.H., McKnight, R.D., et al., 1992. A study to develop clinical decision rules for the use of radiography in acute ankle injuries. Annals of Emergency Medicine 21 (4), 384–390.

Stovitz, S., Johnson, R., 2003. NSAIDs and musculoskeletal treatment. What is the evidence? The Physician and Sports Medicine 31 (1), 35–41.

Summers, A., 2005. Recognising and treating Colles' type fractures in emergency care settings. Emergency Nurse 13 (6), 26–33.

Tsai, A.K., Ruiz, E., 1995. The elbow joint. In: Ruiz, E., Cicero, J.J. (Eds.), Emergency Management of Skeletal Fractures. Mosby, St Louis.

Van Onselen, E.B.H., Karim, R.B., Joris Hage, J., et al., 2003. Journal of Hand Surgery (British and European Volume 28B (5), 491–495.

Vinnars, B., Pietreanu, M., Bodestedt, A., et al., 2008. Nonoperative compared with operative treatment of acute scaphoid fractures – A randomized clinical trial. The Journal of Bone and Joint Surgery, American volume 90 (6), 1176–1185.

Wang, Q.C., Johnson, B.A., 2001. Fingertip injuries. American Family Physician 63, 1961–1966.

Ward, W., 1999. Key issues in nurse requested X-rays. Emergency Nurse 6 (9), 19–23.

Wickham, N., 1997. Pressure area care in A&E: Part Two. Emergency Nurse 5 (4), 25–29.

Wilkins, K.E., 2002. Changes in the Management of Monteggia Fractures. Journal of Pediatric Orthopaedics 22 (4), 548–554.

Winter, M., Balaguer, T., Bessière, C., et al., 2007. Surgical treatment of the boxer's fracture: transverse pinning versus intramedullary pinning. Journal of Hand Surgery European Volume 32 (6), 709–713.

Wyatt, J.P., Illingworth, R.N., Clancy, M.J., Munro, P., Robertson, C.E., 1999. Oxford Handbook of Accident and Emergency Medicine. Oxford University Press, Oxford.

Yuen, M.C., Yap, P.G., Chan, Y.T., et al., 2001. An easy method to reduce anterior shoulder dislocation: the Spaso technique. Emergency Medicine Journal 18 (5), 370–372.

Zacchilli, M.A., Owens, B.D., 2010. Epidemiology of shoulder dislocations presenting to emergency departments in the United States. The Journal of Bone and Joint Surgery (American) 92 (3), 542–549.

Zagorski, J.B., Latta, L.I., Zych, G.A., et al., 1988. Diaphyseal fractures of the humerus treatment with prefabricated braces. Journal of Bone and Joint Surgery 70A, 607–610.

Spinal injuries

Mike Paynter

CHAPTER CONTENTS

Introduction

Spinal cord injury (SCI) is one of the most disabling and catastrophic outcomes of injury in a person's life. The annual incidence of SCI in the UK is about 10–15 per million of the population, with the majority of patients male, usually below the age of 40 years, with a quarter of all cord-injured patients being below the age of 20 (Gallagher 2005). Many of these patients are left with permanent disabilities. The overall physical, emotional and financial consequences of disability are devastating for those injured, and for their families and friends (Zhang et al. 2013). The average Emergency Department (ED) serving a population of 250 000 is likely to receive fewer than four new spinal cord injured patients per year (El Masri 2010). All emergency care clinicians need to be familiar with the initial management of these patients.

Although the effect of the initial injury is irreversible, the spine and spinal cord are at further risk from secondary insult either by accidental ill-handling at the incident scene or by subsequent poor management in the ED. This chapter explores the identification and management of spinal cord injuries in the ED.

Anatomy and physiology

The vertebral column is a series of stacked bones that support the head and trunk and provide the bony encasement for the spinal cord. It comprises 33 vertebrae: 7 cervical (C1–7), 12 thoracic (T1–12), 5 lumbar (L1–5), 5 fused sacral and usually 4 rudimentary coccygeal vertebrae. With the exception of the atlas (C1) and the axis (C2), all vertebrae are anatomically alike but different in size and function (Fig. 7.1).

The human vertebral column enables people to assume an upright position. It provides a base of muscle attachments, protects the spinal cord and vital organs in the thorax, and allows for body movements to occur. A vertebral body consists of the body, a vertebral arch, and a vertebral foramen. The arch of the vertebra is composed of two pedicles, two laminae, four facets, two transverse processes and the spinous process, which can be palpated. Intervertebral cartilaginous discs provide cushioning and shock absorption between vertebral segments.

The spinal cord lies protected within the spinal canal, which is a hollow tunnel extending the length of the vertebral column. The spinal cord descends from the medulla oblongata near the atlas to the level of the second lumbar vertebra. The spinal cord is nearly circular in section and about 1 cm in diameter, with two enlargements. On cross-section, the spinal cord has a grey matter appearing in the form of the letter H. The grey matter consists of nerve cells

http://dx.doi.org/10.1016/B978-0-7020-4315-4.00007-3

Atlas Axis

Cervical curve

Thoracic curve

Lumbar curve

Sacral curve

Cervical vertebrae (7)

Thoracic vertebrae (12)

Lumbar vertebrae (5)

Sacral vertebrae (5)

Coccygeal vertebrae (4)

Figure 7.1 ● Anatomy of spinal vertebrae.

that act as relay stations for nerve impulses transmitted up and down the spinal cord. White matter surrounds the grey matter and contains longitudinal myelinated fibres organized in tracts or bundles to carry information to and from the brain. Ascending tracts are sensory, and descending tracts are motor (Bickley et al. 2005).

Pathophysiology

The cervical vertebrae are the most mobile part of the spine, so this area is the most frequent site of injury. The rib cage keeps the vertebrae from T1 and T10 stable and relatively immobile. The second most common site of injury is the thoracolumbar junction at T11 to L2. This is a transition area between the rigid thoracolumbar region and the more mobile lumbar region (Semonin-Holleran 2003). Force applied to the cervical spine (c-spine) does not always result in localized vertebral damage, however, because the flexibility of the region and the ability of the neck to move in *anteroposterolateral* directions, can help transfer the force downwards to the thoracic spine where there is little or no flexibility (Sheerin 2005).

Vertebral column injury, with or without neurological deficits, must always be sought and excluded in a patient with multiple trauma. Any injury above the clavicle should prompt a search for a c-spine injury. Approximately 15% of patients

sustaining such an injury will have an actual c-spine injury. Approximately 55% of spinal injuries occur in the cervical region, 15% in the thoracic region, 15% at the thoracolumbar junction, and 15% in the lumbosacral area. Approximately 5% of patients have an associated spinal injury, while 25% of spinal injury patients have at least a mild head injury (American College of Surgeons 2008).

Approximately 8–10% of patients with a vertebral fracture have a secondary fracture of another vertebra, often at a distant site. These secondary fractures are usually associated with more violent mechanisms of injury, such as ejection or rollover. Owing to the mechanism of injury, many patients with spinal injury often have other associated injuries, including head, intrathoracic or intra-abdominal injuries, which may alter priorities in management (Lowery et al. 2001). Falls account for 46%, road traffic accidents (RTAs) account for 34% and sports-related incidents account for 10% of spinal injuries in the UK (Harrison 2004). The forces involved in RTAs can cause such severe damage to vertebrae C1 and C2 that the cord is affected, so that the person involved cannot self-ventilate. In such circumstances, death is the most common outcome (Greaves & Porter 2007).

The majority of spinal cord injuries are closed. Table 7.1 outlines the specific categories of movement that may result in spinal cord injury.

Table 7.1 Categories of movement that may result in spinal cord injury	
Category	**Mechanism of injury**
Hyperextension	The head is forced back and the vertebrae of the cervical region are placed in an over-extended position
Hyperflexion	The head is forced forward and the vertebrae are placed in an over-flexion position
Axial loading	A severe blow to the top of the head causes a blunt downward force on the vertebral column
Compression	Forces from above and below compress the vertebrae
Lateral bend	The head and neck are bent to one side, beyond the normal range of motion
Over-rotation and distraction	The head turns to one side and the cervical vertebrae are forced beyond normal limits

(After Semonin-Holleran R (2003) Spinal trauma. In: Newberry L, ed. Sheehy's Emergency Nursing: Principles and Practice, 5th edn. St Louis: Mosby.)

The most common type of injury mechanism is excessive flexion. This usually occurs following RTAs when the patient's head strikes the steering wheel or windscreen and the spine is forced into hyperflexion with the chin thrown forward to the chest. Rupture of the posterior ligaments results in forward dislocation of the spine (Fig. 7.2).

Axial loading or compression-type injuries can occur when the head strikes an object and the weight of the still-moving body bears against the now stationary head, such as when the

Figure 7.2 • Spinal flexion injury. • (After Jaworski MA, Wirtz KM (1995) Spinal trauma. In: Kitt S, Selfridge-Thomas J, Proehl JA, Kaiser J, eds. Emergency Nursing: A Physiological and Clinical Perspective. Philadelphia: WB Saunders.)

Figure 7.3 • Spinal compression injury. • (After Jaworski MA, Wirtz KM (1995) Spinal trauma. In: Kitt S, Selfridge-Thomas J, Proehl JA, Kaiser J, eds. Emergency Nursing: A Physiological and Clinical Perspective. Philadelphia: WB Saunders.)

head of an unrestrained car passenger is flung into the windscreen or during a dive into shallow water. Vertebral bodies are wedged and compressed, and the burst vertebral fragments enter the spinal canal, piercing the cord (Jaworski & Wirtz 1995) (Fig. 7.3).

Rotational injuries (Fig. 7.4) can result from a number of causes. Disruption of the entire ligamentous structure, fracture and fracture-dislocation of spinal facets may occur. Flexion-rotation injuries are highly unstable fractures.

Distraction, or over-elongation of the spine, occurs when one part of the spine is stable and the rest is in longitudinal motion. This 'pulling apart' of the spine can easily cause stretching and tearing of the cord. It is a common mechanism of injury in children's playground accidents and in hangings (Pre-Hospital Trauma Life Support Committee 2006).

Patient assessment

History-taking

The importance of obtaining the patient's history and establishing the mechanism of injury cannot be overemphasized. Obtaining an accurate history represents 90 % of the diagnosis (American College of Surgeons 2008). A fully documented pre-hospital history should be obtained from the ambulance personnel, police officers and others involved in the pre-hospital phase of patient care. If the patient has been injured as the result of an RTA, digital pictures of the incident scene and the damage sustained to vehicles can provide valuable information about the mechanisms involved. If taken, these photographs should be printed off and included in the patient's hospital notes (Greaves et al. 2005).

A high index of suspicion is needed if patients are to be managed correctly (Caroline 2007).

SCI should be suspected with any of the following:

- a history of significant trauma and altered mental status from intoxication
- a history of seizure activity since the accident

Figure 7.4 ● Spinal rotation injury.

- any complaint of neck pain or altered sensation in the upper extremities
- a complaint of midline neck tenderness
- a history of loss of consciousness
- an injury above the clavicle
- a fall greater than three times the patient's height
- a fall that results in a fracture of the heels
- an unrestrained (no seat belt) person with a facial injury
- significant injuries in a RTA that result in chest and intra-abdominal injuries.

The patient may complain of a feeling of 'electric shock' or 'hot water' running down his back. A history of incontinence before arrival in the ED may be reported (Semonin-Holleran 2003). Failure to suspect a spinal injury will lead to failure in its detection, with potentially devastating consequences for the patient.

The patient's ability to walk should not be a factor in determining whether he needs to be treated for spine injury. Not all patients will have a dramatic entrance into the ED; in one North American study 17 % of patients who required surgical repair of unstable spine injuries were found 'walking around' at the incident scene or walked into the ED in the local hospital (McSwain 1992). A nod of the head or a sneeze in such patients could easily push an unstable fragment of vertebra against the spinal cord. Therefore an unstable spine can only be ruled out by careful physical assessment, radiographic imaging or a lack of any potential mechanism.

Spine immobilization

When the patient arrives in the emergency department, extreme care is required in the transfer from the ambulance stretcher to the trauma trolley: total spinal immobilization is the goal. The use of a backboard is ideal for the transfer of such patients.

Once the patient is on the trauma trolley, protection of the c-spine should be given the same priority as the airway (American College of Surgeons 2008). All emergency personnel involved in caring for the patient must be continuously aware that imprudent movement of the spine has the potential to cause secondary injury. The patient must have the c-spine immobilized in a semi-rigid well-fitting cervical collar, have sandbags either side for lateral stabilization and have the forehead taped to the trauma trolley. Collars do reduce movement of the neck, but even correctly fitted ones allow over 30° of flexion, extension and rotation, this is improved by the use of sandbags and tape, which on their own provide better cervical protection than a collar alone (James et al. 2004). Cervical spine injury should be suspected in the presence of head injury, but cervical collars significantly increase intracranial pressure (Ho et al. 2002).

It should also be noted that in children the head is large and the posterior musculature is not well developed. If placed on a rigid board or trolley, a child's head is typically moved to severe flexion. When immobilizing children, significant padding under the torso is usually necessary to maintain the immobilization (Pre-Hospital Trauma Life Support Committee 2006).

One member of the ED team must remain at the patient's head and ensure total in-line immobilization of the spine and airway patency. This team member should communicate with the patient, explaining what is happening and why. The patient is in an unnatural environment, probably surrounded by strangers, and is likely to feel out of control of his situation because of carer interventions. Reassurance and support are therefore vital in gaining the patient's cooperation. If the patient is confused, agitated and restless, it is advisable to leave only the semi-rigid cervical collar on and not to use forcible restraint. Otherwise the patient will be liable to twist and thrash, causing unwanted movement of the neck and trunk and a possible total transection of a partially transected spinal cord. Once the patient has become settled, full immobilization can be initiated.

Airway

Obstruction of the airway is an ever-present threat in managing patients with suspected c-spine injuries. Normal efforts used for maintaining airway patency are liable to exacerbate the injuries. If the patient can talk in a normal voice and give appropriate answers to questions, the airway is patent and the brain is being perfused (American College of Surgeons 2008), however, high-flow oxygen should be given. In an unconscious patient, potential problems come from the tongue falling back against the posterior pharyngeal wall and causing an obstruction. Foreign bodies, such as loose teeth and broken denture plates, and the risk of regurgitation and aspiration all put the airway at risk.

Obstruction caused by the tongue is corrected by the chin lift. The airway can then be maintained by the insertion of an oropharyngeal airway (Greaves & Porter 2007). To perform the chin lift, place the fingers of one hand under the mandible and gently lift the chin upward; the thumb of the same hand lightly depresses the lower lip to open the mouth. The chin lift is the method of choice for the patient with a suspected spinal injury, since it does not risk aggravating a possible fracture.

The jaw thrust is another technique. This is performed by grasping the angles of the lower jaw, one hand on each side; forward displacement of the mandible will open the airway. Again, great care must be taken not to flex or extend the neck. All debris, such as broken teeth or loose denture plates, must be removed in order to prevent potential problems. These can be removed using Magill forceps under direct vision.

Blood and vomit must be removed immediately. A rigid wide-bore suction device, with head-down tilt of the trauma trolley, will help to prevent aspiration. The semi-prone recovery position is contraindicated, since it involves cervical rotation. Endotracheal intubation with a cuffed tube is the definitive method of securing a patent airway, preventing aspiration and aiding ventilation, oxygenation and suctioning. If intubation is required, it must be performed by a suitably skilled and experienced member of the team (Greaves & Porter 2007). During intubation, in-line c-spinal immobilization must be maintained. Cricoid pressure can be applied through the aperture in the front of the semi-rigid collar. Stimulation of the oropharynx during intubation or suctioning may cause a vagal discharge, resulting in profound bradycardia. The heart rate should be closely monitored during intubation and supported if necessary with intravenous atropine.

Breathing

Ventilation may be affected by the level of the cord injury, aspiration and presence of primary lung injury. In the absence of major airway obstruction and flail chest, the presence of paradoxical breathing is considered highly suggestive of c-spine injury. Paradoxical breathing occurs because of loss of motor tone and paralysis of thoracic muscle innervated by thoracic spinal segments. Diaphragmatic action results in a negative intrapleural pressure. As a consequence of chest wall paralysis the tendency is for the soft tissues of the thorax to 'cave in', producing paradoxical chest movement. The diaphragm needs to undertake the full work of breathing, including overcoming added resistance to ventilation caused by paradoxical chest wall movement. In addition to standard respiratory status assessment, continuous pulse oximetry and assessment of vital capacity are necessary. Early intubation should be considered if vital capacity is inadequate or falling (Wassertheil 2004).

Circulation

Complete injuries above T1, and perhaps T4, can be expected to have clinically significant manifestations of neurogenic shock. The clinical signs are bradycardia, peripheral vasodilatation and cessation of sweating. Priapism in a trauma is due to penile vasodilatation from parasympathetic nervous system stimulation and loss of sympathetic nervous system

control. It is highly suggestive of SCI, especially if the patient is unconscious.

Circulatory status is best assessed by conscious state, urine output and venous pressure monitoring. In the early phases of management, close urine output monitoring is of major importance. Early insertion of a urinary catheter not only allows measurement of urinary output but may also assist in identifying occult renal tract injury, and also prevent bladder distension.

Disability

Spinal cord injury has an association with significant head trauma (Wassertheil 2004). In patients with an altered conscious state due to head trauma, brief mental assessment and pupillary reflexes are important.

Once the patient has a safe patent airway and full c-spine precautions are in place, further examination can proceed. All clothing needs to be removed to facilitate examination; this should cause minimum discomfort and not aggravate potential injuries. Under no circumstances must the neck or trunk be flexed, extended or rotated during this process as a SCI must be assumed until proven otherwise. Extending the arms to the side or elevating them above the head causes angulation of the shoulder girdle and substantial movement of the c-spine. Therefore, to ensure no disruption to the cervical immobilization, it is often safest to cut away clothing. Clothing that remains under the patient can be removed during the later log roll.

Once the airway and c-spine are protected, a full set of baseline vital signs must be recorded:

- the patient's neurological status
- respiratory rate
- pulse
- blood pressure
- temperature
- blood glucose levels
- 12-lead electrocardiograph.

In patients who are potentially haemodynamically unstable, cardiac monitoring and measurement of oxygen saturation should be mandatory.

Secondary survey and the log roll

As part of the secondary survey, the patient's back must be fully examined. Obviously this involves turning the injured patient. Without losing control of the in-line c-spine immobilization, this can be safely accomplished by using the log roll technique. Four members of the team are required to safely execute this procedure (Fig. 7.5). The senior team member assumes manual control of the c-spine; only then are tapes and sandbags removed. The remaining three members of the team take responsibility for the chest, pelvis and legs (Griffiths & Gallimore 2005). The senior person at the patient's head coordinates the roll. The person holding the

Figure 7.5 • Log rolling the spinal patient. (A) Initial position; (B) patient on side during roll. • (From Greaves I, Hodgetts T, Porter T (2005) Emergency Care: A Textbook for Paramedics, 2nd edn. London: WB Saunders.)

leg keeps the lateral malleolus in line with the hip, preventing adduction. The patient is then smoothly rolled in a well-coordinated move, avoiding any rotational movements of individual spinal segments.

The cervical, thoracic and lumbar spines are all examined for areas of deformity, grating crepitus, haematomas and areas of increased pain on palpation. An assessment for paraesthesia is made, noting the location and level. Finally a rectal examination is performed, the aim of which is to assess rectal sphincter tone, and thereby the sacral nerves. If voluntary sphincter contraction occurs, the spinal injury is classified as incomplete (Jaworski & Wirtz 1995). Before the patient is returned to the supine position, all remaining clothing that may have been left under the patient can be removed at this stage. Debris such as windscreen glass fragments can easily be cleared away with the aid of a portable car vacuum, thus minimizing further risk to the patient's skin and pressure areas.

Once full posterior examination of the patient has been performed, the person holding the head gives the command for all members of the team to return the patient to the supine position. Once returned, sandbags and tape are reapplied and manual immobilization can then be discontinued.

The risk of pressure sores on long spinal boards is very high and they can develop in less than two hours. The spinal board should be used as a pre-hospital extrication or transfer device, and should therefore be removed at the earliest opportunity once in hospital (McCarthy 2011).

Cervical spine fractures

The c-spine is the most mobile part of the entire vertebral column and as such is liable to considerable injury. Sudden violent forces can move the spine beyond its normal range of movement, either by impacting on the head and neck or by pushing the trunk out from under the head. Since extreme forces are required to damage the c-spine, patients will often present with severe head and maxillofacial wounds. Despite what may look like horrific injuries, the ATLS principles of patient care should be applied: airway and c-spine management is first and foremost, followed by breathing and circulatory support as appropriate.

Good-quality radiographs are essential for accurate diagnosis of spinal injury (Raby et al. 2005). There are only three radiographs that are mandatory in the resuscitation room and these can be obtained as soon as life-threatening problems have been identified and controlled. The first is a lateral c-spine view, which will detect 85% of significant c-spine injuries, and the other two are of the chest and pelvis. The lateral c-spine views can be obtained without interrupting immobilization.

All seven cervical vertebrae, C1 to the C7/T1 junction, must be identified on the lateral views. If problems are encountered viewing C7, the application of downwards traction on the arms will pull the shoulders down and should make viewing easier. Sometimes this proves impossible. If this is the case, a 'swimmer's view' of the lower c-spine and upper thoracic areas can be obtained. Occasionally 'trauma oblique' views may be required, by angulation these views project the shoulders out of the way, and the view is no longer lateral, but may be sufficient to confirm normal alignment and integrity of the vertebrae (Begg 2005, Sakthieval-Wainford 2009). At least 70% of fractures, dislocations or subluxations will be visible on the lateral radiograph with most common injuries around the C1–C2 articulations and between C5 and C7 (Raby et al. 2005).

The type of vertebral injury most likely to produce neurological damage is a fracture-dislocation. Approximately 5% of cervical trauma X-rays are misinterpreted and 50% of missed c-spine fractures are due to incomplete reviews (McCarthy 2011). Inadequate or misinterpreted radiographs of the c-spine are potentially devastating for the patient. It is vital that the ED nurse insists on continued c-spine immobilization until all radiographs have been reviewed and C1 to C7 have been cleared of abnormality. Clinical history and examination must always take precedence over apparently normal radiographs; important neck injuries may still be present despite normal-looking plain radiographs. Spinal cord injury without radiological abnormality (SCIWORA) can occur and may be due to ligamentous damage with instability or other soft tissue injuries such as central disc prolapsed (Grundy 2002). SCIWORA is relatively common in injured children because the greater mobility of the developing spine affords less protection to the spinal cord.

All c-spine fractures should be treated as unstable in the emergency department and, depending upon neurological examination, be referred to the orthopaedic, neurosurgical or specialist spinal unit teams (McRae & Esser 2008). That noted, most of these cases are alert and stable adults and <1% have a c-spine fracture (Stiell et al. 1997) and, increasingly, nurses' clearance of c-spine injuries is taking place in EDs. This means the patient does not need to have prolonged periods of unnecessary immobilization (Clement et al. 2011).

Thoracolumbar spine fractures

Fractures of the thoracic spine between T2 and T10 are usually the result of hyperflexion which produces a wedge compression of one or more vertebrae. Wedge compression fractures of the thorax are rarely unstable because the rib cage provides fairly rigid support; however, these fractures can be rendered unstable if there are associated fractures of the ribs and sternum. Fractures of the thoracic vertebrae tend to be more common in elderly patients, where they are often associated with a degree of osteoporosis and can sometimes occur with minimal trauma (van der Jagt-Willems 2012). In younger patients, severe trauma is required to cause these fractures (McRae & Esser 2008). Fractures of the thoracolumbar region are frequently due to the relative immobility of the thoracic spine compared with the lumbar spine. The mechanism of injury is usually acute hyperflexion and rotation, and hence these fractures are commonly unstable.

Falling from a height and landing on the feet can result in compression and axial loading. Typically, falls from a height are from second- or third-storey levels (National Spinal Injuries Unit 2005). The individual falls and the fall is broken by contact with a solid barrier causing a sudden change in the velocity of the body to 0 mph. On impact, an equal and opposite force is created and meets the impacting individual. If the person falls on their feet, the two forces travel longitudinally along the vertebral column, which causes 'axial loading', and meet at a point where the forces are concentrated. This can compress vertebrae and the spinal cord, cause burst fractures, and force bone fragments to enter the spinal canal. There may also be fractures to the lower extremities. If the person falls on the buttocks, a hyperflexion injury to the lumbar area may result, again with compression fractures (Sheerin 2005).

The impact of landing forces the weight of the head and thorax down against the lumbar vertebrae, while the sacral vertebrae remain stationary. Fractures of the lumbar vertebrae are reasonably common, especially at the T12/L1 and L4/S levels (McRae & Esser 2008); 20% of falls greater than 15 feet involve associated fractures of the lumbar vertebrae.

Isolated sacral fractures are uncommon and are frequently associated with much more serious fractures of the pelvis. As with c-spine injuries, the patient must be kept in the neutral position and complete spinal immobilization maintained. The log roll must be employed to facilitate examination of the back.

Spinal cord injury

The main risk factor associated with spinal fractures is damage to the spinal cord. If the fracture is stable, the cord is safe, but if the fracture is unstable the possibility of cord injury is present. Stable fractures are not likely to displace further than at the time of injury; an unstable fracture or dislocation is, however, liable to further displacement, therefore posing considerable risk to the spinal cord with some 16% of SCI patients dying before they reach hospital (McCarthy 2011) (Box 7.1).

The spinal cord is the communication pathway between the brain and the body. A transection of the cord will render all nerves distal to the injury useless. A conscious patient will be able to identify pain at the site of the injury but have no sensation below it; from the moment of injury the patient feels cut in two. Voluntary movement below the level of the cord injury is lost immediately and the muscles become flaccid. The bladder and rectum are paralyzed; however the bladder sphincter subsequently recovers and causes acute urinary retention.

The position of the cord injury has a direct effect on the patient's prognosis. Complete transection of the cord at levels C1, C2 or C3 is incompatible with life. Damage to the cord at this level causes both intercostal and diaphragmatic movement to cease, and only intermittent positive pressure ventilation (IPPV) will keep the patient alive. Lower cervical cord damage may leave the phrenic nerve sufficiently intact to maintain diaphragmatic breathing. Diaphragmatic breathing only, provided from C4 to T6, is liable to reduce vital capacity and a subsequent compensatory tachypnoea will develop. If tidal volume and vital capacity are reduced, consideration must be given to intubating and providing IPPV (Wassertheil 2004) (Table 7.2).

Box 7.1

Summary of statistics associated with spinal cord injury (McCarthy 2011)

Causes of SCI

- Motor vehicle collision 38–50 %
- Falls 18–22 %
- Violence 11–25 %
- Sports 7–10 %

Level of SCI

- Cervical 50–64 %
- Thoracic 17–19 %
- Thoracolumbar 15 %
- Lumbar 15–24 %

Type of SCI

- Complete tetraplegia 19 %
- Incomplete tetraplegia 30 %
- Complete paraplegia 29 %
- Incomplete paraplegia 22 %

Other spinal injury facts

- 16 % of SCI patients will die prior to hospitalization
- Neurological deterioration is seen in up to 50 % of cases where there is a missed diagnosis or mismanagement of SCI
- 50 % of SCI patients have a complete injury at the time of presentation
- 85 % of SCI patients who survive the first 24 h after injury will still be alive 10 years post-injury
- 25 % of SCI patients will have a head injury

(After McCarthy M (2011) Spinal injury. In J Smith, I Greaves, K Porter (Eds.). Oxford Desk Reference: Major Trauma. Oxford, Oxford Medical Publications.)

Table 7.2 Assessing level of spinal injury

Muscle group	Nerve supply	Reflex
Diaphragm	C3, C4, C5	
Shoulder abductors	C5	
Elbow flexors	C5, C6	Biceps jerk
Supinators/pronators	C6	Supinator jerk
Wrist extensors	C6	
Wrist flexors	C7	
Elbow extensors	C7	Triceps jerk
Finger extensors	C7	
Finger flexors	C8	
Intrinsic hand muscles	T1	
Hip flexors	L1, L2	
Hip adductors	L2, L3	
Knee extensors	L3, L4	Knee jerk
Ankle dorsiflexors	L4, L5	
Toe extensors	L5	
Knee flexors	L4, L5, S1	
Ankle plantar flexors	S1, S2	Ankle jerk
Toe flexors	S1, S2	
Anal sphincter	S2, S3, S4	Bulbocavernosus reflex Anal reflex

(After Szilagyi PG, Bickley LS (2004) Bates' Guide to Physical Examination and History Taking, 8th edition. Philadelphia, Lippincott Williams & Wilkins.)

If the patient is unconscious, the following clinical findings will indicate a cervical cord injury:

- diaphragmatic breathing
- weakness or paralysis
- hypotension with bradycardia
- flaccidity
- loss of bulbocavernosus reflex and anal tone
- evidence of painful stimuli above the clavicles
- ability to flex, but not extend, the elbows
- priapism.

Since the urinary bladder is paralyzed when the cord is damaged, acute urinary retention will occur. Insertion under strict aseptic technique of an indwelling urinary catheter will be required to decompress the bladder in order to monitor the patient's haemodynamic status. Short periods of local pressure result in pressure sores. It is essential that all clothing and debris are removed from under the patient at the earliest opportunity, ideally during the secondary survey log roll procedure. Loss of gastrointestinal tone will result in the cessation of peristaltic activity with subsequent gastric distension and a paralytic ileus, necessitating the use of a nasogastric tube.

Early correct management in the emergency department can do much to reduce later complications in the cord-injured patient. Rehabilitation after cord injury requires on-going multidisciplinary commitment to reducing the morbidity from the physical and psychological problems associated with cord injury, long after the patient has left the care of the ED (El Masri 2010).

Neurogenic shock

Neurogenic shock is often confused with spinal shock even though they are different entities. Neurogenic shock is most often associated with acute spinal cord disruption from trauma or spinal anaesthesia. Other causes include brain injury, hypoxia, depressant drug actions and hypoglycaemia associated with insulin shock. It results from impairment of the descending sympathetic pathways in the cord between T1 and L2, resulting in the loss of vasomotor and cardiac sympathetic tone. Loss of vasomotor tone causes vasodilatation and a pooling of blood in the lower extremities, resulting in hypotension. Loss of cardiac tone produces a bradycardia

(American College of Surgeons 2008). Priapism is seen in male patients and rectal and bladder sphincter control is absent (Chapman 2009).

Patients presenting to the emergency department may have extensive injuries that would normally be associated with a hypovolaemic shock state; bradycardia with hypotension – not tachycardia and hypotension – and this should increase suspicion of SCI. The peripheral skin is generally warm and dry because of peripheral vasodilatation and may be either flushed or pale. Fluid resuscitation is required if circulatory volume is to be restored (Grundy 2002); therefore patients may require a small bolus of crystalloid (up to 500 mL i.v.) to correct hypotension. No further fluid should be given if SCI is the sole injury. Overloading the patient who is in purely neurogenic shock can precipitate pulmonary oedema, and therefore all patients must have careful monitoring of their vital signs in order to detect the physiological response to fluid resuscitation. Insertion of an indwelling catheter will drain the dysfunctional bladder and provide information about overall tissue perfusion. Central venous pressure monitoring also provides an accurate method of determining response. Improved cardiac output may be indicated by a heart rate above 50 beats/min and a systolic pressure of greater than 100 mmHg.

Spinal shock

Spinal shock (or cord shock) is a temporary neurological condition that occurs after injury to the cord above the T6 level. The signs are a loss of all motor, sensory, reflex and autonomic responses below the site of the injury. There will be flaccidity and a positive Babinski sign, i.e., dorsal flexion of the first toe instead of plantar flexion, although all areas below the level of injury will not necessarily be permanently destroyed (Bickley et al. 2005). Hypotension, bradycardia and hypothermia,

because of the loss of sympathetic control and tone, are classic signs of spinal cord shock that occur immediately after injury.

Spinal shock does not resolve abruptly but rather in a series of phases extending over a few hours to several weeks, depending on the segmental level and extent of the cord injury (Ditunno et al. 2004). In areas where no function has returned, flaccid paralysis becomes spastic with increased tone. The diagnosis of spinal shock can only be formally made retrospectively. The immediate management in the emergency department is the same as for any cord-injured patient.

Conclusion

Spinal injuries are not a common cause of presentation to emergency departments but their consequences can be devastating. Whatever associated injuries coexist, the priorities – airway with c-spine control, breathing and circulatory support – remain unchanged, as hypoxia from an upper airway obstruction or transection of the upper cervical cord will kill before hypoperfusion.

The nurse should always listen carefully to the pre-hospital history to find out the mechanism of injury, maintain a high index of suspicion and if in doubt initiate full spinal immobilization (Dickinson 2004). A semi-rigid cervical collar alone will not provide adequate immobilization; sandbags and tape must be used. The initial damage from the injury has already occurred, and ED staff must prevent secondary injury by careful handling of the patient – one false move could result in quadriplegia or paraplegia. Almost all complications following SCI are preventable or can be minimized; sadly many are iatrogenic (El Masri 2010). Failure to suspect spinal injury can lead to failure in its detection. All vertebral fractures should be treated as unstable in the emergency department until fully evaluated by senior emergency medicine clinicians.

References

American College of Surgeons, 2008. Advanced Trauma Life Support, eighth ed. American College of Surgeons, Chicago.

Begg, J.D., 2005. Accident and Emergency X-rays. Churchill Livingstone, Edinburgh.

Bickley, L.S., Bates, B., Szilagy, P.G., 2005. Bates' Guide to Physical Examination and History Taking, nineth ed. Lippincott, Williams and Wilkins, Philadelphia.

Caroline, N., 2007. Emergency Care in the Streets, sixth ed. Little Brown, Boston.

Chapman, C.A., 2009. Shock emergencies. In: Newberry, L. (Ed.), Sheehy's Emergency Nursing: Principles and Practice, ninth ed. Mosby, St Louis.

Clement, C.M., Stiell, I.G., Davies, B., et al., 2011. Perceived facilitators and barriers to clinical clearance of the cervical spine by emergency department nurses: A major step towards changing practice in the emergency department. International Emergency Nursing 19, 4–52.

Dickinson, M., 2004. Understanding the mechanism of injury and kinetic forces involved in traumatic injuries. Nursing Standard 12 (6), 30–34.

Ditunno, J.F., Little, J.W., Tessler, A., Burns, A.S., 2004. Spinal shock revisited: A four-phase model. Spinal Cord 42, 383–395.

El Masri, W.S., 2010. Management of traumatic spinal cord injuries: Current standard of care revisited. Advances in Clinical Neuroscience and Rehabilitation 10 (1), 37–39.

Gallagher, S.M., 2005. Spinal trauma. In: O'Shea, R.A. (Ed.), Principles and Practice of Trauma Nursing. Elsevier Churchill Livingstone, Edinburgh.

Greaves, I., Porter, K., 2007. Oxford Handbook of Pre-Hospital Care. Oxford University Press, Oxford.

Greaves, I., Hodgetts, T., Porter, T., 2005. Emergency Care: A Textbook for Paramedics, second ed. WB Saunders, London.

Griffiths, H., Gallimore, D., 2005. Positioning critically ill patients in hospital. Nursing Standard 19 (42), 56–64.

Grundy, D., 2002. ABC of Spinal Cord Injury, fourth ed. BMJ Publications, Bristol.

Harrison, P., 2004. Spinal cord injury incidence update: UK database summary 2001. Spinal Cord Injury Link 3 (2), 4.

Ho, A.M., Fung, K.Y., Joyant, G.M., et al., 2002. Rigid cervical collar and intracrainial pressure of patients with severe head injury. Journal of Trauma, Injury, Infection and Critical Care. 53 (6), 1185–1188.

James, C.Y., Riemann, B.L., Munkasy, B.A., Joyner, A.B., 2004. Comparison of cervical spine motion during application among 4 rigid immobilization collars. Journal of Athletic Training 39 (2), 138–145.

Jaworski, M.A., Wirtz, K.M., 1995. Spinal trauma. In: Kitt, S., Selfridge-Thomas, J., Proehl, J.A., Kaiser, J. (Eds.), Emergency Nursing: A Physiological and Clinical Perspective. WB Saunders, Philadelphia.

Lowery, D., Marlena, M., Browne, B., Tiggs, S., et al., 2001. Epidemiology of spine injury victims. Annals of Emergency Medicine 38, 12–16.

McCarthy, M., 2011. Spinal injury. In: Smith, J., Greaves, I., Porter, K. (Eds.), Oxford Desk Reference: Major Trauma. Oxford Medical Publications, Oxford.

McRae, R., Esser, M., 2008. Practical Fracture Treatment, fifth ed. Elsevier, Edinburgh.

McSwain, N., 1992. Advanced Emergency Care. JB Lippincott, Philadelphia.

National Spinal Injuries Unit, 2005. NSIU Database. Mater Misericordiae University Hospital, Dublin.

Pre-Hospital Trauma Life Support Committee, 2006. PHTLS: Basic and Advanced Pre-Hospital Trauma Life Support. Mosby Lifeline, St Louis.

Raby, N., Berman, L., de Lacey, G., 2005. Accident and Emergency Radiology. Elsevier Saunders, Philadelphia.

Saktheivel-Wainford, K., 2009. Axial Skeletal Musculoskeletal Trauma X-rays. M&K Publishing, London.

Semonin-Holleran, R., 2003. Spinal trauma. In: Newberry, L. (Ed.), Sheehy's Emergency Nursing: Principles and Practice, fifth ed. Mosby, St Louis.

Sheerin, F., 2005. Spinal injury: Causation and pathophysiology. Emergency Nurse 12 (9), 29–38.

Stiell, I.G., Wells, G.A., Vandemheen, K., et al., 1997. Variation in emergency department use of cervical spine. radiography for alert, stable trauma patients. Canadian Medical Association Journal 156, 1537–1544.

Szilagyi, P.G., Bickley, L.S., 2004. Bates' Guide to Physical Examination and History Taking, eighth ed. Lippincott Williams & Wilkins, Philadelphia.

van der Jagt-Willems, H.C., van Hengel, M., Vis, M., et al., 2012. Why do geriatric outpatients have so many moderate and severe vertebral fractures? Exploring prevalence and risk factors. Age and Ageing 41 (2), 200–206.

Wassertheil, J., 2004. Spinal trauma. In: Cameron, P., Jelinek, G., Kelly, A.M., Murray, L., Brown, A.F.T., Heyworth, J. (Eds.), Textbook of Emergency Medicine, second ed. Churchill Livingstone, Edinburgh.

Zhang, S., Wadhwa, R., Haydel, J., et al., 2013. Spine and Spinal Cord Trauma: Diagnosis and Management. Neurologic Clinics 31 (1), 183–206.

Thoracic injuries

8

Richard Smith

Introduction

Thoracic injury is one of the most serious types of trauma, second only to central nervous system injuries and may result in disruption of the airway, breathing or circulation. It is responsible for approximately 25 % of trauma-related deaths and approximately 33 % of patients presenting with blunt trauma will have a thoracic injury (Kiraly & Schreiber 2010). Although many of these deaths occur immediately from the combined effects on respiratory and haemodynamic function, namely hypoxia, hypercarbia and acidosis (Rooney et al. 2000), there is a significant group of patients who, having sustained thoracic trauma, may survive with simple prompt effective systematic assessment and management. The management of patients with chest injuries can, therefore, be challenging and rewarding.

Mechanisms of injury

The Emergency Department (ED) nurse is likely to be the first contact with the patient on arrival at the hospital. It is therefore imperative that the nurse obtains all available information about the patient and the incident. When recording the history and clinical findings, forensic and medico-legal aspects need to be remembered. It is important to remember that serious intrathoracic injury can occur without obvious external damage to the chest wall. The mechanism of injury is an essential part of the history and can give crucial diagnostic clues to aid patient assessment. The main consideration when obtaining this history is whether the chest injury was caused by blunt or penetrating trauma as this will give some insight as to the types of injuries to be expected. In addition, an estimate of the velocity (speed) causing the injury may be gleaned from evidence of intrusion or vehicle damage, seat belt usage and steering wheel damage. Known high-velocity trauma, the presence of other seriously injured or dead people, ejection from a vehicle or fall from a great height are indicative of the potential for serious injuries to be present.

Blunt and penetrating mechanical energy transfers are the most common causes of thoracic trauma (Legare & Sawatzky 2010). Blunt chest trauma commonly results from rapid deceleration of the chest wall against a solid object. Typically, this is seen following road traffic collisions (RTCs) in which the chest strikes the vehicle steering wheel, causing a high-velocity blunt chest injury. Superficial tissues are mostly affected; however, as the energy transfer increases in direct-force injuries, deeper tissues become involved, producing contusions, haemorrhages, organ ruptures and fractures. RTCs represent the most common cause of blunt thoracic trauma (Kiraly & Schreiber 2010). However blunt chest trauma can also result from a fall from a height. Shearing forces make organs and tissue planes move relative to each other, resulting in tearing of the communicating structures and blood vessels. This type of chest trauma may be associated with injuries to the great vessels, major airways, lung parenchyma and myocardium, as well as diaphragmatic rupture and fractures to the ribs and/or sternum. Crush injuries are second only to RTCs as a major cause of blunt trauma, this includes chest compressions during cardiopulmonary resuscitation efforts which may also lead to cardiac injury (El-Chami et al. 2008). Frequently, fractured ribs and cardiac and pulmonary contusion may ensue. Other causes of blunt chest trauma include blast injury and low-velocity impact from direct blows to the chest. Penetrating injuries, such as stabbings or gunshot wounds, cause 7.9% of major trauma in the US compared to 4% in Europe (Edwards et al. 2007, Glance et al. 2010). There is no longer such a large gap (15%) between the two continents where penetrating trauma is concerned.

Penetrating trauma to the chest can be subdivided depending on the energy transfer involved. Stab wounds and impalements are a cause of low-energy chest trauma and cause direct damage along a straight track (cavitation). Medium- and high-energy chest wounds are determined by a number of variables, which determine how much energy is transferred to the tissues and how rapidly. These variables depend on the projectiles' physical makeup, the speed, range and characteristics of their flight and the nature of the tissue impacted; they generally produce a much larger cavity than lower-energy mechanisms therefore causing much more damage than is initially apparent.

Although this chapter deals predominantly with thoracic injuries, it is imperative that the chest is not viewed in isolation, as other life-threatening injuries outside the chest may be present. While chest trauma may occur in isolation, it is more common in patients with multiple injuries. Ingestion of alcohol or drugs is particularly noteworthy in patients with chest trauma because the pattern, depth and rate of respiration may be affected.

Anatomy of the chest

Chest injury occurs when there is damage to the thoracic cage or its contents. The thoracic cage comprises ribs and intercostal muscles. It is divided by the central mediastinum, which acts as a partition between the lungs. The outer surface of each lung is covered by the visceral pleura and this is reflected onto the chest wall as the parietal pleura (Fig. 8.1). The two pleural layers are effectively sealed together by a film of pleural fluid that exerts a strong surface tension force that prevents separation of the membranes. This enables the lungs to cling tightly to the thorax wall, which forces them to expand and recoil passively as the volume of the thoracic cavity alternately increases and decreases during breathing (Marieb & Hoehn 2007). If the pleura is breached, e.g., as a result of penetrating trauma, the integrity of this system is disrupted and the lung will collapse.

The mediastinum forms the central part of the thorax and extends from the sternum to the vertebral column. The mediastinum contains the trachea, oesophagus and major blood vessels, such as the aorta. It also encases the heart. It is important in the assessment of a trauma patient because disruption of its shape, such as widening, is indicative of damage to one of the structures within it, most commonly the aorta.

The heart lies above the diaphragm at the base of the thoracic cavity, with two-thirds of its bulk to the left of the body's midline. The outer surface of the heart is covered by the visceral pericardium. This is reflected onto the surrounding fibrous sac to form the parietal pericardium. A thin film of fluid separates these pericardial surfaces, allowing the heart to move freely, only being anchored by the great vessels (Fig. 8.2). This potential space can become filled with blood (haemopericardium) following trauma or myocardial infarction. As the fibrous pericardium is unable to distend, any fluid collecting within the potential space (pericardial cavity) will exert pressure on the heart and impair filling.

Below the level of the fourth intercostal space, the thoracic cage surrounds the upper abdominal region, particularly

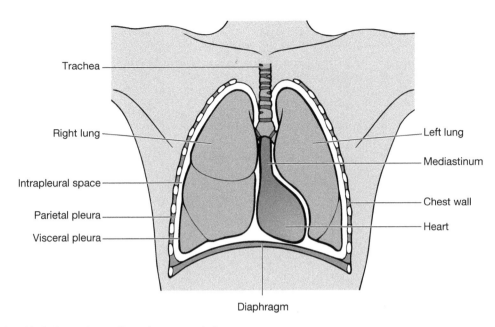

Figure 8.1 • Relationship between lungs, thoracic cage and pleurae.

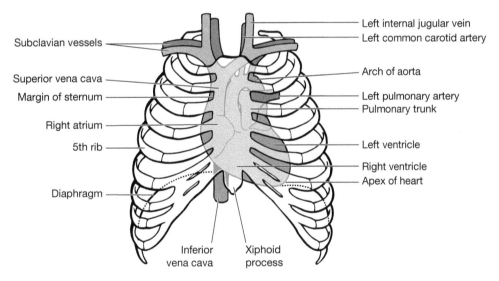

Figure 8.2 • Location of the heart and associated blood vessels in the thoracic cavity.

when the diaphragm elevates during expiration. Any injury to the ribs at or below this level should alert the nurse that an intra-abdominal injury, specifically to the liver, spleen or diaphragm, may also be present.

The physiology of respiration

The key functions of respiration are oxygen uptake and carbon dioxide elimination. To enable this to happen, air is conveyed through the respiratory tract – this is called ventilation (Fig. 8.3).

In addition, an adequate blood volume must circulate through the pulmonary capillaries. This is called perfusion. The exchange of oxygen and carbon dioxide between the alveoli and capillaries is called diffusion. Gases move from an area of high partial pressure to one of low partial pressure. When leaving the lungs via the alveolar capillaries and into the pulmonary veins, blood has its highest partial pressure of oxygen (PO_2) (Marieb & Hoehn 2007).

Oxygen diffusion requires:

- a high concentration of oxygen in the alveolus
- a low blood concentration of oxygen
- solubility of the gas
- membrane thickness that the gas has to cross
- perfusion pressure
- alveolar ventilation.

Damage to either system leads to hypoxia or hypercapnia, which in turn threatens homeostasis. The ratio between ventilation and perfusion is fundamental to the success of respiratory function (Fig. 8.4).

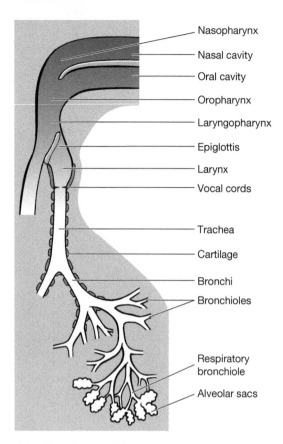

Figure 8.3 • Organization of the airways.

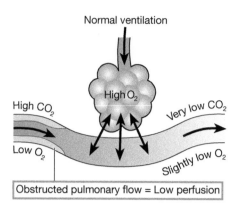

Figure 8.5 • Ventilation greater than perfusion.

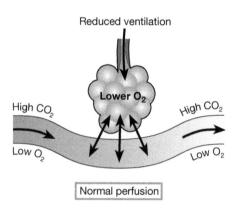

Figure 8.6 • Ventilation lower than perfusion.

Although the ventilation/perfusion ratio varies in different parts of the lung, a high ratio in one area will not offset a low ventilation/perfusion ratio in another. This is because of the reduction in haemoglobin saturation. In the trauma patient, particularly where chest injury has occurred, maintaining adequate ventilation is crucial in preventing hypoxia. Oxygen should be administered in high-inspired concentrations (preferably via face mask) to all patients as soon as they are placed on the bed (Curtis et al. 2010). Acidosis, which results from impaired ventilation associated with chest injury, activates the respiratory centre to increase respiratory rate and depth, which eliminates more CO_2 (Marieb & Hoehn 2007). Metabolic acidosis results from inadequate tissue perfusion secondary to airway, breathing and circulatory problems, further compounding the patient's condition.

Principles of care

The trauma team

Each hospital should have its own activation criteria based on its individual patient population. This may also be dependent on the size of emergency department, and some major trauma centres now have a tiered response to the multiple injured patients (Curtis & Asha 2010). Many EDs have established a system of care for seriously injured patients based on a team approach that utilizes Advanced Trauma Life Support (ATLS) principles and incorporates well-established objectives

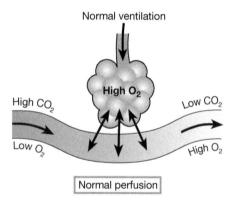

Figure 8.4 • Normal ventilation/perfusion ratio.

If a problem occurs with pulmonary flow, most commonly a low circulatory volume in trauma, adequate oxygen cannot be taken up. This is because less blood passes the alveoli and there is subsequently less haemoglobin take-up of oxygen. This results in a decrease in tissue perfusion. Unbound oxygen is expired. This results in a high ventilation/perfusion ratio (Fig. 8.5).

If ventilation decreases, most commonly with an obstructed airway, the amount of oxygen reaching the alveoli is reduced. When perfusion is normal this results in more blood and haemoglobin passing the alveoli than can be saturated with oxygen. As a result, the blood leaving the lungs has a low oxygen content. This is a low ventilation/perfusion ratio (Fig. 8.6).

of trauma management (American College of Surgeons 2008) (see Chapter 2). The team leader is responsible for the coordination of care and the appropriate delegation of roles whilst maintaining an overview of the situation. The use of a standardized systematic approach not only expedites patient care, but also offers a format enabling less-experienced staff to focus their activities in a predetermined order. Some hospitals have established trauma teams in which each member has a specific role.

Clearly, the ED nurse's role is dynamic and directly related to the patient's needs. The key components of the nursing role when caring for patients with chest trauma are outlined in Box 8.1. The number and experience of other team members may influence the nurse's actual activities, but the needs of the patient and their family/friends must remain paramount. Ideally, a member of the care team will be allocated to care for and liaise with the patient's family and/or friends (see Chapter 14 for guidance on this issue).

Box 8.1

The role of the ED nurse
- Prepare the environment for receiving the patient
- Perform a systematic, rapid assessment using the ABC approach
- Prioritize and initiate appropriate interventions and care, continually evaluating their effectiveness
- Function as an effective member of a multidisciplinary team
- Act as an advocate for the patient who may be incapacitated
- Ensure patient and staff safety at all times
- Coordinate holistic patient care from receipt to transfer or definitive care

Assessment of chest injury

The immediate management of the patient with chest injury should follow the principles laid down in the ATLS guidelines (American College of Surgeons 2008). A primary survey should be carried out to identify and treat any immediately life-threatening conditions (Box 8.2; the management of specific conditions will be discussed later in the chapter). In the stable patient, a secondary survey or head-to-toe examination should then be carried out to identify any other injury.

The Trauma Nursing Core Course (Emergency Nurses Association 2007) and similar such courses recommend pre-hospital

Box 8.2

Immediately life-threatening conditions of the chest
- Airway obstruction
- Tension pneumothorax
- Open chest wound
- Massive haemothorax
- Flail chest
- Cardiac tamponade

information should be obtained before the patient's arrival to ED, e.g., a tension pneumothorax may have been decompressed. The sequence of questions in the hand-over to the hospital care can be remembered as 'MIST': Mechanism of injury, Injuries found and suspected, Signs (respiratory rate, sPO₂, blood pressure), Treatment given pre-hospital.

Nursing assessment of the patient's overall condition is part of the overall progress towards definitive care. Nursing observations should include:
- the rate and depth of respiration
- chest wall movement
- blood pressure
- pulse oximetry
- pulse rate and pressure
- pain assessment
- level of consciousness
- urine output.

Additional investigations may include:
- cardiac monitoring
- chest X-ray/lateral cervical spine and pelvis (trauma series)
- ECG
- blood gas analysis
- blood chemistry (may include CPK and CK-MP, troponin I and troponin T; however, no specific blood test for myocardial injury following trauma exists)
- full blood count and cross-match
- ultrasound/echocardiography/Focussed Assessment with Sonography for Trauma (FAST)
- computed tomography/magnetic resonance imaging
- angiography (aortic disruption)
- thorascopy: direct or video assisted if not contra-indicated.

A specific chest injury assessment is listed in Box 8.3.

Initial management of chest injury

Airway and breathing

Management of chest injury should include high-flow oxygen as described above. The method of delivery depends largely on the patient's condition; in a conscious patient without obvious compromise, use of a tight-fitting mask (NB: be aware of possible parallel facial injuries) and non-rebreathing bag is the method of choice. If the patient is unable to maintain their airway, as is common after chest injury, supportive methods should be found (Box 8.4).

Airway compromise occurs either because of damage to the airway, resulting in oedema, compression, bleeding, foreign body obstruction, displaced facial bones or suspected cervical spine injuries, or through a deterioration in the patient's consciousness level, resulting in the loss of the gag reflex. If breathing is absent, the airway should be assumed to be blocked. Noisy breathing (stridor) may be indicative of partial upper airway obstruction or laryngospasm. If the patient is able to give a verbal response, then the airway can be assumed to be patent for the present time (Box 8.5).

Box 8.3

Specific assessment of the chest

Visual inspection
- Wounds, bruises, surface trauma
- Symmetry of chest expansion
- Rate, rhythm and depth of respiration
- Use of accessory muscles
- Intercostal recession
- Paradoxical chest movement

Auscultation
- Breath sounds – check rate, quality, type
- Heart sounds

Percussion
- Resonant (normal)
- Hyper-resonance
- Dullness

Palpation
- Subcutaneous emphysema
- Pain
- Swelling
- Masses
- Pulsation
- Crepitus
- Step defects
- Apex beat
- Tracheal deviation and tracheal tug (late sign)

Box 8.4

Assessing and securing the airway in a trauma patient

1. Seek verbal response from patient, by asking, for example, 'Are you all right?', while giving O₂ and stabilizing the cervical spine. Steps 2, 3 & 4 *should be simultaneous*
2. Look for chest movement – for 10 seconds minimum
3. Listen for breath sounds – for 10 seconds minimum (check simultaneously with chest movement)
4. Feel for expired air – for 10 seconds minimum
5. If the airway is compromised → chin lift or jaw thrust (avoiding hyperextension of the neck)
6. Reassess and if airway remains compromised repeat steps 2–4
7. Clear mouth of obvious debris, such as blood, vomit, broken teeth, ill-fitting dentures
8. Reassess and if airway remains compromised, repeat steps 2–4
9. Intubation with assisted ventilation and reassess

The tongue slipping back and occluding the oropharynx causes a significant number of airway obstructions. These can be simply resolved by using a chin lift or jaw thrust manoeuvre (always observing the potential for a cervical spine injury). This will pull the tongue forward in the mouth and remove the obstruction. The mouth should be inspected with adequate light to identify any debris, which should be removed

Box 8.5

Indicators of airway obstruction
- Apnoea
- Tachypnoea
- Increased respiratory effort
- Intercostal recession
- Use of accessory muscles
- Tracheal tug
- Stridor/noisy breathing
- Pallor/cyanosis (late sign)

Box 8.6

Indications for endotracheal intubation
- Poor airway maintenance with other methods due to injury
- Loss of gag reflex with high risk of aspiration
- Compromised respiratory function due to chest injury
- Need for mechanical ventilation
- Anticipation of airway obstruction, such as increasing oedema
- Raised intracranial pressure (GCS <8)

carefully with suction or angled forceps. It is important not to stimulate the gag reflex during suction because this can induce vomiting.

The nasopharyngeal airway can be used in patients with an intact gag reflex, trismus or oral trauma (Roberts et al. 2005). The airway is inserted via the nostril to the pharynx. This type of adjunct should not be used where a base of skull fracture is suspected or where facial injuries prevent its use. The tube should never be forced. If oedema or potential haemorrhage is likely, alternative airway support should be used.

If the gag reflex is absent, the patient needs endotracheal intubation; however, an oropharyngeal or Guedel airway can provide temporary support. This will prevent the tongue from occluding the pharynx and provide an artificial airway. If simple airway management fails to secure a patent airway, because of either injury or vomiting, endotracheal intubation should be performed (Box 8.6). It is important to stress the need for in-line immobilization of the cervical spine. This is addressed in detail in Chapter 7.

The effectiveness of all airway management should be assessed by:

- looking at chest movement
  - is it symmetrical bilateral?
  - is there sufficient chest expansion?
- listening to breath sounds
  - are they present?
  - is there stridor or gurgling from debris?
- feeling for expired air.

Thoracic injuries which compromise breathing will be discussed later in this chapter.

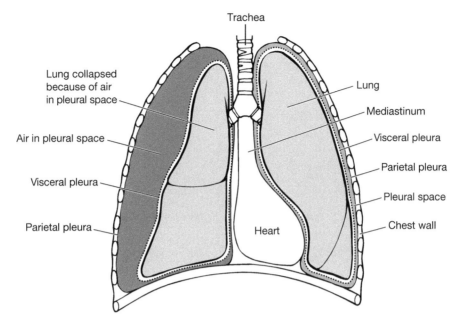

Figure 8.7 • Right-sided pneumothorax, normal left lung.

Circulation

The patient's circulatory status should be assessed by:

- pulse rate and volume
- the speed of capillary return
- skin colour or pallor.

All patients should have i.v. access established with two wide-bore cannulae and a fluid regime appropriate to circulatory status. Some facilities may treat the patient hypotensively (permissive hypotension) and trauma courses like ATLS and TNCC are starting to advocate the judicious use of fluid infusion and blood pressure increase, particularly in penetrating torso trauma and uncontrolled bleeding (Rezende-Neto et al. 2010). Blood should also be taken for cross-matching, baseline full blood count and urea and electrolytes during initial management.

Disability

The hypoxic patient may be confused initially and could become combative. Primary head injury could also cause an altered mental state, and this will be compounded by hypoxia or hypercarbia. It is essential that the patient receives adequate oxygen, particularly for potential brain-injured patients because hypoxia decreases cerebral oxygenation, leading to secondary brain injury (McNett et al. 2010).

Exposure

The patient should be fully exposed to identify any further injuries that may not have been identified earlier in the assessment. These may range from small abrasions to life-threatening injuries covered by clothing. Once the patient has been exposed they should be covered again immediately to preserve body warmth as the trauma patient is prone to becoming hypothermic very quickly. The nurse should be aware of the importance of the clothing for evidence in victims of crime.

Immediately life-threatening chest injuries

Pneumothorax

A pneumothorax can be caused by blunt or penetrating trauma. One or more lacerations to the visceral pleura from the sharp edges of fractured ribs can cause a pneumothorax in blunt trauma and direct pleural laceration from knives, bullets, etc., in penetrating trauma (Curtis et al. 2007). Pneumothorax occurs when the fluid seal between the parietal and visceral pleura is broken. Once the seal is broken, air rushes in, expands the space and the existing negative pressure is lost. The resulting positive pressure in the expanded intrapleural space is exerted onto the adjacent lung. This may result in partial or total collapse of the lung, and serious impairment of gaseous exchange. Because the pleural layers are separated by the mediastinum, the opposite lung continues to move with the chest wall and functions normally, unless it becomes compressed by the volume of air accumulating on the injured side (Fig. 8.7).

Pneumothoraces are classified in Box 8.7.

Box 8.7

Classification of pneumothoraces

- **Simple** – occurs spontaneously or as a result of blunt trauma. It is not initially life-threatening but has the potential to develop into a tension pneumothorax. A simple pneumothorax may compromise respiratory function, particularly on mild exertion
- **Open** – results from a penetrating injury, where the integrity of the chest wall is breached and air is sucked into the pleural cavity
- **Tension** – results from blunt or penetrating trauma, mechanical ventilation or from a simple pneumothorax. It occurs when air enters the pleural space and becomes trapped. The volume of air increases and causes compression of other organs

Tension pneumothorax

This is an immediately life-threatening chest injury and should be dealt with as soon as it is identified in the primary survey. Tension pneumothorax can result:

- from blunt or penetrating trauma
- from baro-trauma associated with positive pressure ventilation
- where chest injury such as rib fracture exists
- following invasive procedures, such as insertion of a central line
- as a complication of a simple pneumothorax.

It is imperative that the ED nurse remains vigilant, as a tension pneumothorax can occur at any stage of the patient's treatment.

A tension pneumothorax is a clinical diagnosis. It occurs when air is sucked into the pleural space, either from the lung or from outside the chest wall. The pleura acts as a one-way valve, trapping air in the pleural space, therefore allowing air in to, but not out of, the cavity. The pressure of this causes a total collapse of the lung on the affected side. As the intrathoracic pressure increases, the mediastinum and trachea shift towards the unaffected side, causing impaired venous return and cardiac compression. This results in reduced cardiac output and severe hypotension. The increasing pressure also causes compression of the adjacent lung, compounding the patient's already compromised ventilation, systemic hypotension, shock and, ultimately, cardiac arrest (Curtis et al. 2007). A tension pneumothorax is a condition of rapid onset and demands immediate decompression of the pleural space to maintain life. Time should not be wasted by attempting to obtain a chest X-ray (Fig. 8.8).

Assessment

Priorities for care of the patient with a tension pneumothorax lie with correct identification of the condition. A conscious patient will be very distressed due to the rapid worsening of the dyspnoea. Hypoxia may also make the patient confused, agitated and restless. Specific clinical features are highlighted in Box 8.8.

A tension pneumothorax can expand rapidly. This increase in size correlates with a decrease in functional lung space. Therefore, as the condition worsens, the patient's dyspnoea, respiratory function and tissue oxygenation all deteriorate.

Immediate management

Immediate management entails maintaining oxygenation. This is a twofold activity. First, oxygen intake must be maintained either through a high-flow mask with oxygen reservoir or with assisted manual or mechanical ventilation. The second life-saving intervention is to remove the 'tension' from the pneumothorax to reduce further loss of lung capacity. This is achieved by providing an artificial escape route for the trapped air. To facilitate this, a needle thoracentesis is performed. While this is a rapid and simple procedure which buys time for the resuscitation team, it is not definitive treatment.

A

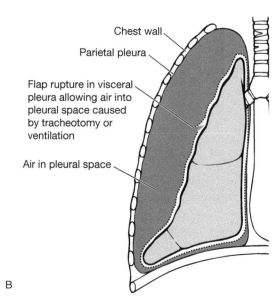

B

Figure 8.8 • Tension pneumothorax.

Box 8.8

Clinical signs of tension pneumothorax

- Tachypnoea
- Tachycardia
- Shock
- Decreased or absent air entry to affected side
- Hyper-resonance on affected side
- Distended neck veins – if the patient is not hypovolaemic (late sign)
- Tracheal deviation away from affected side (late sign)
- Cyanosis (late sign)

Chest decompression by needle thoracentesis is carried out by inserting a wide-bore cannula into the pleural space. The largest calibre needle typically used for this purpose is a 14 gauge 5 cm needle with a sheath length of 4.5 cm (Zengerink et al. 2006). The cannula is inserted in the second intercostal space mid-clavicular line over the superior aspect of the third rib. The cannula is attached to a one-way valve to prevent it becoming an open pneumothorax, and once in situ, the rapid release of air confirms initial diagnosis. This procedure should dramatically reduce the patient's discomfort and clinical symptoms.

At this stage, it is important to obtain intravenous access as bleeding may lead to hypovolaemia. A chest drain will facilitate the removal of remaining air from the pleural cavity. The chest drain can be inserted in front of the mid-axillary line anywhere between the second and seventh intercostal space depending on what is to be drained from the pleural space. Air tends to be around the second to fifth intercostal space, and blood etc., from the fifth to seventh intercostal space. The fifth intercostal space is generally used for trauma patients. The drainage tube is connected to an underwater sealed system that allows air out of the pleural space, but not back in. Fluid levels in the drainage system should swing back and forth on inspiration and expiration (Sullivan 2008). While a chest X-ray will verify the presence of collapsed lung and demonstrate a mediastinal shift towards the unaffected lung, if the patient has clinical signs and a high suspicion that tension pneumothorax exists, immediate treatment should be instituted without obtaining a chest X-ray.

Open pneumothorax

Open pneumothorax may occur following penetrating trauma in which the chest wall is pierced. When chest wall integrity is breached, e.g., by a stab wound, air can enter the pleural space creating a pneumothorax. This occurs because of a loss of negative pressure and an equalling of atmospheric and intrathoracic pressures. If the external damage to the chest wall is large enough, i.e., greater than two-thirds of the diameter of the trachea, air will enter the pleural cavity via the wound rather than via the normal respiratory tract, because air tends to follow the path of least resistance.

It is for this reason that an open pneumothorax is often referred to as a 'sucking chest wound', as air can be heard entering the pleural space on inspiration. As air enters the thoracic cavity by this route, respiratory efficiency is rapidly decreased. This is because of alveolar hypoventilation despite increased respiratory effort. This results in a low ventilation/perfusion ratio and tissue hypoxia.

Assessment

The mechanism of injury is the main factor in assessment. The patient will have a history of penetrating trauma and may or may not have an impaled object in situ, this object should not be removed. On examination, the patient will be tachypnoeic and tachycardic and may be hypotensive. Breath sounds may be decreased or absent on the affected side. The chest wound will have an audible sucking sound on inspiration. Bubbles often occur around the wound as air escapes through the blood; there may also be subcutaneous emphysema as air escapes under the skin. The actual size of the wound does not give significant indication of the extent of intrathoracic damage. Treatment is aimed at returning normal ventilation and closing the wound (Yamamoto et al. 2005).

Immediate management

This is a potentially life-threatening condition and should be treated in the resuscitation phase of the primary survey. Initial management is relatively simple; it involves maintaining oxygen intake and temporary closure of the chest wound. Oxygen intake is supported by the use of high-flow oxygen via a mask and reservoir bag. If the patient is unable to maintain breathing, artificial ventilation is indicated. The chest wound is covered with a sterile occlusive dressing taped down on three sides to create a flutter valve. During inhalation, the dressing is sucked against the chest wall and acts as a seal, which prevents any further air from entering the pleural space. On expiration, the open side of the dressing pushes away from the patient's skin, allowing air to escape from the pleural space.

A dressing sealed on all sides would result in a tension pneumothorax, as air would enter the pleural space but would have no means of escape. If the patient has any signs of respiratory distress and a tension pneumothorax is suspected, the occlusive dressing should be temporarily removed to allow air to escape (Yamamoto et al. 2005).

Any impaled object should not be removed as this significantly increases the risk of respiratory compromise and circulatory collapse. After establishing i.v. access, a chest drain should be inserted through a surgically created hole, not via the wound, to facilitate decompression of the pleural space. Prophylactic antibiotics and anti-tetanus will be necessary. The majority of patients with an open pneumothorax require surgical closure of the wound once their overall condition has been stabilized. It is at this stage that any impaled objects are usually removed.

Massive haemothorax

Haemothorax can result from penetrating trauma or blunt injury where an intercostal vessel or internal mammary artery has been ruptured. A massive haemothorax is usually defined as a rapid accumulation of blood, greater than 1500 mL in the pleural cavity or 200 mL/h from the chest drain (Yamamoto et al. 2005). The incidence of haemothorax or haemopneumothorax is as high as 30–40 % of patients with blunt injuries and 70–90 % of patients with penetrating injuries (Wise et al. 2011) (Fig. 8.9).

Assessment

The patient will present with tachypnoea, tachycardia and hypovolaemic shock. Specifically, chest examination will reveal decreased or absent breath sounds on the affected

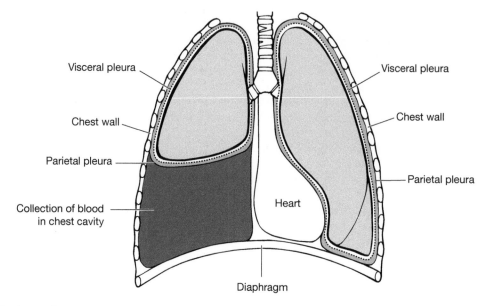

Figure 8.9 • Massive haemothorax.

side. On percussion, dullness will be detected over the haemothorax due to the density of blood. Internal jugular veins should be observed; jugular venous pressure (JVP) may be elevated as a result of pressure in the thoracic cavity because of the accumulation of blood, or other associated injury, such as tension pneumothorax or cardiac tamponade. Conversely, neck veins may be collapsed as a result of hypovolaemia. To observe the JVP is difficult at the best of times, so in a trauma situation it is often difficult to observe and is therefore unreliable.

Immediate management

Initial management is by the simultaneous restoration of blood volume and decompression of the chest cavity. The patient should be given high-flow oxygen via a mask and reservoir bag. Intravenous access using large-bore needles should be established and fluid resuscitation commenced. Once fluid replacement begins, a chest drain should be inserted to drain blood from the thoracic cavity and allow the lung to reinflate. Before a chest drain is inserted, a ruptured diaphragm should be excluded as the cause of reduced breath sounds and dull resonance. This can be done by careful history-taking of the mechanism of injury and listening to the chest for bowel sounds. A chest drain should always be inserted by blunt dissection, so that any herniated abdominal organs can be felt with a finger prior to the insertion of a drainage tube, thus preventing further injury. Bleeding to the lung parenchyma usually stops once the lung is reinflated because of the drop in pulmonary perfusion (Driscoll & Skinner 2007). An early thoracotomy is indicated if 1500 mL are immediately evacuated; however, some patients who have an initial volume output of less than 1500 mL may require a thoracotomy. This decision is based on the patient's haemodynamic status, signs of exsanguination and not just on continuing blood loss (200 mL/h for 2 to 4 hours) (Yamamoto et al. 2005). The patient should

ideally have a central venous line placed in order to monitor right-sided cardiac filling pressure.

Flail chest

Flail chest usually results from blunt trauma, most commonly RTCs (Borman et al. 2006, Kilic et al. 2011). It is defined as a compromise of the integrity of the thoracic rigid cage and a segment, its size depending on the number of fractured ribs or costal cartilages, loses its continuity with the rest of the thoracic cage and moves paradoxically during spontaneous respiration (Borman et al. 2006). A flail segment can result from the fracture of as little as two or more adjacent ribs in two places, therefore disconnecting them from the rest of the thoracic cage (Fig. 8.10).

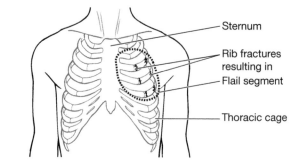

Figure 8.10 • Flail chest.

This paradoxical movement on inspiration reduces tidal volume, and therefore compromises ventilation. While this carries a risk of hypoxia, the primary danger to the patient stems from underlying lung injury. Lung contusion or penetrating injury can cause profound hypoxia, and rib fractures cause significant hypovolaemia, particularly if there is sternal involvement.

Assessment

Rib fractures are extremely painful and the conscious patient will complain of severe chest pain and difficulty in breathing. The patient will be tachypnoeic with shallow breaths, tachycardic and will show early signs of hypoxia. Examination of the chest usually reveals a paradoxical segment not expanding with the rest of the chest wall on inspiration. Palpation of the area will reveal crepitus and instability of the rib cage. Splinting from chest wall muscular spasm may mask the paradoxical movement, and the diagnosis is not uncommonly delayed until the muscles relax, due to exhaustion or when paralysing drugs are given. The possibility of central flail chest should be particularly considered in patients who have sustained steering-wheel injuries.

Assessment should include careful monitoring for hypoxia. This should include rate and respiratory effort, tachycardia, skin colour, oxygen saturation and arterial blood gases. Arterial blood gas values may aid in diagnosis by reflecting respiratory failure, however this should not be solely relied upon.

Management

Management involves the restoration of respiratory function. Pain is a significant threat to respiratory function as it reduces respiratory effort, resulting in shallow breathing and reduced tidal volume. In addition, pain inhibits coughing, allowing bronchial secretions to build up, further jeopardizing respiratory function. Adequate pain control is essential to recovery; often the method of choice is an intercostal nerve block, which is performed as part of definitive care. Other treatments are also being utilized, including operative stabilization which although not widely adopted, has successfully been used for almost four decades with encouraging results (Bottlang et al. 2010); it is also recommended that larger studies are undertaken (Kiraly & Schreiber 2010).

Both ventilation and perfusion are vital to respiratory function, so initial management should include adequate oxygenation and restoration of circulatory volume. Fluid replacement should be managed carefully, measured by heart rate, capillary refill and urine output. An injured lung is sensitive to underperfusion, which reduces the diffusion rate of oxygen. It is equally sensitive to circulatory overload, which can rapidly cause a raised central venous pressure (CVP) and left ventricular failure.

Unless profound hypoxia is present, many patients with a flail chest maintain their own ventilation, supported with high-flow oxygen via a mask and reservoir bag. The need for mechanical ventilation is determined by respiratory function and the level of hypoxia, not necessarily by the size of a flail segment (Box 8.9). Continuous positive pressure (CPAP) may be indicated for some patients.

Cardiac tamponade

Cardiac tamponade is a life-threatening cardiac injury that occurs most often with a penetrating injury (Emergency

Box 8.9

Indications for mechanical ventilation

- Respiratory rate of >30 breaths/min
- Exhaustion
- Falling PaO_2 <10.5 kPa on O_2
- Rising $PaCO_2$ >6.0 kPa on O_2
- Associated head injuries (GCS <8)
- Respiratory rate <10 breaths/min

Nurses Association 2007). It can also result from blunt trauma if the heart or great vessels have been damaged. Cardiac tamponade can be a rare complication of an expanding, untreated tension pneumothorax that causes mediastinal shift and eventually cardiac compression. Tamponade occasionally results from a myocardial infarction. The pericardium anchors the heart to the mediastinum, diaphragm and sternal wall. The risk of tamponade in trauma occurs because the pericardium is non-elastic and inflexible. This allows the heart to move without causing friction. The heart wall, consisting of myocardium and endocardium, lies beneath the pericardium and forms the muscle needed for cardiac function (Fig. 8.11).

Cardiac tamponade occurs when injury to the heart or disruption of its blood vessels results in bleeding into the pericardial cavity. Because there is no elasticity in the pericardium, it only requires a small amount of fluid to compress the cardiac wall and chamber. This is primarily because filling capacity is reduced during diastole, and therefore venous pressure is elevated and there is a fall in stroke volume.

Assessment

The mechanism of injury should alert the trauma team to suspect a cardiac tamponade. If a penetrating injury has occurred to the thoracic area, anteriorly, posteriorly or to the left lateral aspect, tamponade should be excluded as part of the primary survey. A patient with cardiac tamponade will be shocked, and therefore assessment of pulse and respiration are important. Specifically, patients will show signs of falling arterial pressure, because of reduced cardiac output, and increased venous pressure, because of cardiac compression. As tamponade worsens the patient exhibits air hunger, agitation and deterioration in the level of consciousness. Venous pressure can be assessed by venous distension; time should not be spent inserting CVP lines in the initial stages of management (Driscoll & Skinner 2007).

Venous pressure is also influenced by hypovolaemia, and therefore absence of distended neck veins does not exclude cardiac tamponade. Pulsus paradoxus, a decrease in blood pressure >10 mmHg with inspiration may be found with tamponade but is a difficult sign to elicit. Beck's triad is another diagnostic tool that can be a sign of cardiac tamponade, however it does not have sufficient sensitivity and specificity alone to indicate tamponade (Mullins & Harrahill 2010) (Box 8.10).

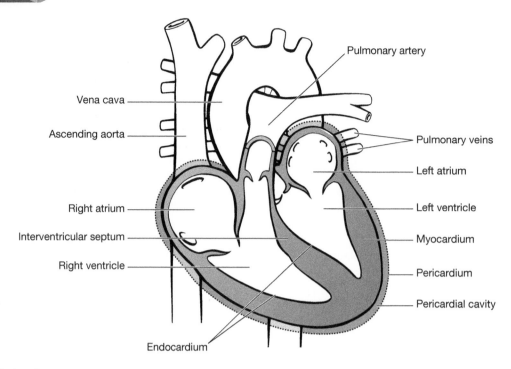

Figure 8.11 • The heart.

Box 8.10

Beck's triad

1. *Raised CVP* – due to impaired venous return because of cardiac compression
2. *Hypotension* – low arterial pressure because of poor cardiac output
3. *Decreased, muffled heart sounds* – due to fluid in pericardial cavity

A 12-lead ECG trace is useful. It may indicate damage to myocardium, seen as ST elevation in the affected area. Continuous cardiac monitoring is recommended to detect any rhythm changes, commonly ventricular ectopics.

Management

Similar to all trauma patients, those with cardiac tamponade should be given high-flow oxygen through a mask and reservoir bag. Initial attempts should be towards circulatory resuscitation to correct hypovolaemia. If there is no improvement in the patient's condition, pericardiocentesis should be performed to relieve the tamponade. This is a mechanism for draining fluid from the pericardial cavity and reducing cardiac compression.

Pericardiocentesis is performed by inserting a wide-bore cannula, at least 15 cm in length, into the pericardial cavity. This is done 1–2 cm left of the xiphochondral junction at a 45° angle, aiming the needle towards the tip of the scapula. The cannula should be attached to a three-way tap and syringe. Continuous aspiration should take place during insertion. When blood flows freely into the syringe, the insertion should stop. Blood removed from the pericardial sac will generally not clot (because blood is defibrinated from agitation during systole), and the haematocrit will be lower than venous blood (Emergency Nurses Association 2007).

Continuous ECG monitoring is imperative during this procedure for a number of reasons. First, if the needle is inserted too far, myocardial irritation (seen as ventricular ectopics on the ECG monitor) or myocardial damage (seen as QRS complexes or ST segment changes) can occur. Should this happen, the needle should be withdrawn gradually until the ECG returns to normal. Second, as blood is removed on aspiration, cardiac decompression occurs and the myocardium expands back into its usual position.

Once blood has been withdrawn from the pericardial cavity, the cannula should be firmly taped in position in case further aspiration is required. If blood has clotted in the pericardial cavity it is impossible to relieve symptoms of tamponade by pericardiocentesis. If the results of pericardiocentesis reveal blood in the pericardial cavity, or if there is a strong clinical suspicion of tamponade, the patient should undergo urgent surgical exploration.

Cardiac compression severely compromises circulatory activity and will lead to cardiac arrest if unchecked. However, by reducing cardiac compression, internal cardiac pressure is increased and profound haemorrhage can occur because the tamponade effect is lost. Some EDs recommend emergency thoracotomy in ED should cardiac arrest occur. Survival from this is rare unless cardiothoracic back-up is available and cardiac bypass can be quickly established.

Box 8.11

Serious chest injuries
- Pulmonary contusion
- Blunt cardiac trauma
- Aortic rupture
- Ruptured diaphragm
- Tracheobronchial injury
- Oesophageal rupture

Box 8.12

Indications for mechanical ventilation in patients with pulmonary contusion
- Hypoxia and worsening respiratory function
- Impaired level of consciousness
- Progressive fall in PaO_2
- Progressive increase in $PaCO_2$
- Pre-existing chronic lung disease
- Imminent surgery for associated injuries
- Other systems failure, e.g., renal failure
- Prior to transfer to another hospital

Serious chest injuries

The following injuries can be potentially life-threatening and should be diagnosed as part of the secondary survey and treated definitively (Box 8.11).

Pulmonary contusion

Pulmonary contusion commonly occurs following a rapid deceleration injury. For example, a restrained passenger in an RTC may come to an abrupt stop on impact, but soft viscera such as the lung remain in motion, causing stretching, tearing and shearing. The resultant bruising and pain cause an insidious onset of respiratory distress, with decreased lung compliance and, rarely, increased airway resistance. It may also occur as a result of primary blast injuries (Harrison et al. 2009).

Assessment

Pulmonary contusion tends to evolve over several hours and signs and symptoms can develop up to 48 hours after the initial injury; therefore the mechanism and the time elapsed can give some clues to pulmonary contusion. It also underlines the importance of regular observation, and of recording and reporting vital signs (Taylor & Dawood 2005, Wyatt et al. 2005). Primarily, the ED nurse should assess the respiration rate and depth. Patients will classically demonstrate an increasing tachypnoea and increasingly shallow breathing. Initially, the work of breathing is manifested by accessory muscles and intercostal recession. Because ventilation is poor, an imbalance in the ventilation/perfusion ratio occurs. This is demonstrated by a fall in PaO_2; serial arterial blood gas monitoring should take place. The nurse must look for any marks, e.g., abrasions or bruising on the chest wall, following the original injury. These may indicate pulmonary contusion.

Assessment is aided by chest X-ray; contusions can evolve over several days on an X-ray. A CT scan has been demonstrated to have superior sensitivity and specificity for the diagnosis of pulmonary contusion (Kiraly & Schreiber 2010). Pulse oximetry and ECG monitoring are also useful.

Management

Management principles entail maintaining respiratory function. High-flow oxygen should be given and the oxygen saturation carefully monitored. Adequate pain control aids respiratory function. Careful fluid balance is imperative to prevent secondary lung damage from pulmonary oedema, as a result of fluid overload, and to ensure fluid replacement is not underestimated; this would cause hypovolaemia and a subsequent reduction in pulmonary perfusion, compounding existing hypoxia. The ED nurse should be aware that patients with pulmonary contusions may need mechanical ventilation.

Indications for mechanical ventilation are shown in Box 8.12.

Blunt cardiac trauma

Blunt cardiac trauma can result in myocardial muscle contusion, valvular disruption or cardiac chamber rupture. This usually results from RTCs and is exemplified by a driver who sustains an impact with the vehicle steering wheel, causing a deceleration injury. It is a commonly undiagnosed condition, sometimes with fatal consequences. Compression of the heart results in bleeding into the myocardium and ischaemia. The coronary arteries become occluded because of spasm or oedema. The physiological effect of this is similar to a myocardial infarction: the heart becomes ischaemic and, if not treated, necrosis and infarction occur. Chest pain in patients following blunt cardiac trauma should be assessed like any other cardiac pain. A large percentage of these injuries are overlooked because pain is attributed to chest wall injury, e.g., with rib or sternal fractures.

Assessment

It is imperative to obtain a thorough trauma history as well as a physical examination, as these will give the ED nurse an index of suspicion for cardiac injury (Cook & Gleason 2009). Blunt trauma is associated with sternal fracture and wedge fracture of the thoracic vertebrae. Assessment should follow the same pattern as the assessment of a patient with a non-traumatic cardiac pain.

Baseline observations should be obtained and the patient should be observed on a cardiac monitor; troponins are used as part of diagnostic algorithms as an adjunct to the ECG to rule out clinically significant blunt cardiac injury (Curtis & Asha 2010). The ECG may show a similar pattern to that of an evolving myocardial infarct (see also Chapter

28). However, myocardial damage can occur without ECG changes. Sinus tachycardia and arrhythmias, such as ventricular ectopics and atrial fibrillation, are indicators of a 'stressed' myocardium.

Management

The priorities for management are to maintain adequate oxygenation and cardiac output. The patient should be given high-flow oxygen through a mask and reservoir bag, and oxygen saturation levels should be monitored. Pain control is important and intravenous morphine is the drug of choice, unless other injuries contraindicate its use. The patient should be managed by giving symptomatic support, i.e., treating dysrhythmias and maintaining blood pressure with drug therapy if necessary.

Aortic rupture

The descending thoracic aorta is particularly susceptible to rupture in rapid deceleration injury. Ninety per cent of patients die immediately (Driscoll & Skinner 2007). Those who survive do so because they have an incomplete laceration near the ligamentum arteriosum. Continuity is maintained by the adventitial layer of the aorta that contains the haematoma, which has a tamponade effect, preventing massive haemorrhage. Survival depends on rapid diagnosis and surgical repair.

Assessment

The history of deceleration injury should lead the ED nurse to suspect a possible aortic rupture. Because of the tamponade effect, patients with this injury may have lost less than 500 mL of circulating volume, so they may not appear clinically shocked. The patient may complain of chest pain or pain between the scapulae, often described as unrelenting and severe. Other symptoms include dyspnoea or respiratory distress (Yamamoto et al. 2005). If aortic injury is suspected, the pulse should be checked in all limbs. Patients with an aortic injury will have higher pulse pressure in upper limbs than in lower limbs. Blood pressure may also vary between arms. Chest X-ray may show a widened mediastinum because of the tamponade effect. Conclusive assessment should include CT scan, angiography and/or transoesophageal echocardiography to show the extent and location of the tear.

Management

Initial management involves stabilizing and resuscitating the patient in preparation for theatre. Definitive management demands rapid surgical repair of the aorta by grafting. Thoracic aortic surgery is carried out at a cardiothoracic centre, so many patients need to be transferred to alternative sites for surgery. Patients should always be intubated prior to transfer and adequate fluid and analgesia should be available. In order to prevent the flimsy adventitial layer from rupturing and leading to fatal haemorrhage, the systemic blood pressure should be kept below 100 mmHg.

Ruptured diaphragm

A ruptured diaphragm can be caused by blunt or penetrating trauma. Generally, penetrating injuries are smaller and less serious; blunt injury, however, can cause large tears. It is uncommon to injure both hemispheres of the diaphragm. The impact of large-scale tearing, particularly rupture to the left side, is that the abdominal viscera herniates into the thoracic cavity. These patients often present with a clinical picture similar to a haemothorax, but if a ruptured diaphragm cannot be excluded, diagnosis should be confirmed on X-ray.

Assessment

The mechanism of injury will give a high index of suspicion that a ruptured diaphragm has occurred. This is important because some patients will be asymptomatic, which hampers diagnosis. More commonly, patients will present with respiratory difficulty and tachypnoea due to decreased lung capacity as a result of abdominal contents in the thoracic cavity. In addition to chest pain, patients may complain of dysphagia and dyspepsia because of shifting gastric contents, and shoulder tip pain because of phrenic nerve irritation (Kehr's sign). Chest auscultation will reveal reduced breath sounds on the affected side and bowel sounds may be present. A chest X-ray will complete assessment.

Management

The management priority is to maintain respiratory function. High-flow oxygen should be given via a mask with a reservoir bag. Unless contraindicated because of other injuries, a nasogastric tube should be inserted to decompress the stomach and give symptomatic relief. Chest drain insertion is by blunt dissection because of the risk of rupture to organs such as the liver or spleen. Early surgical repair is the treatment of choice; this minimizes damage to lung tissue from gastric contents if gastric rupture or aspiration has occurred.

Tracheobronchial injuries

Injury to the major airways occurs following both severe blunt trauma and obvious penetrating trauma. Trauma to the major airways is rare, but in the case of blunt trauma it can be difficult to detect. It usually results in some degree of rupture to the airway at one of three anatomical levels.

The larynx

Injury results from RTCs where impact with the steering wheel or dashboard has occurred, or from direct blows from a fist or foot. Attempted hanging can sometimes result in a fractured larynx.

Assessment

In addition to pain and dyspnoea, the classic indications of laryngeal damage include hoarseness, crepitus and subcutaneous emphysema around the neck, because of air leaking into tissues.

Initial management entails the establishment and maintenance of a patent airway. Usually a formal tracheostomy is required.

The trachea

Mechanisms of injury are similar to those of laryngeal injury.

Assessment

Penetrating injury is usually obvious, but blunt trauma is more difficult to assess, particularly in a multiply injured patient. Respiratory distress is usually the only sign to guide the ED nurse towards an airway injury. The patient may also have haemoptysis if conscious. Obstruction occurs in the airway because of oedema and bleeding.

Initial management is to maintain a patent airway. This normally requires endotracheal intubation. In penetrating injury this can sometimes be achieved through the wound site. Where available, bronchoscopy is useful both to confirm diagnosis and to remove tissue debris and blood. Early surgical repair is required.

The bronchi

The proximal bronchi are anatomically fairly immobile and therefore susceptible to rapid deceleration injury, which results in partial or complete tearing. Patients often have associated lung injuries and the outside hospital mortality rate is >30% (Gomez-Caro et al. 2006).

Assessment

The patient will show signs of severe respiratory distress, have haemoptysis and surgical emphysema. The patient may also have a pneumothorax on the injured side. Bronchoscopy will help to determine the extent of injury.

Initial management is similar to that in tracheal injury, except that oral intubation may be difficult because of oedema. If an adequate airway can be maintained, patients are often managed conservatively. If there is a complete bronchial tear, then surgical intervention is indicated.

Oesophageal injury

Penetrating trauma can cause a rupture to the oesophagus. Oesophageal injury may also be caused by gastric contents creating a tear from inside the oesophagus, often as a result of a blow to the stomach forcing gastric contents up the oesophagus under pressure. The gastric contents then leak into the mediastinum and can erode into pleural cavities.

Assessment

Specific signs include severe pain and shock which is not consistent with other injuries, pneumothorax without fractures, and gastric contents in chest drainage.

Management

This involves maintaining adequate ventilation, pain control and surgical repair of the oesophagus.

Sternum, rib and scapular injuries

The ribs, sternum and scapula are most commonly damaged by blunt trauma. Such injuries may follow a direct blow to the chest, crushing or rapid deceleration as epitomized by RTCs. Typically, rib and sternal fractures occur on impact with a steering wheel. In comparison with injuries to the scapulae, rib injuries are much more common. Rib fractures are often associated with other injuries and therefore this suspicion should always be borne in mind. A fragment of a fractured rib may pierce the lung, pleura, pericardium or skin. Thus, subsequent complications include pneumothorax and haemothorax. Fracture of the first or second rib and/or scapula often occurs concurrently with serious head, neck, lung, great vessel and spinal cord injury and therefore is of great significance. Lower rib fractures are associated with spleen and liver injuries.

Although rib injuries vary in severity, they are all significant because of the associated pain with chest movement which may cause splinting of the chest and impair ventilation. Furthermore, this may lead to pneumonia and atelectasis. The mechanism of injury, together with chest wall contusions and bruising, should raise suspicion of rib or sternal fractures. The patient may be dyspnoeic and will have pain, localized tenderness, crepitus and deformity. Suitable analgesia to ensure adequate ventilation and deep-breathing exercises are an essential part of the management of fractured ribs. An intercostal nerve block may be used and is often the most effective way of reducing pain and facilitating adequate inspiration.

Since seat-belt legislation was introduced, an increasing number of patients with seat-belt-related sternal fractures have been reported; however, mortality from RTCs has reduced. As a great deal of force is required to fracture the sternum, underlying injury to the heart and great vessels should be suspected. Monitoring for cardiac dysrhythmias is required for patients with fractured sternum as there may be significant cardiac contusion. The majority of these patients will require a short admission to the hospital to establish an adequate analgesic regimen, which should initially include the liberal administration of parenteral narcotics in most cases, and to monitor for the early signs and symptoms of respiratory failure (Ursic & Curtis 2010).

Analgesia

Chest injuries cause hypoxaemia directly through lung damage, but also indirectly through reduced chest expansion secondary to pain. Adequate analgesia is therefore essential. The choice of analgesia in trauma care is the use of opiates and these should be used as required in thoracic trauma, remembering that opiates can reduce ventilation and the clearing of secretions.

Localized pain strategies are varied and include intrapleural blocks, intercostal blocks, paravertebral blocks, epidural blocks and transdermal local anaesthetics (Kiraly & Schreiber 2010). For long-term relief in patients who are admitted with chest trauma, epidural infusions of local anaesthetic may be used.

Conclusion

In the ED the main focus for care of patients with chest injury must be to ensure a patent airway, adequate breathing and maintenance of a viable circulation. Essentials of nursing care include early administration of high-flow oxygen, careful monitoring of vital signs and judicious fluid resuscitation. Only when these fundamental elements have been secured can more specific management ensue.

References

American College of Surgeons, 2008. Advanced Trauma Life Support, eighth ed. American College of Surgeons, Chicago.

Borman, J.B., Aharonson-Daniel, L., Savitsky, B., et al., 2006. Unilateral flail chest is seldom a lethal injury. Emergency Medicine Journal 23 (12), 903–905.

Bottlang, M., Helzel, I., Long, W.B., et al., 2010. Anatomically contoured plates for fixation of rib fractures. The Journal of Trauma Injury, Infection and Critical Care 68 (3), 611–615.

Cook, C.C., Gleason, T.G., 2009. Great Vessel and Cardiac Trauma. Surgical Clinics of North America 89 (4), 797–820.

Curtis, K., Asha, S., 2010. Blunt cardiac injury as a result of a motor vehicle collision: A case study. Australasian Emergency Nursing Journal 13 (4), 124–129.

Curtis, K., Ramsden, C., Friendship, J. (Eds.), 2007. Emergency and Trauma Nursing. Mosby Elsevier, Sydney.

Driscoll, P.A., Skinner, D., 2007. ABC of Major Trauma, fourth ed. BMJ, London.

Edwards, A., Di Bartolomeo, S., Chieregato, A., et al., 2007. A comparison of European trauma registries. The first report from the EuroTARN Group. Resuscitation 75 (2), 286–297.

Emergency Nurses Association, 2007. Trauma Nursing Core Course, sixth ed. Emergency Nurses Association, Illinois.

El-Chami, M.F., Nicholson, W., Helmy, T., 2008. Blunt cardiac trauma. The Journal of Emergency Medicine 35 (2), 127–133.

Glance, L.G., Osler, T.M., Dick, A.W., et al., 2010. The Survival Measurement and Reporting Trial for Trauma (SMARTT): Background and study design. The Journal of Trauma Injury, Infection and Critical Care 68 (6), 1491–1497.

Gomez-Caro, A., Ausin, P., Moradiellos, F.J., et al., 2006. Role of conservative medical management of tracheobronchial injuries. The Journal of Trauma Injury, Infection and Critical Care 61 (6), 1426–1435.

Harrison, C.D., Bebarta, V.S., Grant, G.A., 2009. Tympanic membrane perforation after combat blast exposure in Iraq: A poor biomarker of primary blast injury. The Journal of Trauma Injury, Infection and Critical Care 67 (1), 210–211.

Kilic, D., Findikcioglu, A., Akin, S., et al., 2011. Factors affecting morbidity and mortality in flail chest: comparison of anterior and lateral location. Thoracic Cardiovascular Surgery 59 (1), 45–48.

Kiraly, L., Schreiber, M., 2010. Management of the crushed chest. Critical Care Medicine 38 (9) suppl, 469–477.

Legare, C., Sawatzky, J.V., 2010. Dyspnea in the thoracic patient: A human response to illness. Journal of Trauma Nursing 17 (1), 36–42.

Marieb, E.N., Hoehn, K., 2007. Human Anatomy and Physiology, seventh ed. Pearson Benjamin Cummings, San Francisco.

McNett, M., Doheny, M., Sedlak, C.A., et al., 2010. Judgments of critical care nurses about risk for secondary brain injury. American Journal of Critical Care 19 (3), 250–260.

Mullins, J., Harrahill, M., 2010. Blunt cardiac trauma. Journal of Emergency Nursing 36 (6), 597–598.

Rezende-Neto, J.B., Rizoli, S.B., Andrade, M.V., et al., 2010. Permissive hypotension and desmopressin enhance clot formation. The Journal of Trauma Injury, Infection and Critical Care 68 (1), 42–51.

Roberts, K., Whalley, H., Bleetman, A., 2005. The nasopharyngeal airway: Dispelling myths and establishing facts. Emergency Medicine Journal 22, 394–396.

Rooney, S., Westaby, S., Graham, T., 2000. Chest injuries. In: Skinner, D., Driscoll, P., Easlam, R. (Eds.), ABC of Major Trauma, third ed. BMJ, London.

Sullivan, B., 2008. Nursing management of patients with a chest drain. British Journal of Nursing 17 (6), 388–393.

Taylor, I., Dawood, M., 2005. Terrorism: The reality of blast injuries. Emergency Nurse 13 (8), 22–25.

Ursic, C., Curtis, K., 2010. Thoracic and neck trauma: Part Two. International Emergency Nursing 18 (2), 99–108.

Wise, D., Chalkley, S., Ahmed, K., 2011. Massive haemothorax. In: Smith, J., Greaves, I., Porter, K. (Eds.), Oxford Desk Reference: Major Trauma. Oxford Medical Publications, Oxford.

Wyatt, J., Illingworth, R., Robertson, C., et al., 2005. Oxford Handbook of Accident and Emergency Medicine, second ed. Oxford University Press, Oxford.

Yamamoto, L., Schroeder, C., Beliveau, C., 2005. Thoracic trauma the deadly dozen. Critical Care Nursing Quarterly 28 (1), 22–40.

Zengerink, I., Brink, P.R., Laupland, K.B., et al., 2008. Needle thoracostomy in the treatment of a tension pneumothorax in trauma patients: What size needle?. The Journal of Trauma Injury, Infection and Critical Care 64 (1), 111–114.

Abdominal injuries

9

Valerie Small

CHAPTER CONTENTS

Introduction

Abdominal injuries are common in patients who sustain major trauma: approximately one-fifth of all trauma patients requiring operative intervention have sustained an injury to the abdomen (Feliciano et al. 2008, Jansen et al. 2008). Unrecognized abdominal injury continues to be the biggest cause of preventable death after truncal trauma (American College of Surgeons 2008); the resulting mortality rate in patients with abdominal trauma is reported at 13–15% (Emergency Nurses Association 2007).

Identification of serious intra-abdominal pathology is often challenging, as mechanisms of injury often result in other associated injuries that divert attention from potentially life-threatening presentations (Barry et al. 2003, American College of Surgeons 2008). Patients sustaining significant blunt torso injury from a direct blow or deceleration, or a penetrating torso injury, must be considered to have an abdominal visceral or vascular injury (Barry et al. 2003, Alarcon & Peitzman 2007). Significant amounts of blood may be present in the abdominal cavity without outward changes in the appearance of the abdomen and with no obvious signs of peritoneal irritation (American College of Surgeons 2008, Jansen et al. 2008). Evaluation and stabilization of individuals with traumatic injury utilizing the advanced trauma life support protocols provide a paradigm for patient assessment and management that prioritizes trauma resuscitation, leading to an improvement in quality of care provided by all practitioners involved in the care of patients with trauma (Sikka 2004, Alarcon & Peitzman 2007).

In this chapter specific issues related to mechanism of injury, patient assessment, physical examination and diagnostic tests will be outlined, and nursing care priorities for managing patients with abdominal injuries will be discussed.

Anatomy and pathophysiology

External anatomy of abdomen

Anterior abdomen

As the abdomen is partially enclosed by the lower thorax, the anterior abdomen is defined as the area between the transnipple line superiorly, inguinal ligaments and symphysis pubis inferiorly, and the anterior axillary lines laterally.

Flank

This is the area between the anterior and posterior axillary lines from the sixth intercostal space to the iliac crest. The thick abdominal wall musculature in this location, rather than the much thinner aponeurotic sheaths of the anterior abdomen, acts as a partial barrier to penetrating wounds, particularly stab wounds (Claridge & Croce 2007).

Back

This is the area located posterior to the posterior axillary lines from the tip of the scapulae to the iliac crests. Similar to the abdominal wall muscles in the flank, the thick back and paraspinal muscles act as a partial barrier to penetrating wounds.

Internal anatomy of the abdomen

The abdomen has three distinct anatomic compartments – the peritoneal compartment, the retroperitoneal space and the pelvic cavity. The pelvic cavity contains components of both the peritoneal cavity and the retroperitoneal spaces.

Peritoneal cavity

For convenience the peritoneal compartment may be divided into two parts, upper and lower. The upper peritoneal cavity is covered by the bony thorax and includes the diaphragm, liver, spleen, stomach and transverse colon; it is often referred to as the thoracoabdominal component of the abdomen. The diaphragm rises to the level of the fourth intercostal space on full expiration, which allows for injury to abdominal viscera from lower rib fractures and penetrating wounds below the nipple line. The lower peritoneal cavity contains the small bowel, parts of the ascending and descending colon, sigmoid colon and, in women, the organs of reproduction (Fig. 9.1).

Retroperitoneal space

The retroperitoneal space is the area posterior to the peritoneal lining of the abdomen, and contains the abdominal aorta, inferior vena cava, the pancreas, kidneys, adrenal glands, ureters, duodenum, and the posterior aspects of the ascending and descending colon and the retroperitoneal components of the pelvic cavity. Detecting injuries to the retroperitoneal viscera is difficult and may be delayed due to the obscurity of physical examination and the delay in appearance of signs and symptoms of peritonitis. Diagnostic peritoneal lavage does not sample this space and is therefore an unreliable test for injury to this area of the abdomen (Sikka 2004, Emergency Nurses Association 2007, American College of Surgeons 2008).

Pelvic cavity

The pelvic cavity is surrounded by the pelvic bones; it contains the rectum, bladder, urethra, prostate gland, iliac vessels and, in women, internal reproductive organs. Examination of the pelvic structures is compromised by the overlying bony framework.

Mechanism of injury

Many injuries may not manifest during the initial assessment and treatment period, resulting in an undiagnosed or missed injury. The most common errors in the initial assessment of a patient with trauma are an inadequate primary and secondary survey and a low index of suspicion of significant injury. Both of these clinical failures may be attributed to an under-appreciation of and for the mechanism of injury and history of the traumatic episode (Sikka 2004, American College of Surgeons 2008, Weber et al. 2010).

Missed injury is defined as an injury that is not discovered during the initial evaluation and workup in the emergency department (ED) or operating room (Sikka 2004). The incidence of missed traumatic injuries (all injuries) has been broadly estimated to be 1–18% in the paediatric population and 1–65% in the adult population. More specifically, missed intra-abdominal injuries are common and carry an additional risk as delays in diagnosis are associated with additional surgery with mortality greater than 50% (Jansen et al. 2008, Williams et al. 2009, Malinoski et al. 2010).

Intra-abdominal injuries are classically divided into blunt and penetrating trauma and will be described separately.

Right upper quadrant

Right lobe of liver
Gallbladder
Pylorus
Duodenum
Head of pancreas
Upper right kidney

Right lower quadrant

Lower right kidney
Cecum
Appendix
Ascending colon
Right fallopian tube (female)
Right ovary (female)
Right ureter
Bladder (distended)

Left upper quadrant

Left lobe of liver
Spleen
Stomach
Left kidney
Body of pancreas
Splenic flexure of colon

Left lower quadrant

Descending colon
Sigmoid colon
Left fallopian tube (female)
Left ovary (female)
Left ureter
Bladder (distended)

A

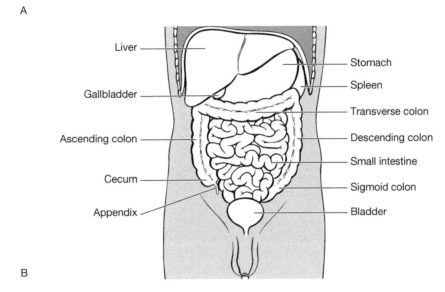

Liver
Gallbladder
Ascending colon
Cecum
Appendix

Stomach
Spleen
Transverse colon
Descending colon
Small intestine
Sigmoid colon
Bladder

B

Figure 9.1 • (A) Abdominal contents. (B) Gastrointestinal structures. • ((A) After Stillwell S (1996). Mosby's Critical Care Nursing Reference Guide, 2nd edn. St Louis: Mosby; (B) After Seidel HM et al. (1995) Mosby's Guide to Physical Examination. 3rd edn. St Louis: Mosby.)

Blunt trauma

Blunt abdominal trauma is a leading cause of morbidity and mortality among all age groups (Jansen et al. 2008, Malinoski et al. 2010). Injury to intra-abdominal structures can be classified into two primary mechanisms of injury: compression forces and deceleration forces. Compression or concussive forces may result from direct blows or external compression against a fixed object (lower rim of steering wheel, lap belt, spinal column). Most commonly these crushing forces cause tears and subcapsular haematomas to the solid viscera. These solid viscera, which cannot change shape or stretch, are therefore vulnerable to damage, although they are protected by the thoracic skeleton. When great force is applied, they may be crushed between the lower ribs and the anterior vertebral column or the para-vertebral muscles (American College of Surgeons 2008, Rushings & Britt 2008). Fractures of the lower ribs should create a high level of suspicion of associated visceral damage or diaphragmatic injury (Guitron et al. 2009).

Lap-belt marks have been correlated with rupture of small intestine and increased incidence of other intra-abdominal injury (Barry et al. 2003, Rushings & Britt 2008).

Although more commonly injured as a result of penetrating trauma, the pancreas may also be injured by crushing against the anterior spine. These forces may also deform hollow organs and transiently increase intraluminal pressure, resulting in rupture; this is a common mechanism of blunt injury to the small bowel.

Sudden-deceleration injuries may be the result of motor vehicle trauma or falls from a height. The abdominal organs move at the same speed as the external framework of the body. The external framework may decelerate suddenly, as in the case of a car driver hitting the steering wheel, dashboard or windscreen during a high-velocity collision. The driver's abdominal organs will continue at the pre-collision velocity, putting strain on or disrupting their points of attachment, until they meet another structure such as the abdominal wall.

Deceleration forces cause stretching and linear shearing between relatively fixed and free objects. Longitudinal shearing forces tend to rupture supporting structures at the junction between free and fixed segments (Rushings & Britt 2008). Classic deceleration injuries include hepatic tear along the ligamentum teres, intimal injuries to renal arteries and injuries to the arch of the aorta. Thrombosis and mesenteric tears can occur as a result of loops of bowel travelling from their mesenteric attachments.

Frequency

The true frequency of abdominal injury due to blunt trauma is unknown. According to the American College of Surgeons (2008), in patients undergoing laparotomy for blunt trauma the organs most frequently injured are the spleen (40–55%), liver (35–45%) and small intestine (5–10%). In addition, there is a 15% incidence of retroperitoneal haematoma in patients undergoing laparotomy for this type of injury.

Review of adult trauma databases in the US reveals that blunt trauma is the leading cause of intra-abdominal injury and that motor vehicle collisions are the leading mode of injury. Blunt injuries account for approximately two-thirds of all injuries, with a male to female ratio of 60:40. Peak incidence occurs in persons aged 14–30 years (Burkitt & Quick 2007, American College of Surgeons 2008).

Penetrating trauma

Throughout history, humans have created easily concealed personal weaponry designed initially for self-defense. Penetrating injuries are caused as a result of stabbing, accidental impalement, or high- or low-velocity projectiles, such as bullets or debris resulting from blast explosions. Each class of instrument or wounding source is associated with a different injury pattern of tissue damage by laceration or cutting. Abdominal organs are vulnerable to penetrating injuries not only through the anterior abdominal wall but also through the back, flank and chest below the fourth intercostal space, which may result in additional penetration of the abdomen through the diaphragm (Emergency Nurses Association 2007, Jurkovich & Wilson 2008).

Stab wounds

Stab wounds traverse adjacent abdominal structures and most commonly involve the liver (40%), small intestine (30%), diaphragm (20%) and colon (15%) (American College of Surgeons 2008). Only 33% of stab wounds penetrate the peritoneal envelope, however, and of these peritoneal violations only 50% require intervention (Barry et al. 2003, Jurkovich & Wilson 2008). Knowledge of anatomic site, number of wounds, and type, size and length of blade will aid in determining the likely path and whether the peritoneum was breached (Fig. 9.2). Lacerated hollow organs result in haemorrhage and leakage of contained fluids into the peritoneal or retroperitoneal space, resulting in poorly defined and localized somatic pain. Pain radiating to the back or shoulder may provide a valuable clue to the presence of intraperitoneal blood, clots or air. Kehr's sign is described as severe left shoulder pain caused by irritation of the left diaphragm and

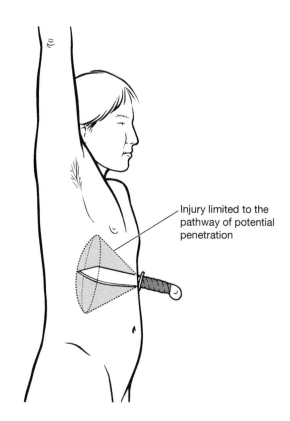

Figure 9.2 • Path of knife blade penetration in patient. • (After McSwain N (2003). The Basic EMT: Comprehensive Prehospital Patient Care. 2nd Edn. St Louis: Mosby.)

Injury limited to the pathway of potential penetration

phrenic nerve, which is induced by laying the patient in a supine position and is indicative of free intra-abdominal blood and clots (Aitken & Niggemeyer 2007). Ecchymosis around the umbilicus (Cullen's sign) or Grey-Turner's sign, which is described as a bluish discoloration at the lower abdominal flanks and lower back, may appear with retroperitoneal bleeding originating in the kidney or with pelvic fractures. These signs may occur some hours or even days after initial injury but may be observed during nursing assessment in the ED (Aitken & Niggemeyer 2007, Bacidore 2010, Blank-Reid & Reid 2010).

Gunshot injury

Gunshot injuries to the abdomen involve high energies and may damage organs remote from the site of penetration into the abdomen. It is important to establish the type of weapon used, whether handgun, shotgun or rifle, and the distance between the patient and the gun. Gunpowder around the bullet entry site will suggest firing at close range and is usually associated with an increase in injury severity. Up to 95% of gunshot wounds to the abdomen result in visceral injury and require a surgical procedure (Feliciano et al. 2008). The amount of energy released is proportional to the mass and velocity of the bullet and also depends on the density of tissue involved. A low-velocity bullet from a handgun will release less energy and cause less injury than a high-velocity bullet from a rifle. Similarly, a high-mass bullet will cause more

High-velocity wound profile

Low-velocity wound profile

Figure 9.3 • Potential injury path of high- and low-velocity bullets.
• (After Neff JA, Kidd PS (1993). Trauma Nursing: the Art and Science. St Louis: Mosby.)

damage than a low-mass bullet of similar velocity. An accurate history involving the type of weapon used and the range at which it was fired is essential in order to assess the likely magnitude of visceral injury (American College of Surgeons 2008).

A bullet will release its energy in the abdomen in two ways: first, by direct contact with organs in its path. Bullets may take a non-linear path through the abdomen. A simple, straight line connecting entry and exit wounds may not indicate the actual path of the bullet. In cases where there is no exit wound, X-rays will locate the bullet. Second, bullets transfer energy in the form of pressure waves. These pressure waves may disrupt many organs not in the actual path of the bullet. Pressure waves result in cavitation, extending the diameter of injury to many times the actual diameter of the bullet. A low-velocity missile, from a gun travelling at 1000–3000 ft/s, creates a cavity 2–3 times the diameter of the missile (Feliciano et al. 2008). High-velocity missiles, i.e., those travelling at more than 3000 ft/s, create a cavity that may be 30–40 times the diameter of the bullet (Dickinson 2004, Blank-Reid & Reid 2010) (Fig. 9.3).

Dense, solid viscera are more susceptible to cavitation than hollow organs. The sudden formation of a cavity increases intra-abdominal volume, creating a negative pressure, which may suck debris, such as clothing in through the entry wound resulting in gross intra-abdominal contamination. Gunshot wounds most commonly involve the small bowel (50%), colon (40%), liver (30%), and abdominal vascular structures (25%) (Barry et al. 2003, American College of Surgeons 2008).

Frequency

The frequency of penetrating abdominal injury across the globe relates to the industrialization of developing nations and, significantly, to the presence of military conflicts. The death rate from penetrating abdominal trauma spans the entire spectrum (0–100%), depending on the extent of injury. Patients with violation of the anterior abdominal wall fascia without peritoneal injury have a 0% mortality and morbidity rate. An average mortality rate for all patients with penetrating abdominal trauma is approximately 5% (Barry et al. 2003, Burkitt & Quick 2007).

Blast injuries

In general, most blast injuries managed in EDs tend to be accidental. They include firework mishaps, unintended occupational or industrial fuel eruptions, and unforeseen mine explosions. In many parts of the world, however, the reality persists of deadly, dormant, non-detonated, military incendiary devices such as land mines and hand grenades. Such devices cause significant numbers of civilian casualties years after local hostilities cease. During wartime, injuries arising from explosions frequently outnumber those from gunshots; many victims are innocent civilians. Blast injuries caused by terrorist bombings are also a growing part of the landscape in which people now live their lives.

The sudden, massive and catastrophic changes of pressure associated with blasts or explosions may damage the air-filled 'hollow' viscera of the gastrointestinal tract. The air within the viscera will transmit the force of the blast equally in all directions, leading to a general disruption or 'bursting' effect (Fig. 9.4).

Mannion & Chaloner (2005) categorize blast injuries into four categories: primary, secondary, tertiary, and quaternary. A patient may be injured by more than one of these mechanisms.

- Primary blast injury is caused solely by the direct effect of blast overpressure on tissue. Air is easily compressible, unlike water. As a result, a primary blast injury almost always affects air-filled structures such as the lung, middle ear and gastrointestinal (GI) tract. Other injuries include rupture of the eye and concussion without signs of head injury.
- Secondary blast injury is caused by flying objects that strike people. Injuries include penetrating ballistic or blunt injuries and eye penetration that can be occult.
- Tertiary blast injury is a feature of high-energy explosions. This type of injury occurs when people fly through the air and hit fixed objects such as walls. Fracture and traumatic amputations and closed and open brain injury are common with tertiary blast injuries.
- Quaternary blast-related injuries encompass all other injuries caused by explosions. For example, the collision of two jet airplanes into the World Trade Center on 11 September 2001 created a relatively low-order pressure wave, but the resulting fire and building collapse killed thousands (Arnold et al. 2004). The range of injuries from quaternary blasts includes flash, partial and full-thickness

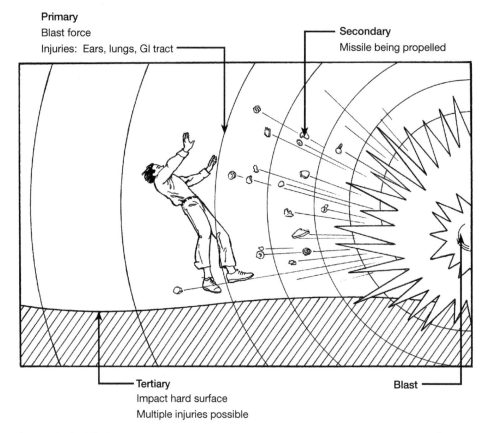

Primary
Blast force
Injuries: Ears, lungs, GI tract

Secondary
Missile being propelled

Tertiary
Impact hard surface
Multiple injuries possible

Blast

Figure 9.4 • Effects of an explosive blast. • (From ENA & Newberry: Sheehy's Emergency Nursing: Principles and Practice, 5th edn, Mosby 2002, with permission.)

burns, crush injuries, closed and open brain injury, asthma or other breathing-related problems from dust, smoke or toxic fumes, angina, hyperglycaemia, hypertension, etc. (Taylor & Dawood 2005).

Frequency

Internationally, the incidence of blast injury is sporadic and infrequent and is dependent on the political (terrorism, occupational health and safety priorities) stability of the region. Mortality rates vary widely and are increased when explosions occur in closed or confined spaces (Owers et al. 2011). The presence of tympanic membrane rupture indicates that a high-pressure wave (at least 40 kPa, 6 psi) was present and may correlate with more dangerous organ injury. Table 9.1 provides an overview of explosion-related injuries.

Assessment of abdominal trauma

The aim of assessment is to rapidly establish whether an intra-abdominal injury exists, not what the specific injury is. Evidence of intra-abdominal injury mandates urgent surgical exploration of the abdomen, at which time an accurate diagnosis may be made. Assessment is made on the basis of a history, the results of a primary survey, the victim's response to treatment started as a result of that primary survey, a secondary survey including an abdominal examination, and the results of any diagnostic tests such as focused assessment

sonogram for trauma (FAST), diagnostic peritoneal lavage (DPL) or computed tomography (CT) scan. The emergency nurse plays a key role in the initial and continuous assessment and monitoring of the injured patient and may be the first member of the trauma team to identify subtle but significant changes in the patient's condition.

History

An accurate history of the events leading to injury is crucial to identifying possible serious intra-abdominal pathology and can direct potential therapeutic priorities. The emergency nurse plays a vital role in gathering and collating information from a number of sources and disseminating that information to members of the trauma team (Cole et al. 2006). Information can be provided by the patient if alert, or by bystanders, police and emergency medical personnel. Pertinent information in assessing the patient injured in a motor vehicle collision includes the speed of the vehicle, type of collision (frontal or lateral impact, rear impact or rollover), vehicle intrusion into the passenger compartment, types of restraint, deployment of air bag, the patient's position in the vehicle and status of passengers (American College of Surgeons 2008). The history surrounding a patient with penetrating trauma is also important, as it provides clues to the likely injury complex. Clues are gleaned from the injury location and from determination of the associated weapon

Table 9.1 Overview of explosion-related injuries

System	Injury or condition
Auditory	Tympanic membrane rupture, ossicular disruption, cochlear damage, foreign body
Eye, orbit, face	Perforated globe, foreign body, air embolism
Respiratory	'Blast lung', haemothorax, pneumothorax, pulmonary contusion or haemorrhage, arteriovenous fistulae acting as sources of air embolism, airway epithelial damage, aspiration, pneumonitis sepsis
Digestive	Bowel perforation, haemorrhage, ruptured liver or spleen, sepsis, mesenteric ischaemia from air embolism
Circulatory	Cardiac contusion, myocardial infarction from air embolism, shock, vasovagal hypotension, peripheral vascular injury, air-embolism-induced injury
Central nervous injury	Concussion, closed and open brain injury, stroke, spinal cord injury, air-embolism-induced injury
Renal	Renal contusion or laceration, acute renal failure due to rhabdomyolysis, hypotension, hypovolaemia
Extremities	Traumatic amputation, fractures, crush injuries, compartment syndrome, burns, cuts, lacerations, acute arterial occlusion, air-embolism-induced injury

(After Taylor I, Dawood M (2005) Terrorism: the reality of blast injuries. Emergency Nurse, 13(8), 22–25; Centers for Disease Control (CDC) (2003) Explosions and Blast Injuries: A Primer for Clinicians. Atlanta: CDC.)

Box 9.1

History-taking for stabbing or for gunshot injuries impalement

- The size, shape and length of the weapon
- The number of stabbing attempts made
- Blood loss at scene and in transit
- Angle of penetration
- Height of assailant
- Sex of assailant (males tend to stab upwards) (Luckmann & Sorenson 1987)
- The type of weapon involved
- High/low velocity and bullet size
- Weapon to victim distance
- Number of shots fired

(e.g., gun, knife) or injury-causing object. The number of gunshots heard, times stabbed, and position of the patient at the time of injury help describe the trajectory and path of the injuring object. Range also is important when assessing gunshot wounds. A careful history that assesses secondary and multi-cavity injuries is vital, as many victims sustain a blunt assault or fall from various heights after sustaining a penetrating trauma (Barry et al. 2003) (Boxes 9.1, 9.2).

Box 9.2

Useful information specific to blunt injuries

- Motor vehicle speed, or height of fall
- Was the victim ejected from the vehicle on impact?
- Damage caused to vehicle and position of victim in vehicle
- Was the victim restrained by a seatbelt?
- The impact configuration

Blood loss at the scene should be quantified as accurately as possible to help determine transfusion needs. The character of the bleeding (e.g., arterial pumping, venous flow) helps determine whether major vascular injury has occurred. The initial level of consciousness or, for moribund patients, the presence of any signs of life at the scene (e.g., pupillary response, respiratory efforts, heart rate or tones) is vital to determine the prognosis and to guide resuscitative efforts. Particularly important is the patient's response to therapy en route to the emergency department.

Primary survey

The primary survey and resuscitation are examined in detail in Chapter 2. Assessment priorities relevant to abdominal trauma are outlined here:

- *airway maintenance* with cervical spine control
- *breathing*, ventilation, and oxygenation: injuries to the diaphragm or penetrating injuries involving the intra-thoracic abdomen and chest may compromise breathing
- *circulation* with haemorrhage control: gross external haemorrhage from the abdomen is rare. The abdomen, however, is a potential reservoir for a large volume of occult haemorrhage. Uncontrolled haemorrhage from damaged abdominal organs and vessels will cause hypovolaemia and death. Haemorrhage may remain uncontrolled because it is not detected. Early detection of haemorrhage is therefore essential for survival in any case of abdominal injury. Any hypovolaemia is treated with an intra-venous fluid challenge
- *disability:* neurological status
- *exposure*: completely undress the patient; care should be taken not to cut clothes across stab or bullet holes as this may destroy crucial forensic evidence. Hypothermia must be prevented by the use of overhead heaters or a warm-air heating system which can be easily controlled and adjusted according to the patient's temperature
- *adjuncts to primary survey and resuscitation*: obtain arterial blood gas analysis and ventilatory rate, monitor exhaled CO_2.

The insertion of gastric and urinary catheters is frequently performed as part of the resuscitation phase once problems with airway, breathing and circulation are corrected.

The goal of inserting a gastric tube is to relieve acute gastric dilatation, decompress the stomach before physical examination or performing a DPL (if indicated) and remove gastric contents, thus removing risk of aspiration (American College of Surgeons 2008). Special consideration should be given in circumstances where there is severe facial trauma or a suspicion of cribriform plate fracture, in which case the gastric tube may be inserted through the mouth.

Similar goals apply to the insertion of a urinary catheter in this phase, such as decompression of the bladder prior to DPL, in preparation for an abdominal examination and possible surgical entry into the abdomen and to allow monitoring of urinary output as an index of tissue perfusion. Haematuria if present raises a high index of suspicion of genitourinary trauma. Contraindications for urinary catheterization are blood at the urethral meatus, and the presence of a scrotal haematoma, both of which may indicate urethral injury. A disruption to the urethra may require a supra-pubic catheter to be inserted. A urinalysis is carried out on all patients and a urine pregnancy test is indicated in all females of childbearing age (American College of Surgeons 2008).

Radiological examination should not delay patient resuscitation and should be used judiciously. The anteroposterior (AP) chest film and an AP pelvis may provide important information about patients with blunt trauma. A lateral cervical spine X-ray that demonstrates an injury is an extremely important finding and will dictate the patient's management in the secondary survey. Negative or inadequate X-ray does not exclude cervical spine injury and spinal cord protection should continue until further radiological investigation is carried out in the secondary survey.

Diagnostic studies such as DPL and abdominal ultrasound are useful tools for detecting occult intra-abdominal haemorrhage and may be considered at this stage; however, such tests require the skills of an experienced practitioner and may be performed as part of the secondary survey. The indications, advantages and disadvantages of these studies are discussed in further detail in this chapter.

Secondary survey

The secondary survey does not begin until the primary survey (ABCDEs) has been completed, resuscitation is initiated and the patient is demonstrating normal vital functions (American College of Surgeons 2008). The secondary survey is a head-to-toe evaluation of the trauma patient and includes a complete history and physical examination of all systems and a reassessment of vital signs. A physical examination of the abdomen is performed as part of a complete secondary survey of the patient.

History

The AMPLE history is often useful as a mnemonic for remembering key elements of the history:

A – allergies, age and alcohol?
M – medications currently used
P – past, pertinent medical history
L – last meal, low temperature?
E – events/environment related to injury.

Physical examination

Abdominal injuries must be identified and treated aggressively; a normal initial examination of the abdomen does not exclude a significant intra-abdominal injury. Close evaluation and frequent re-evaluation of the abdomen preferably by the same observer in conjunction with close monitoring of vital signs is important when dealing with blunt abdominal trauma.

Inspection

The anterior and posterior abdomen as well as the lower chest and perineum should be inspected; injury patterns that suggest a potential for intra-abdominal trauma should raise suspicion (lap-belt abrasions or ecchymosis, steering wheel-shaped contusions). Obvious abnormalities including distension and asymmetry along with contusions, abrasions, penetrating wounds or exposed viscera should be noted and documented accurately (Blank-Reid & Reid 2010, Talley & O'Connor 2010).

Auscultation

Auscultation of the abdomen may be carried out to confirm the presence or absence of bowel sounds; however, this may prove difficult in a noisy ED. Auscultation should take place before percussion and palpation because these examinations can change the frequency of bowel sounds. Visceral injury may release blood or enteric contents into the peritoneal cavity, resulting in irritation of the bowel which may produce a paralytic ileus, and thus an absence of bowel sounds. If bowel sounds are heard in the chest it is an indication of diaphragmatic rupture with herniation of stomach or small bowel into the thoracic cavity (Bacidore 2010, Talley & O'Connor 2010).

Percussion

Percussion, or gentle tapping of the abdomen, produces a slight movement of the peritoneum. In the normal abdomen, percussion elicits dull sounds over solid organs and fluid-filled structures such as a full bladder and tympani over air-filled areas such as the stomach. If the peritoneum is injured, or irritated by free fluid released as a result of injury to viscera, this movement will cause pain. This is an unequivocal sign of intra-abdominal injury. Percussion may elicit subtle signs of peritonitis or isolate acute gastric dilatation by producing tympanic sounds or dullness due to haemoperitoneum. Percussion tenderness constitutes a peritoneal sign and mandates further evaluation and surgical consultation (Sikka 2004).

Palpation

Palpation is carried out to elicit and localize superficial, deep or rebound tenderness. The presence of a pregnant uterus, as well as estimation of foetal age, can also be determined at this stage of assessment. Involuntary guarding, rigidity, pain or spasm during palpation indicates peritoneal irritation. These signs may be absent, however, if the patient has competing pain from another injury, a retroperitoneal injury, a spinal cord injury, has ingested alcohol or narcotics or has a decreased level of consciousness.

Log roll and cervical spine immobilization

The patient should be cautiously log-rolled, maintaining cervical spine immobilization. This is necessary for complete assessment of the posterior chest, flank and back. Evidence of penetrating injury, surface ecchymosis, grazing or tenderness over the thoracolumbar spine may indicate possible retroperitoneal organ injury.

While the patient is in a lateral position, a rectal examination should be performed. Bony fragments felt on rectal examination may indicate a fractured pelvis. Fresh blood in the rectum suggests a disrupted colon or rectum. A high-riding or absent prostate, in the male, may indicate a urethral transection, and contraindicates urinary catheterization. A vaginal examination is necessary in the female patient. Fractures of the pelvis may be discovered by direct palpation, and the integrity of the vaginal wall can be assessed. Examination of the gluteal region which extends from the iliac crests to the gluteal folds should also be carried out. Penetrating injuries to this area are associated with up to 50% incidence of significant intra-abdominal trauma and mandate a search for intra-abdominal injury (American College of Surgeons 2008).

Radiological studies

A lateral cervical spine X-ray, an AP chest and a pelvic X-ray are the screening radiographs obtained in the patient with multisystem blunt trauma and continue to be important adjuncts to the primary survey. Jansen et al. (2008) argue that plain abdominal radiography has no role in the assessment of blunt abdominal trauma as it does not visualize abdominal viscera or detect free fluid and therefore cannot provide direct evidence of organ injury or indirect evidence of injury. Abdominal X-rays (supine, upright, lateral decubitus) may be useful in the haemodynamically stable patient to detect extra-luminal air in the retroperitoneum or free air under the diaphragm, both of which mandate urgent laparotomy (American College of Surgeons 2008). CT is regarded as the imaging modality of choice for evaluating the haemodynamically stable patient as it is 92–97.6% sensitive and 98.7% specific for detecting injuries which include the retroperitoneum and diaphragm (Hom 2010, Jansen et al. 2008).

The haemodynamically unstable patient with a penetrating abdominal wound does not require radiological screening in the ED. An upright chest X-ray is useful in the patient who is haemodynamically stable with penetrating injury above the umbilicus or who has a suspected thoracoabdominal injury.

Chest X-ray can detect an associated pneumothorax or haemopneumothorax, or isolate air in the peritoneum. Supine abdominal X-ray may be useful to determine the track of a missile or bullet or the presence of retroperitoneal air; however, obtaining an abdominal X-ray is strongly discouraged as it delays more useful investigations (Raby et al. 2005).

Subsequent action

The management of blunt and penetrative trauma to the abdomen that follows the completion of the secondary survey is determined by the results of the physical examination and the circulatory status of the patient, i.e., whether there is any hypovolaemia, and the nature of the response to any fluid challenge measured by frequent recordings of vital signs. All blunt traumas should carry an associated high index of suspicion of intra-abdominal injury. Constant reassessment of the patient is necessary as it may take several hours for symptoms to develop, particularly splenic or duodenal injuries (Eckert 2005).

A three-stage response to abdominal examination exists:

1. *No immediate action – observation only:* a negative abdominal examination with no hypovolaemia. The abdominal examination should be repeated at frequent intervals.
2. *Special diagnostic studies urgently required:* an equivocal or unreliable abdominal examination in a multiply injured patient.
3. *Immediate surgical exploration of the abdomen required:* the need for urgent laparotomy is determined by history, findings on examination, and the results of investigations.

The following indications are commonly used to facilitate the decision-making process and are described by the American College of Surgeons (2008):

- blunt abdominal trauma with hypotension and clinical evidence of intraperitoneal bleeding
- blunt abdominal trauma with positive DPL or FAST
- hypotension with penetrating abdominal wound
- gunshot wounds traversing the peritoneal cavity or visceral/vascular retroperitoneum
- organ evisceration
- bleeding from the stomach, rectum, or genitourinary tract from penetrating wounds
- presenting or subsequent peritonitis
- free air, retroperitoneal air, or rupture of the hemidiaphragm
- contrast-enhanced CT demonstrates ruptured gastrointestinal tract, intraperitoneal bladder injury, renal pedicle injury or severe visceral parenchymal injury after blunt or penetrating trauma.

Special diagnostic studies

If there are early or obvious indications that a trauma patient will be transferred to another facility, time-consuming tests such as DPL, CT, contrast urologic and gastrointestinal studies should not be performed (American College of Surgeons 2008).

Diagnostic peritoneal lavage

Diagnostic peritoneal lavage was first described in 1965 (Schulman 2003, Jansen et al. 2008) and has been a primary diagnostic method of evaluation of abdominal injury. Although its application in practice has decreased significantly (Badger et al. 2009), DPL is a rapidly performed invasive procedure that is considered 95 % sensitive for detecting intraperitoneal haemorrhage (Emergency Nurses Association 2007). While DPL is a highly sensitive test it lacks specificity for evaluating the severity and identifying the location of the injured organ. It has a complication rate of approximately 1 % from mechanical injury to viscera during incision, or during insertion of the catheter (Schulman 2003). Bleeding from the incision, dissection or catheter insertion can cause false-positive results that may lead to unnecessary laparotomy (American College of Surgeons 2008, Jansen et al. 2008).

It is recommended that the procedure should be carried out by the surgical team caring for the haemodynamically unstable patient with multiple blunt injuries. The procedure may also be carried out in haemodynamically stable patients when ultrasound or CT is unavailable.

The preferred procedure involves an open or semi-open technique that is performed in the infra-umbilical area. In pregnant patients or patients with pelvic fracture an open supra-umbilical technique is preferred to avoid entering a pelvic haematoma or damaging the enlarged uterus. The procedure is performed under local anaesthetic, with lignocaine and adrenaline (epinephrine) to constrict the blood supply to the incised area. A catheter is inserted into the peritoneal cavity through the incision: free aspiration of blood, gastrointestinal contents, vegetable fibres or bile through the lavage catheter in the haemodynamically unstable patient mandates an urgent laparotomy. If gross blood (>10 mL) is not aspirated, lavage is performed with a litre of warmed Ringer's lactate solution (10 mL/kg in a child). Following adequate mixing of peritoneal contents with fluid by compressing the abdomen and log rolling the patient, the effluent is allowed to free drain by gravity and is sent to the laboratory for analysis. A positive test is indicated by the presence of more than $100\,000$ RBC/mm^3, or more than 500 WBC/mm^3, or a Gram stain with bacteria present (American College of Surgeons 2008).

The indications for carrying out DPL are outlined in Box 9.3.

An absolute contraindication to DPL is an existing indication for immediate laparotomy. The disadvantages of DPL include utilizing an invasive technique and requiring the patient to have a gastric tube and indwelling catheter in place to avoid accidental perforation of bladder or stomach. Additional limitations include the inability of DPL to identify retroperitoneal or diaphragmatic injury as well as detecting hollow viscous injuries (Chughtai et al. 2009). The time required for laboratory test analysis and the relative

---

Box 9.3

Diagnostic peritoneal lavage

Indications

- Altered sensorium – brain injury, alcohol or drug ingestion
- Spinal cord injury
- Injury to adjacent structures – lower ribs, pelvis, lumbar spine
- Equivocal physical examination
- Prolonged loss of contact with patient anticipated (lengthy X-ray studies in haemodynamically unstable or stable patient)
- Lap belt sign with suspicion of bowel injury

Contraindications

Absolute contraindication

- Obvious need for surgery, for instance, due to gunshot wound to abdomen

Relative contraindications

- Previous abdominal surgery
- Pregnancy
- Abdominal wall haematoma
- Obesity
- Distended abdomen

---

contraindications in patients with prior abdominal surgery, obesity, advanced cirrhosis of the liver or patients in the third trimester of pregnancy may suggest consideration of other diagnostic tests such as FAST.

Focused abdominal sonography for trauma

The use of ultrasound in the evaluation of abdominal injury has been practised since the early 1970s and has grown in popularity as a diagnostic tool in the ED setting particularly since the 1990s (Schulman 2003, Raby et al. 2005, Jansen et al. 2008).

Ultrasound can be used to detect with 98 % accuracy the presence of haemoperitoneum and visceral injury and it has 98–100 % specificity in locating the site of injury (Schulman 2003, Jansen et al. 2008). FAST provides a rapid, non-invasive, accurate and inexpensive means of diagnosing haemoperitoneum that can be repeated frequently (Raby et al. 2005, Kirkpatrick 2007). Even if ultrasonography reveals no obvious aetiology, it can facilitate diagnosis by excluding potentially life-threatening conditions. Emergency abdominal ultrasonography is indicated for the evaluation of aortic aneurysm, appendicitis, and biliary and renal colic, as well as of blunt or penetrating abdominal trauma (Chen et al. 2000, Richards et al. 2002, Kirkpatrick 2007).

The use of FAST is not intended to replace CT or DPL; rather, it is recommended as an adjunct diagnostic tool for rapid screening for potential abdominal injuries during the initial physical examination. It can be performed in the resuscitation room at the bedside while simultaneously performing other diagnostic or therapeutic procedures (Kirkpatrick 2007, Jansen et al. 2008).

Fast examination

Identification of haemoperitoneum by ultrasound is based upon experience and understanding of abdominal anatomy, therefore specific equipment in experienced hands is a requirement for utilizing such a tool. Current literature recommends that the use of FAST should be limited to clinicians who have completed a special training programme (Schulman 2003, American College of Surgeons 2008, Jansen et al. 2008).

FAST can demonstrate the presence or absence of pericardial fluid, abdominal fluid, and some parenchymal injuries in a two to three minute examination.

A hand-held transducer is positioned on four key areas to evaluate fluid collection:

- to screen for life-threatening accumulation of pericardial fluid the transducer is placed left of the lower sternum and angled under the costal margin towards the patient's shoulder
- to visualize the spleen and perisplenic area the transducer is placed between the 10th and 11th ribs on the left posterior axillary line
- to evaluate the perihepatic region, the transducer is placed between the 10th and 11th ribs on the right axillary line
- as blood may accumulate in dependent areas of the abdomen and pelvis, the transducer is placed above the symphysis pubis.

False negatives may result if FAST is performed early on in the patient's care; at least 100 mL of fluid are needed to be detectable on scan (Schulman 2003).

Advantages of FAST include rapid access, quick performance time, non-invasive testing, easy repetition, and no requirement for patient transport (Eckert 2005, Kirkpatrick 2007). Unlike DPL, ultrasound is capable of locating the injury, testing is not compromised by previous laparotomy or contraindicated in pregnancy and it can be used on patients with clotting disorders. Performance of the test by a trained surgeon or emergency physician eliminates the waiting time for technicians. Reported studies have found that the use of ultrasound has reduced the need for CT (from 56 % to 26 %) and DPL (17 % to 4 %) and reduced overall hospital admission rates by 38 % (Branney et al. 1997).

A limitation of ultrasound is in detecting intestinal injury and estimating the amount of haemoperitoneum present. Interpretation of test results may be limited depending on the expertise of the operator and interpreter; it may also be unreliable in patients with obesity, ascites and subcutaneous emphysema. It is important that ultrasound is not used as the single diagnostic tool in evaluating patients with abdominal injury; rather it should be utilized in conjunction with serial physical examinations, DPL, CT scanning and re-evaluation by ultrasound (American College of Surgeons 2008, Jansen et al. 2008). The emergency nurse should be aware and anticipate the use of FAST in the early diagnostic phase of trauma patient care and understand the limitations of such a diagnostic test so that continued vital-sign monitoring and vigilance in patient assessment is maintained to avoid missed life-threatening injuries.

Computed tomography

Computed tomography (CT) scanning is a non-invasive radiological examination and since its introduction in the 1990s, CT has become increasingly important in trauma care (Sierink et al. 2012). It is considered the best method for identifying specific sites and amounts of bleeding, but may miss mesenteric or hollow-organ injury; also some specific injuries to the diaphragm and pancreas may be missed (Schulman 2003, Khan & Garner 2011). Although CT scanning is the most sensitive diagnostic tool for most abdominal injuries, it is costly and requires time to prepare and execute. It also greatly increases radiation exposure which, with liberal use, imparts a small but finite risk of later cancer, especially in younger patients (Kirkpatrick 2007). In most hospitals, the patient must be transported to the radiology department, which is contraindicated in the haemodynamically unstable patient. However turnaround times are decreasing as a result of new-generation multidetector helical scanners with faster image acquisition and also an increasing trend to locate scanners in or close to emergency departments (Jansen et al. 2008). CT may require the administration of intravenous or oral contrast, which can prove problematic where information on allergies is unknown. Additional limitations of CT include inability to perform the scan on an uncooperative patient (Table 9.2).

Specific intra-abdominal injuries

Diaphragmatic injury

Diaphragmatic injury in blunt trauma is relatively rare. It is estimated that it is seen in 3–5 % of all patients with blunt trauma who survive long enough to be admitted to hospital (Guitron et al. 2009). The diaphragm is integral to normal ventilation and injuries can result in significant compromise. A history of respiratory difficulty and related pulmonary symptoms may indicate a diaphragmatic disruption. The mechanism of diaphragm rupture is related to the pressure gradient between the pleural and peritoneal cavities. Lateral impact from a motor vehicle collision is three times more likely than any other type of impact to cause a rupture, since it can distort the chest wall and shear the ipsilateral diaphragm (Rushings & Britt 2008, Chen et al. 2010). Frontal impact from a motor vehicle collision can cause an increase in intra-abdominal pressure, which results in long radial tears in the posterolateral aspect of the diaphragm, its embryologic weak point. The majority (70–80 %) of diaphragmatic injuries occur on the left side, with 20–30 % occurring on the right side and 5–10 % occurring bilaterally (Chen et al. 2010).

Diaphragmatic tears do not occur in isolation; patients often have associated thoracic and/or abdominal injury or a concomitant head or extremity injury. Symptoms and signs of diaphragmatic rupture such as respiratory distress, cardiac disturbances, deviated trachea and bowel sounds in the chest are present in only a minority of patients initially assessed (Guitron et al. 2009, Chen et al. 2010). The less common right-sided ruptures are associated with more severe injuries such as tears of the juxtahepatic vena cava and hepatic veins

Table 9.2 Comparison of DPL versus FAST versus CT in blunt abdominal trauma

	DPL	FAST	CT scan
Indication	• Provide evidence of bleeding if hypotensive	• Provide evidence of fluid if hypotensive	• Provide evidence of organ injury if BP normal
Advantages	• Early diagnosis • All patients • Performed rapidly • 98 % sensitive • Detects bowel injury • No transport required	• Early diagnosis • All patients • Non-invasive • Performed rapidly • Repeatable • 86–97 % accurate • 98–100 % specificity • No transport required	• Most specific for injury • Sensitive: 92–98 % accurate
Disadvantages	• Invasive • Low specificity • Misses injury to diaphragm and retroperitoneum	• Operator-dependent • Bowel gas and subcutaneous air distortion • Misses diaphragm, bowel, pancreatic and solid organ injuries	• High cost • Time-consuming • Misses diaphragm and some pancreatic injuries • Transport required

(Adapted from American College of Surgeons (2008) Advanced Trauma Life Support, 8th edn. Chicago: American College of Surgeons.)

as well as laceration of the liver. When herniation occurs on the right the liver is always present and the colon occasionally; such injuries result in haemodynamic instability and hypovolaemic shock. Reports on an autopsy series revealed that left- and right-sided diaphragmatic ruptures occurred almost equally; however, the more severe injuries associated with right-sided rupture caused more deaths and thus a lower rate of patient survival until diagnosis in hospital.

The rates of associated injury are: pelvic fractures 40 %, splenic rupture 25 %, liver laceration 25 %, thoracic aortic tear 5–10 %. Diagnosis may not be obvious and is made pre-operatively in only 40–50% of left-sided and 0–10 % of right-sided blunt ruptures. If diagnosis is not made in the first four hours it may be delayed for months or years; thus 10–50 % of injuries are diagnosed in a latent phase which occurs as a result of gradual herniation of abdominal contents into the pleural cavity. Diagnosis may be made later still in a third phase which is characterized by bowel or visceral herniation, causing obstruction and/or strangulation of stomach and colon. If herniation causes significant lung compression it can lead to tension pneumothorax, while cardiac tamponade has been described from herniation of abdominal contents into the pericardium (Chen et al. 2010). The incidence of diaphragmatic injury increases each decade as a result of increased occurrence of high-speed motor-vehicle accidents. Improved survival rates are likely to be due to improvements in pre-hospital and emergency care and earlier recognition and treatment of severe injury.

Duodenum

Duodenal injury is a rare condition and is typically associated with a direct blow to the epigastrium due to a traffic accident or sports injury. Delay in diagnosis is common because the duodenum lies in the retroperitoneum and often combines with other severe injury such as fractures or other organ injury. The incidence of traumatic duodenum injury, however, is lower than other abdominal injury, with reported rates of 3.5–12 % (Aherne et al. 2003). Morbidity is more dependent on other associated injuries than on the degree of the duodenal injury. Bloody gastric aspirate or retroperitoneal air on X-ray or abdominal CT scanning will raise suspicion for this injury (American College of Surgeons 2008) and will require further investigation. Treatment is often simple surgical repair but is dependent on the extent and nature of injury to the duodenum and other concomitant injuries.

Solid organ injury

Injuries to the liver, spleen or kidney that result in shock, haemodynamic instability or evidence of continued bleeding remain indications for urgent laparotomy. Isolated solid organ injury in the haemodynamically stable patient can often be managed conservatively but will require evaluation by a surgeon and admission to hospital for observation.

Spleen

Injury to the spleen is most commonly associated with blunt trauma. Fracture of ribs 10 to 12 on the left should raise suspicion of spleen injury, which ranges from laceration of the capsule or a non-expanding haematoma to ruptured subcapsular haematoma or parenchymal lacerations. The most serious types of injury are a severely fractured spleen or vascular tear that causes splenic ischaemia and massive blood loss; however, shock and hypotension are present in as few as 30 % of patients with splenic trauma (Bacidore 2010).

Liver

Hepatobilary and pancreatic trauma represent a significant management challenge for emergency clinicians. These injuries require a high index of suspicion, rapid investigation, and well-defined management protocols to ensure an optimal outcome with minimal long-term consequences (Oniscu 2006, Badger et al. 2009). Due to its size and location the liver is the most commonly injured solid intra-abdominal organ (Oniscu et al. 2006). Severity ranges from a controlled subcapsular haematoma and lacerations of the parenchyma to hepatic avulsion or a severe injury to the hepatic veins. Because liver tissue is very friable and the liver's blood supply and storage capacity are extensive, a patient with liver injury can haemorrhage profusely and may need surgery to control bleeding. Prior to 1990, most blunt injuries were treated surgically to ensure haemostasis. It is now widely accepted that 50–80% of liver injuries stop bleeding spontaneously and therefore a conservative approach is effective and relatively safe in haemodynamically stable patients who can be closely monitored (Oniscu et al. 2006, Badger et al. 2009).

Pancreas

Although less common than liver trauma, pancreatic injuries should be suspected in any patient with penetrating trauma to the trunk or following blunt compression of the upper abdomen. As with liver trauma, CT scanning is the main diagnostic procedure used to detect pancreatic trauma (Oniscu et al. 2006).

Genitourinary

Direct blows to the back or flank resulting in contusions, ecchymosis or haematoma are markers for potential underlying renal injury and warrant evaluation of the urinary tract (American College of Surgeons 2008). Contusion is the most common kidney injury and should be suspected in posterior rib fracture or fracture to the lumbar vertebrae. Other renal injuries include lacerations or contusion of the renal parenchyma, the deeper a laceration the more serious the bleeding. Deceleration forces may damage the renal artery: collateral circulation in that area is limited, therefore any ischaemia is serious and may trigger acute tubular necrosis.

Pelvic injury

The pelvis protects the organs within the pelvic compartment, transmits weight from the trunk to the lower limbs and has attachment points for muscles. A stable pelvis can withstand vertical and rotational physiological forces, but either fractures or ligamentous injuries can disrupt pelvic stability. Pelvic blood supply comes primarily from the iliac and hypogastric arteries, which run at the level of the sacroiliac joints. Those arteries are supplemented by a rich associated network, including the superior gluteal artery, which is susceptible to injury in posterior fractures, and the obturator and internal pudendal arteries, which can be injured in fractures of the ramus (Frakes & Evans 2004).

Road traffic accidents cause about 60% of pelvic fractures; most of the remainder result from falls (Frakes & Evans 2004, O'Sullivan et al. 2005). Pelvic fracture is said to contribute to traumatic death but is not the primary cause. For patients with pelvic fracture who die, hypotension at the time of admission is associated with increased mortality (42% vs 3.4% with stable vital signs), as are head injuries requiring neurosurgery (50% mortality); abdominal injuries requiring laparotomy (52% mortality); concomitant thoracic, urological or skeletal injuries (22% mortality). Survival is poorer for patients with open pelvic fractures and for pedestrians struck by cars (Frakes & Evans 2004, O'Sullivan et al. 2005). Genitourinary injuries are seen in association with 15% of all pelvic fractures. The bladder, rectum and vagina may be punctured by fracture fragments, or the bladder may be ruptured by a direct blow if full of urine. The male urethra that passes through the prostate is relatively immobile; the rest of the urethra passes through the urogenital diaphragm, which is attached to the pubic rami. If the pelvis is fractured, this portion may shear from the rest at the apex of the prostate and the prostate is then displaced upwards. Injuries to the female urethra are rare.

Pelvic fractures can be accurately diagnosed through physical examination but a high index of suspicion for a fracture based on the mechanism of injury is essential. Abrasions, contusions, isolated rotation of the lower extremity and discrepancy in limb length may alert the emergency nurse to the presence of pelvic fracture (Frakes & Evans 2004, Bailey 2005). Gentle compression of the iliac crests is advised to assess for tenderness, crepitus and stability of the pelvic ring. Rocking the pelvis and repeated examination is contraindicated where pelvic fracture is suspected or diagnosed. Repeated examination and excessive or unnecessary movement can aggravate bleeding, displace a fracture or disrupt a pelvic haematoma (Frakes & Evans 2004, Bailey 2005, American College of Surgeons 2008). Immobilization tools and techniques range from a sheet wrapped around the pelvis causing internal rotation of the lower limbs, a commercially available pelvic splint and external fixation devices which may be inserted by the orthopaedic surgeon in the resuscitation room in order to limit blood loss (Tile et al. 2003, Emergency Nurses Association 2007) (see also Chapter 6).

Abdominal injuries in children

Injury continues to be the most common cause of death and disability in childhood (Rothrock et al. 2000, Wise et al. 2002, Advanced Life Support Group 2005) and injury morbidity and mortality surpass all major diseases in children and young adults (American College of Surgeons 2008). At least 25% of children with multisystem injury have significant abdominal injury although most are due to blunt trauma, most frequently from motor-vehicle collisions. The priorities of assessment and management of the injured child are the same as in the adult although physically, emotionally, intellectually and socially they differ greatly from adults. Only the differences related to abdominal injuries are considered in this section.

Specific anatomy in children

Children are vulnerable to abdominal injury for a number of reasons. Children are small; therefore any blunt trauma is likely to affect more body systems than in a similar incident involving an adult. The abdominal wall is thin, and offers little protection to its contents. Children have relatively compact torsos with smaller anterior–posterior diameters, which provide a smaller area over which the force of injury can be dissipated. The ribs are more elastic, decreasing protection to the spleen, liver and kidneys. The diaphragm lies more horizontally, lowering and further exposing these organs, which are relatively larger than in adults, with less overlying fat and weaker abdominal musculature. The kidneys are also more mobile, and not shielded by perinephretic fat, as in adults. The bladder is superior to the protection of the pelvis, and therefore more vulnerable. Finally, abdominal injuries may cause diaphragmatic irritation and splinting, compromising ventilation (Day & Rupp 2003, Advanced Life Support Group 2005, Fleisher & Ludwig 2010).

Types and patterns of abdominal injury in children

The majority of abdominal injuries in children are caused by blunt trauma. Penetrating injuries are rare but the hypotensive child who sustains a penetrating abdominal injury requires prompt surgical intervention (Advanced Life Support Group 2005). Motor vehicle trauma, bicycle handlebar injuries, falls and non-accidental injury are the most common causes of abdominal injuries (Williams et al. 2009, Browne et al. 2010). As in adults, the spleen, liver and kidneys are the most commonly injured organs in the child victim of blunt trauma. The mortality of blunt abdominal trauma in children is directly related to the level of involvement: it is less than 20% in isolated liver, spleen, kidney or pancreatic trauma; increases to 20% if the gastrointestinal tract is involved; and increases to 50% if major vessels are injured (Day & Rupp 2003, Williams et al. 2009).

Assessment of abdominal trauma in children

The primary survey is carried out as in adults, with the same priorities and aims. An examination of the abdomen is carried out as part of the secondary survey. The examination is the same as that for adults, with the following special considerations. Care should be taken to be gentle on palpation, as any pain will produce voluntary guarding, making assessment difficult. Children swallow air when crying and upset; this produces distension of the stomach, which makes assessment difficult, and may mimic the rigidity and distension found in intra-abdominal injury. A nasogastric or orogastric tube (in infants and patients with maxillofacial trauma) should be placed in the resuscitation phase before abdominal examination (American College of Surgeons 2008). Gastric decompression will facilitate abdominal examination and prevent aspiration of gastric contents if vomiting occurs (Saladino & Lund 2010). A urinary catheter of appropriate size should always be passed, unless contraindicated, in order to decompress the bladder and facilitate abdominal evaluation and close monitoring of urinary output (American College of Surgeons 2008).

Repeated, serial examinations are necessary in children with abdominal trauma because life-threatening abdominal injury may not be apparent upon the initial examination. Severe intra-abdominal haemorrhage in children can be masked by their ability to maintain normal blood pressure with large-volume blood loss. Abdominal injury can be obscured by concurrent extra abdominal injury such as head injury, thoracic trauma or fracture of the extremities (Day & Rupp 2003, Advanced Life Support Group 2005).

Children in whom intra-abdominal injury is suspected on the basis of mechanism of injury or physical examination findings should undergo emergent computed tomography (CT) scanning of the abdomen without waiting for laboratory results.

In the remainder of children (e.g., those with mild to moderate blunt abdominal trauma who are haemodynamically stable, awake, alert and cooperative), laboratory testing can occasionally identify unsuspected injury. The presence of haematuria (>5 red blood cells per high-powered field) or elevation of serum transaminases (ALT >125 U/L or ALT >200 U/L) may be the only indication of intra-abdominal injury in these children.

Diagnostic tests

Abdominal CT is the preferred diagnostic imaging modality to detect intra-abdominal injury in haemodynamically stable children who have sustained blunt abdominal trauma. CT is sensitive and specific in diagnosing liver, spleen and retroperitoneal injuries, which may be managed non-operatively. CT scanning is more frequently used in children because it and will confirm renal perfusion, can evaluate solid organs and the intestines (Advanced Life Support Group 2005, Hom 2010).

Ultrasonography is useful when available for the rapid, early evaluation of children with blunt abdominal trauma who are stable; in such patients it might provide an indication for immediate laparotomy (Wise et al. 2002).

The indications for diagnostic peritoneal lavage are the same as in adults; however, its use has been rendered virtually obsolete in the trauma setting by modern imaging modalities. The usefulness of the test is questioned in the presence of solid organ injury where little or no peritoneal fluid may be present (Advanced Life Support Group 2005). Advanced trauma life support protocol suggests that only the surgeon who will care for the injured child should perform the diagnostic peritoneal lavage (American College of Surgeons 2008).

Non-operative management

Surgical intervention is not always warranted for haemodynamically stable children with solid organ injuries. Non-surgical observation of selected solid organ injuries in children is a safe practice that improves patient outcome and resource utilization (Wise et al. 2002, Advanced Life Support Group 2005). Approximately 90 % of children with liver and spleen injuries can be managed non-operatively as haemorrhage associated with these injuries is often self-limiting (Advanced Life Support Group 2005). In contrast, approximately 50 % of children with pancreatic injuries require surgical intervention (Wise et al. 2002). When non-operative management is selected as the treatment option, care must be delivered in a paediatric intensive care facility where staff have the skill to carry out frequent repeated examination and the expertise available to intervene immediately should the child's condition deteriorate (Fleisher & Ludwig 2010).

Conclusion

The challenge for nursing the patient with abdominal trauma in the emergency department lies in the rapid stabilization and assessment of the patient leading to early detection of life-threatening abdominal injury.

Training in the systematic assessment and resuscitation of victims of trauma, such as that offered by an Advanced Trauma Nursing Course, Advanced Paediatric Life Support or Trauma Nursing Core Course, should be a basic requirement for all emergency nurses.

This training enables emergency nurses to effectively participate as members of the multidisciplinary team, ensuring that a systematic, protocol-driven method of clinical assessment, continuous monitoring and re-evaluation of the injured patient will detect early signs of serious intra-abdominal injury and expedite the need for urgent surgical intervention.

References

Advanced Life Support Group, 2005. Advanced Paediatric Life Support, fourth ed. British Medical Journal Publishing Group, London.

Aherne, N.J., Kavanagh, E.G., Condon, E.T., et al., 2003. Duodenal perforation after a blunt abdominal sporting injury: the importance of early diagnosis. Journal of Trauma 54, 791–794.

Aitken, L.M., Niggemeyer, L., 2007. Trauma Management. In: Elliott, D., Aitken, L., Chaboyer, W. (Eds.), ACCCN'S Critical Care Nursing, third ed. Elsevier, Sydney.

Alarcon, L.H., Peitzman, A.B., 2007. Initial assessment and early resuscitation. In: Britt, L.D., Trunkey, D.D., Feliciano, D.V. (Eds.), Acute Care Surgery: Principles and Practice. Springer, New York.

American College of Surgeons, 2008. Advanced Trauma Life Support, eighth ed. American College of Surgeons, Chicago.

Arnold, J.L., Halpern, P., Tsai, M.C., et al., 2004. Mass casualty terrorist bombings: a comparison of outcomes by bombing type. Annals of Emergency Medicine 43 (2), 263–273.

Bacidore, V., 2010. Abdominal and genitourinary trauma. In: Howard, P.K., Steinmann, R.A. (Eds.), Sheehy's Emergency Nursing: Principles and Practice, sixth ed. Mosby, St Louis.

Badger, S.A., Barclay, R., Campbell, P., et al., 2009. Management of liver trauma. World Journal of Surgery 33 (12), 2522–2537.

Bailey, M.M., 2005. Staying on your toes when managing pelvic fractures. Nursing 35 (10), 32–34.

Barry, P., Shakeshaft, J., Studd, R., 2003. Abdominal injuries. In: Sherry, E., Triou, L., Templeton, J. (Eds.), Trauma. Oxford University Press, Oxford.

Blank-Reid, C., Reid, P.C., 2010. Epidemiology and mechanism of injury. In: Howard, P.K., Steinmann, R.A. (Eds.), Sheehy's Emergency Nursing: Principles and Practice, sixth ed. Mosby, St Louis.

Branney, S., Moore, E., Cantrill, S., et al., 1997. Ultrasound-based key clinical pathway reduces the use of hospital resources for the evaluation of blunt abdominal trauma. The Journal of Trauma: Injury, Infection and Critical Care 42, 1086–1090.

Browne, G.J., Noaman, F., Lam, L.T., Soundappan, S.V., 2010. The nature and characteristics of abdominal injuries sustained during children's sports. Pediatric Emergency Care 26 (1), 30–35.

Burkitt, H.G., Quick, C.R.G., 2007. Essential Surgery: Problems, Diagnosis and Management, fourth ed. Churchill Livingstone, London.

Centers for Disease Control (CDC), 2003. Explosions and Blast Injuries: A Primer for Clinicians. CDC, Atlanta.

Chen, S.C., Wang, H.P., Hsu, H.Y., et al., 2000. Accuracy of ED sonography in the diagnosis of acute appendicitis. American Journal of Emergency Medicine 18 (4), 449–452.

Chen, H.W., Wong, Y.C., Wang, L.J., et al., 2010. Computed tomography in left-sided and right-sided blunt diaphragmatic rupture: experience with 43 patients. Clinical Radiology 65 (3), 201–212.

Chughtai, T., Sharkey, P., Lins, M., et al., 2009. Update on managing diaphragmatic rupture in blunt trauma a review of 208 consecutive cases. Canadian Journal of Surgery 52 (3), 177–181.

Claridge, J.A., Croce, M., 2007. Abdominal Wall. In: Britt, L.D., Trunkey, D.D., Feliciano, D.V. (Eds.), Acute Care Surgery: Principles and Practice. Springer, New York.

Cole, E., Lynch, A., Cugnoni, H., 2006. Assessment of the patient with acute abdominal pain. Nursing Standard 20 (38), 56–64.

Day, M., Rupp, L., 2003. Children are different; pediatric differences and the impact on trauma. In: Czerwinski, S.J., Maloney-Harmon, P.A. (Eds.), Nursing Care of the Pediatric Trauma Patient. Saunders, St Louis.

Dickinson, M., 2004. Understanding the mechanism of injury and kinetic forces involved in traumatic injuries. Emergency Nurse 12 (6), 30–34.

Eckert, K.L., 2005. Penetrating and blunt abdominal trauma. Critical Care Nurse 28 (1), 41–59.

Emergency Nurses Association, 2007. Trauma Nursing Core Course. Provider Manual, sixth ed. ENA, Chicago.

Feliciano, D.V.B., Mattox, K.L., Moore, E.E., 2008. Trauma, sixth ed. McGraw-Hill, New York.

Fleisher, G.R., Ludwig, S., 2010. Textbook of Pediatric Emergency Medicine, sixth ed. Lippincott, Williams and Wilkins, Philadelphia.

Frakes, M.A., Evans, T., 2004. Major pelvic fractures. Critical Care Nurse 24 (2), 18–30.

Guitron, J., Howington, J., LoCicero, J., 2009. Diaphragmatic injuries. In: Sheilds, T.W., LoCicero, J., Reed, C.E., Feins, R.H. (Eds.), General Thoracic Surgery, seventh ed. Lippincott, Williams & Wilkins, Philadelphia.

Hom, J., 2010. The risk of intra-abdominal injuries in pediatric patients with stable abdominal trauma and negative abdominal computed tomography. Academic Emergency Medicine 17, 469–475.

Jansen, J.O., Yule, S.R., Loudon, M.A., 2008. Investigation of blunt abdominal trauma. British Medical Journal 336 (7650), 938–942.

Jurkovich, G.J., Wilson, A.J., 2008. Patterns of penetrating injury. In: Peitzman, A.B., Rhodes, M.C., Schwab, W.C., Yealy, D.M., Fabian, T.C. (Eds.), The Trauma Manual: Trauma and Acute Care Surgery, third ed. Lippincott, Williams and Wilkins, Philidelphia.

Khan, M.A., Garner, J.P., 2011. Investigations outside the resuscitation room. In: Smith, J., Greaves, I., Porter, K. (Eds.), Oxford Desk Reference: Major Trauma. Oxford Medical Publications, Oxford.

Kirkpatrick, A.W., 2007. Clinician-performed focused sonography for the resuscitation of trauma. Critical Care Medicine 35 (5), 162–172.

Luckman, J., Sorenson, K.C., 1987. Medical-Surgical Nursing. Saunders, Philadelphia.

McSwain, N., 2003. The Basic EMT: Comprehensive Prehospital Patient Care, second ed. Mosby, St Louis.

Malinoski, D.J., Patel, M.S., Yaker, D.O., et al., 2010. A diagnostic delay in 5 hours increases the risk of death after blunt hollow viscus injury. Journal of Trauma-Injury Infection and Critical Care 69 (1), 84–87.

Mannion, S.J., Chaloner, E., 2005. Principles of war surgery: ABC of conflict and disaster. British Medical Journal 330 (7506), 1498–1500.

Neff, J.A., Kidd, P.S., 1993. Trauma Nursing: the Art and Science. Mosby, St Louis.

Oniscu, G.C., Parks, R.W., Garden, O.J., 2006. Classification of liver and pancreatic trauma. HPB (Oxford) 8 (1), 4–9.

O'Sullivan, R.E.M., White, T.O., Keating, J.F., 2005. Major pelvic fractures: identification of patients at high risk. Journal of Bone and Joint Surgery 87 (4), 530–534.

Owers, C., Morgan, J.L., Garner, J.P., 2011. Abdominal trauma in primary blast injuries. British Journal of Surgery 98 (2), 168–179.

Raby, N., Berman, L., deLacey, G., 2005. Accident and Emergency Radiology: A Survival Guide, second ed. Elsevier Saunders, Philadelphia.

Richards, J.R., Schleper, N.H., Woo, B., et al., 2002. Sonographic assessment of blunt abdominal trauma: a 4-year prospective study. Journal of Clinical Ultrasound 30 (2), 59–67.

Rothrock, S.G., Green, S., Morgan, R., 2000. Abdominal trauma in infants and children: prompt identification and early management of life-threatening injuries. Part 1: Injury patterns and initial assessment. Paediatric Emergency Care 16 (2), 106–115.

Rushings, G.D., Britt, L.D., 2008. Patterns of blunt trauma. In: Peitzman, A.B., Rhodes, M.C., Schwab, W.C., Yealy, D.M., Fabian, T.C. (Eds.), The Trauma Manual: Trauma and Acute Care Surgery, third ed. Lippincott, Williams and Wilkins, Philidelphia.

Saladino, R.A., Lund, D.P., 2010. Abdominal Trauma. In: Fleisher, G.R., Ludwig, S. (Eds.), Textbook of Pediatric Emergency Medicine, sixth ed. Lippincott, Williams and Wilkins, Philadelphia.

Schulman, C.S., 2003. A FASTer method of detecting abdominal trauma. Nursing Management 34 (9), 47–49.

Seidel, H.M., Ball, J.W., Dains, J.E., Benedict, G.W., 1995. Mosby's Guide to Physical Examination, third ed. Mosby, St Louis.

Sierink, J.C., Saltzherr, T.P., Reitsma, J.B., et al., 2012. Systematic review and meta-analysis of immediate total-body computed tomography compared with selective radiological imaging of injured patients. British Journal of Surgery 99 (S1), 52–58.

Sikka, R., 2004. Unsuspected internal organ traumatic injuries. Emergency Medicine Clinics of North America 22 (4), 1067–1080.

Stillwell, S., 1996. Mosby's Critical Care Nursing Reference Guide, second ed. Mosby, St Louis.

Talley, N.J., O'Connor, S., 2010. Clinical Examination: A Systematic Guide to Physical Diagnosis, sixth ed. Churchill Livingstone, Edinburgh.

Taylor, I., Dawood, M., 2005. Terrorism: the reality of blast injuries. Emergency Nurse 13 (8), 22–25.

Tile, M., Helfet, D.L., Kellem, J.F., 2003. Fractures of the Pelvis and Acetabulum. Lippincott, Williams & Wilkins, Philadelphia.

Weber, J.M., Jablonski, R.A., Penrod, J., 2010. Missed opportunities: Under-detection of trauma in elderly adults involved in motor vehicle crashes. Journal of Emergency Nursing 36 (1), 6–9.

Williams, B.G., Hlaing, T., Aaland, M.O., 2009. Ten-year retrospective study of delayed diagnosis of injury in pediatric trauma patients at a level 11 trauma center. Pediatric Emergency Care 25 (8), 489–493.

Wise, B.V., Spears, S., Wilson, M.E., 2002. Management of blunt abdominal trauma in children. Journal of Trauma Nursing 9 (1), 6–14.

Maxillofacial injuries

Jenni Ward

10

CHAPTER CONTENTS

Introduction

Maxillofacial injuries range from the simple isolated laceration to massive facial trauma involving airway obstruction, respiratory distress, haemorrhage, and accompanying multisystem involvement. The injuries can involve the soft tissues, bones, nerves and blood vessels of the face, mouth and ears. This chapter focuses on those maxillofacial injuries commonly seen in the Emergency Department (ED). It will provide an overview of anatomy and physiology, describe how these injuries are sustained, discuss assessment and outline management. After initial resuscitation and stabilization of the patient, management is aimed at restoration of normal function and cosmetic appearances. These injuries can often be dramatic and for the patient are frequently disfiguring, leading to considerable psychological damage.

Anatomy and physiology

The face contains special structures and centres for airway, breathing, smell, speech, vision, hearing, mastication and facial expression (Parkins 2005) (Box 10.1, Fig. 10.1). Branches of the seventh cranial (facial) nerve provide sensory, parasympathetic and motor innervation to the face (Marieb 2001, Bickley et al. 2005) (Fig 10.2). Due to the location and superficial distribution of the facial nerve branches, these are often damaged in maxillofacial trauma. The face is highly vascular with the blood supply derived from branches of the internal and external carotid arteries. Venous drainage of the face, head and neck is collected through branches of the external and internal jugular veins and the vertebral vein (Marieb 2001, Bates et al. 2005). The face is vulnerable to a wide variety of injuries that can compromise the airway, cause haemorrhage, disrupt the appearance and impact on the ability to express emotions.

The diagnosis and treatment of maxillofacial injuries depends on the type of injury involved; therefore it is crucial to understand the anatomy and physiology of the injured area and mechanism of injury.

Mechanism of injury

Maxillofacial injuries result from blunt or penetrating trauma. Blunt injuries are more common and are caused by motor vehicle crashes, interpersonal violence (including domestic violence), sport activities, occupational trauma and falls (Macken 2009). Penetrating injuries are less common and include motor vehicle crashes, gunshot wounds, stabbings and explosions (Taylor & Dawood 2006, McQuillan & Thurman 2009). Mass, density and shape of the striking object, as well as speed of impact, directly affect the type and severity of facial injury. The amount of force required to fracture various facial bones may be classified as high impact (greater than 50 times force of gravity [g]) or low impact (less than 50g) (Box 10.2).

Box 10.1

The facial bones

The skeleton of the face is formed by 14 bones including the frontal bones.

Zygomatic – the two bones commonly referred to as the cheek bones

Maxilla – forms the upper jaw, the anterior part of the roof of the mouth, the lateral walls of the nasal cavities and part of the floor of the orbital cavities

Nasal – the paired bones form part of the bridge of the nose. The lower and major part of the nose consists of cartilage

Lacrimal – two thin bones that roughly resemble a fingernail in size and shape. They are the smallest bones of the face

Palatine – two L-shaped bones form the posterior portion of the hard palate

Turbinate – two scroll-like bones which project into the nasal cavity. Their function is the filtration of air before it passes into the lungs

Vomer – roughly resembles a triangle in shape and forms the lower and back part of the nasal septum

Box 10.2

Force of gravity (g) impact required for facial fracture

High impact
- Supraorbital rim: 200g
- Symphysis mandible: 100g
- Midline maxilla: 100g
- Frontal–glabellar: 100g
- Angle of mandible: 70g

Low impact
- Zygoma: 50g
- Nasal bone: 30g

It is generally accepted that the greater the speed of the motor vehicle the greater the maxillofacial injury. A history of a broken windscreen, damaged dashboard, and steering wheel deformity is associated with head, facial and laryngotracheal injuries. Although airbags and seatbelts have reduced the incidence and severity of maxillofacial injuries in motor vehicle crashes, facial lacerations, abrasions and burns are now more common with airbag deployment (Leslie & Skapetis 2007).

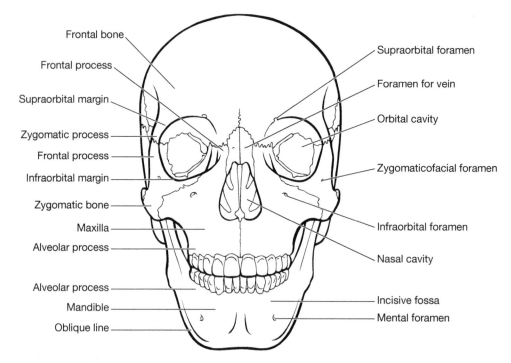

Figure 10.1 • Normal facial/skull anatomy.

Parotid gland

Branches of
facial nerve

Figure 10.2 • Anatomy of facial and trigeminal nerves.

Helmets are found to be effective in reducing head injuries, facial injuries and death in motorcycle crashes when compared with wearing no helmet; however, full-face helmets do not appear to have a significant effect on facial injuries when compared with open-faced helmets (Liu et al. 2009). Maxillofacial injuries caused by interpersonal violence account for many emergency department attendances. Studies in the US, Western Europe and Australia show that the majority of facial injuries occur in young males in the late teens to early 20s age group (Parkins 2005, Leslie & Skapetis 2007). The diagnosis and treatment can often be made more complex as alcohol intoxication plays a major part in many altercations; however, injuries tend to be less severe than those following road traffic accidents (Magennis et al. 1998, Elder et al. 2004).

The facial bony structures and sinus cavities offer protection to the brain and will collapse under force, expending energy away from the brain. The attachments of facial muscles also assist to expend this energy away by exerting downwards and backwards force to the maxilla. The mandible is often described as one of the strongest bones of the body; however, the condylar necks are frequent fracture sites as they absorb energy forces directed towards the brain. The incidence of maxillofacial injuries are less common in children, representing approximately 5–10 % of all cases, with the rate increasing with age. This is due in part to the resilience and elasticity of paediatric facial tissues and the usually protected, supervised environment given to younger age groups (Simpson & McLean 1995). When injury does occur, the pattern differs from adults as the relatively large cranium of the child protects the facial bones.

Airway assessment and management

Assessment of the patient requires a systematic approach such as advocated by the Advanced Trauma Life Support (ATLS)

principles to identify and treat early any life-threatening injuries (Edwards 2005, American College of Surgeons 2008).

A thorough history is essential, with emphasis on those components that may impact on the assessment and subsequent management of the facial injuries and include, i.e., the mechanism of injury, alteration in mental status or loss of consciousness, if the patient has any allergies, their medical history and current medications (including prescription, nonprescription and recreational drugs), and last time the patient ate and drank (Hutchinson et al. 1996).

Initial airway assessment involves a rapid but thorough examination of the face, mouth and throat to identify any cause of obstruction such as foreign material, burns, lacerations and fractures (American College of Surgeons 2008). Obstruction may occur instantaneously or slowly, as oedema, secretions and bleeding progressively occlude the airway. Upper-airway obstruction is most commonly due to the tongue and foreign bodies, including vomitus, blood, dislodged teeth, broken dentures, oedema of the area surrounding the epiglottis and, uncommonly, injury to the larynx. During unconsciousness, tone is lost in the muscles that normally hold the tongue away from the pharyngeal wall. Abnormal or prolonged relaxation of these muscles will allow the tongue to prolapse back, obstructing the upper airway. Signs and symptoms of airway obstruction including agitation, combativeness, the use of accessory muscles, intercostal retractions, dyspnoea, stridor, gurgling, cyanosis, and a SaO_2 less than 96% (Keane 2007, American College of Surgeons 2008).

Airway obstruction can be alleviated by either the chin-lift manoeuvre or the jaw-thrust manoeuvre to move the mandible anteriorly and thereby lifting the tongue. Both manoeuvres should not hyperextend the neck or compromise possible cervical spine fractures (American College of Surgeons 2008). Intubation may be inevitable where the patient has a decreased level of consciousness (Glasgow Coma Score of 8 or less), has poor gag, swallowing or coughing reflexes, or has difficulty in maintaining a patent airway or adequate oxygenation. Intubation is often difficult as the head must be maintained in a neutral position with in-line immobilization of the spine during the procedure. Performance of nontraumatic intubation is vital, as traumatic insertion causes increased intracranial pressure, which underlines the need to obtain experienced specialist help. The nasopharyngeal route should normally be avoided unless basilar skull fracture has been excluded. If attempts at intubation are unsuccessful, a cricothyrotomy or tracheostomy may be undertaken (American College of Surgeons 2008). While suctioning remains the primary method of clearing secretions, extreme care is needed so as not to stimulate the gag reflex or aggravate existing injuries. Where appropriate, the fully conscious patient may be allowed to hold their own suction catheter, thereby controlling the build up of secretions and eliminating the risk of over stimulation.

Examination

If there is no airway obstruction and the patient is haemodynamically stable, a systematic examination of the head and face can be performed (Box 10.3). Careful inspection and palpation of the scalp is undertaken for injuries and foreign bodies (such as glass and dirt) hidden by the hair. The head and face are inspected and palpated for bleeding, crepitus, bony irregularity, tenderness and soft tissue swelling. Visual acuity and extraocular movements are assessed to detect cranial nerve damage, globe rupture and extraocular muscle injury or entrapment. Diplopia may indicate the presence of an orbital floor fracture (Box 10.4).

The ears and mastoid areas are inspected for ecchymosis (Battle's sign), lacerations, bleeding or discharge. Perforation of the eardrum, bloody or serous otorrhoea, haemotympanum and bilateral periorbital haematomas ('panda' or 'raccoon' eyes) are

Box 10.3

Assessment of facial injuries

- Adequate airway
- Cervical spine injury
- Bleeding
- Level of consciousness
- Scalp injuries
- Asymmetry of facial structures
- Difficulty in swallowing or talking
- Decreased hearing or tinnitus
- Missing or broken teeth
- Malocclusion of the mandible
- Cerebrospinal leak from eyes, ears, mouth and/or nose
- Visual acuity
- Numbness or tingling on the face

(After LeDuc Jimmerson C, Lomas G (1994) Facial, ophthalmic and otolaryngeal trauma. In: Driscoll PA, Gwinnutt CL, LeDuc Jimmerson C, Goodall O, eds. Trauma Resuscitation: The Team Approach. Basingstoke: Macmillan.)

Box 10.4

Examination of eyes following facial trauma

- Visual acuity – can the patient count four fingers? Can he or she read print?
- Limitation of eye movements, diplopia and unequal pupillary levels. If one or more of these is present suspect trauma of the orbital floor and wall with entrapment of periorbital tissues
- Direct, consensual and accommodation reflexes. Examination of these may help detect a rise in intracranial pressure, but be aware of false-positive signs caused by trauma to the globe
- Proptosis (or exophthalmos). This suggests haemorrhage within the orbital walls
- Enophthalmos, the sinking of the eye globe, suggesting fracture of an orbital wall – usually the floor or medial wall
- If periorbital swelling is present, fracture of the zygoma or maxilla should be suspected
- If subconjunctival ecchymosis is present, direct trauma to the globe or a fractured zygoma should be suspected

(After Hutchinson I, Lawlor M, Skinner D (1996) Maxillofacial injuries. In: Skinner D, Driscoll P, Earlam R, eds. ABC of Major Trauma, 2nd edn. London: BMJ Publishing Group.)

suggestive of a basilar skull fracture (Criddle 1995, McQuillan & Thurman 2009). The nose is examined for alignment, deformity, pain, swelling, ecchymosis, septal haematoma, epistaxis, rhinorrhoea and difficulty in breathing. The presence of bleeding and leakage of cerebrospinal fluid (CSF) are also suggestive of a basilar skull fracture. Thin, watery, nasal discharge should be considered CSF leakage until proven otherwise and the halo or dextrostix test should be undertaken. Nasal endotracheal and nasogastric tubes should not be inserted in the presence of a basilar skull fracture due to the risk of these being lodged intracranially or further aggravating the fracture.

The mouth is examined for fractures, subluxations and avulsions of the teeth as well as lacerations and contusions. Jaw malocclusion is assessed by checking for pain, malalignment, range of motion and loss of strength (Parkins 2005, Macken 2009).

Facial motor and sensory motor function is assessed preferably before analgesia or anaesthetics are administered. Assessment of the facial nerve includes testing for muscle strength, symmetry and taste sensation on the anterior two-thirds of the tongue (Criddle 1995). Motor function of the facial nerve is checked by having the patient wrinkle his or her forehead, frown, smile, bare the teeth and close the eyes tightly. All three major branches of the trigeminal nerve are tested by determining sensation on each side of the face including the upper and lower lips. Loss of sensation in any one of these areas may imply a fracture in the vicinity of that nerve branch (see Fig. 10.2).

Positioning of the patient with facial injuries is crucial as 10% have a cervical spine injury and 10% an ocular injury (Ali et al 2012). After cervical spine injury has been eliminated by clinical examination, CT or lateral cervical X-ray, the fully conscious patient may be allowed to adopt a suitable position for both adequate airway management and comfort. Elevation of the trolley head between 15° and 30° will assist drainage of blood and secretions from the nasopharynx and lessen the amount of oedema (LeDuc Jimmerson & Lomas 1994).

Additionally, while extensive superficial lacerations do not usually require a transfusion, there is danger in overlooking the continuous trickle of fresh blood from a puncture wound. Prophylactic antibiotics depend on the mechanism of injury, the type and extent of injury and the patient's immune status. Antibiotics need to be prescribed with extensive soft tissue injuries, contaminated wounds, open fractures, and fractures involving sinuses, the mouth and basilar skull. Antibiotic choices are determined by local institution guidelines and may include amoxicillin or cephalexin (Macken 2009).

Le Fort fractures

In 1901, Rene Le Fort classified patterns of mid-face fractures following experiments with 35 cadavers in whom force was applied to parts of the face from different directions and energy levels. Although the Le Fort classification of maxillary fractures is commonly used, most midface fractures may be a combination of various types (Fig. 10.3). Le Fort fractures account for approximately 10–20% of all facial fractures, with the adult male:female ratio being 3:1. The predominant mechanisms of injury are motor vehicle accidents, followed by altercations and falls. Maxillary fractures are rare in children due to the soft, spongy and elastic nature of their maxilla, proportionally large frontal bone and mandible, underdeveloped sinuses and unerupted teeth. As with all maxillofacial traumas, cases should be followed using ATLS guidelines (Ali et al. 2012).

Le Fort I is a horizontal fracture across the lower third of the maxilla, palate and pterygoid plate, at the level of the nasal fossae. As a consequence, the body of the maxilla separates from the base of skull and face (Dunn et al. 2010). The separation may be unilateral or bilateral, with the mobile segment involving the upper teeth and lower maxilla (Leslie & Skapetis 2007).

Le Fort II is a pyramidal fracture that passes through the lateral orbital rim, zygomatic arches, roof of the nose and high in the pterygoid plates. The fracture line is tripod shaped with the nose being at the apex (Leslie & Skapetis 2007, Lewis 2009).

Le Fort III fracture line passes through the lateral orbital rim, zygomatic arches, roof of the nose and high in the pterygoid plates. It results in complete separation of the facial skeleton from the cranial skeleton (craniofacial disassociation) resulting in a mobile maxilla and zygoma (Dunn et al. 2010). It is not unusual for patients to sustain different combinations of these fractures, such as a Le Fort II on one side with a Le Fort III on the other.

LeFort I #

LeFort II #

LeFort III #

Figure 10.3 • Le Fort I, II and III fractures.

Clinical evidence

As the force required to create a Le Fort fracture is quite significant, patients with these fractures need to be assessed for associated head injuries, such as basilar skull fractures, mandible fractures and cervical spine injuries. Clinical findings associated with Le Fort fractures include pain, oedema, periorbital ecchymosis, nasopharyngeal bleeding, flattening and/or elongation of the facial features, tenderness, diplopia and malocclusion with the patient describing the teeth as feeling different (Cascarini et al. 2012). Anaesthesia of the cheek, caused by damage to the infraorbital nerve, is also a common finding. A cerebrospinal fluid leak may occur in 25–50 % of Le Fort II and III fractures and indicates the presence of an open fracture (Leslie & Skapetis 2007). Patients with Le Fort III fractures tend to have massive facial oedema, ecchymosis, conjunctival haemorrhage, infraorbital paraesthesia and occasionally suffer airway obstruction either as a result of the posterior and inferior displacement of the facial skeleton, or secondary to a haematoma into the palate, pharyngeal wall or tonsillar pillars (Lewis 2009).

Management

This is initially directed at maintaining the airway, providing adequate ventilation and controlling haemorrhage. Airway obstruction may be due to haemorrhage, accumulation of vomit or other foreign material within the mouth, oedema of the lips, tongue or pharynx.

Conscious patients should be positioned upright and leaning forward (if other injuries permit and the cervical spine has been cleared) allowing any blood and secretions to drain and assist in reducing swelling (Leslie & Skapetis 2007). It may be necessary to pass an endotracheal (ET) tube to secure the patient's airway. If the airway remains obstructed, a tracheostomy or cricothyroidotomy may be required.

Control of bleeding may involve cold packs to the face, applying direct pressure to the wound, packing the anterior and posterior nasal cavity and around the ET tube following intubation, insertion of a balloon catheter (Foley), reduction of Le Fort fractures and suturing of lacerations. Ongoing bleeding may require an angiogram with vascular embolization and ligation of vessels (Dunn et al. 2010).

Where there is a CSF leak, nasal packing, nasal intubation (with a gastric or endotracheal tube) and blowing of the nose should be avoided (Sherwood & McQuillan 2009). Prophylactic antibiotics as per individual institution guidelines are commenced if a CSF leak is suspected or present to prevent meningitis (Ali et al. 2012).

Definitive treatment of Le Fort fractures is usually delayed for several days until the patient is stabilized, any life-threatening injuries are treated and the facial oedema subsides. Wound care can commence as soon as possible and facial lacerations repaired within 24 hours. Application of cold packs will also assist in minimizing oedema formation and aid in pain relief and can be considered as soon as practicable. Adequate analgesia is to be administered as prescribed (Lewis 2009).

Mandibular fractures

Mandibular fractures are the second most common facial fracture after nasal fractures. The majority of mandibular fractures occur in the adolescent or young adult population and are due to intepersonal violence, sports injuries, road traffic accidents and falls (Jones 1997). The prominent position of the mandible at the lower part of the face predisposes it to trauma. Due to its shape and the articulations at the temporomandibular joints, the mandible often fractures in two or more places, either at the site of impact or the opposite side (Lewis 2009) (Fig. 10.4).

The most common sites for fracture are at the mandible's weak and thin areas, i.e., the condyle, angle and body at the first and second molar (Parkins 2005). The severity of the fracture may depend upon the mechanism of injury and the dentition of the jaw, as the more teeth there are, the less severe the fracture. Displacement of the fragments depends

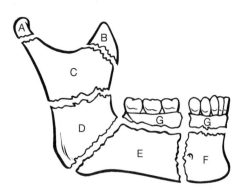

Figure 10.4 • Mandibular fracture sites. A, Condyle; B, coronoid process; C, ascending ramus; D, angle; E, body; F, symphysis; G, alveolar process.

on the shape of the fracture and the action of muscles. It is important not to underestimate the degree of force required to break a jaw. The mandible is the densest bone in the body so the cranium will have absorbed considerable force, therefore it is important to rule out head injury (Cascarini et al. 2012).

Clinical evidence

Although clinical manifestations of mandibular fractures will vary depending on the location, assessment usually reveals malocclusion of teeth, broken or loose teeth, pain, trismus, difficulty in speaking, swallowing and opening and closing the mouth, with decreased range of motion, facial asymmetry, swelling and localized paraesthesia. Haematoma, ecchymosis and oedema of the floor of the mouth are highly suggestive of mandibular fracture. Mandibular injuries are classified as open or closed. A fracture is considered open if it passes through a tooth-bearing segment, where there is bleeding at the gum line, or there is communication with the skin surface (Parkins 2005).

Evaluation of the malocclusion is the most important aspect of the mandibular examination. Patients with only mild pain and full range of motion, including lateral motion, a normal bite and no loss of strength are unlikely to have a mandibular fracture (Criddle 1995). Radiographic diagnosis of a fracture is most easily made with a dental panoramic X-ray film, but regular films will detect most fractures. Fractures in the area of the condyles may be visible only on CT scan. The importance of correct diagnosis of mandible fractures cannot be more stressed, particularly in the case of children. If mismanaged or undetected, they may lead to gross asymmetry of growth or ankylosis of the joint.

Management

Management of mandibular fractures begins with clearing and maintaining a patent airway as described for Le Fort fractures (Roberts et al. 2000). Application of cold packs to reduce swelling, wound care and repair of oral lacerations as soon as possible to prevent contamination by saliva are important considerations. Antibiotics are indicated if the fracture is compound or includes a tooth-bearing area. Mandibular fractures are generally more painful than other facial fractures so the patient requires adequate and regular analgesia (Dunn et al. 2010). Most mandibular fractures require some form of immobilization for approximately six weeks to promote both healing and comfort. Fixation is usually delayed until the patient is stable and may consist of intermaxillary wiring for simple fractures with open reduction and interosseous wiring for more complex fractures.

Orbit floor fractures (blow-out fracture)

Orbital floor fractures (blow-out fractures) may occur as an isolated injury or in conjunction with other facial fractures. These fractures result from a sudden increase in intraorbital hydraulic pressure caused by a high-velocity object, such as a ball or fist that impacts the globe and upper eyelid. Kinetic energy is transmitted via the globe to the periocular structures resulting in the bone of the orbital floor giving way under pressure of the eyeball with herniation of the inferior oblique and inferior rectus muscles and some periorbital fat through the fracture into the maxillary antrum (Maartens & Lethbridge 2005) (Fig. 10.5).

the administration of analgesia, and recording of vital signs and neurological observations are an important part of nursing management. To avoid further haemorrhage, the patient should be made aware of the need to avoid blowing the nose. Surgical elevation of the orbital floor may be required after the release of any trapped nerves. As the patient may be acutely anxious about the loss of vision, they need reassurance and information about the treatment and care plans.

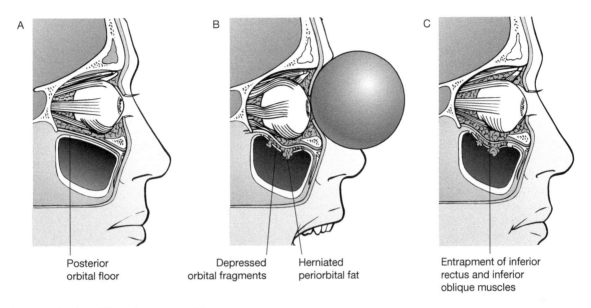

Figure 10.5 • Mechanism of injury in a blow-out fracture.

Clinical evidence

Entrapment of nerves and muscles produces the signs and symptoms associated with this injury. On examination, enophthalmus may be detectable. If more than 2 mm of enophthalmus exists, this can create a noticeable imbalance. Patients may describe decreased visual acuity, blepharoptosis, binocular vertical or oblique diplopia and impaired upward gaze. They may complain of pain, infraorbital paraesthesia and subconjunctival haemorrhage. Epistaxis and eyelid swelling may occur following nose blowing (Macken 2009).

Wilkins & Havins reported a 30% incidence of a ruptured globe in conjunction with orbital fractures, with vision loss present in 8% of patients (Tintinalli et al. 1996). Pain, periorbital bruising and subconjunctival haemorrhage are regarded as reliable signs of a blowout fracture. The only evidence of a blow-out fracture on an X-ray may be a 'tear drop' of soft tissue hanging down into the antrum. CT scanning has supplanted radiographs and is needed to fully define orbital fractures (Macken 2009).

Management

Treatment includes the application of cold packs and elevating the patient's head, once the cervical spine has been cleared, to reduce oedema formation and provide pain relief (Nayduch 2009). Antibiotic cover to prevent orbital cellulitis,

Frontal sinus fractures

Frontal sinus fractures frequently occur as a result of motor vehicle crashes, interpersonal violence, sports, industrial accidents and falls. They are frequently depressed and can be compound or closed.

Clinical evidence

Frontal sinus fractures constitute 5–15% of maxillofacial fractures, with motor vehicle accidents being the most common and sports injuries the second most common cause of these injuries (Yavuzer et al 2005). The patient with a frontal sinus fracture will often present with forehead and nasal pain, tenderness and swelling at the site of the injury. Periorbital ecchymosis and severe lateral, subconjunctival haemorrhage, with forehead paraesthesia and deformity are often present. Physical examination is usually hampered by oedema, and these injuries are notorious for appearing insignificant until the oedema resolves. Related injuries to the face, eyes, brain and skull with CSF rhinorrhoea may be evident.

Management

Initial management is dependent on any associated life-threatening injuries and the patient's overall clinical condition.

Management includes wound care and ice packs to reduce swelling. Antibiotic cover will be required if the fracture is compound and where there is a CSF leak. Surgical treatment of sinus fractures may be delayed due to any associated life-threatening injuries or haemodynamic instability. The aim of surgical interventions is to stop any CSF leakage, reduce the incidence of infection, restore normal sinus function where possible, and repair any cosmetic deformities (Lipschitz & Oleksy 2009). Elevation of any depressed fractures will be required when the patient's condition is stable. The patient needs to be instructed to avoid blowing the nose or sneezing as these increase sinus pressure and can result in pneumocephalus (Nayduch 2009).

Nasal fractures

The nose is the most common site for facial fractures and is frequently associated with other fractures of the middle third of the face. Nasal fractures are usually the result of blunt trauma because of their prominence, the lack of supportive structures, and being thin and fragile (Parkins 2005). Traumatic disruption of the nasal bones and cartilages can result in significant external deformity and airway obstruction. The type and severity of nasal fracture are dependent on the force, direction and mechanism of injury (Fig. 10.6).

Nasal bones may be displaced laterally or posteriorly depending on the direction of the traumatic force. Lateral nasal trauma is most common and may result in the fracture of one or both nasal bones. This is often accompanied by dislocation of the nasal septum off the maxillary crest. Septal dislocation can result in an S-shaped nasal dorsum, tip asymmetry and airway obstruction. Direct frontal trauma to the nose often results in the depression and widening of the nasal dorsum with associated nasal obstruction. More severe injuries may result in comminution of the entire nasal pyramid. If these injuries are not properly diagnosed and treated, the patient will have significant cosmetic and functional problems (Rubeinstein & Strong 2000).

Clinical evidence

Patients with nasal fractures usually present with oedema, tenderness, pain on palpation, ecchymosis, deformity and nasal obstruction. Periorbital haematoma, subconjunctival haemorrhage and epiphora (tearing) may also be evident. Epistaxis may or may not be present and is usually minor and may be due to bleeding from Little's area or the pharynx (Lipschitz & Oleksy 2009). It is important to examine the inside of the patient's nose for the presence or absence of a septal haematoma. The presence of CSF rhinorrhoea indicates fractures of the cribriform plate with torn dura (Leslie & Skapetis 2007). Diagnosis of a nasal fracture is usually based on physical examination findings as X-rays are often unreliable (Macken 2009). CT scans are not routinely indicated unless the patient is suspected of having more significant facial injuries.

Management

Bleeding can be controlled with direct pressure by compressing the nostrils and applying ice packs to the nose and back of the neck. Anterior or posterior nasal packing with tampons, or a balloon catheter (Foleys) may be required if direct pressure is not effective. Septal haematomas need to be drained urgently to prevent nasal airway obstruction and septal cartilage necrosis (Lipschitz & Oleksy 2009, Nayduch 2009). If haemorrhage is severe or persistent, then vital signs and haemoglobin level should be checked.

Displaced nasal fractures causing significant cosmetic deformity and/or compromise function may be reduced within the first 2–3 hours following injury. However, reduction can be performed within 7–10 days to allow nasal

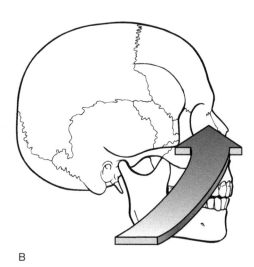

A   B

Figure 10.6 • Mechanism of injury in nasal fractures. (A) Tangential forces displace nasal bones laterally. (B) Posteriorly directed blows displace fracture fragments into other facial structures. • (After Criddle LM (1995) Maxillofacial trauma and ear, nose and throat emergencies. In: Kitt S, Selfridge-Thomas J, Proehl JA, Kaiser J, eds. Emergency Nursing: A Physiologic and Clinical Perspective. 2nd edn. Philadelphia: WB Saunders.)

swelling to subside. There is no treatment required for undisplaced fractures; however, the ENT department may wish to see the patient 5–10 days post injury when any swelling has resolved and before the fracture has united. The patient can be given analgesics and advised to apply cold packs to the nose regularly for comfort.

Temporomandibular joint (jaw) dislocation

Temporomandibular joint (TMJ) dislocations are caused by yawning, chewing, laughing, trauma to the face and in whiplash injuries (Leslie & Skapetis 2007) (Fig. 10.7). The patient presents with pain and inability to close their mouth. Swelling involving the temporomandibular joint may be evident on examination. X-rays are required to confirm dislocation of the mandible and exclude fracture (Dunn et al. 2010). The dislocation is usually reduced in the emergency department with the patient given a light sedation such as midazolam with analgesia. Rarely, the patient may require a general anaesthesia or open reduction. In simple dislocations, when the mandibular condyles have been dislocated for less than two hours, it may be possible to reduce the condyle into its correct position without any specific medication (Hutchison et al. 1998).

Reduction is accomplished by sitting the patient up in bed or on a chair. A physician or nurse practitioner with gloved thumbs stands directly in front of the patient and places his or her thumbs on the posterior molars of the mandible, with the fingers curled under the symphysis of the mandible. Downward pressure is applied on the molars with slight upward pressure on the symphysis to lever the condyles downward. As soon as the condyles are past the articular eminence, the jaw muscles will cause the mandible to shut into the normal closed position. If there is bilateral dislocation one side is relocated at a time.

Figure 10.7 • Dislocation of the temporomandibular joint dislocation.

Post-reduction X-rays are taken to ensure the mandible is in the correct position. The patient should be advised to avoid yawning or opening the jaw widely for several weeks and to take a soft diet for a few days to reduce the risk of further dislocations (Dunn et al. 2010).

Facial wounds

Soft tissue injuries of the face include lacerations, abrasions, contusions, avulsions and burns (Macken 2008). As the face is highly vascular, most wounds, even when contaminated, heal well if careful wound management is carried out. Infection is usually rare, but haemorrhage can be severe and may involve arteries such as the facial artery, superficial temporal artery, the angular artery or a combination of these. Bleeding can usually be controlled by direct pressure and if necessary blood vessels ligated or clipped. However, the patient may require a transfusion if the blood loss is significant.

Wounds should be assessed regularly for blood loss and thoroughly irrigated and explored for foreign bodies and debris. As road traffic accidents are frequently the cause of facial wounds, glass may be present therefore soft tissue X-rays may be taken before any attempt is made at wound closure (Reynolds & Cole 2006).

Simple lacerations may be repaired in the emergency department. Small wounds with irregular skin edges need to be trimmed, and dirty abrasions scrubbed thoroughly. As facial wounds heal faster than wounds elsewhere on the body, fine monofilament nylon or polypropylene, which causes less tissue reaction, should be used and removed after approximately four days. If required, adhesive strips may be applied when the sutures have been removed. This provides a little extra support and eliminates the risk of scarring caused by suture marks.

Repair of complicated wounds may require the skills of an experienced plastic surgeon whenever possible. Soft tissue injuries that involve significant tissue loss, nerve, glands, ducts, are contaminated, or require exact anatomical closure, or where the patient is not compliant, usually need to be repaired in operating theatre under a general anaesthetic (Macken 2009). Wound care is examined in detail in Chapter 24.

Eyelids

Wounds of the lids frequently occur but are rarely dangerous. Nevertheless, patients with eyelid lacerations need to be examined for any ocular and nasolacrimal duct injuries. Eyelid wounds caused by a fall or that are the result of a penetrating injury may create complications and should be referred to an ophthalmic or plastic surgeon.

Lips

A blow on the lip can sometimes split it cleanly against the teeth, but if the blow is angled it can cause a shearing of the lip from its attachment to the gum. It is particularly important that perfect alignment of the mucocutaneous junction of the lip is achieved in order to avoid a step resulting in the lip margin (vermilion border). It is possible for injected local anaesthetic to cause distortion of the tissues and the picture may be confused as a result. However, careful attention by an experienced senior doctor or plastic surgeon can produce excellent results. Any tissue loss from the lip requires a plastic surgeon for reconstructive surgery (Leslie & Skapetis 2007).

Infection is common where a penetrating wound is caused by the teeth when both sides of the lip have been involved. It is important that the laceration be repaired inside and out. Careful examination is required where broken teeth are present to eliminate any fragments which may be retained within the lip. Small monofilament sutures are used to close lacerations and are removed after 4–5 days to avoid suture marks (Dunn et al. 2010).

Eyebrows

Eyebrows are *never* to be shaved as they may not regrow properly, can hinder proper alignment of the wound during closure and result in unnecessary distress (Thaker & Blumetti 2009). As with the treatment of the lip, careful assessment of the type, size and location of wound is required in order to achieve alignment and closure. Methods of wound closure include the use of tissue adhesive in addition to sutures.

Ears

Simple lacerations without cartilage involvement can usually be sutured in the emergency department. Local anaesthetic with adrenaline (epinephrine) should be avoided on the ear due to its vasoconstriction effect on the local blood supply. Lacerations involving cartilage need ENT referral for careful reconstruction, with suturing of the skin not the cartilage. Avulsion of the pinna is common in interpersonal altercations. If there is adequate blood supply in the flap which is formed, then the cartilage can be tucked back in and the skin sutured (Farnsworth 2007).

Subperichondrial haematomas (cauliflower or rugby player's ear) require urgent aspiration, followed by pressure pads bandaged or strapped to press the ear against the head. This procedure may need to be carried out frequently to prevent re-accumulation of blood, and allow the perichondrium to grow back onto the cartilage. If this is not achieved then it will die and shrivel, resulting in scar deformity known as a cauliflower ear (Farnsworth 2007, Thaker & Bumetti 2009).

Rupture of the eardrum can occur from sustaining a blow to the side of the head. The patient should be warned not to allow water into the meatus. The ear does not need packing or ear drops. Referral to an ENT clinic is necessary (see Chapter 32).

Teeth

Teeth may be fractured, dislocated (subluxated) or avulsed from the socket. Fractured teeth may range from only involving the enamel through to involving the root and pulp of the tooth. Although trauma to the teeth is not life threatening, associated maxillofacial injuries can compromise the patient's airway. Airway management therefore is the first priority in dental injuries due to the possibility of obstruction due to teeth fragments or swelling from associated injuries (Parkins 2005, Farnsworth 2007, Nayduch 2009). Care must be taken not to miss any inhaled or ingested teeth, and if in any doubt a chest X-ray is required to exclude teeth in the lungs or oesophagus.

Teeth sockets which continue to bleed may require packing with adrenaline-soaked gauze. Failure to arrest the haemorrhage may result in suturing and/or packing of the socket, with surgical referral to a dentist.

If a patient presents with a broken tooth, the ideal storage medium is either milk or the patient's own saliva; however, normal saline can be used. The tooth should not be kept dry or soaked in tap water for any length of time. If the socket is full of blood clot, it can be gently irrigated with normal saline to clear the clot. The tooth can be reimplanted up to 60 minutes if it has been stored in Hank's solution, milk or normal saline. The tooth should be gripped by its crown the correct way round and re-implanted firmly into the socket. Local anaesthetic may be needed into the local gingival. After reimplantation, the patient may be fitted with a mouth guard or a splint such as glass ionomer cement or 'Blu Tack' if available, to hold the tooth in place (Hutchison 1998, Leslie & Skapetis 2007). Avoid reimplanting avulsed primary teeth due to the risk of fusion to alveolar bone with resultant facial deformities (Farnsworth 2007).

Injuries to inside the mouth and tongue

These are most commonly seen in children after a fall when the teeth penetrate the tongue. Small lacerations can be left untouched as they will heal quickly. Larger lacerations often result in prolonged haemorrhage and can be distressing to both patient and parent. Airway management is the first priority due to the bleeding and swelling from any contusions (Nayduch 2009). Suturing of the wound is often necessary, especially if there is gaping or the edge of the tongue is involved (Dunn et al. 2010). Absorbable suture material is often used, thereby reducing the need for a return visit for removal. However, this procedure is frequently difficult in children and uncooperative patients and occasionally general anaesthesia is required if optimum results are to be achieved.

Advise the patient or parent of the need to adopt meticulous oral hygiene care when there is injury to the tongue or inside the mouth. Antibiotics may be prescribed due to the large amount of bacteria present in the oral cavity.

Fauces

Injury to the tonsillar fossa is often the result of a child falling while holding an object in his or her mouth. As the internal carotid artery is close by and traumatic thrombosis can ensue, this situation should be taken seriously from the outset. The patient needs to be closely observed for signs of developing retropharyngeal abscess post-injury.

Conclusion

All maxillofacial injuries should be treated as a head injury; therefore neurological and vital signs should be checked and recorded at regular intervals (see Chapter 5).

Detailed initial assessment of the patient with maxillofacial injuries is crucial and will consequently influence the final outcome. Correct airway management is essential and continuous monitoring of the patient is imperative if a satisfactory outcome is to be achieved. The patient is likely to be very anxious and the nurse will play a major part in the early provision of both physical and psychological care due to the distressing nature of the maxillofacial injuries. Ideally, severe injuries should be managed by an experienced maxillofacial surgeon if the patient is to receive the best possible care with the best possible outcome.

References

Ali, F., Gwanmesia, I., Simmons, J., 2012. Maxillofacial trauma. In: Hettarchy, S.P., Griffiths, M., Ali, F., Simmons, J. (Eds.), Plastic Surgery: A problem based approach. Springer Verlag, London.

American College of Surgeons, 2008. Advanced Trauma Life Support, eighth ed. American College of Surgeons, Chicago.

Bickley, L.S., Bates, B., Szilagy, P.G., 2005. Bates' Guide to Physical Examination and History Taking, nineth ed. Lippincott, Williams and Wilkins, Philadelphia.

Cascarini, L., Schilling, C., Gurney, B., et al., 2012. Oxford Handbook of Oral and Maxillofacial Surgery. Oxford University Press, Oxford.

Criddle, L.M., 1995. Maxillofacial trauma and ear, nose and throat emergencies. In: Kitt, S., Selfridge-Thomas, J., Proehl, J.A., Kaiser, J. (Eds.), Emergency Nursing: A Physiologic and Clinical Perspective, second ed. WB Saunders, Philadelphia.

Dunn, R., Dilley, S., Brookes, J. (Eds.), 2010. fifth ed. The emergency medicine manual, vol. 2. Venom, Adelaide.

Edwards, G.J., 2005. Airway management. In: Sheehy's Manual of Emergency Care, sixth ed. Elsevier Mosby, St Louis.

Elder, R.W., Ryan, G.W., Shults, R.A., et al., 2004. Alcohol related emergency department visits among people ages 13 to 25 years. Journal of Studies on Alcohol 65, 297.

Farnsworth, L., 2007. Dental, ear, nose and throat emergencies. In: Curtis, K et al., (Eds.), Emergency and Trauma Nursing, Elsevier, Sydney.

Hutchinson, I., Lawlor, M., Skinner, D., 1996. Maxillofacial injuries. In: Skinner, D., Driscoll, P., Earlam, R. (Eds.), ABC of Major Trauma, second ed. BMJ Publishing Group, London.

Jones, N., 1997. Facial fractures. In: Jones, N. (Ed.), Craniofacial Trauma. Oxford University Press, Oxford.

Keane, C., 2007. Laboratory, imaging, investigations and analysis. In: Curtis, K et al., (Eds.), Emergency and Trauma Nursing. Elsevier, Sydney.

LeDuc Jimmerson, C., Lomas, G., 1994. Facial, ophthalmic and otolaryngeal trauma. In: Driscoll, P.A., Gwinnutt, C.L., LeDuc Jimmerson, C., Goodall, O. (Eds.), Trauma Resuscitation: The Team Approach. Macmillan, Basingstoke.

Leslie, J., Skapetis, T., 2007. Faciomaxillary trauma. In: K Curtis, K. (Edset al.,), Emergency and Trauma Nursing. Elsevier, Sydney.

Lewis, A.M., 2009. Facial, ocular, ENT, and dental trauma. In: Kunz Howard, P., Steinmann, R.A. (Eds.), Sheehy's Emergency Nursing: Principles and Practice, sixth ed. Mosby Elsevier, St Louis.

Lipschitz, A., Oleksy, B., 2009. Facial fractures I: Upper facial skeleton. In: Eastman AL, A.L., Rosenbaum, D., Thal, E. (Eds.), Parkland Memorial Hospital: Parkland Trauma Handbook, third ed. Elsevier Mosby, Philadelphia.

Liu, B., Ivers, R., Norton, R., et al., 2009. Helmets for preventing injury in motorcycle riders: review. Cochrane Database. CD004333, 2009. Cochrane collaboration, Oxford.

Maartens, N., Lethbridge, G., 2005. Head and neck trauma. In: O'Shea, R. (Ed.), Principles and Practice of Trauma Nursing. Elsevier, Edinburgh.

Macken, L., 2009. Facial trauma. In: Cameron, P et al., (Eds.), Textbook of Adult Emergency Medicine, third ed. Churchill Livingstone Elsevier, Edinburgh.

Magennis, P., Shepherd, J., Hutchison, I., et al., 1998. Trends in facial injury. British Medical Journal 316, 325–326.

Marieb, E.N., 2001. Human Anatomy and Physiology, fifth ed. Benjamin Cummings, San Francisco.

McQuillan, K.A., Thurman, P.A., 2009. Maxillofacial trauma. In: Whalen, E., McQillan, K.A., Flynn Makic, M.B. (Eds.), Trauma Nursing: From Resuscitation Through Rehabilitation, fourth ed. Saunders Elsevier, St Louis.

Nayduch, D., 2009. Nurse to Nurse: Trauma Care Expert Interventions. McGraw Hill, New York.

Parkins, D.R., 2005. Maxillofacial trauma. In: O'Shea, R. (Ed.), Principles and Practice of Trauma Nursing. Elsevier, Edinburgh.

Reynolds, T., Cole, E., 2006. Techniques for acute wound closure. Nursing Standard 20 (21), 55–64.

Roberts, G., Scully, C., Shotts, R., 2000. ABC of oral health: Dental emergencies. British Medical Journal 321, 559–562.

Rubenstein, B., Strong, E.B., 2000. Management of nasal fractures. Archives of Family Medicine 9, 738–742.

Sherwood, S.F., McQuillan, K.A., 2009. Maxillofacial trauma. In: Whalen, E., McQillan, K.A., Flynn Makic, M.B. (Eds.), Trauma Nursing: From Resuscitation Through Rehabilitation, fourth ed. Saunders Elsevier, St Louis.

Simpson, D.A., McLean, A.J., 1995. Epidemiology. In: David, D.J., Simpson, D.A. (Eds.), Craniomaxillofacial Trauma. Churchill Livingstone, Edinburgh.

Taylor, I., Dawood, M., 2006. The reality of blast injuries. Emergency Nurse 13 (8), 22–25.

Thaker, H., Blumetti, J., 2009. Soft tissue injuries of the face. In: Eastman AL, A.L., Rosenbaum, D., Thal, E. (Eds.), Parkland Memorial Hospital: Parkland Trauma Handbook, third ed. Elsevier Mosby, Philadelphia.

Tintinalli, B., Stapczynski, J.S., Ma, O.J., et al., 1996. Emergency Medicine: A Comprehensive Study Guide. McGraw-Hill, New York.

Yavuzer, R., Sari, A., Kelly, C.P., et al., 2005. Management of frontal sinus fractures. Plastic Reconstructive Surgery 115 (6), 79e–93e.

Burns

11

Tamsin Attenburrow

Introduction

Despite legislative attempts to improve safety and increase public awareness, patients with burn injuries remain a significant proportion of trauma patients attending emergency departments (EDs) (Herndon 2007). Each year in the UK, it is estimated that 175 000 people visit EDs with acute burn injuries and some 13 000 of them need admission to hospital (Dunn 2000). Add to this the number of individuals treated as outpatients and in community and primary care settings, and the scale of the problem becomes apparent (Moss 2010). Although the chances for survival following the massive trauma of a major burn have improved steadily over the last 25 years, there are still 300 deaths in hospital each year in the UK (National Audit Office 2010, NHS Clinical Advisory Group 2010).

The care provided in the first few hours after injury is crucial (Wiebelhaus & Hansen 2001) and without pertinent and urgent treatment the chances of surviving a major burn are greatly reduced. Burn injuries should be thought of as more than 'skin deep': they represent a complicated assault on the body's vital organs and systems. Management of major burn injuries must reflect this, and through effective organization and prioritization of care, potentially life-threatening problems can be dealt with successfully, or in some cases avoided in the first instance.

http://dx.doi.org/10.1016/B978-0-7020-4315-4.00011-5

This chapter aims to unravel some of the complexities of burn injury management. Mechanisms of injury with specific first-aid measures, implications of a burn injury in the assessment of airway, breathing and circulation, and immediate psychological care needs will all be covered in detail. The chapter will also consider burn wound management, treatment of more minor injuries and indications for transfer to specialist burns units.

Assessment

First aid can overlap the initial ED management of burn injuries, especially when first aid has not been commenced at the scene of the incident. Decisions and treatment received at the scene, particularly the quality of first aid, often have a profound effect on mortality and morbidity (Dunn 2000). In a stressful situation confusion often exists over what constitutes safe first aid, particularly for the layperson.

Appropriate action can be summarized as:

- safe removal from the source of the burn – rescuers should be aware of any potential risk or immediate danger from the environment, to themselves, before attempting to remove the casualty
- maintenance of airway
- arresting the burning process by application of cold water to reduce residual heat in body tissues or to remove corrosive substances
- reduction of pain
- protection of damaged skin from desiccation and infection.

During this period it is important to obtain a brief, accurate history of the event (Settle 1995). Establishing what, where, when, why and how injuries happened will enable appropriate, prioritized care to be commenced promptly.

This can be taken from the patient, relatives or ambulance crew (Box 11.1).

The principles of Advanced Trauma Life Support (ATLS), primary and secondary survey, should be applied to the assessment and immediate care of patients with major burn injuries. During the primary survey thorough assessment of the ABCs should be performed.

Box 11.1

Information about patient/incident

- Circumstances of the incident (e.g., explosion, road traffic accident or fire)
- Time of injury, to allow accurate estimation of circulatory fluid loss
- First aid measures undertaken
- Distribution of burns
- Presence of other injuries: fractures, head injury
- Relevant medical history, including tetanus status and current drug therapy

---

Airway and breathing

The first priority in the management of a burn-injured patient is immediate assessment of the patient's airway for patency and maintenance (Jones 2003). Inhalation injury and respiratory complications are two of the leading causes of fatality in the early period following burn injury (Zassan et al. 2010). The early detection and treatment of airway or breathing problems must be paramount in the patient's overall management. Thermal inhalation (direct heat) and chemical inhalation injuries pose the greatest threat to airways and breathing with an incidence of 20–30% and at least 30% of patients with inhalation injury die (Smith et al. 1994). A direct heat injury will be evident soon after injury. Unless steam inhalation has occurred, the damage is usually limited to the upper airway. Direct heat injury causes face, neck and intraoral burns and leads to a rapid development of oedema, resulting in complete airway obstruction within hours (Wilding 1990).

Chemical inhalation usually involves the by-products of combustion. The most worrying toxins are those that asphyxiate patients, depriving them of oxygen, carbon monoxide (CO) and cyanide (Jones 2003). The chemicals affect the lower airways, causing alveolar damage, pulmonary oedema and surfactant insufficiency. They reduce the circulatory availability of oxygen because carbon monoxide has a much greater affinity for haemoglobin (Hb) than oxygen, and subsequently induce acidosis. Chemical inhalation should be suspected following a loss of or altered consciousness, history of fire within an enclosed or confined area, the presence of intraoral burns and soot in the mouth, nose and sputum, and where a confirmed history of smoke inhalation exists.

Acute airway obstruction is diagnosed by the presence of dyspnoea, wheezing, hoarseness, stridor, loss of voice and even minimal evidence of laryngeal swelling. Once this has been detected, early intubation is essential to allow effective airway management. If in doubt, intubate; intubation is much more difficult once the patient's airway is swollen.

During the airway assessment, also check for cervical spine injury and take appropriate precautions. If you need to open the airway and you suspect a cervical spine injury, use a combined jaw thrust and spine immobilization manoeuvre. Apply a hard cervical collar if indicated, even if it goes over the burn (see also Chapter 7).

In less severe cases, where there is no direct evidence of airway involvement, close and careful observations should be continued as symptoms may become apparent over the next 24 to 48 hours (Muehlberger et al. 1998). The ED nurse should not be misled by the apparent mildness of symptoms. This is often an inaccurate indicator of the degree of damage occurring, and the patient's condition should be continually reviewed for increasing shortness of breath, feelings of tightness, wheezing or hoarseness. The patient's chest should be adequately visualized for respiratory effort and bilateral movement. Percussion and auscultation should be performed to determine adequate air entry, and to detect wheezing, signs of pulmonary oedema and lower airway obstruction.

All patients with suspected inhalation injuries should be given high-flow 100% oxygen as soon as possible (McParkland 1999). The administration of high levels of oxygen, via either mask or endotracheal tube, greatly reduces the half-life of carboxyhaemoglobin (COHb) and increases its rate of elimination from the body. This reduces systemic hypoxia. Measuring this can prove difficult in the ED, because the usual methods such as oxygen saturation monitoring are rendered ineffective as they do not distinguish between oxy- and carboxyhaemoglobin (Wiebelhaus & Hansen 2001). The actual diagnosis of an inhalation injury is often difficult to confirm in the initial stages of care. Investigations include immediate arterial blood gas analysis as a baseline for the evaluation of the patient's pulmonary status, with sequential arterial blood gas measurements to confirm CO elimination (Campbell 2000). Oxygen saturation monitoring should not be used until blood gas analysis reveals that COHb concentrations have reached a normal level.

Measurement of COHb and cyanide levels is important, but results are not always immediately available to ED staff. Fibre-optic bronchoscopy is valuable as a secondary investigation to confirm the presence of soot in the lower respiratory tract (Muehlberger et al. 1998). Because of the difficulty in diagnosis, objective observation and reporting of respiratory changes by the emergency nurse provide the subtle indicators needed to decide the treatment needed. Burn injuries result in a significant increase in respiratory tract secretion as part of the histamine response. If the patient has a compromised airway or is intubated, regular suctioning may be necessary to clear the airway of excessive secretions. Circumferential full-thickness burns to the neck and chest may compromise the mechanism of breathing and necessitate emergency escharotomy (Settle 1995). Chest X-rays are usually obtained, but they do not often show early signs of respiratory problems, although they may highlight other injuries.

Circulation

The patient with major burns will develop severe hypovolaemic shock within 3–4 hours from the time of injury, unless adequate fluid resuscitation measures are initiated (Settle 1995). Damage to the capillary network in the skin leads to loss of water, proteins and electrolytes from the circulation into the interstitial compartment (Hettiaratchy & Dziewulski 2004). There are three reasons for this: wound secretion, evaporation and localized oedema. In severe cases, generalized oedema in surrounding, apparently uninjured, areas also occurs. The oedema occurs because of changes in permeability of capillaries and tissues affected by heat. Fluid consists mostly of dilute plasma, which increases the viscosity of the remaining intravascular fluid and slows or stops blood flow to capillaries. Poor tissue perfusion increases the extent of the burn because of low oxygen (Cook 1997). If this process is left unchecked, severe shock is likely, but given the predictability of fluid loss, the principal aim of care is to anticipate it and compensate with fluid resuscitation (Settle 1995). The greatest amount of fluid loss in burn patients is in the first 24 hours after injury.

Loss of circulating volume always occurs following a major burn injury. Cardiac output is reduced by about a third within the first hour of injury (Cook 1997). Normal compensatory mechanisms allow homeostasis to be maintained initially, but fluid resuscitation is vital if this is to be maintained. Rapid initial transfusion may result in little improvement. It does, however, reduce the impact of a further reduction of cardiac output around six hours post-injury. Although haemoglobin becomes more fragile and has a shorter lifespan following a significant burn injury, blood transfusion is not recommended in initial management as it may increase the viscosity of intracellular fluid. Haemolysis will occur in transfused blood, therefore reducing its effectiveness.

Fluid replacement

Intravenous (i.v.) access with large-calibre i.v. lines must be established immediately in a peripheral vein (American College of Surgeons 2008). If possible, place two large-bore i.v. devices through unburned skin. If placement of the i.v. cannula is in a burned area, ensure the cannula is correctly and securely inserted into the vein, as swelling will push the hub out and may cause infiltration.

To accurately determine the amount of fluid required, it is necessary to assess the area of body surface damaged by burn injury. The 'rule of nines' (Fig. 11.1) is a convenient tool for a quick initial assessment. The rule of nines cannot be used for children because a child's body has different proportions. The Lund–Browder (1944) assessment guide (Fig. 11.2) enables a

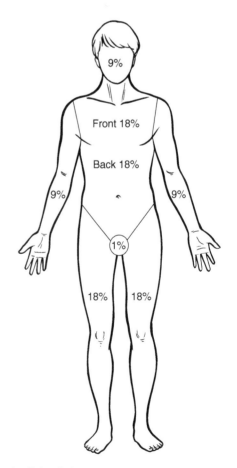

Figure 11.1 • Rule of nines.

NAME _____   WARD _____   NUMBER _____   DATE _____
AGE _____   ADMISSION WEIGHT _____

LUND AND BROWDER CHARTS

IGNORE SIMPLE ERYTHEMA

Partial thickness loss (PTL)

Full thickness loss (FTL)

REGION	%	
	PTL	FTL
HEAD		
NECK		
ANT. TRUNK		
POST.TRUNK		
RIGHT ARM		
LEFT ARM		
BUTTOCKS		
GENITALIA		
RIGHT LEG		
LEFT LEG		
TOTAL BURN		

RELATIVE PERCENTAGE OF BODY SURFACE AREA AFFECTED BY GROWTH

AREA	AGE 0	1	5	10	15	ADULT
A = ½ OF HEAD	9½	8½	6½	5½	4½	3½
B = ½ OF ONE THIGH	2¾	3¼	4	4½	4½	4¾
C = ½ OF ONE LEG	2½	2½	2¾	3	3¼	3½

Figure 11.2 • Lund–Browder (1944) assessment chart.

more accurate assessment, as it allows for surface area variations with age. If the surface area burned exceeds 15% in adults or 10% in children and the elderly, intravenous fluid resuscitation is indicated: over 20% and this resuscitation becomes urgent (Wiebelhaus & Hansen 2001). It is also possible to estimate the patient's likelihood of survival based on the percentage area of body burned (Table 11.1).

Fluid replacement is calculated from the time the burn is sustained, rather than the time resuscitation begins. The most commonly used and favoured resuscitation formula is the Parkland formula, a pure crystalloid formula. It is favoured by the British Burns Association over The Muir and Barclay Formula, which is described for albumin as the resuscitation fluid, because it has the advantages of being easy to calculate and the rate is titrated against urine output.

The Parkland formula

This calculates the amount of fluid required in the first 24 hours. Children require maintenance fluid in addition to this (Boxes 11.2, 11.3).

As stated above, the starting point for resuscitation is the time of injury, not the time of admission. Any fluid already given should be deducted for the calculated requirement.

At the end of the 24 hours, colloid infusion is begun at a rate of:

0.5 mL × (total burn surface area (%) × (body weight (kg)

and maintenance crystalloid is continued at a rate of:

1.5 mL × (total burn surface area (%) × (body weight (kg)

Table 11.1 Statistical values of mortality with age and percentage area of body burned

Area of body burned (%)	Age (years)								
	0–4	5–14	15–24	25–34	35–44	45–54	55–64	65–74	75+
93+	1.0	1.0	1.0	1.0	1.0	1.0	1.0	1.0	1.0
83–92	0.9	0.9	0.9	0.9	1.0	1.0	1.0	1.0	1.0
73–82	0.7	0.8	0.8	0.9	0.9	1.0	1.0	1.0	1.0
63–72	0.5	0.6	0.6	0.7	0.8	0.9	1.0	1.0	1.0
53–62	0.3	0.3	0.4	0.5	0.7	0.8	0.9	1.0	1.0
43–52	0.2	0.2	0.2	0.3	0.5	0.6	0.8	1.0	1.0
33–42	0.1	0.1	0.1	0.2	0.3	0.4	0.6	0.9	1.0
23–32	0	0	0	0.1	0.1	0.2	0.4	0.7	1.0
13–22	0	0	0	0	0	0.1	0.2	0.4	0.7
3–12	0	0	0	0	0	0	0.1	0.2	0.4
0–2	0	0	0	0	0	0	0	0.1	0.3

01 = 10% mortality; 0.9 = 90% mortality.

(After Bull, JP. (1971) Revised analysis of mortality due to burns. The Lancet, 298 (7734), 1133 – 1134.)

Box 11.2

Parkland formula for burns resuscitation:

Total fluid requirement in **24 hours** =
4 mL × (total burn surface area (%)) × (body weight (kg))
50 % given in first **8 hours**
50 % given in next **16 hours**

Children receive maintenance fluid in addition, at hourly rate of:
4 mL/kg for first 10 kg of body weight *plus*
2 mL/kg for second 10 kg of body weight *plus*
1 mL/kg for >20 kg of body weight

Box 11.3

Example of Parkland fluid replacement formula

Adult

A 60-kg woman with 20% burn was admitted at 3 p.m. Her burn occurred at 2 p.m.
1. *Total fluid replacement for first 24 hours*
   4 mL × (20% total burn surface area) × (60 kg) = 4800 mL in 24 hours.
2. *50 % in first 8 hours, 50 % over the next 16 hours*
   2400 mL during 0–8 hours and 2400 mL during 8–24 hours.
3. *Remember to subtract any fluid already received from amount required for first 8 hours*
   Has already received 1000 mL from ambulance services. So need:
   2400 – 1000 = 1400 mL in first 8 hours.
4. *Calculate hourly infusion rate for first 8 hours*
   Divide amount of fluid calculated in (3) by time left until it is 8 hours **after burn**
   Burn occurred at 2 p.m., so 8-hour point is 10 p.m. It is now 3 p.m., so need:
   1400 mL/7 hours = 200 mL/h from 3 p.m. to 10 p.m.
5. *Calculate hourly infusion rate for next 16 hours*
   Divide figure in (2) by 16 to give fluid infusion rate, so need:
   2400/16 hours = 150 mL/h from 10 p.m. to 2 p.m. next day.
   Remember children need maintenance fluid in addition

A fluid resuscitation formula can help to reduce inaccuracies in fluid replacement, particularly when assessment has to be made by inexperienced staff, but these formulae only act as a guideline for infusion. Actual amounts of fluid administered should reflect the condition of the patient. The amount of fluid given should be continuously adjusted according to the individual patient's response, to maintain a urinary output of 0.5–1 mL/kg/h (adult) or 1–1.5 mL/kg/h (child) (American College of Surgeons 2008) and other physiological parameters (pulse, blood pressure and respiratory rate) (Fig. 11.3).

There is no agreement on the type of fluid that should be used for resuscitating the burn-injured patient. Colloids have no advantage over crystalloids in the initial management to maintain circulatory volume (Heittiaratchy & Papini 2004). In the UK, Hartmann's solution (sodium chloride 0.6%, sodium lactate 0.25%, potassium chloride 0.04%, calcium chloride 0.027%) is the most commonly used crystalloid. Crystalloids are given to supplement that used by metabolic requirements, which tend to increase following injury. In adults, 50 mL/h of sodium base crystalloid should be given to maintain metabolic function. In children, fluid replacement should be titrated by the child's weight (Wilson 1997) (Box 11.2). Colloid use is controversial. However, a lot of protein is lost through the burn wound, so there is a need to replace this: some units introduce colloid after 8 hours, as the capillary leak begins to shut down; others wait 24 hours. Fresh frozen plasma is often used in children and albumin in adults (Heittiaratchy & Papini 2004).

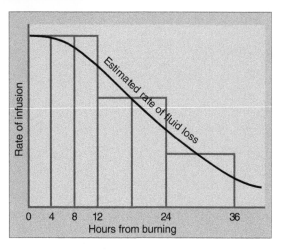

Figure 11.3 • Estimated rate of fluid loss (after Bosworth 1997).

Disabilities

The last step of the primary survey is to look for any obvious disabilities and assess changes in the patient's level of consciousness.

Secondary survey

The secondary survey should follow that of the primary. In the secondary survey, expose and examine the patient from head to toe, looking for any minor associated injuries. Care should be taken at this stage to prevent hypothermia in an already compromised patient. Obtain an AMPLE history:

- *Allergies*
- *Medications*
- *Past medical history*
- *Last meal*
- *Events surrounding the injury.*

In the resuscitation phase, even seemingly well patients with a major burn should be kept nil by mouth because of the risk of developing paralytic ileus. If this occurs, gastric aspiration via nasogastric tube may be necessary to prevent persistent vomiting. During resuscitation, frequent monitoring is necessary to detect changes and to attempt to maintain the patient's stability. By using several indicators to give a picture of the patient's overall condition, appropriate clinical decisions can be made.

Pulse, respiration and blood pressure

These give an indication of changes to the patient's homeostasis, level of pain and anxiety. Any increase in pulse or respiratory rate should be closely monitored and its cause established. Changes to blood pressure are a late sign in most cases of haemodynamic compromise, but monitoring is still valuable.

Altered level of consciousness

This can have a variety of causes, from primary injury to substance abuse, but hypoxia and hypovolaemia should not be disregarded. A sudden onset of restlessness, particularly in children, should be treated with suspicion and other indicators of stability should be checked. Using the AVPU mnemonic (Alert and orientated, responds to Verbal stimulus, responds to Painful stimulus, Unresponsive) is recommended to determine a child's level of consciousness.

Skin colour

This is used to detect shock, as well as the level of injury to specific areas. A pink skin tone is indicative of a well-perfused patient, whereas pallor indicates arteriole constriction and a blue skin tone indicates venous stagnation consistent with severe shock.

Skin and core temperature

This is useful for determining the level of vasoconstriction — the greater the difference, the poorer the level of perfusion. In a well person, this difference is between 18 and 48°C.

Urinary output

Patients with major burn injuries should be catheterized at an early stage, unless specific contraindications exist. Urine output will vary in early resuscitation because of hormones secreted as part of the stress response to injury. As previously stated, adequate fluid resuscitation should yield 0.5–1 mL/kg of body weight per hour (adults). Less than this indicates inadequate resuscitation and large volumes of low-concentration urine indicate over transfusion.

Central venous pressure

Although this is useful in the monitoring of most cases of major trauma, its value for the burns patient is limited. Changes to central venous pressure are gradual and the risk of infection is high (Copley & Glencorse 1992).

Frequent laboratory analysis of haematocrit level

This gives an indication of the ratio of red cells to plasma volume. An increased haematocrit level indicates a low plasma volume and therefore inadequate fluid replacement.

Specific burn injuries

Thermal burns

These account for a large percentage of minor burn injuries, and a significant proportion of major burn injuries. They can be subdivided into three groups (Box 11.4).

Box 11.4

Thermal burns

Scalds

Injuries from hot fluids, such as tea, bath water, kettles, etc., are the most common causes of all burns. Most of these cause skin damage or loss and are extremely painful. Exposure to water at 60°C (140°F) for 3 seconds can cause a deep partial-thickness or full-thickness burn. If the water is 69°C (156°F), the same burn occurs in 1 second. As a comparison, freshly brewed coffee is about 82°C (180°F). Steam can cause deeper injuries because of its heat. Hot fat also causes more severe injury because of its temperature and, usually, a more prolonged contact with skin.

Contact

The most commonly treated are injuries from contact with hot objects, such as irons, ovens, hot metal or bitumen. Friction contact, e.g., with road surfaces, causes more superficial burn injuries.

Flame

Ignition of clothing by petrol, barbecues, bonfires, house fires etc. causes severe injury because of the prolonged contact of the source with the patient's skin. Flash burns from lightning or other electrical sources cause brief exposure to very high temperatures and therefore can result in significant injury (Thayre 1995).

Pre-hospital management

Remembering the safety of the rescuer, the source of the burn should first be removed, i.e., flames should be extinguished and contact with hot substances reduced. Cold running water at 15°C applied to the affected area for approximately 20 minutes to dissipate heat and relieve pain is associated with an initial improvement in re-epithelialization and decreased scar tissue after six weeks (Cuttle et al. 2010). Ice should not be used as it can cause blood vessels to constrict and produce further damage (Hudspith & Rayatt 2004). Cooling should not exceed 20 minutes because of a significant risk of hypothermia, and the patient should be protected from environmental heat loss. Care should be taken if removing molten clothing, as the risk of devitalizing healthy tissue is high. Adherent material, such as nylon clothing, should be left on. Tar burns should be cooled with water, but the tar itself should not be removed (Hudspith & Rayatt 2004).

Chemical burns

Patients with chemical burns represent only 3 % of all burns, however they present with an important morbidity – nearly 55 % of them require surgery – commonly involve cosmetic body areas, e.g., the face, thorax and hands, and some series carry approximately 30 % of burns death (Palao 2010). Common injuries occur from contact with acids and alkalines, as well as domestic substances, e.g., bleach and cleaning agents. The severity of the burn injury will be determined by the:

* type of chemical
* concentration
* duration of skin contact
* penetration
* mechanism of action.

Chemical injury is classified either by the mechanism of action on skin or by chemical class of the agent.

Pre-hospital management

The treatment priority lies with removal of caustic chemicals from the patient's skin. After rapid removal of soaked clothing, the patient should be showered by large amounts of running water to dilute and remove the chemical. Dry powders should be brushed off before decontamination with water commences (Wiebelhaus & Hansen 2001). Water has advantages over specific neutralizing solutions. The principal aim of decontamination is to minimize the period of contact between the contaminant and the skin. Time taken searching for particular antidotes leads to deeper levels of injury. More importantly, do not attempt to neutralize a chemical burn; this could cause exothermic reaction and further injury (Wiebelhaus & Hansen 2001). In most cases, adequate dilution reduces the risk of further damage.

Litmus testing of wet skin will indicate acidity or alkalinity, and a neutral buffer solution can be applied, if necessary, once the chemical is diluted sufficiently. In extensive chemical burns, absorption can have systemic effects, including alteration of the blood's acid–base and electrolyte balance, together with renal and hepatic damage. Where possible, the identity of the chemical should be established and local poison unit facilities contacted to provide information on specific reactions and antidotes (Settle 1995).

Chemical eye injuries require immediate attention (Gerard et al. 2002). Signs and symptoms include:

* pain
* oedema and irritation of the eyelids
* reddened sclera
* loss of or blurred vision.

Periorbital skin irritation or damage should always increase suspicion of eye problems. Alkaline injuries are more serious than those involving acids because they rapidly penetrate the conjunctiva through to the cornea, causing significant long-term damage. In all chemical injuries, the eyes should be irrigated, with water initially, with the eyelids held open until the contaminant is removed. This can be checked by gently placing litmus paper into the conjunctival sac. Insertion of a buffer neutralizing solution may be necessary to halt the injury process.

Ensure contact lenses are removed prior to irrigation to prevent a film of contaminant remaining between lens and cornea. The use of a local anaesthetic will relieve pain, reduce anxiety and allow easier examination and treatment. Once decontamination has been completed, antibiotic ointments should be prescribed and applied to reduce corneal scarring. All chemical eye injuries must be referred for specialist ophthalmological opinion (see also Chapter 31).

Electrical burns

These are sometimes more serious than they first appear, as there may be little superficial tissue loss; however, massive muscle injury may be present beneath normal-looking skin. Contact with high-voltage cables can lead to propulsion injuries. Domestic injury, although of lower voltage, can also cause significant damage. The electrical current takes the path of least resistance through the body, usually through the blood vessels, exiting through the earth contact. Small entry and exit points on the skin's surface may belie the amount of damage to the blood vessels, muscles and bone tissue beneath. In addition to direct heat damage caused by the progression of the current, injury can be sustained by blood vessel necrosis, severe tetany of muscles, conductivity problems in the myocardium, and the force of propulsive impact, often severe enough to cause bone fractures. These patients often suffer secondary 'flash' burns.

Following electrical injury, cardiac monitoring should be used to detect possible arrhythmias. Depending on the path of the current, a 12-lead ECG should be performed to detect myocardial damage, which may occur at the time of injury or several hours afterwards as myocardial tissue breaks down. In serious cases, where there are ECG abnormalities or a loss of consciousness, 24 hours of monitoring is advised (Hettiaratchy & Dziewulski 2004). Jenkins (2005) suggests that while cardiac dysrhythmias may initially be seen, they may also be delayed for up to 24 hours. These include sinus bradycardia, right bundle branch block and focal ectopic dysrhythmias. Sutcliffe (1998) notes that ST elevation and QT elongation are other non-specific changes associated with severe burns.

Close attention should also be paid to renal function, which will be severely impaired by the release of proteins (myoglobin) from massive tissue breakdown. Hourly urine output should be observed after insertion of a urinary catheter. Darkened urine indicates that myoglobin is present and warrants immediate action to maintain renal function, including intravenous fluid therapy and possibly mannitol to create a high urine output and quickly flush out proteins from the kidneys (Settle 1995).

Cold burns (frostbite)

Frostbite is a thermal injury that can occur when temperatures drop low enough for tissue to freeze (Grieve et al. 2011). Although relatively uncommon in the UK, frostbite can be seen in individuals who have had prolonged exposure to extreme cold conditions. Immediate management of the patient concentrates on the monitoring and gradual increase of core body temperature. The extreme cold causes the formation of ice crystals and disrupts cell membranes; vasoconstriction of blood vessels leads to tissue necrosis and an increase in blood viscosity impairs capillary blood flow. This occurs most commonly on exposed extremities such as fingertips, ear lobes and toes. With superficial frostbite, the frozen part is waxy white and does not blanch or show capillary refilling after mild pressure. The tissue below is soft and

resilient on pressure and the affected part is anaesthetized. Rewarming is usually painful, and afterwards the appearance is initially erythematous and oedematous, progressing to a mottled purple colour. Blisters appear, lasting approximately 5–10 days, and eventually dry out leaving a black eschar associated with pain. Demarcation and separation occur over the next month, leaving a delicately epithelialized area that is the site of long-term hypersensitivity.

Deep frostbite occurs when the temperature of a limb is lowered. The frozen part is waxy white and does not blanch or show capillary refilling after mild pressure. The tissue below is hard and cannot be compressed. The affected part is numb. Rewarming is often painful and afterwards the appearance is usually mottled blue (Mills et al. 1995). Frostbitten areas should be protected from further trauma, quickly reheated in warm water (around 38°C), dried and maintained at room temperature. Thawing frozen tissue is extremely painful, so intravenous analgesia may be given. Heparin therapy may be commenced together with intravenous Dextran 40 to improve peripheral blood flow. Swelling of the whole limb occurs or appears at the demarcation line several weeks later. If necrosis has occurred, the areas are usually allowed to demarcate before amputation surgery is carried out. The extent of the tissue loss reflects the severity of the cold exposure and includes factors such as temperature, duration, wind chill, altitude, and systemic hypothermia (Grieve et al. 2011).

Radiation

These are most commonly caused through over exposure to sunlight or sunbeds. The burns are usually superficial but slow to heal due to injury thromboangitis. More serious injury occurs from exposure to nuclear substances or accidents in radiotherapy. Acute radiation syndrome is a symptom complex that occurs following whole-body irradiation. It varies in nature and severity depending on dose, dose rate, distribution and individual susceptibility.

Pre-hospital management

Decontamination is necessary in cases of nuclear exposure. If the patient's condition permits, this should be initiated at the scene. Ambulance personnel should wear protective clothing, including rubber gloves and shoe covers. The patient's clothing should be removed and placed in plastic bags and, if possible, soap and water cleansing of exposed skin should be performed. Performing these tasks will minimize contamination of the ambulance and emergency department, most of which are not currently well designed for decontamination patients.

Assessment and management

The receiving hospital should be given as much information as possible about the numbers and types of patients involved in a radiation exposure incident, as a decision will need to be made regarding implementation of a full disaster plan versus a limited response. Ideally, contaminated patients should enter the department through a separate, protected entrance. All healthcare personnel should wear protective, disposable clothing, including surgical gloves and shoe covers. If not already done, the patient should be immediately undressed and washed and all clothing placed in sealed containers labelled 'radioactive waste'. If the patient has open wounds, the surrounding skin should be decontaminated by scrubbing with soap and water. Wounds should be irrigated with copious amounts of saline. The normal principles of wound closure should be followed. No danger to healthcare personnel should exist if proper precautions are carried out.

Non-accidental injury

Detecting these injuries is important as it is estimated that 3–10% of paediatric burns are due to non-accidental injury (NAI) (Hettiaratchy & Dziewulski 2004). As with other NAIs, the history and the pattern of injury may arouse suspicion.

Assessment and management

Initial treatment of the physical burn injury is paramount. The team should also carry out the following:

- examine for other signs of abuse
- photograph all injuries
- obtain other medical information (from general practitioner, health visitor)
- interview family members separately about the incident to check for inconsistencies and together to observe interaction (Hettiaratchy & Dziewulski 2004).

Any suspicion of NAI should lead to immediate admission of the child to hospital, irrespective of the burn injury, and notification to social services (see also Pre-school children).

Burn wound care

Initial management of burn wounds

The aims are:

- to limit further damage with appropriate first aid measures
- to assess the depth of injury, in order to determine treatment plan
- to maintain perfusion and protect damaged tissue from desiccation and infection.

Measurement of burn depth

Burns can be divided into two categories: partial- and full-thickness skin damage. Partial-thickness burns are subcategorized into superficial and deep.

Superficial burn injuries involve skin loss from epidermis only (Fig. 11.4). The dermal capillaries dilate and fluid leaks

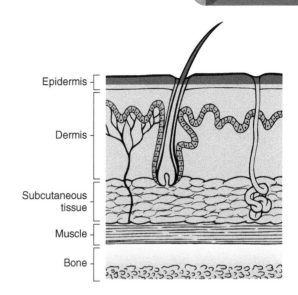

Figure 11.4 • Superficial burn.

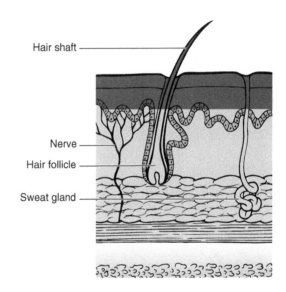

Figure 11.5 • Deeper partial-thickness burn.

into the surrounding tissues. This causes increased pressure on intact nerve endings, which results in a reddened painful wound, with good capillary refill. Pain and swelling usually subside within 48 hours and it will heal by epithelialization over a period of about 7 days. These burns usually leave no scarring.

Deeper partial-thickness burns involve both epidermal and dermal damage of varying depths (Fig. 11.5). Capillary destruction occurs, which results in fluid escaping to form blisters or a shiny wet wound surface. The wound appears less red than a superficial injury and may have some white avascular areas. Nerve supply is sometimes damaged and generally these wounds are less painful than superficial wounds. Sensation is not lost and the patient should be able to distinguish between blunt and sharp. These burns heal by regeneration, usually within 14 days.

Figure 11.6 • Full-thickness burn.

Full-thickness burns involve the entire dermal layer and may involve underlying structures such as muscle, tendon and bone (Fig. 11.6). The upper skin layers are destroyed, the wound is avascular and appears white or charred, capillary return is absent, and wound exudate is minimal. Sensation is reduced or absent in full-thickness burns. These injuries heal by granulation. Because of the vascular damage, blood supply is reduced and so necrosis and infection are common. Full-thickness burns often require surgical debridement.

Protection of wound

Asepsis is of paramount importance with burn injuries because of the inherent infection risk. Wounds should be cleaned by irrigation with saline. Irrigation reduces the risk of tissue damage when compared with other cleaning methods, and is less painful for the patient. As saline is isotonic, it is unlikely to cause irritation to tissue. Burned clothing, dirt and devitalized tissue should be carefully removed as part of the cleaning process. Controversy exists over the management of blisters. Although the fluid contained in blisters promotes healing, and the roof of the blister provides an effective cover of protection and, from a practical perspective, many patients find it extremely painful to have a blister de-roofed in the first day or two following burn injury (Cole 2003), it is thought the size and weight of the blister creates a risk of traumatic shearing that can increase the extent of the wound (Collier 2000). To remove this risk, larger blisters should be de-roofed and dead skin removed with sterile scissors (Hudspith & Rayatt 2004). The optimum approach is to aspirate blister fluid, removing the shearing risk and leaving the blister roof in place to act as a natural dressing.

Exposed wounds have a faster rate of fluid loss than covered wounds. Wound care should focus on reinstating the functions lost by the destruction of skin, control of body temperature, maintenance of fluid balance and providing a barrier to infection (Collier 2006). For major burn wounds, the replacement of skin functions is the only reason for dressings; they should be simple and not include creams or lotions.

The initial treatment of choice is PVC cling film (Allison 2002). It reduces evaporative fluid loss and provides a protective barrier to infection. It is also transparent, allowing continual visual inspection of the wound. Cling film can be used next to skin or over wet compresses. It is easy to apply and painless to remove. Cling film should not be applied to the face for obvious reasons. The patient needs additional protection against heat loss. It is important to check the patient's tetanus status and administer tetanus toxoid if the patient is not covered. Systemic antibiotics have not proven effective in preventing wound infections. They should not be used as a prophylactic measure because they increase the risk of resistant bacteria developing (Lawrence 1992).

Pain control

Most patients with burn injuries will experience pain and, after immediate life-saving interventions, pain control should be treated aggressively (Esfahlan 2010). The psychological response to burn injury should not be underestimated when assessing a patient's pain. The euphoria of survival and ignorance or denial of the full impact of injury can result in a transient period of little or no pain. Fear and insight into potential outcomes can also have an effect on the extent and type of pain the patient feels. It is imperative that the ED nurse recognizes psychological influences and uses both pharmacological and psychological methods to achieve pain control.

Assessment of pain should include:

- psychological state
- verbal responses
- facial expression
- mobility
- protecting injured areas
- posture.

It is uncommon for an injury to be solely full-thickness (Settle 1995). It is more likely that the wound will be of mixed depth, and therefore some nerve endings will be intact, causing pain. Pain relief starts with the application of cold water and the burn wound being covered from the air.

Initial treatment in the ED can include the use of inhaled nitrous oxide (Entonox) in the conscious patient unless associated injuries prevent this. Nitrous oxide has a rapid effect and gives the patient control over their own pain relief. Because it is self-administered, there is an inherent safeguard against overdose.

For major burn injuries, patients should be given small, frequent doses of intravenous opioids until pain relief is achieved (Copely & Glencorse 1992). Intramuscular or subcutaneous routes are inappropriate because of hypovolaemia, which causes reduced peripheral circulation and results in poor absorption of the drug and inadequate pain control. Intramuscular and subcutaneous routes also carry the risk of respiratory or CNS depression. This is because a delayed absorption of the drug takes place as circulation improves. Because this happens rapidly, an overdose effect can occur (Singer & Dagum 2008).

Assessment of pain should include the observation of non-verbal behaviour, such as facial expressions, distorted posture, splinting and impaired mobility, in addition to verbal responses. This may also give an indication of other traumatic injuries, especially if the patient has been involved in an road traffic accident, explosion or high-voltage injury (see also Chapter 25).

Escharotomies

Escharotomies are carried out where circumferential full-thickness burns occur around limbs, chest, neck, digits or penis. As oedema develops in the tissue beneath, the relatively inflexible full-thickness injury cannot compensate for the increase in tissue volume and exerts a tourniquet effect. If the increasing pressure is not released at an early stage, usually within three hours, ischaemic damage will occur in tissues distal to the burn (Settle 1995). In the case of the chest and neck, the rigidity compromises the expansion of the lungs (Judkins 1992).

The procedure is carried out by making longitudinal incisions with a sterile blade through the burned skin to bleeding tissue. The release of tension forces the wound to gape open. An absorbent haemostatic dressing, such as calcium alginate, can be placed into the wounds to arrest bleeding. Because the burns are full-thickness in nature, relatively little analgesia is required. Although they are an urgent procedure, escharotomies are best done in an operating theatre by experienced staff. Initially, at-risk limbs should be observed for signs of impaired circulation, looking at perfusion, capillary refill, temperature and sensation (Molter & Greenfield 1997). Rings, watches, restrictive clothing and tight dressings should be removed and the limbs elevated above heart level to reduce swelling. Controversies surrounding escharotomies are not new and alternatives should be considered in the management of acute burns (Burd et al. 2006).

Psychological considerations

Burn injuries produce highly emotive responses because of their association with loss of life, pain and scarring. The psychological impact can be devastating for the patient, relatives and those required to deal with the aftermath.

The patient

Initial reactions vary, and some patients will exhibit 'shock', bewilderment and disorientation, with an apparent denial of injury linked to internal defense mechanisms to reduce the anxiety associated with severe injury. Many patients also experience an initial euphoria associated with survival (Copley & Glencorse 1992). Often the significance of injury is not appreciated, particularly where full-thickness damage is involved or where respiratory complications have not had time to develop. Others may be distressed because of pain and anxiety caused by an awareness of the seriousness of their condition. Askey & Patterson (2008) found that high pain scores were significantly related to poorer adjustment one month after the burn.

Relatives

The fact that the patient is alert, able to talk and not in any great distress can often lead friends and family into a false sense of security, reinforcing a denial that serious injury has taken place (Konigova 1992). For some, the sight of the patient in pain or with facial or hand burns can be very distressing and cause relatives to fear much worse consequences than will actually be the case. Honest, informative support from experienced ED staff is necessary.

Staff

Burn injuries, particularly those as a result of fires, have characteristics that are not shared with other forms of trauma. The smell of burned skin and degree of suffering witnessed, especially where death occurs, can be very upsetting even to experienced staff. Staff support is crucial; however, the nature of support needs to be tangible and flexible in order to respond to individual needs (Regel 1997) (see also Chapter 13).

Transfer to specialist units

Although policies for admission vary, Box 11.5 lists the types of burn injury considered serious enough to warrant specialist attention (National Burn Care Review 2001).

> **Box 11.5**
>
> **Burn injuries requiring transfer to specialist units. (from Kemble & Lamb 1987)**
>
> - Major burns – partial- or full-thickness burns involving more than 5% of the total body surface area in babies, 10% in children or 15% in adults
> - Burns involving inhalation injury
> - Full-thickness burns – greater than 2.5 cm in diameter, where skin grafting or flap reconstruction will be necessary to facilitate healing and improve scarring
> - Electrical and chemical burns – both are often more serious than they at first appear and require specific care
> - Burns involving specific problematic areas – these include the hands and feet, face, perineum and major joints
> - Burns in those with other problems – e.g., diabetes, epilepsy, the elderly or where child buse is suspected

Burns units offer a concentration of resources in terms of experienced staff and specialized facilities. Each unit tends to be highly individualized, with its own protocols for admission. For this reason it is difficult to draw up a definitive etiquette for transferring burn-injured patients. It might, however, be useful to consider the following points when planning a transfer. And remember: *safety is more important than speed.*

Any attempt at transfer must not be considered until the patient is in a stable condition and prepared in such a way that any risk of deterioration in transit is greatly reduced. While it would seem logical to assume that transport by air is quicker than by land, Chipp et al. (2010) argue that the additional time in mobilizing and landing the aircraft means that this is not necessarily true. It has been shown that helicopters are faster than land transport only at distances greater than 45 miles (72 km) (Diaz et al. 2005).

The airway must be fully assessed and measures must be taken to maintain a patent airway during transfer to reduce the risk of obstruction. An experienced escort, including an anaesthetist where there is airway and respiratory involvement, is essential and the transfer vehicle must be suitably furnished with oxygen, suction and resuscitation equipment. Intravenous access must be established using two wide-bore cannulas. Adequate fluid replacement should be commenced and sustained throughout transfer and the patient should be catheterized with accurate measurement and recording before and during transfer. Similar attention must be paid to analgesia. If the patient has suffered electrical injury, myoglobins/haemoglobins in the urine may lead to catheter blockage so should be observed carefully. The patient should be transferred in a warm vehicle, well insulated with blankets, and equipment should have batteries, including spares, sufficient for the journey. Wet dressings are not necessary at this stage (Ellis & Rylah 1990).

Although the initial referral is carried out by medical staff, verbal communication between nursing personnel in the emergency department and receiving burns unit, prior to transfer, is essential. It is worth drawing up a list of local units and their telephone numbers for ease of reference. Confirm with the nurse in charge that a bed is available. Give preliminary verbal information including:

- the name and age of the patient
- relevant medical record
- brief history and time of the incident
- causative agent, petrol, electricity, chemical, etc.
- extent, i.e., percentage area involved
- nature of other injuries sustained, particularly any inhalation involvement
- time of accident to commencement of first aid
- time of accident to commencement of fluid resuscitation
- time of departure and estimated arrival time
- whether the patient should be transferred directly to the burns unit or the receiving hospital emergency department.

It is difficult to convey large amounts of complex information by verbal means alone. Therefore, when handing over to burns unit staff, the escorting nurse must have clearly written details, documenting the points outlined above and specifically:

- the patient's clinical observations
- fluid input and urine output, including that during the transfer
- laboratory results, including FBC, U&E, coagulation screen
- blood gas and COHb results
- tetanus status
- any medications given
- GP details
- next of kin and relevant social history
- contact name and number of investigating police officers if involved.

Accurate and effective communication improves the continuity of care and allows burns unit specialists to make early decisions about the future course of treatment. It may prove useful to obtain constructive feedback from the burns unit about the transfer procedure and the patient's recovery. This information can be used either to improve the department's future performance or to confirm to those involved that they fulfilled their roles to a satisfactory standard (see Chapter 4).

Minor burn wound care

Minor burns tend to be classified as those that can be treated on an outpatient basis. The injury usually represents less than 5% of the body surface area and excludes some of the problematic body areas (Duncan & Driscoll 1991) (Box 11.6).

The patient's social circumstances should be considered and their level of support/aid assessed before a decision to discharge is taken. The initial burn injury causes significant disruption to normal skin function. Heat causes cellular injury, resulting in a breakdown of the skin's protective barrier and a susceptibility to infection. The wound itself is initially controlled by the body's natural inflammatory response. Oedema and exudate are rapidly produced, which can to some extent be minimized by cooling the wound and reducing further cellular damage (Cole 2003).

The area of the injury has three specific parts (Rylah 1992) (Fig. 11.7):

- zone of necrosis – this is non-viable, or dead, tissue usually found at the centre of the wound

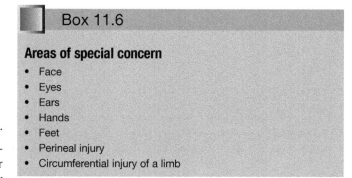

Box 11.6

Areas of special concern
- Face
- Eyes
- Ears
- Hands
- Feet
- Perineal injury
- Circumferential injury of a limb

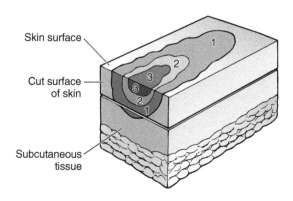

Figure 11.7 ● Pathophysiology of a burn wound. 1, Zone of hyperaemia; 2, zone of stasis; 3, zone of necrosis.

- zone of stasis – this is the area of the wound that is most vulnerable and potentially salvageable; it consists of viable tissue, but is at risk of ischaemic damage because of reduced tissue perfusion
- zone of hyperaemia – this is the area immediately surrounding the damage (outermost zone), which is undergoing the inflammatory phase to injury; the tissue itself is undamaged and develops an increased blood flow in an attempt to control the extent of injury.

The healing of a burn wound depends very much on the depth of injury. Superficial and partial-thickness burns involving the epidermis and upper dermal layers will only heal spontaneously by epithelialization and regeneration over a period of 7–14 days. It is this group of injuries which are best treated on an outpatient basis. Deeper partial-thickness burns, with damage to all but the deep dermal layers, will heal much more slowly over a period of 3–4 weeks. Full-thickness burns heal by granulation, a process which can take several weeks or months depending on the size of the injury, its site and the patient's general health and age. This group of patients benefit from referral to specialist units for excision and grafting of wounds.

For those patients who can be discharged, wound care and appropriate advice are paramount. The primary aim is to foster an environment that is appropriate to the healing needs of the wound at a particular stage (Table 11.2).

Wound cleaning, as discussed above, should be as rigorous for small or minor wounds as for major burns. Differences in management occur in the assessment of wound dressings needed (Edwards 2006). Most major injuries will not have their full extent and depth assessed for 48 hours until oedema begins to subside. For smaller wounds, the aims of burns dressings are to prevent colonization by bacteria, to provide a warm, moist environment for cellular reconstruction, to absorb exudate and to protect the area from further injury.

Dressing care for burns patients may vary according to local policy. However, ED care usually focuses around the inflammatory stage where copious exudate is present, and the destructive phase where autolysis demands a moist environment. Initially, a multiple layer of paraffin tulle-type dressing, applied under copious padding and bandages, will provide a warm non-adherent, protective dressing for the inflammatory phase. The disadvantage with this method is that, if the dressing soaks through, a tract for infection is created and the patient will need to return to ED for renewal. These types of dressing should be changed at least daily. Antibacterial agents such as silver sulfadiazine cream or an advanced silver dressing such as Acticoat® (Smith & Nephew) are useful in preventing Gram-negative or *Pseudomonas* infections in the initial stages. For the cream to remain effective, it should be reapplied daily for the first three days (Holt 1998). The reapplication of the cream and the removal technique, which requires manual cleansing of the wound over exposed nerve endings, are undoubtedly a painful experience. Adequate analgesia for the patient should be considered before and during dressing changes (Varas et al. 2005). In comparison, the benefit of the newer advanced silver dressings is that the often painful dressing changes associated with the cream are avoided as the dressing can be left intact for 3 days. For usage of either product, the manufacturer's guidelines should be followed.

After 48 hours, as the wound enters the destructive phase, exudate begins to reduce and the wound benefits from less-frequent dressing changes. Hydrocolloid dressings are most effective for this stage of healing. They provide a warm and moist environment that facilitates autolysis and natural debridement of the wound. For maximum effectiveness, these dressings should be left in situ for 4–7 days depending on the site and extent of the wound. Hydrocolloid dressings are also valuable in the treatment of granulating wounds.

Facial burns

Facial burns should be referred to a specialist unit, unless the injury is simple, e.g., sunburn. Burns to facial areas should be kept moist with soft paraffin ointment and left exposed. Antibacterial creams should not be used as they can cause skin staining when in contact with oxygen. Ears are the exception to this. Nanocrystalline silver dressings should be applied. This is because the risk of complications from infection includes ear deformity and internal structural damage.

Hands and feet

One of the treatment priorities is to maintain movement. For this reason, wounds are treated with antibacterial cream and covered with polythene bags or gloves. This allows for observation of the wound as well as movement of digits. Wounds treated in this way require daily dressing changes. Unfortunately, dressings applied to the burnt hand and individual fingers are often bulky (Kok et al. 2006). For further information on wound care see Chapter 24.

Discharge information should include advice about wound care and when to return to ED, but should also include advice on:

- nutrition to promote wound healing
- exercise regimes to restore normal function
- wound progress and scarring.

Table 11.2 Stages of wound healing	
Stage	**Features of healing**
Inflammatory (0–3 days)	Initial response to injury causes redness, heat, pain and swelling with copious exudate
Destruction (2–5 days)	Clearing of devitalized tissue and bacteria and development of fibroblasts
Proliferation (3–24 days)	Production of collagen and granulation tissue which fills the wound space. Although it may look 'healed' the wound remains very fragile
Maturation (24 days–1 year)	This focuses on restructuring scar tissue; vascularity decreases and redness fades. The wound area strengthens and by 6 weeks scar tissue has about 50% of the tensile strength of uninjured skin
Contraction (4 days onwards)	Process whereby the wound naturally reduces in size. Usually only occurs in large wounds with considerable tissue loss

Psychological support should also be provided at this time, by allowing the patient to express fears or uncertainty about management of the injury as well as to ask any general questions he may have about care.

Conclusion

Caring for a patient with burn injuries represents a multifocal challenge to ED staff. Priorities of care must be with the systematic assessment and implementation of life-saving activities, such as airway management and fluid resuscitation. Protection of burn wounds is imperative if secondary injury and infection are to be prevented. The initiation of wound care and patient education are important for those with minor injuries. All patients need time and psychological support to come to terms with their injury, as even minor wounds create high levels of anxiety about scarring. However, the emergency nurse can do much to alleviate the physical and psychological suffering of the burns patient.

References

Allison, K., 2002. The UK pre-hospital management of burn patients: current practice and the need for a standard approach. Burns 28 (2), 135–142.

American College of Surgeons, 2008. Advanced Trauma Life Support, eighth ed. American College of Surgeons, Chicago.

Askay, S.W., Patterson, D.R., 2008. What are the psychiatric sequelae of burn pain? Current Pain Headache Reports 12, 94–97.

Bull, J.P., 1971. Revised analysis of mortality due to burns. The Lancet 298 (7734), 1133–1134.

Burd, A., Noronha, F.V., Ahmed, K., et al., 2006. Decompression not escharotomy in acute burns. Burns 32 (3), 284–292.

Campbell, A., 2000. Hospital management of poisoning in victims suffering from smoke inhalation. Emergency Nurse 8 (4), 12–16.

Chipp, E., Warner, R.M., McGill, D.J., 2010. Air ambulance transfer of adult patients to a UK regional burns centre: Who needs to fly? Burns 36, 1201–1207.

Cole, E., 2003. Wound management in the A&E department. Nursing Standard 17 (46), 45–52.

Collier, M., 2000. Expert comment on managing burn blisters. Nursing Times 96 (4), 20.

Collier, M., 2006. The use of advanced biological and tissue-engineered wound products. Nursing Standard 21 (7), 68–76.

Cook, D., 1997. Pathophysiology of burns. In: Bosworth, C. (Ed.), Burns Trauma: Management and Nursing Care. Baillière Tindall, London.

Copley, J., Glencorse, C., 1992. The nursing management of burns. Care of the Critically Ill 8 (6), 246–251.

Cuttle, S., Kempf, M., Pei-Yun, L., et al., 2010. The optimal duration and delay of first aid treatment for deep partial thickness burn injuries. Burns 36, 673–679.

Diaz, M.A., Hendey, G.W., Bivins, H.G., 2005. When is the helicopter faster? A comparison of helicopter and ground ambulance transport times. Journal of Trauma 58 (1), 148–153.

Duncan, D.J., Driscoll, D.M., 1991. Burn wound management. Critical Care Clinics of North America 3 (2), 255–267.

Dunn, K.W., 2000. Standards and Strategy for Burn Care: A Review of Burn Care in the British Isles. National Burn Care Review Committee Report, London.

Edwards, S.L., 2006. Tissue viability: Understanding the mechanisms of injury and repair. Nursing Standard 21 (13), 48–56.

Ellis, A., Rylah, L.T.A., 1990. Transfer of the thermally injured patient. British Journal of Hospital Medicine 44 (3), 200–206.

Esfahlan, A.J., Mojgan Lotfi, M., Zamanzadeh, V., et al., 2010. Burn pain and patients' responses. Burns 36, 1129–1133.

Gerard, M., Merle, H., Chiambaretta, F., et al., 2002. An amphoteric rinse used in the emergency treatment of a serious ocular burn. Burns 28, 670–673.

Grieve, A.W., Davis, P., Dhillon, S., et al., 2011. A clinical review of the management of frostbite. Journal of Royal Army Medical Corps 157 (1), 73–78.

Herndon, D., 2007. Total Burn Care. Saunders, Philadelphia.

Hettiaratchy, S., Dziewulski, P., 2004. Pathophysiology and types of burns. British Medical Journal 328, 1427–1429.

Hettiaratchy, S., Papini, R., 2004. Initial management of a major burn: assessment and resuscitation. British Medical Journal 329, 101–104.

Holt, L., 1998. Assessing and managing minor burns. Emergency Nurse 6 (2), 14–16.

Hudspith, J., Rayatt, S., 2004. First aid and treatment of minor burns. British Medical Journal 328, 1487–1489.

Jenkins, L., 2005. Care of the patient with major burns. In: O'Shea, R.A. (Ed.), Principles and Practice of Trauma Nursing. Churchill Livingstone Elsevier, Edinburgh.

Jones, R., 2003. Smoke inhalation: assessing and managing patients. Emergency Nurse 11 (7), 18–23.

Judkins, K.C., 1992. Burns and respiratory system injury. Care of the Critically Ill 8 (6), 238–241.

Kok, K., Georgeu, G.A., Wilson, V.Y., 2006. The acticoat glove: an effective dressing for the completely burnt hand. Burns 32 (4), 487–489.

Konigova, R., 1992. The psychological problems of burned patients: The Rudy Hermans Lecture 1991. Burns 18 (3), 189–199.

Lawrence, J.C., 1992. Infective complications of burns. Care of the Critically Ill 8 (6), 234–236.

Lund, C., Browder, N., 1944. Estimation of areas of burns. Surgery, Gynaecology & Obstetrics 79, 352–358.

McParkland, M., 1999. Carbon monoxide poisoning. Emergency Nurse 7 (6), 18–22.

Mills, K., Morton, R., Page, G., 1995. Colour Atlas and Text of Emergencies, second ed. Mosby-Wolfe, London.

Molter, N.C., Greenfield, E., 1997. Burns. In: Hartshorn, H.C., Sole, M.I., Lamborn, M.L. (Eds.), Introduction to Critical Care Nursing, second ed. WB Saunders, Philadelphia.

Moss, L., 2010. Treatment of the burn patient in primary care. Advances in Skin and Wound Care (23), 517–524.

Muehlberger, T., Kunar, D., Munster, A., et al., 1998. Efficacy of fibreoptic laryngoscopy in the diagnosis of inhalation injuries. Archives of Otolaryngology Head & Neck Surgery 124 (9), 1003–1007.

National Audit Office, 2010. Major Trauma Care in England. The Stationery Office, London.

National Burn Care Review, 2001. National burn injury referral guidelines. In: Standards and Strategy for Burn Care. NBCR, London.

National Health Service Clinical Advisory Group, 2010. Regional Networks for Major Trauma. NHS Clinical Advisory Groups Report, London, NHS.

Palao, R., Monge, I., Ruiz, M., 2010. Chemical burns: Pathophysiology and treatment. Burns 36 (3), 295–304.

Regel, S., 1997. Staff support on the burns unit. In: Bosworth, C. (Ed.), Burns Trauma: Management and Nursing Care, Baillière Tindall, London.

Rylah, L.T.A., 1992. Critical Care of the Burned Patient. Cambridge University Press, Cambridge.

Settle, J.A.D., 1995. Burns: The First Five Days. Smith and Nephew, Romford.

Singer, A., Dagum, A., 2008. Current management of acute cutaneous wounds. New England Journal of Medicine 359, 1037–1046.

Smith, D.L., Cairns, B.A., Ramadan, F., et al., 1994. Effect of inhalation injury, burn size, and age on mortality: a study of 1447 consecutive burn patients. Journal of Trauma 37 (4), 655–659.

Sutcliffe, A.J., 1998. Electrical injuries and the critical care physician. Care of the Critically Ill 14, 102–105.

Thayre, K., 1995. Lightning strike injuries. Emergency Nurse 3 (3), 16–18.

Varas, R.P., O'Keeffe, T., Namias, N., et al., 2005. A prospective randomized trial of acticoat versus silver sulfadiazine in the treatment of partial-thickness burns: which method is less painful? Journal of Burn Care & Rehabilitation 26 (4), 344–347.

Wiebelhaus, P., Hansen, S.L., 2001. What you should know about managing burn emergencies. Nursing 31 (1), 36–41.

Wilding, P.A., 1990. Care of respiratory burns: hard work can bring spectacular results. Professional Nurse 5, 412–420.

Wilson, D., 1997. Management in the first 48 hours following burn trauma. In: Bosworth, C. (Ed.), Burns Trauma: Management and Nursing Care. Baillière Tindall, London.

Zassan, Z., Wong, J.K., Bush, J., et al., 2010. Assessing the severity of inhalation injuries in adults. Burns 36 (10), 212–216.

PART 3

Psychological dimensions

Aggression

Barbara Neades

CHAPTER CONTENTS

Introduction

Violence and aggression is recognized as a major hazard for staff within the healthcare sector (Chuo et al. 2012a). The fields of mental health, learning disability and emergency care, unsurprisingly, report the highest incidence of verbal and physical threats to staff (Health & Safety Commission Advisory 1997). The regular occurrence of violence within the NHS has been frequently documented (Crilly et al. 2004, Whittington & Winstanley 2008). A review of the management of work-related violence by the Royal College of Nursing (2008) suggested that the impact of work-related violence and aggression is not only physical in terms of injuries sustained by an individual, but can also result in psychological harm that may lead to stress, burn-out, anxiety and depression. These effects can, in turn, lead to a diminished job satisfaction, lower commitment to work and increasing levels of absence for the individual, which clearly impacts on the NHS as an organization.

While far from being the only area within the general hospital setting to see a rise in aggression and violence, the growing level of aggression witnessed within the emergency care setting is also well documented (Atawnehet al. 2003,

Crilly et al. 2004). Standing & Nicolini (1997) argued that the highest risks of violence at work are associated with:

* dealing with the public
* providing care or advice
* working with confused older people
* working with those who have mental health problems
* alcohol or drug misuse
* working alone
* handling valuables or medication
* working with people under stress.

In a study of the psychological impact of violence on staff, Hislop & Melby (2003) found that emergency nurses who had experienced violence in their departments expressed feelings of frustration, anger and fear as a result of this. The Scottish Government recognized the growing number of aggressive and violent incidents being perpetrated against emergency care staff, introducing new legislation, the Emergency Workers (Scotland) Act (2005) aimed at offering some protection for staff in this area. Although prevention of aggression and violence in the Emergency Department (ED) is the aim, it may not always be possible to stop this occurring. Aggression and violence in the ED develops as a result of a wide variety of factors, some of which can be identified and managed within the clinical setting. Others are unfortunately beyond the control of the emergency care staff; however, their awareness of these factors and the appropriate strategies to manage these issues is vital to maintain a safe environment for both staff and patients. This chapter will discuss the problem from these perspectives and offer some suggestions to assist the emergency nurse to resolve this increasing difficulty.

Assessing the problem

If staff are to attempt to resolve aggression in the ED, it is necessary to assess and manage the problem from a holistic and caring viewpoint, maintaining the safety and dignity of everyone involved. The ED can appear a very hostile and threatening place to a patient or relative in an emotionally charged state. Brennan (1998), in examining the range of theories of aggression and violence, suggested that providing satisfactory definitions or an explanation as to where or how these behaviours originate is a complex task.

From a psychological perspective the occurrence of a sudden crisis resulting from a serious illness or accident, with the hurried removal of an individual to an ED, can often trigger strong emotions (Hildegard et al. 1987). These emotions of fear, anxiety, confusion and loss of control often result in stress reactions within the patient or relative and can be displayed in a variety of ways, sometimes displayed as aggression. Many individuals view the ED as an anxiety-provoking and hostile environment. In these situations adrenaline (epinephrine) is released, and the classical 'flight or fight' response triggered. Freud (1932) argued that aggression was an innate, independent, instinctive tendency in humans. In contrast, Bandura (1973) identified the way in which children learn aggressive responses by role modelling what they had observed in adults. Bateson (1980) further argued that an individual is only aggressive when assessed in relation to the other people or surroundings affecting that individual. Dollard et al. (1939) suggested the hydraulic type model of aggression where he viewed the need to release built-up frustration as a natural event similar to that of a pressure cooker effect. The frustration of prolonged waiting times in ED can also trigger an aggression (Derlet & Richards 2000), however Crilly et al. (2004) found that 67% of patients who exhibited violent behaviour had been in the departments for less than 1 hour.

In reviewing the theories underpinning the development of aggression, Brewer (2007) identified a synthesis model of aggression within which the individual's general level of aggression is determined by the combination of three types of factors; the individual, group and social (Fig. 12.1). In this model, physiological factors and neurochemical changes in the individual may combine with perceptions of other people's behaviour to influence their response to an event or a situation. In this interpretation of factors that influence a person's

aggressive response, family or peer group views of acceptable levels of aggression or violence may also influence the individual's response. Finally, this model acknowledges the impact of social factors such as the frequency of aggression portrayed on televions and the acceptability by society.

The major contribution made by physiological factors in the development of aggression in the ED has been identified as being the high consumption or withdrawal from alcohol or drugs (Jenkins et al. 1998). Intoxication with these drugs not only reduces the individual's capacity to understand and interpret events, but also reduces inhibitory responses in times of stress. Violent incidents in the ED are more likely to occur within the hours of 00.00–07.00 with alcohol being identified as a major cause of violent behaviour (Schnieden & Marren-Bell 1995, Jenkins et al. 1998). Other organic reactions seen in acute confused states, e.g., metabolic disorders (diabetes or hypoxia resulting from respiratory or head injuries) or pain, may result in altered perceptions for the patient. These alterations in perception may also result in a confused aggressive patient arriving in the ED. When admitting these patients, the nurse may have to utilize very well-developed communication skills in order to make themself understood. In this condition the patient also may experience major problems in perceiving what is happening.

From an organizational viewpoint, the location of the ED, e.g., near to the public street, and 24-hour access may also attract a number of hostile individuals (Lyneham 2000). Distressed or psychologically disturbed patients often attend ED aware of the immediate access to medical and nursing care for crisis intervention. Their confused or distressed state may also result in aggressive responses to the ED staff. The ED itself can also influence the level of aggression displayed by patients and relatives who attend. The frustration that results from unrealistic expectations of the service may produce conflict and confrontation between the nurse and the patient or relative. Brewer (2007) suggests that the negative perceptions of the NHS often portrayed in the media may also impact upon the level of aggression demonstrated towards NHS staff. Lack of information and long waiting times for treatment as a result of

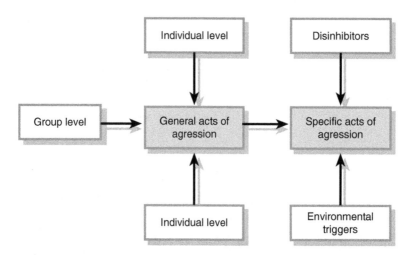

Figure 12.1 • The synthesis model to explain aggression. • (After Brewer K (2007) Analysing aggression. Emergency Nurse 15 (4) 8-9.)

poor staffing levels can also lead to frustration and anger (Jenkins et al. 1998). Poor waiting environments with lack of stimulation have also been suggested as being influential in developing aggression.

Judgmental attitudes and behaviours adopted by staff can result in confrontation between the nurse and the patient or relative. The lack of self awareness in the staff's responses and behaviours in an aggressive situation can cause further aggression, and can also lead to non-therapeutic behaviours been adopted by NHS staff:

- defensiveness
- condescension
- avoidance.

Further research suggests that less-experienced staff who demonstrated a more authoritarian attitude were potentially more at risk of assault (Breakwell & Rowett, 1989). Studies also identify that certain characteristics might be associated with some assaulted staff, which made them more prone to being assaulted (Lanza et al. 1991). The key element in all these studies is the nurse's ability to communicate in a positive and caring manner with the patient or client. The importance of the nurse's verbal and non-verbal communications with the patient or relative is demonstrated to be very important in conveying a caring, understanding attitude to an individual in times of stress or crisis, and in averting confrontation or aggression. It is acknowledged, however, that it may be difficult for the nurse to mask their underlying negative views on a patient and prevent negative non-verbal cues from being transmitted.

Inadequate resources, low staffing levels and inappropriate skill mix may form significant contributory factors. Poor staffing, especially where there is a considerable workload, can contribute to an atmosphere of tension. In these conditions, the nurse may be under pressure to care for a large number of patients at any given time. This lack of time to care for the patient adequately may convey an impression of lack of interest in the patient and relatives, resulting in negative non-verbal cues from the nurse and provoking aggressive confrontations.

Identifying and recording the incidence of violence and aggression in the ED

Many authors suggest that aggressive incidents within healthcare and the ED are not recorded, and it is therefore difficult to measure the problem accurately (Forrester 2002, Pawlin 2008). This may be as a result of the lack of appropriate strategies and structures with which to recognize and record these incidents that occur all too regularly in ED. The Royal College of Nursing (2008) identifies a growing need for NHS staff to have access to the appropriate tools to identify the nature of the problem of violence and aggression in the workplace. They also recognize the lack of knowledge and information held by individuals, teams and organizations in relation to this issue, identifying a structure for risk assessments that should be undertaken to assess the problem. For staff, one of these risk assessments may require a

review of the particular factors that influence aggression and violence in this particular environment, identifying practical measures within the emergency setting to address these factors.

The physical environment into which the patient or relative is received can have a major effect on the response to the stressful events experienced. Poor communication between staff and patients on admission, and inadequate waiting areas with little or no facilities for stimulation or refreshments can cause frustration in both the patient and relatives. Lack of information and increasing waiting times to see a doctor or an emergency nurse practitioner can often trigger aggressive confrontations between the nurse and the patient or relative. The communication and healthcare information supplied or interventions undertaken on behalf of the patient and relative whilst they wait for treatment or decisions to be made relating to their care is therefore very important in the prevention of aggression. Simple measures that provide the patient or relative with information, such as clear displays of waiting times and comfortable surroundings in which to wait can relieve the anxiety and tension that may result in aggression.

Careful consideration of seating arrangements and decor of ED can help to reduce stress in those waiting to be treated. Other measures such as providing up-to-date reading material and a television or radio within the waiting area can reduce the boredom and frustration so often experienced while waiting in ED. The use of videos/DVDs explaining the organization of the ED or providing healthcare information can reduce tension and anxiety in the waiting area. These measures can also be employed to provide health promotion advice to the public. The provision of information is easily the most important issue to stressed relatives and friends, with other environmental factors also impacting on the level of anxiety and frustration experienced by the patient or relative (Box 12.1).

Box 12.1

Reducing the risk of violence

Environmental factors

- All areas should look clean and welcoming, paying special attention to reception areas
- There should be adequate warmth and ventilation
- Noise should be minimized, e.g., by keeping the television volume at a comfortable level
- Designated separate smoking areas as appropriate
- Overcrowding as far as possible should be avoided
- Natural daylight and fresh air should be maximized
- Privacy for staff and patients must be provided
- Clear directional signage

Providing a secure environment

- There should be a safe room for severely disturbed people as appropriate
- Consider the weight, size and construction of movable objects
- Allow unimpeded sightlines with access points in sight of staff
- Install alarm, communication and monitoring systems where appropriate
- Clinical areas should be lockable to prevent intruders

The increasing number of triage systems has been invaluable in improving the communication between the nurse and the public in the ED. During triage the patient can be assessed by the nurse and gain information with regard to their illness or injury and the expected waiting times. This initial assessment allows a relationship to be formed between the nurse and the patient and can provide an opportunity for the nurse to reduce the stress experienced by the patient. Access to the triage nurse keeps patients or relatives in constant communication with their progress through the department, further reducing stress and anxiety (Dolan 1998, Pich et al. 2011). The provision of adequate numbers of medical and nursing staff in the ED prevents long waiting times and allows good communication and the development of good patient–staff relationships. Less aggression is usually demonstrated if the patient or relative is satisfied with the level of care provided and good patient–staff relationships are formulated. This cannot occur in areas where patients and staff are under-resourced and under pressure. Dolan et al. (1997) found that the use of emergency nurse practitioners in the ED helped to reduce waiting times, assisting in a reduction in aggressive incidents at the times when nurse practitioners were on duty. In some inner city EDs it has been necessary, however, to provide increased security measures to limit the risk of aggression to staff. These measures have included the provision of security screens for reception staff, closed circuit security cameras, security guards, direct links to police stations via panic buttons and personal attack alarms (Cooke et al. 2000). Although these measures are not often conducive to conveying a caring, trusting attitude to the public, in some instances they have been required to protect the staff from injury.

Managing aggression in the ED

Managing aggression needs to be a planned and organized process. The nurse needs to have an awareness of the contributing factors in the development of aggression. In addition, the nurse must also have the ability to spot physical signs of impending aggression in order to measure the potential risk and manage it successfully. Aggressive outbursts rarely occur without warning and are almost always preceded by clear indications that the individual is becoming agitated or aggressive. Examination of behaviours immediately prior to an assault suggests that there are often 'normal signs' of impending aggression, both verbal and non-verbal, which if left to go unheeded may result in violent outbursts (Whittington & Patterson 1996). In the patient or relative, these signs include:

- approaching the victim rapidly
- using intrusive gestures
- starting to yell
- prolonged eye contact
- speaking loudly
- invasion of other patients' or staffs' personal space
- frowning
- making threatening gestures.

The ED nurse may not be the intended object of the aggressive individual's outburst, but merely an obstacle in the path of the patient or a vehicle for releasing pent-up emotions. This, however, may be of little comfort to the nurse who experiences an aggressive outburst or who is injured by an agitated patient or relative. The nurse therefore has a responsibility to develop an awareness of the patient's or relative's emotional status through good communication, in order to prevent potentially aggressive incidents occurring.

Inexperience and lack of skill in some nurses in dealing with aggression may result in their avoidance of the agitated person until a violent situation occurs. Indeed, not all nurses are equipped or able to deal with aggressive or violent individuals. Defusing or de-escalating aggression is a complex process. Self-efficacy can be a major factor in the success of resolving an aggressive situation (Lee 2001). This perception of ourselves can help guide our behaviour and prevent escalation of an aggressive incident. Good verbal communication with the aggressive individual is vital in defusing the situation. A calm, confident non-threatening but assertive attempt to engage the individual in conversation is viewed as the first step to restoring order to the situation. This low-level approach to communication with the aggressor may prevent them from viewing the nurse as the aggressor. Lowe (1992) offers advice on how to manage the aggressive individual during this important stage:

- inform colleagues prior to your approach
- use confirming messages, expressing the person's worth
- model personal control, and the ability to stay calm during the expression of anger and resentment towards you
- use honesty, expressing your feelings congruently
- if it is safe to do so, suggest a quieter area of the department
- set limits and clear guidelines that are consistently exerted
- use structure to let people know in advance what is expected of them
- monitor and learn to recognize patterns of behaviour
- timely and calmly intervene (de-escalation), helping the person to work through their anger, thereby breaking the aggressive cycle
- facilitate expression, allow people to express anger and fear somewhere safely
- use non-verbal skills, avoiding threat, and promoting calm and maintaining openness.

Encouraging the patient to discuss the problem may assist in defusing the tension of the moment. If the aggressive individual is confused or under the influence of alcohol or drugs, the nurse may have to repeat the message several times, before being understood. Intoxicated thinking often proceeds by association rather than logic. Key phrases such as 'let us work together' are recommended. Conversely, negative phrases such as 'you're not going to fight or give us trouble' are generally inflammatory as the patient may associate with the words 'fight' and 'trouble' (Taylor & Ryrie 1996). Nothing will be gained by the nurse responding to the patient or relative negatively, despite the provocation from the aggressor. The nurse should listen carefully to the complaint and attempt to offer an explanation or agree a plan of action with the individual to resolve the situation. The use of solutions that are unachievable and the use of inaccurate information to pacify the individual are to be avoided. When these promises are not forthcoming, aggression is more likely. Self-awareness should also relate to the nurse taking appropriate measures to anticipate potential violence and initiate appropriate behaviours to avoid this.

Engaging in communication with large groups of people in an attempt to defuse aggression is not recommended with aggression being amplified by large groups of people. The aggressive individual should be interviewed in a quiet area, offering privacy and dignity to the patient or relative and, allowing them to express the source of their grievance. The approach of the nurse to caring for the aggressive individual is vital in resolving the problem and protecting the nurse from the danger of physical injury. Non-verbal communication with the patient via body language is an important factor in reducing tension.

The nurse should also be aware of personal space and stand at least two arms lengths away from the individual, allowing the opportunity and means of escape should it be required. Turning slightly side-on to the person, positioning the feet slightly apart with the body weight evenly distributed will assist in presenting a non-threatening and reasonably protective stance, and offer a useful position to promote a quick escape. Direct eye contact with the individual can also be interpreted as being provocative by the aggressive individual; however eye contact is an important aspect of communication. It is recommended that staff try to maintain their 'normal' level of eye contact, and use discreet glances to the aggressor's shoulder area, to create a subtle break in potentially prolonged eye contact. Attentive facial expressions suggest interest to the individual and allow good peripheral vision for the nurse.

It is also important for the nurse to be aware of the danger in being trapped in an enclosed area while this conversation is in progress. The nurse should always ensure that there is a clear method of exit should it be required. The room where the interview is conducted should be as free as possible of objects that could be used as weapons against the nurse. It is important to bear in mind that all unsecured objects have the potential to be used as weapons. Objects carried by the nurse, such as scissors or pens, can be easily grabbed and used against them. Neck chains, ties and an inappropriately draped stethoscope can all quickly become weapons against the nurse. These should all be removed before approaching the individual. In today's society, aggressive individuals can use weapons such as knives and guns. The nurse should be aware of suspicious bulges in clothing that may be concealed weapons.

Managing the violent individual

Managing the violent individual can be very distressing for staff and result in an acute crisis within the ED. As previously highlighted, many departments now employ security guards to assist in dealing with violent incidents and issue staff with personal attack alarms to reduce the risks to their person. This support is certainly useful to staff, but if a caring approach is to be adopted towards all individuals, the nurse cannot discharge the responsibility of managing the violent patient or relative to other colleagues. Learning to deal with this challenging and stressful situation is not easy. The appropriate knowledge and skills must result from a combination of

role modelling of good management strategies and education (Paterson et al. 1999).

If violence does erupt while the nurse is alone with the patient, it is unwise to attempt to restrain the individual. Assistance from other departmental staff, security or local police should be summoned via agreed methods. Until assistance is available, the nurse should make every attempt to avoid physical contact, even if this means there is some damage to property. If assistance is not forthcoming, it is better for the nurse to withdraw to a safe distance and, if possible, observe the individual rather than to engage that person alone. This can only be done if other patients and staff are not put at risk. If a member of staff is attacked, there should be an attempt made to break away, endeavouring not to put anyone else at risk in doing so. If the situation escalates and restraint is required to contain the aggressive individual, this should be carried out in a coordinated manner with a minimum of three staff.

Whilst some question the use of physical restraint in patient care, Section 13.5 of the Code of Practice for the appropriate application of the Mental Capacity Act 2005 (Public Guardians Office 2005) suggests that restraint is acceptable when it is: 'Necessary to protect the person who lacks capacity from harm and in proportion to the likelihood and seriousness of that harm'.

When approaching an aggressive individual it should be as a member of a three-person team with an identified lead person. Prior to the approach it should have been decided at which point in the response physical restraint is to be used and how the leader will signal this. In addition they offer the following advice on how the aggressive individual should be approached should the crisis point arise:

- ensure that all staff are trained in crisis management
- remain calm and non-threatening in manner avoiding counter transference
- assess the person's position and possible mode of attack – adjust response as necessary
- approach safely and gradually – do not be rushed
- move to a side-on position reducing exposure to assault and minimizing the appearance of threat
- one person should be responsible for verbal communication
- keep talking and negotiating on a non-physical alternative
- do not make promises or make offers which you cannot keep
- provide at least one face-saving opportunity
- the team should all be aware of the safe distance threshold
- if negotiation fails be decisive about reacting as a team
- when the individual is secured, move them to a resting position in a chair, to a trolley or on the floor
- allow the person time to relax
- ensure that only one team member communicates with the person
- use appropriate measures to screen the individual from the rest of the department maintaining dignity at all times
- when the individual is calm move to a quieter area with less stimulation.

The method of restraint will vary, depending on the incident. There are a variety of systems of physical intervention skills designed specifically for use in healthcare settings. It is strongly recommended that all staff that may be expected to implement restraint should be fully trained in carrying out these and other related procedures. In any type of restraint, it is essential that the individual being held is not compromised in their ability to breathe adequately. During restraint procedures, one team member must take responsibility for monitoring the individual's airway, breathing and circulation. At no point in any restraint should pressure be applied to the throat, neck, chest, back or abdomen. Physical restraint should be used for the minimum amount of time required to control the situation, and the level of force used should be no greater than that required to achieve safety and control. This may include sedation or observation and counselling of the individual by staff. The decision to release the individual must be made by the team and carried out in a controlled, coordinated fashion to minimize the risk of injury to the violent individual and staff.

At the earliest opportunity, senior medical and nursing staff should examine the aggressive individual so that a fuller assessment of the individual's condition may be undertaken. The psychiatric or psychological response of the aggressive individual may help to determine whether they are calm enough to be released, if they require further intervention, e.g., a psychiatric assessment, or whether they are to be released into the custody of the police.

It is acknowledged that in extreme instances the degree of reasonable force necessary to control a violent individual may be of concern to the staff involved. In line with the requirement to treat people as individuals and respect their dignity highlighted in the Nursing and Midwifery Council (2008) Code of Conduct, the degree of force should be the minimum required to control the violence in a manner appropriate to calm rather than provoke further violence (Ferns 2005). Staff injured in the attempt to restrain the violent individual must also be reviewed by a doctor at the earliest opportunity and be made aware of their entitlement to criminal injuries compensation, if appropriate.

Follow-up care after an aggressive violent incident

In accordance with good professional practice, any aggressive or violent incidents should be reported to the senior nursing, medical and management teams and recorded appropriately within the documentation. In recognition of the growing levels of violence in the ED, most departments now require completion of an incident form specifically designed to record verbal or physical abuse of the staff. In making the report it is important to provide as much detail as possible about the circumstances of the incident. Pawlin (2008) reports the development of a data-recording tool used to capture incidences of violence and abuse directed towards staff in the ED. Analysis of this information may be useful in the prevention of further incidents, safeguarding future patients and staff. Box 12.2 identifies some of the information that should be documented following an aggressive or violent event.

Box 12.2

Information to be recorded on the Aggression Incident Form

- When and where the incident occurred
- The names, addresses and status of the people involved
- A brief factual account of the incident, including the main direction of the aggression
- Type of aggression/abuse
- The action taken to resolve the incident
- The names of all additional people bearing professional responsibility
- Observations on the mental state of the aggressive individual involved
- Any injury or damage that occurred
- Outcomes as a result of the incident
- Impact of the incident on the staff and patients involved
- Any additional comments

Box 12.3

Components of the Welsh National Assembly's education programme on violence and aggression

Module A: Introduction and Awareness Raising
Module B: Theory of personal safety and de-escalation
Module C: Breakaway
Module D: Physical Intervention Training

(From Welsh Assembly Government (2004) All Wales Violence and Aggression Training Passport and Information Scheme. Cardiff: WAG.)

In addition to the care of the aggressive individual, the nurse also has a responsibility for the psychological care of the staff and patients who may have been involved in or witnessed the incident. Distressed staff or patients/relatives should be afforded an opportunity to discuss their fears and anxieties arising from the incident, not least as one study found that nearly a third of post-violent incident reports indicated that there were no warning signs prior to the violent incidents (Chuo et al. 2012b). In some cases following extreme events, individuals involved in incidents of aggression or violence may require post-traumatic counselling. It is not a sign of weakness or failure for a nurse to admit the need for this support to overcome the trauma of such incidents. Critical incident stress debriefing should also be available for involved members of staff (Whitfield 1994) (see also Chapter 13).

Clearly, education in the risk factors that may lead to aggression and violence in the ED, the prevention and management of aggression, together with the skills in de-escalation strategies and breakaway techniques should violence occur, is vital for the nurse in the emergency care setting. In acknowledging this the Welsh Assembly Government (2004) has recently developed a new education programme for all NHS staff, the All Wales Violence and Aggression Training Passport and Information Scheme, designed to equip staff with the knowledge and skills to manage this problem (Box 12.3). This comprehensive programme will be available to all NHS staff and particularly aimed at the staff within the ED.

Conclusion

There should be a coordinated approach to dealing with aggression and violence in the ED, similar to the coordinated approach adopted in dealing with a critically ill patient or a cardiac arrest situation. Planning and resourcing for the prevention of aggression and violence in the ED should, therefore, be as detailed as the planning and resources provided for the prevention of death from cardiac arrest. For this to be achieved there must be a planned policy of response to a violent or aggressive outburst, which is known to all the staff within the department and practised on a regular basis. This policy should address key components such as a risk assessment, prevention strategies, training for staff, together with acceptable methods of managing violence and aggression (Hardin 2012).

The purpose of this response must be to control the violent or aggressive outburst as efficiently as possible, thereby minimizing the danger to the aggressive individual, other patients or relatives and to the staff involved. The achievement of this objective has staffing and educational implications for the ED management team. To respond to aggressive or violent incidents requires the provision of adequate levels of staff. Failure to provide the staffing levels renders any policy to deal with aggression redundant.

The knowledge and skills required by the nurse to deal with such incidents are not commonplace among emergency care setting nurses. These skills must be developed through experience and by undertaking specialist training designed to inform the nurse and build confidence in coping professionally with these challenging incidents for the betterment of the staff and patients. Opportunities must be provided for all staff in the ED to undertake suitable education programmes and to practise the acquired knowledge and skills regularly. By undertaking these measures, the problem of aggression in the ED will not be totally eradicated, but nurses will have the means to deal with the situation in a professional and appropriate manner.

References

Atawnehet, F.A., Zahid, M.A., AL-Sahlawi, K.S., et al., 2003. Violence against nurses in hospitals: Prevalence and effects. British Journal of Nursing 12 (2), 102–107.

Bandura, K., 1973. Aggression: A Social Learning Analysis. Prentice-Hill, Englewood Cliffs, New Jersey.

Bateson, G., 1980. Mind and Nature. Fontana, London.

Breakwell, G., Rowett, C., 1989. Violence and social work. In: Archer, J., Browne, K. (Eds.), Human Aggression Naturalistic Approaches. Routledge, London.

Brennan, W., 1998. Aggression and violence: Examining the theories. Emergency Nurse 6 (2), 18–21.

Brewer, K., 2007. Analysing aggression. Emergency Nurse 15 (4), 8–9.

Chuo, J.B., Magarey, J., Wiechula, R., 2012a. Violence in the emergency department: An ethnographic study (part 1). International Emergency Nursing 20 (2), 69–75.

Chuo, J.B., Magarey, J., Wiechula, R., 2012b. Violence in the emergency department: An ethnographic study (part 1). International Emergency Nursing 20 (4), 126–132.

Cooke, M.W., Higgins, J., Bridge, P., 2000. The Present State Emergency. Medicine Research Group Warwick. University of Warwick.

Crilly, J., Chaboyer, W., Creedy, D., 2004. Violence towards emergency department nurses and patients. Accident and Emergency Nursing 12, 67–73.

Derlet, R.W., Richards, J.R., 2000. Overcrowding in the nation's emergency departments: Complex causes and disturbing effects. Annals of Emergency Medicine 35 (1), 63–68.

Dolan, B., 1998. Waiting times (Editorial). Emergency Nurse 6 (4), 1.

Dolan, B., Dale, J., Morley, V., 1997. Nurse practitioners: Role in A&E and primary care. Nursing Standard 11 (17), 33–38.

Dollard, J., Doob, L.W., Miller, N.E., et al., 1939. Frustration and Aggression. Yale University Press, New Haven, Connecticut.

Emergency Workers (Scotland) Act 2005. Edinburgh, Scottish Parliament.

Ferns, T., 2005. Terminology, stereotypes and aggression dynamics in the accident and emergency department. Accident and Emergency Nursing 13 (4), 238–246.

Forrester, K., 2002. Aggressions and assault against nurse in the workplace: Practice and legal issues. Journal of Law and Medicine 9 (4), 386–391.

Freud, S., 1932. The Complete Psychological Works of Sigmund Freud. Hogarth Press, London.

Hardin, D., 2012. Strategies for nurse leaders to address aggressive and violent events. Journal of Nursing Administration 42 (1), 5–8.

Health & Safety Commission Advisory, 1997. Committee on Violence and Aggression to Staff in the Health Services. HSE Books, London.

Hildegard, E.R., Hildegard, R., Atkinson, R.C., 1987. Introduction to Psychology. Harcourt Brace Jovanovich, New York.

Hislop, E., Melby, V., 2003. The lived experience of violence in accident and emergency. Accident and Emergency Nursing 11 (1), 5–11.

Jenkins, M.G., Rocke, L.G., McNicholl, B.P., et al., 1998. Violence and verbal abuse against staff in A&E departments: Survey of consultants in the UK and the Republic of Ireland. Journal of Accident and Emergency Medicine 15 (4), 262–265.

Lanza, M.L., Kayne, HL.C., Hicks, C., et al., 1991. Nursing staff characteristics related to patients assault. Issues in Mental Health Nursing 12 (3), 253–265.

Lee, F., 2001. Violence in A&E: The role of training in self-efficacy. Nursing Standard 15 (46), 33–38.

Lowe, T., 1992. Characteristics of effective nursing interventions in the management of challenging behaviour. Journal of Advanced Nursing 17, 1226–1232.

Lyneham, J., 2000. Violence in New South Wales emergency departments. Australian Journal of Advanced Nursing 18, 8–17.

Nursing and Midwifery Council, 2008. The Code: Standards of Conduct Performance and Ethics for Nurses and Midwives. NMC, London.

Paterson, B., McCormish, A.G., Bradley, P., 1999. Violence at work. Nursing Standard 13 (21), 43–46.

Pawlin, S., 2008. Reporting violence. Emergency Nurse 16 (4), 16–21.

Pich, J., Hazelton, M., Sundin, D., et al., 2011. Patient-related violence at triage: A qualitative descriptive study. International Emergency Nursing 19, 12–19.

Public Guardians Office, 2005. Code of Practice for the Appropriate Application of the Mental Capacity Act 2005. PGO, London.

Royal College of Nursing, 2008. Work-related Violence: an RCN Tool to Manage Risk and Promote Safer Working Practices in Health Care. RCN, London.

Schnieden, V., Marren-Bell, U., 1995. Violence in the A&E department. Accident and Emergency Nursing 3 (2), 74–78.

Standing, H., Nicolini, D., 1997. Review of Workplace Related Violence. HSE Books, London.

Taylor, R., Ryrie, I., 1996. Chronic alcohol users in A&E. Emergency Nurse 4 (3), 6–8.

Welsh Assembly Government, 2004. All Wales Violence and Aggression Training Passport and Information Scheme. WAG, Cardiff.

Whitfield, A., 1994. Critical incident debriefing in A&E. Emergency Nurse 2 (3), 6–9.

Whittington, R., Patterson, P., 1996. Verbal and non-verbal behaviour immediately prior to aggression by mentally disordered people: enhancing risk assessment. Journal of Psychiatric and Mental Health Nursing 3, 47–54.

Whittington, R., Winstanley, R., 2008. Commentary on Luck L, Jackson D, Usher K (2008) Innocent or culpable? Meanings that ED nurses ascribe to individual acts of violence. Journal of Clinical Nursing 17 (16), 2235–2237.

Stress and stress management

13

Heather Josland

CHAPTER CONTENTS

Introduction

Emergency nursing is generally regarded as stressful. Scenarios that confront emergency staff include patients in severe pain, unpredictability of presentations, trauma victims, dying patients and physically demanding work (Curtis 2001, Cameron et al. 2009). The International Council of Nurses (2000) recognizes the emotional, social, psychological and spiritual challenges that nurses engage within such complex environments. This chapter will provide an understanding of stress and stress management that may assist the Emergency Department (ED) nurse to cope in a busy and sometimes chaotic environment. Highlighted topics are stress and coping theories, including stressors specific to ED nursing. Contemporary issues contributing to stress take account of workload, nursing shortage, overcrowding, delayed discharge, patient expectations and violence. Crucial to this subject is an overview of stress management strategies that includes demobilizing, defusing and debriefing along with emphasis on care and support for ED nurses.

Stress theory

Multiple theories exist on stress and coping in application to physical, cognitive, emotional and behavioural characteristics. Selye (1976) defined stress as the physical body's non-specific response to any demand made on it. The stress response is elicited when an individual perceives a threat to their self, whether real or imagined. Cognitive appraisal of a stressor determines mental as well as physical aspects of emotion. The sympathetic nervous system activates the release of adrenaline (epinephrine) and then synthesizes and secretes corticosteroids. The distribution of cortisol into the circulatory system causes raised blood glucose levels, increased heart rate, blood pressure, respirations, peripheral constriction, dilated pupils and a state of arousal or mental alertness (Tortora & Derrickson 2009).

This is what Cannon (1935) called the 'flight-or-fight response', describing an inbuilt mechanism that enabled our forebears to battle assailants or flee from wild animals. Matsakis (1996) has expanded this to fight, flight or freeze, explaining that contemporary stressors are different from the

http://dx.doi.org/10.1016/B978-0-7020-4315-4.00013-9

wild animals or battles facing earlier generations. Immobility or freezing of physical or mental capacities may occur during modern stressful situations. Exhibited behavioural responses of impaired physical or emotional function may include inadequate skills or poor communication.

Selye's (1976) general adaptation system (GAS) is described as alarm where the body attempts to adjust; secondly, the resistance stage where the body attempts to manage the situation; and finally, the exhaustion stage where resources have been drained. Cannon (1935) examined the body's ability to maintain and correct body systems, including regulation of temperature, nervous system, fluid–electrolyte balance and the immune response. Cannon coined the term homeostasis as the body's attempt to re-establish equilibrium. He linked stress to be a cause of disease, explaining that the fight response is the body's attempt towards restoration. When the body faces continued stress, illness can occur. Selye (1976) asserted that if illness were a consequence of being *dis* at *ease*, then it would be prudent to utilize preventive measures rather than temporarily patch up or mask disease states.

Exposure to stress is more commonly evidenced by the first and second stages. Selye explained that through recurring experiences individuals learn to adapt and return to a state of homeostasis. He maintained that the ability to adapt to stressful situations and regain homeostasis was an exceptional attribute of humans. The body's attempt to re-establish homeostasis via a higher or lowered level of physiological function has been more recently identified by McEwen (2007) as allostasis. However, a continued period of physiological adaptation due to exposure to chronic stress is problematic. McEwen refers to allostatic loading as an exacerbation of the 'flight-or-fight' response to stress. The ED nurse who experiences chronic stress may adapt over time to wear and tear on the body and perform with a physiological adjusted 'allostatic load'. However, adverse manifestations of excess allostatic loading include disease states such as hypertension, neurological or immune dysfunctions. Less commonly, a severe threat or continued demand on individual adaptation resources including allostasis may result in the third and most damaging stage of the GAS, which is exhaustion.

Coping

In general terms coping refers to the processes or skills used to deal with situations that are out of the ordinary. Some authorities identify coping more readily in the context of crisis or in adjustment to adverse conditions. Wolfe (1950) referred to stress as a process of altered internal dynamics of an individual caused by interaction with external energy from the environment. The person's internal response as they interacted with the environmental pressure was considered by Wolfe to be influenced by prior experiences.

Lazarus's (1966) work developed a three-phase approach to stress theory that involved a cognitive process of appraisal, coping and outcome. Primary appraisal consists of the initial evaluation of the stressor and the extent to which the threat is considered to be hazardous. Secondary appraisal considers the availability of coping strategies or resources. Lazarus describes stress as disruption of meaning, while coping is defined as the way in which an individual deals with the disruption resulting in the third phase which may be a positive or negative outcome.

Subsequently, Lazarus & Folkman (1984) differentiated ways of coping as strategies that are both behavioural and psychological. Efforts to reduce a stressful situation involve problem-focused coping or emotion-focused coping. A problem-focused coping method would be to confront or retreat from the perceived threat. While the psychological or emotion-focused approach would be to reduce stress by reframing the individual's view and response to the stressor. Lazarus & Folkman state that the value of either mechanism determines the effect of the stressor on the individual. It is individual style that dictates the strategy applied. Vernarec (2001) adds that factors influencing the stress response consist not only of individual interpretation of the stressor, but also of the amount of perceptible support and a person's overall health. It is unimportant whether the final outcome is helpful or unhelpful, only that the effort of coping has occurred (Lazarus & Folkman 1984).

Stress and distress

It is likely that all nurses experience stress in some form, even those who will not admit it. Workplace stress and its effects on job performance are major concerns from both a human and economic perspective (Noblet & LaMontagne 2006, Bright & Crocket 2011). Selye (1976) described eustress as good stress that motivates people to go to work, while distress is the bad stress that can create anxiety and illness through, for example, overwork. Aspects of emergency work necessitate that ED nurses will experience both distress and eustress. Experienced ED nurses may rely on instinct composed of a mixture of knowledge, skills and experience necessary to effectively cope with a variety of situations. Stimuli in the internal environment may arise in terms of thoughts, feelings and physical illness.

Research suggests a vulnerability to adverse effects of stress in a study of Singapore ED nurses. A study by Yang et al. (2002) found ED nurses to have lower levels of lysozome in saliva samples than general ward nurses, correlating with higher levels of perceived stress. Excessive release of glucocorticoids inhibits secretion of immunoglobin A and lysozomes, both of which affect immunity levels. This correlated with questionnaires measuring a perceived level of stress scale. Because ED nurses are exposed to significant pressures they should be aware of the signs and symptoms of increasing stress.

Signs and symptoms of stress

Stress may be observed in colleagues or friends before the affected nurse is actually aware. Stress can subtly influence professional and personal relationships, and is often manifested in forms of physical, emotional, behavioural and mental expression as seen in Table 13.1.

Table 13.1 Signs and symptoms of stress

Mental	Physical	Behavioural	Emotional
Insomnia	Headaches	Distancing	Frequent crying
Poor communication	Fatigue	Cynical	Anxiety
Decreased decision-making	Excessive thirst	Increased ETOH	Frustration
Decreased concentration span	Increased pulse	Increased escape activities	Anger
Memory lapse	Muscle tension	Errors	Depression
Unpleasant dreams	Shortness of breath	Ill temper	Irritability

Stressors in ED nursing

For even the most competent ED nurse, continued exposure to particularly difficult and emotionally draining situations can result in crisis. Key stressors or demands identified in the literature include nursing shortage, workload, overcrowding, violence, shift work, environmental factors, communication problems and burnout (Maslasch et al. 1996). A literature review by Chang et al. (2005) identified common nursing stressors to be:

- high work demands with little support
- poor control over workload
- shortage of resources – human and equipment
- excessive duties to perform.

The subject of this review is the implications of stress on the nurse, the organization and the ensuing relationship between role stress and nursing shortages.

Workload and nursing shortage

Workload for ED nurses includes additional stressors, with unexpected numbers and type of patient presentations; rapidly changing status of patients; response to traumatic incidents; and patient violence (Yang et al. 2002). ED nurses have the stress of sudden and unpredictable arrivals of complex presentations without time for preparation. Increasing patient numbers and intensity increase the work of the nurse. The consequences include increased reliance on EDs and lengthening waits (National Audit Office 2004). Chang et al. (2005) blame workload underscored by work stress as the major contributor to an exodus from nursing.

Unsafe nurse:patient ratios can be accentuated in the ED where unstable patients may be vulnerable to incomplete or incompetent care (Lyneham et al. 2008). ED nurses working under pressure are at risk of compromising not only the quality of care to patients, but compromising their own job satisfaction and level of health. High ED attendance is compounded when overcrowding or bed block occurs.

Overcrowding and delayed discharge

When the number of unwell patients in an overcrowded ED exceeds the number of resources to provide competent and safe care, staff in the ED become stressed (Ardagh & Richardson 2004). Commonly thought reasons for overcrowding include an increasing ageing population, non-urgent attendees and the incline of patient admissions with existing co-morbidities. However, the chief reason for ED overcrowding appears to be a lack of hospital resourced beds (Richardson & Mountain, 2009).

Delayed discharge, also termed bed block or gridlock, refers to the unavailability of hospital beds to which ED patients would normally be transferred or admitted to (Capolingua 2008, Lyneham et al. 2008). The aging population increasingly present as high-acuity patients that negatively impacts on the ED's maximum capacity (Cowan & Trzeciak, 2005). Despite being fully worked up and ready for admission to a ward, these patients are kept within the confines of the ED. The impact of this extra load on EDs is possibly most felt by the ED nurse (Ardagh & Richardson 2004, Cowan & Trzeciak 2005). Identified problems are not only the physical lack of space, health and safety issues, such as infection control and cluttered environment, but also the lack of privacy and dignity for patients that can contribute to moral distress for ED nurses (Kilcoyne & Dowling 2008). The astute ED nurse will focus on absolute prioritizing of key nursing cares and patient safety, yet may experience moral distress due to an inability to provide other less vital but caring tasks. An attempt to improve nursing numbers however, does not always result in a mix of equally skilled nurses.

Skill mix

Overcrowding of EDs is acknowledged by Derlet & Richards (2000) to be a critical problem accentuated not only by bed shortages but also by staffing shortages who are already dealing with increasing patient presentations and severity. Poor skill mix where staffing is supplemented with less experienced or new ED nurses impacts heavily on EDs, where senior and more experienced nurses are allocated the most complex patients as well as supervising less experienced nurses (Emergency Nurses Association 2006). Lack of experienced ED nurses and work pressure is compounded by difficulties in communicating with aggressive patients (Walsh et al. 1998). A multitude of cultural and language variations further challenge communication stressors. Iltun (2002) underlines the importance of being aware of one's own values, cultural differences and biases in order to avoid ineffective communication. The underlying danger exists that skill mix with a low ratio of qualified nurses can impact negatively on quality of care and patient expectations.

Patient expectations

Patients have high expectations of health care and an awareness of their rights due to increased information from the health services, media and internet. Newly highlighted successful treatments may be demanded against recommendations of standard procedures offered by nurses. Nurses can feel unappreciated and disillusioned in their attempts to provide good nursing care. Patients sometimes arrive at the ED with the expectation that they will be seen immediately. Individuals may express opinions that their needs and conditions are the most important and it is their right to do so. Building resentment in patients may be displaced onto the ED nurse who then may become a target for violent outbursts.

Violence

It is common for the ED nurse to witness or be exposed to verbal or physical violence, and was found by Healy & Tyrell (2011) to be the second most common cause of stress for ED nurses and doctors. Multiple reasons exist for exacerbated stress in patients. Pain, fear, prolonged waiting and exposure to unpleasant stimuli may trigger violent outbursts in patients (Presley & Robinson 2002). Noxious smells, sights and sounds in EDs can distress patients and visitors, which may then be displaced to nurses. Possible contributors to violence must also take into account social factors, intoxicants, withdrawal, psychoses, dementias, brain injuries and seizures or post-ictal status (Bakes & Markovchick 2010). Some stressed nurses acknowledge contributing to violent reponses from mental health patients through rude or confrontational comments or behaviours (Spokes et al. 2002). Despite stress, the ED nurse is obliged ethically and morally to respond appropriately to offensive situations by utilizing effective communication skills (Inoue et al. 2006). Presley & Robinson (2002) advise the ED nurse to manage difficult situations through psychological control, e.g., gaining trust, or physical control, e.g., ensuring seclusion or restraint through administering prescribed pharmacological sedation (see also Chapter 12).

Implications of stress

Patients and families are not usually prepared for managing the intensity of emotions that accompany a traumatic event (Emergency Nurses Association 2002). The ED nurse may be expected to deal with a complex mixture of physical, social, emotional and even spiritual patient requirements. Some patients or events may connect on a personal level with the nurse, initiating feelings and emotions that would normally be contained. Demands on the nurse may seem insurmountable at times and lead to dissatisfaction and fatigue. ED nurses can face acute and chronic stressors that may accumulate over time from dealing with multiple incidents.

The altruistic nature of nursing lends a vulnerability where attempts to demonstrate high levels of care sprinkled with compassion leave the nurse emotionally and physically exhausted. Consequences of stress can be indicated by cognitive, physical, emotional or behavioural changes. Nurses may experience fatigue, loss of enthusiasm and energy, sleep disturbance, job dissatisfaction and escape activities such as alcohol or drugs (Spence-Laschinger et al. 2001). A stressed nurse may impose consequences onto patients such as inadequate care, increased waiting times, inattention, impatience and cynicism (Maslach et al. 1996). Poor performance behaviours are indicated by distancing or avoiding the patient, ignoring the patient's feelings, concentrating on equipment instead of the patient, forgetfulness or incompletion of tasks. Maladaptive responses or ineffective coping mechanisms can result in depression and physical illness (Selye 1976).

A study of 43 000 nurses from 700 hospitals in five countries, i.e., England, Scotland, Germany, USA and Canada, identified low morale, job dissatisfaction and burnout as consequences of stress (Aiken et al. 2001). A major concern was reported as inadequate time to complete nursing responsibilities. Inadequate nursing resources were linked to adverse events such as increased patient morbidity and even mortality. Health institutions suffer consequences of stressed nurses revealed by tardiness, absenteeism, errors, workplace conflict, high staff turnover and patient dissatisfaction, all leading to increased cost (Spence-Laschinger et al. 2001, Johansen 2012). The diversity of ED work, although valued by the nurses, can be difficult to tolerate, especially as it covers such a wide range of conditions and can unexpectedly lead to burnout.

Burnout

Maslach (1982) termed the word burnout as an occupational reaction to stress caused by the physical and emotional demands of care for patients. The Maslach Burnout Inventory (MBI) defines characteristics such as emotional fatigue, depersonalization, and feelings of decreased personal worth or accomplishment (Maslach et al. 1996). Emotional exhaustion was evidenced by a depleted emotional reservoir as occurs under high pressure and patient demands. Depersonalization may occur in the development of negative attitudes towards colleagues or patients. This can lead to workers isolating themselves from others. Poor personal accomplishment can result in self-criticism or feelings of insufficiency. All are indicators for burnout.

Burnout is evident through unrealistic expectations, inflexibility towards change, resentment and suspicion, intolerance, being judgemental, lack of direction or goals, physical and mental exhaustion, an insensitive attitude towards others, a feeling of being unappreciated, diminished energy, pessimism, inefficiency, increased absenteeism, low morale, low self-esteem and frequent illness (Demerouti et al. 2000, Iltun 2002, Jackson 2004). Successful coping includes enduring or alleviating stress, upholding worthwhile personal relationships, maintaining self-esteem and value regardless of setbacks, and meeting necessary aspects of stressful duties.

Burnout may be symptomatic not simply of work stress but of unmanaged stress from excessive demands on workers (Iltun 2002). Some research found the gap between reality and expectations does affect nurses' energy levels, job satisfaction and overall health, and that personal beliefs play a role in perceived levels of burnout (Iltun 2002).

In a study using the MBI, Walsh et al. (1998) found that participants in the study were on the borderline between moderate and high levels of depersonalization, one of the three components of burnout. They also showed nurses experienced moderate levels of emotional exhaustion. This was reflected in the fact that about half the 134 nurses in the sample reported feeling used up at the end of the day, frustrated by their job and emotionally drained at least once a week.

Accumulation of burnout is insidious, leaving nurses drained and exhausted with lowered tolerance and immunity (Maslach 1982). Maslach warns that burnout leads to impaired work ability. Decreased work satisfaction can spill over to decreased life satisfaction and affect relationships outside of work. The unfortunate consequence of caring for trauma victims or critically ill patients is that the stress can be transferred onto the nurse, often referred to as secondary traumatic stress (STS) (Figley 2002, Dominguez-Gomez & Rutledge 2009). One study found 85% of ED nurses reported symptoms of STS, frequently reporting examples such as memory or sleeping problems, intrusive thoughts, irritability, and emotional numbness. Figley (2002) terms this compassion fatigue (CF) likened to battle fatigue experienced by soldiers in war-time.

Exploring and defining the phenomenon of CF within nursing has only recently been attempted (Coetzee & Klopper 2010). Risk factors are similar to those that predispose nurses to burnout. The final accumulation of prolonged or intense caring for patients without adequate rest or relief may result in a loss of the nurse's ability to provide meaningful care.

The opposite concept is compassion satisfaction, where a nurse feels awarded with a sense of fulfillment and pleasure in providing competent skills and care (Coetzee & Klopper 2010). Compassion satisfaction may be the reason ED nurses are able to thrive and provide competent skills and genuine caring despite difficult situations.

The fatigue factor influences attitudes that become apparent in unsuccessful communication with colleagues. Communication problems can create havoc in the often chaotic environment of emergency areas. Insomnia and escape activities such as increased smoking, alcohol consumption and unhealthy diets have often been linked to burnout (Walsh et al. 1998). Research exploring job satisfaction among nurses and therapists cited stress as a commonly cited reason for absenteeism and emphasized the need for training and support for front-line staff (Webb et al. 2002). Burnout could be considered a potential hazard, with warning signs evident in physical, emotional and behavioural changes (Vernarec 2001). This determines a need to encourage a good quality of work life for ED nurses, prevent illness and burnout, enhance patient care and decrease costs to the health provider. Phillips (2011) and Hooper et al. (2010) urge that nurse leaders should be alert to the symptoms and take steps to address nursing compassion fatigue and burn-out.

Stress management

The best form of stress management is prevention. However, due to the insidious nature of distress, adverse psychological or physiological effects may occur before the ED nurse is aware themselves. An understanding of acute critical incidents and chronic stress may help the ED nurse to be aware of signs and symptoms of stress and take appropriate actions towards prevention or restoration.

Critical incident stress (CIS)

Exceptional clinical events have the potential to elicit emotions that are so intense they may impact on the individuals' ability to function during the event or later. Mitchell & Everly (1995) refer to this as a normal response to an abnormal event. Emotional responses may be suppressed while cognitive functioning allows knowledge and skills to be utilized as the ED nurse manages an airway and draws up drugs in preparation for an emergency intubation. It is after the incident when the patient has left the department that the cognitive subsides and the emotions can then surface, leaving the emergency nurse with a feeling of overwhelming sadness or emotional exhaustion. A more serious condition can occur from significant events or untreated stress in the form of post-traumatic stress disorder (PTSD).

Described as a catastrophic occurrence, PTSD may severely disrupt a person's equilibrium (Ochberg 1993). A study by O'Connor & Jeavons (2003) reported emergency nurses to have higher exposure to critical stress than ward nurses. The most stressful situation for nurses was identified as dealing with the assault or death of a child, while the most frequent was the responding to a sudden arrest. Recognized strategies include defusion, demobilization and critical incident stress debriefing (Human Resources Branch Department of Human Services 1997).

Defusion

Defusion may best be described as a short type of crisis intervention. It is intended to bring some psychological closure to the event. This should ideally be carried out before staff leave the shift or within 48 hours (Mitchell 2004). This is an informal talk that allows reflection of thoughts and feelings, often over tea or coffee.

The facilitator maintains a low profile and ensures a safe environment and conditions for the defusing to occur in a healthy manner. In the case of a momentous event, a person trained in debriefing may be required. General rules dictate that only people directly involved in the event are in attendance. Participants are reminded of confidentiality and again support is to be clearly demonstrated. This session is not an evaluation of behaviour, but individuals are encouraged to express feelings and thoughts. Individuals are to be cautioned that some may feel worse when confronting their emotions. It should reduce tension, focus on strengths and skills and assist staff to regain emotional control.

Ideally people will go over the details of the event naturally and spontaneously. Details of other events or other information will not be shared until the entire story has unfolded. Any attempts to curtail disclosure of a critical incident will cause it to emerge later. Time and attention to those involved will, on the other hand, allow the incident to be laid to rest or ended more appropriately (Wright 1993).

Demobilization

Demobilization provides staff with a structure to end a duty. While many people end the shift at the same time, some, because of workload or altered shift, may leave at different times. Their needs should not be ignored. Large-scale incidents benefit most from this approach. A room will be needed to hold large numbers of staff. The group should be multi-disciplinary. The time is approximately 15 minutes and should be within their working day. It is recommended that it is carried out as soon as possible following the incident.

The team leader should have factual information regarding the whole event from the beginning to the present time. Wright (1993) stresses that all involved people should have obligatory attendance, emphasizing that demobilization is not just for the sensitive or vulnerable or those who think they need it; the whole team must attend to acknowledge that the issue affects everyone. The time may permit questions that enable a clarification of circumstances. Aims of the demobilization are:

- to regain emotional control and cognitive functioning and to reduce tension
- to focus on strengths and skills, to re-evaluate the incident and to receive some factual information
- to begin the recovery process and leave behind some of the stress
- to begin to be educated by the incident.

The difference between a demobilization and defusion is that although they have similar aims, the demobilization is clearly time-limited and focused. Different members of staff will have worked in different aspects of the incident but will generally not be aware of the entire event. For this reason, information regarding the whole incident may be useful.

Information may be given regarding the possibility of adverse reactions after the event. Staff needs may be assessed at this time and advice made available on any required assistance. Demobilization should be ended with thanks extended to every staff member that acknowledges their contribution during a difficult and demanding event. The purpose of the organizational demobilization is to demonstrate support, plan for the immediate future and restore organizational function. A more difficult approach to expedite is that of critical incident debriefing, which permits a deeper exploration of an event.

Critical Incident Stress Debriefing (CISD)

Debate exists on debriefing, and although sessions are not routinely offered, many ED nurses feel it is useful (Ross-Adje et al. 2007). A formal type of debriefing is CISD, which is expected to be carried out within 24–48 hours after the event. Some authorities recommend that debriefing should be directed only by an experienced person trained in stress management (Human Resources Branch Department of Human Services 1997, Mitchell 2004). The goal of CISD is to assist staff to transfer from a state of high arousal to a state of normalization after a significant event. The time is used to allow staff a chance to ventilate feelings such as anger, disappointment or sadness. A possible format for CISD could consist of three 1-hour sessions to be held within two weeks.

Each ED will have its own view on the decided course of action regarding any need or procedure for CISD. Some EDs have teams represented by peer support from all emergency personnel. Interventions were proposed by Mitchell & Everly (1995) to be carried out in seven stages, listed as:

- introductions
- facts
- thoughts
- reaction
- symptoms
- teaching
- re-entry phase.

The first session may cover mainly facts and individual's roles in the event. Session two encourages the person or persons to consider thoughts and feelings around the event. The person may be assisted in confronting the more disturbing aspects of the incident. The last session is educational and largely involves natural stress responses and putting strategies in place to avoid further difficulties. This session aims to bring individuals back as much as possible to normal function. Some goals or plan may be established to assist the re-entry.

The rationale behind debriefing is to shed some light around the event, mobilize resources and utilize problem-solving skills that may improve future planning. Support for the individual and group is again paramount. Controversy exists around the proposed benefits of critical incident stress debriefing. Deahl & Bisson (1995) argue that the benefits of debriefing are not scientifically proven. Further research using longitudinal studies is needed to establish proven benefits. Ochberg (1993), a long-term authority on PTSD, values therapeutic debriefing. Indeed a 'do nothing' attitude could be considered cruel and may ignore the possibility that a serious incident may induce a strong stress response in a person or persons. The ED nurse without adequate coping strategies or basic support to deal with this could be at risk for psychological and/or physical illness.

Approaches to support and care

Self-support groups

Jackson (2004) cited social support as the most useful coping mechanism for nurses. Groups that meet regularly to discuss cumulative stress have been found to be useful. Good social support has been associated with lower levels of work-related stress. Establishment of positive social support systems at work and home provide effective coping mechanisms to help maintain physical and psychological wellness (Jonsson & Halabi 2006). Nursing managers and ED supervisors who demonstrate positive behaviours play a pivotal role in monitoring and assisting nurses to manage critical or cumulative stress (Lewis et al. 2010).

When the perceived source of stress is the patient, the ED nurse concerned may find it helpful to request a change of patient or, at least, some time out to regain some level of restored equanimity. Such actions as listening are basic and simple responses and should not be underestimated. Talking and sharing with colleagues are well-used and caring responses. Trust is imperative, as self-disclosure is involved and insight into the person behind the nursing role will increase the value of sharing (Wright 1992).

Balance and self-care

Maintaining basic health rules of adequate sleep, nutrition, exercise and relaxation or recreational activities outside work will assist the nurse to maintain a healthy sense of balance. Self-care strategies identified by Badger (2001) comprise self-monitoring and reflection, and maintaining realistic goals and expectations. ED nurses cognizant of coping strategies will be able to contribute more meaningfully to care of themselves, their colleagues and ultimately their patients. Jackson's (2004) alternative vision for nurses is to create healing communities where a holistic approach enables healing for the mind, body and spirit. Her suggestion is for EDs to pipe soothing music in the hope of decreasing stress levels. Other suggestions include aromatherapy, massage, reflexology and even art. If nurses maintain high levels of wellness themselves, they may be in a position to offer equally therapeutic treatment for their patients. Although idealistic and improbable for most EDs, Jackson's suggestions do remind nurses of the importance of quality time out for self-care.

Education

This book acknowledges the variety of specialties that the ED nurse is expected to encounter, including respiratory, cardiology, orthopaedics, and nephrological emergencies to obstetrical and gynaecological emergencies. Ongoing and updating of education is imperative for ED nurses who are expected to have a sound nursing knowledge and skill level encompassing a wide range of medical and surgical conditions across the lifespan. Bailey et al.'s (2005) review of literature and survey of nurses revealed a need for health-care organizations to provide education opportunities for emergency nurses.

Increased knowledge was found to enhance nurse's confidence in clinical practice, and produce greater respect amongst colleagues. Possible follow-on effects are stated to be increased job satisfaction, a positive effect on nurse retention and increased patient care and satisfaction. Education on dealing with grieving relatives (Curtis et al. 2007) as well as training for mass casualty or large-scale incidents will also help prepare the ED nurse (Ross-Adjie et al. 2007).

Education on stress management that encompasses recognition of stressors, stress symptoms and effective strategies to reduce stress may assist ED nurses which work with their individual personality traits. It is not known whether personal attributes to coping well with stress are inherent or can be taught. More recently, advice encourages strategies to 'banish burnout' by encouraging workers to engage with the environment (Leiter & Maslach 2005); however according to Bennet & Lowe (2008) ED nurses generally feel they manage coping well. It is possible that many ED nurses are attributed with a personality trait deemed by Kobasa (1979) as the hardiness factor. Hardiness is the ability to bounce back from difficult situations after a relatively short period. The hardiness factor is characterized by commitment (to engage with environment), challenge (willingness to adapt and change) and control (belief in one's own influence in a situation). This enables the ability to view one's work as meaningful. More recently, research has explored the relationship between emotional intelligence (EI), work stress and nurses' health (Augusto et al. 2008). Findings reveal health benefits in terms of protection against stress in nurses who have what is referred to as high clarity and high emotional repair. These components of EI are described as an ability to perceive and manage not only one's own emotions but a capacity to detect and interpret the emotions of others.

Education and practice for nurses to care for themselves and one another may help build and maintain the resources necessary to offer quality care for others. A desirable goal is for the nurse to regularly update with current trends and practice that will impact positively on patients. A novel approach to stress management found evidence that humour education is beneficial as an effective antidote to stress. Wooten (1997) found nurses to have decreased levels of cortisol following laughter training. The important thing is for people to laugh with one another not at one another. Further research is needed to decide on effectiveness of stress-management interventions. The goal is for the ED nurses to harness resources that protect them from burnout and to be in the best position to facilitate quality care of patients, mobilizing the nurse towards healthy adaptation and rewarding interpersonal relationships. Some may argue that the most stressful situations are those which promote the greatest level of satisfaction. This implies then that ED nurses will enjoy adequate levels of eustress that motivate and maintain their commitment to this vital area of nursing.

Conclusion

The unique stressors that ED nurses face daily may challenge even the most competent ED nurse. Adrenaline-fuelled efforts to provide good care may be part of the thrill of the work. Nonetheless, it is important for nurses to ensure that they do not expose themselves repeatedly to a state of exhaustion without adequate rest periods. Despite effective coping mechanisms, the continued exposure to pain, suffering, stress and trauma makes the ED nurse susceptible. The literature suggests a need to prevent job stress through encouragement of individual and organizational awareness to address causes rather than symptoms. Departmental policies that address the issues of defusion, demobilization and debriefing make a clear statement that it is the department's philosophy to care for its staff and acknowledge the difficulty of the work. The emphasis is on education that may help emergency nurses recognize signs and symptoms of stress and a range of ways to respond and manage stress effectively. When supported in maintaining their own health within a positive work environment, the ED nurse may possess the necessary resources to facilitate quality health in meeting the wide-ranging needs of their patients.

References

Aiken, L., Clark, S., Sloane, D., et al., 2001. Nurses' reports on hospital care in five countries. Health Affairs 20 (3), 43–54.

Ardagh, M., Richardson, S., 2004. Emergency department crowding: Can we fix it? The New Zealand Medical Journal 117 (1189), 1–6.

Augusto, J., Lopez-Zafra, E., Berrios-Martos, M., et al., 2008. The relationship between emotional intelligence, occupational stress and health in nurses: A questionnaire survey. International Journal of Nursing Studies 45, 888–901.

Badger, J., 2001. Understanding secondary traumatic stress. American Journal of Nursing 101 (7), 26–32.

Bailey, K., Swinger, M., Bard, M., et al., 2005. The effectiveness of a specialised trauma course in the knowledge base and level of job satisfaction in emergency nurses. Journal of Trauma Nursing 12 (1), 10–15.

Bakes, K., Markovchick, V., 2010. The agitated or violent patient. In: Wolfson, A. (Ed.), Harwood Nuss' Clinical Practice of Emergency Medicine, fifth ed. Walters, Lippincott, Williams, London.

Bennett, P., Lowe, R., 2008. Emotions and their cognitive precursors: Responses to spontaneously identified stressful events among hospital nurses. Journal of Health Psychology 13 (4), 537–546.

Bright, D., Crockett, A.B., 2011. Stressed out! Strategies for enhancing performance. Journal of Nursing Administration 42 (10), 50–54.

Cameron, P., Jelinek, G., Kelly, A., Murray, L., Brown, A. (Eds.), 2009. Textbook of Adult Emergency Medicine, third ed. Elsevier, Edinburgh.

Cannon, W., 1935. Stresses and strains of homeostasis. American Journal of Medical Sciences 189 (1), 1.

Capolingua, R., 2008. AMA Public Hospital Report Card. Australian Medical Association.

Chang, E., Hancock, K., Johnson, A., et al., 2005. Role stress in nurses: review of related factors and strategies for moving forward. Nursing and Health Sciences 7, 57–65.

Coetzee, S., Klopper, H., 2010. Compassion fatigue within nursing practice: A concept analysis. Nursing and Health Sciences 12, 235–243.

Cowan, R., Trzeciak, S., 2005. High acuity patients and limited capacity for inpatient admissions resulting in the ED exceeding maximum capacity. Ageing population. Clinical review: Emergency department overcrowding and the potential impact on the critically ill. Critical Care 9, 291–295.

Curtis, K., 2001. Nurse's experience of working with trauma patients. Nursing Standard 16 (9), 33–38.

Curtis, K., Friendship, C., Ramsden, J., 2007. Emergency and trauma nursing. Mosby, Marrickville, NSW Australia.

Deahl, M.P., Bisson, J.I., 1995. Dealing with disasters: does psychological debriefing work? Journal of Accident and Emergency Medicine 12 (4), 255–258.

Demerouti, E., Bakker, A., Nachreiner, F., 2000. A model of burnout and life satisfaction amongst nurses. Journal of Advanced Nursing 32 (2), 454–463.

Derlet, R., Richards, J., 2000. Overcrowding in the nation's emergency departments; complex causes and disturbing effects. Annals of Emergency Medicine 35 (1), 63–68.

Dominguez-Gomez, E., Rutledge, D., 2009. Prevalence of secondary traumatic stress among emergency nurses. Journal of Emergency Nursing 35 (3), 199–204.

Emergency Nurses Association, 2002. Trauma Nursing Core Course Provider Manual, fourth ed. ENA, Chicago.

Emergency Nurses Association, 2006. ENA 2005 National Emergency Department Benchmark Guide. ENA, Des Plaines. Illinois.

Figley, C., 2002. Compassion fatigue: psychotherapists chronic lack of self care. Journal of Clinical Psychology 58 (11), 1433–1441.

Healy, S., Tyrell, M., 2011. Stress in emergency departments: experiences of nurses and doctors. Emergency Nurse 19 (4), 31–37.

Hooper, C., Craig, J., Janvrin, D.R., et al., 2010. Compassion satisfaction, burnout, and compassion fatigue among emergency nurses compared with nurses in other selected inpatient specialties. Journal of Emergency Nursing 36, 420–427.

Human Resources Branch Department of Human Services, 1997. Resource Guide for Critical Incident Stress and Debriefing in Human Service Agencies. Government Department of Human Services, Melbourne: Victoria.

Iltun, I., 2002. Burnout and nurses' personal and professional values. Nursing Ethics 9 (3), 269–278.

Inoue, M., Tsukano, K., Muraoka, M., et al., 2006. Psychological impact of nurses working in psychiatric departments. Psychiatry and Clinical Neurosciences 60, 29–36.

International Council of Nurses, 2000. Occupational Health and Safety for Nurses. ICN Position Statement. International Council of Nurses, Geneva.

Jackson, C., 2004. Healing ourselves, healing others. Holistic Nurse Practitioner 18 (4), 199–210.

Johansen, M.L., 2012. Keeping the peace: conflict management strategies for nurse managers. Journal of Nursing Administration 43 (2), 50–54.

Jonsson, A., Halabi, J., 2006. Work related post traumatic stress as described by Jordanian emergency nurses. Accident and Emergency Nursing 14, 89–96.

Kobasa, S., 1979. Stressful life events personality and health: an inquiry into hardiness. Journal of Personality and Social Psychology 37 (1), 1–11.

Kilcoyne, M., Dowling, M., 2008. Working in an overcrowded accident and emergency department: nurse's narratives. Australian Journal of Advanced Nursing 25 (2), 21–27.

Lazarus, R.S., 1966. Psychological Stress and the Coping Process. McGraw-Hill, New York.

Lazarus, R.S., Folkman, S., 1984. Stress, Appraisal and Coping. Springer, New York.

Leiter, M., Maslach, C., 2005. Banishing Burnout: Six Strategies for Improving your Relationship with Work. Jossey-Bass, San Francisco, CA.

Lewis, R., Yarker, J., Donaldson-Feilder, E., et al., 2010. Using a competency-based approach to identify the management behaviours required to manage workplace stress in nursing: A critical incident study. International Journal of Nursing Studies 47, 307–313.

Lyneham, J., Cloughessy, L., Martin, V., 2008. Workloads in Australian emergency departments: A descriptive study. International Emergency Nursing 16, 200–206.

Maslach, C., 1982. Burnout, the Cost of Caring: Burnout in Health Professionals. Prentice Hall, New Jersey.

Maslach, C., Jackson, S., Leiter, M., 1996. Maslach Burnout Inventory, third ed. Consulting Psychologists Press, Palo Alto CA.

Matsakis, A., 1996. I Can't Get Over It: A Handbook for Trauma Survivors, second ed. New Harbinger Publication, Oakland, California.

McEwen, B., 2007. Physiology and neurobiology of stress and adaptation: Central role of the brain. Physiology Review 87, 873–904.

Mitchell, J., 2004. Characteristics of successful early intervention programs. International Journal of Emergency Mental Health 6 (4), 175–184.

Mitchell, J., Everly, G., 1995. Critical Incident Stress Debriefing: an Operational Manual for the Prevention of Traumatic Stress Among Emergency Services Workers. Chevron Publishing Corporation, Elliot City.

National Audit Office, 2004. Improving Emergency Care in England. NAO, London.

Noblet, A., LaMontagne, A.D., 2006. The role of workplace health promotion in addressing job stress. Health Promotion International 21 (4), 346–353.

Ochberg, F., 1993. Posttraumatic therapy. In: Wilson, J., Raphael, B. (Eds.), International Handbook of Traumatic Stress Syndromes. Plenum Press, New York.

O'Connor, J., Jeavons, S., 2003. Nurse's perceptions of critical incidents. Journal of Advanced Nursing 41 (1), 43–62.

Phillips, J., 2011. Hardiness as a defense against compassion fatigue and burnout. Journal of Emergency Nursing 37 (2), 125.

Presley, D., Robinson, G., 2002. Violence and assault in the emergency department. The Nursing Clinics of North America Emergency Nursing 37 (1), 161–169.

Richardson, D., Mountain, D., 2009. Myths versus facts in emergency department overcrowding and hospital access block. Medical Journal of Australia 190 (7), 369–374.

Ross-Adjie, G., Leslie, G., Gillman, L., 2007. Occupational stress in the ED: What matters to nurses? Australian Emergency Nursing Journal 10, 117–123.

Selye, H., 1976. The Stress of Life, second ed. McGraw-Hill, New York.

Spence-Laschinger, H., Shamian, J., Thomson, D., 2001. Impact of magnet hospital characteristics on nurses' perceptions of trust, burnout, quality of care, and work satisfaction. Nursing Economics 19 (5), 209–219.

Spokes, K., Bond, T., Lowe, J., et al., 2002. HOVIS: The Hertfordshire/Oxfordshire Violent Incident Study. Journal of Psychiatric and Mental Health Nursing 9 (2), 199–209.

Tortora, G., Derrickson, B., 2009. Principles of Anatomy and Physiology, twelveth ed. Wiley, Hoboken, New Jersey.

Vernarec, E., 2001. How to cope with job stress. Registered Nurse 64 (3), 44–46.

Walsh, M., Dolan, B., Lewis, A., 1998. Burnout and stress among A&E nurses. Emergency Nurse 6 (2), 23–30.

Webb, Y., Stear, A., Pettybridge, J., et al., 2002. Nursing the nurses: why staff need support. Nursing Times 98 (16), 36–37.

Wolfe, H., 1950. Life Stress and Bodily Diseases. Williams & Wilkins, Baltimore.

Wooten, P., 1996. Humour: Antidote for stress. Holistic Nurse Practitioner 10, 49–56.

Wright, B., 1992. Communication Skills: Skills for Caring. Churchill Livingstone, Edinburgh.

Wright, B., 1993. Caring in Crisis, second ed. Churchill Livingstone, Edinburgh.

Yang, Y., Doh, D., Ng, V., et al., 2002. Self perceived work related stress and the relation with salivary IgA and lysozome among emergency department nurses. Occupational and Environmental Medicine 59 (12), 836–841.

Care of the bereaved

14

Brian Dolan

CHAPTER CONTENTS

Introduction

It is estimated that there are some 25 000–30 000 resuscitation attempts in the UK every year (Resuscitation Council 1996, Royal College of Nursing 2002). Dealing with the suddenly bereaved in Emergency Departments (ED) is difficult for all staff, no matter how much experience they have. This chapter will consider approaches to the management of sudden death in ED. It will examine the literature surrounding this subject, before exploring the process of care for those who have been suddenly bereaved. It will also outline the care of staff that have cared for the suddenly bereaved.

Background

The literature surrounding the subject of sudden death is vast (Royal College of Nursing 2002, Mushtaq & Ritchie 2005, Moons & Norekval 2008, Kingsnorth-Hinrichs 2009). Death is the permanent cessation of all vital functions, the end of human life, an event and a state. Dying is a process of coming to an end: the final act of living (Thompson 1994). Wright (1996) defined sudden deaths as those occurring without warning – the unexpected death. Deaths that result from acute disease, accidents, suicides and homicides fall into this category. It is these sudden deaths that are most frequently encountered in ED.

The Royal College of Nursing and British Association for Accident and Emergency Medicine (1995), in the largest study of its kind, considered the facilities in ED for the bereaved. A questionnaire was sent to all 267 ED in England and Wales to identify the systems, facilities and training provided. Of the 248 (93%) departments that responded, it was possible to estimate that two to three attendances per 1000 new attendances involved relatives who were bereaved following a patient dying in the ED. Forty per cent of the departments that responded stated they had two to three deaths per week, with a further 25% having four to five deaths per week. In terms of workload and impact on the average ED, sudden death can be significant for staff as well as for relatives.

The concept of a trajectory of death was developed by Glaser & Strauss (1965, 1968) to refer to the pattern of death. They distinguish between 'quick' and 'slow' dying trajectories. Generally, in ED, the patients have a 'quick' death trajectory, which is unexpected by the family, even when it is the result of a longstanding medical condition, such as heart disease. Lindemann (1944), in a classic study of bereavement, suggested that people who fear the death of a loved one often begin the process of grieving before any loss actually occurs. The acute reactions to loss include an initial period of shock followed by intense emotional pangs of grief. Lindemann identified the following symptoms of normal grief:

- somatic distress, such as feelings of tightness in the throat or chest
- preoccupation with the image of the deceased
- guilt

- hostile reactions
- loss of patterns of conduct.

These symptoms will be familiar to ED staff who have looked after recently bereaved relatives. Lindemann's work stemmed from a fire at the Coconut Grove nightclub in 1942 that claimed the lives of 474 people. He found that the fire resulted in a crisis for all individuals closely involved, including staff. Scott (1994) suggested that caring for distressed relatives following a sudden death is perhaps one of the most emotionally draining of nursing interventions. Wright (1996), in a study of relatives' responses to sudden death, found nine common emotional responses identified by nurses as difficult to manage, including:

- denial
- withdrawal
- anger
- acceptance
- isolation
- bargaining
- crying, sobbing, weeping.

It is noteworthy that five of the emotional responses that cause difficulties for ED nurses also correspond with what Kubler-Ross (1973) described as the stages of grief, i.e., denial, anger, isolation, bargaining and acceptance. Kubler-Ross was careful to point out that these stages do not happen in a particular order, and can occur side by side. These stages do not just affect dying patients but, as can be seen above, affect relatives and staff as well.

There is, however, debate regarding the usefulness of identifying emotions in an attempt to define the manifestation of grieving as this may lead people to think of grief in a simplistic way. Thus the theories and emotions attributed to grief should only be used as a guide to inform the possible reactions experienced by those who are bereaved (Kent & Dowell 2004, Oman & Duran 2010). That noted, people experiencing the sudden unexpected death of a loved one are at risk of more pronounced and prolonged grief reactions than those who had been expecting death. There is also a higher morbidity rate among these people in the following two years after the death (Kent & Dowell 2004).

Preparing for receiving the patient and relatives

With growing improvements in communications technology, staff are increasingly informed of the impending arrival of critically ill or injured patients by ambulance control or the ambulance crew en route from the scene. This enables staff to prepare the resuscitation room and contact the on-call medical, paediatric and anaesthetic teams as appropriate. In accordance with advanced life-support principles, staff should be designated specific roles for the management of the patient (see also Chapter 2).

The 5–10 minutes' forewarning also serve to mentally prepare staff for the arrival of patients and their relatives. This time can also be used to provide support and guidance for more junior staff about what they might expect. A member of staff should be allocated to receive relatives. This nurse

should not have any clinical responsibilities in the management of the resuscitation (Box 14.1).

When anxious relatives arrive, they should be met by a named link nurse and not be kept waiting around at reception for the department's communications to be established (Purves & Edwards 2005, Oman & Duran 2010). While the term 'relatives' is used throughout this chapter, it is important to note that in some instances close friends or partners of either sex may be severely distressed and should be handled in the same way as the relatives.

Witnessed resuscitation

Witnessed resuscitation, the practice of enabling relatives to stay in the resuscitation room while their loved one is being resuscitated, remains controversial (Boyd & White 1998, Royal College of Nursing, British Medical Association and Resuscitation Council 2002, Emergency Nurses Association 2009, Kingsnorth-Hinrichs 2009, Oman & Duran 2010). In a review of 117 studies into family presence, as witnessed resuscitation is also known, the Emergency Nurses Association (2009) found the following:

- there is some evidence that patients would prefer to have their family members present during resuscitation
- there is strong evidence that family members wish to be offered the option to be present during invasive procedures and resuscitation of a family member
- there is little or no evidence to indicate that the practice of family member presence is detrimental to the patient, the family or the healthcare team
- there is evidence that family member presence does not interfere with patient care during invasive procedures or resuscitation
- there is evidence that healthcare professionals support the presence of a designated healthcare professional assigned to present family members to provide explanation and comfort
- there is some evidence that a policy regarding family member presence provides structure and support to healthcare professionals involved in this practice
- family member presence during invasive procedures or resuscitation should be offered as an option to appropriate family members and should be based on written institution policy.

Dolan (1997) has argued that 'enabling witnessed resuscitation is about having enough faith in ourselves as carers to show we are not afraid of others seeing us losing the battle for someone's life', and Connors (1996) suggests that the advantages of allowing relatives to be present in the resuscitation room appear to outweigh any potential disadvantages. Boxes 14.2 and 14.3 outline healthcare professionals' concerns about allowing relatives into resuscitation rooms as well as reasons why relatives should be allowed in the resuscitation room.

Witnessed resuscitation was first documented by the Foote Hospital Michigan, after they introduced the system in 1982 following two incidents when family members insisted on being present (Doyle et al. 1987). They questioned

Box 14.1

Principles of best practice when caring for the suddenly bereaved in ED

Contacting relatives or friends (see also Box 14.7)

- Communicate by telephone
- Speak to the most significant relative or friend, state own name and position held. If this is not the significant relative, it is important to ascertain where this person can be found
- The caller should state his name, designation and the hospital from which he is calling
- Give the patient's full name
- If there is doubt about the identity of the patient, state it is believed to be this person
- After giving this information, the caller should check that the relative is clear about:
  - Which hospital
  - How to get there
  - What has been said
- The relative should be advised:
  - To get someone to come out to the hospital with them
  - To drive carefully, and preferably get someone else to drive
  - To inform other close relatives or friends where they are heading
- Check understanding
- Records of the time of the call, who made the call, who responded, and how, are important. After a death, some relatives may want to clarify details

Arrival of relatives or friends

- Allocate one support nurse to the family or friends
- Meet them on arrival
- Take relatives or friends to an appropriately furnished private sitting room

Resuscitation

- Inform relatives or friends of the situation, assure them that every effort is being made to save the patient
- Provide an honest update every 10–15 minutes (support nurse)
- Encourage relatives or next of kin to witness resuscitation if they wish

Informing relatives or friends of the death

- Inform relatives or friends promptly of the death, using clear unambiguous language
- Sit at the same level as the relatives/friends when breaking bad news
- Express care and concern, support bereaved relatives and friends whatever their reaction
- Allow time to talk, listen and answer questions
- In the case of a paediatric death, challenge any unrealistic expectations parents may have about their roles. Remind the parents there was no way to protect their child from this death, unless this is not the case (Chan 2009)

Viewing the body

- Present the deceased person to look as peaceful as possible
- Encourage relatives or friends to see, touch and talk to the deceased person
- Allow time alone with the body
- Allow relatives or friends to participate in the last offices
- Provide the opportunity to see the place of death

The deceased person's belongings

- Fold clothing, place in a specially designed container; avoid plastic clothing bags
- Explain soiled or cut clothes, place a note with clothing stating same

Concluding procedures

- Accommodate, wherever possible, cultural or religious rituals
- Discuss organ or tissue donation
- Inform relatives and friends about the post-mortem
- Provide information on arranging a funeral, registering a death and bereavement support groups
- Retain photograph or lock of hair, as appropriate

Follow-up

- Provide a hospital contact number and name of support nurse or doctor
- Ideally provide follow-up care in the week following the death by telephone or written note

(After Kent H, McDowell J (2004) Sudden bereavement in acute care settings. Nursing Standard, 19(6), 38–42.)

recently bereaved relatives and found that 72% would have liked to have witnessed the resuscitation attempt. As a result, a programme of witnessed resuscitation began; however, there was resistance from many staff members. In an audit three years later, staff were questioned about their views and 71% endorsed the practice even though some felt it had incurred an increased stress level, largely because the patient undergoing resuscitation becomes 'more human' in the presence of family members. In a follow-up paper, Hanson & Strawser (1992) argued that in their nine years of facilitating acceptance of death and grieving by this method, staff members continued to find it a humanizing and workable experience.

A UK study by Robinson et al. (1998) found there were no adverse psychological effects among relatives who witnessed

resuscitation, all of whom were satisfied with the decision to remain with the patient. The trial was discontinued when the clinical team involved became convinced of the benefits to relatives of allowing them to witness resuscitation if they wished. Psychological follow-up at three and six months found fewer symptoms of grief and distress in the group who had witnessed resuscitation than in the control group. Of the patients who survived, none believed that their confidentiality had been compromised.

Witnessed resuscitation is becoming more common and relatives will, in future, increasingly insist on being present. It is already seen as good practice by the working group of the Royal College of Nursing and British Association for Accident & Emergency Medicine (1995) as well as recommended practice by the Royal College of Nursing, British

Box 14.2

Healthcare professionals' concerns about allowing relatives in resuscitation rooms

- Family members' uncontrollable grief would disrupt smooth functioning of the resuscitation team
- Family members would become physically involved in the resuscitation attempt
- The team's emotions would be too strongly evoked by family presence
- Fear that some observed action or remark by the medical or nursing staff may offend grieving family members, such as use of humour as a stress reliever (Jezierski 1993)
- Witnessing a resuscitation is an experience that is non-therapeutic and traumatic enough to haunt the surviving family members as long as they live (Osuagwn 1993)
- There would not be enough adequately trained staff to implement a supportive role for all families (Back & Rooke 1994)
- The relatives may become cardiac arrest victims themselves (Osuagwn 1993)
- Fear that allowing observation of the activity and procedures would increase the legal risk (Hanson & Stawser 1992)
- Relatives may feel pressured into attending a resuscitation

Box 14.3

Reasons why relatives should be allowed in the resuscitation room

- There is some evidence that patients would prefer to have their family members present during resuscitation (Emergency Nurses Association 2009)
- The relative is able to see rather than being told that everything possible is being done. This comes from the belief that the reality of the resuscitation room is far less horrifying than the fantasy
- The relative is able to touch the patient while she is still warm – to the general public, warm means alive (Connors 1996)
- Relatives can say whatever they need to while there is still a chance that the patient can hear them
- The grieving process is long and hard enough without eliminating any elements that might help adjustment (Martin 1991)
- The family is viewed more as part of a loving family and less as a clinical challenge
- Closer relationships are formed between nursing staff and patients' relatives (Hanson & Strawser 1992)
- Reduces the legal risk as families can see for themselves that no-one is trying to hide anything (Renzi-Brown 1989)
- The relatives feel that they are doing something in a hopeless situation
- There is strong evidence that family members wish to be offered the option to be present during invasive procedures and resuscitation of a family member (Emergency Nurses Association 2009)

Medical Association and Resuscitation Council (UK) (2007), Emergency Nurses Association (2009) and European Resuscitation Council (Nolan et al. 2010). Nurses should anticipate the changing needs of the community and plan this change carefully. Hampe (1975) found that family members expressed three main needs:

- to be with the dying patient
- to be kept informed
- to know that the dying person was not in pain.

It was also found that the least supportive measure was to remove the family members from the bedside. Given that resuscitation attempts are unsuccessful in 70–98% of cases and death ultimately is inevitable (Nolan et al. 2010), causing those who have been bereaved to feel left out, uninformed and helpless may lead to feelings of anger that can result in unnecessary despair during the grieving process (Kent & Dowell 2004).

For staff who have, or wish to develop, a witnessed resuscitation policy, Box 14.4 offers guidance on what to say to relatives prior to witnessing a resuscitation. Box 14.5 provides guidance for the team leader, doctors and nurses on how to stop an arrest with relatives present.

Breaking bad news

For relatives who are waiting in the 'sitting room' or 'relatives' room', it should be sensitively decorated, bright and well lit (Box 14.6). Frequent updates on the patient's condition are important. The link nurse should liaise with staff in the resuscitation room to maintain communication between the relatives and the resuscitation team. Concise terms such as 'critical', 'serious', 'good' and 'fair' appear to be reasonably understood by lay people and professionals alike.

In the event of cessation of resuscitation, if relatives are not present when the patient dies, or if they arrive after the death, staff will have to break the news to them. McLauchlan (1996) suggested that breaking bad news has to be tailored to the situation and particular relatives; however, the following principles apply:

- on leaving the resuscitation room, the breaker of bad news, who is usually a doctor but may also be a nurse, should take a moment to gather his composure. Removal of plastic aprons, stethoscopes around the neck and other obviously clinical paraphernalia is recommended
- it is important to confirm that the correct relatives are being addressed. It can be a simple but traumatic mistake to inform the wrong people of the death of a relative. If there is more than one victim, assign one staff member to each group of survivors/relatives (Chan 2009)
- on entering the relatives' room, it is important for the nurse and doctor to introduce themselves and also establish those in the room and their relationship to the patient. Sitting down to talk with relatives gives the impression that the bearers of bad news are not in a rush to leave
- during the interview, it may be helpful and natural to touch or hold the hand of the bereaved relative(s). While various social and cultural factors may influence the appropriateness of this, if it feels appropriate then it probably is right
- getting to the point quickly is important.

When providing information and answering questions, keep it honest, direct and simple. Phrases like 'dead', 'death' and

Box 14.4

Suggested guidelines for staff on what to say to relatives prior to witnessing a resuscitation

- Relatives should be informed that their loved one is very ill and that at present their heart has stopped, so the doctors and nurses are having to breathe for the patient and artificially make her heart pump by pressing on her chest wall. If there is any signs that the heart is starting to function again, then the team may have to give an electrical shock to try to kick start the heart again
- Relatives should be informed that the prognosis is very grim and it is very unlikely that their loved one will live. Should the patient come out of this event then the next 24 hours will be critical and there is the likelihood that this event will recur
- Relatives should be given the choice of going into the resuscitation room; they should never be made to feel they must go in
- The link nurse should describe the patient's appearance, treatment, jargon and equipment in use and where they can stand in the resuscitation room
- Relatives should be informed that it is acceptable for them to come in for a couple of minutes at a time and leave whenever they wish
- Relatives should be informed that even though their loved one cannot respond to them it is possible that she might be able to hear them. This information should only be given to relatives who have decided to enter the area
- Relatives should be informed that no more than two to three relatives are allowed into the resuscitation room at any one time, as more might distract or hamper the resuscitation attempt. This number is suggested as it would be very difficult and distressing to the relatives to allow two out of three attending the department into the resuscitation area. The third person would then be lacking in support
- Relatives should be informed that the doctors, radiographers etc. may ask them to wait outside while some investigations, such as X-rays or invasive procedures, are carried out
- Relatives should be informed that at some point the team will feel that they have done everything possible to regain life, and that unfortunately their loved one is going to die. When this decision has been reached, the carer should say something like, 'We're going to stop soon, we've tried everything and nothing is helping'
- Before all attempts have ceased, the team should try to accommodate the relatives and give them the opportunity to be able to get close to their loved one to say 'goodbye' etc.

 Box 14.5

Guidance for team leader, doctors and nurses on how to stop an arrest with relatives present

- The relatives must be supported by an experienced trained nurse, and this must be this nurse's only role. The relatives should have been informed before entering the scene that the prognosis is very poor and that the chances of successful resuscitation are very slim
- The decision to stop resuscitation should be made quietly. All staff involved should be consulted and, if feasible, the relatives should be included in this
- The team leader with the help of the support nurse, will inform relatives that the resuscitation attempt has failed and that they are about to stop
- Gradually, one by one, staff should leave the scene, those with no active involvement leaving first. The team leader should stay to support the relatives and nurse looking after them. When most of the staff have left, the staff member carrying out cardiac massage should stop and leave quietly. The anaesthetist should then turn off the ventilator and cardiac monitor and, when possible, remove the ET tube, stop all i.v. lines and then leave the area
- When ready, the nurse should then escort the relatives out of the area and follow the local bereavement guidelines
- The team leader will talk to the relatives in the relatives' room, answering any questions that may arise. The support nurse should still be with the relatives
- All staff should be involved in the debriefing

Box 14.6

Facilities for the bereaved in the emergency department

In the room there should be:
- Comfortable, domestic chairs and sofas. In recognition of people with special needs, for example, the elderly, appropriate furniture should be provided
- Tissues
- Ashtrays
- A telephone with direct dial access for incoming and outgoing calls
- Telephone directories
- A washbasin, with soap, towel, mirror and freshen-up pack
- TV/radio available, but not prominent
- Hot and cold drinks should be available. A fridge and kettle point enable independence, and are convenient for staff. A non-institutional tea/coffee set should also be available
- Toys and books should be available

'died' should be used as they are unambiguous. Giving the news thoughtfully and showing concern will enable the relatives to understand the event as reality.

- if a language barrier exists, attempt to obtain a translator from outside the family and prepare the translator. If a family member is the only translator, it is important to acknowledge how difficult a task it is to hear bad news about a loved one and to explain the news to someone else
- euphemisms should be avoided at all costs. Table 14.1 outlines phrases that should not be used when breaking bad news
- after breaking the bad news, allow time and silence while the facts sink in, re-emphasizing them if

appropriate. Sometimes, just listening to someone who is distressed, or sitting in silence with them, witnessing their grief, may be the most important service a nurse or doctor can provide for someone who is bereaved (Casarett 2001)

- be prepared for a variety of emotional responses or reactions. Some may appear unmoved, while others will sob and wail. These reactions are not the fault of the bearer of bad news, but are a reaction to the news itself
- offer the relatives the opportunity to view the deceased.

Table 14.1 Phrases to be avoided when breaking bad news

What is said	What the relative may understand
We have lost him	He has gone missing in the hospital
She has passed on	She has been transferred to another ward
He has slipped away	He has sneaked out of the department
She has suffered irreversible asystole	Nothing!

Communication is a dynamic, complex and continuous exchange (Winchester 1999). Frequently, however, the person communicating the bad news feels that it has been done badly. In a health profession which still sees death as a failure, this is not surprising, especially when it is compounded with the powerful feelings evoked by sudden death. Thayre & Hadfield-Law (1995) noted that, when preparing to give bad news, it is essential that the nurse is aware that increasing urbanization, advances in medical technology and skills, and the declining size and importance of the extended family have all decreased people's experience of close death. In addition, changing cultural and religious practices mean that nurses may not always be aware of family needs in this respect. It is also important to stress that when breaking bad news the medical facts are less important than the compassion shown to relatives.

Telephone notification

Where possible, telephone notification of bereavement should be avoided as it can cause acute distress to the receiver as well as to the person delivering the news. Wright (1993) noted that the feelings of a person receiving information over the telephone frequently include the following:

- 'they knew more than they said'
- 'I am not sure what they said'
- 'it cannot be as bad as they say'
- 'I am not sure what they want me to do'
- 'it does not make sense'.

Fears of the individual giving information over the telephone may include:

- 'I hope I have identified and am speaking to the right person'
- 'what if they collapse when I tell them, and they are alone?'
- 'panic may prevent them hearing me'
- 'what will I say if they ask me outright if their relative is dead?'
- 'people just should not hear this over the phone'.

Thayre & Hadfield-Law (1995) suggested that information given over the telephone should be in small units. Following the shock of bad news, people tend to respond only to simple questions or instructions and may be slow to take in involved explanations. Jones & Buttery (1981) found that relatives only rarely asked over the telephone whether their loved one was dead. Box 14.7 outlines the information that should be given to those who ring or are contacted about death or critical illness of a relative.

Box 14.7

Information to give to relatives over the telephone

- Clear, concise communication is vital
- The caller should state his name, designation and the hospital from which he is calling
- If this is not the significant relative, it is important to ascertain where this person can be found
- Give the name of the ill or injured person and her condition
- If there is doubt about the identity of the patient, tell the relative it is believed to be this person
- After giving this information, the caller should check that the relative is clear about:
  - Which hospital
  - How to get there
  - What has been said
- The relative should be advised:
  - To get someone to come out to the hospital with them
  - To drive carefully, and preferably get someone else to drive
  - To inform other close relatives or friends where they are heading
- Records of the time of the call, who made the call, who responded and how, are important. After a death, some relatives may want to clarify details

Viewing the body

The opportunity to see the dead person should always be offered and gently encouraged (Haas 2003). While some well-meaning friends or relatives may discourage this act, it is an important part of accepting the reality of the situation and can facilitate grieving and ease feelings of guilt after sudden death. Jones & Buttery (1981) found that relatives of sudden-death victims who spent time with the body in the ED concluded that the viewing process was helpful.

The environment in which the relatives view the body should be made as non-clinical as reasonably possible. Monitors should always be switched off. Drips and invasive treatment aids, such as ET tubes, catheters and cannulas, should be removed. Before allowing viewing, blood should be wiped from the patient's body, eyes should be closed and a blanket should cover the patient up to the upper shoulder. Leaving the deceased person's arm(s) over the covers and respectful washing of the face and combing of the hair should be done before relatives attend. Religious insignia can be added as appropriate. Sufficient chairs should be available for relatives to sit down. Reluctant or unwilling family members should be reassured that viewing is a highly personal decision and that a decision *not* to view the deceased person may be best for many people. What is essential is enabling relatives to have the *choice* to view or not view the deceased person.

When the dead person is disfigured or mutilated, the relatives' wishes are paramount. Gentle, honest explanations beforehand can inform the relatives' decision about whether they wish to see the dead person (Davies 1997). The relatives should be encouraged to touch, hold, kiss, hug or say goodbye to their loved one. When speaking of the dead person, use the person's name, 'him' or 'her', but never 'body' or 'it'. Warn the family that the patient may look different from their expectations. Unless there are suspicious circumstances and the police wish to remain with the body, the relatives may also like to be left alone with the body and must be given permission to stay as long as they wish or as is practically possible (Morgan 1997). As Boucher (2010) notes, relatives should not be regarded as complications, but as extensions of the patient's lives and their need to say goodbye their loved ones should not be underestimated.

Organ donation

Body organs, e.g., the kidneys, heart, liver, pancreas and corneas, and tissues may be donated by the patient for availability for transplant. There is, however, a great shortage of organs for transplant, which continues to limit transplant efforts. The demand is growing at a much greater rate than the supply with more than 10 000 people in the UK currently needing a transplant. Of these, 1000 will die each year waiting as there are not enough organs available (Sque & Galasinski 2013, Department of Health 2011). Currently only 28 % of the UK population are on the organ donation register (Vincent & Logan 2012). The usage of potential organs from emergency departments is very low.

Donation after circulatory death (DCD) describes the retrieval of organs for the purpose of transplantation that follows death confirmed using circulatory criteria. DCD represents approximately one third of all deceased organ donors, and usually all found in ED (Manara et al. 2012). The majority of transplants use organs from heartbeating donors after brain death (DBD). DBD are more likely to donate multiple transplantable organs (mean 3.9 organs vs 2.5 for DCD in the UK) (NHS Blood and Transplant 2011), and are currently the only reliable source for cardiac transplants (McKeown et al. 2012).

Wellesley et al. (1997) noted that the organs that can be donated from ED include corneas, heart valves and, in certain departments, kidneys. For heart valves there must be no congenital valve defect, no systemic infection, no hepatitis B or C, and the donor must not be HIV positive. For corneas, there are even fewer contraindications: no scarring of the cornea, no infection in the eye and no invasive brain tumours. Both organs are very successfully transplanted, with at least 85 % success for corneas and even higher for heart valves, due to the absence of rejection problems. Currently, most transplants follow multiple organ retrieval from heartbeating brain-dead organ donors (McKeown et al. 2012).

Consent from the coroner may be a limiting factor to tissue retrieval in the ED. Unless a doctor is prepared to sign a death certificate to state that a patient died of natural causes then the coroner must give consent prior to removal of any organ or tissue, as stated in the Human Tissue Act 2004.

Many nurses believe relatives should not be approached about organ donation in the ED, feeling that they have been through enough (Coupe 1990). However, a recent small-scale study by Wellesley et al. (1997) highlighted that 27 (72.9 %) of the 37 recently bereaved respondents to a questionnaire would not have minded being asked about organ donation following a sudden death. They suggested that the subject could be broached by having leaflets in the room where relatives are given the bad news, as a way of introducing this delicate subject and providing more information. They believe the interview with bereaved relatives needs to be carried out sensitively by senior nurses, registrars or, in some cases, the consultant, who have been appropriately trained and who have access to staff support within the ED (see also Chapter 39).

Legal and ethical issues

Contact with the coroner's officer may occur in the ED or in the home when the notification of the death and identification of the body are established. It is important to distinguish between a coroner's officer who gathers and records details related to the death, e.g., by attending postmortems, and the coroner, usually a doctor or lawyer, who responds to the results of the details by concluding on the circumstances of the death and reaching, if necessary, a verdict at inquest.

Scott (1995) suggested that relatives are often devastated by the news of the death and that these feelings are intensified at the thought of the purposeful mutilation of the body at autopsy. In fact, the autopsy is a legal requirement for most deaths that occur in the ED (Box 14.8). This information needs to be conveyed to patients in a dignified, sensitive way.

Controversy exists over whether personal possessions, and in particular jewellery and precious metals, should be given to relatives. Should relatives wish to remove any rings or special belongings, they should be enabled to do so. Legally, a witnessed signature is sufficient to corroborate the act of handing over or retaining property and this may be obtained from another nurse, doctor or coroner's officer (Cooke et al. 1992). Clothing should be carefully folded and itemized along with any other possessions such as jewellery and money. The nurse should seek permission

Box 14.8

Criteria for investigation of a death by a coroner

The coroner is a doctor or lawyer responsible for investigating death in the following situations:

- The deceased was not attended by a doctor during the last illness or the doctor treating the deceased had not seen her after the death or within 14 days of the death
- The death was violent or unnatural or occurred under suspicious circumstances
- The cause of death is not known or is uncertain
- The death occurred in prison or in police custody
- The death occurred while the patient was undergoing an operation or the patient did not recover from the anaesthetic
- The death was caused by an industrial disease

from the family to dispose of badly damaged clothing. This should be recorded in the patient's notes.

Advanced care directives

An advance care directive (ACD), sometimes called a 'living will', is a document that describes one's future preferences for medical treatment in anticipation of a time when one is unable to express those preferences because of illness or injury (New South Wales Department of Health 2004). For many years it has been a general principle of both common law and medical practice that people have a right to refuse treatment.

The guidance on 'Advance Decisions to Refuse Treatment' (National Council for Palliative Care and Department of Health 2008) acknowledges that it is a general principle of law and medical practice that people have a right to consent to or refuse treatment. The courts have recognized that adults have the right to say in advance that they want to refuse treatment if they lose capacity in the future – even if this results in their death. A valid and applicable advance decision to refuse treatment has the same force as a contemporaneous decision. This has been a fundamental principle of the common law for many years and it is now set out in the Mental Capacity Act 2005. Sections 24–26 of the Act set out when a person can make an advance decision to refuse treatment. This applies if:

- the person is 18 or older, and
- they have the capacity to make an advance decision about treatment.

Healthcare professionals must follow an advance decision if it is valid and applies to the particular circumstances. If they do not, they could face criminal prosecution, i.e., they could be charged for committing a crime, or civil liability, i.e., somebody could sue them.

Healthcare professionals will be protected from liability if they:

- stop or withhold treatment because they reasonably believe that an advance decision exists, and that it is valid and applicable
- treat a person because, having taken all practical and appropriate steps to find out if the person has made an advance decision to refuse treatment, they do not know or are not satisfied that a valid and applicable advance decision exists.

People can only make an advance decision under the Act if they are 18 or over and have the capacity to make the decision. They must say what treatment they want to refuse, and they can cancel their decision – or part of it – at any time.

If the advance decision refuses life-sustaining treatment, it must:

- be in writing – it can be written by someone else or recorded in healthcare notes
- be signed and witnessed
- state clearly that the decision applies even if life is at risk.

To establish whether an advance decision is valid and applicable, healthcare professionals must try to find out if the person:

- has done anything that clearly goes against their advance decision
- has withdrawn their decision
- has subsequently conferred the power to make that decision on an attorney, or
- would have changed their decision if they had known more about the current circumstances.

ACDs will become increasingly common in EDs, partly in response to changing social structures, demography and demands. Respecting the desires of the patient and their family, plus enabling individuals to achieve a sense of control of their own health reflects best care at a particularly difficult time in people's lives.

Sudden infant death syndrome

This issue is addressed in detail in Chapter 16.

Staff support

Cudmore (1998) believes that ED nurses are 'at risk' of developing post-traumatic stress reactions because of their exposure to traumatic events as a routine part of their job, which for most people would be outside the range of human experience. Walsh et al. (1998) argued that if stress is the main cause of burnout, then understanding coping mechanisms is the key to minimizing the problem. Coping strategies employed by those working with trauma include the following:

- suppressing emotions and feelings
- mutual staff support
- promoting a sense of unreality
- mental preparation for tasks
- feeling competent and capable
- regulating exposure to the event
- having a sense of purpose
- humour.

Box 14.9 outlines the effects of traumatic events on carers. The following are methods that staff working with dying people can use to improve their coping skills:

- the encouragement of personal insight to understand and acknowledge one's own limits
- a healthy balance between work and outside life
- the promotion of a team approach to care
- an ongoing support system within work and outside work
- for those working in isolation, continuing guidance and support, from peers and superiors.

Nykiel et al. (2011) stress the importance of ongoing education on the relevance of family presence and its benefits through in-service training and meetings.

(Defusion, demobilization and critical incident debriefing skills for staff are discussed in detail in Chapter 13.)

Box 14.9

The effects of traumatic events such as failed resuscitation attempts on carers

- *Emotional effects* – anxiety, depression, anger, guilt, irritability and feelings of helplessness
- *Cognitive effects* – memory/concentration changes, nightmares, intrusive thoughts and imagery
- *Behavioural effects* – alters use of drugs, alcohol, nicotine, caffeine, etc., social withdrawal and loss of interest in usual activities
- *Relationship effects* – changes in work, social, intimate and sexual relationships through irritability, inability to share feelings, isolation and conflict of loyalty between work and home
- *Somatic effects* – changes in sleeping and eating habits, altered energy levels, an increase in accidents and physical health problems
- *Motivational effects* – viewing life from a different perspective, often as more tenuous. Values may be reoriented to less materialistic ones

Conclusion

Sudden death, by whatever cause, is a stressful and distressing event for staff as well as for patients' relatives.

While EDs may be geared towards saving lives, death should not be seen by staff as a failure. No matter how confident or experienced the practitioner, it is never easy to tell relatives or friends that a loved one has died (Kendrick 1997). In relation to the needs of relatives, Dolan (1995) argued that:

> '… in so many respects, it seems worth the effort and distress of the trip to know that everything that could be done was done. The tacit transfer of responsibility from patient and family to health carers highlights that while caring costs, our compassion must never get sacrificed as the cost of our caring.'

This chapter has highlighted the process of care for those who have been suddenly bereaved. Within an ageing society, it is likely that more people will require the resuscitative efforts of ED staff; however, many will not survive. Their relatives are particularly vulnerable in this traumatic situation and require the nurse to advocate for them at this time, enabling them to witness the resuscitation if they wish and receive the news of death with compassion and understanding. For ED personnel, training and ongoing support will enable them to deal with the challenges of caring for such vulnerable people. The unexpected end of one person's life is the beginning of someone else's grief. ED nurses are in a key position to enable a relative's last memory of a loved one to become a lasting memory of compassionate support and care.

References

Back, D., Rooke, V., 1994. The presence of relatives in the resuscitation room. Nursing Times 90 (30), 34–35.

Boucher, M., 2010. Family witnessed resuscitation. Emergency Nurse 18 (5), 10–14.

Boyd, R., White, S., 1998. Does witnessed cardiopulmonary resuscitation alter perceived stress levels in Accident and Emergency staff? Journal of Accident and Emergency Medicine 15, 109–111.

Casarett, D., et al., 2001. Life after death: a practical approach to grief and bereavement. Annals of Internal Medicine 134 (3), 208–215.

Chan, G.K., 2009. Palliative and end-of-life care in the emergency department. In: Kunz Howard, P., Steinmann, R.A. (Eds.), Sheehy's Emergency Nursing: Principles and Practice, sixth ed. Mosby Elsevier, St Louis.

Connors, P., 1996. Should relatives be allowed in the resuscitation room? Nursing Standard 10 (44), 44–46.

Cooke, M.W., Cooke, H.W., Glucksmann, E.E., 1992. Management of sudden bereavement in the accident & emergency department. British Medical Journal 304, 1207–1209.

Coupe, C., 1990. Donation dilemmas. Nursing Times 86 (27), 34–36.

Cudmore, J., 1998. Critical incident stress management strategies. Emergency Nurse 6 (3), 22–27.

Davies, J., 1997. Grieving after a sudden death: the impact of the initial intervention. Accident and Emergency Nursing 5 (4), 181–184.

Department of Health, 2011. Driving up Organ Donations. Department of Health, London.

Dolan, B., 1995. Drama within a crisis: Relatives in the resuscitation room. Journal of Clinical Nursing 4 (5), 275.

Dolan, B., 1997. Editorial. Underlining compassion in casualty. Emergency Nurse 5 (2), 1.

Doyle, C.J., Post, H., Burney, R.E., et al., 1987. Family participation during resuscitation: An option. Annals of Emergency Medicine 16, 673–675.

Emergency Nurses Association, 2009. Emergency Nursing Resource: Family Presence During Invasive Procedures and Resuscitation in the Emergency Department. ENA, Des Plaines, Il.

Glaser, B.G., Strauss, A.L., 1965. Awareness of Dying. Aldine Press, Chicago.

Glaser, B.G., Strauss, A.L., 1968. Time for Dying. Aldine Press, Chicago.

Haas, F., 2003. Bereavement care: seeing the body. Nursing Standard 17 (28), 33–37.

Hampe, S.O., 1975. Needs of the grieving spouse in a hospital setting. Nursing Research 24, 113–120.

Hanson, C., Strawser, D., 1992. Family presence during CPR: Foote Hospital Emergency Department's nine-year perspective. Journal of Emergency Nursing 18 (2), 104–106.

Jezierski, M., 1993. Foote Hospital emergency department: Shattering a paradigm. Journal of Emergency Nursing 19 (3), 266–267.

Jones, W.H., Buttery, H., 1981. Sudden death: survivors' perceptions of their emergency department experience. Journal of Emergency Nursing 7 (1), 14–17.

Kendrick, K., 1997. Sudden death: walking in a moral minefield. Emergency Nurse 5 (1), 17–19.

Kent, H., McDowell, J., 2004. Sudden bereavement in acute care settings. Nursing Standard 19 (6), 38–42.

Kingsnorth-Hinrichs, J., 2009. Family presence during resuscitation. In: Kunz Howard, P., Steinmann, R.A. (Eds.), Sheehy's Emergency Nursing: Principles and Practice, sixth ed. Mosby Elsevier, St Louis.

Kubler-Ross, H., 1973. On Death and Dying. Macmillan, New York.

Lindemann, E., 1944. Symptomatology and management of acute grief. American Journal of Psychiatry 101, 141–148.

Martin, J., 1991. Rethinking traditional thoughts. Journal of Emergency Nursing 17 (2), 67–68.

Manara, A.R., Murphy, P.G., O'Callaghan, G., 2012. Donation after circulatory death. British Journal of Anaesthesia 108 (S1), i108–i121.

McKeown, D.W., Bonser, R.S., Kellum, J.A., 2012. Donation after circulatory death. British Journal of Anaesthesia 108 (S1), i96–i107.

McLauchlan, C.A.J., 1996. Handling distressed relatives and breaking bad news. In: Skinner, D., Driscoll, P., Earlam, R. (Eds.), ABC of Major Trauma, second ed. BMJ, London.

Moons, P., Norekval, T.M., 2008. European nursing organizations stand up for family presence during cardiopulmonary resuscitation: A joint position statement. Progress in Cardiovascular Nursing 23 (3), 136–139.

Morgan, J., 1997. Introducing a witnessed resuscitation policy to ED. Emergency Nurse 5 (2), 13–17.

Mushtaq, F., Ritchie, D., 2005. Do we know what people die of in the emergency department? Emergency Medicine Journal 22, 718–721.

National Council for Palliative Care and Department of Health, 2008. Advance Decisions to Refuse Treatment: A Guide for Health and Social Care Professionals. Department of Health, London.

New South Wales Department of Health, 2004. Using Advance Care Directives (NSW). NSW Department of Health, Sydney.

NHS Blood and Transplant, 2011. Activity report 2010–2011. NHS Blood and Transplant, London.

Nolan, J.P., Soar, J., Zideman, D.A., et al., 2010. Section 1. Executive summary. Resuscitation. European Resuscitation Council Guidelines for Resuscitation 81, 1219–1276.

Nykiel, L., Denicke, R., Schneider, R., et al., 2011. Evidence-based practice and family presence: paving the path for bedside nurse scientists. Journal of Emergency Nursing 37 (1), 9–16.

Oman, K.S., Duran, C.R., 2010. Health care providers' evaluations of family presence during resuscitation. Journal of Emergency Nursing 36 (6), 524–533.

Osuagwn, C.C., 1993. More on family presence during resuscitation. Journal of Emergency Nursing 19 (4), 276–277.

Purves, Y., Edwards, S., 2005. Initial needs of bereaved relatives following sudden and unexpected death. Emergency Nurse 13 (7), 28–34.

Renzi-Brown, J., 1989. Legally, it makes good sense. Nursing 19 (3), 46.

Resuscitation Council, 1996. Should Relatives Witness Resuscitation? Resuscitation Council, London.

Robinson, S.M., Campbell-Hewson, G.L., Egelston, C.V., et al., 1998. The psychological impact on relatives of witnessing resuscitation. Lancet 352 (9128), 614–617.

Royal College of Nursing, 2002. Witnessed Resuscitation. RCN, London.

Royal College of Nursing and British Association for Accident and Emergency Medicine, 1995. Bereavement Care in A&E Departments: Report of a Working Group. RCN, London.

Royal College of Nursing, British Medical Association and Resuscitation Council, 2002. Decisions Relating to Cardiopulmonary Resuscitation: A Joint Statement from the British Medical Association, Resuscitation Council (UK) and the Royal College of Nursing. BMA, London.

Royal College of Nursing, British Medical Association and Resuscitation Council (UK), 2007. Decisions relating to cardiopulmonary resuscitation: A joint statement from the British Medical Association, the Resuscitation Council (UK) and the Royal College of Nursing. BMA, London.

Scott, T., 1995. Sudden death in A&E. Emergency Nurse 2 (4), 10–15.

Sque, M., Galasinski, D., 2013. 'Keeping her whole': Bereaved families' accounts of declining a request for organ donation. Cambridge Quarterly of Healthcare Ethics 22 (1), 55–63.

Thayre, K., Hadfield-Law, L., 1995. Never going to be easy: giving bad news. Nursing Standard (RCN Nursing Update supplement) 9 (50), 3–8.

Thompson, D., 1994. Death and dying in critical care. In: Burnard, P., Millar, B. (Eds.), Critical Care Nursing. Baillière Tindall, London.

Vincent, A., Logan, 2012. Consent for organ donation. British Journal of Anaesthesia 108 (S1), i80–i87.

Walsh, M., Dolan, B., Lewis, A., 1998. Burnout and stress among A&E nurses. Emergency Nurse 6 (2), 23–30.

Wellesley, A., Glucksmann, E.E., Crouch, R., 1997. Organ donation in the accident and emergency department: a study of relatives' views. Journal of Accident and Emergency Medicine 14, 24–25.

Winchester, A., 1999. Sharing bad news. Nursing Standard 13 (26), 48–52.

Wright, B., 1993. Caring in Crisis, second ed. Churchill Livingstone, Edinburgh.

Wright, B., 1996. Sudden Death: A Research Base for Practice. Churchill Livingstone, Edinburgh.

Mental health emergencies

15

Caroline Delaforce and Brian Dolan

Introduction

It is estimated that 1–2% of clients presenting to an Emergency Department (ED) require a formal mental-state assessment (Andrew-Starkey 2004). At any one time, common mental health disorders, including depression and anxiety disorders, can be found in around one in six people in the community. Of these, around half have significant symptoms that would warrant intervention from healthcare professionals (National Institute for Health and Clinical Excellence 2011).

The prevalence of individual common mental health disorders varies considerably. The 1-week prevalence rates from the Office of National Statistics 2007 national survey (McManus et al. 2007) were 4.4% for generalized anxiety disorder, 3.0% for post-traumatic stress disorder (PTSD), 2.3% for depression, 1.4% for phobias, 1.1% for obsessive-compulsive disorder (OCD), and 1.1% for panic disorder. Estimates of the proportion of people who are likely to experience specific disorders during their lifetime are from 4–10% for major depression, 2.5–5% for dysthymia, 5.7% for generalized anxiety disorder, 1.4% for panic disorder, 12.5% for specific phobias, 12.1% for social anxiety disorder, 1.6% for OCD and 6.8% for PTSD.

More than half of people aged 16 to 64 years who meet the diagnostic criteria for at least one common mental health disorder experience co-morbid anxiety and depressive disorders (National Institute for Health and Clinical Excellence 2011). This does not include major psychiatric disturbances such as schizophrenia, which has a prevalence of approximately 1% of the population. A psychiatric emergency is any disturbance in the client's thoughts, feelings or actions for which immediate therapeutic intervention is necessary.

EDs play a critical role in the assessment and management of people presenting with mental health disorders (Nicholls et al. 2011). People who come to the ED range from those with specific requests for help to those who are brought in against their will for reasons they do not understand. In either case, the client or carers may believe that the client is no longer able to maintain coping abilities at his usual level of functioning.

The reasons why many of these clients attend ED are multifactorial. A primary reason, however, is the deinstitutionalization of the mentally ill, due to the introduction of psychotropic medication in the 1950s and the changing focus on treatment, rehabilitation and least restrictive practices within the community. As a consequence, for many in society, their only access to healthcare is through ED.

For the ED nurse who deals with various life-threatening emergencies on a routine basis, these needs may not appear to be true emergencies; however, it is a crisis that brings the mental health client to the ED and the nature and degree of a crisis are defined by the person experiencing it. It is also to be seen as an opportunity, because prompt and skilful interventions may prevent the development of serious long-term disability and allow new coping patterns to develop (Richards 2001, Guidelines and Audit Implementation Network 2010).

Aetiology of mental illness

It is recognized that genetic, biological and biochemical dyscrasias play a significant role in the causes of major psychiatric illness. It is therefore difficult to discuss psychiatric disorders as having a purely organic or functional basis. However, for the purpose of this chapter organic disorders will be considered as those disorders that have a grossly identifiable and potentially reversible physiological cause, such as endocrine and metabolic disorders, neurological causes and drug-induced states. Functional disorders will be considered as those disorders without a grossly identifiable physiological cause.

Assessment of mental health clients

The goals of ED psychiatric evaluation are to conduct a rapid assessment, including diagnosis of any underlying medical problems, to provide emergency treatment and to arrange appropriate disposition. These goals will be hampered by various obstructions and restrictions, such as time and space, departmental milieu, inability to obtain a history from a disturbed or distressed client and experience of staff. Information collected must be concise and methods of assessment flexible enough to take into consideration the client's and the unit's needs. Relevant details must be documented accurately, as they may be the only recorded evidence of symptoms displayed by the client in the acute phase. This forms the baseline for the management and treatment plan. Records are also important for medico-legal reasons. The nurse should make full use of any collateral information available, such as family, escorts, ambulance personnel, community staff, police, hospital notes and other staff who may know the client from previous attendances or admissions. Once an assessment is made, the client should be given the appropriate triage category employed by the unit, e.g., Manchester Triage guidelines (Mackway-Jones et al. 2005).

History

History is usually initiated by the triage/assessment nurse, who must speedily determine the urgency of the crisis for which the person is seeking care and his capacity to wait. The nurse at this time has to determine how much of a risk the client poses to himself and to others, such as violent tendencies, suicide, self-mutilation, impaired judgement, etc. The history should include:

* reason for attendance
* history of presenting illness to include onset, course, duration and precipitants
* past general medical/psychiatric history
* social history including occupation, marital status, children and current social situation
* family history especially family history of mental illness.

The triage/assessment nurse may be the client's first contact with the healthcare system, and an attitude of acceptance, respect and empathy, with a desire to help, should be conveyed to the client. This first contact may significantly influence the client's acceptance of emergency care and his receptivity to future treatment. Ward (1995) suggested the following as a reasonable focus to begin with:

* what does the client want?
* who is in danger?
* what has caused this behaviour?

And, if the client is already known:

* what has happened in previous situations like this?
* what did this mean to the client the last time it happened?

Mental state examination

Examination of the mental state in psychiatry is analogous to the physical examination in a general medical or surgical practice (Andrew-Starkey 2004). It consists of historical and observational data. At a minimum the nurse should note:

- appearance and general behaviour – especially if the client is disturbed and no history is available. Assess the state of the client's clothes, cleanliness, facial expressions and interaction with the interviewing clinician. Describe motor behaviour, impulse control, orientation, eye contact, attention/concentration, rapport and posture
- affect and mood – mood is the clients internal subjective state, what the client describes is the objective external expression blunting/flattening of affect, agitation, hypomania, diurnal mood variation (depressed in the mornings, but feeling brighter in the evenings or vice versa), sleep pattern, appetite, weight loss/gain
- speech and thought – this assessment should include form and content of speech, rate and rhythm, anxieties, suicidal/future references, evidence of formal thought disorder, thought broadcasting, thought insertion, pressure of speech, ideas of reference, delusions (for glossary of terms see Box 15.3)
- abnormal perceptions and related experiences – hallucinations, derealization, depersonalization
- cognitive state – if an organic diagnosis is suspected, a more formal and detailed examination is required
- insight and judgement – does the client recognize that he is ill and in need of assistance? Is he able to make rational judgements?
- impulse control – is the client capable of controlling sexual, aggressive or other impulses? Is he a potential danger to himself or others? Is this as a result of an organic mental disease or of psychosis or chronic character traits?
- physical assessment – a complete physical assessment is required to rule out a physical cause. This will include neurological observations, blood sugar level (BSL), glucose, U&Es, FBC, LFT(DAX), thyroid function tests, ECG etc.

Formulating and agreeing a nursing and medical management framework of aims and objectives are important, i.e.:

- main features of presenting complaint
- physical examination and consultation
- investigations undertaken
- provisional and differential diagnosis, e.g., organic cause, acute functional psychosis (schizophrenia, affective states), neurosis, personality disorders
- any immediate intervention taken.

If admission is not recommended or required, the ED nurse should be aware of local services and agencies that the client may be referred to, such as:

- chemical dependency/alcohol, tobacco, other drug (ATODs)
- outclients
- crisis telephone numbers
- day hospital facilities
- social services
- facilities available for the homeless
- hostels
- ethnic minority advisory groups
- interpreters
- sexual assault counselling centres
- needle exchanges
- sexual health and associated conditions services
- police/probation officers.

Acute organic reactions

Frequently, acute organic reactions present to the ED as psychiatric emergencies when the aetiology is unknown and there is loss of behavioural control (Box 15.1). The most consistent symptom of an acute organic reaction is impairment in the consciousness, worsening symptoms at night, and good premorbid personality.

Nursing and medical management

A treatment plan, both nursing and medical/psychological, will be based on the cause and presenting behavioural disturbance. If possible, medication should be withheld, as this may mask or distort neurological signs, unless the client's presenting behaviour warrants it.

A physical examination should be performed on all clients presenting with a psychiatric crisis in order to rule out common physical illnesses that mimic psychiatric disorder (Box 15.2). People with mental health problems have a higher morbidity rate for physical illness than the general population, so their physical symptoms and complaints need to be taken seriously and investigated (Gournay & Beadsmore 1995). Diagnostic tests to confirm or rule out physical conditions masking psychiatric disorders or vice versa should be performed as necessary.

Acute psychotic episode

Psychotic clients experience impaired reality testing as they are unable to distinguish between what is real and what is not. Their thought processes are often disordered and often characterized by hallucinations, delusions, ideas of reference, thought broadcasting and thought insertion (Kaiser & Pyngolil 1995) (Box 15.3). It is essential that the ED nurse is able to differentiate between a psychosis with an organic cause, e.g., delirium, and a functional psychosis, e.g., schizophrenia. Psychotic clients may present to the ED on an emergency basis when it is:

- an acute psychotic episode, first presentation
- the exacerbation of a chronic state
- a long-term problem where the client is requesting admission, support or medication
- a catatonic excitement/stupor.

Box 15.1

Causes of acute organic reactions

- Trauma
- Infection – local
  - cerebral abscess
  - meningitis
  - encephalitis
  - syphilis
  - cerebral malaria
- Infection – general
  - systemic infection
  - septicaemia
  - typhus
  - typhoid
- Cerebrovascular
  - cerebrovascular accident
  - transient ischaemic attack
  - subarachnoid haemorrhage
  - subdural haemorrhage
  - hypertensive encephalopathy
  - systemic lupus erythematosus
  - cervical arteritis
- Epilepsy
- Tumour
  - primary and secondary metastatic effects
- Organ failure
  - renal, cardiac, hepatic, respiratory
- Anaemia
- Metabolic
  - U&E imbalance
  - acid–base imbalance
  - uraemia
- Endocrine
  - hypo/hyperthyroidism
  - hypo/hyperparathyroidism, hypopituitarism
  - hypo/hyperglycaemia
- Deficiency disorders
  - thiamine, nicotinic acid, folic acid, vitamin B_{12}
- Toxic causes
  - drug overdose
  - alcohol withdrawal
  - lead, arsenic, carbon monoxide/disulphide, mercury

Box 15.2

Organic illnesses or conditions that mimic psychiatric symptoms

- Thyrotoxicosis
- Hypoparathyroidism
- Hypoglycaemia
- Phaeochromocytoma
- Carcinoid syndrome
- Brain tumours or bleeding
- Head trauma
- Seizure disorders, such as, epilepsy
- Drug ingestions or poisoning
  - amphetamines
  - hallucinogens
  - lead poisoning
  - steroid toxicity
  - atropine
- Myxoedema
- Cushing's syndrome
- Porphyria
- Hyperparathyroidism
- Addison's disease
- Systemic lupus erythematosus
- Carcinoma

The distinction between subtypes will be based on a full assessment and is less relevant in ED.

The 'first rank' symptoms of schizophrenia are rare in other psychotic illnesses, e.g., mania or organic psychosis. The presence of only one of the following symptoms is strongly predictive of the diagnosis of schizophrenia:

- auditory hallucinations, especially the echoing of thoughts, or a third-person 'commentary' on one's actions, e.g., 'Now he's taking his jacket off'
- thought insertion, removal or interruption – delusions about external control of thought
- thought broadcasting – the delusion that others can hear one's thoughts
- delusional perceptions – i.e., abnormal significance for a normal event, e.g., 'The sun shone and I knew it was a sign from God'
- external control of emotions
- somatic passivity – thoughts, sensations and actions are under external control (see Box 15.3).

These acute symptoms may be superimposed on those of a chronic illness, e.g., apathy, impaired social network, etc. Personal hygiene in the psychotic client is frequently neglected. He may be incontinent and have a poor diet intake.

Long-term clients frequently attend the ED as a 24-hour walk-in service for requests of admission, social support or medication. Often these clients are in need of reassurance and support. If the delusions or hallucinations are a re-emergence in a long-term client, the client may be referred to outclients for adjustment of medication. It is important to ensure that the client's consultant and community team are

Schizophrenia

Schizophrenia is the commonest form of psychosis and, while it can develop at any age, it most commonly starts in late adolescence and the early twenties. It has a prevalence of approximately 1% worldwide and is highest in inner cities (Boydell et al. 2003).

Clinical features

Clinical features will depend to a certain extent on the type of schizophrenia – paranoid, hebephrenic, simple or catatonic.

Box 15.3

Acute psychotic episode symptoms

- Ideas of reference
  - referring to him in their gestures, speech, mannerisms
- Delusions, delusional mood
  - a fixed false idea or belief held by the client which cannot be corrected by reasoning and is not consistent with client's level of intelligence or cultural identity
- Hallucinations
  - apparent perception of external object not actually there involving any of the special senses, e.g., visual, auditory, third person auditory, voices arguing, commenting, commanding, gustatory, tactile, olfactory
- Disorder of experience of thought
  - *thought insertion:* client believes others are inserting, placing thoughts into his mind
  - *broadcasting:* person believes his thoughts are being broadcasted and that all are aware of what he is thinking
  - *blocking:* interruption of a train of speech as a result of the person losing his train of thought
- Experience of passivity
  - a delusional feeling that the person is under some outside control and therefore must be inactive
- Disturbance of speech
  - *tangential speech:* a style of speech containing oblique or irrelevant responses to questions asked, e.g. the person will talk about world hunger when asked about his breakfast
  - *poverty of content:* restriction of speech, so that spontaneous speech and replies to questions are brief and without elaboration
  - *word salad:* a characteristic of schizophrenia – a mixture of words that lack meaningful connections
- Emotional disturbance
  - *emotional flattening:* without normal 'highs' or 'lows' of feelings
  - *inappropriate affect:* incongruous responses to situations, e.g., laughing at hearing sad news
- Motor disturbance
  - excitement; bizarreness, in response to hallucinations; stupor

aware of his attendance and changes, and that appropriate referrals are made.

Kaiser & Pyngolil (1995) suggested that the following therapeutic principles be used in guiding the ED nurse caring for clients who are experiencing distortions in thought content and perception (that are often associated with great fear):

- attempt to establish a trusting relationship. The nurse should reassure the client that she wants to help and that the client is in a safe place and will not be harmed
- attempt to determine whether there was a precipitating event that triggered the psychotic episode. If so, evaluate it accordingly
- if an organic, reversible cause is identified, reassure the client that his feelings and thoughts are temporary
- minimize external stimulation. Psychotic people may be having trouble processing thoughts and often hear voices.

By decreasing external stimulation, the nurse may decrease sensory stimulation to which the client may be responding

- do not attempt to reason, challenge or argue the client out of his delusions or hallucinations. Often these clients need to believe their delusions in order to decrease their anxiety and maintain control
- the nurse should not imply that she believes the client's hallucinations or delusional system in an attempt to win his trust. Statements to the effect that the nurse does not hear these things the client is hearing but is interested in knowing about them are recommended
- do not underestimate the significance of a client's psychotic thoughts. They are very real to the client, and he cannot just 'put them aside'
- unless restraint is required, physical contact with psychotic clients or sudden movements should be avoided, as they may induce or validate the client's fears.

Puskar & Obus (1989) suggested the following questions be asked when assessing a possibly schizophrenic client:

- do your thoughts make sense to you?
- do you have ideas that come into your head that do not seem to be your own?
- do you worry about what other people think about you?
- do you think other people know what you are thinking?
- do you hear your own thoughts spoken out loud?
- do you sometimes feel that someone or some outside influence is controlling you, or making you think these things?

Once an organic cause has been ruled out, admission from ED will generally be required if the client is disturbed, suicidal/homicidal or experiencing command hallucinations telling him to harm himself. The prognosis with schizophrenia varies widely, as with any chronic disorder. Approximately 14–20 % will recover completely from an acute episode of psychosis. Others will improve but have recurrences (National Collaborating Centre for Mental Health 2010). There may be suicidal ideation; about 10 % of clients with schizophrenia will commit suicide within 5 years of the onset of their illness and about 30 % of people with schizophrenia attempt suicide at least once. Male clients and those who are unemployed, socially isolated, or recently discharged from hospital are most at risk (Doy et al. 2006, McAllister 2009).

Depression

Depression is a period of impaired functioning associated with low mood and related symptoms, including sleep and appetite changes, psychomotor changes, impaired concentration, fatigue, feelings of hopelessness, helplessness and suicide (Kaplan & Sadock 1993). Although estimates vary, approximately 20 % of women and 10 % of men will suffer from depression at some point in their lives. Community surveys indicate that 3–6 % of adults are suffering from depression at any one time (Merson & Baldwin 1995). While it is a condition that can affect any individual at any time of life, Barker (1999) suggests that it is most prevalent in the working age population. The prevalence is approximately 2–3 times higher in women than men.

Clinical features

Clinical features may include many of the following: depressed mood and affect; feelings of hopelessness, helplessness and worthlessness; guilt and inappropriate self-blame; suicidal ideation and intent; decreased energy and activity; agitation/stupor; psychomotor retardation; anorexia; weight loss; and early morning wakening/difficulty getting to sleep. In more severe cases the client may have somatic delusions and/or auditory hallucinations.

Nursing and medical management

Kaplan & Sadock (1993) proposed the following guidelines for evaluation and management of depression in the ED:

- treat any medical problems that may have resulted from suicide attempts or gestures
- maintain a safe environment for the client
- rule out organic and pharmacological causes of depression
- make an assessment of the severity of depression to determine the client's disposition.

It is important to convey an attitude of compassion, empathy and understanding to the depressed client (Moore & McLaughlin 2003). It is also worth reassuring the client that depression is reversible. However, it is pointless attempting to talk the client out of depression as he cannot snap out of it any more than he could snap out of a diabetic coma. The client's social networks should be identified and mobilized where appropriate. The client should be placed in a safe room, especially if he is at high risk of suicide. The room should be free of any objects that can be used to self-harm, e.g., glass, telephone cords etc. The client will need admission if he is suicidal, stuporous, hyper-agitated or lacks social support (De Gioannis & De Leo 2012). Referral to the psychiatric outclient department or other services should be arranged if the client does not require admission, and his GP and/or community psychiatric nurse (CPN) should be informed of the attendance at ED. The outlook for depression varies with the severity of the condition. For major depression approximately 80% of people who have received psychiatric care for an episode will have at least one more episode in their lifetime, with a median of four episodes. The outcome for those seen in primary care also seems to be poor, with only about a third remaining well over 11 years and about 20% having a chronic course (Anderson et al. 2000, King et al. 2008).

Antenatal and postnatal mental health problems

Mental disorder during pregnancy and the postnatal period can have serious consequences for the mother, her infant and other family members. ED nurses may be the first contact the pregnant woman may have with services in both the antenatal and postnatal periods. The assessing nurse should ask questions about past or present severe mental illness including schizophrenia, bipolar disorder, severe depression and psychosis in the postnatal period. Any previous treatment by a psychiatrist or specialist mental health team and whether there is a family history of mental illness (Heron et al. 2005, Lewis 2007, National Collaborating Centre for Mental Health 2007).

The assessing nurse should also ask the following two questions to identify possible depression:

1. during the past month, have you been bothered by feeling down, hopeless or depressed?
2. during the past month, have you been bothered by having little interest or pleasure in doing things?

If the woman answers yes to both the initial questions, the nurse should consider the following question:

- is this something you feel you need or want help with?

Women requiring psychological treatment should be referred for co-care between obstetric and mental health services and should be seen for treatment normally within one month of initial assessment. This is because of the lower threshold for access to psychological therapies during pregnancy and the postnatal period arising from the changing risk–benefit for psychotropic medication at this time.

In the postnatal period, the client may present with:

- acute organic reaction
- affective psychosis
- schizophreniform psychosis.

Affective puerperal disorder episodes may range from 'the blues' to a clinical depression severe enough to require admission.

Symptoms for *puerperal psychosis* may occur within two weeks to approximately nine months following the birth of a child. Postnatal depression is common; it has been estimated to affect 13% of women in the first year following the birth of their child, which equates to 70 000 women annually in the UK (Warner et al. 1996, Jones & Smith 2009). There may be clouding of consciousness, perplexity, delusions and hallucinations.

Management

If after assessment in ED the client can be managed on an outclient basis, adequate home support should be initiated and the presenting complaint treated as appropriate. Generally, clients presenting with puerperal psychosis or severe clinical depression will require admission from ED, and arrangements should be made for both mother and baby. Medication in the ED will need to be selective to prevent drugs being prescribed that are secreted in breast milk if the mother is breast-feeding. Although some cases of postnatal depression last less than three months, 30–50% may last for more than six months. If a mother develops postnatal depression in her first pregnancy, then she is at a 30% risk of recurrence with subsequent pregnancies.

Hypomania/mania/acute or chronic mania

Hypomania is the term used to describe a syndrome involving sustained and pathological elevation of mood, accompanied by other changes in function, such as disturbances of physical energy, sleep and appetite. Mania is a similar syndrome in which the client additionally holds delusional ideas, i.e., he is psychotic (Merson & Baldwin 1995). The client who frequently attends the ED does so when he has become too disruptive for family life. He may have a history of mania or depression, with his behaviour becoming increasingly disruptive over a few days. As a result, if mania is not controlled, the client is at risk of harming himself or others. Drugs such as steroids and amphetamines may also trigger mania.

Clinical features

The key component of manic disorders is a persistent elevation of mood. However, these feelings of euphoria and elation may vacillate with feelings of irritability and hostility. The client may experience racing of thoughts and pressure of speech and it may be very difficult to sustain conversations with clients in a manic state due to the constant pressure of bubbling and exciting ideas. Grandiose delusions are common and can lead to dangerous activities by the client; for instance, he may believe he (and others) can fly and want to jump off a building. Such clients are therefore at high risk of suicide or homicide and should be assessed accordingly.

Nursing and medical management

Nursing care of these clients must centre on protecting them and others from injury while measures to control mania are instituted. If the client has a history of mania, he is likely to be prescribed lithium carbonate. This is a metallic salt, identified as controlling mood swings in the 1970s. It has the ability to stabilize mood, thus reducing the possibility of elation and severe depression. If the client has had two or more episodes of mania in five years or less, it is likely he is on lithium therapy, and the levels and dosage may require adjustment as necessary (Dinan 2002). Lithium toxicity usually occurs at greater plasma concentration levels of 1.5 mmol/L Li$^+$, although it can occur at therapeutic levels (0.4–1.0 mmol/L Li$^+$).

Toxic levels may result from deliberate overdose, inappropriate usage or non-compliance. It can lead to electrolyte disturbance through water loss, diarrhoea, vomiting and polyuria. Early symptomatology also includes nausea, sweating, tremor and twitching. With plasma concentrations above 2.0 mmol/L (severe overdosage), symptoms displayed include convulsions, oliguria/renal failure and hypokalemia. ECG changes (inverted/flat T wave) may also be present. Lithium should be stopped and urea and electrolytes checked. The client should be admitted and haemodialysis or peritoneal dialysis may be required. In acute overdose much higher serum concentrations may be present without features of toxicity, and measures to increase urine production are necessary (Cipriani et al. 2005).

The manic client requires patience in handling and tolerant, tactful, kindly authority to make it as restful and unstimulating as is reasonably possible. It is essential to make appropriate arrangements to provide close observation and to protect the client from danger and over-exhausting himself. As this kind of close observation can be quite exhausting for staff, one-to-one nurse contact is advised, with each nurse taking turns for a maximum of 30 minutes each. The ED nurse must provide fluids and snacks of high calorific value for this client, in order to reduce the risk of dehydration and hypoglycemia.

Management of a manic client outside hospital is only possible when the client is sufficiently insightful to comply with treatment and where there is considerable and dependable informal support. Admission to hospital is usually indicated.

Bipolar disease

This is a major mental illness characterized by mood swings, alternating between periods of excitement and an overwhelming feeling of sadness, misery, gloom and despondency. Management in the ED is directed towards presenting symptoms (National Collaborating Centre for Mental Health 2006, Duffy et al. 2009, Saunders & Goodwin 2010, Elanjithara et al. 2011).

Anxiety states

Anxiety is an emotional sense of impending doom, a mental sense of unknown terror or fear of losing one's mind (Kaiser & Pyngolil 1995). The client may present to the ED when symptoms are no longer tolerable or when there is a marked deterioration in ability to carry out day-to-day activities. Clients may also present with panic attacks.

Clinical features

Anxiety is characterized by both psychological and physiological features (Merson & Baldwin 1995):

- psychological symptoms and signs
  - apprehensiveness
  - unfounded worrying
  - fearfulness
  - inner restlessness
  - irritability
  - exaggerated startle response
- physiological features
  - autonomic in origin, e.g., palpitation, breathlessness, epigastric discomfort, diarrhoea and urinary frequency
  - musculoskeletal, e.g., tension, stiffness and tremor.

Clients may be brought to ED with an acute anxiety attack, exhibiting signs associated with sympathetic nervous system stimulation, such as tachycardia, palpitations, sweaty palms and hyperventilation (Meuret & Ritz 2010). This change in respiration can produce serious biochemical changes due to the lowering in blood CO_2 levels that occurs with overbreathing. This in turn upsets the pH balance, making the blood more alkaline, which in turn upsets the calcium balance, causing muscle spasm (tetany) and tingling in the fingers. There is a characteristic carpopedal spasm of the fingers and abdominal cramps that are associated with hysterical hyperventilation. The effect is to make the client even more anxious and therefore more likely to hyperventilate. The solution is to reassure the client and encourage him to use a rebreathing bag to increase the CO_2 levels to normal as he rebreathes exhaled CO_2. After about 15 minutes, the respiratory rate will be back to normal and the muscle cramps will resolve (Walsh & Kent 2001).

Tachycardia is a common feature of anxiety attacks; however, in attempting to rule out organic causes of anxiety, it should be noted that tachycardia in clients experiencing anxiety attacks usually does not exceed 140 beats/min, whereas in paroxysmal supraventricular tachycardia the heartbeat is usually above 140 beats/min. In addition, supraventricular tachycardia is more likely to respond to vagal stimulation than tachycardia due to anxiety.

Nursing and medical management

The client may respond to explanation, reassurance and a feeling of security. Admission may be required to break the cycle; if medication is required, 10 mg diazepam i.v. is usually given. If admission is not required, the aim should be for symptomatic relief and psychological support. Reassure the client and allow him to discuss problems at his own pace. Arrange follow-up appointments for further treatment as appropriate.

Alcohol-related emergencies

Around 90% of the adult population drink alcohol at some time, 28% of men and 11% of women exceed safe levels of consumption, 1–2% of the population have alcohol problems and there are 200 000 dependent drinkers in the UK. Every year, the adverse effects of alcohol consumption lead to an estimated 1.2 million assaults, result in 150 000 hospital admissions and costs the NHS £1.7 billion (Smith & Allen 2004, Bellis et al. 2005, Fuller et al. 2009, National Collaborating Centre for Mental Health 2011).

Alcoholic clients may present with a variety of problems:

- intoxication
- withdrawal states – delirium tremens
- morbid jealousy
- alcoholic hallucinations
- physical consequences of alcohol abuse, e.g., tuberculosis, gastrointestinal bleed.

It is dangerous and unrealistic to attempt to conduct a satisfactory psychiatric interview when someone is intoxicated. While this may occasionally leave ED staff feeling frustrated, on-call psychiatrists or community psychiatric nurses (CPNs) will rarely attend ED while the client is intoxicated on the grounds that no meaningful psychiatric interview can take place. Clinical management of clients with alcohol intoxication is often confounded by the potentially disruptive and violent behaviour associated with intoxication.

Alcohol is a central nervous system (CNS) depressant. Measures of alcohol are described in units, with one unit being equal to half a pint of ordinary beer, one standard glass of wine or one-sixth of a gill of spirit (a pub measure) at 40% alcohol concentration. Blood alcohol concentration (BAC) is a measure of the amount of alcohol (mg) present in the bloodstream (per 100 mL), with a standard unit containing approximately 15 mg of alcohol. As with any drug, the effect of a certain dose will vary with the physical and psychological condition of the user (Kennedy & Faugier 1989). Degrees of intoxication may be classified as mild, moderate or severe.

Mild intoxication occurs in individuals with a BAC of up to 80 and is usually achieved with between one and five units. The typical reaction in an emotionally stable person is a feeling of warmth and cheerfulness accompanied by impairment of both judgement and inhibition. Apart from an increased susceptibility to accidents and the risk of post-intoxication headache and mild gastritis there is negligible health risk from a single episode of intoxication at these levels.

Moderate intoxication occurs in individuals with a BAC of between 80 and 150, who will exhibit a loss of self-control, slurred speech, double vision and memory loss. This is usually achieved with doses of up to 10 units. These symptoms are similar to those of raised intracranial pressure, diabetic hypoglycaemia and drug overdose. These and other possible aetiologies must therefore be excluded prior to such behaviour being ascribed purely to alcohol intoxication.

Accurate assessment and diagnosis of a client's condition at this level of intoxication may be confounded due to alcohol's desensitizing effect on pain response and its disruption to levels of consciousness. Other health problems from this level of intoxication include vomiting, severe gastritis, pancreatitis, hepatitis and interactions with medication and/or existing medical problems (Taylor & Ryrie 1996).

A BAC of between 200 and 400 leads to sleepiness, oblivion and coma, with possible cough reflex depression and airway obstruction from vomit or tongue. Such clients require constant neurological observation and may well require airway and cardiovascular support.

With a BAC of more than 400, death from severe CNS depression, particularly respiratory depression, is possible. Full emergency resuscitation with endotracheal intubation and cardiovascular support may be necessary. Stomach lavage should be considered with extreme caution since chronic alcohol abuse may result in peptic ulceration and/or oesophageal varices. In very severe alcohol poisoning, some clients may require transfer to intensive care units for haemodialysis or haemoperfusion. A BAC of over 600 is usually fatal and is generally only achieved by ingestion of large amounts of spirits.

Nursing management

Due to the behavioural component of moderate intoxication, these clients have the potential to become uncooperative, disruptive and violent, making assessment and treatment very difficult. Ballesteros et al. (2004) recommend a variety of behavioural management techniques that ED staff may employ in such situations. As with any client, a friendly interest and recognition as a person are essential. Staff are also advised to pace their interactions to suit the impaired cognitive processing of the client, allowing him to comprehend what is required or suggested. Intoxicated thinking often proceeds by association rather than logic. Key words such as 'let us work together' or involving the client in actions such as helping with dressings is recommended. Conversely, negative phrases such as 'you're not going to fight or give us trouble' are generally inflammatory, as the client may associate with the words 'fight' and 'trouble'. In addition, adopting a non-authoritarian but confident manner, acting calmly and quietly, separating opposing groups and removing the injured person from his accompanying friends are valuable approaches.

Levels of intoxication are not static but exist on a time continuum line in relation to blood concentration of the drug. Alcohol is metabolized at approximately one unit or 15 mg of blood alcohol per hour, which is slower than most people drink alcohol. Nurses should therefore be aware that clients can move rapidly from mild to life-threatening intoxication while in the ED as they absorb previously ingested alcohol and/or drugs. Conversely, the aforementioned behavioural problems associated with moderate intoxication may follow treatment for the physical effects of severe intoxication.

The easiest way to determine risk levels is to ask clients how much they drink. While there is a general belief that people are reluctant to accurately disclose their drinking patterns, there is good evidence to suggest this is not so and that information on the whole is sufficiently truthful (Watson 1996). Information should be sought in a sensitive but matter-of-fact way when asking about other lifestyle factors such as diet and smoking. Patterns of consumption are also important since a man who drinks 21 units on 1 or 2 days a week is likely to experience different problems from someone who drinks as much, but in smaller amounts, on a more regular basis.

A more subjective approach to assessment, which provides information on an individual's experience of his alcohol use, is the CAGE questionnaire, which includes the following four questions:

- have you ever felt you had to **C**ut down your alcohol intake?
- have you ever become **A**nnoyed by someone criticizing the amount of alcohol you drink?
- have you ever felt **G**uilty about how much alcohol you drink?
- have you ever used alcohol as an **E**ye-opener in the morning?

A positive response to two or more of these questions is considered to indicate an unhealthy attitude towards drinking that warrants some form of intervention (Kennedy & Faugier 1989).

Management of acute alcohol intoxication, the identification of potential problem drinkers and the provision of brief interventions do not require the skills of the specialist practitioner. Some basic knowledge and specific nursing actions are necessary, which may be employed as part of standard ED service provision; however, there is evidence to suggest that the profession, while acknowledging its role in the detection and management of alcohol-related problems, often fails to address such issues adequately (Watson 1996, Drummond et al. 2005).

Munchausen's syndrome and Munchausen's syndrome by proxy

This is characterized by a client frequently and repeatedly seeking admission, usually travelling to out-of-area ED units. Munchausen's syndrome and Munchausen's syndrome by proxy are characterized by a person simulating physical or mental illness, either in himself or, in the case of Munchausen's by proxy, in a third person, e.g., a child. The carer, usually the mother or both parents, fabricates symptoms or signs and then presents the child to hospital. There is an overlap with other forms of child abuse (see also Chapter 17).

The symptoms are supported by a plausible history and convincing physical signs. Motivation derives from a desire for attention. Physical examination may reveal multiple scars. Walsh (1996) identified five broad types of presentation by clients with Munchausen's syndrome:

- The *acute abdominal type* – these clients will manifest acute abdominal symptoms and swallow objects, including safety blades and safety pins, in order to obtain the surgery and hospitalization they crave. Nuts, bolts, coins and other paraphernalia are also swallowed. In well-documented cases, individuals have obtained well over 100 admissions and laparotomies in double figures.
- The *haemorrhagic type* – this presentation is characterized by complaints of bleeding from various orifices. One eye-watering approach is for the client to insert a coat hanger or needle into the penis, causing trauma and bleeding to the urethra. The positive test for haematuria, along with proclaimed symptoms of renal colic, usually leads to an injection of the desired analgesic agent. Presentations of haemoptysis and haematemesis are also lent further credibility by self-inflicted wounds to the back of the tongue with needles or razor blades.
- The *neurological type* – this type of the syndrome is characterized by clients presenting with convincing (and not so convincing) epileptic fits or complaints of migraine. Men more frequently present with pseudo-fits than women. The practice of sternal rubs and squeezing the nail bed with a biro smacks of punishment and cannot be condoned under any circumstances. A more humane and equally effective means of assessing a pseudo-fit is to gently stroke the eyelashes in an unsuspecting 'unconscious' client. It is difficult for them not to reflexively flicker their eyes, an action which would not occur in the genuinely unconscious client (Dolan 1998).
- The *cardiac type* – here, the client will present with a classic, textbook display of central chest pain, sometimes described as cardiopathia fantastica (Mehta & Khan 2002). Many such clients will be aware that intravenous morphine is administered for cardiac-related chest pain, hence their behaviour.
- The *psychiatric type* – in some instances, clients will imitate various forms of mental illness in order to gain admission to psychiatric units and hospitals.

Clinical features and management

The diagnosis is generally not apparent at first presentation, although characteristic features may be noticeable in retrospect:

- the client may be unwilling to provide significant personal details, such as an address or that of the next of kin
- clients may claim to be in transit and offer elaborate and seemingly implausible explanations for their movements (pseudologia fantastica)
- the presentation of symptoms may be classical, reflecting careful rehearsal, leading to retrospective opinions among professionals that symptoms were 'too good to be true'
- there may be signs of recent i.v. sites or cut-downs. Multiple abdominal scars should rate a very high probability of Munchausen's, especially if the first two points are present
- the client's manner and behaviour, especially when he thinks he is not being observed, give cause for suspicion (Walsh 1996)
- the client may have significant links with the healthcare profession, either through family connections or a paramedical occupation or as a result of prolonged hospital stays earlier in life (Merson & Baldwin 1995).

Management within the ED is usually difficult due to time restrictions on obtaining a full history. The client/carer, when confronted with the fictitious nature of the symptoms (his own or a third person's), usually discharges himself. Communication with other ED units and mobilization of services are required, e.g., the health visitor or GP.

Suicide and deliberate self-harm

Suicide occurs when a person knowingly brings about his own death. There are approximately 4000 suicides in England and Wales each year, equivalent to one death every two hours, and it is the third most common cause of death in people aged 15–30 years. In England the death rate from suicide is 8.6 deaths per 100 000 population. The majority of suicides continue to occur in young adult males, i.e., those under 40 years. In relation to women of the same age, younger men are more likely to commit suicide. The peak difference is the 30–39 age group, in which four males commit suicide to each female. Although women are more likely to be admitted to hospital following a suicide attempt, men complete suicide in considerably greater numbers with around three to four men completing suicide for every woman. While the suicide rate for women shows a gradual increase with age, men's suicide rate first peaks in middle adulthood, showing a marginal decline until the dramatic increase for the 75+ age group (Care Services Improvement Partnership/National Institute for Mental Health in England 2006a, National Collaborating Centre for Mental Health 2010, Da Cruz et al. 2011, Office for National Statistics 2011, De Gioannis & De Leo 2012). Among those with mental health problems, suicide is the single largest cause of premature death; 10 % of people with psychosis will ultimately kill

Box 15.4

High-risk factors associated with suicidal behaviour

Demographic factors
- Adolescence or older than 45 years
- Male
- White
- Protestant
- Separated, divorced or widowed
- Living alone
- Unemployed

Antecedent life circumstances
- Previous suicide attempts
  - recent attempt(s) with serious intent
  - previous attempt(s) with resultant physical or mental sequelae
  - previous attempt(s) that did not effect desired response(s)
- Family history of suicide or suicide attempts
- Inadequate or unavailable support systems
- Major life changes
  - major losses, e.g., spouse, job, money
  - major illness (of self or others)

Psychiatric conditions
- Depressive illnesses
- Alcoholism
- Schizophrenia

themselves, two-thirds within the first 5 years (Wiersma et al. 1998). Around the time of emerging psychosis, young females have a 150-times higher and young males a 300-fold higher risk for suicide than the general population (Care Services Improvement Partnership/National Institute for Mental Health in England 2006b, Bergen et al. 2010, Gwashavanhu 2010).

Deliberate self-harm (DSH), formerly known as parasuicide, is a non-fatal act of self-injury or the taking of substances in excess of the generally recognized or prescribed therapeutic dose. The incidence of self-harm, of which 90 % of cases involve self-poisoning, now accounts for 100 000 admissions to hospital per year, making DSH the most common reason for acute medical admission among women aged under 60 years (Crawford 2001).

Although potentially lethal drugs are regularly consumed, the overall hospital mortality rate is less than 1 %. Ryan et al. (1996) noted that there is a significant association between suicide and previous attendance at ED with deliberate self-harm. It is now commonly held that those who commit suicide and those who undertake acts of deliberate self-harm are two distinct groups (Vaughan 1985). Box 15.4 outlines the high-risk factors associated with suicidal behaviour; Box 15.5 highlights Beck's suicide scale, which has been used to identify the seriousness of suicidal intent; and Boxes 15.6 and 15.7 provide assessment tools of suicidal ideas and risk (Hughes & Owens 1996).

The risk of suicide is increased by a factor of 100 compared with that in the general population where there is both

Box 15.5

Beck's suicide risk scale

Preparation
- Act planned in advance
- Suicide note written
- Action in anticipation of death, for example, writing a will

Circumstances of the act
- Client was alone
- Timed such that intervention was unlikely
- Precautions taken against discovery

Sequelae of the act
- Did not seek help
- Stated wish to die
- Stated belief that the act would be proven fatal
- Sorry the act failed

(After Beck AT, Morris JB, Beck A (1974) Cross-validation of the suicidal intent scale. Psychological Reports, 34(2), 445–446.)

Box 15.6

The assessment of suicidal ideas: progressively specific questions
- How do you see the future?
- Do you ever feel hopeless, like giving up?
- Do things ever seem so bad that you feel you cannot go on?
- Have you ever wished you could go to sleep and not wake up?
- Have you ever thought of doing anything to harm yourself?
- Have you made any plans for that?
- Have you done anything about it?

Box 15.7

Assessing suicidal risk following deliberate self-harm
- What happened before and during the self-harm event?
- Did the client intend to die?
- Does the client still intend to die?
- Does the client have a psychiatric disorder?
- What are the client's problems?
- What are the client's resources for dealing with this crisis?

a recent history of deliberate self-harm and persistent, distressing suicidal ideation. Many of the suicide intent scales depend on the balance between lethality and rescuability (Pritchard 1995). Lethality is the medical danger to life; methods such as shooting and jumping from a high building have high lethality values, whereas a tranquillizer overdose will have a lower lethality value. Conversely, someone who takes an overdose of tranquillizers and alcohol and then disappears into the sea has a low likelihood of rescuability. The person who is drunk and attempts to take a large number of tablets in front of their partner has a high likelihood of rescue. The overall level of intent depends on the balance between lethality and rescuability (Jones 1995).

Obtaining a history from a client following a suicide attempt is frequently very difficult. The client may also give false information to avoid embarrassment. A client has the right to refuse treatment, and any treatment which is enforced on a client is considered assault or battery (Dimond 2004). Under common law, treatment can be given without the consent of the client in cases of necessity: circumstances in which immediate action is required and necessary to preserve life or prevent a serious or immediate danger to the client or others. The treatment or physical restraint used must be reasonable and sufficient only to the purpose of bringing the emergency to an end. Medical treatment should be administered under the specific direction of a medical practitioner (Hughes & Owens 1996). This duty is imposed by statute and the Nursing and Midwifery Council (2008) *Code: Standards of conduct, performance and ethics* and is underpinned by the principles of civil law relating to negligence, including the Mental Capacity Act 2005 (Gertz et al. 2006).

The feelings of ED staff towards clients with self-inflicted injuries appear to be predominantly negative (Celenza 2004). Ward (1995) recommends that the nurse seeks to make sense of the client's behaviour from the client's point of view, rather than the nurse's. The key to a successful nurse/client relationship lies in establishing a positive rapport from the initial assessment. A strategy for achieving this was suggested by Burnard (1990) in relation to interviewing technique. He proposed the acronym 'SOLER' to remind the interviewer of the following:

- *s*it squarely opposite the client, not behind a desk, and avoid distraction
- *o*pen positioning, feet apart and palms resting on thighs
- *l*ean forward towards the client
- *e*ye contact – show attention and give feedback. This helps to establish a relationship. No staring or glaring
- *r*elax – tension or fidgeting may convey impatience or lack of interest.

This position helps to make the nurse appear warm and empathetic. By adopting this strategy the nurse should be able to dissociate herself from prejudicial feelings, and the client is more likely to feel accepted and worthwhile.

If the client is determined to be at continued risk, the nurse should not leave him alone. If the client is considered to be at high risk and is not willing to accept hospitalization, involuntary admission will be necessary. If doubt exists, caution should be exercised and admission arranged.

Self-mutilation

Destructive acts against the self, such as putting a fist through a window and wrist cutting, may occur as behaviour secondary to personality problems. Clients are usually in their 20s or 30s and may be single or married. Most clients who cut themselves have a history of self-injury. The wrists, arms and thighs are common sites, and instruments such as razor blades, knives, broken glass or mirrors may be used. The wounds are usually relatively superficial and the client may describe how the act brings relief of tension and depersonalization. Clients who self-mutilate tend to have low self-esteem but the lethality of the intent is usually low.

Nursing management

Treatment in ED should revolve around immediate care of the injury, evaluating the risk of suicide, protecting the client from further self-harm and assisting in crisis resolution (Repper 1999). Clients who attend regularly following acts of deliberate self-harm may leave staff feeling frustrated and hostile towards them. However, such beliefs and attitudes must not be allowed to interfere with the care of the client. The environment of care should be supportive and non-confrontational for clients who deliberately self-harm, and care should be delivered non-judgementally. Given the degree of aggression that is channelled internally into acts of deliberate self-harm, the ED nurse should also exercise caution when caring for these clients as the aggressive tendencies exhibited may be directed towards staff. Referral to appropriate agencies, such as CPNs, is encouraged so that the client can ventilate and discuss feelings and explore other ways of coping more appropriately (Brookes & Leach 2004).

Individuals at odds with society (sociopathy)

Sociopathy refers to a group of well-defined anomalies or deviations of personality that are not the result of either psychotic or any other illness. Numerous theories have been put forward as to why this disorder should develop (Bowlby 1965, Cleckly 1967).

The client may present to the ED with depression, suicidal gestures, abuse of drugs, alcohol and sex, or as a result of aggressive and violent behaviour and lack of impulse control, etc. Management requires a complete history to be taken to exclude epilepsy, hypoglycaemia or any other acute organic reaction. Treatment is directed at managing the presenting condition with a firm and consistent approach. Reference to mental health teams is as appropriate.

Violent clients

Violence or threats of violence may be associated with a variety of disorders, e.g., psychosis, chemical intoxication, sociopathy, etc., or with a specific situation, such as lack of communication. The nurse should be alert for violence, particularly if the client has a previous history of violent behaviour or poor impulse control, if he has been brought in by the police or if he is verbally or physically threatening.

There are several management points in the ED:

- always manage the client with the required number of staff to do so appropriately and beware of uniform limitations

- be familiar with the alarm/security system
- if entering a room, do so letting a colleague know where you are; see the client in a non-isolated room and leave yourself and the client an exit
- maintain a quiet, calm but firm approach; avoid any contact which may be misinterpreted
- monitor both your own and the client's reactions.

Management

If circumstances allow, try to establish whether a psychiatric disorder is present: is the client demanding; is conscious level fluctuating? If a psychiatric disorder is present, assess the need for admission and suitability of facilities available. Give medication as appropriate.

If no clinical reason for admission is elicited and the client remains disruptive, security and/or the police should be contacted (see also Chapter 12).

Learning disability clients and mental health problems

Clients with learning disabilities may present with:

- self-mutilation
- depression
- schizophrenia
- anxiety.

The client should be assessed as appropriate and a history taken from the escort. If admission is not required, referral to local learning disability services and social services may be required to provide an emergency service. If behaviour is disturbed and the client requires medications, low doses of neuroleptics should be given because of susceptibility to side-effects (see also Chapter 33).

Elderly clients presenting to the ED with mental health problems

Psychiatric emergencies arising de novo or superimposed upon dementia include:

- acute confusional states
- mania (usually a history of bipolar disease is present)
- depression and deliberate self-harm
- paranoid disorder.

In healthcare for the elderly, the decision as to whether to admit a client is usually made after careful assessment. Ideally, problems presented by the elderly client will be assessed by the healthcare for the elderly team (mental health) on a domiciliary visit. In reality, elderly clients may be referred or present directly to the ED. Therefore the nurse must be alert to social admission. Dementia per se is not a sole reason for admission.

Assessment should be directed towards:

- evidence of an acute organic reaction, such as recent confusion, disorientation etc.
- in the absence of an acute organic reaction, whether mental illness is present, e.g., clinical depression, paranoid psychosis
- strength of family support, if any; respite need
- whether behaviour is disturbed.

If admission is necessary, the appropriate team should be contacted. If immediate treatment is required, medication should be limited to low doses, particularly if there is evidence of renal or hepatic improvement (see also Chapter 22).

Child and adolescent psychiatry

Children and adolescents will present to ED as emergency referrals. The ED nurse should be familiar with the procedure to contact the duty child and adolescent mental health team and management should be discussed with them. Any child or adolescent present with psychiatric pathology should be taken as seriously as any other age group and managed according to the presenting condition (Kaplan 2009).

Common psychiatric presentations include:

- chemical abuse
- suicidal behaviour/deliberate self-harm
- depression – reactive and endogenous
- early schizophrenia
- adolescent behavioural disorders
- eating and nutrition disorders.

Management

Management is based on the following:

- assess, treat and admit as appropriate
- referral to child psychiatric team
- support and reassurance for the client and family
- institute appropriate follow-up.

Clients attending the ED with eating disorders

The most common of eating disorders are:

- anorexia nervosa
- bulimia nervosa
- compulsive eating/food addiction – severe overweight.

Clients with eating disorders may present to the ED with problems such as osteoporotic fractures, collapse, infection, dehydration, oedema, cardiac failure, fatigue, cyanosis, bradycardia, hypotension, weight loss, obesity, hypoglycaemia, hypocalcaemia/kalaemia, infertility, amenorrhoea, constipation and vomiting, or may be referred by dental practitioners for dental problems. In addition, they may present with agitation, depression or acopia.

Management

Treatment is aimed at the presenting symptoms and includes a complete physical work-up. Admission in the acute phase is usually required. In the ED, basic nursing care as well as care of malnutrition/dehydration needs to be addressed.

Social problems

Some people tend to use ED as a crisis walk-in clinic, e.g., someone who has become acutely disturbed or who is blamed as the cause of a crisis and is brought to ED as the client (Brookes & Leach 2004). Although these incidents may not be true psychiatric emergencies, the ED is seen as a 24-hour emergency unit when no other help or assistance is perceived to be available. The presence of an impartial observer and environment may enable the client and his family/carers to discuss the problems for the first time. Referral to agencies for follow-up is required, e.g., to counselling services in general and/or for specific needs, such as HIV, rape, social worker or probation officer.

Other social problems that may present to the ED are those people searching for a trolley, bed, shelter or food, often with no apparent psychiatric or medical illness. These clients can be very difficult or manipulative and require limit-setting and firm handling. The opportunity to discuss problems may help but the nurse should attempt to clarify what type of assistance the person requires and be familiar with telephone numbers of agencies able to help, such as crisis centres, social security, local hostels, emergency social workers, etc.

Acute stress reaction

This is a common, normal response to an unwanted situation and may last days to weeks and may be triggered by exposure to a traumatic event. It may develop into a more severe disorder such as simple/complex PTSD. Simple or complex PTSD can manifest itself both physically and mentally and may present with a variety of symptoms that usually appear within 6 months of the traumatic event and/or co-morbidity, e.g., alcohol/chemical dependency, sleep problems, fear and anxiety, tearfulness, sadness, helplessness, anger, irritability, guilt, concentration/memory problems, body pains, avoidance/numbness and unpleasant intrusive thoughts/flashbacks/nightmares and hypervigilance.

The onset of a stress response is associated with specific physiological actions in the sympathetic nervous system, both directly and indirectly through the release of epinephrine and to a lesser extent nor-epinephrine from the medulla of the adrenal glands. The release is triggered by acetylcholine released from pre-ganglionic sympathetic nerves. These catecholamine hormones cause an immediate physical reaction by triggering increases in heart rate and breathing, peripheral vasoconstriction or vasodilatation (see Chapter 23). In the ED, management will depend on the presenting symptoms and referral for cognitive behavioural therapy may be appropriate (National Institute of Health and Clinical Excellence 2006) (see Chapter 13).

Iatrogenic drug-induced psychosis

Non-specific psychosis may occur, including mania, delirium, schizophreniform psychosis or depression in clients on maintenance therapy for a physical condition, e.g., Cushing's syndrome. If a client's condition precludes reducing the dose of medication, antipsychotic agents can be administered concurrently to control symptoms.

Psychotropic drugs have served to revolutionize the treatment and care of the mentally ill. However, these drugs can also have side-effects which may require management in the ED. All antipsychotic agents may produce acute dystonias, akathisia, parkinsonism, and akinesia.

Acute dystonia

Symptoms usually occur one hour to five days after commencement of antipsychotic medication, especially with high-potency neuroleptics such as haloperidol or trifluoperazine. Dystonic reactions are prolonged tonic contractions of muscle groups. When the muscles of the neck, tongue and jaw are involved, this is called torticollis. Torticollis combined with contractions of the extraocular muscles, whereby the eyes are rolled upwards with the head turned to one side, is called occulogyric crisis.

Although these muscle contractions can be very frightening for the client, they can usually be easily reversed with the intramuscular administration of 2 mg of benztropine mesylate or 10 mg of procyclidine. The nurse should stay with the client and provide reassurance that the reaction can be reversed usually within 5–20 minutes of injection.

Akathisia

Symptoms of akathisia usually occur within 2–3 months of commencement of medication. The client complains of an inability to sit still, pacing and fidgeting. While this is not an emergency, it can be distressing for the client and be mistaken for agitation associated with the client's primary disorder. Anti-parkinsonian agents such as benztropine mesylate provide relief.

Akinesia

Akinesia is an extrapyrimidal reaction characterized by signs and symptoms of decreased motor activity. The client experiences fatigue and muscle weakness. It can easily be controlled with an anti-parkinsonian agent (Kaiser & Pyngolil 1995).

Monoamine oxidase inhibitors (MAOIs)

MAOIs inhibit monamine oxidase, therefore causing an accumulation of amine neurotransmitters. The metabolism of some amine drugs and tyramine found in some foods may cause a dangerous rise in the blood pressure. MAOIs also interact with opiates, lithium and tricyclic antidepressants. The danger of interaction persists for up to 14 days after treatment with MAOIs is discontinued.

Hypertensive crisis may occur if MAOIs are taken in combination with:

- amphetamines
- appetite suppressants
- dietary amines, cheese, marmite, broad beans, chocolate, bananas, Chianti wine, whisky, beer, caffeinated tea or coffee
- proprietary cold and allergy remedies containing sympathomimetics, e.g., adrenaline, phenylephrine.

Hypertensive crisis is characterized by the sudden onset of severe throbbing headache, nausea, vomiting and dizziness. The client's blood pressure can be as high as 350/250 mmHg, and chest and neck pain, palpitations and malignant hyperthermia, the usual cause of death in clients experiencing hypertensive crisis, may occur.

Nursing and medical management

Hypertensive crisis is an emergency, and therefore the client's vital signs should be monitored closely and 12–15 L of oxygen administered via a tight-fitting reservoir mask. Intravenous phentolamine 5–10 mg should be given to reduce the client's blood pressure and repeated as necessary. Supportive measures include forced diuresis, and therefore urine output should be monitored. Hypertensive crisis should resolve 1–3 hours after initiation of treatment.

Serotonin syndrome is a rare but potentially life-threatening adverse drug reaction that results from intentional self-poisoning, therapeutic drug use or inadvertent interactions between drugs. It is a consequence of excess serotonergic activity in the central nervous system and peripheral serotonin receptors. This excess serotonin activity produces a specific spectrum of clinical findings which may range from barely perceptible to being fatal (Boyer et al. 2005, Prator 2006).

Serotonin syndrome can arise from other drug interactions that do not involve MAOIs. Selective serotonin reuptake inhibitors (SSRIs) are a class of antidepressant medication that is widely prescribed for the use of depression and anxiety, these include paroxetine, fluoxetine, sertraline and cipramil. These alone can cause serotonin syndrome or more commonly if taken in combination with other drugs:

- antidepressants – MAOIs, mirtazapine, paroxetine, fluoxetine
- analgesics – pethidine, fentanyl, oxycodone, tramadol
- anti-emetics – metoclopromide and ondansetron

- illicit drugs – cocaine, MDMA, LSD, amphetamine and methamphetamine.

There is no laboratory test for serotonin syndrome, so diagnosis is by symptom observation and the client's medical and pharmaceutical history. It may go unrecognized as it can be mistaken for a viral illness, anxiety, neurological disorder or worsening psychiatric condition.

Symptoms are often described as a clinical triad of abnormalities:

- cognitive effects; mental confusion, hypomania, hallucinations, agitation, headache, coma
- autonomic effects; hyperpyrexia, shivering, sweating, fever, hypertension, tachycardia, nausea, diarrhoea; late-stage presentation may include rhabdomyolosis, metabolic acidosis, seizures, renal failure and disseminated intravascular coagulation
- somatic effects: muscle twitching (myoclonus/clonus), hyperreflexia, and tremor.

There is no antidote to the condition itself and management involves removing the precipitating drug and the initiation of supportive therapy (control of agitation, autonomic instability, hyperthermia) and the administration of serotonin antagonists.

The clinical features of neurolepetic malignant syndrome and serotonergic syndrome are very similar, thus making diagnosis very difficult. Features that classically present in narcoleptic malignant syndrome that are useful for differentiating the two syndromes are: fever and muscle rigidity (Inott 2009).

Conclusion

Psychiatric emergencies present a particular challenge to ED nurses as they may be a result of physical or functional disorders and increasingly present for the first time to EDs for initial management. There has been a recent increase in the number of liaison psychiatric nurses working within the ED. Among other responsibilities, referrals may be made to them for assessment of clients attending the ED with non-life-threatening deliberate self-harm injuries. They also have a major role in the assessment and management of behaviourally disturbed clients who are referred to the ED or are self-referrals. They have particular skills on advising on the management of psychotic or suicidal clients and can advise the ED team appropriately. This chapter has considered the more common psychiatric emergencies and identified a range of interventions for nurses to employ when caring for these distressed and frequently distressing clients. Recognizing and understanding these emergencies will help the nurse meet the challenges of psychiatric emergency care in the ED.

References

Anderson, I.M., Nutt, D.J., Deakin, J.F., 2000. Evidence-based guidelines for treating depressive disorders with antidepressants: a revision of the 1993 British Association for Psychopharmacology guidelines. British Journal of Psychopharmacology 14 (1), 3–20.

Andrew-Starkey, S., 2004. Mental State Examination. In: Cameron, P., Jelinek, G., Kelly, A.M., Murray, L., Brown, A.F.T., Heyworth, J. (Eds.), Textbook of Emergency Medicine, second ed. Churchill Livingstone, Edinburgh.

Ballesteros, J., Gonzales-Pinto, A., Querejeta, I., et al., 2004. Brief interventions for hazardous drinkers delivered in primary care are equally effective in men and women. Journal of Addiction 99 (1), 3–20.

Barker, P., 1999. Therapeutic nursing of the person in depression. In: Clinton, M., Nelson, S. (Eds.), Advanced Practice in Mental Health Nursing. Blackwell Science, Oxford.

Beck, A.T., Morris, J.B., Beck, A., 1974. Cross-validation of the suicidal intent scale. Psychological Reports 34 (2), 445–446.

Bellis, M.A., Hughes, K., McVeigh, J., et al., 2005. Effects of nightlife activity on health. Nursing Standard 19 (30), 63–71.

Bergen, H., Hawton, K., Waters, K., et al., 2010. Psychosocial assessment and repetition of self-harm: The significance of single and multiple repeat episode analyses. Journal of Affective Disorders 127 (2010), 257–265.

Bowlby, J., 1965. Child Care and the Growth of Love. Penguin, Harmondsworth.

Boydell, J., Van Os, J., Lambri, M., et al., 2003. Incidence of schizophrenia in south-east London between 1965 and 1997. British Journal of Psychiatry 182, 45–49.

Boyer, E.W., Shannon, M., 2005. Current concepts: The Serotonin Syndrome. The New England Journal of Medicine 352 (11), 1112–1122.

Brookes, J.G., Leach, D.S., 2004. Crisis intervention in the emergency department. In: Cameron, P., Jelinek, G., Kelly, A.M., Murray, L., Brown, A.F.T., Heyworth, J. (Eds.), Textbook of Emergency Medicine, second ed. Churchill Livingstone, Edinburgh.

Burnard, P., 1990. Learning Human Skills: an Experiential Guide for Nurses. Heinemann, Oxford.

Care Services Improvement Partnership/ National Institute for Mental Health in England, 2006a. National Suicide Prevention Strategy for England: Annual Report on Progress 2005. Care Services Improvement Partnership, London.

Care Services Improvement Partnership/ National Institute for Mental Health in England, 2006b. 10 High Impact Changes for Mental Health Services. Care Services Improvement Partnership, London.

Celenza, A., 2004. Deliberate self harm/suicide. In: Cameron, P., Jelinek, G., Kelly, A.M., Murray, L., Brown, A.F.T., Heyworth, J. (Eds.), Textbook of Emergency Medicine, second ed. Churchill Livingstone, Edinburgh.

Cipriani, A., Pretty, H., Hawton, K., et al., 2005. Lithium in the prevention of suicidal behavior and all-cause mortality in patients with mood disorders: a systematic review of randomized trials. American Journal of Psychiatry 162, 1805–1819.

Cleckly, B., 1967. The Mask of Sanity. Basic Books, New York.

Crawford, M., 2001. Psychological management following deliberate self harm. Clinical Medicine 1 (3), 185–187.

Da Cruz, D., Pearson, A., Saini, P., et al., 2011. Emergency department contact prior to suicide in mental health patients. Emergency Medicine Journal 28, 467–471.

De Gioannis, A., De Leo, D., 2012. Managing suicidal patients in clinical practice. Open Journal of Psychiatry 2 (1), 49–60.

Dimond, B., 2004. Legal Aspects of Nursing, fourth ed. Prentice Hall, Hemel Hempstead.

Dinan, T.G., 2002. Lithium in bipolar mood disorder. British Medical Journal 324 (7344), 989–990.

Dolan, B., 1998. The hospital hoppers. Nursing Times 94 (30), 26–27.

Doy, R., Blowers, E.J., Sutton, E., 2006. The ABC of Community Emergency Care: 16 mental health. Emergency Medicine Journal 23, 304–312.

Drummond, D.C., Oyefeso, N., Phillips, T., et al., 2005. Alcohol Needs Assessment Research Project: The 2004 National Alcohol Needs Assessment for England. Department of Health, London.

Duffy, A., Alda, M., Hajek, T., et al., 2009. Early course of bipolar disorder in high-risk offspring: prospective study. British Journal of Psychiatry 195, 457–458.

Elanjithara, T.E., Frango, S., McGuire, P., 2011. Treatment of the early stages of bipolar disorder. Advances in Psychiatry 17, 283–291.

Fuller, E., Jotangia, D., Farrell, M., 2009. Alcohol misuse and dependence. In: McManus, S., Meltzer, H., Brugha, T. (Eds.), Adult Psychiatric Morbidity in England, 2007 Results of a Household Survey. NHS Information Centre for Health and Social Care, Leeds.

Gertz, R., Harmon, S., Laurie, G., et al., 2006. Developments in medical law in the United Kingdom in 2005 and 2006. European Journal of Health Law 13, 143–158.

Gournay, K., Beadsmore, A., 1995. The report of the Clinical Standards Advisory Group: standards of care for people with schizophrenia in the UK and implications for mental health nursing. Journal of Mental and Psychiatric Nursing 2, 359–364.

Guidelines and Audit Implementation Network, 2010. Guidelines on caring for people with a learning disability in general hospital settings. GAIN, Belfast.

Gwashavanhu, C., 2010. Demographics of people who self harm deliberately. Emergency Nurse 18 (8), 28–32.

Heron, J., Craddock, N., Jones, I., 2005. Postnatal euphoria: Are 'the highs' an indication of bipolarity? Bipolar Disorders 7, 103–110.

Hughes, T., Owens, D., 1996. Management of suicidal risk. British Journal of Hospital Medicine 56 (4), 151–154.

Inott, T.J., 2009. The dark side of SSRIs selective serotonin reuptake inhibitors. Nursing Management 40 (11), 44–46.

Jones, L., 1995. Assessing suicide risk in A&E. Emergency Nurse 2 (4), 7–9.

Jones, I., Smith, S., 2009. Puerperal psychosis: Identifying and caring for women at risk. Advances in Psychiatric Treatment 15 (6), 411–418.

Kaiser, J., Pyngolil, M.J., 1995. Psychiatric emergencies. In: Kitt, S., Selfridge-Thomas, J., Proehl, J.A., Kaiser, J. (Eds.), Emergency Nursing: a Physiologic and Clinical Perspective, second ed. WB Saunders, Philadelphia.

Kaplan, H.I., Sadock, B.J., 1993. Pocket Handbook of Emergency Psychiatric Medicine. Wilkins & Wilkins, Baltimore.

Kaplan, T., 2009. Emergency Department Handbook: Children and adolescents with mental health problems. RCPsych Publications, London.

Kennedy, J., Faugier, J., 1989. Drug and Alcohol Dependency Nursing. Heinemann Nursing, Oxford.

King, M., Walker, C., Levy, G., et al., 2008. Development and validation of an international risk prediction algorithm for episodes of major depression in general practice attendees: The PredictD study. Archives of General Psychiatry. 65, 1368–1376.

Lewis, G., (Ed.), 2007. The Confidential Enquiry into Maternal and Child Health (CEMACH). Saving Mothers' Lives: Reviewing Maternal Deaths to Make Motherhood Safer–2003–2005. In: The Seventh Report on Confidential Enquiries into Maternal Deaths in the United Kingdom. RCOG Press, London.

Mackway-Jones, K., Marsden, J., Windle, J., 2005. Emergency Triage, second ed. Blackwell Publishing, Oxford.

McAllister, M., Billett, S., Zimmer-Gembeck, M., 2009. 'I can actually talk to them now': qualitative results of an educational intervention for emergency nurses caring for clients who self-injure. Journal of Clinical Nursing 18, 2838–2845.

McManus, S., Meltzer, H., Brugha, T., et al., 2007. Adult Psychiatric Morbidity in England, 2007: Results of a Household Survey. The Information Centre for Health and Social Care, Leeds.

Mehta, N.J., Khan, I.A., 2002. Cardiac Munchausen syndrome. Chest 122 (5), 1649–1653.

Merson, S., Baldwin, D., 1995. Psychiatric Emergencies. Oxford University Press, Oxford.

Meuret, A.E., Ritz, T., 2010. Hyperventilation in panic disorder and asthma: Empirical evidence and clinical strategies. International Journal of Psychophysiology 78 (1), 68–79.

Moore, K., McLaughlin, D., 2003. Depression: the challenge for all healthcare professionals. Nursing Standard 17 (26), 45–52.

National Collaborating Centre for Mental Health, 2006. Bipolar Disorder: The Management of Bipolar Disorder in Adults, Children and Adolescents. Primary And Secondary Care. The British Psychological Society and The Royal College of Psychiatrists, London.

National Collaborating Centre for Mental Health, 2007. Antenatal and Postnatal Health. The British Psychological Society and The Royal College of Psychiatrists, London.

National Collaborating Centre for Mental Health, 2010. Schizophrenia: Core Interventions in the Treatment and Management of Schizophrenia in Adults in Primary and Secondary Care (updated edition). The British Psychological Society and The Royal College of Psychiatrists, London.

National Collaborating Centre for Mental Health, 2011. Alcohol-Use Disorders: Diagnosis, Assessment and Management of Harmful Drinking and Alcohol Dependence. The British Psychological Society and The Royal College of Psychiatrists, London.

National Institute of Health and Clinical Excellence, 2006. Computerized Cognitive Behaviour Therapy for Depression and Anxiety. NIHCE, London.

National Institute for Health and Clinical Excellence, 2011. Common Mental Health Disorders: Identification and Pathways to Care. NIHCE, London.

Nicholls, D., Gaynor, N., Shafei, T., et al., 2011. Mental health nursing in emergency departments: the case for a nurse practitioner role. Journal of Clinical Nursing 20, 530–536.

Nursing and Midwifery Council, 2008. Code: Standards of Conduct, Performance and Ethics. Nursing and Midwifery Council, London.

Office for National Statistics, 2011. Suicide rates in the United Kingdom 2000–2009. Office for National Statistics, London.

Prator, B., 2006. Serotonin syndrome. Journal of Neuroscience Nursing 38 (2), 102–106.

Pritchard, C., 1995. Suicide – The Ultimate Rejection? A Psychosocial Study. Open University Press, Buckingham.

Puskar, K.R., Obus, N.L., 1989. Management of the psychiatric emergency. Nurse Practitioner 14 (7), 9–10, 12, 14, 16, 18, 23, 26.

Repper, J., 1999. A review of the literature on the prevention of suicide interventions in accident and emergency departments. Journal of Clinical Nursing 8 (1), 3–12.

Richards, M., Maughan, B., Hardy, R., et al., 2001. Long-term affective disorder in people with mild intellectual disability. British Journal of Psychiatry 179, 523–527.

Ryan, J., Rushdy, A., Perez-Avilla, C.A., et al., 1996. Suicide rate following attendance at an accident and emergency department with deliberate self harm. Journal of Accident and Emergency Medicine 13, 101–104.

Saunders, K.E.A., Goodwin, G.M., 2010. The course of bipolar disorder. Advances in Psychiatric Treatment 16, 318–328.

Smith, C., Allen, J., 2004. Violent Crime in England and Wales. Home Office, London.

Taylor, R., Ryrie, I., 1996. Clinical management of acute and chronic alcohol use in A&E. Emergency Nurse 4 (3), 6–8.

Vaughan, P., 1985. Suicide Prevention. PEPAR, Birmingham.

Walsh, M., 1996. Accident & Emergency Nursing: A New Approach, third ed. Butterworth Heinemann Ltd, London.

Walsh, M., Kent, A., 2001. Accident & Emergency Nursing: A New Approach, fourth ed. Butterworth Heinemann Ltd, London.

Ward, M., 1995. Nursing the Psychiatric Emergency. Butterworth-Heinemann, Oxford.

Warner, R., Appleby, L., Whitton, A., Faragher, B., 1996. Demographic and obstetric risk factors for postnatal psychiatric morbidity. British Journal of Psychiatry 168 (5), 607–611.

Watson, H., 1996. Minimal interventions for problem drinkers. Journal of Substances Misuse for Nursing, Health and Social Care 1 (2), 107–110.

Wiersma, D., Nienhuis, F.J., Slooff, C.J., et al., 1998. Natural course of schizophrenic disorders: a 15-year follow-up of a Dutch incidence cohort. Schizophrenia Bulletin 24, 75–85.

PART 4

Life continuum

Infants

16

Samantha Minett and Matthew Stuart

CHAPTER CONTENTS

Introduction

The emergency care of infants requires specific knowledge and skills that can only be gained through study, training and experience. Infancy is defined as the first year of life, with 0–28 days being the neonatal period. Whilst there are some commonalities for assessing patients across all age ranges, it is essential to recognize that infants present with a different range of illnesses and injury patterns from older children and adults. This is due to anatomical and physiological differences and immaturity of the immune system; consequently, different management is required (Table 16.1). There can be little doubt that sick or injured infants are one of the most challenging patient cohorts presenting to the Emergency Department (ED) and parental anxiety can contribute significantly to the challenge. In a typical year up to 50 % of infants will attend an ED (Department of Health 2004). Parental concern should always be taken seriously and the emergency nurse should seek to reassure the accompanying adults by displaying a calm, confident and efficient demeanour, being attentive to their concerns and addressing them accordingly. Infants presenting to the ED with a worrying history may appear quite well at the time they are assessed. Parents should never be

Table 16.1 Emergency nurse considerations for the care of infants

Factor	Nursing considerations
Airway	
Infants <6 months are obligate nose breathers	Airway is easily obstructed by nasal secretions – saline drops and the judicious use of suctioning may assist
Large tongue	Airway is easily obstructed by tongue; jaw-thrust manoeuvre may be needed to lift tongue forward in obtunded patients
Soft palate is easily compressible	Requires care during airway opening manoeuvres/bag-valve-mask ventilation
Narrower airways	Small amounts of mucus or swelling easily obstruct the airways; the smaller the airway the greater the resistance to airflow
Cartilage of larynx and trachea are softer than in adults	Airway of infant can be compressed if neck is flexed or hyperextended
Cricoid cartilage is narrowest portion of trachea which is funnel-shaped	Foreign body may become lodged at this point. Provides a natural seal for endotracheal tube
Breathing	
Sternum and ribs are cartilaginous; chest wall is soft and pliable	A significant force may result in an injury to underlying structures (e.g., liver/lungs) without rib fracture. Infant's chest wall prone to recession when lung compliance is decreased
Diaphragm is the primary muscle of respiration	Respiratory rate is best measured by observation of abdominal movement
Higher metabolic rate	Respiratory rates are faster to meet increased demand
Circulation	
Infant's circulating blood volume is greater per unit of body weight, but absolute volume is relatively small	Blood loss considered minor in an adult may lead to shock in an infant
70–80% of a newborn's body weight is water, compared to 50–60% of an adult body weight, about half of this volume is extracellular	Decreased fluid intake or increased fluid loss quickly leads to dehydration
Infants compensate against hypovolaemia by increasing the heart rate and peripheral vascular resistance	Tachycardia, poor peripheral perfusion and delayed CRT are indicative of compensating shock. Hypotension is a late sign of deterioration
Thermoregulation	
Proportionately greater body surface area and less subcutaneous tissue for heat insulation. Infants have immature thermoregulatory centre	Infants quickly lose heat when exposed
Other	
The liver is more anterior and less protected by the ribs	
The kidneys are more mobile and not protected by fat	
The head is heavier and larger in relation to the rest of the body	Increased risk of head and neck trauma (spinal cord injury without radiological abnormality – SCIWORA)

criticised for bringing their child to the ED and the provision of comprehensive discharge advice including written information, if available, prior to departure will ensure the most appropriate use of primary and secondary healthcare.

Infant mortality rates in England and Wales have reduced significantly since 1980 due in part to improvements in living conditions, antenatal screening, the childhood vaccination programme and the provision of emergency care (Advanced Life Support Group 2011, Office of National Statistics 2011). Thanks to vaccinations against diphtheria, pertussis and *Haemophilus influenzae* type b (Hib), many previously common life-threatening diseases affecting infants in the UK are now thankfully rare. It is important that the emergency nurse remains alert to infants whose parents have not had access to, or chosen not to take-up these public health measures. It is suggested there is still scope to further reduce infant mortality rates by improving emergency care to bring the UK in line with other developed countries (Advanced Life Support Group 2011).

Development of the normal infant

The emergency nurse must have a reasonable understanding of normal cognitive, behavioural, motor, anatomical and physiological development of the infant. The first year of

Table 16.2 A brief outline of developmental milestones

Age	Stage of development
4–6 weeks	Smiles to social stimuli
2 months	Smiles and vocalizes when talked to Eyes follow moving person/object
3 months	Holds a rattle when placed in hand Turns head to sounds on level with ear
5 months	Laughs aloud Pulled to sit – no head lag Able to reach and grasp objects
6 months	Sits on floor with support Rolls prone to supine Begins to imitate, for example, cough Held in standing position puts weight on legs
9 months	Crawls on front Stands holding onto furniture
10 months	Waves goodbye Helps parent/carer when being dressed, for example, by holding arms for coat Pincer grip used to pick up fine objects
12 months	Walks holding onto furniture or with one or two hands held Speaks two or three words with meaning

life is a time of rapid growth and development. The average full-term infant in the UK weighs approximately 3.5 kg and by 12 months has almost tripled this to an average of 10 kg (Advanced Life Support Group 2011). Development from a 'babe in arms' to being able to stand unaided and maybe even taking a few steps at 12 months proves an outstanding year of growth. Incorporate into this a couple of meaningful words, a wave goodbye and progressing from an exclusive milk diet to eating solids and you have an impressive period of advancement. Rolling for the first time off an elevated changing table or parental bed reminds parents that each day their baby is growing in ability. Recognizing that infants develop stranger anxiety at around eleven months will also help the emergency nurse to adapt their approach to this exceptionally challenging group.

Developmental tables offer a useful guide to infant's cognitive, behavioural and motor development that may assist the emergency nurse to identify the infant who is failing to thrive, not reaching developmental milestones or behaving inappropriately (Table 16.2).

Airway and breathing

The infant's airways differ from those of adults and older children in a number of ways that impact upon the response to infection, inflammation and foreign body inhalation. These differences also impact upon the emergency management of the infant's airway and the equipment used to provide support and stabilization. The infant lungs are immature and have a relatively small surface area for gas exchange. The narrower airways of the infant are at greater risk of compromise even from relatively small amounts of inflammation, secretions and bronchospasm. This is because 'resistance to airflow is inversely proportional to the fourth power of the airway radius (halving the radius increases the resistance 16-fold)' (Advanced Life Support Group 2011). Being obligate nose breathers renders infants less than around 6 months old susceptible to airway obstruction from nasal secretions. The trachea of the infant is soft and therefore prone to compression from both flexion and extension of the neck. A collapsed or exhausted infant may need a folded towel or pillowcase placing under the shoulders to prevent flexion of the neck caused by the large occiput.

The soft cartilaginous ribs and pliable chest wall of the infant allows recession when the airway is partially obstructed. Recession indicates inefficiency of breathing as the infant's effort to move the chest wall is not matched by the volume of air inspired. Sternal recession is more significant than subcostal and intercostal recession due to amount of effort required to move the larger sternum. The primary muscle of inspiration in the infant is the diaphragm and not the costals as in adults. Rib movement therefore contributes relatively little to chest expansion in infants. Consequently it is easier to determine the respiratory rate by direct observation of the abdomen and not the chest. Infants with respiratory distress are at risk of exhaustion having little respiratory reserve.

Circulation

The relative circulating volume is much higher in infants than in adults (80 mL/kg vs 50 mL/kg), however, the total volume is small in comparison. Therefore seemingly small amounts of blood loss can result in the rapid development of hypovolaemic shock. Cardiac output is the product of heart rate and stroke volume. Since the stroke volume in infants is relatively fixed, cardiac output can only be increased to meet metabolic demand by increasing the heart rate. Tachycardia is a compensatory mechanism to ensure oxygen and metabolite delivery to the tissues, such as in respiratory distress, sepsis or dehydration. The emergency nurse should be mindful that tachycardia can also be induced by excitement or anxiety and the aim should be to minimize distress.

Significant tachycardia is not sustainable and will eventually lead to decompensation. During the decompensatory phase of shock the heart rate will begin to fall and a normal heart rate in a seriously unwell infant may be misinterpreted as an improvement in condition. Bradycardia is a pre-terminal sign. Close attention to heart rate and rhythm, skin colour and temperature, capillary refill time (CRT) and mental status are key to early recognition of compensated shock. A CRT of >2 seconds indicates poor perfusion, although this may be influenced by a number of factors, particularly cold. Capillary refill should be recorded serially to monitor the response of any measures undertaken to improve circulatory status and is recognized as a better indicator of tissue perfusion than systolic blood pressure (Salter & Maconochie 2005).

Box 16.1

Assessment of the infant

- Rapid cardiopulmonary assessment – ABC
- Conscious level – AVPU
- Details of the current illness/injury, including changes in feeding and sleeping patterns
- Past medical history including birth history
- Immunization status
- Prescribed/over-the-counter medication
- Known allergies
- General appearance, cleanliness, interaction/response to accompanying adult

Table 16.3 Vital signs in infants

Age (months)	Average weight (kg)	Normal BP	Heart rate	Respiratory rate
1	4	60–90/45–60	120–160	30–60
3	5	74–100/50–70	120–160	30–60
6	7	74–100/50–70	120–160	30–60
9	9	74–100/50–70	120–160	30–60
12	10	80–112/50–80	90–140	24–40

Disability

By far the most useful source of information regarding change to the infant's normal abilities, posture and tone are the parents, and their concerns should be held in high regard. Modified paediatric Glasgow coma scores (GCS) are available and very useful, however, the AVPU score provides a quick and simple tool to assess whether the infant is *a*lert, responsive to *v*oice, responsive to *p*ain, or is *u*nresponsive. A child who only responds to pain or who is unresponsive has an equivalent GCS of 8 or less. Babies who are floppy, drowsy or difficult to rouse, irritable on handling and/or have a high-pitched cry should be treated with a high index of suspicion for a neurological problem and have a full set of neurological observations measured and recorded. It is important to obtain an accurate history to illicit details of potential trauma or poisoning and any relevant past medical history. Infants, especially neonates, are particularly sensitive to hypoglycaemia and the emergency nurse should always remember 'DEFG' – *'don't ever forget glucose'*. Heel-prick testing is preferred and training is required to select the appropriate sites, which include the lateral and medial edges of the heel and not the centre.

Assessment

To carry out a full assessment of the sick or injured infant requires specific skills and equipment as well as knowledge of the acceptable parameters for vital signs and factors that affect them (Box 16.1). Normal parameters for an infant's vital signs change with age (Table 16.3). The measurement of vital signs is more challenging than in older children and certain aspects, such as obtaining oxygen saturations and blood pressure readings can require some persistence and patience (Box 16.2). The assessment should begin from the moment of first visualizing the infant, noting whether he/she is a healthy colour, is awake and alert, sleeping or not responsive and as always followed with a rapid assessment of ABC.

In most cases the first part of the assessment can be performed with the infant on the parent's lap to minimize distress to both parent and child and provide more accurate readings and is especially important in certain conditions such as croup. If the child is not alert or looks obviously sick the assessment should rapidly move to a trolley/bed/cot where

Box 16.2

Practical tips for measuring vital signs in infants

It is essential to follow the manufacturer's advice in the use of monitoring equipment and to confirm that it is suitable for use on infants. The emergency nurse must be familiar with monitoring equipment used for measuring infants' vital signs and must be trained and competent in its use.

Body temperature is best measured by use of an electronic thermometer placed in the axilla. It is essential to select the 'paediatric axillary' mode if this is available. Tympanic thermometry should never be used in neonates. In post neonatal infants, correct positioning requires manipulation of the external ear downwards and not 'up and back' as in adults and older children to straighten the ear canal.

Heart rate should be measured by auscultation over the apex of the heart for a whole minute. Use of electronic monitoring should always be verified manually. The brachial pulses are far easier to detect than either radial or carotid pulses in infants.

Respiratory rate should also be counted over a whole minute and is best observed with the chest and abdomen exposed to detect other signs of respiratory distress. Observation for rise and fall of the abdomen is often easier.

Oxygen saturation can be measured using adhesive 'wrap-around' probes on either the lateral edge of the foot or big toe in larger infants. In smaller infants the ulnar aspect of the hand may also be used. Good contact of both the LED and the sensor is necessary to ensure an accurate reading and movement will grossly affect the reading. A regular waveform must be seen before readings can be relied upon.

Capillary refill time is best measured on the sternum or forehead. Sufficient pressure should be applied to blanch the skin by pressing gently onto the sternum or forehead for five seconds. Upon release of the pressure, the time taken for the colour to return is the capillary refill time. Peripheral capillary refill is measured by gently squeezing the tip of a digit or the hand/foot between the index finger and the thumb for five seconds – the limb should be held above the level of the infant's heart.

Blood pressure is best measured on the infant's upper arm, but the lower leg may be used. Selection of the correct cuff size is essential to obtain an accurate reading. The cuff should cover 80% of the length of the upper arm or lower leg and the inflatable bladder should cover at least 40% of the circumference of the limb. The first reading of automated devices should not be used.

(Advanced Life Support Group 2011, Royal College of Nursing 2007)

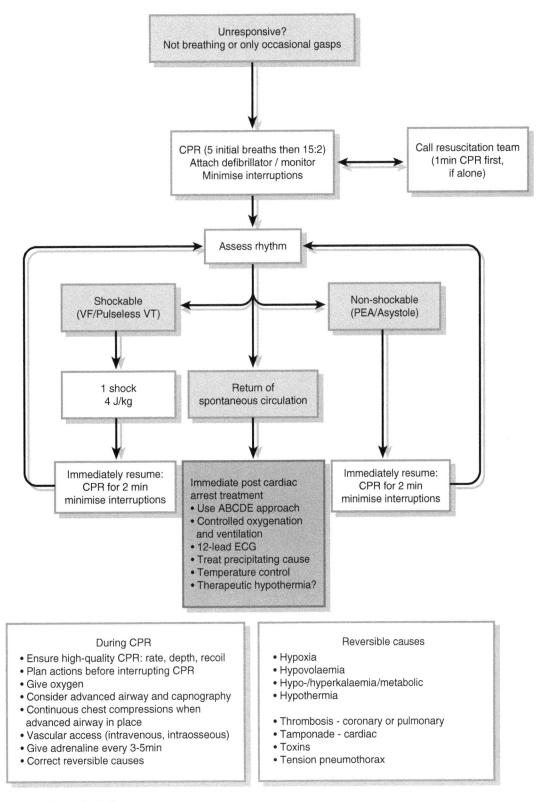

Figure 16.1 • Advanced paediatric life support.

he can be quickly undressed and examined more thoroughly. A degree of common sense must be applied in assessing infants who are obviously sleeping normally, which presents the opportune time to record resting respiratory and heart rate and accurate pulse oximetry; but if there is any doubt regarding responsiveness, immediate attempts should be made to rouse the child. If the child cannot be roused, immediate assistance must be summoned in line with paediatric life support algorithms before assessment of the ABC, with intervention as problems are identified (Fig. 16.1).

The assessment of any infant cannot be deemed complete until he/she has been examined naked to check for rashes, mottling, bruises, mongolian blue spots, injuries, limb deformities, skin temperature, central and peripheral capillary refill time and, wherever possible, an accurate weight obtained. The importance of weighing the infant naked should not be underestimated. All infants and children under 2 years old should be weighed naked in baby scales (Royal College of Nursing 2010). This provides an opportunity to observe the infant's condition and alert the emergency nurse to any safeguarding concerns such as poor hygiene, bruising and unusual markings. It is also necessary for accurate medication administration, almost all of which given in hospital is calculated according to weight (British National Formulary 2011). The formula: '½ age in months + 4' may be used to estimate an infant's weight in kilograms in an emergency. Accurate weighing is the only *objective* measure of dehydration (Advanced Life Support Group 2011) and poor weight gain or weight loss may indicate chronic or serious illnesses such as cystic fibrosis or congenital cardiac abnormalities. It is always worth plotting the infant's weight on the centile chart in the parent held record and noting the general trend in weight gain.

The order in which vital signs are measured in routine assessments where urgent intervention is unnecessary is dependent largely on opportunity and the nature of the presenting complaint. As a minimum, the assessment should include measuring the temperature, heart rate, respiratory rate, oxygen saturation, CRT and conscious level. Local guidance should be followed regarding triage tools and paediatric assessment scores which are becoming increasingly popular, however, sound clinical judgement cannot be substituted for such scoring methods and it is much safer to seek senior advice early when there is doubt regarding the accuracy of the score. Where such early warning tools are used staff should be given specific training in their use and limitations (Royal College of Nursing 2007).

Pain assessment

Pain is often under-recognized and under-treated in the ED (Todd et al. 2002). This can be particularly difficult in infants. The emergency nurse should be trained in the use of pain assessment tools specific to infants and treatment given according to the determined severity. One such tool is the FLACC tool that scores *f*acial expression, *l*eg movement, *a*ctivity, *c*onsolability and *c*rying on a scale of 0–2, the combined total providing a score out of ten (Table 16.4 and Box 16.3). The crying/screaming infant should be presumed to be in pain when none of the usual parental comforting methods such as feeding and rocking are effective. Specific signs such as drawing-up the legs indicating abdominal pain or reluctance to move a particular limb should guide the assessment. Oral sucrose solution and non-nutritive sucking can be used in young infants to provide analgesia during painful procedures such as intravenous cannulation. Consideration of opioid analgesics should be discussed with experienced paediatric-trained staff when simple oral analgesia such as paracetamol and ibuprofen are insufficient.

Table 16.4 The FLACC behavioural pain assessment scale

Categories	Scoring		
	0	**1**	**2**
Face	No particular expression or smile	Occasional grimace or frown; withdrawn, disinterested	Frequent constant frown, clenched jaw, quivering chin
Legs	Normal position or relaxed	Uneasy, restless, tense	Kicking or legs drawn up
Activity	Lying quietly, normal position, moves easily	Squirming, shifting back and forth, tense	Arched, rigid, or jerking
Cry	No cry (awake or asleep)	Moans or whimpers, occasional complaint	Crying steadily, screams or sobs; frequent complaints
Consolability	Content, relaxed	Reassured by occasional touching, hugging, or being talked to; distractible	Difficult to console or comfort

Each of the five categories is scored from 0–2, resulting in a total score of between 0–10

(Reprinted from Merkel SI et al. (1997) The FLACC: A behavioral scale for scoring post-operative pain in young children. Pediatric Nursing, 23(3):293–297. The FLACC scale was developed by Sandra Merkel, MS, RN, Terri Voepel-Lewis, MS, RN, and Shobha Malviya, MD, at C.S. Molt Children's Hospital, University of Michigan Health System, Ann Arbour, MI. © 2002, The Regents of the University of Michigan.)

Respiratory assessment

The infants' pattern of breathing must be assessed in terms of rate, rhythm and effort. The number of breaths should be counted for 60 seconds (Royal College of Nursing 2007); this is best achieved by observing abdominal movement. Quick count methods (30- or 15-second counts) or using electronic monitors have been shown to be inaccurate as often as 62% of the time (Lovett et al. 2005). Worryingly, bradypnoea is almost always missed even though it is indicative of hypoxia and is pre-terminal (Advanced Life Support Group 2011). Tachypnoea may be difficult to count, as often the smaller 'panting' breaths are missed (Aylott 2006a). In these circumstances auscultation is necessary. Other clinical signs of respiratory distress include nasal flaring, use of accessory muscles, head-bobbing, intercostal/subcostal/sternal/supraclavicular recession and tracheal tug. See-sawing, which is the paradoxical movement of the chest and abdomen (i.e., the chest falls and abdomen rises during inspiration), represents extremely inefficient breathing and results from significant airway obstruction. Added breath sounds such as grunting, stridor and wheezing may be heard. Grunting is often a sign of significant respiratory or metabolic disease. This is caused

Box 16.3

How to use the FLACC

In *patients who are awake*: observe for 1 to 5 minutes or longer. Observe legs and body uncovered. Reposition patient or observe activity. Assess body for tenseness and tone. Initiate consoling interventions if needed.

In *patients who are asleep*: observe for 5 minutes or longer. Observe body and legs uncovered. If possible, reposition the patient. Touch the body and assess for tenseness and tone.

Face

- Score 0 if the patient has a relaxed face, makes eye contact, shows interest in surroundings
- Score 1 if the patient has a worried facial expression, with eyebrows lowered, eyes partially closed, cheeks raised, mouth pursed
- Score 2 if the patient has deep furrows in the forehead, closed eyes, an open mouth, deep lines around the nose and lips

Legs

- Score 0 if the muscle tone and motion in the limbs are normal
- Score 1 if patient has increased tone, rigidity, or tension; if there is intermittent flexion or extension of the limbs
- Score 2 if patient has hypertonicity, the legs are pulled tight, there is exaggerated flexion or extension of the limbs, tremors

Activity

- Score 0 if the patient moves easily and freely, normal activity or restrictions
- Score 1 if the patient shifts positions, appears hesitant to move, demonstrates guarding, a tense torso, pressure on a body part
- Score 2 if the patient is in a fixed position, rocking; demonstrates side-to-side head movements or rubbing of a body part

Cry

- Score 0 if the patient has no cry or moan, awake or asleep
- Score 1 if the patient has occasional moans, cries, whimpers, sighs
- Score 2 if the patient has frequent or continuous moans, cries, grunts

Consolability

- Score 0 if the patient is calm and does not require consoling
- Score 1 if the patient responds to comfort by touching or talking in 30 seconds to 1 minute
- Score 2 if the patient requires constant comforting or is inconsolable

Whenever feasible, behavioural measurement of pain should be used in conjunction with self-report. When self-report is not possible, interpretation of pain behaviours and decisions regarding treatment of pain require careful consideration of the context in which the pain behaviours are observed.

Each category is scored on the 0–2 scale, which results in a score out of 0–10:

0 = Relaxed and comfortable
1–3 = Mild discomfort
4–6 = Moderate pain
7–10 = Severe discomfort or pain or both

by the infant breathing out against a partially closed glottis in order to generate positive end expiratory pressure (PEEP) to prevent alveolar collapse. Wheezing is a high-pitched, musical, expiratory sound indicative of lower airway pathology such as in bronchiolitis and other viral infections. It is caused by turbulent airflow through very narrow airways (Aylott 2006b). Wheezing may also be heard in cardiac failure. Stridor is a harsh, low-pitched, usually inspiratory noise indicative of upper airway obstruction, for example in croup or foreign body obstruction.

Cardiovascular assessment

The heart rate in infants should be measured for a full minute by auscultation of the apex beat and electronic measurements should be verified manually (Royal College of Nursing 2007). The apex beat can be heard over the 5th intercostal space in the left, mid-clavicular line. This should be consistent with the brachial pulse, which is palpated on the medial aspect of the upper arm. The carotid and radial pulses are not used routinely in infants as they are difficult to locate. The skin colour and temperature should be consistent over the trunk and limbs; however, when assessing the patient consider the ambient temperature. Decreased skin perfusion can be an early sign of shock. Clinical signs of poor perfusion include peripherally cool skin, pallor, mottling and peripheral cyanosis. CRT is very useful in assessing perfusion. The sternum or forehead are preferred sites (Maconochie 1998) as ambient temperatures can affect peripheral sites. Sufficient pressure to cause the skin to blanch should be applied for five seconds and the length of time for normal colour to return recorded (Castle 2002). Normal capillary refill time is <2 seconds in post-neonatal infants and <3 seconds in neonates. When recording blood pressure, the size of cuff should be at least two-thirds of the length of the upper arm (or lower leg) and the inflatable portion should cover the entire circumference of the limb. This is essential to obtain an accurate reading. It is usually best to leave this measurement to last as it is the least useful data in most cases and tends to be distressing. The first automated blood pressure measurement should be disregarded (Royal College of Nursing 2007). Enquiring about fluid input and output, i.e., drinking well, vomiting, diarrhoea, frequency of wet nappies and observing for moist mucous membranes are all aspects of the cardiovascular assessment.

Advanced paediatric life support

Cardiopulmonary arrest in infants and children is seldom a sudden event and rarely due to a primary cardiac event. It is often the end result of progressive deterioration in respiratory and circulatory function. It usually results from a period of hypoxia and acidosis, which has been caused by respiratory and/or circulatory failure. If pulseless cardiac arrest occurs the outcome is bleak. Early recognition and treatment of decompensating shock to prevent cardiopulmonary arrest is fundamental to successful resuscitation. Thus cardiopulmonary arrest can often be prevented if the clinical signs of respiratory failure and shock are recognized promptly (Wilmhurst & Graydon 2012).

Establish basic life support (Resuscitation Council (UK) 2010a). Oxygenate and ensure the provision of positive pressure ventilation with high-concentration oxygen. Attach a defibrillator or monitor. Look for signs of life. Assess the cardiac rhythm as either non-shockable or shockable:

- non-shockable: asystole or pulseless electrical activity (PEA)
- shockable: VF or pulseless VT.

The most common cardiac arrest rhythms in infants are non-shockable. This is usually due to hypoxia and associated acidosis following a period of respiratory or circulatory failure. This leads to a profound bradycardia which rapidly deteriorates to asystole, although PEA can occur. The treatment of asystole/PEA is effective basic life support and the administration of adrenaline (epinephrine) $10\,\mu g/kg$ ($0.1\,mL$ of the $1:10000$ solution) by the intravenous or intraosseous routes or $100\,\mu g/kg$ via the endotracheal route. Four minutes of basic life support at a ratio of 2 ventilations to 15 chest compressions (at a rate of $100–120/min$) should be carried out between doses of adrenaline, with the monitor checked every two minutes to confirm asystole/PEA. Repeating the cycle at least twice more is encouraged to aid the circulation of drugs and the correction of hypoxia and acidosis. Consider and treat reversible causes.

Shockable rhythms are less common in paediatric life support but the nurse must always be aware of the possibility of treating this arrhythmia rapidly and effectively. Place the defibrillator paddles on the chest wall; one just below the right clavicle, the other at the left anterior axillary line; for infants, when using this method of monitoring, it may be more appropriate to apply the pads to the front and back of the infant's chest. Defibrillate the heart with one defibrillation shock at $4\,J/kg$ followed by two minutes of CPR. Chest compressions should be re-commenced immediately after shocks. After two minutes, pause briefly to check the monitor. If VF/VT is still present a second shock at $4\,J/kg$ should be delivered followed immediately by a further two minutes of CPR without pausing to recheck the rhythm. If VF/VT is still present a third shock at $4\,J/kg$ should be delivered followed immediately by a further two minutes of CPR, then adrenaline ($10\,\mu g/kg$) and amiodarone $5\,mg/kg$. After a further two minutes of CPR pause briefly to check the monitor. If the rhythm is still VF/VT, continue giving shocks every two minutes with a dose of adrenaline after every other shock (Advanced Life Support Group 2011). After the fifth shock a second and final dose of amiodarone $5\,mg/kg$ should be given. There are various causes of VF/VT in children but drug overdose, hypokalaemia and hypothermia should be actively considered (Resuscitation Council (UK) 2010b).

Causes of respiratory difficulty

Bronchiolitis

Bronchiolitis is the most common lower respiratory tract infection in infants (Nair et al. 2010). It is most prevalent in autumn and winter and respiratory syncytial virus (RSV) is the most common underlying cause (Ducharme 2011). Bronchiolitis is often precipitated by an upper respiratory tract infection. The virus causes an inflammatory response in the bronchioles, thus causing constriction of the smaller airways. The resultant secretions begin to accumulate as exudate cannot be easily expectorated because of damage to ciliated cells. This results in impaired gaseous exchange.

Infants generally present with a history of 'runny nose', low-grade pyrexia, wet cough, shortness of breath, wheezing worsening over a period of a few days. However, infants under six months, or those born prematurely may present with a history of apnoea. On assessment, there may be signs of respiratory distress with tachypnoea, recession, use of accessory muscles and nasal flaring. The disease is generally most severe in smaller infants, especially those born pre-term and is particularly dangerous for infants with certain co-existing heart and lung diseases. High-risk patients may be treated with RSV prophylaxis in the form of monthly injections of palivizumab (RSV antibody therapy) throughout the bronchiolitis season.

Nursing interventions include reassurance of parents/carers and maintenance of a calm environment. The degree of clinical intervention depends on the severity of respiratory distress, oxygen requirements and the infant's ability to feed adequately. The vast majority of infants with bronchiolitis require no specific treatment and may be discharged home with clear advice on when to seek further assistance, preferably reinforced in writing. Where treatment is required this is largely supportive and includes oxygen therapy and assistance with feeding. In the most severe cases, nasal continuous positive airway pressure is often effective in preventing deterioration and the subsequent need for intubation and ventilation. Inhaled bronchodilators may be of benefit to a small cohort and are worth considering. If oxygen saturations are below 93%, supplementary oxygen is required and should be administered by the least distressing route, i.e., via nasal cannulas or a facemask.

Infants with suspected bronchiolitis should be nursed away from other babies and stringent cross-infection measures should be employed as RSV is particularly contagious (SIGN 2006).

Viral croup

Viral croup, or laryngotracheobronchitis, is a common upper airway infection that is characterized by coryzal symptoms, low-grade fever and a harsh 'barking' cough. Other causes of upper airway obstruction include foreign body inhalation, epiglottitis and tracheitis but these can be differentiated by onset of symptoms and clinical picture. Foreign body inhalation presents with a sudden onset with no prodromal features such as coryza or fever. Both epiglottitis and tracheitis present with shock, high-grade fever and drooling, and in the case of epiglottitis a soft inspiratory stridor is usually present. If either of these presentations is suspected senior anaesthetic and ENT assessment are required as both conditions are life-threatening. The same is true in cases of severe croup. There are many croup scores available to determine the severity of the illness and local guidelines should be followed. As a general rule, the degree of respiratory distress is a good indicator of severity and inspiratory stridor at rest is suggestive of significant upper airway obstruction.

As with all cases of upper airway obstruction, the approach should be cautious and interventions minimized to avoid distressing the infant. The parent should be encouraged to hold and reassure the infant and assessment carried out in the parents' arms in all but obtunded patients. Crying can stimulate laryngospasm and precipitate a significant decline in the patient's condition to the point of airway occlusion; therefore keeping a symptomatic infant calm by avoiding distressing procedures is important (Zoorob et al. 2011). If oxygen is required this should be administered by face-mask as close as the infant will tolerate. Treatment is not required if respiratory distress is absent or minimal. In cases of moderate respiratory distress, treatment consists of oral dexamethasone or inhaled budesonide and in severe cases inhaled adrenaline can be used as a temporary measure to buy time for the onset of action of steroid therapy or planned intubation.

Inhalation of foreign body

Although more common in toddlers than infants, inhalation of a foreign body should always be considered if a baby presents with a sudden onset of cyanosis, stridor or choking. Timely treatment will prevent severe complications. The Heimlich manoeuvre or abdominal thrusts are not recommended in infants as they may cause intra-abdominal injury (Advanced Life Support Group 2011). Blind finger sweeps to remove foreign bodies may convert a partial obstruction of the upper airway to a total obstruction, as the foreign body can pass from the upper part of the larynx to obstruct the airway completely at the level of the cricoid cartilage (Salter & Maconochie 2005).

Infants with an ineffective cough should be placed head down and prone across the rescuer's lap, with their head being well supported by the bony angles of the mandible and not soft compressible tissues that may further occlude the airway. Five back blows should be given in succession to relieve the obstruction. If this does not expel the foreign body, the infant should be placed supine along the rescuer's forearm with the occiput supported in the palm or on a firm surface if this is not possible, and five chest thrusts administered. These are delivered as with chest compressions but sharper and at a slower rate (Resuscitation Council UK 2010a) (Fig. 16.2).

Apparent life-threatening events

The term apparent life-threatening events or ALTEs is used to describe a combination of signs and symptoms and is not in itself a diagnosis. ALTEs are a common cause for infants to present to the ED and are defined as an episode that is frightening to the observer and that is characterized by some combination of apnoea (central or occasionally obstructive), colour change (usually cyanotic or pallid but occasionally erythematous or plethoric), marked change in muscle tone (usually marked limpness), choking or gagging. In some cases the observer fears that the infant has died. There are many potential causes of ALTEs, including gastro-oesophageal reflux, seizure, respiratory tract infections, urinary tract infection, and sepsis, ranging between the extremes of severity. In many cases no cause is found. Despite the apparent severity of the witnessed event, these infants are frequently fully recovered and appear quite well by the time of arrival in the ED. Given the sheer range of possible causes and difficulty ascertaining whether the ALTE is benign or due to serious illness it is especially important that the emergency nurse conducts a thorough assessment of the

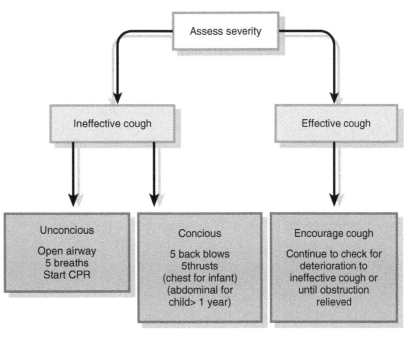

Figure 16.2 • Paediatric choking algorithm.

infant and demonstrates to the parents that their concerns are being taken seriously. By definition, ALTEs are extremely distressing for the parents and the emergency nurse should be mindful of this when assessing a seemingly well infant. The observations and investigations carried out at the time should be guided by the history and as a minimum include obtaining a full set of vital sign measurements. The infant should be fully undressed and examined, including a careful look for bruises, petechiae, rash and injury (Lockwood 2009). It may also be useful to obtain a capillary blood gas if this facility is available and consider whether a urine sample is required as this can take time to obtain and may be diagnostic. It is usually prudent to involve the paediatricians as further investigations and admission to the children's ward or a short-stay facility for a period of observation is often required to exclude serious illness.

Cardiac emergencies

The termination of the placental blood supply to the infant shortly after birth requires the newborn to adapt rapidly. The fluid-filled foetal lungs expand with the first few breaths and circulatory changes are required. Consequently, the heart has to redirect the flow of oxygen-depleted blood to the lungs before it returns to be pumped to the rest of the body. These changes begin in the first few minutes of life and may take several hours, days and weeks to *reach completion*. It is in these first few days and weeks that congenital cardiac anomalies, which are not always detectable during routine antenatal ultrasound scans, may present to the ED.

There are a number of significant differences between the foetal and 'adult' circulation which reflect that the foetus receives oxygenated blood from the placenta and not the lungs (Fig. 16.3). The process of change from foetal to adult circulation begins shortly after the infant's first breath to redirect blood to the now inflated lungs for gas exchange. The change involves the closure of the foramen ovale and the ductus arteriosus. In the foetus, the foramen ovale is a flap-like opening that allows much of the foetal blood to pass from the right to left atrium without entering the right ventricle and therefore bypassing the uninflated lungs. The ductus arteriosis connects the pulmonary artery and the

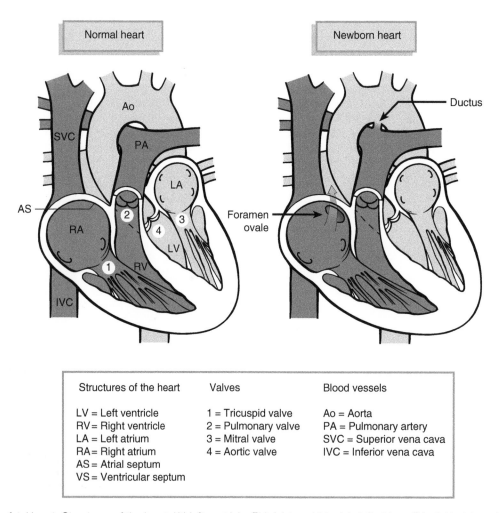

Figure 16.3 • The fetal heart. Structures of the heart: LV, left ventricle; RV, right ventricle; LA, left atrium; RA, right atrium; AS, atrial septum; VS, ventricular septum. Valves: 1, tricuspid valve; 2, pulmonary valve; 3, mitral valve, 4, aortic valve. Blood vessels: Ao, aorta; PA, pulmonary artery; SVC, superior vena cava; IVC. inferior vena cava.

aorta. This duct allows much of the blood that reaches the right ventricle to escape from the pulmonary vein directly into the aorta and then around the body. Under normal circumstances the ductus arteriosus closes within thirty minutes of the infant's first breath and the foramen ovale is closed by an increase in pressure in the left atrium. However, in infants with 'duct-dependent congenital heart disease' the ductus arteriosus must remain patent to permit adequate circulation of oxygenated blood to enter the aorta. As not all cases of duct-dependent congenital heart disease are detected in routine ultrasound scans in the antenatal period, affected infants may present to the ED within the first few weeks of life with a range of signs and symptoms. Such symptoms include respiratory distress, mottling or discolouration of the lower limbs indicating poor blood supply, failure to thrive, and feeding problems. The most important consideration for the emergency nurse is that the administration of high-flow oxygen can precipitate closure of the ductus arteriosus leading to a paradoxical decrease in oxygen saturations and significant deterioration in the patient's condition that may rapidly result in cardiopulmonary arrest. In this small population, the emergency nurse should titrate the administration of oxygen to the minimum required to achieve optimal oxygen saturation. Senior paediatric assistance must be sought in all suspected cases.

The febrile infant

Fever is one of the most common reasons for infants and young children to present to the emergency department. Fever is almost always due to an infective process and in the majority of cases this illness will be a self-limiting viral infection requiring no medical intervention (National Institute for Health and Clinical Excellence 2007a). However, fever is of particular concern in young infants and may be the presenting feature of serious bacterial illnesses such as meningitis, septicaemia, urinary tract infections and pneumonia. It is essential to enquire about immunization status as well as recent foreign travel as this may assist the diagnosis.

Fever is a cause of considerable concern for parents and can be a diagnostic challenge for healthcare professionals (National Institute for Health and Clinical Excellence 2007a). The priority for the emergency nurse should be to identify and treat any life-threatening features using the ABC approach and establish the likely severity of the illness. The *Feverish Illness in Children* guidelines (National Institute for Health and Clinical Excellence 2007a) provide a useful 'traffic light' tool to identify risk of serious illness (Table 16.5). The need for antipyretic therapies should be

Table 16.5 Traffic light tool

	Green: low risk	Amber: intermediate risk	Red: high risk
Colour	Normal colour	Pallor reported by parent/carer	Pale/mottled/ashen/blue
Activity	Responds normally to social cues Content/smiles Stays awake or awakens quickly Strong normal cry/not crying	Not responding normally to social cues Wakes only with prolonged stimulation Decrease in activity No smile	No response to social cues Appears ill to a healthcare professional Unable to rouse or if roused does not stay awake Weak, high-pitched or continuous cry
Respiratory		Nasal flaring Tachypnoea: RR >50 breaths/min age 6–12 months RR >40 breaths/min age >12 months Oxygen saturation ≤95 % in air Crackles	Grunting Tachypnoea: RR >60 breaths/min Moderate or severe chest indrawing
Hydration	Normal skin and eyes Moist mucous membranes	Dry mucous membrane Poor feeding in infants CRT ≥3 seconds Reduced urine input	Reduced skin turgor
Other	None of the amber or red symptoms or signs	Fever for ≥5 days Swelling of a limb or joint Non-weight bearing/not using an extremity A new lump >2 cm	Age 0–3 months, temperature ≥38 °C Age 3–6 months, temperature ≥39 °C Non-blanching rash Bulging fontanelle Neck stiffness Status epilepticus Focal neurological signs Focal seizures Bile-stained vomiting

CRT, capillary refill time; RR, respiratory rate.

(Reprinted from National Institute for Health and Clinical Excellence (2007a) Feverish Illness in Children: Assessment and Initial Management in Children Younger than 5 Years. National Institute for Health and Clinical Excellence: London.)

considered only after determining the severity of illness and intervening appropriately. Routine use of antipyretics to reduce body temperature in a febrile infant who appears comfortable and well are not required as fever is a normal physiological response that may aid the immune response. There is no evidence to suggest that preventative administration of agents such as paracetamol or ibuprofen offer prophylaxis against febrile convulsions. These should only be administered if the infant appears distressed or miserable. The ability to control fever with antipyretic agents should not be relied upon to determine the seriousness of illness. The use of cooling methods such as removal of clothing, tepid sponging and fan therapy are not beneficial and are no longer recommended.

The height of the fever alone does not indicate severity; however, serious bacterial illness (SBI) is more likely in infants aged less than 3 months with a body temperature of 38°C or higher and infants aged 3–6 months with a body temperature of 39°C or higher. Infants less than 3 months old are approximately fourteen times more likely to develop an SBI than other children less than 5 years old (National Institute for Health and Clinical Excellence 2007a). Therefore, any infant less than 3 months old presenting with a fever should be treated with extreme caution. All of these infants should have blood taken for culture, full blood count and C-reactive protein, and urine obtained for urgent microscopy. If respiratory symptoms are present a chest X-ray is required and if diarrhoea is present a stool sample should be obtained for culture. A lumbar puncture should be performed on all neonates with a fever and febrile infants aged 1–3 months who appear unwell or have abnormally high or low white blood cell counts (<5 or $>15 \times 10^9$/litre) if this is not contraindicated. Signs and symptoms of specific illnesses should be sought; however, a significant proportion of infants present with no obvious focus of infection such as upper respiratory tract infection or gastroenteritis. Obtaining urine for testing is mandatory for all febrile infants with no obvious cause, this should preferably be a clean catch specimen into a sterile container; see also National Institute for Health and Clinical Excellence (2007b) *Urinary Tract Infection in Children*.

Parents of infants being discharged must be given verbal and written advice of when to seek further medical attention. This should include deterioration, parental concern or fitting.

Febrile convulsions

Febrile convulsions are seizures that occur in a child with a febrile illness. They are common, but usually benign events occurring in infants, toddlers and young children. Witnessing a convulsion is, however, extremely distressing for parents. Approximately 2–4% of all children are affected (Waruiru & Appleton 2004). The seizures are generalized, of tonic–clonic nature, usually lasting less than 10 minutes and complete recovery usually occurs within one hour. The onset of a febrile convulsion is often the first sign that an infant is unwell, as seizures usually occur near the onset of a fever rather than

after prolonged fever. The peak incidence occurs between 8 and 20 months; febrile seizures are uncommon after 5 to 6 years (Zukin et al. 1998).

A comprehensive review of the literature by Armon et al. (2003) identified the conditions usually associated with febrile convulsions. In order of decreasing frequency these are:

- viral infections
- otitis media
- tonsillitis
- urinary tract infection
- gastroenteritis
- lower respiratory tract infection
- meningitis
- post-immunization.

Most febrile convulsions are self-limiting; however, a fit lasting longer than 10 minutes demands treatment with intravenous lorazepam, buccal midazolam or rectal diazepam after the initial management of ABC and administration of high-flow oxygen. There are guidelines on the management of status epilepticus that should be followed to terminate fitting for example the APLS algorithms and parenteral antibiotic treatment must be administered if there is suspicion that the fitting is due to serious bacterial illness.

Parents and carers need a lot of support and reassurance that simple febrile convulsions do not harm their child and that they are not the same as epilepsy that emerges only in very few cases. Immunization is still advised after a febrile convulsion, even if, as rarely happens, the febrile convulsion followed an immunization (Waruiru & Appleton 2004).

All infants presenting after a febrile convulsion should be referred for a paediatric opinion. The priority should be to identify and treat the *cause* of the fever. Before discharge parents need to be advised how to manage any further convulsions and when to seek further medical attention.

Bacterial meningitis and septicaemia

As mentioned above, serious bacterial infections are far more common in young infants than in other age groups. These include urinary tract infection, pneumonia, meningitis and septicaemia. Survival rates and likelihood of full recovery are greatly improved with early recognition and effective treatment. This is especially so of meningococcal septicaemia as the disease progresses rapidly and can quickly prove fatal. Diagnosis of these conditions is especially difficult in infants as specific signs and symptoms are often not present. The classic signs of meningitis – neck stiffness, bulging fontanelle and high-pitched cry – are often absent in infants and nonspecific signs such as fever, irritability, vomiting, rapid deterioration and level of parental concern should be considered carefully (National Institute for Health and Clinical Excellence 2010).

Common causes of bacterial meningitis are *Streptococcus pnuemoniae, Neisseria meningitidis* and *Haemophilus*

Box 16.4

Signs and symptoms of bacterial meningitis

Non-specific signs and symptoms
- Drowsiness
- Irritability
- Off feeds
- Distressed when handled
- Vomiting
- Pyrexia

Specific signs and symptoms
- Neck stiffness
- Tense bulging fontanelle
- Purpuric or petechial rash
- Mottled appearance
- Hypothermic

Late signs and symptoms
- High-pitched moaning cry
- Reduced level of consciousness/coma
- Neck retraction/arched back
- Shock
- Widespread haemorrhagic rash

influenzae, the latter being reduced by the introduction of the Hib vaccine in childhood immunizations. Protocols for the management of suspected bacterial meningitis and septicaemia will aid rapid treatment; these should be agreed with the paediatric department and made readily available to ED staff. The nurse will usually be the first person to assess an infant, therefore accurate and thorough assessment is vital. Signs of shock should be sought, which include tachycardia, pallor, cold extremities, altered conscious level, prolonged capillary refill time, respiratory symptoms and breathing difficulty and poor urine output. Where present, shock should be treated with high-flow oxygen via a non-rebreathe mask, boluses of intravenous fluids, which should initially be 20 mL/kg of 0.9 % saline solution. Infants should be thoroughly examined for rashes, especially unexplained non-blanching spots including petechiae, which are red, pinprick-sized lesions. The presence of larger non-blanching lesions is of particular concern and should immediately trigger suspicion of meningococcal disease. Bacterial meningitis or septicaemia should be considered as a potential diagnosis in all febrile infants who appear unwell to experienced healthcare professionals. Signs and symptoms of bacterial meningitis are given in Box 16.4. Infants with signs of meningitis or septicaemia require immediate treatment with intravenous antibiotics. In most cases of bacterial meningitis a broad-spectrum cephalosporin (cefotaxime or ceftriaxone) should be administered. These cover *Neisseria meningitidis*, *Streptococcus pneumoniae* and *Haemophilus influenzae*. Ampicillin or amoxicillin should be added in infants less than 3 months old to cover *Listeria* (National Institute for Health and Clinical Excellence 2010). The National Institute for

Health and Clinical Excellence (2010) guidelines on bacterial meningitis and meningococcal septicaemia in children states that a lumbar puncture should be performed as a primary investigation on all infants who have suspected meningitis or meningococcal disease unless contraindicated by: reduced or fluctuating conscious level, relative bradycardia or hypertension, focal neurological signs, abnormal posture, abnormal 'doll's eye' movements, pupillary response, papilloedema, shock, extensive or spreading purpura, post-fitting, clotting abnormalities, respiratory distress or infection at lumbar puncture site.

The continuing treatment of the child or the infant with bacterial meningitis or septicaemia will depend upon the severity of illness. Infants with persistent shock following fluid boluses of > 40 mL/kg should be discussed with a paediatric intensivist and will probably require intubation and inotropic therapy and retrieval to a paediatric intensive care setting.

Dehydration in infants

Dehydration occurs when fluid loss exceeds fluid intake over a period, leaving the body in negative fluid balance and at risk of hypovolaemic shock. Infants, particularly those less than 6 months old, along with those who were a low birth weight are at an increased risk of dehydration (National Institute for Health and Clinical Excellence 2009). Other factors that increase the risk of dehydration in this high-risk age group are infants who have stopped breastfeeding because of illness or those who have not been offered or have not been able to tolerate supplementary fluids; those with signs of malnutrition; those who have passed more than five diarrhoeal stools in the previous 24 hours or children who have vomited more than twice in the past 24 hours (National Institute for Health and Clinical Excellence 2009).

The severity of clinical dehydration is indicated by an increasing number of signs and symptoms clearly illustrated in Table 16.6. The presence of any red flag symptom demands close attention through monitoring for potential deterioration into clinical shock (National Institute for Health and Clinical Excellence 2009).

History

Gaining a clear history from the parent/carer is essential:

- elicit the time of onset of symptoms such as diarrhoea, vomiting or both and its character (i.e., presence of bile, blood or mucus)
- is there a history of constipation?
- what is the oral intake in the last 24 hours?
- what is their normal fluid intake?
- are they refusing to drink or do they appear thirsty?
- when was the last normal wet nappy?
- has the baby felt hot/have the parents recorded a pyrexia?
- do they have a recent weight?

Physical assessment

This should be thorough, including all routine observations allowing the determination of any signs or symptoms of clinical dehydration with particular attention to the presence of any red flag symptoms. Sunken eyes may well be pointed out by the parent as a change in appearance, reduced skin turgor is established if skinfold return is greater than one second.

Hypernatraemic dehydration, reflecting loss of water, may be suspected if there are any jittery movements, increased muscle tone, hyper-reflexia or convulsions, drowsiness or coma. Enteral rehydration therapy is considered the safest approach.

Treatment

Oral rehydration solutions are an easily metabolized fluid and electrolyte replacement, and significantly reduce admission rates from the emergency department (Boyd et al. 2005). The method of administration and amount given is vital in ensuring the best possible outcome. The suggested protocol for

rehydration volume is 50 mL/kg in addition to normal maintenance allowance over 4 hours. 'Little and often' really does work in most cases, and parents/carers should be encouraged to persevere. Providing a simple fluid chart for the parents to complete may foster compliance. If the infant does not tolerate oral fluid because of poor feeding or persistent vomiting, he/she may be admitted for intravenous fluid replacement. On discharge parents should be advised regarding fluid maintenance and monitoring with accompanying written advice.

The vomiting infant

Vomiting is a common symptom of many presentations of infants in ED. The most common cause of vomiting is acute gastroenteritis. Other infections include urinary and respiratory tract infections, ear infections and tonsillitis. Poor feeding techniques or excessive feeding may also lead to vomiting. Management of infantile vomiting should focus on correcting fluid deficits as well as identification and definitive treatment of the underlying cause. Most well-hydrated infants with a

Table 16.6 Assessment of dehydration and shock

	Increasing severity of dehydration →		
	No clinically detectable dehydration	**Clinical dehydration**	**Clinical shock**
Symptoms (remote and face-to-face assessment)	Appears well	‡Appears to be unwell or deteriorating	–
	Alert and responsive	‡Altered responsiveness (e.g., irritable, lethargic)	Decreased level of consciousness
	Normal urine output	Decreased urine output	–
	Skin colour unchanged	Skin colour unchanged	Pale or mottled skin
	Warm extremities	Warm extremities	Cold extremities
Signs (face-to-face assessment)	Alert and responsive	‡Altered responsiveness (e.g., irritable, lethargic)	Decreased level of consciousness
	Skin colour unchanged	Skin colour unchanged	Pale or mottled skin
	Warm extremities	Warm extremities	Cold extremities
	Eyes not sunken	‡Sunken eyes	–
	Moist mucous membranes (except after a drink)	Dry mucous membranes (except for 'mouth breather')	–
	Normal heart rate	‡Tachycardia	Tachycardia
	Normal breathing pattern	‡Tachypnoea	Tachypnoea
	Normal peripheral pulses	Normal peripheral pulses	Weak peripheral pulses
	Normal capillary refill time	Normal capillary refill time	Prolonged capillary refill time
	Normal skin turgor	‡Reduced skin turgor	–
	Normal blood pressure	Normal blood pressure	Hypotension (decompensated shock)

‡Symptoms and signs with the (red) flag may help in the identification of an infant at risk of developing clinical shock.

(Reproduced from National Institute for Health and Clinical Excellence (2009) Diarrhoea and Vomiting in Children: Diarrhoea and Vomiting Caused by Gastroenteritis: Diagnosis, Assessment and Management in Children Younger than 5 years. London, National Institute for Health and Clinical Excellence.)

self-limiting problem can usually be discharged home with appropriate advice regarding feeding.

Gastroenteritis

Infective gastroenteritis is characterized by the sudden onset of diarrhoea and/or vomiting that is often accompanied by fever. Acute gastroenteritis lasting less than 10 days is one of the most common medical illnesses of childhood. Parents bring their child to the ED in varying stages of ill health, the majority of which can be managed at home. An accurate history should be taken to rule out chronic illness. The following information should be gathered:

- when the illness commenced
- diet and fluids taken
- episodes of vomiting since onset
- episodes of diarrhoea since onset
- urine output
- relevant medical history
- note any recent visits abroad
- prescribed medication or over-the-counter medication.

The priority is to assess for dehydration (see Table 16.6) and rehydrate as necessary. The risk of cross infection is high and strict hand washing is essential (National Institute for Health and Clinical Excellence 2007a). Written discharge advice such as that suggested by National Institute for Health and Clinical Excellence should be provided.

Gastro-oesophageal reflux

Asymptomatic, infrequent reflux of gastric contents is physiological. Reflux is most common in young infants, who effortlessly regurgitate milk. While the vast majority remain well, infants may present with failure to gain weight or weight loss, feeding problems or anaemia (Meadow & Newell 2002). Gastro-oesophageal reflux can also result in recurrent pulmonary disease due to the aspiration of gastric acid. The most likely presentation to the ED is of a young infant who appears in pain and cries excessively.

Pyloric stenosis

Pyloric stenosis is a disorder that usually becomes apparent during the 2–8 weeks after birth and rarely beyond three months. The incidence is 3/1000 and falling and much lower in Afro-Caribbean and Asian children and less frequent in breast-fed babies (Davies & Lindley 2010). There is progressive hypertrophy of the pylorus causing partial or total obstruction of the pyloric sphincter. Typically, the infant has poor weight gain or weight loss due to the projectile vomiting that occurs after feeds. The infant is excessively hungry and shows a willingness to feed immediately after vomiting. This can be very distressing for parents, particularly those caring for their first baby. Many parents blame their feeding technique, and careful intervention from the ED staff is needed to establish the diagnosis and reduce feelings of anxiety or guilt the parents may have.

Pyloric stenosis does have a familial incidence so parents of a second or subsequent baby may already suspect what is wrong, and come to the ED seeking confirmation and action from staff. The infant may or may not be dehydrated on attendance but this largely depends on the duration and severity of the stenosis. A test feed is indicated to help establish diagnosis. As the stomach fills, waves of peristalsis become visible until the infant vomits. These babies will be admitted to hospital and undergo surgery once rehydrated and stable.

Intussusception

Intussusception is a telescoping of a portion of the intestine and is the most common cause of intestinal obstruction in infants and children (Weihmiller et al. 2012). The onset is sudden and typically occurs in males aged 3–8 weeks (Brown 2002), however, any young child, especially if aged between 2 months and 2 years, presenting with rectal bleeding, vomiting, abdominal pain or a mass or cardiovascular compromise should have the diagnosis of intussusception considered (Rogers & Robb 2010). It causes severe intermittent attacks of screaming and abdominal pain, often with associated drawing up of the legs, vomiting and pallor. The infant is irritable or lethargic with paroxysms of colicky pain. Diarrhoea is mucus-laden and blood-stained 'red currant jelly' stools are passed. An infant presenting with this history should be seen as a matter of urgency; however, classic symptoms are absent in up to half of babies with intussusception (Barkin & Rosen 1994).

The infant with intussusception is extremely unstable; therefore, intravenous access should be established and referral to a paediatric surgeon should be swift. An air-reduction enema is the definitive treatment of choice for this condition. It should only be undertaken once the child has been resuscitated and stabilized. Absolute contraindications to radiological reduction are evidence of peritonitis or perforation.

Failure to thrive

This is a general descriptive term applied to poor growth in early life. As previously mentioned, poor weight gain or weight loss may be indicative of serious acute and/or chronic illness. Consideration should be given to excluding serious illness and ensuring the infant is adequately hydrated. Referral to a paediatrician is necessary to investigate the cause and ensure appropriate follow up.

The injured infant

The infant is totally dependent on his or her parents/carer, and accidents that occur to infants are a reflection of this fact. As the infant develops, his or her mobility increases together with a growing susceptibility to injury. Constant supervision of infants is not always possible. Parental behaviour and education can help reduce the serious consequences of injury.

Assessment of the injured infant

Parents are often distressed and anxious, and may feel guilty or responsible for the infant's injury. Assessment, therefore, needs to be done carefully if a therapeutic relationship is to be established. The following information should be collected;

- time elapsed since injury
- was the accident witnessed?
- cause and mechanism of injury
- accident environment or whether indoors or outdoors
- examine wound/injury
- analgesia
- relevant medial history, immunization status, medications.

This assessment gives the nurse an insight into the history leading to injury and the family dynamics and should highlight any areas of concern relating to the family's psychosocial set-up, as well as determining the actual severity of the injury. The ED nurses must remain vigilant for possible or evident non-accidental injuries (see also Chapter 17). The majority of injuries to infants are minor, requiring a one-off visit to the ED. On discharge, written advice to support nursing and medical intervention should be given. Information regarding the attendance of all infants should be communicated with their Health Visitor and GP and local procedures must be in place to facilitate this.

Head and neck injuries

Head injury in infancy is most commonly the result of a fall from a surface such as a baby changer, bed, sofa or work surface or by being dropped accidently. Occasionally a high-impact event such as involvement in a road traffic accident (RTA) may result in attendance, although the use of car seats has significantly reduced this. Infants are predisposed to head and neck injuries as a result of their proportionately large heads and poor neck control and relatively mobile cervical spine. As a result of this seriously injured infants may present with spinal cord injury without radiological abnormality (SCIWORA) following an RTA. Determination of this by means of MRI is then indicated. Non-accidental cause of head injury must be considered carefully in this age group as they are rarely able to cause significant injury to themselves due to their relative immobility.

Initial assessment with neurological observations should occur within 15 minutes of arrival. As always the priority is to establish A(c), B and C where 'c' denotes cervical spine immobilization as indicated. The baby who is too small for a hard neck collar should be manually immobilized throughout (Advanced Life Support Group 2011). As a minimum, neurological observations must include paediatric GCS, respiratory rate, pulse, blood pressure, temperature, oxygen saturation and pupil response. The aim of this assessment is to establish the likelihood of having a clinically significant brain/neck injury which should inform further management and clinical priority (Box 16.5).

CT scanning is recommended if any one of the CHALICE predictions apply (National Institute for Health and Clinical

Box 16.5

Assessment of head-injured infant

Physical Assessment

Airway with **C**-spine immobilization if necessary

Breathing

Circulation

Disability - neurological observations with AVPU/Paediatric GCS

    Inspect the head for evidence of injury – lacerations, haematomas, contusions, bleeding or CSF leak from nose or ears

    Palpate for tenderness, bony deformity and check the anterior fontanelle

    Examine for any other signs of injury

History

How did the injury occur? (RTA, fall – onto what surface/from what height, high-velocity impact)

When and where did the injury occur?

Was the incident witnessed?

Has there been reduced conscious level, e.g., unresponsive/ drowsiness?

Has the infant had a seizure?

Did the infant cry immediately?

Has there been any vomiting and how many times?

Box 16.6

CHALICE Prediction Rules (applicable to infants)

- Witnessed loss of consciousness for longer than five minutes
- Abnormal drowsiness
- Three or more discrete episodes of vomiting
- Suspicion of non-accidental injury
- Seizure with no history of epilepsy
- Paediatric GCS less than 15 in the emergency department
- Suspicion of open or depressed skull injury or tense fontanelle
- Sign of basal skull fracture
- Focal neurological deficit (including motor, sensory, coordination or reflex abnormality)
- Bruise, swelling or laceration greater than 5 cm on the head
- Dangerous mechanism of injury including high-speed RTC, fall from a height greater than 3 m or high-speed impact from a projectile

If none of these variables are present then the risk of significant brain injury is considered to be *low*.

(From National Institute for Health and Clinical Excellence (2007c) Head Injury: Triage, Assessment, Investigation and Early Management of Head Injury in Infants, Children and Adults. Methods, Evidence & Guidance. London, National Institute for Health and linical Excellence.)

Excellence 2007c) (Box 16.6). Observations should be recorded every 30 minutes, until the GCS returns to 15. At this point or if presentation is with a GCS of 15 observations following initial assessment observations should be repeated half hourly for the next 2 hours, hourly for 4 hours and then 2 hourly thereafter. Local guidelines should be followed regarding paediatric and surgical/neurosurgical involvement.

The vast majority of infants that attend the ED are determined to be of low risk and are discharged home with verbal and written advice for the accompanying adult. This advice should include instructions to seek further medical attention if the infant vomits more than once, is difficult to rouse, develops poor feeding, irritability, unusual behaviour or parental concern. See also Chapter 5.

Child protection

While child protection issues span the whole of childhood, this issue is addressed in detail in Chapter 17.

Infant death

Infant mortality statistics prove that the incidence of deaths over the past 30 years has fallen by nearly two thirds, from 12 deaths per 1000 live births in 1980 to a rate of 4.5 deaths per 1000 live births in 2009. This equates to 3191 infant deaths in 2009 (Office for National Statistics 2011). There are a number of causes for the death of an infant. In the neonatal period (0–28 days) prematurity, low birth weight and congenital abnormalities remain the most significant causes. During the post-neonatal period to 1 year causes such as congenital cardiac conditions, metabolic disorders, neoplasms, infection, injuries from accidents including road traffic incidents and non-accidental causes are recorded. However, the most significant cause (over 50%) is attributed to sudden unexpected death in infancy (SUDI) where post mortem fails to determine a cause. The terms sudden infant death syndrome (SIDS) or cot death are still commonly used.

In 2008, 312 deaths were attributed to cot death, the majority occurring during the first year of life (Foundation for Study of Infant Deaths 2009). The launch of the 'Reduce the Risk' campaign in England and Wales in 1991 has had a huge impact, reducing the number of sudden and unexpected infant deaths by approximately 70%. The risk factors identified include being male, having a teenage mother, parental smoking during pregnancy and smoking around the baby, low income, low birth weight (<2500g), maternal age <20 and sharing the parental bed (Foundation for Study of Infant Deaths 2009, Ball et al. 2012). Health promotion advice on prevention of cot death should be offered to all parents (Box 16.7).

Rapid response

Cardiopulmonary resuscitation will always have been initiated unless clearly inappropriate. It will usually have been started by paramedics and/or parents but by time of arrival in the ED the outcome of asystolic cardiac arrest is extremely bleak. Out-of-hospital arrest carries a very high mortality rate with only 1–2% surviving to hospital discharge and only about 25% of the survivors having a favourable neurological outcome (Gerein et al. 2006, Wilmhust & Graydon 2012).

Resuscitation should be continued until a senior doctor, usually a consultant paediatrician, has made a decision to

---

Box 16.7

How to reduce the risk of sudden unexpected death in infancy (cot death)

- Put the baby in a cot on their back to sleep, with feet at the bottom end of the bed
- Prevent overheating. Keep baby's head uncovered
- Avoid bed sharing, especially if either parent smokes, has drunk alcohol, taken any potentially sedating medication or drugs or feels very tired, baby was premature or of low birth weight. Do not sleep on a sofa or armchair with the baby
- Settle baby to sleep with a dummy/pacifier
- Breastfeed the baby
- Avoid parental smoking in pregnancy. Do not allow anyone to smoke in the same room as the baby

(Adapted from Foundation for the Study of Infant Deaths (2009) Reduce the Risk of Cot Death. Department of Health, London.)

---

discontinue resuscitation attempts. Ideally an experienced nurse should remain with the parents, accompanying them in the resuscitation room if they wish to be present in order to provide support and explanations.

It is a legal requirement that, in all but the rarest of circumstances, infants who die suddenly and unexpectedly at home or in the community must be transferred to the ED to allow for a thorough process of investigation to be commenced (The Children Act 1989). Since 2006, Local Safeguarding Children Boards (LSCBs) must coordinate 24-hour rapid response teams. This team of professionals usually includes a paediatrician, health visitor or social worker, police officer and any other relevant professional/organizational member. The responsibility of the team is to investigate the circumstances around the death, aiming to minimize duplication and ensure that the lessons learnt contribute to safeguarding and promoting the welfare of children in the future (Department for Education 2010).

Following declaration of the infant's death the baby should be examined by the attending consultant. A detailed history of events leading up to and following the discovery of the child's collapse should be taken from the parents/carers. The Department of Education *Every Child Matters* website provides national templates for collecting such information. The templates are specific to the circumstances surrounding the death, i.e., SUDI, drowning, road traffic collisions, etc. The purpose of obtaining clear, relevant information at this point is to identify any potential cause of death and identify any suspicious circumstances. LSCB guidelines should be agreed with the coroner to determine any samples or investigations after death has been declared. A skeletal survey may be indicated if there is suspicion of trauma or non-accidental injury. The Royal College of Pathologists and Royal College of Paediatric and Child Health (2004) recommend the collection of the following samples:

- serum venous or arterial blood for toxicology screening
- arterial or venous blood for aerobic and anaerobic culture
- lithium heparin for cytogenetics
- Guthrie card blood test for inherited metabolic diseases
- cerebrospinal fluid for microscopy, culture and sensitivity

- nasopharyngeal aspirate for virology and microbiology
- swabs from any lesions
- urine for toxicology and inherited metabolic diseases.

Additional samples may include:

- skin biopsy for fibroblast culture
- muscle biopsy if history is suggestive of mitochondrial disease.

Care of the bereaved family

The death of an infant is infrequent but the emergency nurse must be prepared for managing this tragic event. Bereavement training should ideally be provided to emergency nurses to facilitate effective and sensitive communication with the infant's parents and family. The training should be concerned mainly with communication skills, such as the breaking of bad news, sympathetic listening, responding to questions, non-verbal communication and dealing with anxiety, grief and anger (Lawrence 2010). During this highly emotional time, parents are especially sensitive to the attitude of hospital staff who should remain open-minded and not be perceived to apportion blame. Careful thought should be given to the choice of language and terminology used as this may impact upon the grieving process and be remembered for many years to come. The infant should always be referred to by name. Staff should display empathy but remain wholly professional at all times in order to provide effective support and guidance.

Support should be offered to the family, including where available, a bereavement counsellor, hospital chaplain or other faith leader. The hospital team should offer to contact any relatives or friends to support the parents at this time. The parents should be allowed to spend as much time as they wish with the child and any examination of the child or further investigations should where possible be carried out in a manner that causes least disruption to the family. Mementos such as a photograph, lock of hair, or hand and footprints should be offered to the family, in agreement with the coroner. Following the unexpected death of an infant, it is usually appropriate to allow the parents to spend time with and hold their child, provided this does not interfere with preservation of evidence. This should be facilitated by the hospital staff and rapid response team, with a quiet, designated area provided for the family. In most situations the parents will have already handled their child after the death, and allowing them to hold their child will not in any way interfere with the investigation into the cause of death. A nurse must maintain a discreet presence at all times. Families may wish to remain in the department for a substantial period of time and consideration must be given to their cultural and religious customs and beliefs. If the mother is breast-feeding she will need immediate advice on suppression of lactation. If the baby was a twin, the surviving twin should be admitted to hospital for full assessment and monitoring. If non-accidental causes are suspected the safety of siblings must be addressed.

Discharge advice and information

It is important to explain the coroner's duty to investigate all sudden deaths. Parents should be provided with sensitive but factual verbal and written information regarding the post-mortem examination and what will happen next. Little of what is said may actually be heard and retained by the grief-stricken parents or family. The family should be provided with details of where to obtain further support e.g., child bereavement charity, FSID, health visitor and GP. The GP and midwife or health visitor should be informed as soon as possible. Between one and three months after the death, the parents should be offered an appointment to see a relevant consultant in order to explain the medical facts and after support (Royal College of Paediatrics & Child Health 2007).

Staff care

The impact of a baby's death on the ED staff is enormous. The provision of bereavement care to parents is demanding and stressful and staff should be given time to reflect on their experiences. It is important to realize that such events are traumatic and may stretch or exceed the emergency nurse's ability to cope. Occupational health departments can be an excellent source of support at this time and the emergency nurse should be encouraged to access these services. A facilitated opportunity to discuss events may be of benefit to some individuals, but is by no means mandatory.

Conclusion

This chapter discusses the major differences between infants and older children and outlines a number of common presentations specific to stages of development within the first year of life. The key to success is thorough assessment, recognition of the acutely sick or injured baby and timely intervention. Parental anxiety is to be expected and the best way to minimize this is through a confident, knowledgeable approach and effective communication.

References

Advanced Life Support Group, 2011. Advanced Paediatric Life Support: The Practical Approach. West Sussex, Wiley-Blackwell.

Armon, K., Stephenson, T., Hemingway, P., et al., 2003. An evidence and consensus based guideline for the management of a child after a seizure. Emergency Medicine Journal 20 (1), 13–20.

Aylott, M., 2006a. Observing the sick child: Part 2a: Respiratory assessment. Paediatric Nursing. 18 (9), 38–44.

Aylott, M., 2006b. Observing the sick child: Part 2c: Respiratory auscultation. Paediatric Nursing. 19 (3), 38–45.

Ball, H.L., Moya, E., Fairley, L., et al., 2012. Infant care practices related to sudden infant death syndrome in South Asian and White British families in the UK. Paediatric and Perinatal Epidemiology 26 (1), 3–12.

Boyd, R., Busuttil, M., Stuart, P., 2005. Pilot study of a paediatric emergency department oral rehydration protocol. Emergency Medicine Journal 22 (2), 116.

British National Formulary, 2011. BNF for Children 2011–2012. Pharmaceutical Press, London.

Brown, A.F.T., 2002. Accident and Emergency: Diagnosis and Management. Arnold, London.

Castle, N., 2002. Paediatric resuscitation: advanced life support. Nursing Standard 17 (11), 47–52.

Davies, B.W., Lindley, R., 2010. The vomiting infant: pyloric stenosis. Surgery 28 (1), 43–46.

Department for Education, 2010. Working together to Safeguard Children: A guide to Inter-agency Working to Safeguard and Promote the Welfare of Children. Department for Education, London.

Department of Health, 2004. Ill Child Standard, National Service Framework for Children, Young People and Maternity Services. HMSO, London.

Ducharme, F.M., 2011. Management of acute bronchiolitis. British Medical Journal 342, 1658.

Foundation for the Study of Infant Deaths, 2009. Reduce the Risk of Cot Death. Department of Health, London.

Gerein, R.B., Osmond, M.H., Stiell, I.G., et al., 2006. What are the etiology and epidemiology of out-of-hospital pediatric cardiopulmonary arrest in Ontario, Canada? Academic Emergency Medicine 13 (6), 653–658.

Hay, P., 1996. Care of the infant with bronchiolitis. Emergency Nurse 4 (3), 19–22.

Lawrence, N., 2010. Care of bereaved parents after sudden infant death. Emergency Nurse 18 (3), 22–26.

Lockwood, S., 2009. Emergency care of the infant and child. In: Crouch, R., Charters, A., Dawood, M., Bennett, P. (Eds.), Oxford Handbook of Emergency Nursing, Oxford University Press, Oxford.

Lovett, P.B., et al., 2005. The vexatious vital: Neither clinical measurement by nurses nor an electronic monitor provides accurate measurements of respiratory rate in triage. Annals of Emergency Medicine. 45 (1), 68–76.

Maconochie, I., 1998. Capillary refill time in the field – it's enough to make you blush! Pre-Hospital Immediate Care 2, 95–96.

Meadow, R., Newell, S., 2002. Paediatrics. Blackwell Science, Oxford.

Merkel, S.I., Voepel-Lewis, T., Shayevitz, J.R., Malviya, S., 1997. The FLACC: A behavioural scale for scoring post-operative pain in young children. Pediatric Nursing 23 (3), 293–297.

Nair, H., Nokes, D.J., Gessner, B.D., et al., 2010. Global burden of acute lower respiratory infections due to respiratory syncytial virus in young children: a systematic review and meta-analysis. Lancet 375, 1545–1555.

National Institute for Health and Clinical Excellence, 2007a. Feverish Illness in Children: Assessment and Initial Management in Children Younger than 5 years. National Institute for Health and Clinical Excellence, London.

National Institute for Health and Clinical Excellence, 2007b. Urinary Tract Infection in Children: Diagnosis, Treatment and Long-term Management. Clinical Guidelines. National Institute for Health and Clinical Excellence, London.

National Institute for Health and Clinical Excellence, 2007c. Head Injury: Triage, Assessment, Investigation and Early Management of Head Injury in Infants, Children and Adults. Methods, Evidence & Guidance. National Institute for Health and Clinical Excellence, London.

National Institute for Health and Clinical Excellence, 2009. Diarrhoea and Vomiting in Children: diarrhoea and Vomiting Caused by Gastroenteritis: Diagnosis, Assessment and Management in Children Younger than 5 Years. National Institute for Health and Clinical Excellence, London.

National Institute for Health and Clinical Excellence, 2010. Bacterial Meningitis and Meningococcal Septicaemia in Children. National Institute for Health and Clinical Excellence, London.

Office of National Statistics, 2011. Childhood, Infant and Perinatal Mortality in England and Wales, 2009. ONS Statistical Bulletin. Newport, ONS.

Resuscitation Council (UK), 2010a. Paediatric Basic Life Support. Resuscitation Council (UK), London.

Resuscitation Council (UK), 2010b. Paediatric Advanced Life Support. Resuscitation Council (UK), London.

Rogers, T.N., Robb, A., 2010. Intussesception in infants and young children. Surgery (Oxford) 28 (8), 402–405.

Royal College of Nursing, 2007. Standards for Assessing, Measuring and Monitoring Vital Signs in Infants, Children and Young People. RCN, London.

Royal College of Nursing, 2010. Standards for the Weighing of Infants, Children and Young People in the Acute Health Care Setting. RCN, London.

Royal College of Paediatrics & Child Health, 2007. Report of the Intercollegiate Committee for Services for Children in Emergency Departments. Royal College of Paediatrics and Child Health, London.

Royal College of Pathologists and the Royal College of Paediatric and Child Health, 2004. Sudden Unexpected Death in Infancy. RCPath & RCPCH, London.

Salter, R., Maconochie, I., 2005. Paediatric emergencies. In: O'Shea, R.A. (Ed.), Principles and Practice of Trauma Nursing. Elsevier Churchill Livingstone, Edinburgh.

SIGN (Scottish Intercollegiate Guidelines Network), 2006. Bronchiolitis Guide. SIGN, Edinburgh.

The Children Act (1989). London: HMSO.

Todd, K.H., Sloan, E.P., Chen, C., et al., 2002. Survey of pain etiology, management practices and patient satisfaction in two urban emergency departments. Canadian Journal of Emergency Medicine 4 (4), 252–256.

Waruiru, C., Appleton, R., 2004. Febrile seizures: an update. Archives of Disease in Childhood 89 (8), 751–756.

Weihmiller, S.N., Monuteaux, M.C., Bachur, R.G., 2012. Ability of pediatric physicians to judge the likelihood of intussusception. Pediatric Emergency Care 28 (2), 136–140.

Wilmhurst, S.L., Graydon, C., 2012. Aetioloy and outcome of paediatric cardiopulmonary arrest. Paediatric Critical Care 13 (1), 11–14.

Zoorob, R., Sidani, M., Murray, J., 2011. Croup: an overview. American Family Physician 83 (9), 1067–1073.

Zukin, D.D., Grisham, J.E., Saulys, A., et al., 1998. Fever in children. In: Rosen, P. (Ed.), Emergency Medicine: Concepts and Clinical Practice, Mosby Year Book, St Louis.

The pre-school child

Amy Lamb

17

CHAPTER CONTENTS

Introduction

More than 3 million children aged 0–16, the equivalent of 28% of all children in England, attended Emergency Departments (EDs) in 2006/7 accounting for 25% of all patients seen in EDs across the UK (Royal College of Paediatrics and Child Health and Royal College of Nursing 2010). As many as four out of five children attend with minor injuries, with one in five attendances resulting from parental concern about acute illness (Department of Health 2004). Findings from the Children's

http://dx.doi.org/10.1016/B978-0-7020-4315-4.00017-6

National Service Framework 2004 (Department of Health 2004) indicate that 70% of children attending rural EDs have accidental injuries and in inner city EDs 70% of attendees are for acute medical illness. Recent figures suggest that children attending EDs often require an episode of care without an overnight stay, on average, an increase of 15%, highlighting the importance of community-based facilities competent in the assessment, treatment and observation of children (NHS Institute for Innovation and Improvement 2008). In the younger age group 1 child per 1000 of the population is in hospital with acute illness on any given day (Department of Health 2003a). Only a small percentage, less than 0.25%, of all children attending the ED will require a paediatric intensive care bed.

Changing patterns of illness in children have shown a decrease in many of the acute presentations to the ED. This is felt to be due in part to the revision of immunization programmes, increased awareness of health promotion and the introduction of new technologies. Health promotion and early preventive measures have improved the management of some children's conditions such as asthma. However, there is an increase in recognition of emotional/behavioural problems across childhood, including deliberate self-harm and harm to others (Department of Health 2003a).

Recent times have seen a shift in attitudes towards children and their needs and development, and considering the child as an individual in their own right rather than a 'little adult' is now more likely to be the norm. The concepts of children as people with rights are now also reflected in everyday policy and debate such as in the National Service Framework (Department of Health 2004), UNICEF (1990) and the UN Convention on the Rights of the Child (United Nations 1989). The Royal College of Paediatrics and Child Health and Royal College of Nursing (2010) have indicated the number of registered children's nurses working within the ED setting is insufficient despite reports as far back as the 1950s stipulating that children in hospital must be cared for by staff trained in caring for children (Ministry of Health 1959); however, it is equally as important to recognize that emergency care skills are something conventional children's nurse training does not offer (Royal College of Paediatrics and Child Health 2007a).

The visit to the ED is often a child's first experience of hospital, thus making the whole incident doubly traumatic. Young children have insatiable curiosity about their surrounding environments, creating greater vulnerability by being generally unaware of the imposing dangers. Between 1 and 4 years a child's physical and mental development is very rapid, with 50% of the child's mental capacity developed before the age of 5 years (Brain & Martin 1989). Coupled with substantial leaps in acquisition of language and multi-skills, such quick development can prove the danger for unsuspecting parents/carers. It can come as a surprise when the child is first able to scramble up the stairs and reach up to a work surface or has the strength to pull over a chair. Pre-school children usually arrive in accident and emergency as a result of accidental injury. The challenges of climbing furniture, stairs, the opening of all manner of containers, sampling even the most unpalatable of agents all increase the likelihood of a small child suffering falls, minor injury and poisoning (Mead & Sibert 1991).

Normal development

This chapter will consider normal childhood development and some of the common reasons for ED attendances within this age group.

The child in the age range of 3 months to 1 year is termed an infant; 1 to 3 years a toddler; and 3 to 4 years a pre-school child. In the context of this chapter, all children above the age of 1 will be considered pre-school children. The pre-school child, unlike the infant, has begun to develop his own identity. From about the age of 2 years the child discovers that he can control what happens around him; motor skills develop rapidly and a child able to walk, run, climb and jump uses the newfound skills to explore his environment. The child strives for autonomy and self-esteem. However, he also needs to know the safety limits of behaviour in a given environment. For example when climbing the stairs with a parent the child may feel good because of the praise for his achievement, but this needs to be tempered so the child is aware that it is not good to climb over the stair gate and attempt to climb the stairs alone.

Pre-school children perceive the world differently from adults. The 2-year-old is egocentric and will perceive that he is the centre of his world, being unable to identify with anybody else's point of view. The child may believe that it is he who is responsible for events that we know to be out of his control. Throughout this pre-operational phase of development, memory and imagination are developing rapidly. There is a tendency to mix fact with fantasy and a belief that the child's thoughts can control events. There is an intuitive, magical quality to their thoughts (Hall & Elliman 2003).

Children often perceive illness and injury as a punishment for something they did or failed to do. Illness and hospitalization deprive children of opportunities to play with other children and other children may even reject or taunt an ill child because of physical differences and limitation.

The child under stress

The pre-school child is more vulnerable and traumatized when separated from his parents than at any other age. Bowlby (1953), in his famous study *Child Care and the Growth of Love*, shows how a child suffers maternal deprivation when separated from his significant carers, the male or female person who supplies love, care, protection and comfort.

Since then, many seminal reports have confirmed the importance of keeping parents and child together (Ministry of Health 1959, Department of Health 2004, Royal College of Paediatrics and Child Health and Royal College of Nursing 2010). This is particularly important in EDs where events leading to attendance will have caused some stress (Box 17.1). Injured/unwell children, despite their parents' presence, may become clingy or dependent (regress) while in the hospital setting.

Effective nursing interventions at this early stage can do a lot towards developing a rapport with the child and family, and to alleviate stress and fear. Acknowledging the child's

Box 17.1

Categories of children's worries

- Physical harm or bodily injury in the form of discomfort, pain, mutilation and death
- Separation from parent or absence of trusted adult
- A strange unknown environment
- Uncertainty about limits and expected acceptable behaviour
- Loss of control, autonomy and competence

(After Visintainer MA, Wolfer JA (1975) Psychological preparation for surgical pediatric patients: The effects on children's and parents' stress responses and adjustment. Pediatrics. 56(2), 187-202.)

suffering and putting it into context using toys or pictures can be helpful, as is prompt pain relief. Parental input from the outset is essential not only to reduce stress and induce normality in the child but also to reduce stress in the parents/carers themselves. Encouraging parents/carers to undress their child and to help them with the examination as well as to be there to give reassurance to their child reinforces the parents' importance in the treatment and helps to allay their fears.

The environment in which a child is cared for has come under much scrutiny in recent years (Bentley 2004, National Audit Office 2004). Facilities for children are best provided in an environment away from adult patients. Children should have their separate waiting area geared towards their needs with appropriate toys, books, television, video and electronic games. Treatment areas should also be child-oriented not only in décor and furnishings but also in equipment so time is not wasted hunting for appropriate items such as child-size blood-pressure cuffs or pulse oxy-sensitivity probes.

Parental anxiety

Parents and carers have their own anxieties, which can in turn increase the anxiety of the child. Parents often feel incredibly guilty about accidents and injuries that their children suffer. These anxiety feelings often overwhelm parents so much so that they are less aware of the child's need for support and reassurance.

Parents/carers frequently experience a lack of confidence in their judgement when their child is ill and often remain anxious and concerned, having to manage their sick child at home even after reassurance from a medical professional. In situations like this it has been shown that parents/carers do not know how to contact health services when their child has not improved (Neill 2000). It is easy in circumstances following an accident for the parents to feel inadequate or lose confidence in their own ability. This must be addressed in the ED constructively and without proportionate blame, to enable the parents to support their child. Reassurance, information and what the parents/carers can do to help their child should be clearly communicated. Poor handling of parents in the ED can have a long-term effect on both the child and the family's recovery (Mead & Sibert 1991).

The term 'family-centered care' is frequently used in children's nursing and aims to evoke the inclusion of parental participation in child health and shared care decisions ensuring both the needs of the child and family are paramount (Hughes & Lyte 2009). Working within the ED setting, this concept is no different. The ED nurse's attitude should be family oriented when dealing with children. Parents are often under a great deal of stress, feel guilty and are very anxious. These negative emotions can have a profound effect on the child. The parents need reassurance and a chance to relay their fears and guilt to the nurse (Bentley 2004).

A critical attitude from nursing and medical staff will only reinforce the guilt and inadequacy the parent is likely to experience. An anxious parent will make the child feel anxious. Keeping the parent informed and building the bond between the family and staff will help the child.

Communicating with the child and family

Effective communication is central to nursing any patient of any age. A key factor in reducing stress and relieving anxiety is the way by which we communicate with the child and family. The value of effective communication is not only dependent on the nursing staff but also on the multi-disciplinary team. Good communication is the basis of forming a trusting relationship with the child and family and Maguire & Pitceathly (2002) suggest that this aids the practitioner in identifying the child or family members' problem resulting in greater patient/family satisfaction.

With a pre-school child the use of non-verbal communication in the way that we express ourselves is as equally important as speech. Children of this age might appear shy, withdrawn or outgoing. Whatever impression they give, they will have an awareness of facial expressions, gestures, eye contact, watching and waiting in anticipation. This should be borne in mind when communicating with children; get down to the child's level, as towering above them is intimidating. Address the child by their name, talking in a soft tone, and bring the level of conversation to things that are familiar to the child, such as the topic of a television programme or television characters.

Understanding illness

To a young child, illness is remote and viewed as an external process. There is a tendency to believe this has something to do with magic or is a punishment. Pre-school children do not fully understand internal body processes. In this pre-operative phase (Piaget 1990), children are only just developing their thought processes in relation to internal body organs. They have little concept of where internal organs lie, other than the heart, which lies in the middle of their chest and is used for loving and caring. When talking with pre-school children they often describe tummy ache and at the same time point to their head or equally they will say they have headache and point to their tummy. A child of this younger age is concerned with external injury and very often frightened of seeing blood, small cuts and marks. The external aspect of his environment such as light, equipment, uniforms and noise will affect the child much more than an explanation of what is going on in his/her body.

Play is a very important aspect of the child's care and is at the very centre of a healthy child's life (Webster 2002). Children can express fear and anxiety through play, so a playful environment will help reduce stress and anxiety. Watching a child play gives a fair assessment of social and multi-skills. Playing with children during examination and assessment will help the child understand treatment and procedures. Play specialists in EDs often have little or no time to plan play or distraction therapies because of the unpredictability of the setting and speed at which interventions are required (Knight & Gregory 2009) and therefore must have the skills to adapt to this situation quickly. Dolls and teddy bears come in very useful when trying to demonstrate what is about to be done to a child. Through play children are able to learn both the sensory and concrete information they need in preparation for some clinical procedures.

Asthma

There are approximately 5.2 million people in the UK with asthma, nearly 1 million of whom are children (National Institute for Health and Clinical Excellence 2007). During the past two decades, many scientific advances have improved the understanding of asthma and ability to manage and control it effectively. Since the late 1990s admission rates have declined (Shabu et al. 2007). However, recommendations for asthma care need to be adapted to local conditions, resources and services (Bateman et al. 2008). Asthma is acknowledged to be the most common long-term childhood condition and although mortality as a result of asthma is rare, the condition can have a significant impact on the child's quality of life. Regardless of medical advances and technological improvement in asthma management confidential enquiries into asthma deaths have often indicated that the fatality could have been avoided if there had been better preventive measures, better recognition and help in avoiding delay during the final attack and in receiving earlier emergency care. Younger children with asthma are particularly vulnerable because they rely on others to react to the severity of their condition and to act on their behalf. Children in the 0–4-year age range have the most frequent health consultations with GP and out-of-hours services for asthma conditions.

When a young child attends the ED with breathing difficulties, it is important that he/she is not unnecessarily distressed any further. Practical steps to prevent distress include not separating the child from the parents or carer, behaving in a calm and friendly manner, and assessing the child promptly in an appropriate environment. If a child does become upset, the extra energy and oxygen needed when crying can be enough to turn a moderate asthma attack into a severe one.

Assessment

The overall clinical picture is developed from the combination of history, physical assessment and clinical investigations. If the child has obvious breathing difficulty, oxygen and nebulized bronchial dilators should be commenced immediately, prior to detailed history-taking from the parents/carers. Children under the age of five cannot adequately use a peak flow meter so peak expiratory flow is not recommended for this age group. Questions which should be asked in establishing a history of the event and the child's general health are given in Box 17.2.

Box 17.2

Establishing history of asthma attack

- How long has this episode lasted?
- Is the child getting better or worse?
- What medication has been given prior to ED attendance and what was the effect?
- Is there an identifiable trigger to the episode?
- Is the child on regular medication? If so, what is it?
- Has the child had previous serious asthma episodes requiring steroids or hospital?
- How frequent are the asthma symptoms?
- Does the child have any other illness?

Physical assessment

Initial observation of the child will allow the nurse to observe respiratory rate, rhythm and effort (Aylott 2007). The respiratory rate and depth should be established first as this correlates to the severity of asthma. Normal breathing is effortless and quiet. The use of accessory muscles such as those in the neck and shoulders is described as laboured and requires substantial effort (Brooker & Nicol 2003). Intercostal and sternal recession is an indication of moderate to severe respiratory difficulty. As the child's ability to speak is an indication of respiratory function, the nurse should know if the child can speak in full sentences using more than a few words or not at all. Parents are invaluable in assessing difficulties in the child's normal pattern of speech, as ability to converse varies with this age group.

Respiratory assessment should be conducted and interpreted in association with other clinical assessment; therefore a rise pulse rate may be indicative of increasing hypoxia, but must be considered within context (Aylott 2007) such as if the child is upset, pyrexial or on beta agonists such as salbutamol, a tachycardia would be expected. Although wheezing is a classic symptom of bronchospasm, it is unreliable in detecting the severity of an episode. At assessment, any audible wheeze or wheeze on auscultation should be recorded and used as baseline. It is important to remember that if air is not being moved effectively in and out of the lungs, no wheeze will be present. Signs of respiratory distress, e.g., nasal flaring, grunting, wheezing, recession, use of accessory and intercostal muscles, chest shape and movement should be noted by looking and listening (Royal College of Nursing 2007).

Peak flow measurement is considered an important indication of the severity of an asthma episode; however, Scullion (2005) notes that young children can also be confused by the exhalation method required to use a peak flow meter. Exercise testing, by getting a child to run around for about six minutes, may therefore be more suitable for younger children. Peak flow measurement should therefore only be attempted in children who have previously and regularly used a peak flow meter.

Pulse oximetry is one of the most useful diagnostic aids in the under-five age group. It is non-invasive and the monitor can be a distraction for the child. Pulse oximetry will identify reductions in oxygen saturation, which may not be obviously clinical. The lower the oxygen saturation, the more severe the impact of the attack on the child, so it is important to ensure oximetry reading is accurate. Poor contact, excessive movement and temperature of the child's skin can all affect the accuracy of the reading. The ED nurse can check the validity of the oxygen reading by matching the peaks of recording, bleeps or monitored pulse rate to the child's actual pulse rate. These should be the same if the oxygen saturation level is to be considered accurate. In severe asthma, arterial blood gases should be measured; however this is often taken as a capillary sample in children in order not to distress or cause the child pain. Such tests act as an indication of the level of respiratory distress and possible need for alternative treatments or possible artificial ventilation.

Management

In cases of life-threatening asthma (Box 17.3) these children need immediate high-flow oxygen via a non-rebreathing mask, and a nebulized beta agonist such as salbutamol. Preparation should be to establish i.v. access for the administration of medications. Children in this age group both deteriorate and respond to treatment rapidly. The nurse must be vigilant for any changes and equipment should be at hand for intubation and ventilation.

Rapid oxygen therapy and nebulized bronchial dilators should be commenced and in cases of severe asthma (Box 17.4) an oxygen saturation of at least 95% should be the aim (British Thoracic Society and Scottish Intercollegiate Guidelines Network 2011). It is important not to distress the child unnecessarily as this significantly increases the work of breathing. Intravenous access should be considered particularly if the child does not respond rapidly to nebulizer therapy.

Compliance with treatment is crucial to the successful management of this group of children. It is important to be calm and to keep the parents/carers informed of treatment plans to enable them to assist in the care of their child. Initial management involves inhaled bronchial dilators (short-acting and long-acting) and cortical steroids are the drugs of choice. The administration of beta agonists such as salbutamol (dose dependent on age) is the first-line treatment for acute asthma and they can be given by a variety of devices. For the mild to moderate asthma a spacer with mask can be ideal for the younger age group. However, with severe asthma it is advisable to use a nebulizer. It is important that the nurse explains what is being done first and uses toys and play where appropriate. Alternative devices such as a mouthpiece nebulizer can be more successful. If the child is very upset it is sometimes better to get a parent to hold the nebulizer by the child's mouth than to increase the level of distress by attaching the mask to the child. If the child responds well to nebulizer treatment, they should be observed in the ED as per local policy post-nebulizer, to ensure that the response is not transient – ideally 2–4 h (British Thoracic Society and Scottish Intercollegiate Guidelines Network 2011). If the response is not maintained, the child should be admitted for treatment and continued assessment.

When planning the discharge of a young child from ED it is important that parents understand and are happy with ongoing treatment plans. Although a child may appear well after nebulizer therapy for an acute episode of asthma, the small airways obstruction can persist for several days. Parents must be able to administer supportive therapy at home. Many devices exist to assist young children in the inhalation of bronchial dilators. Spacers are commonly used for children under the age of five (British Thoracic Society and Scottish Intercollegiate Guidelines Network 2011). These create an enclosed space between an aerosol inhaler and the child's mouth allowing him to work at his own pace without the need for hand-breathing coordination that an aerosol would demand.

The early use of steroids for acute asthma can reduce the need for hospital admission and prevent a relapse in symptoms after initial presentation. A short course of oral steroids can speed up the race for recovery from an acute episode of small airways obstruction. Prednisolone 1-2 mg/kg for three days or longer if necessary (Royal Pharmaceutical Society 2010) is recommended for children who have not responded to regular home treatment over a period of 24 hours or more prior to ED attendance. Children regularly on inhaled steroids may also benefit from this boost.

Box 17.3

Life-threatening asthma signs

- Silent chest on auscultation
- Oxygen saturation less than 92%
- Poor respiratory effort
- Hypotension
- Cyanosis
- Exhaustion
- Reduced level of consciousness or confusion
- Coma

Box 17.4

Severe asthma signs

- Agitated
- Respiratory rate >30 (>5 years old) or >40 (2–5 years old)
- Recession
- Oxygen saturation less than 90%
- Pulse >125 (>5 years old) or >140 (2–5 years old)
- Unable to talk in sentences

Box 17.5

Moderate asthma signs
- Alert and oriented
- Tachypnoea
- Able to speak normally
- Audible wheeze

As well as advice on drug therapy, it is important that parents and carers are able to detect their child's worsening condition and know when and where to seek help (Box 17.5). Parents/carers should be advised to return to the emergency department if:

- the respiratory rate increases
- recession becomes apparent
- the child is unable to feed
- the ability to speak deteriorates
- the positive response to inhaled bronchodilators reduces
- the child becomes agitated and is not behaving as normal for a child.

Follow-up should be arranged for all children discharged from ED; this can usually be done via children's community nurse teams and/or the child's own GP.

Acute laryngotracheobronchitis (viral croup)

Croup is a broad term used to describe an infection, usually viral in nature, of the upper airway and vocal chords. Croup is a common childhood illness, with the majority of children presenting with symptoms including acute onset of barking cough, low-grade fever and stridor. The stridor is made worse by crying, agitation and coughing. The most important thing to remember is to keep the child as happy as possible with as little or no intervention as possible (Bjornson & Johnson 2007). Croup is more common in boys than in girls, usually occurs between 6 and 36 months of age, and peaks during the second year of life (Zoorob et al. 2011). Croup most commonly occurs in damper weather of late autumn, winter and early spring. Typically the symptoms are worse between 18.00 and 06.00 and peak around the second or third night.

Pathophysiology

Croup encompasses a range of upper respiratory inflammations, mostly viral in nature. The most common source is acute laryngotracheobronchitis caused by the parainfluenza virus. This inflammation spreads through the bronchus and results in:

- mucosal oedema
- inflammation of the subglottic area
- increased mucus production, which can affect the entire respiratory tract.

The increase in mucus together with the pharyngeal irritation results in the hoarse cough. Obstruction to airflow through the upper airway causes stridor and difficulty in breathing, and can progress to hypoxia. Hypoxia with mild obstruction indicates involvement of the lower airway, where obstruction causes ventilation perfusion mismatching. Later, hypercapnia occurs as hypoventilation progresses with obstruction (Dykes 2005). Less common symptoms of croup are highlighted in Box 17.6.

Box 17.6

Other causes of stridor
- Inhalation of a foreign body, which has become lodged in the laryngeal region. This should be considered in all cases of stridor, as inhalation is often witnessed in small children
- Tonsillitis can present with stridor or hoarse cough when there is tonsillar enlargement which may be associated with glandular fever
- Angioneurotic oedema resulting from an acute anaphylactic reaction
- Bacterial: tracheitis is an unusual cause of croup but has a high mortality rate if not treated. These children look toxic, like those with epiglottitis, but are differentiated by their croupy cough. Intubation and antibiotic therapy are required promptly
- Diphtheria is uncommon in the UK but should be considered in children with croup symptoms who have not been immunized against diphtheria

Assessment

History

The ED nurse can quickly put together a picture of viral croup by asking the parents/carers about the lead up to attendance such as:

- duration
- symptoms – are they worse at night?
- is the child drinking?
- is the child talking normally?
- past medical history.

The nurse can expect to find a history of illness worsening over several days. Viral croup usually starts with a coryzal illness (common cold) and is followed after 48–72 hours by a sudden and often frightening onset of stridor and barking cough. At this stage children are commonly brought to ED. Unlike epiglottitis, children with croup are able to drink, although they complain of a sore throat. The ED nurse should expect these children to be able to talk but their voices will have varying levels of hoarseness. Significant past medical history is uncommon but previous airways disease or recurrent croup should be noted.

Physical assessment

Assessment of the child in ED should focus on determining the degree of threat to the respiratory function. The work of breathing should be assessed in terms of the child's colour, level of consciousness, respiratory rate, use of accessory muscles, nasal flaring and intercostal recessions. The degree of stridor is significant; the nurse should know whether the stridor is inspiratory, which usually indicates a supraglottic cause, or expiratory, which usually comes from the trachea. In severe cases inspiratory and expiratory stridor may be present. The loudness of the stridor is not an indication of its severity, but often influences the degree of anxiety. It is important to establish whether stridor is present at rest or only when the child becomes agitated or exerts him- or herself.

Heart rate should be regularly monitored. Tachycardia, particularly if it co-exists with agitation, restlessness or altered consciousness, is associated with an increase in hypoxia. Oxygen saturation should be measured in children with increased respiratory rates and tachycardia and saturation levels below 95% should be treated with oxygen therapy. By assessing a child with viral croup the ED nurse would expect to find a clinical picture of moderate fever, with a child unwell for a few days with a sudden onset of a harsh, dry and barking cough. As croup is often associated with fever, if none is present, a foreign body in the airway should also be considered. The child will usually be active, but irritable and easily upset. The key to successful management lies with accurate assessing and responding to the level of respiratory compromise. In the event of severe croup, summon anaesthetic support immediately. The child should always be nursed in the position that is most comfortable for him. This is usually semi-upright, cradled in his parent's or carer's arms. As anxiety and psychological distress have a detrimental effect on respiratory function, every effort should be made by the ED team to keep the child calm and accommodate his wishes.

Having assessed the severity of the croup, the first line treatment is dexamethasone 0.15 mg/kg orally (Sparrow & Geelhooed 2006) if this is ineffective or if the child is assessed as having moderate to severe croup then the administration of an adrenaline (epinephrine) nebulizer 5 mL 1 in 1000 is the next step. This is best administered by a parent holding the nebulizer in front of the child, as face masks and mouthpieces can be frightening and considerably increase the child's distress. Adrenaline acts both as a bronchodilator and suppresses histamine, thereby reducing mucous secretions and relieving airway obstructions. The effects of adrenaline nebulizers are relatively short-acting but often quick-acting. Should the child's condition be deteriorating then a repeat adrenaline nebulizer 5 mL 1 in 1000 should be administered while preparations for intubation are underway with the support and presence of an anaesthetist. However, if the child is showing signs of improvement then further assessment should be taken 30 minutes post-nebulizer. Clinical investigations, such as blood tests and chest and neck X-rays, do little to alter the management plan but do much to increase the child's distress and anxiety. For this reason investigations of this nature should not form part of the initial management (Box 17.7).

If the child continues to improve then a period of observation should be carried out, usually a minimum of two hours. Further medical treatment is unlikely to be required and

Box 17.7

Priorities in the treatment of croup

- Rapid and accurate assessment of airway impairment
- Keep the child calm. Nurse in a comfortable position; involve parents/carers
- Give nebulized adrenaline (epinephrine) 0.5 mg/kg of 1:1000 preparation up to 5 mL maximum
- Give oral dexamethasone 0.15 mg/kg or if the child is unable to take give nebulized steroids budesonide 2 mg
- Maintain hydration
- Monitor oxygen saturation levels; intubate if child has unresolved, worsening hypoxia

should the child remain stable and continue to be seen to be improving, discharge home with advice; children's community nursing support would be advisable. A child who is no better but remains stable should be admitted at this stage to a children's inpatient unit.

Children should have oxygen saturation levels monitored and there should be vigilant observation for clinical signs of hypoxia. In children who are not hypoxic, oxygen therapy is considered unnecessary and sometimes unhelpful as it makes the child distressed. Hypoxia in children with croup is usually a late sign and should be treated seriously. It usually indicates a need for medical intervention in airway management and in the case of a fatigued child intubation is often necessary. All children with hypoxia should be nursed in high-dependency or resuscitation areas and appropriate airway maintenance should be available.

Hydration is an important and sometimes overlooked area of care in the child with croup: many are reluctant to drink because of a painful throat and some, particularly younger children, find it difficult to take fluids because of dyspnoea. Parents should be encouraged to give frequent small amounts of clear fluid where possible. This not only prevents dehydration, but also helps to reduce tenacity of secretions. If a child is too short of breath to take fluids or is clinically dehydrated intravenous fluid replacement should be considered after initial symptoms have been relieved. Antibiotics are not considered useful as croup is predominantly of viral origin.

Criteria for admission

All children with moderate to severe croup should be admitted for observation. This can be determined by poor or transient response to treatment, persistent stridor at rest, oxygen saturation level below 92% and any degree of hypoxia. Admission should also be considered for any child who is clinically dehydrated, social circumstances should also be considered when making a decision to admit or discharge the child. If the family live a long distance from healthcare facilities or do not have transport admission should be considered.

Discharge advice

If, after a period of observation, the child is considered well enough to be discharged, the parents/carers should be given clear advice on home care, which should be supported with written information. The advice should include the following:

- stay with the child and observe the breathing pattern, as a worsening obstruction will not always wake the child from sleeping
- if the croup returns look after the child in a warm humidified environment, e.g., a steamy bathroom (made so with a hot shower running for five to ten minutes)
- if there is no improvement or the child worsens return to ED. There is no evidence to support this, however practice and experience tell us this is so.

Epiglottitis

Aetiology

Epiglottitis is a bacterial infection caused by *Haemophilus influenzae* type b (Hib) and is a relatively uncommon but life-threatening condition. Unlike laryngotracheobronchitis, it has no winter peak of incidence, nor is it more common in the evening or at night (Table 17.1). It can occur at any time of the day, throughout the year. People of all age groups are at risk of contracting epiglottitis, but it is most common in the age group 2–7 years old. Among children the incidence of epiglottitis has been reduced due to vaccination against Hibl; however this reduction in the incidence is not apparent in adults (Mathoera et al. 2008).

Table 17.1 Differentiation of croup from epiglottitis

Symptom	Croup	Epiglottitis
Age	6 months–3 years	2–5 years
Season	Winter	All year
Worst time of day	Evening/night	Any time
Aetiology	Parainfluenza virus	*Haemophilus influenzae*
Onset	Over days	Over hours
Proceeding illness	Yes	No
Fever	<38.50°C	>38.50°C
Sore throat	Sometimes	Yes
Drooling	No	Yes
Cough	Harsh barking	No
Stridor	Inspiratory and expiratory	Soft expiratory
Voice	Hoarse	None
Wheeze	Often present	None
Position	Varied, active	Upright with neck extended

Pathophysiology

Epiglottitis is a serious life-threatening condition because *Haemophilus influenzae* infection causes a rapid inflammatory infection in the epiglottis, vallecula, arytenoids and aryepiglottic folds; the tissues swell downward and over the glottic opening, making breathing difficult.

Assessment

History

Acute epiglottitis is a rapidly progressive airway emergency that progresses to complete airway obstruction within hours in the absence of prompt diagnosis and treatment (Atik & Krilis 2012). Obtaining an accurate history from parents/carers is imperative, as physical examination of the child is restricted when epiglottitis is suspected. Finesilver (2003) states physical examination only reinforces the diagnosis derived from the history, as diagnosis is often made well before examination on this basis.

Duration of the child's illness is an important factor in determining the likelihood of epiglottitis. Illness is rapid in onset, with respiratory symptoms occurring in a matter of hours. Despite this, other accompanying infections are common with epiglottitis, usually otitis media or lymphadenitis. Because of the urgent need for treatment, the ED nurse should simultaneously perform a physical inspection of the child if epiglottitis is suspected. This should differentiate between inhalation of a foreign body and epiglottitis. Additionally, croup is a common misdiagnosis in young children; however, patients with epiglottitis do not have the distinctive, barking cough that patients with croup have.

Physical assessment

It is essential the child is kept calm and that repeated attempts to examine the throat are not made. Such examination can lead to a complete obstruction of the airway by pushing the epiglottis onto the larynx (Reynolds 2004). For these reasons, assessment is a hands-off visual activity. Children with epiglottitis usually prefer to sit up leaning forward, often with their neck extended forwards and their elbows on their knees, the so-called tripod position. This allows the maximum use of their compromised airway. Most children will have a soft inspiratory stridor without an associated cough. Most children are reluctant to speak but those who do usually have a muffled voice. Drooling is a strong indication of epiglottitis because swallowing is painful, due in part to a sore throat (Tanner et al. 2002). The child usually has significant pyrexia in excess of 38.5°C. Stridor is frequently present.

Management

If epiglottitis is suspected the most important action is to summon specialist help. The child's epiglottis needs to be examined under anaesthesia in theatre and an artificial airway established in a controlled environment. While waiting for this the ED nurse should keep the child and parent/carers calm, ensuring that the child is in the most comfortable position for him and is given oxygen if possible. If the child is upset by oxygen therapy then it should not be pursued.

As any child with epiglottitis is at risk of airway obstruction at any time the ED nurse should always have equipment available to establish artificial ventilation; because of the position and degree of swelling of the epiglottis intubation in emergency can be extremely difficult. It is often necessary to perform a cricothyroidotomy. Once an artificial airway has been successfully established and the child is haemodynamically stable, other investigations and definitive management can take place, usually in the paediatric intensive care unit. This includes blood screening and cultures, the initiation of antibodies and maintenance of hydration.

Accidental injury

Accidental injuries are a major health problem throughout the UK. They are the commonest cause of death in children over one year of age. Children aged 0–4 are most likely to have an accident in the home (Royal Society for Prevention of Accidents 2008). Over 1 million children under the age of 15 experience accidents in and around the home every year, some are taken to the ED but many more are treated by general practitioners and by parents and carers (Audit Commission 2007). Falls account for the majority of non-fatal accidents, while the highest number and proportion of deaths (46%) are due to house fires (Office for National Statistics 2002).

The causes of accidents involving pre-school children are varied. Young children are vulnerable because they rely on their parents to provide a safe environment for them and to keep a careful watch on them while they explore and play. The role of the ED nurses is not just associated with treatment; they are also in a position to help educate the public and prevent further accidents from occurring. Despite all these opportunities, comparison of the home accident statistics for 1999 and 2002 indicates that even with the increased awareness and health promotion and a commitment to prevent home accidents the overall incidence of home accidents continues largely unabated (Royal Society for Prevention of Accidents 2006).

Aetiology

The factors that increase a child's risks of accidental injury are similar to agents that may increase the incidence of non-accidental injury. Bennet & Muir (2010) describe how children from lower social classes have a death rate from injury five times higher than that of children living in a higher social class. Environmental stress in the family such as illness, shortage of money and paternal tension leads to an increase in the incidence of childhood accidents.

Management

In ED, the main focus of care has traditionally been to diagnose and treat the child's injury. Nurses are very good at providing parents/carers with information about how to look after the child's injury at home, but less good at actively engaging in health promotion. Timely intervention by ED staff can prevent further accidents and ease the impact of family tension or stress. This intervention may be in the form of actual advice on accident prevention either written or verbal and/or referral to other professionals such as school nurse health visitor or if necessary social services for further assessment and support. The health visitor also has the advantage of knowing the family and can follow up the ED attendances of pre-school children under the age of five years with supportive information and active accident prevention. Parents respond better to familiar health visitors who can give relevant one-to-one advice specific to that child and family.

Trampoline injuries

Trampoline sales have rocketed over the last few years and along with it so have children attending the ED with associated injuries. It is a misguided conception that parents believe injury will only occur through falling from the trampoline, and therefore apply safety netting. However Wootton & Harris (2008) found as many as 68% of the injuries incurred are sustained without leaving the confines of the trampoline. Due to the smaller size of the pre-school child, accidents often happen because two or more smaller children are using the trampoline at a time, which may result in collision and unnecessary falls. Trampoline accidents happen when children try different stunts such as somersaults, bouncing at the sides of the trampoline, jumping off the trampoline sustaining limb injuries or crouching underneath the trampoline and equipment. Limb injuries are most common, with neck and head injuries being the most serious (Royal Society for Prevention of Accidents 2005).

Accidental poisoning

Under the age of five years, children explore their environment around them and frequently place objects in their mouths as part of this process, resulting in a large number of calls to poisons services, but a relatively low rate of serious poisoning (Bateman 2012a). Over 28 000 children receive treatment for poisoning, or suspected poisoning accidents every year (Royal Society for Prevention of Accidents 2008). More boys than girls take poisons accidentally, and it has a higher incidence in families with existing stresses such as illness, pregnancy or recent birth, absence of one parent, a house move or anxiety/depression in a parent. Some children die from poisoning each year, but the number of deaths has fallen over recent years, probably because of better treatment and because of the child-resistant container regulations. There are also fewer tricyclic antidepressants prescribed (Lyons et al. 2008).

The most commonly digested poisons are childhood medicines such as paracetamol elixir or cough mixture, oral contraceptives and vitamin supplements. Household products such as detergents, bleach, disinfectant, perfume and cosmetics are also commonly ingested (Boxes 17.8, 17.9 and 17.10). The Royal Society for Prevention of Accidents (2006) has suggested that the provision of a secure cupboard within the home should be provided as part of the built-in provision of any new homes that are built. The best location for the cupboard would be within the kitchen at a height of 1.5 metres above floor level so that smaller children cannot gain access.

Box 17.8

Non-toxic agents
- Most cosmetics – beware of alcohol in perfumes
- Non-leaded paint
- Inks
- Most antibiotics
- Vitamins
- Oral contraceptives

Box 17.9

Toxic drugs
- Paracetamol
- Salicylate and aspirin
- Tricyclic antidepressants
- Narcotics
- Iron

Box 17.10

Toxic household products
- Bleach
- Caustic soda
- Detergent
- Disinfectant
- Antifreeze
- Alcohol

Assessment

History

Establishing a clear history can often prove challenging for the ED nurse. Parents and carers and the child are very often distressed and the information may be scanty. The nurse must try to find out:

- what has been taken – the container is a useful aid to active ingredients
- how much has been ingested – the container will give useful clues to the amount left, as will the appearance of the child if spillage is possible
- parents and carers should be asked about spillages at home

- description of child's behaviour or symptoms since ingestion: vomiting is of particular significance as it reduces the likelihood of absorption
- any pre-existing illness should be noted as should any medication the child is currently taking: unless clear evidence to the contrary exists the ED nurse should assume and treat the child as if he has ingested the maximum amount of poison available.

The majority of children who have ingested the common poisons noted above will show no immediate physical signs. As a baseline the following should be established:

- respiration rate and depth
- pulse and circulatory status
- consciousness level
- pupil size and reaction
- skin condition evidence of irritation/burn particularly around or in the mouth
- weight of the child.

Management

Specific management of a poison can be aided by gaining specialist advice from a regional poisons unit or via Toxbase (www.toxbase.org). Common principles of care exist: for most poisonous substances information and clinical management can be easily downloaded from specialist advice centres.

Gastric lavage has limited effectiveness in children because of the small size of tube used. For this reason it is not recommended except in varying consciousness levels when gastric emptying is considered essential. In those circumstances, intubation and anaesthetic cover are essential before insertion of the gastric tube takes place.

In the majority of cases of accidental poisoning, the potential toxicity is low and therefore enforced emesis is considered unnecessary. In these cases activated charcoal is used as a binding agent to absorb toxins. A single dose of activated charcoal in most cases should be given within one hour of ingestion. The dose by weight is calculated at 1 g/kg or a dose by age 25–50 g (Royal College of Paediatrics and Child Health 2003). Because of the risk of aspiration, charcoal should never be given in the absence of a gag reflex or where there is impaired consciousness unless the airway is first protected by an endotracheal tube.

The decision whether to admit a child under 5 years of age can be made solely on the circumstantial history and the presence or absence of symptoms. If the child is thought to have ingested a toxic agent, such as aspirin, paracetamol, a tricyclic antidepressant, an opioid or an iron-containing compound, hospital observation is invariably required, at least for a few hours, to allow appropriate analytical measurements or more intensive monitoring (Vale & Bradberry 2012). Parents should be constructively offered advice and support, as many will have found the child's accidental poisoning very distressing.

With narcotic drugs, clinical symptoms are similar with all types of opiate drug and the nurse should suspect ingestion of narcotics if the child has pinpoint pupils. Sometimes an accurate history can be difficult to obtain, particularly if the drug is an illegal substance. Narcotic drugs often cause respiratory depression for several hours after ingestion and have a sudden onset. If the child shows signs of respiratory depression or is unconscious intravenous naloxone should be given. Children should always be admitted following narcotic poisoning.

Iron ingestion

Although used as a dietary supplement, an excess of iron is extremely toxic, causing severe gastric haemorrhage. Any symptoms the child may have should be treated on admission; i.v. access should be established at an early stage and fluid resuscitation commenced if necessary. Intramuscular desferrioxamine (15 mg/kg/h) should be given, and may be necessary over a 24-hour period depending on the severity of symptoms. Administration should be stopped when improvement occurs. The iron desferrioxamine complex (ferrioxamine) is excreted in the urine, which becomes orange-red, and may be eliminated by dialysis if renal failure develops (Bateman 2012b).

As a general rule emetics should not be given as a first-line treatment; milk can be given. Advice specific to the substance should be sought from the poison centre.

alcohol ingestion

Young children accidentally ingest alcohol in drinks or in perfumes/aftershave. Small amounts of alcohol can result in hypoglycaemia in children. A blood sugar level should be established and intravenous dextrose-based fluids given to the child if the child is significantly intoxicated or hypoglycaemic. Drowsy or unconscious children need airway management and close observation. Alcohol needs time to be excreted from the body and care in the ED revolves around maintaining homeostasis during this time. Once the child is alert and aware of his surroundings he can be discharged. Parents should be advised to increase the fluid intake over 12 hours after discharge and return if the child shows signs of gastric discomfort. If the parent/carer offers a history inconsistent with the child's condition or offers no explanation of poisoning the possibility of deliberate poisoning by a parent or a third party should be considered. It is often difficult to establish deliberate poisoning conclusively but a long and vague medical history of the child and frequent hospitalizations may raise suspicions.

Paracetamol/acetophinomen overdose

This is one of the most common drugs that children accidentally ingest however, unlike in adults, it is very rare that death or hepatotoxicity results from such ingestion (Penna & Buchanan, 1991). In children <5 y acute paracetamol/acetophinomen toxicity is usually due to accidental ingestion, in the older child this may be the result of attempted suicide (Hickson et al. 1989). It is a simple, effective analgesic, with few side effects when taken as per the recommended dose.

Paracetamol/acetophinomen poisoning is however potentially fatal (Bronstein et al. 2010).

Assessment (Box 17.11)

History

The history is crucial, and the ED nurse must ascertain dose taken, time taken and any past medical history that may make the patient more susceptible than average to the toxic effects of paracetamol (Fenner et al. 2011).

Box 17.11

Risk factors
- Malnourished
- Eating disorders
- Failure to thrive
- AIDS
- Cachexia
- Long term treatment with enzyme inducing drugs such as carbamazepine

Management

Investigations are the timed serum paracetamol concentration, liver and kidney functions and prothrombin time. Paracetamol concentration in blood should be obtained between 4 and 16 hours of ingestion to enable patient risk to be determined. The standard treatment of choice for patients who have taken a potentially toxic dose of paracetamol is the antidote acetylcysteine. The optimal dosage of acetylcysteine and the appropriate dose adjustment for body weight remain unclear and are difficult to study in patients (Ferner et al. 2011), where necessary advice should be taken from senior staff and the clinical toxicology database of the National Poisons Information Service of the relevant jurisdiction.

Safeguarding children

The nature of the work of safeguarding children is complex, multifaceted and uncertain (Smith 2010). Whether working directly with children and young people or with adults whose lives impact on children, a health professional can make all the difference.

The earliest organized professional response to child abuse in the UK was the British Society against Cruelty to Children in 1883, which led to the National Society for the Prevention of Child Cruelty (NSPCC) being established in 1890 (Royal College of Paediatrics and Child Health 2007b). The legislative framework for child protection is enshrined in the Children's Act (Department of Health 1989) and the Children (Scotland) Act (Scottish Office 1995). Over the years, the recognition and handling of child abuse has come a long way. Lessons already learnt have frequently been as a result of tragedies leading to public enquiries, such as that of the death of Marie Colwell in 1974, Jasmine Beckford in 1985, Kimberly Carlile in 1987 and more recently the violent deaths of Victoria Climbié in 2000 and that of Baby P in 2007. In the UK, the death of Victoria Climbié in 2000 brought child protection to the forefront of people's mind, public and professionals alike. The subsequent report by Lord Laming with 108 recommendations, 27 of which related to healthcare aimed to reshape and reorganize individual practice in child protection (Royal College of Paediatrics and Child Health 2007b).

Lord Laming identified five key messages from the Victoria Climbié inquiry. These were:

- communication
- written documentation
- working with each other
- training
- recognition of child abuse.

It may be that a child is seen just once and yet the record of the event could help to save a life. Victoria had no fewer than five 'unique' hospital reference numbers. Often it is only when many apparently unrelated factors are pieced together that practitioners can identify a case of child abuse. Good record-keeping is always factual, clear, accurate, accessible and comprehensive (Royal College of Nursing 2007). Write down all observations and discussions as they happen, include details of communications with other healthcare agencies notified. Seek guidance from Trust policy and senior colleagues, liaising with a designated named child protection nurse, always dating and timing any actions. Confidentiality must not be confused with secrecy. Information should always be shared on a 'need to know' basis when it is in the best interest of the child. The intercollegiate committee services for children in EDs, recommends that all staff, whether clinical or non-clinical, must receive training in safeguarding children appropriate to their posts (Royal College of Paediatrics and Child Health 2007b).

Following on from Lord Laming's original report, The Victoria Climbié Enquiry (Department of Health 2003c), and as a result of the recent Baby P investigations, Ministers announced to the UK Parliament in late 2008 that Lord Laming had once again been asked to prepare an independent report on the progress being made nationally to deliver and implement effective child protection and also identify any possible barriers and how these could be overcome. In March 2009, Lord Laming produced 'The Protection of Children in England: A Progress Report' in which he highlighted the progress that had been made over the previous 5 years in implementing the legislation and guidance outlined in documents such as Every Child Matters (Department for Education and Skills 2004) and the interagency working that had occurred as a result of guidance in the document Working Together to Safeguard Children (Department for Children, Schools and Families 2010), both of which provided a sound framework for promoting and ensuring the welfare of the child. However,

he also made very clear the new challenges ahead in protecting children from significant harm and neglect with one of the main challenges being to ensure leaders of local services effectively translate policy, legislation and guidance into day-to-day practice on the frontline of every service (Lord Laming 2009).

Prevalence

The true incidence of child abuse is difficult to ascertain. In 2004, there were 26 000 children on the child protection register, 41 % were considered to be at risk due to neglect, 19 % due to physical abuse, 18 % due to emotional abuse and 9 % due to sexual abuse (Royal College of Paediatrics and Child Health 2007b). As a result of recommendations by Lord Laming in 2003, child protection registers were phased out in England in 2006 and instead children are made subjects of child protection plans under guidance from Working Together to safeguard Children (Department for Children, Schools and Families 2010).

Because of differing perceptions of child abuse, and hence changing definitions, as well as difficulties in ascertainment, it is impossible to build up a full picture of its incidence of abuse (Royal College of Paediatrics and Child Health 2007b). The first national survey of all types of abuse and neglect was conducted in the UK for the NSPCC (Cawson et al. 2000). In the study, 2869 young adults between the ages of 18 and 24 years were interviewed. There were no definitions of abuse and neglect but respondents were asked if they had experienced specific behaviours.

The prevalence figures obtained were as follows:

- serious physical abuse (violence used regularly over the years, or which had caused physical injury or frequently led to physical effects): 7 %
- serious absence of physical care (behaviours that carried a high risk of injury or long-term harmful effects): 6 %
- serious absence of parental supervision (staying home alone without supervision overnight under 10 years of age or staying out overnight without parents knowing their whereabouts under 14 years of age): 5 %
- serious emotional maltreatment (control and domination (psychological and/or physical), humiliation, withdrawal, antipathy, terrorizing and proxy attacks): 6 %
- sexually abused (contact and non-contact – against their wishes or under the age of 13 years): 16 %
- sexually abused (contact – against their wishes or under the age of 13 years): 11 %.

First-born children are more likely to be affected and it is not uncommon to find one child is abused while other siblings are free from abuse. Young children of pre-school age are more at risk because they cannot seek help. Most children are abused by a parent; but in this context a not uncommon scenario is a co-habitant living in the house who is not the child's biological parent. Statistically, the younger the parents, the more likely it is that they will abuse their children. Child abuse is also seen across all layers of society. The acknowledgement that child abuse exists and is quite common is an important start for ED staff; however, in order to enable detection the nurse needs to keep an open and enquiring mind. It is also worth noting that children who are subjected to maltreatment are unlikely to have one type of abuse (Browne 2002) (Box 17.12).

Box 17.12

Types of child abuse
- Physical
- Neglect
- Emotional
- Social
- Sexual

The definition taken from *Working Together to Safeguard Children* (Department for Children, Schools and Families 2010) of child abuse is as follows: 'Abuse and neglect are forms of maltreatment of a child. Somebody may abuse or neglect a child by inflicting harm, or by failing to act to prevent harm. Children may be abused in a family or in an institutional or community setting; by those known to them or, more rarely, by a stranger. They may be abused by an adult or adults or another child or children.' These forms of abuse are described as below. Common physical and non-physical indicators of child abuse are given in Box 17.13.

Physical

Most commonly, physical abuse is inflicted on the child under the guise of punishment or when an adult loses control. It usually involves violence, often of a short duration but repetitive. Physical abuse includes poisoning and suffocation. A study of non-accidental drowning's found that there were no cases of accidental bath drowning over the age of 18 months, and in all cases over this age the child drowned due to abuse or epilepsy (Kemp et al. 1994). Similarly, Barber & Sibert (2000) suggest that it is very rare for children over the age of 3 years to present with non-accidental bruising or fractures, in contrast to accidental causes. Besharou (1990) notes that deliberately inflicted burns can be distinguished by their severity and area. For instance, burns resulting from deliberate immersion in hot water have distinct lines around them and no splash marks (Joaghim 2003). In the absence of a clinical or plausible accidental explanation, these types of injuries are highly suggestive of abuse.

Neglect

Neglect is the persistent and severe failure to provide love, care, food, shelter or the physical circumstances to allow for

Box 17.13

Common indicators of child abuse

Physical indicators
- Alterations in skin integrity
- Abrasions to palms, elbows, or knees from being pushed down
- Burns resulting from:
  - cigarettes and cigars
  - curling tongs, clothes iron
  - chemicals
  - friction – being dragged on the ground
  - immersion in hot liquid or 'dunking' injury patterns
  - splashes
- Bite marks – human are crest-shaped
- External genitalia lacerations or abrasions
- Vaginal bleeding, discharge or infections
- Penile bleeding, discharge or infections
- Rectal bleeding, discharge or infections
- Patterned bruises such as from a whip, belt or other implement
- Bruises in various stages of healing

Alterations in musculoskeletal system
- Multiple fractures
- Fractures in various stages of healing
- Spiral or midshaft fractures of long bones
- Fractured ribs – uncommon in young children
- Skull fractures

Neurological impairment
- Acute onset of paresis
- Post-concussion symptoms
- Intracranial haemorrhage
- Visual impairment resulting from retinal detachment

Non-physical indicators
- Conflicting histories obtained from parent(s) or adult(s) and child regarding the nature of the child's injuries
- Children who are not allowed by the parent(s) or adult(s) to verbalize a history despite the fact that they are developmentally and chronologically old enough to do so
- A history given by the parent(s) or adult(s) that does not fit the nature of the presenting injuries
- Children who display fearful body language, e.g., guarding when a sudden movement is made
- A delay in bringing the child to ED for treatment of an injury or illness that indicates abuse or neglect

(After Sheridan MS (2003) The deceit continues: an updated literature review of Munchausen Syndrome by Proxy. Child Abuse & Neglect. 27(4), 431-51.)

normal development (Box 17.14). It also includes willfully exposing a child to any kind of danger. Neglect can lead to failure to thrive, manifest by a fall away from initial centile lines in weight, height and head circumference, which is why repeated growth measurements are crucially important in primary care. Signs of malnutrition include wasted muscles and poor condition of skin and hair. It is important not to miss an organic cause of failure to thrive; if this is suspected, further investigations will be required.

Box 17.14

Common indicators of child neglect

Physical indicators

- Poor hygiene and/or clothing that does not protect a child from weather
- Chronic signs of malnutrition and dehydration
- Poor oral hygiene or untreated dental problems
- Failure to receive immunizations
- Child abandonment
- Delays in seeking prompt medical care for an acute injury or illness
- Failure to give child a prescribed medication, which results in the child developing more severe symptoms
- Failure to thrive in infants

Emotional and behavioural indicators

- Delay or absence of age-appropriate behaviours, especially in infants and young children
- Constant hunger
- Poor personal hygiene
- Lethargy in the absence of illness
- Social withdrawal or depression
- Relentless attention-seeking behaviour
- Minimal response to painful medical interventions
- Suicidal ideation or attempts
- Poor state of clothing
- Emaciation
- Untreated medical problems
- No social relationships
- Compulsive scavenging

(After Sheridan MS (2003) The deceit continues: an updated literature review of Munchausen Syndrome by Proxy. Child Abuse & Neglect. 27(4), 431-51.)

Emotional abuse

Emotional abuse is the persistent emotional ill-treatment of a child such as to cause severe and persistent adverse effects on the child's emotional development. It may involve conveying to children that they are worthless or unloved, inadequate, or valued only in so far as they meet the needs of another person; having age or developmentally inappropriate expectations imposed on children; causing children frequently to feel frightened; or the exploitation or corruption of children (Department of Health 2003b). All abuses involve some emotional ill-treatment. Iwaniec (1997) argued that parents and carers who persistently criticize, shame, threaten, humiliate, induce fear and anxiety and who are never satisfied with the child's behaviour and performance, and do so deliberately, are emotionally abusive and cruel. Children suffering from emotional abuse may be withdrawn and emotionally flat. One reaction is for the child to seek attention constantly or to be over-familiar. Lack of self-esteem and developmental delay are again likely to be present.

Sexual abuse

This is discussed in a separate section further on.

The parents

The vast majority of child abuse involves at least one of the child's parents. Approximately one-third of parents who were abused as children are at risk of abusing their own children. As abused children, they may have been subjected to marked negative reinforcement and an inability to get their needs met, have little practice in problem-solving, and no basis for trusting others. As a consequence they may lack empathy with their children as little was directed towards them and a self-perpetuating cycle then begins (Tercier 1992). The parents may present as hostile or exhibit a lack of concern or guilt or may show a lack of interest or disturbed interaction with the child and seem more interested in their own problem than the child's, for example, how they are going to get home. That noted, it is important to acknowledge the crisis and distress that investigation and intervention cause to the child and family and that there may be conflicting interests between the needs of the child and those of the parents; however, it is also important to stress that under the Children Act (Department of Health 1989) the child's welfare is paramount.

The child

These children have a number of characteristics that predispose them to victimization. They are often the unwanted child of unplanned pregnancies, illegitimate births, and the opposite sex from that desired by the parents, born in periods of crisis or from a former relationship. The children themselves may have problems that make them difficult to rear, being poor feeders, or with challenging behaviours, abnormal sleep patterns, excessive crying and hyperactivity. The child may present as passive, withdrawn and uncomplaining during dressings, or may present hyperactive, angry or rebellious behaviour. There may be obvious signs of neglect.

Management of suspected child abuse

Every ED should have an agreed procedure for the management of suspected child abuse and nurses need to be acquainted with this procedure. All such cases of suspected abuse should be reported to senior medical staff and consultant paediatricians for further investigation and intervention where necessary. Suspicions of child abuse start at initial assessment; an astute nurse will pick up discrepancies in the history of the incident, incompatibilities between the alleged mechanism of injury and the actual injury, and the usual interactions between the child and his carer (Saines 1992). All life-threatening conditions must be given immediate attention; however, while the nursing care and treatment of the child's physical needs remain paramount, the emotional needs of the child must also be addressed. When clinicians are suspicious of child abuse they have a duty to inform the parents of the need to inform and notify a child protection agency. Local guidelines for child protection should be followed and the child and family should be supported and cared for in a private but safe area during their stay in ED (Department of Health 2003b).

The health worker's attitude can have a great impact on the child. It is imperative that the health carer appears non-judgemental and is not disgusted by findings or revelations. These should be handled with diplomacy to prevent a difficult situation from becoming inflamed; however, it should be acknowledged that abused cases of any kind could foster feelings amongst staff of hostility and anger towards the alleged perpetrators. Nevertheless, for nursing to be effective, staff must control these feelings. Team leaders and members should monitor each other's emotional and physical well-being and provide support for those who appear to be affected by an incident (Cudmore 1998).

Careful documentation is critical in cases of suspected child abuse. For the nurse taking a history, the single most important factor is the history of the incident as told by the child. It is important to write exactly, or as closely as possible, any allegations of abuse or neglect, noting who made them and who was present. The veracity and accuracy of information recorded should be exact.

Evidence

No child should be discharged into the custody of parents or carers if staff feel that there is a risk to the child's health and welfare. Where parents are unwilling to cooperate the protection of the Children Act (Department of Health 1989) may need to be applied to bring an Emergency Protection Order. In most instances, however, where non-judgemental approaches are used and open communication prevails parental agreement will be forthcoming.

Consent for photographs should be sought before any photographs of injuries are taken, as they may play an important part in subsequent legal proceedings as well as providing valuable clinical evidence.

Sanders & Cobly (2005) note that there is a culture of under-reporting of suspected non-accidental injury in children in EDs, which is largely to do with the fact that a significant proportion of medical and nursing staff receive no formal training in identifying potential indicators of child abuse and because they have no rapid access to a paediatric opinion. Additionally, bureaucratic and inter-professional barriers to accessing confidential information about children from social services registers also lead to long delays in the ability of clinicians to obtain a rapid assessment of each suspected case of abuse.

The reforms arising out of Lord Laming's inquiry into the death of Victoria Climbié, who died of abuse at the hands of her aunt and her aunt's partner, present an ideal opportunity to encourage clinicians to be alert to the possibility of non-accidental injury and address the current culture of under-reporting (Department of Health 2003c). The recommendations from this report and the subsequent review are reshaping the way child protection cases are managed and have influenced the children's national service frameworks (Department of Health 2003c, Welsh Assembly Government 2004).

Sexual abuse

This occurs when dependent, developmentally immature children are forced to participate in sexual activity. Although sexual abuse may occur at any age, peaks tend to occur between the 2–6 years and 12–16 years (Tercier 1992). Perhaps the most difficult area of abuse to detect in ED is sexual abuse, primarily because sexually abused children often display no physical signs and it is therefore necessary to be alert to the behavioural and emotional factors that may indicate abuse.

Various degrees and forms of sexual abuse include molestation, touching or fondling of the child's genitalia, masturbation of the perpetrator by the child, combination of oral-genital contact, attempted or actual anal or vaginal intercourse, exhibitionism, voyeurism and exploitation of children in the preparation of pornographic materials. Sexual abuse differs from other forms of child abuse in that it is not used as a form of punishment. However, while violence is seldom a factor, coercion and threats are common (Tercier 1992). Hobbs & Wynne (2001) suggest that physical abuse and sexual abuse are thought to be closely related; however, the two can occur independently of each other. This relationship is based on power: the threat of physical abuse gives the perpetrator the power to ensure the compliance of the child and allows them to guarantee that the child keeps the sexual abuse a secret (Chudleigh 2005).

Sexual abuse may present to ED staff in a number of different ways:

- physical complaints: for example, abdominal pain, urinary tract infection, per rectum and per vaginal bleeds
- parental accusations; this should always be taken seriously where one parent or carer accuses another
- request by the child for help; children do not fabricate stories of sexual activity
- physical abuse; children who have been physically abused may present with evidence of sexual abuse; careful examination may reveal trauma or infection
- emotional or psychological problems; these may present as bed-wetting, night terrors and developmental regression
- sexually transmitted diseases; any sexually transmitted disease in a child should be considered evidence of sexual abuse until proven otherwise.

Management

The management of children who are suspected of being sexually abused is similar to that for child abuse. Establishing rapport and trust is critical, using language that is appropriate for the child's age and development stage: it is important to stress that children have short attention spans and therefore a prolonged interview will not be tolerated. Children must be constantly reassured that it is alright to share their secrets with the nurse and for this reason it is best to interview the child away from the family members, even those not initially believed to be involved in the abuse or neglectfulness (Sheridan 1995). Once there is significant indication that sexual abuse may have occurred, arrangements should be made for a physical examination to be completed. Forensic examination should be completed first to ensure that evidence is not destroyed therefore a joint examination in conjunction with an experienced paediatrician may be appropriate to save the child from repeated examination.

A number of key facts need to be established in gaining a history of sexual abuse. These are presented in Box 17.15.

All too often ED staff do not hear the outcomes of particularly difficult cases of suspected child sexual abuse. It is good practice to promote inter-disciplinary team meetings for a period review and updating of such cases to provide feedback, support and opportunities to further improve protocols.

Box 17.15

Sexual abuse history

- Date and time of assault
- Place of assault(s)
- Number of people involved and relationship to abused
- Physical characteristics
- Use of restraints
- Use of sexual aids
- Use of lubricants, powders or other chemicals
- Statements made during assault
- Use of photographs or videotaping
- Removal of locks of hair or other 'artifacts'
- Form of assault, i.e., vaginal, anal or oral intercourse
- Occurrence of ejaculation
- Oral manipulation of breasts or other body parts
- Use of condom
- Bath, douche or clean mouth after assault
- Last bowel movement and last urination
- Last menstrual period, if appropriate
- Use of contraceptive pill or IUD, if appropriate
- Use of tampons or pads, if appropriate

Box 17.16

Characteristics of fabricated illness

- Persistent or recurrent illnesses that cannot be explained or are very unusual
- Laboratory results or physical findings that are at variance with the general health of the child
- Symptoms that only occur when the child is in the presence of the caretaker
- A caretaker who appears overly attentive, with prolonged visiting or living in with the child in the hospital
- Standard treatments that are not tolerated, e.g., i.v. lines that always come out, vomiting of medications
- A caretaker who does not seem as concerned about the child's illness as the medical or nursing staff
- A caretaker with previous medical experience or education
- Atypical episodes of seizures, near-miss SIDS or SIDS, apnoeic or cyanotic episodes occurring only in the presence of the caretaker and which do not seem to respond to standard therapy
- A history of multiple resuscitations in a child with no recognizable cardiopulmonary abnormalities

List of behaviours exhibited by carers with parenting responsibilities (Department for Education and Skills 2004)

- Deliberately inducing symptoms in children by administering medicines or other substances, or by means of suffocation
- Interfering with treatments by overdosing, not administering, or interfering with medical equipment
- Obtaining specialist treatments or equipment for children who don't require them
- Exaggerating symptoms, causing professionals to undertake investigations and treatments which may be invasive, are unnecessary and therefore harmful and possibly dangerous
- Claiming the child has symptoms which are unverifiable unless obviously directly, such as pain, frequency of passing urine, vomiting, or fitting, claims result in unnecessary investigations and treatments which present secondary physical problems
- Alleging psychological illness in a child

(After Meadow R (1982) Munchausen syndrome by proxy. Archives of Diseases of Childhood 57(2), 92-98.)

Fabricated illness

Fabricated illness in babies and children by a parent/carer is often referred to by any number of different terms, most commonly Munchausen's syndrome by proxy (MBP), factitious illness by proxy or illness induction syndrome (Department of Health 2004). Professor Roy Meadows (1977, 1997) who first described Munchausen by proxy (Box 17.16), however, in 2001, following continuing contention regarding the existence, application and definition of the term MBP and many complaints by parents/carers claiming to be falsely accused of child abuse, the Department of Health developed guidance for child protection professionals attempting to give credibility and validity to MBP and introduced the new term 'fabricated illness' (Department of Health, Home Office, Department of Education and Skills, Welsh Assembly Government 2004). Munchausen by proxy is now the term reserved for the disorder whereby there are two elements, one indicating a behaviour in the parent/carer for a particular

self-serving psychological need and secondly a diagnosis in the child who has been harmed by the parent/carer (Schreier 2002). Fabrication and induction of illness is a broad term to describe a group of behaviours by parents, or those 'in loco parentis', that cause harm to children. The behaviours have a wide range, from those causing immediate, direct physical harm (inductions), to verbal fabrications of symptoms that are more indirectly and chronically dangerous in both physical and emotional ways. There are many in-between variants. The illnesses fabricated include any medical, surgical or psychiatric conditions, and may extend to fabrication of special educational needs and disabilities (Royal College of Paediatrics and Child Health 2007b).

Fabrication of illness or illness induction should be considered whenever a baby or child presents with unusual signs and symptoms that are not easily explained physiologically. The fabrication of illness is usually manifested in one of three ways:

- induction of illness or injury by a variety of means
- falsification of signs and symptoms that may include fabrication of past medical history
- falsification of specimens of bodily fluids, falsification of hospital record charts, letters and documents.

The variety of diseases mimicked or produced is alarmingly diverse and limited only by the parent's imagination and insanity. The child, who is usually under 5 years old, is most commonly presented with problems related to one body system such as blood in urine or recurrent seizures. The illness story is related consistently by the carer, who in 90% of cases is the child's natural mother. Events relating to the illness episode only start in her presence. While ideal parenting behaviours may be demonstrated, the mother is often inappropriately calm in relation to the gravity of the child's illness.

Fabricated illness can be difficult to detect and may go unrecognized for long periods (Eminson 2000). Parents who fabricate or induce illness in >80% of cases, are mothers. McClure et al. (1996) found that 6% of children died as a direct result of extreme fabricated illness, with 12% requiring paediatric intensive care. Up to 35% of children from reported incidents suffer major physical problems as a result of the abuse, with as many as 50% of children experiencing long-term morbidity. Child welfare concerns arise when the patterns of presentation in the child are not consistent and incongruent and the conjunction of unobserved parental access and deterioration in the child's health occurs. At all times, nurses must have a high index of suspicion and while it is possible that there are any number of explanations for any of these circumstances, each will require careful consideration (Box 17.17). When concerns are such that a positive explanation for the child's presentation is that of fabricated illness then referral to a senior paediatrician and social services should be made.

Personal information about the child and family held by professionals is subject to a legal duty of confidence and should not be discussed inappropriately without the consent of the subject. Notwithstanding this, the law of disclosure of confidential information is necessary to safeguard children in the public interest: that is, the public interest in maintaining confidentiality (Department of Health, Home Office, Department of Education and Skills, Welsh Assembly Government 2004). Without exception children are entitled to the same duty of confidence as adults.

Despite the understandable feelings of anger and frustration of clinical staff in these situations, the need for non-judgemental care remains paramount, as is the continuing need for vigilance to safeguard children. Support and

> ## Box 17.17
>
> ### Child welfare concerns
> - Reported signs and symptoms found on assessment are not explained by any medical condition the child might be suffering from; or
> - Physical examinations and results of diagnostics do not explain symptoms and signs on examination; or
> - There is an inexplicably poor response to prescribed medication and treatment; or
> - New symptoms are reported on resolution of previous ones; or
> - Reported symptoms and found signs are not observed independently of the carer; or
> - The child's normal, daily life activities are being curtailed beyond what might be expected for any known medical disorder from which the child might be suffering
>
> (After Department for Education and Skills (2004) Quality Protects: The Finch Report on Delay in Public Law Children Act Proceedings. DFES, London.)

debriefing should be made available for staff, including all the multidisciplinary team who have been involved in the care of abused children and who have been affected by fabricated or induced illness (Dolan 1998).

Conclusion

Children of pre-school age are more likely than others to attend for emergency treatments, because of their vulnerability to accidents and illness. EDs can be developed to become more child-oriented, helping to reduce children's anxieties. The emergency nurse should appreciate the importance of supporting and reassuring a child's family.

Through helping them, the nurse will help the child and increase their cooperation. It is important that professionals working with children have fundamental knowledge of normal development stages, both physiological and cognitive, enabling the consultation to be pitched at the appropriate level for the child and family.

A trip to the ED is usually the young child's first experience of hospital. Every effort should be made to make the experience as little upsetting as possible. Avoid separation from parents/carers, explain simply what is wrong, and if and how it can be amended, in a language that is easily understandable to the child. On this first visit to the hospital, it is the emergency nurse's responsibility to ensure the experience is as positive as can be.

References

Atik, A., Krilis, M., 2012. Epiglottis in a vaccinated child: A life-saving diagnosis. Hong Kong Journal of Emergency Medicine 19 (2), 138–140.

Audit Commission, 2007. Better safe than sorry: Preventing unintentional injury in children. Audit Commission, London.

Aylott, M., 2007. Observing the sick child. Paediatric Nurse 19 (1), 38–45.

Barber, M.A., Sibert, J.R., 2000. Diagnosing physical child abuse: The way forward. Postgraduate Medical Journal 76, 743–749.

Bateman, D.N., 2012a. The epidemiology of poisoning. Medicine 40 (2), 42–44.

Bateman, D.N., 2012b. Iron. Medicine 40 (3), 128–129.

Bateman, E.D., Hurd, S.S., Barnes, P.J., et al., 2008. Global strategy of asthma management and prevention. European Respiratory Journal 31 (1), 143–178.

Bennet, C., Muir, N., 2010. Prevention of unintentional injury in the community setting. Nursing Standard 24 (42), 50–56.

Bentley, J., 2004. Distress in children attending A&E. Emergency Nurse 2 (4), 20–26.

Besharou, D., 1990. Recognising Child Abuse: A Guide for the Concerned. Free Press, London.

Bjornson, C., Johnson, D., 2007. Croup in paediatric emergency departments. Paediatric Child Health 12 (6), 473–477.

Bowlby, J., 1953. Child Care and the Growth of Love. Penguin, London.

Brain, J., Martin, M.D., 1989. Child Care and Health for Nursery Nurses, third ed. Stanley Thornes and Hulton, Cheltenham.

British Thoracic Society and Scottish Intercollegiate Guidelines Network, 2011. British Guideline on the Management of Asthma: A National Clinical Guideline. BTS/SIGN, Edinburgh.

Bronstein, A.C., Spyker, D.A., Cantilena, L.R., et al., 2009. Annual Report of the American Association of Poison Control Centres (NPDS) 27th Annual Report Clinical Toxicology 48, 978–1178.

Brooker, C., Nicol, M., 2003. Nursing Adults The Practice of Caring. Mosby, London.

Browne, K., 2002. Child abuse: defining, understanding and intervening. In: Wilson, K., James, A. (Eds.), (2002) The Child Protection Handbook, second ed. Baillière Tindall, London.

Cawson, P., Wattam, C., Brooker, S., et al., 2000. Child Maltreatment in the United Kingdom: A Study of the Prevalence of Abuse and Neglect. NSPCC, London.

Child Accident Prevention Trust, 2011. Cycle Safety Factsheet. CAPT, London.

Chudleigh, J., 2005. Safeguarding children. Paediatric Nursing 17 (1), 37–42.

Cudmore, J., 1998. Critical incident stress management strategies. Emergency Nurse 6 (3), 22–27.

Department for Children, Schools and Families, 2010. Working Together to Safeguard Children. London: Department of Health. Department for Education and Skills (2004) Every Child Matters. The Stationery Office, London.

Department for Education and Skills, 2004. Quality Protects: The Finch Report on Delay in Public Law Children Act Proceedings. DFES, London.

Department of Health, 1989. The Children Act. HMSO, London.

Department of Health, 2003a. The Ill Child Module Ambulatory Care Sub Group Children's National Service Framework. Department of Health, London.

Department of Health, 2003b. What To Do If You're Worried A Child Is Being Abused. Department of Health, London.

Department of Health, 2003c. The Victoria Climbié Inquiry: Report of an Inquiry by Lord Laming. Cmnd 5730. The Stationery Office, London.

Department of Health, 2004. The National Service Framework for Children, Young People and Maternity Services. Department of Health, London.

Department of Health, Home Office, Department of Education and Skills, Welsh Assembly Government, 2004. Safeguarding Children in which Illness is Fabricated or Induced. Department of Health, London.

Dolan, B., 1998. The hospital hoppers. Nursing Times 94 (30), 26–27.

Dykes, J., 2005. Managing children with croup in emergency departments. Emergency Nurse 13 (6), 14–19.

Eminson, D.M., 2000. Background. In: Eminson, D.M., Postlethwaite, R.J. (Eds.), Munchausen Syndrome by Proxy Abuse: A Practical Guide. Arnold, London.

Fenner, R.E., Dear, J.W., Bateman, N., 2011. Management of paracetamol poisoning. British Medical Journal 342, 2218.

Finesilver, C., 2003. Pulmonary Assessment: what you need to know. Progress in Cardiovascular Nursing 18 (2), 83–92.

Hall, D., Elliman, D., 2003. Health for all Children, fourth ed. Oxford University Press, Oxford.

Hickson, G.B., Altemier, W.A., Martin, E., 1989. Parental administration of chemical agents: a cause of apparent life-threatening events. Paediatrics 83 (5), 772–776.

Hughes, J., Lyte, G., 2009. Developing Nursing Practice with Children and Young People. Wiley Blackwell, Oxford.

Hobbs, C.J., Wynne, J.M., 2001. Physical Signs of Child Abuse. WB Saunders, London.

Iwaniec, D., 1997. The Emotionally Abused and Neglected Child. John Wiley, Chichester.

Joaghin, V., 2003. Working together for child protection in A&E. Emergency Nurse 11 (7), 30–37.

Kemp, A., Mott, A.M., Sibert, J.R., 1994. Accidents and child abuse in bathtub submersions. Archives of Diseases in Childhood 70, 435–438.

Knight, S., Gregory, S., 2009. Specialising in play. Emergency Nurse 16 (10), 16–19.

Lord Laming, 2009. The Protection of Children in England: A Progress Report. The Stationery Office, London.

Lyons, R., Goldsmid, J.M., Kibel, M.A., et al., 2008. Accidents, poisoning and SIDS. In: McIntosh, N., Helms, P., Smyth, R., Logan, S. (Eds.), Forfar & Arneil's Textbook of Paediatrics. Elsevier, Edinburgh.

McClure, R.J., Davis, P.M., Meadow, S.R., Sibert, J.R., 1996. Epidemiology of Munchausen syndrome by proxy, non-accidental poisoning, and non-accidental suffocation. Archives of Diseases in Childhood 75, 57–61.

Maguire, P., Pitceathly, C., 2002. Key communication skills and how to acquire them. British Medical Journal 325, 697–700.

Mathoera, R., Wever, P., Van Dorsten, F., et al., 2008. Epiglottitis in the adult patient. The Journal of Medicine 66 (9), 373–377.

Mead, D., Sibert, J., 1991. The Injured Child: An Action Plan for Nurses. Scutari, London.

Meadow, R., 1977. Munchausen syndrome by proxy: The hinterlands of child abuse. Lancet 2, 343–345.

Meadow, R., 1982. Munchausen syndrome by proxy. Archives of Diseases of Childhood 57 (2), 92–98.

Meadow, R., 1997. ABC of Child Abuse, third ed. British Medical Association, London.

Ministry of Health, 1959. The Welfare of Children in Hospital (The Platt Report). HMSO, London.

NHS Institute for Innovation and Improvement, 2008. Children and Young People Emergency Care Pathway. NHS Institute for Innovation and Improvement, Warwick.

National Audit Office, 2004. Improving Emergency Care in England. NAO, London.

National Institute for Health and Clinical Excellence, 2007. Management and Guidelines on Asthma in Children. NICE, London.

Neill, S.J., 2000. Acute childhood illness at home: the parents' perspective. Journal of Advanced Nursing 31 (4), 821–832.

Office for National Statistics, 2002. Mortality Statistics; Injury and Poisoning: England & Wales. Office for National Statistics, London.

Penna, A., Buchanan, N., 1991. Paracetamol poisoning in children and hepatotoxicity. British Journal of Clinical Pharmacology 32, 143–149.

Piaget, J., 1990. The Child's Conception of the World. Little Fields Adams, New York.

Reynolds, T., 2004. Ear, nose and throat problems. Nursing Standard 18 (26), 47–52.

Royal College of Nursing, 2007. Standards for Assessing, Measuring and Monitoring Vital Signs in Infants, Children and Young People. RCN, London.

Royal College of Paediatrics and Child Health, 2003. Medicines for Children. RCPCH, London.

Royal College of Paediatrics and Child Health, 2007a. Maximising Nursing Skills in Caring for Children in Emergency Departments. Royal College of Nursing, London.

Royal College of Paediatrics and Child Health, 2007b. Child Protection Reader. RCPCH, London.

Royal College of Paediatrics and Child Health, 2009. Annual Report. RCPCH, London.

Royal College of Paediatrics and Child Health and Royal College of Nursing, 2010. Maximising Nursing Skills in Caring for Children in Emergency Departments. RCN, London.

Royal Pharmaceutical Society, 2010. BNF for Children. RCPCH Publications, London.

Royal Society for Prevention of Accidents, 2005. Leisure Safety Information: Trampoline Safety. RoSPA, Birmingham.

Royal Society for Prevention of Accidents (RoSPA), 2006. Accidents to Children: Can the Home Ever be Safe? RoSPA, Birmingham.

Royal Society for Prevention of Accidents, 2008. A Short RoSPA Guide to Core Concepts. RoSPA, Birmingham.

Saines, J., 1992. A considered response to an emotional crisis: A&E nurses role in detecting child sexual abuse. Professional Nurse 8 (3), 148–152.

Sanders, T., Cobley, C., 2005. Identifying non-accidental injury in children presenting to A&E departments: an overview of the literature. Accident & Emergency Nursing 13 (2), 130–136.

Schreier, H., 2002. Munchausen by proxy defined. Paediatrics 110 (5), 985–988.

Scottish Office, 1995. Scotland's Children: A Brief Guide to the Children (Scotland) Act (1995). The Stationery Office, Edinburgh.

Scullion, J., 2005. A proactive approach to asthma. Nursing Standard 20 (9), 57–65.

Shabu, A., Carr, M., Crushell, E., et al., 2007. Patterns of asthma admissions in children. Irish Medical Journal 100 (3), 407–409.

Sheridan, M.S., 1995. The descent continues: An updated literature review Munchausen's syndrome by proxy. Child Abuse & Neglect. The International Journal 27 (4), 431–451.

Sheridan, M.S., 2003. The deceit continues: an updated literature review of Munchausen syndrome by proxy. Child Abuse & Neglect 27 (4), 431–451.

Smith, S., 2010. Safeguarding children: Assessment and decision-making. Nursing in Practice 52, 57–60.

Sparrow, A., Geelhoed, G., 2006. Prednisolone versus dexamethasone in croup: A randomized equivalence trial. Archive of Diseases of Childhood 91, 580–583.

Tanner, K., Fitzsimmons, G., Carrol, D., et al., 2002. *Haemophilus influenzae* type b epiglottitis as a cause of acute upper airways obstruction in children. British Medical Journal 325 (7372), 1099–1100.

Tercier, A., 1992. Child abuse. In: Rosen, P., Barkin, R.M., Braen, G. (Eds.), Emergency Medicine: Concepts and Clinical Practice, third ed. Mosby Year Book, St. Louis.

UNICEF, 1990. Office of the United Nations High Commissioner of Human Rights. UNICEF, Geneva.

United Nation, 1989. Convention on the Rights of the Child. United Nations, Geneva.

Vale, A., Bradberry, S., 2012. Management of poisoning: initial management and need for admission. Medicine 40 (2), 65–66.

Visintainer, M.A., Wolfer, J.A., 1975. Psychological preparation for surgical pediatric patients: The effects on children's and parents' stress responses and adjustment. Pediatrics 56 (2), 187–202.

Webster, A., 2002. The facility role of the play specialist. Paediatric Nursing 12 (7), 24–27.

Welsh Assembly Government, 2004. NSF for Children, Young People and Maternity Services. Welsh Assembly Government, Cardiff.

Wootton, M., Harris, D., 2008. Trampolining injuries. Emergency Medicine Journal 26, 728–731.

Zoorob, R., Sidani, M., Murray, J., 2011. Croup: an overview. American Family Physician 83 (9), 1067–1073.

Age 5 to puberty

18

Catherine Sumsky

CHAPTER CONTENTS

Introduction

This chapter considers reasons for Emergency Department (ED) attendance by children between the ages of 5 and 13 years. While this age range is somewhat arbitrary, especially in the context of the decreasing age of puberty, for the purposes of this chapter it will be used as a chronological benchmark between pre-school children and adolescence. Some of the more common injuries and conditions occurring in this age group will be considered, with particular reference to a child's development and the need for a suitable environment and a family-centred approach.

Children's school years are proposed as the best years of their lives, but unfortunately they are also a very dangerous time. Children's maturity and their interests and needs differ from adults. Therefore, simply reproducing injury-prevention strategies that are relevant to adults does not adequately protect children. As children develop, their curiosity and wish to experiment are not always matched by their capacity to understand or respond to danger (World Health Organization 2008). Each year one in five children attends an ED and one in 10–15 children will be admitted to hospital (Department of Health 2005). Once children reach the age of 5 years, unintentional injuries are the biggest threat to their survival. Death in childhood is most prevalent during the first year of life, while the fewest deaths occur between the ages of 5 and 14. Of these deaths trauma and neoplasms are the biggest killers (National Institute for Health and Clinical Excellence 2005, American College of Surgeons 2008). The number of deaths from trauma in this age group has decreased dramatically since 1991; this may be due to an increase in safety awareness or an increase in paediatric resuscitation courses.

Children's deaths following injury are most commonly road traffic accidents (RTAs) followed by drowning, suffocation, fire and falls (Mead & Sibert 1991). About 10 000 children are permanently disabled annually as a result of accidents (Morton & Phillips 1996). Road traffic fatality injury rates (global) per 100 000 children aged 5–14 years, varied between sexes. Boys' injury rates were 22 per 100 000 whilst girls' were 13.8 per 100 000 (WHO 2008). However, the figures do not show the real impact an accident can have on both the child and the extended family. The cost can be enormous in both physical and emotional terms which can have a long-lasting impact on all facets of children's lives: relationships, learning and play. Among those children who live in poverty, the burden of injury is highest, as these children are less likely to benefit from the protective measures others may receive (World Health Organization 2008).

http://dx.doi.org/10.1016/B978-0-7020-4315-4.00018-8

Child development

Children are involved in different types of accident according to their stage of development. At 5 years of age children run confidently, although they frequently fall. As they progress from infant to junior to secondary school, balance and coordination improve, as does their dexterity. Children in this age group become more aware of their bodies and subsequently may be self-conscious during examinations. As children develop, their curiosity and wish to experiment are not always matched by their capacity to understand or to respond to danger. According to World Health Organization (2008) data, boys tend to have both more frequent and more severe injuries than girls; this is evident from the first year of life.

Piaget's theory of the development of causal reasoning (Piaget 1983) demonstrates a systematic progression in children's understanding of illness: this is linked to Piaget's four stages of cognitive development:

- sensori-motor: birth–18 months
- pre-operational: 18 months–7 years
- concrete-operational: 7 years–11 years
- formal-operational: 11 years–adult.

The pre-operational stage is dominated by the perception and direct experiences, while illness concepts are related to phenomenism and contagion. Phenomenism occurs in the younger children in this stage, the cause of illness is believed to be external, such as the sun. Contagion occurs in the older children in this stage: illness is seen to be in objects or people. Colds are caught by someone coming near and transferred by magic. Pre-operational children may see illness or unpleasant procedures as punishment for their naughty behaviour. They are unable to comprehend unpleasant procedures being part of the cure.

In the concrete-operational stage children can apply thinking and reasoning to real objects and events. Contamination children can distinguish from cause and effect, such as bad food will give a tummy ache. However, all illnesses are seen as being caused by contact with the causative agent: if someone has a rash and it is touched then the rash is transmitted. Internalization occurs in the older children in this age group, where illness is seen as internal with an external cause; for example, kissing someone with a cold will cause the germs to go into your mouth and make you ill. Mechanisms of illness remain poorly understood but there is a realization that the body responds to causative agents such as allergens. Children in this age range understand that illnesses are preventable by immunizations and healthcare (Swanwick 1990).

When caring for children, consideration for their conception of illness can ease the path of the child through assessment and treatment to admission or discharge. Be aware of using metaphors when explaining to children as they might confuse or increase fear: for example, white cells 'fighting' infection may give rise to terrifying thoughts of soldiers with guns, missiles and tanks in their bloodstream. Despite this acquired understanding, many children regress in behaviour when they become ill, probably as a coping mechanism for the stress associated with hospitalization (Swanwick 1990).

Childhood is a social construction and is characterized by boundaries that shift with time and place and this has implications for vulnerability to injury. Tasks that may be considered the norm in one country for the child and family can vary enormously in another country where the child may be protected by economic and domestic responsibility (World Health Organization 2008). Childhood and developmental stages need to be seen as being closely linked with age, sex, family, culture and social background.

Children aged between 5 and 7 years have gained some independence, both socially and intellectually, but their behaviour is unpredictable. They become preoccupied when playing, their perceptions of speed and distance are often wrong and therefore they continue to need supervision, particularly on roads etc.

Much of an early school-goers' time is spent under adult supervision at school or in the home. Increasingly, as they get older, children spend their time away from home in parks and playgrounds unsupervised. Being unsupervised can lead to children using unsuitable areas to play in, such as derelict buildings, water or building sites. They can also indulge in dangerous activities, such as playing with fire, increasing the likelihood of injury. The majority of older children drown in open water and dams, followed by public and private swimming pools; 84% were unsupervised and lacked swimming abilities (Candy et al. 2001).

As children approach adolescence they are more likely to attempt to flaunt their independence, resent rules and authority, and take risks. Peer pressure influences children's behaviour in activities that they know to be dangerous but take part in to avoid losing face in front of their friends. Children will often lie about the mechanisms of injury to prevent detection of a dangerous/banned activity or location.

Illness and hospitalization are stressful experiences for child patients and their families. Illness itself can produce stress and when hospitalization is added to illness, that stress is increased. Studies have shown that hospital experiences can seriously influence a child's development. Negative hospital experiences can interfere with a child's rehabilitation and recuperation and can inhibit normal growth and development (Ryan-Wenger & Gardner 2012).

Hospital attendance is stressful at any age; Visintainer & Wolfer (1975) identify five categories that worry a child regarding hospitalization:

1. physical harm
2. fear of the unknown
3. uncertainty
4. separation
5. loss of control.

Both the child's and the parent's previous experiences of hospital/illness/injury as well as the parent/child relationship can have a profound effect on the child's attitude, behavior and recovery.

As well as differences in cognition between the ages in this group, there are also anatomical and physiological considerations that will impact on the child's recovery (Barnes 2003, Advanced Life Support Group 2011).

Environment and family-centred care

The Children and Young People's National Service Framework (NSF) (Department for Education and Skills/Department of Health 2005) and *Children's Charter* (Department of Health 1995) state that EDs caring for children should provide an environment that, as a minimum, has:

- a separate waiting area with play facilities
- a separate treatment area suitably decorated and equipped
- a private room for distressed parents
- at least one registered sick children's nurse (RSCN) or RN (child)
- a liaison health visitor.

Many others, such as the Royal College of Paediatrics and Child Health and Royal College of Nursing (2010), the Royal College of Paediatrics and Child Health (2007, 2009) and the American Academy of Pediatrics (2009), have made similar recommendations regarding the provision of care of children in EDs. While the aim of the ED is to provide 24-hour care by paediatric nurses, this is difficult to achieve and must not detract from the skills and experience that general nurses have in caring for children. Paediatric nurses within EDs augment the expertise of general nurses; the children's nurse acts as a resource, innovator of practice and educator in all things paediatric.

When a child presents to hospital they rarely present alone. A sick or injured child is usually accompanied to the ED by at least one adult, and sometimes by numerous family members and friends, including other children. Family-centred care should be the aim throughout the child's stay, and both the child and her family should be involved in decisions about care wherever possible (Brown et al. 2008). Lee (2001) suggests that Casey's model of partnership could be implemented in the ED environment. Casey's model developed from the philosophy stated as: *'The care of children, well or sick, is best carried out by their families with varying degrees of help from suitably qualified members of the healthcare team whenever necessary'*.

The child may require help to meet his needs in order to function, grow and develop. These needs are met by:

- *family care* – the parents carry out family care to help the child meet his needs; care is given by a nurse if parents are absent or unable
- *nursing care* – the nurse gives extra care related to health needs; care is given by parents, child or significant others with support and teaching (Casey 1993).

Using Casey's partnership model in the ED, the nurse determines whether a parent wishes to be involved in their child's care. Some parents may feel unable to be involved, for instance being unable to be present during suturing. Others would expect to be involved, for example, comforting the child during suturing. Parental involvement is not necessarily a time-saving process, as time is required to enable parental participation. Partnership care may result in quicker discharges from the ED, for instance for a child with constipation and a reduced re-attendance rate, which is of benefit to the child, family and nurse (Lee 2001).

Children usually benefit from a parent or carer being present during examination/investigation, but pressure should not be placed upon parents/carers if they feel unable to be with their child during specific treatments. It is important for ED nurses to reassure parents that their continuing presence is welcome should hospital admission become necessary.

Should a child need critical intervention, such as resuscitation, many parents would wish to stay with their child. The needs of parents must be considered, with the provision of a nurse to support the parents during this time, keeping them informed, giving explanations of treatments/procedures. Both nurses and medical staff may feel stressed by parental presence in an already tense situation, but in aiming for family-centred care, the parents' and the child's wishes should be respected wherever possible. Even if the parents decide not to be at their child's bedside, knowing that they have the option fosters trust and positive communication (Baren et al. 2008).

The majority of children attending the ED do so following injury rather than illness although most will have relatively minor injuries (Hendry et al. 2005). To the child and parents a minor injury may appear catastrophic. A child-friendly environment, including books, toys and hospital play specialist, will distract and provide a sense of normality for the child, thus helping to reduce the emotional impact of injury. The attitude of the multi-professional team, from receptionists to radiologists, towards children and their families plays a large part in reducing the impact of the injury/illness and the ED visit (Nadzam & Westergaard 2008).

Activities and conversation should be related to things included in the child's normal world, such as the current children's films, childhood heroes, pop stars and footballers. Parents and others, especially other children, can be particularly helpful with this. The younger children in this age group appreciate bravery awards and stickers following their treatment.

When planned properly, family presence helps meet the family's needs without disrupting medical care. With time, commitment and support this type of change is possible.

Pain assessment and management

Most children attending the ED will require pain relief in some form. Pain assessment can prove difficult, even in older children, and a long-standing problem in paediatric pain management has been the difficulty of objectively assessing pain. An assessment tool such as QUESTT is designed specifically for the assessment of children's pain (Box 18.1).

The impact of anxiety on a child's pain level should not be underestimated and appropriate measures to reduce anxiety are an important part of pain control (Jeffs et al. 2011). It is imperative that assessment and management of pain are appropriate to the child's understanding and not beyond comprehension. The use of toys and play demonstration is proven to be helpful in reducing anxiety and increasing cooperation in the younger child. The use of play therapy promotes normalization by providing a non-threatening environment and familiar activities in an otherwise unfamiliar and often frightening environment. Through structured play activities children and their carers can be educated about procedures in a manner appropriate to the child's developmental stage. This reinforces the need for the nurse to have an awareness of normal childhood development, so communication is effective and pain assessment accurate.

Pain scales, such as numerical continuums, facial expressions and visual analogues, can be a useful aid to pain assessment (Royal College of Nursing 2009, Bailey et al. 2012) but should not be used in isolation. The use of pain rating scales may be difficult in the ED environment due to anxiety, distress, fear and the unfamiliarity with pain rating scales. Hall (2002) describes a paediatric pain assessment tool designed specifically for the ED comprising a mixture of subjective and objective assessments along with examples of injury. The child is asked to choose both a face and a number most appropriate to their degree of pain. The nurse then circles the most fitting behaviour seen in the child. Twycross (1998) suggests that children's perceptions of pain are frequently established prior to a painful episode, thus making the task of pain assessment in ED more difficult.

For many children, immobilization and support of an injured area comprise the first step in pain control, but this should not be used as a substitute for analgesia. ED nurses must not underestimate actual pain, as opposed to the fear of pain and anxiety, as the cause of the child's distress (Morcombe 1998).

For minor injuries, simple analgesia (paracetamol and ibuprofen and/or Panadol® and codeine combinations) can be administered at an early stage, such as at assessment, thus easing the child's passage through ED. Many departments enable the nurse to administer simple analgesia under Patient Group Directives. The start of the pain assessment and management process is at home with the parents administering simple analgesics. Unfortunately it has been found that where parents do not give children analgesia prior to attending the ED, they cite not having any suitable analgesics or the accident not occurring at home, and the majority felt that it was the hospital's responsibility (Spedding et al. 1999). Aspirin is not to be used in children under 12 because of the risk of Reye's syndrome (Scott & Thompson 2011).

Entonox, which is 50% nitrous oxide, 50% oxygen (and up to 70% nitrous and 30% oxygen in certain procedures) is a useful and rapid analgesia for children who are able to hold the mask or mouthpiece (pleasant-smelling masks are available). Its restrictions for use are the same as for adults. A safe dose is one that can be self-administered, and it should not be used for children with chest and moderate to severe head injury. It is useful for dressings, suturing and prior to cannulation (Bruce & Frank 2000).

Children with significant injuries such as displaced fractures, fractured femurs and burns affecting greater than 5% surface area require opiates. These should be given intravenously due to faster action times, ability to titrate dose according to response and reduced risk of tissue storage associated with muscular injections following significant trauma (Advanced Life Support Group 2011). Intravenous cannulation is not easy in an injured/ill or distressed child and repeated attempts should be avoided: seek more experienced help and/or ask for the paediatric team's assistance. Many departments use intranasal diamorphine, thus negating the need for cannulation for opiate administration.

Anaesthetic is useful for many procedures. Topical substances containing lignocaine are useful prior to non-urgent cannulation and venipuncture. Local anaesthetic for suturing and wound cleansing provides pain relief and thus increases the child's cooperation. Unfortunately infiltration with local anaesthetic can be painful; warming the solution, buffering with sodium bicarbonate or applying topical adrenaline cocaine can reduce pain at infiltration. The use of topical adrenaline cocaine, especially on facial wounds, makes local anaesthetic unnecessary.

In some cases children requiring suturing or other procedure may be unable to cooperate despite all measures of reassurance, hospital play specialist, analgesia etc., or the wound is too large to allow adequate infiltration of local anaesthetic (maximum of 3 mg/kg of 1% lignocaine): these children require general anaesthetic. Some departments advocate the use of sedation for such cases, but this may be problematic in terms of providing adequate staff and resuscitation facilities to ensure the safety of the child, as recommended by the Scottish Intercollegiate Guidelines Network (2002).

Regional nerve blocks are an effective source of pain relief. A femoral block, for example, provides good pain control while X-raying and splinting a fractured femur (Advanced Life Support Group 2011). Children with fractured femurs also require intravenous opiates as the initial pain management.

Where possible, all paediatric medications should be prescribed according to the child's weight; where actual weights are not available a child's weight may be calculated using the formula 2 × age + 4 (Advanced Life Support Group 2011).

It is essential for all EDs to keep a guide to paediatric medications such as the British National Formulary (Joint Formulary Committee 2012) in the children's area and resuscitation room.

Musculoskeletal injuries

As they get older children usually become increasingly competitive, participating in regimented repetitive training, and this creates a potential for serious physical (over-use or acute) and psychological injury. Psychological problems are difficult to measure, whereas acute physical injury can be assessed.

Foster & Kay (2003) suggest that the diagnosis of a musculoskeletal problem is essentially clinical and describe comprehensive assessment skills.

There are three main types of musculoskeletal injury associated with children's sport:

- osteochondritis
- specific injury such as fractures
- stress fracture.

Osteochondritis refers to a group of conditions affecting the growth plate. The disorder results from the stresses produced at the bone/ligament junction or articular surfaces during physical activity. The most commonly affected areas include:

- tibial tuberosity
- metatarsals
- navicular
- lunate
- capitulum
- calcaneum.

Rest is usually sufficient to cure these injuries, but orthopaedic follow-up should be given (O'Brennan et al. 2001).

Extensive training without a proper build-up period can lead to stress fractures. Runners and gymnasts are the most likely to incur these injuries. Sports injuries can be prevented with careful supervision, a gradual increase in training activity, and correction of poor technique or inappropriate use of equipment.

Fractures

The developmental process of the skeletal system is such that children are prone to incomplete fractures, described as greenstick or torus fractures, with dislocations rare (Davies et al. 2003). These are usually a disruption of the bone cortex on one side as opposed to a complete break. Emergency nurses must be prudent when assessing limb injuries in children as often those with greenstick fractures display no visible signs of bruising, swelling or deformity, leading to these fractures remaining undetected. Most greenstick fractures will heal independently; however, it is common practice to immobilize the fracture with plaster for pain relief.

Mechanism of injury is important, as is exact location of pain and extent of movement and pain association. It is often difficult to make this assessment if the child is very distressed, and simple immobilization and simple analgesia may be useful until after X-ray. Some children sustain fractures that are displaced, and these fractures require reduction to allow healing without deformity to the affected limb. It is preferable to carry out the reduction procedure under general anaesthetic.

Although children most commonly sustain greenstick fractures, they are not exempt from other types of fracture. Fractures through a growth plate (epiphysis) are described as Salter–Harris fractures and graded I–V. They require referral to orthopaedic specialists and may need surgical intervention (Davies et al. 2003).

If a child is discharged with a lower limb cast, her developmental dexterity must be considered. Many 5-to-7-year-olds may be unable to mobilize with crutches partly because of balance and partly because of the weight of the cast. In some cases, a Zimmer frame may be a better aid. Crutches use in the older child may also be difficult due to balance, and schooling also needs to be considered as many schools with a large pupil population or stairs may feel that the child on crutches is at risk of further injury. Parents and children should be made aware of the risks and side-effects of an immobilized limb and be aware of local facilities for review and advice (also Chapter 6).

Limping child

Acute non-traumatic limp is a common reason for children to present to the ED. There is a wide differential diagnosis for these patients, and there are certain serious conditions that cannot be missed (McCanny et al. 2012). Diagnoses include fractures, soft tissue injury, osteomyelitis, septic arthritis, irritable hip, juvenile arthritis, Baker's cyst, Perthes' disease and slipped upper femoral epiphysis.

Some children may be systematically unwell presenting with associated symptoms of headaches and vomiting; history of seizures, acute or chronic pain and a febrile illness (Baren et al. 2008). Investigations must exclude infective causes. Investigations may include venipuncture (apply topical anaesthetic cream at triage), X-ray, ultrasound scan and observation. Management of the child in the ED consists of analgesia, support and antipyretics.

Hip disease should be considered in any child with thigh, groin, or knee pain (Baren et al. 2008). Perthes' disease is a condition found in the age range 5–9 years, more commonly in boys, where avascular necrosis of the femoral epiphysis (femoral head) occurs. Physical examination may show a limp secondary to either pain or a leg-length discrepancy. The aetiology is unknown; diagnosis is made by X-ray. Treatment varies from centre to centre and may include immobilization with traction or splints in conjunction with analgesia.

Slipped capital femoral epiphysis (SCFE) is defined as displacement of the femoral epiphysis on the femoral metaphysis (femoral neck). SCFE is often associated with overweight children but can occur in non-obese children. It generally occurs in adolescents during prepubescent growth (10–14 years) and is more common in boys.

SCFE can be classified into two categories, stable and unstable (Baren et al. 2008). Clinically, the child is able to weight-bear with or without crutches with a stable SCFE, but is unable to walk at all with an unstable SCFE despite crutches. Confirmation is by X-ray, and often corrective surgery is required (Baren et al. 2008). The onset can be acute or insidious, with 30% developing the same condition in the opposite limb (Waterson et al. 1997, O'Brennan et al. 2001, Barnes 2003, Davies et al. 2003).

Abdominal pain

Abdominal pain is one of the most common reasons children in this age group often attend EDs (Marin & Alpern 2011). Assessment and accurate diagnosis can sometimes be made difficult, as discussed previously, by the level of cognitive development, pain, effects of hospitalization and level of cooperation by the child.

Children with abdominal pain present with a host of signs and symptoms, including vomiting, altered bowel habits, diarrhoea, constipation, anorexia, not drinking, nausea, frequency of micturition, pain on micturition and pains that may be colicky, continuous or stabbing in nature.

Urinary tract infection, gastroenteritis, constipation, appendicitis, menarche, period pain, renal stone, obstruction, perforation, inflammatory bowel disease, pneumonia, otitis media, diabetes, trauma and psychosomatic pain are all reasons for ED attendance with abdominal pain (Waterson et al. 2000). The history and development of pain provide many clues for diagnosis. Acute pain of sudden onset may indicate obstruction or perforation. A more insidious onset is indicative of appendicitis, and colicky pain is usually associated with intestinal disorders such as gastroenteritis or inflammatory bowel disease.

Assessment of the child with acute abdominal pain, as with all ill/injured children, begins with a rapid assessment of airway, breathing, circulation and disability and any compromise treated immediately as per resuscitation guidelines.

Further assessment and management includes recording of baseline and subsequent observations, urinalysis, pain assessment and appropriate administration of analgesics, and may include venipuncture, cannulation, intravenous fluids and specialist opinion if surgical intervention is considered necessary (Box 18.2).

Box 18.2

Assessment of abdominal pain

The nurse should determine:
- The duration of pain
- The severity of pain
- The exact location and any radiation
- Factors that improve or worsen pain
- The child's overall posture and level of activity
- Associated symptoms, e.g., vomiting, nausea, constipation, diarrhoea, dysuria/frequency and vaginal discharge, should be noted
- Any obvious social influences such as problems at school or family stresses should not be dismissed

Appendicitis

Appendectomy is the most common operation in childhood apart from ear, nose and throat surgery and is common to all age groups. In one-third of children with appendicitis, the appendix ruptures before operative treatment (Smink et al. 2005). If appendicitis cannot be ruled out as the cause of abdominal pain, the child is usually admitted to hospital for observation. The pain often subsides and the child is subsequently discharged with a diagnosis of non-specific abdominal pain.

In appendicitis the child usually gives a history of moderate pain, commencing centrally and moving down to the right iliac fossa. These children are often off their food, but continue to drink. They complain of nausea, and may or may not give a history of vomiting. Altered bowel habits, including constipation and diarrhoea, may be present.

On assessment, children with appendicitis are moderately unwell, the pulse rate may be raised, and the temperature can be normal or raised and usually ranges from 37.5–38.5°C. Abdominal examination will reveal guarding and rebound tenderness in the right iliac fossa area. If appendicitis is suspected, early surgical opinion is indicated. It should be noted, however, that appendicitis can progress to perforation and peritonitis without appropriate treatment.

Constipation

Children with constipation, particularly in the younger part of this age group, often present to the ED with acute abdominal pain or rectal bleeding. This may be a result of the commencement of full-time schooling, a hectic morning household and poor condition of school toilets (Barnes 2003).

They may give a history of infrequent bowel activity, associated with small amounts of hard stools. History may consist of colicky abdominal pain, urinary symptoms including retention, anorexia and nausea. Rectal bleeding is not uncommon as a result of anal fissures. Physical assessment usually reveals no abnormality. Examination of the abdomen reveals a loaded descending colon. Abdominal X-ray is not recommended for the diagnosis of constipation (Royal College of Radiologists 1998). Management of constipation may include relief of acute discomfort, either with suppositories or a micro-enema. Many constipated children can be treated at home with oral medications of stool softeners and stimulants (titrated to response), toileting and dietary advice (Dale 2005). The child and parents should be advised that treatment may be necessary for 6–12 months and therefore continued follow-up by their GP, paediatrician (Dale 2005) or nurse-led clinic, where available, is essential.

Urinary tract infection

Urinary tract infection (UTI) comprises symptoms of infection, together with the presence of pathogenic micro-organisms in the urine, urethra, bladder or kidney. The most common cause of urinary tract infections is from *Escherichia coli*, a bacterium from the gastrointestinal tract (Struthers et al. 2003). UTIs are among the most common bacterial childhood infections and in 7-year-olds have an incidence of 2.8% in boys and 8.2% in girls (Coulthard et al. 1997). Older children and adolescent girls become more prone to urinary tract infections once sexual activity begins.

A UTI should be considered in all children with undiagnosed malaise or pyrexia of unknown origin. Urinalysis is the most effective way to obtain a definitive diagnosis. It should be performed on any child presenting with dysuria, frequency, haematuria, and sudden-onset enuresis, pain in the renal area and suprapubic pain, and any child with pyrexia for which no cause has been established.

Children rarely need admission for UTIs unless they are systemically unwell or unable to tolerate oral antibiotics. Most children can therefore be discharged with oral antibiotics and advice regarding increased fluid intake and supportive care. Paracetamol or ibuprofen relieves pain and high temperature. Parents should also be advised that follow-up from their GP is necessary following a UTI, which may involve radiological imaging and prophylactic antibiotic dependent on the age of the child and local practice (Barnes 2003). Recurrent infections are common, but the clinical significance and long-term sequelae of untreated or recurrent urinary tract infections are unknown (Baren et al. 2008).

Testicular torsion

Testicular torsion is a surgical emergency and refers to the twisting of the spermatic cord (Lopez & Beasley 2012). It requires early recognition and management in order to protect and maintain testicular viability. The majority of boys who present to the ED are adolescents, but testicular torsion can occur at any age (Baren et al. 2008). Boys will typically present with a history of sudden, severe scrotal and lower abdominal pain. Fever is uncommon and it is not uncommon for boys to admit having had prior similar pain episodes that resolved without treatment. Ultrasound is currently the preferred modality of imaging for making a definitive diagnosis. Manual or surgical detorsion is required to relieve testicular torsion.

Delaying or missing the diagnosis of testicular torsion can result in decreased spermatogenesis and testicular atrophy with complete reabsorption of the testis within about 12 hours (Baren et al. 2008).

Consent

Consent/refusal of treatment is a much-debated topic within the field of adult EDs. Consent in paediatrics can also give rise to much discussion and confusion.

Since the Children Act (Department of Health 1989) a child under the age of 16 years of age has been able to consent to treatment if they are deemed Gillick competent or if not Gillick competent a parent can give consent on their behalf (Dimond 2001). Thus some of the children referred to in this chapter may be able to consent to treatment.

In order for a parent or child to give consent they must be given all relevant information and time and opportunity to ask questions, i.e., to offer informed consent. A child who fully comprehends what they are consenting to and the consequences of that consent can be said to be Gillick competent (also known as 'Fraser guidelines') (Waterston et al. 1997, Dimond 2001).

In some much-published cases children have refused treatment such as blood transfusions on religious grounds, but Courts of Appeal have overturned the child's refusal and treatment has continued. In an ED where a child refuses consent to treatment an impossible situation arises whereby the nurse must attempt to obtain consent, with parental participation, giving further explanations regarding the necessity of treatment and consequences of refusing treatment. If the child continues to refuse then the best possible alternative treatment is used with comprehensive documentation in the child's notes.

In a life-threatening situation consent is not necessary if the child is unaccompanied; the welfare of the child is paramount. If parents refuse treatment, e.g., blood transfusion, in a life-threatening situation on the grounds of religious beliefs, professionals who consider the treatment essential acquire consent as for an unaccompanied life-threatening situation.

Many children attend EDs unaccompanied or accompanied by an adult who is not a parent or guardian. Consent can be obtained from those who are:

- Gillick competent
- de facto carers
- from contacting parents to attend ED.

De facto carers include teachers, baby-sitters, step-parents or anyone currently caring for a child; The Children Act (Department of Health 1989) gives such a person the right to make decisions on behalf of the child. Dimond (1996) suggests that ED staff could obtain consent from 'de facto' carers for immediately necessary treatment such as stitches or injections (see also Chapter 39).

Health promotion

Many opportunities exist for health promotion in the ED. The waiting area can be used in a variety of ways to target both parents and children with specific aspects of health promotion and accident prevention. Displays about topical issues such as the prevention of sunburn, safety equipment and meningitis symptoms can provide parents and children with practical commonsense advice. Individual advice supported with written information can help to prevent recurrent accidents, as well as trouble-shooting the specific incident.

Distress is common in children and parents following an accident, even when the physical injury is minor; this is due to the sudden and unexpected nature of the incident, and emotional support may be necessary.

Anecdotal evidence suggests an increase in the number of schoolchildren attending ED following incidents of bullying, even during primary school. Bullying involves persistent, deliberate, unprovoked, physical or psychological harm by a more powerful child or young person or group, against a weaker child or group and a proportion of all ages are faced with bullying daily (Gini 2008, Karatas & Ozturk 2011).

Children who attend the ED frequently with apparently trivial complaints may be being bullied, or the child may disclose bullying at assessment. The nurse must be sensitive/supportive in these cases. Providing information about other agencies such as Kidscape and Childline for ongoing support and management is vital. Bullied children are often reluctant to involve schoolteachers if bullying is occurring in school, but most schools have adopted an anti-bullying policy; gentle persuasion may convince the child that 'telling' will stop the bully and prevent others being bullied. Referral to the school nurse may provide a link within the school environment.

Obese children and young people may be the victims of bullying and as a consequence attend the ED. There is a lack of agreement of the diagnostic criteria for the classification of obesity but studies demonstrate an increased prevalence (Fruhbeck 2000, Ruxton 2004). Childhood obesity may lead to long-term health problems, including hypertension, sleep apnoea, asthma, early puberty, diabetes, back pain and slipped upper femoral epiphysis (Ruxton 2004). Treatment of childhood obesity involves promoting a healthy diet, increased physical activity and a behavioural component (Fruhbeck 2000, Ruxton 2004). In the ED it involves the treatment of the presenting complaint and promotion of a healthy lifestyle.

Parents attending the ED may be victims of domestic abuse. Domestic violence impacts on the child directly and indirectly and is now a recognized form of child abuse.

Effects of domestic violence on a child include:

- actual physical injury to the child
- emotional effects of witnessing abuse of a parent
- potential difficulties in accessing healthcare (Spencer 2002, Evans 2005).

As with bullying, the ED nurse must be sensitive to the needs of the child and abused parent; the ED is for many the first agency the family turns to for help. Physical injuries are cared for and the impact on the child is dealt with as per local child protection policy. The ED nurse should then provide guidance to other agencies such as women's aid groups, the NSPCC, domestic violence units, health visitors and school nurse services.

All children attending the ED are potentially victims of child abuse (Chudleigh 2005, Sanders & Cobley 2005),

domestic violence or bullying. The ED nurse must be conversant with trigger factors to these types of incident and be able to provide support and information and refer to the appropriate agency. Although issues of child protection arise across the whole of childhood and beyond, this issue is considered in detail in Chapter 17.

Conclusion

Children attend EDs following accidents as a result of the environment in which they live; many attend using the department as a primary healthcare. Such patients are often labelled as inappropriate attenders; however, this is frequently both unjust and judgemental. There are often situations that force families to attend for primary care – out of GP hours, referred previously by GP, faith in the ED, time of day, etc. ED nurses are obliged to meet the needs of all attending children, giving them the best possible service.

The needs of children between the ages of 5 and 13 years vary considerably. The ED nurse must have an awareness of the developmental stages of children in order to provide appropriate, safe care. The ED environment is important for meeting the needs of children and their families, as is the attitude of staff to children and their families, especially if they are subsequently admitted from ED. Children's positive or negative memories of their hospitalization experiences may influence their future attitudes toward healthcare, utilization of healthcare services, and even their career decisions (Ryan-Wenger & Gardner 2012). Optimum care results from a family-centred approach, with aftercare advice directed at the child and parent in order to achieve concordance.

References

Advanced Life Support Group, 2011. Advanced Paediatric Life Support: The Practical Approach. Wiley-Blackwell, West Sussex.

American Academy of Pediatrics, 2009. Guidelines for the care of children in emergency departments. Pediatrics 124 (4), 1233–1243.

American College of Surgeons, 2008. Advanced Trauma Life Support, eighth ed. American College of Surgeons, Chicago.

Bailey, B., Gravel, J., Daoust, R., 2012. Reliability of the visual analog scale in children with acute pain in the emergency department. Pain 153 (4), 839–842.

Baren, J., Rothrock, S., Brennan, J., et al., 2008. Pediatric Emergency Medicine. Saunders Elsevier, Philadelphia.

Barnes, K., 2003. Paediatrics: A Clinical Guide for Nurse Practitioners. Butterworth Heinemann, Edinburgh.

Brown, K., Mace, S.E., Dietrich, A.M., et al., 2008. Patient and family-centred care for pediatric patients in the emergency department. Canadian Journal of Emergency Medicine 10 (1), 38–43.

Bruce, E., Frank, L., 2000. Self-administered nitrous oxide (Entonox) for management of procedural pain. Paediatric Nursing 12 (7), 15–19.

Candy, D., Davies, G., Ross, E., 2001. Clinical Paediatrics and Child Health. WB Saunders, Edinburgh.

Casey, A., 1993. Development and use of the partnership model of nursing care. In: Glasper, E.A., Tucker, A. (Eds.), Advances in Child Health Nursing. Scutari Press, Harrow.

Chudleigh, J., 2005. Safeguarding children. Paediatric Nursing 17 (1), 37–42.

Coulthard, M.G., Lambert, H.J., Keir, M.J., 1997. Occurrence of renal scars in children after their first referral urinary tract infection. British Medical Journal 315, 918–919.

Dale, A., 2005. Managing constipation and soiling. The Practitioner 249, 490–500.

Davies, F.C.W., Robson, W.J., Smith, A.K., 2003. Minor Trauma in Children. Arnold, London.

Department for Education and Skills/Department of Health, 2005. Ill Child Standard, National Service Framework for Children, Young People and Maternity Services. Department of Health, London.

Department of Health, 1989. The Children Act. HMSO, London.

Department of Health, 1995. Children's Charter. HMSO, London.

Department of Health, 2005. Improving Responses for Children and Young People Requiring Emergency or Urgent Care. Department of Health, London.

Dimond, B., 1996. The Legal Aspects of Health Care. Mosby, London.

Dimond, B., 2001. Legal Aspects of Consent 8: children under the age of 16. British Journal of Nursing 10 (12), 797–798.

Evans, N., 2005. Domestic violence: recognising the signs. Paediatric Nursing 17 (1), 14–16.

Foster, H., Kay, L., 2003. Examination skills in the assessment of the musculoskeletal system in children and adolescents. Current Paediatrics 13, 341–344.

Fruhbeck, G., 2000. Childhood obesity: time for action, not complacency. British Medical Journal 320, 328–329.

Gini, G., 2008. Associations between bullying behaviour, psychosomatic complaints, emotional and behavioural problems. Journal of Paediatrics and Child Health 44, 492–497.

Hall, J., 2002. Paediatric pain assessment. Emergency Nurse 10 (6), 31–33.

Hendry, S.J., Beattie, T.F., Heaney, D., 2005. Minor illness and injury: factors influencing attendance at a paediatric accident and emergency department. Archives of Diseases of Childhood 90, 629–633.

Jeffs, D., Wright, C., Scott, A., et al., 2011. Soft on sticks: An evidence-based practice approach to reduce children's needlestick pain. Journal of Nursing Care Quality 26 (3), 208–215.

Joint Formulary Committee, 2012. British National Formulary, 63 ed. BMJ Group and Pharmaceutical Press, London.

Karatas, H., Ozturk, C., 2011. Relationship between bullying and health problems in primary school children. Asian Nursing Research 5 (2), 81–87.

Lee, P., 2001. Is partnership in A&E possible? Journal of Child Health 5 (1), 26–29.

Lopez, R.N., Beasley, S.W., 2012. Testicular torsion: potential pitfalls in its diagnosis and management. Journal of Paediatrics and Child Health 48 (2), E30–E32.

Marin, J.R., Alpern, E.R., 2011. Abdominal pain in children. Emergency Medicine Clinics of North America 29 (2), 401–428.

McCanny, P.J., McCoy, S., Grant, T., et al., 2012. Implementation of an evidence-based guideline reduces blood tests and length of stay for the limping child in a paediatric emergency department. Emergency Medicine Journal 29.

Mead, D., Sibert, J., 1991. The Injured Child: An Action Plan for Nurses. Scutari Press, Harrow.

Morcombe, J., 1998. Reducing anxiety in children in A&E. Emergency Nurse 6 (2), 10–13.

Morton, R.J., Phillips, B.M., 1996. Accidents and Emergencies in Children, second ed. Oxford University Press, Oxford.

National Institute for Health and Clinical Excellence, 2005. Improving Outcomes in Children and Young People with Cancer: The Evidence Review. NICE, London.

Nadzam, D., Westergaard, D., 2008. Pediatric safety in the emergency department: Identifying risks and preparing to care for child and family. Journal of Nursing Care Quality 23 (3), 189–194.

O'Brennan, P., Yassa, J.G., Ludwig, S., 2001. Paediatric Emergency Medicine. Manson Publishing, London.

Piaget, J., 1983. Piaget's theory. In: Mussen, P. (Ed.), fourth ed. Handbook of Child Psychology, Vol. 1 Wiley, New York.

Royal College of Nursing, 2009. Recognition and Assessment of Acute Pain in Children: Update of full guideline. RCN, London.

Royal College of Paediatrics and Child Health and Royal College of Nursing, 2010. Maximising Nursing Skills in Caring for Children in Emergency Departments. RCN, London.

Royal College of Paediatrics & Child Health. Report of the Intercollegiate Committee for Services for Children in Emergency Departments. Royal College of Paediatrics and Child Health, London.

Royal College of Paediatrics and Child Health, 2009. Annual Report. RCPCH, London.

Royal College of Radiologists, 1998. Making the Best Use of a Department of Clinical Radiology Guidelines for Doctors, fourth ed. The Royal College of Radiologists, London.

Ruxton, C., 2004. Obesity in children. Nursing Standard 18 (20), 47–55.

Ryan-Wenger, N.A., Gardner, W., 2012. Hospitalised children's perspectives on the quality and equity of their nursing care. Journal of Nursing Quality Care 27 (1), 35–42.

Sanders, T., Cobley, C., 2005. Identifying non-accidental injury in children presenting to A&E departments: an overview of the literature. Accident and Emergency Nursing 13, 130–136.

Scott, S., Thompson, J., 2011. Adverse drug reactions. Anaesthesia & Intensive Care Medicine 12 (7), 319–323.

Scottish Intercollegiate Guidelines Network, 2002. Guideline 58: Safe Sedation of Children Undergoing Diagnostic and Therapeutic Procedures. SINE, Edinburgh.

Smink, D.S., Fishman, S.J., Kleinman, K., et al., 2005. Effects of race, insurance status, and hospital volume on perforated appendicitis in children. Pediatrics 115 (4), 920–925.

Spedding, R.L., Harley, D., Dunn, F.J., et al., 1999. Who gives pain relief to children? Journal of Accident and Emergency Medicine 16, 261–264.

Spencer, D., 2002. Paediatric trauma: when it is not an accident? Accident and Emergency Nursing 10, 143–148.

Struthers, S., Scanlon, J., Parker, K., 2003. Parental reporting of smelly urine and urinary tract infection. Archives of Disease in Childhood 88, 250–252.

Swanwick, M., 1990. Knowledge and control. Paediatric Nursing 2 (5), 18–20.

Twycross, A., 1998. The management of acute pain in children. Professional-Nurse 14 (2), 95–98.

Visintainer, M.A., Wolfer, J.A., 1975. Psychological preparation for surgery paediatric patients: the effects on children's and parents stress responses and adjustment. Paediatrics 56 (2), 187–202.

Waterson, T., Helms, P., Ward-Platt, M., 1997. Paediatrics Understanding Child Health. Oxford University Press, Oxford.

Wong, D., Baker, C., 1988. Pain in children: comparison of assessment scales. Pediatric Nursing 14 (1), 9–17.

World Health Organization, 2008. In: Peden, M., Kayode, O., Ozanne-Smith (Eds.), (2004) World Report on Child Injury Prevention, WHO, Geneva.

Adolescence

19

Lynda Holt

CHAPTER CONTENTS

Introduction

Adolescents represent only a small percentage of the total number of patients seen in Emergency Departments (EDs). Their care, however, needs to be specialized and related to their individual stage of development. This chapter will highlight the common areas of adolescent development, such as risk-taking behaviour, and explore them in relation to ED attendance. Sensation-seeking, leading to potentially deviant behaviour such as violent acts, substance misuse and self-harm, will also be considered, as will the generic effects of illness and injury on adolescents. The impact of caring for adolescents on ED nurses will also be examined. Optimum care environments and appropriate nursing skills will be discussed with regard to the quality of service offered to adolescents attending ED.

Adolescent development

The research on adolescent development is vast (Erikson 1965, Croghan 2005, Lerner & Steinberg 2009). An understanding of adolescent development is essential for ED nurses in their daily practice. Adolescence is a period in the life span where the individual, previously dependent on parents and carers for his values and identity, becomes independent and, in this move towards independence, attempts to establish a new and personal identity. The key factors in this process appear to relate to the onset of puberty, i.e., the physical and emotional changes leading to sexual maturity (Bickley & Szilagyi 2003, Tortora & Grabowski 2003), and the need for independence (Smetana 2011).

Cognitively, adolescents are capable of abstract thought and understand many variables within a situation. They should also be able to understand the consequences of their actions (Bernardo & Schenkel 1995). It is a period where group identity is vital, a time of experimentation with self-image, and a time to question fundamental family values. Adolescents are pushing for independence, testing the boundaries of their existing life and, importantly, hoping to find boundaries that will aid the development of their future identity (Croghan 2005, Damon & Lerner 2008).

Caring for the adolescent in the ED

As a client group, adolescents are considered difficult to care for by the majority of nurses (Holt 1993). In the ED, many causes of adolescent attendance can be viewed as self-inflicted, e.g., as a result of alcohol or substance testing, which may render ED nurses less compassionate towards the patient. Although less an issue than before due to the ageing nursing workforce, caring for adolescents presents a particular challenge, as many nurses are just emerging from adolescence themselves. To the adolescent, these nurses may represent a more realistic role model, enhancing the opportunity for health

http://dx.doi.org/10.1016/B978-0-7020-4315-4.00019-X

education. This is particularly pertinent to ED nurses because there is a greater likelihood of interaction with this age group at a time when they are physically and emotionally vulnerable.

Providing ED nurses with a better idea of the process of adolescence may equip them more satisfactorily to meet their patients' needs, which will enable them to recognize normal behaviour instead of reacting to it (Holt 1993).

Nurses are generally less aware of teenagers' needs than those of other age groups. In the ED, adult care is the most familiar and, because of the associated anxiety, paediatric care is more often discussed or taught. An understanding of adolescent development could help nurses in EDs to provide holistic care. It would also enable nurses to rationalize behaviour such as rebellion, non-conformity, antagonism and paranoia, which is frequently demonstrated in hospital, but is arguably the normal behaviour for an adolescent whose independence has been threatened by illness or injury.

Hospital staff, particularly in EDs, are quick to meet the physical needs of these patients, such as maintaining a safe environment for the drunken teenager or arresting haemorrhage in a patient with slashed wrists, but often with little regard to their emotional needs (Kuykendall 1989). An understanding of these needs, however, could reduce the risk of confrontation and diminish any perceived power struggle. The question for ED nurses is how far these needs can be facilitated within an ED without compromising the care or wellbeing of others in the environment. When young people are asked why they do not use health services they admit to feeling intimidated by both the service and the service providers, they dislike the times and locations, and are concerned about confidentiality and trust (Croghan et al. 2004, Croghan 2005).

As with all patients, initial assessment is the key to forming a therapeutic relationship, and the adolescent's response to illness and possible treatment can be quickly gauged, as well as existing coping strategies. Privacy has an important effect on the adolescent because of the significance of self-image; for instance, a wound assessment takes seconds but can cause great embarrassment. Ensuring privacy increases self-esteem and reinforces the adolescent's importance as an individual. Independence is often threatened by hospitalization, even a short period in ED. Including the patient in the care planning and decision-making reduces non-compliance and aggressive behaviour. Separation is greatly underestimated as a stress for the adolescent. While they demand peer belonging and demonstrate independence, most need and want parental support. Parents themselves often underestimate the support needed and the fears of adolescents. This may be because of swift medical and nursing intervention aimed at promoting physical well-being. While ED nurses are quick to include the parents of a sick child, perhaps, because of the demonstrated independence of adolescents, this inclusion is often overlooked.

The adolescent patient needs to assert his independence, but is not yet ready to cope with the implications of this. In 'crisis' situations, as a visit to an ED is often perceived, the ED nurse may be in a position of setting boundaries for the patient. This is not a negative action as it provides the security the adolescent indirectly seeks. All too often, however, on a busy shift, in a packed waiting room, antagonistic behaviour is allowed to escalate into confrontation, often because cues for boundaries

have not been recognized by ED nurses inexperienced in adolescent development. Consistency among staff is essential. Boundaries for acceptable behaviour should be decided as a matter of policy, and this should be made clear to patients on admission while respecting their independence and individuality. In addition, Knight & Rush (1998) argue that waiting rooms should be made more 'user-friendly' for adolescents, ideally incorporating separate waiting and treatment areas.

Illness or injury often induces developmental regression, forces the adolescent out of his peer group and imposes a fear of rejection. Even in a short admission to ED, nurses need to work towards reducing this anxiety. It is paramount for adolescents to be cared for by staff who are comfortable with them, and can behave as adults, listening to them and respecting their needs. Adolescents are not children and, especially at times of high stress, do not respond well to being railroaded by ED personnel who are threatened or irritated by their behaviour.

Personal fable

Despite the upheaval and trauma of adolescence during this life phase, mortality is at its lowest, with the top cause of death being accident-related (Department of Health 2004). An important cause of accident in adolescence is risk-taking behaviour, not just risky sports, but minor law infringement such as failure to wear a safety belt, exceeding speed limits and experimentation with alcohol and illegal substances (Bellis et al. 2005).

A possible explanation of this is the concept of personal fable (Elkind 1967, Pahlke et al. 2010), a belief that despite risk-taking behaviour they will not be affected by life's difficulties. This has both a positive and a negative function, and represents normal cognitive development. Positively, it allows goals to be believed in and attainable, such as dreams of success. Its negative function is that it induces risk-taking behaviour. Normally, consequences of actions are considered, but personal fable gives the security of invulnerability to consequences. This is not unique to adolescents; witness, for example, smoking and lung cancer in older people (Winkenstein 1992).

Personal fable affects not only conformity with perceived authority, but also with chronic illnesses, such as diabetes. Thinking of himself or herself as the centre of attention, the adolescent comes to believe that it is because he or she is special and unique (Alberts et al. 2007).

It is important for ED nurses to understand this concept in order to intervene in the risk-taking behaviour that can result in an ED attendance. Personal fable is there to protect the self-concept at the vulnerable time of adolescence. It allows conformity with peers despite negative consequences; for instance, the diabetic patient who presents in ED with hypoglycaemia because he has been drinking to conform with peers. The patient can 'blot out' the likely hypoglycaemic attack because being the same is more important. Education and support from ED nurses who understand that this behaviour is not intended to be self-destructive, but is normal adolescent experimentation, can reduce the risk of further occurrence. This perception of invulnerability may contribute to the statistic that the largest cause of adolescent death is from risk-taking – in cars, with fire arms, in water and with toxic substances. Sensitive questioning helps adolescents expose their personal myth, recognize their irrationality and induce a change in behaviour.

Risk-taking behaviour

Most common behaviours evolve from experimentation with alcohol, solvents or drugs, but it can be hard for the busy ED nurse to accept the drunk who is abusive as 'normal' when his behaviour is disruptive and difficult to contain. The majority of adolescents who attend ED with drug- or alcohol-related problems are not abusive, and are there because of an injury or illness related to their risk-taking behaviour. These individuals often present with their peer groups and engage in sensation-seeking behaviour, which can appear threatening to ED nurses. Adequate staffing levels and nurse skill mix, with appropriate back-up such as security officers and an incident alarm, should be available. Sensation-seeking is a normal need for experimentation and new experiences, and adolescents are prepared to take physical and social risks to attain these (Barker 1988). Despite risk-taking and sensation-seeking, most adolescents maintain conventional modes of behaviour and deviants are in the minority. EDs frequently treat adolescents as a result of risk-taking behaviour. A non-judgemental attitude is not always easy to foster, and the ED nurse must be aware of her own vulnerability and biases, as well as understanding adolescent development. This enables the nurse to treat adolescents in an appropriate manner, reduces the risk of confrontation or resentment, and respects the adolescents' rights as individuals.

Not all adolescent risk-taking is because of a low perception of danger. Some revolves around deliberate self-harm. This is usually a cry for help from adolescents who cannot cope with the pressures of growing up. Self-poisoning is the most common reason for hospital treatment (Cook et al. 2008). Only the minority of adolescents take this route, and of these the majority are not clinically depressed. This course of behaviour is not just a result of the strains of adolescence, identity confusion, anger and guilt; it is a way of getting back at those seen as responsible for the torment, such as parents, teachers and peers. Adolescent patients often demonstrate this by a blasé attitude towards their actions. Despite low suicide intent, the danger of real harm is great because of low risk awareness. The prevalence of mental health problems among adolescents is estimated at 10–20%, while the incidence of suicide among young men continues to increase and is linked to lifestyle behaviours such as alcohol and drug misuse, and mental health problems (Marfé 2003). Gunnarsdottir & Rafnsson (2010) found that frequent visits to the ED were significantly associated with suicide and fatal poisoning. However, up to 60% of those who later commit suicide have attended the ED the year before the suicide but did not present themselves as cases of self-harm (Gairin et al 2003). Box 19.1 outlines the risk range for suicide among young people.

Box 19.1

Risk categories for adolescent suicide (Marfé 2003)

The young person at extremely high risk:

- Has made previous attempts at serious self-harm
- Has clear intentions of a wish to die
- Has made a deliberate premeditated suicide attempt
- Has obtained the agent (tablets, etc.) prior to that day
- Believes that the agent or his or her actions would cause significant harm
- Has specifically arranged a time when he or she reckoned to be alone
- Has left a note
- Has failed to tell anyone about his or her self-harm attempt
- Is still planning serious self-harm
- Regrets that he or she was unsuccessful in his or her attempt
- Appears to be extremely depressed or despondent

The young person at high risk:

- Has tried to seriously self-harm him- or herself before
- Gives clear reasons for his or her actions, which still pose a risk
- Made a suicide attempt that was planned or impulsive
- Deliberately bought the agent (tablets, etc.) that day, or previously
- Was aware that the agent was harmful
- Left a note
- Was alone when the attempt was made
- Is still experiencing suicidal feelings
- Is regretful or uncertain about the failed attempt at serious self-harm
- Appears extremely depressed

The young person at moderate risk:

- Has a history of deliberate self-harm, risk taking or impulsive behaviour
- Has a history of poor stress-coping mechanisms
- Has no clear intention or a wish to seriously self-harm
- Has given clear reasons for actions – but they no longer pose an obvious risk
- Has made an attempt to deliberately self-harm, but with no actual suicide intent
- Obtained the agent (tablets, etc.) impulsively that day
- Was not fully aware of the effects of the overdose
- Made the attempt at self-harm while others were in the vicinity
- Informed others of his or her actions
- Is glad he or she did not die
- May still be considering other forms of self-harm (cutting, etc.)

The young person at low risk:

- Has no history of previous deliberate self-harm or risk-taking behaviour
- Has no history of poor stress-coping mechanisms
- Has no intentions of, or a wish to, seriously self-harm
- Has given clear reasons for his or her actions, which were never intended to pose a risk
- Has made his or her self-harm actions known to others appropriately
- Accomplished the self-harm when others were in the vicinity
- Is not planning self-harm of any kind

It is vital that nurses are able to distinguish between normal behaviour and abnormal distress. This can only be achieved by listening to and hearing the adolescent. Nothing should be taken at face value, as the superficial self-confidence and frequent mood changes common to teenagers can mask real and needy patients, as well as making them difficult to nurse. It is recognized that the ED is not the ideal place for in-depth discussion, but it may be the only opportunity available to the adolescent. An understanding of why the event occurred is essential before discharging the patient. The adolescent practice of 'dumping distress' on others via self-harm must be controlled and appropriate coping strategies learned in order to prevent further real harm. The ED nurse has a key role to play by providing constructive advice and follow-up arrangements where appropriate, not by punitive intervention (see also Chapter 15).

Substance misuse

Within the past 30 years, the worldwide drug culture has evolved dramatically, stemming from two developments. First, the major consumer generation has shifted sharply towards the young, especially adolescent and young adult males; and second, the availability of drugs has become much more widespread (Emmett & Nice 1996). While substance misuse is clearly a problem for young adults as well as adolescents, for convenience the subject will be addressed in this chapter.

In addition, the growth of the rave scene in Britain and designer drugs such as ecstasy, which appear to have become accepted by many as an integral part of relaxation and pleasure, have resulted in a culture in which substance misuse is no longer perceived as an antisocial activity, but where penalties for use and supply are severe (Box 19.2 and Table 19.1). While the ED nurse will be aware that alcohol is a major causative factor in attendances, there has been a marked increase in attendances as a consequence of other substance misuse.

The mild, moderate and severe effects of drugs of abuse are outlined in Tables 19.2–19.4 (pages 283-284).

Alcohol

Despite its legal status as a controlled substance, alcohol is the most widely available and commonly used psychoactive substance among adolescents aged 12 to 16 years (Rassool & Winnington 2003). Alcohol is a central nervous system depressant. It is absorbed into the bloodstream and starts to have an effect within 5–10 minutes of drinking. The rate of absorption is affected by sex, weight, duration of drinking, nature of drink consumed, food in the stomach, physiological factors, genetic variation and rate of elimination. Paton (1994) suggested that there are 4 million heavy drinkers in the UK, of whom 800 000 are problem drinkers and 400 000 are alcohol-dependent. In recent years there has been a steady decline in the proportion of 11-to-15-year-olds who drink alcohol. The proportion of pupils who had never drank alcohol rose from 39% in 2003 to 55% in 2010. Less than half (45%) of pupils aged between 11 and 15 years said that they had drunk alcohol at least once in their lifetimes. This increased with age from 10% of 11-year-olds to 77% of 15-year-olds. The proportion of pupils who drank alcohol in the last week fell from a peak of 26% in 2001 to 18% in 2009 (Fuller 2011).

In the UK, alcohol misuse and alcohol-related harm cost the NHS nearly £3 billion in 2006/2007 with an estimated 800 000 alcohol-attributable hospital admissions in 2006/2007 (Purshouse et al. 2010). Concomitant misuse of alcohol is also common among drug misusers. Individuals who are habituated to ethanol may have few symptoms despite massive blood ethanol concentrations. In contrast, teenagers unaccustomed to ethanol may become comatose at more modest blood ethanol concentrations (1000–2000 mg/L) (Vale 2012a). Signs, symptoms and management of alcohol intoxication are addressed in Chapter 15.

Ecstasy

Ecstasy is a synthetic hallucinogenic form of amphetamine. It was first synthesized in Germany in 1910 and patented as an appetite suppressant. It failed commercially and did not reappear until the late 1980s, when it became associated with the 'rave' scene. In its pure form, it is seen as a white powder, but is usually found as tablets or capsules. The colour will depend on any colouring agents that have been added. Ecstasy tablets frequently have images of animals or birds imprinted on them. Ecstasy is generally taken orally and is very rarely injected or smoked.

For most users, ecstasy provides a feeling of euphoria, together with an increase in confidence, emotional wellness, enhanced perception of colours and lights, exhilaration and increased intimacy towards other people (Rogers et al. 2009, Meehan et al. 2010). As an amphetamine derivative, it also provides users with feelings of energy and freedom from hunger. Ecstasy use frequently leads to jaw clenching and teeth grinding (gurning), which causes tooth surface loss (Nixon et al. 2002). While adverse reactions are rare, Halpern et al. (2011) describe the most common manifestations of 52 admissions were restlessness, agitation, disorientation, shaking, high blood pressure, headache and loss of consciousness. More serious complications were hyperthermia, hyponatraemia, rhabdomyolysis, brain oedema and coma. They argue that the image of ecstasy as a safe drug is spurious. Walsh & Kent (2001) suggest that signs that should alert an ED nurse to an ecstasy-induced collapse include admission from a late night party or rave of a previously fit young person who has collapsed for no apparent reason. Some deaths have been related to cerebral oedema secondary to excess water ingestion, because the drug has an antidiuretic effect on the kidney (Braback & Humble 2001).

The control of the patient's temperature is the key to survival, as temperatures of up to 42°C are not uncommon. Cool replacement fluids should be given at as fast a rate as the patient can tolerate and unnecessary clothing should be removed. A brisk fluid-led diuresis should be encouraged; however, if this does not control the rise in temperature then endotracheal intubation, sedation and paralysis will be instituted (Henry et al. 1992). If the temperature continues to rise, dantrolene may be used. This has muscle-relaxant

Box 19.2

Penalties under Misuse of Drugs Act 1971

Class A, schedule one

Simple possession

Maximum penalty on indictment is 7 years' imprisonment together with an unlimited fine

Possession with intent to supply

Possessing a class A, schedule one drug with intent to supply, either by sale or by gift, to another person carries a maximum penalty on indictment of life imprisonment together with an unlimited fine and the seizure of all drug-related assets

Supplying to another

As for possession with intent to supply

Examples of class A, schedule one drugs

- LSD
- Magic mushrooms

Class A, schedule two

Simple possession

Maximum penalty on indictment is 14 years together with an unlimited fine

Possession with intent to supply

Possessing a class A, schedule two drug with intent to supply, either by sale or by gift, to another person carries a maximum penalty on indictment of life imprisonment together with an unlimited fine

Supplying to another

As for possession with intent to supply

Examples of class A, schedule two drugs

- Cocaine
- Crack and freebase cocaine
- Heroin
- Methadone
- Ecstasy

Class B, schedule one

Simple possession

Maximum penalty on indictment is 5 years together with an unlimited fine

Possession with intent to supply

Possessing a class B, schedule one drug with intent to supply, either by sale or by gift, to another person carries a maximum penalty on indictment of 14 years' imprisonment together with an unlimited fine and the seizure of drug-related assets

Supplying to another

As for possession with intent to supply

Example of class B, schedule one drug

- Cannabis

Class B, schedule two

Simple possession

Maximum penalty on indictment is 5 years' imprisonment together with an unlimited fine

Possession with intent to supply

Possessing a class B, schedule two drug with intent to supply, either by sale or by gift, to another person carries a maximum penalty on indictment of 14 years' imprisonment together with an unlimited fine and the seizure of drug-related assets

Supplying to another

As for possession with intent to supply

Examples of class B, schedule two drugs

- Amphetamines
- Methamphetamine

Class B, schedule three

Simple possession

Maximum penalty on indictment is 5 years' imprisonment together with an unlimited fine

Possession with intent to supply

Possessing a class B, schedule three drug with intent to supply, either by sale or by gift, to another person carries a maximum penalty on indictment of 5 years' imprisonment together with an unlimited fine

Supplying to another

As for possession with intent to supply

Example of class B, schedule three drug

- Tranquillizers

Class C

Simple possession

Maximum penalty on indictment is 2 years' imprisonment and/or an unlimited fine

Possession with intent to supply

Possessing a Class C drug with intent to supply, either by sale or by gift, to another person carries a maximum penalty indictment of 14 years' imprisonment and/or an unlimited fine

Supplying to another

As for possession with intent to supply

Examples of class C drugs

- Benzodiazepines
- Temazepam
- Anabolic steroids
- GHB

properties and is used in the treatment of malignant hyperthermia following anaesthetic hypersensitivity (Jones 1993).

A central venous catheter should be inserted to measure and guide the rapid dehydration of the patient, and a urinary catheter to monitor renal function. The colour of the urine should be observed for an orange tinge that is suggestive of rhabdomyolysis, the breakdown of skeletal muscle, due to the toxic effects of released globins. Blood tests for creatinine kinase may be ordered to measure this process. Other blood tests may include regular clotting tests, and the patient should be closely observed for clinical signs of coagulation problems. The picture of disseminated intravascular coagulation, falling

Table 19.1 Language of substance misuse

Word	Meaning	Word	Meaning
Acid	LSD	Hit	To buy or inject drugs
Bad trip	A frightening or unpleasant LSD trip	Jack up	To inject drugs
Banging up	To inject drugs	Jellies	Temazepam in capsule form
Blow	Herbal cannabis	Joint	A hand-rolled cannabis cigarette
Buzzing	Feelings after use of ecstasy	Magic mushrooms	Any of the species of hallucinogenic mushrooms
Chill out	A period of cooling down to reduce risk of overheating from ecstasy use	Main lining	Injecting drugs
Clean	Not using drugs	Marijuana	Herbal cannabis
Coke	Cocaine	Moggies	Mogadon sleeping pills
Crack	Freebase cocaine	Poppers	Amyl/alkyl/butyl nitrate
Cut	To mix other substances with a drug to add bulk and weight	Pot	Cannabis resin
Detox	To withdraw from drugs under medical supervision	Rock	Freebase cocaine
Dope	Resin and herbal cannabis	Score	To purchase drugs
Doves	Ecstasy tablets with dove imprint	Shoot up	To inject drugs
'E'	Ecstasy	Smack	Heroin
Eggs	Temazepam tablets	Snorting	Sniffing cocaine or other drug up the nose
Flashback	Tripping out again sometime after LSD use. Can be days, months or even years later and is usually a bad trip (q.v.)	Speed	Amphetamine
		Stash	An amount of drugs, usually hidden
GBH	Gamma hydroxybutyrate or sodium oxybate, a liquid hallucinogenic stimulant	Trip	A hallucinogenic experience under LSD
Grass	Herbal cannabis	Wacky bacci	Herbal cannabis
'H'	Heroin	Whiz	Amphetamine
Hash	Cannabis resin	Works	Needles and syringes
High	The feeling of elation while under the influence of a drug		

(After Emmett D, Nice G (1996) Understanding Drugs: A Handbook for Parents, Teachers and other Professionals. London: Jessica Kingsley.)

platelet and fibrinogen count, raised partial thromboplastin (PT) and kaolin cephalin clotting time (KCCT) is an ominous sign (Jones 1993).

Cannabis

Cannabis is the most commonly used illegal drug in the world. It is the collective term for all psychoactive substances derived from the dried leaves and flowers of the plant *Cannabis sativa* (Vale 2012b). It may be smoked or eaten in food. If smoked, its effects appear within 10–30 minutes and the effects have a duration of 4–8 hours. If eaten, it takes approximately 1 hour to produce its effects. Cannabis comes in three forms:

- herbal – a dried plant material, similar to coarse cut tobacco and sometimes compressed into blocks
- resin – dried and compressed sap, found in blocks of various sizes, shapes and colours

- oil – this is rare; it is extracted from the resin by the use of a chemical solvent and ranges in colour from dark green or dark brown to jet black with a distinctive smell like rotting vegetation.

After use, cannabis has the effect of creating feelings of relaxation, happiness, increased powers of concentration, sexual arousal, loss of inhibitions, increased appetite and talkativeness (Kalant 2004). Fergusson & Boden (2011) note that until relatively recently, cannabis has been viewed as a relatively harmless drug that has few adverse effects. However, in the last two decades there has been an accumulation of evidence suggesting that cannabis may have multiple harmful effects, with these effects being particularly marked for adolescent users (Hall & Degenhardt 2009). It is believed that the greater vulnerability of adolescent users may be due to the biological effects of cannabis on the developing adolescent brain (Asharti et al. 2009).

Table 19.2 Mild clinical effects of drugs of abuse

Clinical effects	MDMA	Amphetamine	Cocaine	Cannabis	LSD
Gastrointestinal effects	✓	✓	✓	✓	✓ (i.v.)
Dilated pupils	✓	✓	✓	✓ (child)	✓
Dry mouth	✓	✓		✓	
Slurred speech			✓	✓ (high dose)	
Salivation					✓
Appetite stimulation				✓	
Chest discomfort		✓	✓		
Agitation	✓	✓	✓	✓ (high dose)	✓
Relaxation				✓	
Tremor	✓	✓	✓	✓ (child)	✓
Ataxia			✓	✓ (child)	✓
Sweating	✓	✓	✓	✓ (child)	
Mild increase in body temperature	✓	✓	✓		
Trismus (jaw clenching)	✓	✓	✓		
Bruxism (teeth grinding)	✓	✓	✓		

(After Schofield E, Lawman S, Volans G et al. (1997) Drugs of abuse: clinical features and management. Emergency Nurse, 5(6), 17–22.)

Table 19.3 Moderate clinical effects of drugs of abuse

Clinical effects	MDMA	Amphetamine	Cocaine	Cannabis	LSD
Headache	✓	✓	✓	✓	✓ (i.v.)
Hypertonia	✓		✓		✓
Hypotonia				✓	
Hyperreflexia	✓	✓	✓		✓
Hyperventilation	✓	✓	✓		✓ (i.v.)
Incontinence			✓		
Extrapyramidal symptoms	✓		✓		
Tachycardia	✓	✓	✓	✓ (high dose)	✓
Hypertension	✓	✓	✓	✓	
Hallucinations	✓	✓	✓	✓ (high dose)	✓
Paranoia	✓		✓	✓ (high dose)	
Palpitations	✓	✓	✓	✓	
Dehydration	✓	✓			
Hypothermia				✓ (child)	
Drowsiness			✓	✓	

(After Schofield E, Lawman S, Volans G et al. (1997) Drugs of abuse: clinical features and management. Emergency Nurse, 5(6), 17–22.)

Table 19.4 Severe clinical effects of drugs of abuse

Clinical effects	MDMA	Amphetamine	Cocaine	Cannabis	LSD
Pyrexia	✓	✓	✓	✓	✓ (mild)
Delirium	✓	✓	✓		✓
Hypotension	✓	✓	✓	✓ (high dose)	
Convulsions	✓	✓	✓		✓ (i.v.)
Hypoxia	✓		✓		
Coma	✓	✓	✓	✓ (child)	✓
Arrhythmias/dysrhythmias	✓	✓	✓		
Myocardial infarction					
Rhabdomyolysis	✓	✓	✓		✓ (i.v.)
Renal failure	✓	✓	✓		✓ (i.v.)
Disseminated intravascular coagulation (DIC)	✓	✓	✓		✓ (i.v.)
Pulmonary oedema			✓		✓ (i.v.)
Adult respiratory distress syndrome (ARDS)	✓				
Subarachnoid/intra-cerebral haemorrhage	✓	✓	✓		

(After Schofield E, Lawman S, Volans G et al. (1997) Drugs of abuse: clinical features and management. Emergency Nurse, 5(6), 17–22.)

Withdrawal effects include disturbed sleep patterns, anxiety, panic and restlessness. It is with these effects that patients may present to the ED department and they should be managed symptomatically.

Amphetamine

Amphetamines are central nervous system stimulants whose action resembles those of adrenaline (epinephrine). They produce a sensation of euphoria and exhilaration as well as increased energy, stamina and strength. They may be injected intravenously, ingested or smoked. Absorbed by the gastrointestinal tract they may have an effect within 20 minutes of ingestion; however, the effects are immediate if injected and last 4–6 hours. They are most commonly seen in the form of a coarse off-white/pink crystalline powder with an average purity of less than 5%. MDMA, or ecstasy, is a type of amphetamine.

Signs and symptoms of intoxication include tachypnoea, tachycardia, dilatation of pupils, dry mouth, pyrexia, blurring of vision, dizziness, loss of desire to eat or sleep, hypertension and loss of coordination (Vale 2012b). The after-effects of lethargy and fatigue can last for several days. Since tolerance develops rapidly, individual response varies greatly, and toxicity correlates poorly with dose. Amphetamines also suppress appetite and, if used regularly, can lead to substantial weight loss (Bellis et al. 2005). Fatalities are rarely reported but predominantly result from convulsions and intracranial haemorrhage. Sedatives, such as chlorpromazine, and antihypertensive agents may be used for management of the patient.

Cocaine

Cocaine is derived from the leaves of the coca bush, *Erythroxylon coca*, or may be synthesized artificially. It is commonly seen as a white crystalline powder with a sparkling appearance. It is a central nervous system stimulant and is commonly sniffed through the nose or taken by intravenous injection. Effects are felt within a few minutes and last up to half an hour. It may also be neutralized to produce 'crack', which is a potent form of cocaine made by mixing it with baking soda, heating it and then smoking it in cigarettes or a pipe. If smoked or injected, the effects are immediate and last 10–15 minutes. 'Speedballing' or 'snowballing' is a technique particularly prone to fatality and involves mixing cocaine and heroin and injecting the mixture.

The effects of use include feelings of energy, strength, exhilaration, euphoria, confidence and well-being. Users often become very talkative. Adverse effects include agitation, panic and feelings of persecution or threat. Regular use can damage nasal passages and cause exhaustion and weight loss. Tolerance rapidly develops with continued use, and marked physical and psychological addiction occurs.

Snorting cocaine can cause permanent damage inside the nose, and sustained use may lead to frequent nosebleeds and recurrent sinus infections (Bellis et al. 2005). In extreme cases, use leads to exposure of the septal cartilage and nasal bones, with eventual collapse of the nose (Millard & Mejia 2001). Administering cocaine by rubbing it into the gums or other mouth-parts can cause ulcers, lesions and gingival recession (Gandara-Rey et al. 2002). Fatalities may rapidly occur secondary to convulsion, intracranial haemorrhage, intestinal ischaemia, respiratory arrest or cardiac arrhythmias. Sedatives such as haloperidol, diazepam for convulsions and antihypertensive agents may be required as part of the management regime in ED. Active external cooling is required when the patient's temperature exceeds 41°C as cocaine impairs sweating and cutaneous vasodilation. Hypertension and tachycardia also respond to sedation and cooling (Vale 2012b).

Heroin

Opiates such as heroin are analgesics that depress the central nervous system through suppression of noradrenaline (norepinephrine). In its pure pharmaceutical form, heroin is a pure white, fine-grained powder. Medicinally, it is known as diamorphine and is used for severe pain, including chest pain. In its street forms it is coarser and varies in colour from a pinkish cream to dark brown. Heroin can be smoked, sniffed or injected. Intravenous injection (mainlining) results in an almost instantaneous effect ('rush'). It generates feelings of euphoria and inner peace, freedom from fear, worry, pain, hunger and cold, and can last 2–6 hours.

Its adverse effects include depressed breathing, severe constipation, nausea and vomiting. In acute intoxication, symptoms include pinpoint pupils, depression of heart rate and respiration, and suppression of the cough reflex. Severe physical and psychological dependence can occur with continued use. Heroin use carries a high risk of overdose, as the street strength of the drug, which is usually around 20%, can range from 10% to over 60%. In cases of overdose, naloxone is a specific opioid antagonist and is given in a dose of 0.4 mg that can be repeated at intervals of 2–3 minutes up to a maximum of 10 mg.

Methadone

Methadone is a synthetic opiate analgesic which is frequently prescribed by specific medical practitioners, usually GPs or drug clinic physicians. It is used in the treatment of heroin addiction to control withdrawal symptoms. It can be used orally or by injection and generates similar feelings to heroin use, with similar signs, symptoms and management as heroin overdose.

Overdose

About 80% of people who present to EDs following self-harm will have taken an overdose of prescribed or over-the-counter medication (Horrocks et al. 2003). A small additional percentage will have intentionally taken a dangerously large amount of an illicit drug or have poisoned themselves with some other substance. The pattern of the type of drug taken in overdose has changed in recent years, largely with changes in their availability (National Collaborating Centre for Mental Health 2004).

Poisonings can be categorized into three groups: accidental, intentional and iatrogenic. Accidental poisoning most commonly occurs among young children, although death is relatively uncommon. Intentional ingestion includes recreational drug use and suicide attempts. Iatrogenic poisoning usually results from unanticipated drug interactions (Zull 1995). In cases of intentional poisoning the ED nurses should ascertain

which drugs have been taken by asking the patient or attending friends or relatives (Box 19.3). The Children Act gives children under the age of 16 the right to refuse consent to treatment

Box 19.3

Information to be determined when interviewing a patient following drug overdose

- What was ingested? Was anyone present at the time to verify the history? Are there any empty or partially filled bottles at home or elsewhere?
- How much was taken? If pill bottles are available, calculate the number of missing tablets from the initial amount prescribed, taking into account the date on the prescription
- What was time of the ingestion? The nurse must take into account the time at which the person was last seen and when symptoms of intoxication began if the timing is not clear
- What was the route of the poisoning, i.e., oral, intravenous, smoked, inhaled, snorted, subcutaneous?
- Does the patient have a history of substance misuse, depression or schizophrenia?
- What is the patient's medical history, past and present prescription drugs, and allergies?

(Department of Health 2001). Castledine (1994) stressed the importance of establishing a good relationship with the patient, but in all cases a patient must consent if care is to be given or he can sue for assault and battery. Castledine (1994) suggested that if a patient is mentally confused due to the physical effects of illness or as a consequence of mind-altering drugs, the ED nurse could proceed to treat on the basis of urgency and necessity. Careful recording of the patient's details and the nursing and medical staffs' actions are important in such cases.

Conclusion

Adolescent attendance patterns highlight the need for ED nurses to understand the normal processes through which adolescents pass. Nurses can appear judgemental and less sympathetic towards a patient perceived as being responsible for his own illness (Stockbridge 1993). ED nurses can be affected by the apparent lack of compliance from adolescent patients. This can lead to paternalistic or confrontational behaviour that destroys the therapeutic relationship and exacerbates conflict. Adolescents cannot be treated wholly as adults as they lack the emotional maturity to cope with independence and still need the emotional support of parents and other carers. ED attendance is often a result of normal adolescent behaviour and ED nurses should be equipped with the knowledge necessary to provide appropriate support and education. An environment that provides boundaries, privacy and protected independence, with support, and peer support if appropriate, should be developed.

It is important to remember that psychological distress can be just as great as physical illness or trauma. ED nurses have a responsibility to consider the needs of young people as individuals. Perhaps an alteration of attitude is more important than a vast financial outlay in the improvement of adolescent care.

References

Alberts, A., Elkind, D., Ginsberg, S., 2007. The personal fable and risk-taking in early adolescence. Journal of Youth and Adolescence 36, 71–76.

Ashtari, M., Cervellione, K., Cottone, J., et al., 2009. Diffusion abnormalities in adolescents and young adults with a history of heavy cannabis use. Journal of Psychiatric Research 43, 189–204.

Barker, P., 1988. Basic Child Psychiatry. Blackwell, Oxford.

Bellis, M.A., Hughes, K., McVeigh, J., et al., 2005. Effects of nightlife activity on health. Nursing Standard 19 (30), 63–71.

Bernardo, L.M., Schenkel, K.A., 1995. Pediatric medical emergencies. In: Kitt, S., Selfridge-Thomas, J., Proehl, J.A., Kaiser, J. (Eds.), Emergency Nursing: A Physiologic and Clinical Perspective. WB Saunders, Philadelphia.

Bickley, L.S., Szilagyi, P.G., 2003. Bates' Guide to Physical Examination and History Taking, eighth ed. Lippincott Williams & Wilkins, Philadelphia.

Braback, L., Humble, M., 2001. Young woman dies of water intoxication after taking one tablet of ecstasy. Today's drug panorama calls for increased vigilance in health care. Lakartidningen 98 (8), 817–819.

Castledine, G., 1994. Ethics and law in ED. Emergency Nurse 2 (1), 25.

Cook, R., Allcock, R., Johnston, M., 2008. Self-poisoning: current trends and practice in a UK teaching hospital. Clinical Medicine 8 (1), 37–40.

Croghan, E., 2005. Supporting adolescents through behaviour change. Nursing Standard 19 (34), 50–53.

Croghan, E., Johnson, C., Aveyard, P., 2004. School nurses: policies, working practices, roles and value perceptions. Journal of Advanced Nursing 47 (4), 377–385.

Damon, W., Lerner, R.M., 2008. Child and Adolescent Development: An Advanced Course. John Wiley & Sons, Hoboken, NJ.

Department of Health, 2001. Reference Guide to Consent for Examination and Treatment. Department of Health, London.

Department of Health, 2004. The National Service Framework for Children, Young People and Maternity Services. Department of Health, London.

Elkind, D., 1967. Egocentrism in adolescence. Child Development 38 (4), 1025–1034.

Emmett, D., Nice, G., 1996. Understanding Drugs: A Handbook for Parents, Teachers and other Professionals. Jessica Kingsley, London.

Erikson, E., 1965. Childhood and Society. Penguin, Harmondsworth.

Fergusson, D., Boden, J., 2011. Cannabis use in adolescence. In: Gluckman, P. (Ed.), Improving the Transition: Reducing Social and Psychological Morbidity During Adolescence. A Report from the Prime Minister's Chief Science Advisor, Office of the Prime Minister's Science Advisory Committee, Auckland.

Fuller, E. (Ed.), 2011. Smoking, Drinking and Drug Use Among Young People in England in 2010. NHS Information Centre, London.

Gairin, I., House, A., Owens, D., 2003. Attendance at the accident and emergency department in the year before suicide: retrospective study. British Journal of Psychiatry 183, 28–33.

Gandara-Rey, J.M., Diniz-Freitas, M., Gandara-Vila, P., et al., 2002. Lesions of the oral mucosa in cocaine users who apply the drug topically. Medicina Oral 7 (2), 103–107.

Gunnarsdottir, O.S., Rafnsson, V., 2010. Risk of suicide and fatal drug poisoning after discharge from the emergency department: a nested case-control study. Emergency Medicine Journal 27, 93–96.

Hall, W., Degenhardt, L., 2009. Adverse health effects of non-medical cannabis use. Lancet 374, 1383–1391.

Halpern, P., Moskovich, J., Avrahami, B., et al., 2011. Morbidity associated with MDMA (ecstasy) abuse: A survey of emergency department admissions. Human and Experimental Toxicology 30 (4), 259–266.

Henry, J., Jeffreys, K.J., Dawling, S., 1992. Toxicity and deaths from 3,4-methylenedioxymethamphetamine ('ecstasy'). Lancet 340, 384–387.

Holt, L., 1993. The adolescent in accident & emergency. Nursing Standard 8 (8), 30–34.

Horrocks, J., Price, S., House, A., et al., 2003. Self-injury attendances in the accident and emergency department: clinical database study. British Journal of Psychiatry 183, 34–39.

Jones, C., 1993. MDMA: the doubts surrounding ecstasy and the response of the emergency nurse. Accident & Emergency Nursing 1, 193–198.

Kalant, H., 2004. Adverse effects of cannabis on health: an update of the literature since (1996). Progress in Neuropsychopharmacology and Biological Psychiatry 28 (5), 849–863.

Knight, S., Rush, H., 1998. Providing facilities for adolescents in ED. Emergency Nurse 6 (4), 22–26.

Kuykendall, J., 1989. Teenage traumas. Nursing Times 85 (27), 26–28.

Lerner, R.M., Steinberg, L.D., 2009. The Scientific Study of Adolescent Development. In: Lerner, R.M., Steinberg, L.D. (Eds.), Handbook of Adolescent Psychology: Individual Bases of Adolescent Development, third ed. Wiley, Hoboken New Jersey.

Marfé, E., 2003. Assessing risk following deliberate self harm. Paediatric Nursing 15 (8), 32–34.

Meehan, T.J., Bryant, S.M., Aks, S.E., 2010. Drugs of abuse: The highs and lows of altered states in the emergency department. Emergency Clinics of North America 28, 663–682.

Millard, D.R., Mejia, F.A., 2001. Reconstruction of the nose damaged by cocaine. Plastic and Reconstructive Surgery 107 (2), 419–424.

National Collaborating Centre for Mental Health, 2004. Self-harm: The Short-Term Physical and Psychological Management and Secondary Prevention of Self-Harm in Primary and Secondary Care. The British Psychological Society and The Royal College of Psychiatrists.

Nixon, P.J., Youngson, C.C., Beese, A., 2002. Tooth surface loss: does recreational drug use contribute? Clinical Oral Investigations 6 (2), 128–130.

Pahlke, E., Bigler, R.S., Green, V.A., 2010. Effects of learning about historical gender discrimination on early adolescents' occupational judgements and aspirations. The Journal of Early Adolescence 30 (6), 854–894.

Paton, A., 1994. ABC of Alcohol. third ed. BMA Publishing Group, London.

Purshouse, R.C., Meier, P.S., Brennan, A., 2010. Estimated effect of alcohol pricing policies on health and health economic outcomes in England: an epidemiological model. Lancet 375, 1355–1364.

Rassool, G.H., Winnington, J., 2003. Adolescents and alcohol misuse. Nursing Standard 17 (30), 46–52.

Rogers, G., Elston, J., Garside, R., et al., 2009. The harmful health effects of recreational ecstasy: a systematic review of observational evidence. Health Technology Assessment 13 (6), 1–354.

Schofield, E., Lawman, S., Volans, G., et al., 1997. Drugs of abuse: clinical features and management. Emergency Nurse 5 (6), 17–22.

Smetana, J.G., 2011. Adolescents' social reasoning and relationships with parents: Conflicts and coordinations within and across domains. In: Amsel, E., Smetana, J.G. (Eds.), Adolescent Vulnerabilities and Opportunities: Developmental and Constructivist Perspectives. Cambridge University Press, Cambridge.

Stockbridge, J., 1993. Parasuicide: does discussing it help? Emergency Nurse 1 (2), 19–21.

Tortora, G.J., Grabowski, S.R., 2003. Principles of Anatomy and Physiology, tenth ed. John Wiley & Sons, New Jersey.

Vale, A., 2012a. Alcohols and glycols. Medicine 40 (2), 89–90.

Vale, A., 2012b. Drugs of abuse (amfetamines, BZP, cannabis, cocaine, GHB, LSD). Medicine 40 (2), 84–87.

Walsh, M., Kent, A., 2001. Accident & Emergency Nursing: A New Approach, fourth ed. Butterworth Heinemann Ltd, London.

Winkenstein, M., 1992. Adolescent smoking. Journal of Paediatric Nursing 7 (2), 120–127.

Zull, D.N., 1995. Poisoning and drug overdose. In: Kitt, S., Selfridge-Thomas, J., Proehl, J.A., Kaiser, J. (Eds.), Emergency Nursing: a Physiologic and Clinical Perspective, second ed. WB Saunders, Philadelphia.

Young adults

20

Jenni Ward

CHAPTER CONTENTS

Introduction

Young adults encompass the age group 18–39 years. This age group is not homogeneous in its characteristics and patterns, as it encompasses the life cycle from adolescence (experimentation) to full maturity. As young adults mature from adolescence and settle down they may have families, face financial burdens, have challenges in or out of work, and may also lack traditional family support. Partnership, pregnancy and parenthood may bring a sense of stability and responsibility, although these also carry the risk of stress-related illnesses. This chapter considers the range of physical and psychological ailments that affect young adults and bring them to EDs.

Sports injuries

In 2009, approximately 75% of UK adults between 16–24 years and 66% of the 25–44 age group participated in sports and physical activities. The most popular sports activities amongst young adults included walking, gym, cycling, and swimming, followed by football and jogging (Beaumont 2011).

Although the mechanisms of injuries associated with sports injuries are dependent on the type of activities, they are similar to those using motor vehicles, motorbikes and pedal cycles and involve energy and force of impact on the victim (Stewart & Allen 2007, Dandy & Edwards 2009). The incidence of people having sports-related injuries is dependent on geographical location and type of sport involved (Office for National Statistics 2011). Seventy-five per cent of all sporting injuries are classified as minor, with musculoskeletal and limb injuries the most common types. In the young adult, the muscles are the greatest points of weakness. The knee is the most vulnerable point in children under 15; after this and up to the age of 19 the pelvis is the weakest, with avulsion fractures most commonly occurring. From 19 to 30 years of age, the hamstring and quadriceps muscles are especially vulnerable. After the age of 30 the tendons start to degenerate and become weaker than the muscles.

Eighty-two per cent of all patients who present to health services with sporting injuries are treated in the ED, with possible subsequent referral to orthopaedic and /or physiotherapy clinics. The remainder are treated by GPs and sports physiotherapists. Many are overuse injuries and are usually caused by training errors, excessive load on the body, environmental problems, poor equipment, ineffective rules or violent play (Kannus 2000). Overuse injuries have a better chance of full recovery if treated by a clinician experienced in sports medicine, then followed by a correct rehabilitation programme.

The more serious sports injuries involve:

- head injuries
- spinal injuries
- haemothorax, pneumothorax and tension pneumothorax
- blunt and penetrating abdominal trauma
- pelvic injuries
- facial injuries
- musculoskeletal injuries
- compartment injuries.

In the UK, the greatest number of sporting head injuries arise from golf and horse riding. Although serious spinal injuries are rare, approximately 20% of patients in spinal injury units have

http://dx.doi.org/10.1016/B978-0-7020-4315-4.00020-6

sustained their injury as a result of a sporting activity. The most common sports to generate serious spinal injuries are horse riding, diving, rugby and other sports such as gymnastics, skiing and motor sports (Grundy & Swain 1996). These injuries have long-term implications for a young person. Paralysis, brain damage or serious reduction in mobility will almost certainly lead to loss of earnings, relationship and sexual problems, depression and a greatly altered lifestyle.

Most deaths from sport arise from professional boxing, followed by horse riding, skating, gymnastics and swimming. Although rare in the young adult, non-accidental sudden death may also occur during sporting activities. The most likely causes are cardiac myopathy, myocarditis, congenital disorders, arrhythmias and conduction disorders (Hillis 2000).

The priorities of management of sports injuries are the same as for other injuries – to save life and limb, to do no harm and prevent further harm (Gregory 2005). The short-term aims of treatment of minor sporting injuries are pain control, maintenance of range of movements, maintenance of basic strength, and re-establishment of neuromuscular function. After initial first aid, some injuries will require surgery and post-operative rehabilitation (Matthews 2000). Most injuries, however, can be treated conservatively using the following acronym:

P – protection of injured area from further damage using immobilization devices (e.g., slings, strapping, braces)

R – rest of part to avoid further harm and prolonged irritation

I – ice for control of pain, bleeding and swelling

C – compression for support and control of swelling

E – elevation for decreased bleeding and dispersal of oedema

S – support for stabilization of injured part.

There is little benefit gained in prolonging 'PRICES' guidelines past 72 hours post injury or subsequent exacerbation (Gregory 2005).

The administration of non-steroidal anti-inflammatory drugs may slightly speed the recovery from injury and also act as an analgesic. Sporting injuries benefit from physiotherapy with early controlled mobilization and functional rehabilitation. Minor sports injuries are rarely associated with major morbidity, although they are painful and inconvenient to the person involved and the overall cost to society is high due to their frequency (Greaves et al. 2009).

Road traffic accidents

Unintentional injuries are a leading cause of death and disability in the young adult (World Health Organization 2010). Despite dramatic falls in child death rates in the UK throughout the 20th century, young adults remain the largest accident risk group (Social Trends 2000, Department for Transport 2009). In the under-35-year age group, injury is the commonest cause of death and has been described as 'the last great plague of the young' (Skinner et al. 1991).

Many of the more serious injuries of adulthood result from road traffic accidents (RTAs). Road deaths in the UK are now one of the lowest in Europe. In 2000, road deaths equated to 6 adults per 100 000 and 2 children per 100 000; the highest numbers are in Portugal with 33 adult deaths per 100 000 and 8 children per 100 000. By 2009, the number killed had fallen 38%, with the number seriously injured approximately 44% lower (Office for National Statistics 2000, Department for Transport 2009).

While the number of fatal head injuries has begun to decline, a pattern of blunt abdominal trauma has emerged (Cope & Stebbings 1996). The main causes of death from RTAs in young adults are:

• chest, abdominal and pelvic injury
• intracranial injury
• fractures of the skull.

For each fatality on the roads there are over 12 serious injuries and 50 minor injuries: 36% of people with serious spinal injuries receive them as a result of RTAs, predominantly from cars, vans or motorcycles (Grundy & Swain 1996).

The number of pedestrian deaths has remained consistent since 1953. The greatest numbers are among elderly people, with a disproportionately high number also occurring in the age group 1–14 years. The highest number of fatalities for pedal cyclists occurs in the 5–14 age group. Those dying in cars, however, are predominantly young adults, but fatalities from motor vehicles, motorcycles and bicycles in this age group have dropped by about one-third. The introduction of the mountain bike has led to a huge surge in the popularity of cycling, with off-road cycling and safety helmets helping to lessen the number of accidents. Legislation limiting the engine capacity of motorcycles that learners can ride has led to a 40% reduction in those killed or seriously injured on motorbikes. Since the 1980s the imposition of speed restrictions and attention to safer road design has contributed to falling road deaths, as have the recent mandatory use of rear seat belts, crumple zones, anti-brake-lock devices, air bags and seasonal anti-drink–drive campaigns. A disproportionately high number of people involved in RTAs have consumed alcohol, and these people are the most likely to sustain serious injuries. Approximately 17% of all road fatalities are linked to alcohol, with approximately 40% of pedestrians killed in car accidents having blood alcohol levels above the legal driving limit (Department for Transport 2009).

Although some accidents involve environmental and vehicular factors, human error is clearly responsible for most accidents. The number of road accidents in the over-25s declines quickly as experience and social maturity develop. Although legislation and attention to environmental issues have reduced the number of road deaths, the problems of inexperience, immaturity, impetuosity and sometimes lack of control are harder to address.

Alcohol-related attendances

The most popular leisure activity named by young adults is 'going to the pub' (Office for National Statistics 2000). Only 7% of men and 13% of women call themselves non-drinkers. The remaining 80% have widely differing drinking habits, with occupations, genetic and parental influences, life events, race, religion, peer pressure and personality all having an effect on alcohol consumption. The heaviest drinking occurs among young adults in the age range 16–24 years (Royal College of Psychiatrists and Royal College of Physicians 2000). Guidelines recommend that men and women drink no more than four and three units, respectively, in one day. However, one study of nightclubs found men consuming an average of 15 units and women 10 units during a night out (Deehan & Saville 2003). Young women in particular are drinking more, with the percentage of 16- to 24-year-old women exceeding the recommended weekly drinking limits doubling over the past decade (Rickards et al. 2004). The changes in image of pubs to café bars, music pubs, family pubs, nightclubs and rave music venues have all made drinking more accessible to young people. Half of 18–24-year-olds visit pubs at least twice a week and 40% visit nightclubs at least once a fortnight (Mintel 2003).

In the UK, alcohol misuse and alcohol-related harm cost the NHS nearly £3 billion in 2006/2007 with an estimated 800 000 alcohol-attributable hospital admissions in 2006/2007 (Purshouse et al. 2010). More than 600 000 violent incidents occur in or around pubs every year (Simmons et al. 2002) and at least one in ten nightlife assaults involves the threatened use of glasses or bottles (Budd 2003), while an estimated 5000 people are injured every year by glass used as a weapon, with many permanently scarred (Deehan 1999).

In one study, some 10% of ambulance call-outs were alcohol-related (Martin et al. 2012). Alcohol-related attendances in the ED may be prompted by injuries, intoxication, medical problems or antisocial behaviour. The former two reasons are most common in the young adult who has had a single episode of heavy drinking, while the latter two are common in the older, habitual heavy drinker. Alcohol acts as a CNS depressant and, although it stimulates conversation and sociability, it also impairs judgement, slows reflexes and can lead to aggressive and violent behaviour. Moulton & Yates (1999) recommend that, due to the high incidence of trauma in patients with alcohol intoxication, when assessing an intoxicated patient ED staff should be aware of the possibility of non-obvious physical injury, including cervical spine and head injury. They advise the following management of the aggressive drunk patient when considering their possible fitness for discharge:

* observe patient carefully, doing head injury observations and blood alcohol readings
* enquire about possible trauma from bystanders
* examine patient, especially head, without personal risk
* undertake blood glucose readings
* get senior medical advice for further management
* observe in hospital, or
* send home with sensible friends with written, explained head injury instructions, or
* send to police custody with written head injury instructions.

Ten per cent of adults in the UK are classified as 'heavy drinkers', with 1 in 2000 needing admission to psychiatric hospitals for alcohol-related disease (Goodwin 2000). Unconscious patients brought to the ED with acute alcohol intoxication need regular head injury observations, blood sugar readings, fluid replacement of isotonic saline 10 mL/kg in the first hour and airway protection. If there is a possibility of trauma, a cervical spine and CT scan will need to be done. A bottle of spirits may pose no serious problem for the chronic drinker, but for the non-regular drinker with a blood alcohol level of 400 mg/100 mL or over, it can lead to deep coma and death, usually from hypoglycaemia, respiratory depression or aspiration (Vale 2012).

Alcoholic coma can be a serious medical emergency requiring admission to hospital and the emergency nurse should be aware that a patient's condition can move from mild to life-threatening as previously ingested alcohol and/or drugs are absorbed (Shahin 2012). Most deaths occur because of respiratory depression or aspiration. Deep alcoholic coma should be treated aggressively with a cuffed endotracheal tube, oxygen and ventilation. Blood glucose should be determined hourly and the rate of intravenous glucose adjusted accordingly. If blood glucose concentrations decrease despite an infusion of glucose 5–10%, a 50% solution (50 mL intravenously) should be given because hypoglycaemia is usually unresponsive to glucagon (Vale 2012). If low blood sugar levels necessitate glucose, it should be accompanied by intravenous thiamine. Otherwise, when carbohydrate metabolism begins again, low levels of vitamin B1 (thiamine) will precipitate Wernicke's encephalopathy, which consists of ocular muscle palsies, nystagmus, ataxic gait and progressive mental impairment. A patient in alcohol withdrawal is generally dehydrated and orthostatic. Hypoglycaemia, acidosis, hypovolaemia and electrolyte disturbance need treatment with intravenous fluids, CVP line, blood gases, glucose and thiamine.

In addition to correction of dehydration and electrolyte abnormalities, the patient may require sedative therapy. Minimal tremulousness in a patient with normal mental status may not require any tranquilliser therapy. However, the patient who is agitated, hallucinating or having seizures, or who has evidence of autonomic hyperactivity, such as fever and tachycardia, should be calmed rapidly. Benzodiazepine sedatives are the preferred agents and diazepam can be given at 15–30-minute intervals, after which the dose and frequency should be decreased or a switch to an oral route made. Drugs such as haloperidol and chlorpromazine are generally avoided because they may increase the risk of seizures. If seizures occur, i.v. diazepam is usually the treatment of choice.

All EDs will have their own regular patients who are heavy drinkers, many of whom will be in their 20s or 30s. Apart from acute intoxication and trauma, they may present with other medical and psychological problems associated with alcoholic liver disease. The most common of these are gastritis, haematemesis, oesophageal varices and pancreatitis. As the disease progresses fits, dementia, cardiomyopathy, strokes and cancers may develop (Edwards et al. 1997). Psychological problems may include parasuicide, depression and acute anxiety attacks. People dependent on alcohol have a mortality rate four times higher than the rest of the population; half of these deaths will be violent and 7% from suicide (Wasserman 2001). After glucose and thiamine for their hypoglycaemia, i.v. diazepam for their fits and cessation of their gastric bleeding, the desire to return to their existing lifestyle will mean that many of these patients will discharge themselves home before they are admitted to hospital. Many young adults are ill-informed about safe drinking patterns. Alcohol education continues to receive a low priority in both policy and resources and it is believed that isolated campaigns to educate the public are ineffective.

Genitourinary trauma and infections

Many young men and women come to the ED because of sexually related activities and genitourinary trauma. All of these patients need to be treated with tact, dignity, confidentiality and privacy. An undisclosed history of sexual assault, buggery, incest, trans-sexualism or transvestism may be reasons for a patient refusing to remove clothing or declining to see a doctor or nurse of a particular gender.

Sexual intercourse can cause lacerations to the vagina and penis, which often bleed profusely. The young, uncircumcised male may present with a paraphimosis – the inability to return the retracted foreskin to its normal position. Causes of retracted foreskin include post cleaning, secondary to erections and self-infliction such as piercing with a penile ring into the glans. This can normally be reduced using lignocaine gel (without adrenaline), ice or cool packs and analgesia, followed by manipulation of the retracted foreskin. If reduction is not possible, a dorsal incision to the foreskin or circumcision may be needed (Burkitt & Quick 2002, Dunn & Maclean 2010).

Injuries to the penile shaft cause considerable distress to young men and 70% of these arise as a result of sexual practices. The commonest of these injuries is a fracture of the penis. This occurs when the penis is bent acutely during intercourse, sexual play or masturbation. The patient usually reports a 'cracking' or 'popping' sound as the corpus cavernosum ruptures. The patient suffers pain, immediate detumescence with deformity and gross swelling (Simpson et al. 2007, Agarwal et al. 2009). A concomitant urethral injury should be considered until proven otherwise. Management involves immediate surgical repair to decrease risk of complications, improve function and appearance (Simpson et al. 2007, Agarwal et al. 2009). Human bites to the penis can pose a serious problem and are associated with a 50% infection rate. Suturing, with the additional help of ice packs and pressure, will usually stop the bleeding. Because large numbers of both anaerobic and aerobic organisms are found in human saliva, these bites need to be treated with a broad-spectrum antibiotic such as augmentin. It should be noted that suturing is not recommended following human bites. These are usually allowed to repair by secondary intention or delayed closure (Moreira & Marcovchick 2007).

Although not common, patients who suffer electric shocks should be questioned and examined for possible burns to the scrotum and penis, since the electrical discharge has a propensity to exit from the genitalia.

Both male and female patients may present with foreign bodies in their rectum, vagina, bladder or urethra. These are usually inserted for self-exploration, inquisitorial reasons or for sexual pleasure. On other occasions it may be for contraceptive use, drug ingestion, or as a means of deliberate self-harm. Symptoms may include dysuria, haematuria, constipation, discharge or rectal bleeding, or abdominal, suprapubic and perineal pain dependent on location of the foreign body. Fever may also be present if the foreign body has been in situ for a period of time (Tanagho & McAninch 2000, Simpson et al. 2007).

Physical examination may reveal the foreign body palpable in, or protruding from, the urethra, vagina and/or anus. Urine and urethral discharge cultures should be obtained and a broad-spectrum antibiotic prescribed (Jordan 2008). The majority of low-lying objects can be removed in the ED. However, objects above the sacral curve and rectosigmoid junction are difficult to visualize or remove and require operative intervention. Multiple attempts at self-removal can lead to mucosal oedema and muscular spasms making attempts at removal difficult. Other complications involving foreign bodies in the rectum include rectal lacerations and bowel perforations (Simpson et al. 2007).

The most common vaginal foreign body is a lost tampon, which can occur due to a broken string, the insertion of two tampons for heavy loss, or as a result of having sexual intercourse with a tampon in situ. It can easily be removed with the aid of a good light and vaginal speculum. The prolonged use of large, absorbent tampons, and also barrier contraceptives such as the diaphragm may lead to toxic shock syndrome (British Paediatric Surveillance Unit 2010), an infective illness caused by *Staphylococcus aureus* or *Streptococcus pyogenes*. The patient may present with symptoms of a low-grade infection or may be in advanced stages of septic shock. If the latter, their initial treatment will need to encompass a full blood screen, blood cultures, intravenous fluids and antibiotics, oxygen and regular observations. Weekends are a common time for young women presenting to the ED for postcoital contraception ('morning-after pill'), when GP surgeries, family planning clinics and pharmacies are closed. Unprotected intercourse, split condoms or sexual assault may be the reasons for this request. The postcoital contraception is most effective if used as soon as possible within the first 72 hours of unprotected intercourse and is almost 100% effective (Homer & Fry 2007). Further details regarding postcoital contraception and vaginal bleeding can be found in Chapter 30.

Miscarriage occurs in 20% of pregnancies and is a source of great distress to many young women and men who come to the ED. It is important that these patients are afforded as much privacy and compassion as possible. The first consideration of the nurse is to establish that the patient is haemodynamically stable, since blood loss can be profuse. After this, pain relief with a rapid gynaecological referral should take place. It is not appropriate for these distressed patients to wait long periods in the department and a nurse-led fast-track system can provide greatly improved care for these young women (Wilson 2000).

The rates of sexually transmitted infections (STIs) are increasing in most countries including the UK, USA, Australia and New Zealand (Homer & Fry 2007). About 10% of young people in some areas of the UK have chlamydial infections with levels more than doubling between 1995 and 2003 (Bellis et al. 2004). Not all STIs require penetrative sex for transmission; for example, syphilis can be spread through oral sex (Cook et al. 2001). For various reasons, young men and women may prefer to come to the ED with STIs. These patients may be reluctant to go to a GP who is well known to them and their families and so prefer the anonymity of the ED. As STIs are common, they often are underestimated in the ED (Bellis et al. 2004, Homer & Fry 2007). The nurse needs effective communication skills, with increased sensitivity and dignity towards the patients due to the sensitive nature of the condition and collecting the history of the patient's sexual activities and their partners. It is prudent to offer tests to the patient and their consenting partner/s for the other STIs in addition to the human immunodeficiency virus (HIV), due to the similar transmission modes. These patients need referring onto either infectious diseases or the sexual health clinic so that the STIs can be effectively treated.

Binge drinking and recreational drug consumption are associated with an increased risk of unprotected sex. As alcohol and some recreational drugs can induce temporary impotence, anti-impotence drugs have been used to enable or enhance sex (Bellis & Hughes 2004). Bellis et al. (2005) also note that women have been using such drugs to improve orgasms. However, these drugs have a range of contraindications, for instance, hypotension and recent stroke and, in combination with alcohol and other drugs, substantially increase the risk of an adverse reaction.

Psychological illnesses in young adults

Many find the transition from adolescence to adulthood extremely difficult and stress-related illnesses are common. Those without a strong support network may feel overwhelmed by the problems confronting them. The suicide rate rises markedly in the teenage years and it may occur without warning (Lader & Cowen 2001). Three to four times more young men than women successfully commit suicide, making it one of the main causes of death for this age group (World Health Organization 2011). Deaths from suicide in young adults rose between 1950 and 2005 in the UK, Australia and America (World Health Organization 2011). Recent analysis, however, shows a decrease in suicides for both men and women from 1990 in these countries.

The pattern of suicide and parasuicide (usually known as deliberate self-harm) varies between men and women, with men tending to favour more violent ways of killing themselves, such as hanging, gassing, drowning, firearms, use of sharp instrument and jumping from heights, while women tend to use self-poisoning (Bird & Faulkner 2000, Large & Nielssen 2010).

Twenty-four per cent of those who successfully committed suicide are recorded as having used the mental health services within the previous week (Bird & Faulkner 2000): 40–50% of those who succeeded in taking their own lives also had a history of self-harm (McClure 2000, Hawton 2004). Deliberate self-harm (DSH) is 3–4 times more common in women than in men. In England and Wales 100 000 patients a year are referred to hospital as a result of DSH. For every suicide there are 30 other cases of self-harm (Evans 1993). Many of these are young adults who take tablets or who inflict wounds on themselves, with 69% of them having been doing so for over five years. Those who self-injure tend to do so by cutting, scratching or burning. They may do this for a variety of reasons: physical, emotional or sexual abuse, feelings of low esteem, eating disorders or periods of distress.

EDs can be both challenging and varied in their handling of the young adult with suicidal ideology. Many patients have reported that the way they were received in the ED was often crucial, with talking, listening and compassionate care having a very positive effect on their self-esteem (Bird & Faulkner 2000); however, Moore & McLaughlin (2003) argue that when staff are very busy and stressed they can struggle to understand why apparently healthy people have attempted or succeeded in taking their own life. Some will be suicidal while others

will not, but those with a past history of DSH are more likely to successfully take their own lives: 20–25% of people who die had come to hospital with self-harm in the previous year (Foster et al. 1997). The difference between the two groups, suicide and self-harm, is not always clear-cut. Those who commit suicide are a small group who tend to plan the act, take precautions against being discovered, use dangerous methods and, in one-sixth of cases, leave a suicide note. The majority of these patients have given a warning of suicidal intent.

Young adulthood is a time when specific mental illnesses can develop. The one that is probably best known as a disorder of the young is schizophrenia, which has a mean age of onset of 31 years in the male and 41 years in the female. Despite the fact that it is believed that this is a disease more prevalent in men, both men and women have a 1% lifetime risk of schizophrenia (Castle et al. 2000). The nurse may first meet the patient with symptoms of disordered thoughts, inappropriate moods, auditory hallucinations or persecutory delusions. These patients can be frightening and difficult to contain if psychiatric referral takes time. Nurses need to understand that the families of these patients bring with them a huge and varying set of feelings. Some feel total bewilderment, shame, anger, disappointment or grief, while others have still not been able to let go of their hope for a complete cure for the person they love (Jones 2002). The care and nursing management of patients with a psychiatric crisis, including schizophrenia, are considered in detail in Chapter 15.

Several illnesses affect young women in particular. In women under 40, collapse, bradycardia or electrolyte imbalance may arise because of a history of anorexia nervosa or bulimia. Postnatal depression or psychosis may also be seen in the ED when young women may present following an overdose, with acute delusions or after being involved in episodes of harm to their children. Certain individuals who are confronted by stress develop anxiety states that vary greatly in severity. These can be a feature of young adult life and symptoms usually persist for an average of five years before treatment is sought. Symptoms include palpitations, tachycardia and chest pain. It is important to get a full history to rule out organic causes such as pneumothorax, infection or myocardial infarction. Individual stress counselling and relaxation groups run by a psychologist or community psychiatric nurse can be very beneficial to help these patients develop coping mechanisms (Hambly & Murie 1997). Life events such as bereavement, divorce, unemployment, marriage, parenthood and physical illness can precipitate these illnesses.

Conclusion

Young adults use EDs in a different way from children, the middle-aged or the elderly. They may have moved away from the influence and environment of the family and may not be registered with a GP. They rarely have long-term healthcare needs and so tend to use the accident department as a 'drop-in' centre not requiring organized planned appointments.

The commonest reason for ED attendance is accidental injury. The younger patient may lack knowledge of their own bodies and become aggressive or depressed if they have to confront personal injury or disease. They have high levels of anxiety about their body image and a visit to hospital can be an emotionally traumatic time when they become impatient and frightened if they are not treated quickly. This means that the ED nurse needs to be aware that reassurance and explanations are necessary and not be surprised that young people, even in their 20s, want their parents with them. The 18–39-year age range has a diverse group within it and good communication skills, tolerance, flexibility are essential to ensure that all patients receive the appropriate treatments for their specific needs.

References

Agarwal, M.M., Singh, S.K., Sharma, D.K., et al., 2009. Fracture of the penis: A radiological or clinical diagnosis? A case series and literature review. Canadian Journal of Urolology 16 (2), 4568–4575.

Beaumont, J. (Ed.), 2011. Lifestyles and Social Participation: Social Trends 41. Office for National Statistics, London.

Bellis, M.A., Hughes, K., 2004. Sex potions: relationships between alcohol, drugs and sex. Adicciones 16 (4), 251–259.

Bellis, M.A., Hughes, K., Ashton, R., 2004. The promiscuous ten percent? Journal of Epidemiology and Community Health 58 (11), 889–890.

Bellis, M.A., Hughes, K., McVeigh, J., et al., 2005. Effects of nightlife activity on health. Nursing Standard 19 (30), 63–71.

Bird, L., Faulkner, A., 2000. Suicide and Self Harm. Mental Health Foundation, London.

British Paediatric Surveillance Unit, 2010. 24th Annual Report 2009–2010. BPSU, London.

Budd, T., 2003. Alcohol Related Assault: Findings From the British Crime Survey. Home Office, London.

Burkitt, G., Quick, C., 2002. Essential Surgery: Diagnosis, Management. Churchill Livingstone, London.

Castle, D., McGrath, J., Kulkarnie, J. (Eds.), 2000. Women and Schizophrenia. Cambridge University Press, Cambridge.

Cook, P.A., Clark, P., Bellis, M.A., et al., 2001. Re-emerging syphilis in the UK: a behavioural analysis of infected individuals. Communicable Disease and Public Health 4 (4), 253–258.

Cope, A., Stebbings, W., 1996. Abdomen. In: Skinner, D., Driscoll, P., Earlham, R. (Eds.), ABC of Major Trauma. BMJ, London.

Dandy, D.J., Edwards, D.J., 2009. Essential Orthopaedics and Trauma, fifth ed. Churchill Livingstone Elsevier, Edinburgh.

Deehan, A., 1999. Alcohol and Crime: Taking Stock. Home Office, London.

Deehan, A., Saville, E., 2003. Calculating the Risk: Recreational Drug Use among Clubbers in the South East of England. Home Office, London.

Department for Transport, 2009. Reported Road Casualties Great Britain: 2009. HMSO, London.

Dunn, R., Maclean, A., 2010. Genitourinary disorders. In: Dunn, R. (Ed.), fifth ed. The Emergency Medicine Manual, Vol 2. Venom Publishing, Adelaide.

Edwards, G., Marshall, E., Cooke, C., 1997. The Treatment of Drinking Problems. Cambridge University Press, Cambridge.

Evans, M., 1993. Suicide: a target for health. RCN Nursing Update. Nursing Standard 7 (18), 9–14.

Foster, T., Gillespie, K., McLelland, R., 1997. Mental disorders and suicide in Northern Ireland. British Journal of Psychiatry 170, 447–452.

Goodwin, D., 2000. Alcoholism: The Facts. Oxford University Press, Oxford.

Greaves, I., Porter, K., Garner, J. (Eds.), 2009. Trauma Care Manual, second ed. Hodder Arnold, London.

Gregory, P.L., 2005. Sports injuries. In: O'Shea, R.A. (Ed.), Principles and Practice of Trauma Nursing. Elsevier, Edinburgh.

Grundy, D., Swain, A., 1996. ABC of Spinal Cord Injury, third ed. BMJ, London.

Hambly, K., Murie, A.J., 1997. Stress Management in Primary Care. Butterworth/Heinemann, Oxford.

Hawton, K., Harriss, L., Simkin, S., et al., 2004. Suicidal behaviour in England and Wales. In: Schmidtke, A., Bille-Brahe, U., De Leo, D., Kerkhof, A. (Eds.), Suicidal Behaviour in Europe: Results from the WHO/EURO Multicentre Study of Suicidal Behaviour. Hogrefe & Huber, Goöttingen.

Hillis, W.S., et al., 2000. Sudden Death: ABC Sports Medicine. BMJ, London.

Homer, C., Fry, M., 2007. Gynaecological emergencies. In: Curtis, K., Ramsden, C. (Eds.), Emergency and Trauma Nursing. Elsevier, Sydney.

Jones, D., 2002. Myths, Madness and the Family. Palgrave, New York.

Jordan, K.S., 2008. Sexually transmitted infections: A major public health challenge for advanced practice nurses. Advanced Emergency Nursing 30 (1), 63–74.

Kannus, P., 2000. Nature, Prevention and Management of Injury: ABC of Sports Medicine. BMJ, London.

Lader, M., Cowen, P. (Eds.), 2001. Depression. Oxford University Press, Oxford.

Large, M.M., Nielssen, O., 2010. Suicide in Australia: meta analysis of rates and methods of suicide between 1988 and 2007. Medical Journal of Australia 192 (8), 432–437.

Martin, N., Newbury-Birch, D., Duckett, J., et al., 2012. A retrospective analysis of the nature, extent and cost of alcohol-related emergency calls to the ambulance service in an English region. Alcohol and Alcoholism 47 (2), 191–197.

Matthews, N., 2000. Physiotherapy, Sports Injury and the Reacquisition of Fitness; ABC of Sports Medicine. BMJ, London.

McClure, G.M., 2000. Changes in suicide in England and Wales 1960–1997. British Journal of Psychiatry 176, 64–67.

Mintel, 2003. Late Licensing UK. Mintel International Group, London.

Moore, K., McLaughlin, D., 2003. Depression: the challenge for all healthcare professionals. Nursing Standard 17 (26), 45–52.

Moreira, M.E., Markovchick, V.J., 2007. Wound management. Emergency Medicine Clinics of North America 25, 873–899.

Moulton, C., Yates, D., 1999. Emergency Medicine. Blackwell Science, Oxford.

Office for National Statistics (2000). London: Stationery Office.

Purshouse, R.C., Meier, P.S., Brennan, A., 2010. Estimated effect of alcohol pricing policies on health and health economic outcomes in England: an epidemiological model. Lancet 375, 1355–1364.

Rickards, L., Fox, K., Roberts, C., et al., 2004. Living in Britain: Results from the 2002 General Household Survey. The Stationery Office, London.

Royal College of Psychiatrists and Royal College of Physicians, 2000. Drugs, Dilemmas and Choices. Bell and Bain, Glasgow.

Shahin, H., 2012. Alcohol and the head-injured patient. Trauma 3, 233–242.

Simmons, J., Allen, J., Aust, R., et al., 2002. Crime in England and Wales 2001/2002. Home Office, London.

Simpson, A., et al., 2007. Abdominal and genitourinary trauma. In: Curtis, K., Ramsden, C. (Eds.), Emergency and Trauma Nursing. Elsevier, Sydney.

Skinner, D., Driscoll, P., Earlham, R., 1991. ABC of Major Trauma. BMJ, London.

Social Trends (2000). 30. Stationery Office, London.

Stewart, J., Allen, T., 2007. Mechanisms of injury. In: Curtis, K., Ramsden, C. (Eds.), Emergency and Trauma Nursing. Elsevier, Sydney.

Tanagho, E., McAnich, J., 2000. Smith's General Urology. McGraw-Hill, New York.

Vale, A., 2012. Alcohols and glycols. Medicine 40 (2), 89–90.

Wasserman, D., 2001. An Unnecessary Death. Martin Duntz, London.

Wilson, W., 2000. A&E nurses fast-track protocol for miscarriages. Accident and Emergency Nursing 8 (1), 9–12.

World Health Organization, 2010. Young People: Health Risks and Solutions: Factsheet 345. WHO, Geneva.

World Health Organization, 2011. Mental Health: Suicide Prevention. WHO, Geneva.

Middle years

21

Brian Boag

CHAPTER CONTENTS

Introduction

The life continuum is a sequence of physical, psychological and social attributes that an individual may experience, and will have an influence on how individuals develop within a changing society and cope with the associated demands and crises. In this chapter the age range of 35–65 years will be taken as the nominal age range. This in itself presents the first challenge, as the spectrum of health can often mean a well 35-year-old becoming ill over the 30 years. The opposite can also be observed, as due to the nature of 'health' many people in their 40s and 50s become much more aware of their physical being and actively work to ensure they are healthy; therefore one can be a very fit 65-year-old or a 35-year-old whose health status is poor.

For many the move into middle years can present many changes and challenges, the spectrum of years means that those at this life point will see many aspects of their lives differently. The changes include: social, psychological, financial and physical, and each can provoke their issues. It is during these years that they will first encounter 'ill-health' and with it the required life changes to occur.

Single life-changing events can combine to have far-reaching consequences that require a re-adjustment in the lifestyle of the individual. It is therefore necessary for the emergency nurse to be aware of the illness and its co-morbidity. For example, type II diabetes, which is more common in this age group than any other, may be as a consequence of obesity and need a change in diet and lifestyle to compensate. A failure to address this illness may lead to heart disease, renal failure, depression and death.

Chest pain

The first major concern for many in this age group is chest pain as it is a major factor affecting the health of those in the middle year's group. With ischaemic heart disease developing during this age period, many are concerned that they will suffer angina or, worse, myocardial infarctions. Despite health education campaigns cardiac disease remains one of the biggest causes of debilitation in the UK and is the most common cause of premature death in people aged under 75 years in the UK. The British Heart Foundation estimates there are around 146 000 myocardial infarctions and 96 000 new cases of angina each year, and 2.5 million people in the UK have coronary heart disease (Allender et al. 2008, Garner 2012).

The overall cost of caring for angina has been calculated by Stewart et al. (2003) to be around 1 % of the NHS budget, mainly because of hospital bed occupancy and revascularization procedures; however, the burden of chest pain is far greater than the burden of angina. Nilsson et al. (2003) report that 1.5 % of primary care consultations are for chest pain, but only 17 % of these are associated with definite or possible angina. Despite this anyone who suffers a sudden onset of chest pain must be encouraged to seek immediate treatment (National Clinical Guideline Centre 2010). Time is heart muscle and to leave ischemic chest pain untreated for any period can result in catastrophic illness.

http://dx.doi.org/10.1016/B978-0-7020-4315-4.00021-8

The patient presenting to the Emergency Department (ED) complaining of chest pain requires careful assessment to determine the symptoms and subtle features that differentiate chest pain which is cardiac in origin from that which is non-cardiac (Box 21.1). Chest pain can be very frightening for the patient, especially if it is the first episode, and staff need to assess and determine the likely signs of such pain (Gerber 2010). A number of key characteristics may help the assessing nurse to distinguish cardiac pain from that of other causes:

- *location:* the location of the pain can give a big clue to the nature of the cause. Cardiac pain is centrally located and chest pain that is peripheral to the sternum is rarely cardiac in nature

- *radiation:* cardiac pain brought on by ischaemia can often radiate to the jaw, neck and arms. Pain situated over the left anterior chest and radiating laterally may have various causes, such as pleurisy, chest wall injury and anxiety

- *provocation:* angina pain is precipitated by exertion, rather than occurring after it. It disappears a few minutes after the cessation of activity when blood flow can again match the oxygen requirements of the muscle. In contrast, pain associated with a specific movement, such as bending, stretching or turning, is likely to be musculoskeletal in origin

- *character of the pain:* ischaemic pain is often described as 'dull' or like a heavy object sitting on the chest. Chest pain caused by gastric problems can be described as a bloating or full feeling. Conversely pleural pain may be described as 'sharp' or 'catching' (Box 21.2)

- *pattern of onset:* the pain of aortic dissection, massive pulmonary embolism or pneumothorax is usually very sudden in onset (within seconds). Myocardial infarction may build up over several minutes or longer, whereas angina builds in proportion to the intensity of the exertion. Pain which develops over a longer period, such as days or even weeks, is often associated with respiratory illness or muscular damage

- *associated features:* the severe pain of a myocardial infarct, massive pulmonary embolus or aortic dissection is often accompanied by autonomic disturbance, including sweating, nausea and vomiting. If the patient is flushed, it may reflect a pyrexia or it may be stress-related. Pallor may be indicative of inadequate cardiac function or shock. Breathlessness is associated with raised pulmonary capillary pressure or pulmonary oedema in myocardial infarction and

---

Box 21.1

Causes of chest pain

Cardiac

- Angina
- Acute myocardial infarction
- Pericarditis
- Endocarditis
- Genetic abnormality
- Respiratory
- Chest infection
- Embolism
- Pneumothorax
- Asthma
- Chronic conditions

Gastric

- Gastritis
- Ulceration
- Hiatus hernia
- Muscular overuse
- Overuse
- Trauma

Psychosomatic

- Depression
- Bereavement

Box 21.2

Characteristic descriptions of chest pain

Stable angina

Typically constricting, retrosternal pain, radiating to the arms (predominantly to the left), neck or jaw. It often occurs in response to stimuli that increase the oxygen demand of the heart, such as physical exertion or emotion, and is relieved by rest

Unstable angina

As in stable angina, but the periods of pain are prolonged and may occur at rest and have no precipitating factors

Myocardial infarction

Three-quarters of patients present with typically severe, crushing, retrosternal pain that may extend to the arms, jaw or back and which often lasts >30 minutes. It is accompanied by nausea, vomiting and sweating. The onset of pain is not always associated with exertion and is not relieved by rest. Some patients have little or no pain, especially the elderly, those from ethnic minority groups (particularly within the Indian subcontinent) and those with diabetes

Pericarditis

The pain is usually sharp and retrosternal and may be more apparent on inspiration. It is often worse when lying flat but is relieved when sitting up or leaning forwards

Pleuritic pain

The pain is usually sharp, localized pain, which is worse on inspiration and coughing

Pulmonary embolism

The pain is pleuritic in nature and may be associated with haemoptysis and breathlessness. Massive pulmonary embolism may produce pain identical in nature to acute myocardial infarction

Oesophageal pain

Oesophageal pain is usually associated with, or eased by, food and is typically worse when lying flat. Oesophageal rupture is usually preceded by vomiting

Aortic dissection

The patient experiences a 'tearing pain', as opposed to the crushing pain of myocardial infarction. This pain is typically felt in the back

Musculoskeletal pain

Pain due to the spinal or muscular disorders can usually be identified by the effect of movement and position. Unlike the other conditions, the chest wall is tender to touch at the specific locations (Adam & Osborne 1997)

Stress-related

The patient will appear flushed and distressed and may be hyperventilating, which will lead to a sensation of central chest pain may accompany any of the respiratory causes of chest pain. Associated gastrointestinal symptoms may provide the clue to non-cardiac chest pain, such as heartburn, peptic ulceration, diarrhoea and vomiting.

On assessment, it is essential to perform a full set of observations. Temperature, if high, can indicate infection, the rate and depth of the pulse can indicate cardiac damage or arrhythmia, respiration rate can indicate respiratory distress and blood pressure can show cardiac instability. This in conjunction with an ECG can give the assessor a clearer picture as to the nature and cause of the chest pain.

The classic pain of angina pectoris is diffuse and retrosternal and will often diminish after rest. In the case of myocardial infarct, it is localized in the centre of the chest, is usually severe in nature, radiating to the left arm and jaw, and is not relieved by rest. Myocardial infarction and its management will be addressed in Chapter 27.

It is vitally important to take a calm, careful history from the patient who presents complaining of chest pain. While diagnosing angina is not as vital as that of a myocardial infarction, it is crucial to know if the patient is developing it as if not a cardiac event it is an indication that the patient is developing coronary heart disease (Harvey 2004).

The patient should firstly be asked to describe the pain – its intensity, location, duration, what brought it on and whether there is any relevant history (Jerlock et al. 2007). Assessing whether the patient can talk in sentences or whether there is pain on movement can indicate whether the chest pain is respiratory or musculoskeletal in origin. Note also that the fear and anxiety brought on by chest pain can exacerbate symptoms in the patient.

Recording of temperature, pulse and blood pressure and a 12-lead ECG can offer an indication of the likelihood of cardiac-related chest pain. A raised temperature may be a result of the breakdown of cardiac enzymes in response to a myocardial infarct that has happened within the previous few hours or may be a result of underlying infection. Recording of pulse oximetry, which measures arterial oxyhaemoglobin saturation (SpO_2), gives important information about the supply of oxygen to the tissues. However, Nicholson (2004) suggests there is no definitive evidence that oxygen has any effect on cardiac ischaemia. Patients whose oxygen saturation levels are under 95% on air are regarded as hypoxic and should be given high-flow

oxygen via a mask (Table 21.1). Supplementary oxygen intake to increase oxygen saturation levels helps to relieve tachycardia induced by hypoxia, thereby reducing cardiac workload.

In the absence of pain and with the patient at rest, the 12-lead ECG may be normal; therefore the ECG should also be performed during an episode of chest pain. ST-segment and T-wave changes, which occur during spontaneous chest pain and disappear with relief of the pain, are significant. Even without changes, the ECG should be repeated after one hour as the absence of abnormality does not rule out disease. Following myocardial infarction, the levels of some of the myocardial enzymes will rise, and estimation of their serum levels is often of diagnostic importance. In addition, the degree of their elevation may give some indication of the size of the infarct (Pride et al. 2009).

Jeremias & Gibson (2005) note that current guidelines for the diagnosis of non-ST-segment elevation myocardial infarction are largely based on an elevated troponin level. While this rapid and sensitive blood test is certainly valuable in the appropriate setting, its widespread use in a variety of clinical scenarios may lead to the detection of troponin elevation in the absence of thrombotic acute coronary syndromes. Many diseases, such as sepsis, hypovolaemia, atrial fibrillation, congestive heart failure, pulmonary embolism, myocarditis, myocardial contusion and renal failure, can also be associated with an increase in troponin level. These elevations may arise from various causes other than thrombotic coronary artery occlusion. Given the lack of any supportive data at present, patients with non-thrombotic troponin elevation should not be treated with antithrombotic and antiplatelet agents. Rather, the underlying cause of the troponin elevation should be targeted. However, troponin elevation in the absence of thrombotic acute coronary syndromes still retains prognostic value. Thus, cardiac troponin elevations are common in numerous disease states and do not necessarily indicate the presence of a thrombotic acute coronary syndrome. While troponin is a sensitive biomarker to 'rule out' non-ST-segment elevation myocardial infarction, it is less useful to 'rule in' this event because it may lack specificity for acute coronary syndromes (Jaffe et al. 2001).

The other measured cardiac enzymes are creatine kinase (CK), lactate dehydrogenase (LDH) and serum glutamic oxaloacetic transaminase (SGOT or AST) and they are released in the first 24 hours after the onset of a myocardial infarct.

Table 21.1 Oxygen masks, flow rates and approximate concentrations of delivered oxygen

Mask oxygen flow (L/min)	Edinburgh (%)	MC(%)	Nasal cannulas	Hudson (%)
1	25–30	–	25–30	–
2	30–35	30–50	30–35	25–38
4	35–40	40–70	32–40	35–45
6	–	55–75	–	50–60
8	–	60–75	–	55–65
10	–	65–80	–	60–75

(After Jowett NI, Thompson D (1995) Comprehensive Coronary Care, 2nd edn. London: Scutari.)

These enzymes may provide retrospective confirmation of infarction rather than a guide to immediate management (analgesia, aspirin, thrombolysis). If the clinical picture suggests myocardial infarction, the patient should be treated as such; however, these are predominantly undertaken as part of the inpatient workup rather than in the ED.

Pain relief may be achieved by administering sublingual glyceryl trinitrate (GTN) tablet or spray, repeated as necessary. Nitrates relax smooth muscle, mainly in the venous system, to increase capacitance and thus reduce cardiac preload. Arteriolar relaxation also occurs, with a fall in peripheral resistance (afterload). The resulting reduction in blood pressure leads to a reduction in chest pain. For patients suspected of having non-cardiac-related chest pain, magnesium trisilicate may relieve symptoms, suggesting an oesophageal or gastric origin of the pain. The use of antacids to differentiate epigastric pain from cardiac pain is common in emergency care; however, consideration must be given to the patient's history, cardiac risk factors and ECG as well as the patient's response to therapy (Novotny-Dinsdale & Andrews 1995). There must always be a high index of suspicion that any chest pain is cardiac in origin until clinical examination and tests prove otherwise (American College of Emergency Physicians 2000).

Abdominal pain

For many, the onset of abdominal pain occurs for the first time during the middle years and often brings the patient into contact with the ED. These abdominal pains range from reflux gastritis through to gastrointestinal haemorrhage; it is therefore essential that a full and robust history should be taken.

As well as ensuring that the correct cardiovascular observations are taken, the assessment nurse should take a full history. This must include:

- age – some conditions are more likely to occur at different points on the age spectrum
- pain
  - time of onset?
  - was it a gradual onset or a sudden pain?
  - how does the patient describe the pain, is it stabbing, does it radiate through the back, is it burning?
  - location of the pain, does it move?
  - is there any vomiting, what did the vomit look like?
  - when does the pain come, e.g., only after eating, after exercise, at night?
- constipation or diarrhoea – if so, when was the last movement, what was the consistency?
- factors that exacerbate or improve symptoms, e.g., food, antacids, exertion
- medications, e.g., aspirin, non-steroidal anti-inflammatory drugs (NSAIDs)
- menstrual history in women
- temperature – this can rule out infection or appendicitis
- social history – frequent alcohol use, especially binge drinking, can cause ulceration, gastritis, oesophageal varices or liver disease.

If there is any doubt in the assessing nurse's mind then the patient should be regarded as potentially unwell and regular 15-minute observations commenced. Intravenous access should be established and a full examination of the abdomen undertaken (see Chapter 29).

Obesity

Obesity is now a major issue for the NHS from strategic management issues regarding equipment to the care and treatment of the patient presenting with obesity. It is estimated that current spending is around is £1bn per year and likely to get higher as in recent years it has become a major concern for the population of the UK (Shan 2008). While not an emergency condition, its presence can lead to attendance, from joint injury (see Chapter 6) to diabetes, from gastric pain to cardiac injury (Box 21.3).

It is now considered good practice to calculate the body mass index (BMI) on all patients (Box 21.4); this can give an indication of potential underlying developing chronic conditions and can also allow the practitioner an opportunity to make a health-promotional intervention. Obese patients also have significantly higher airway management complications during anaesthesia than those within normal weight ranges (Woodall et al. 2012).

It is necessary for the emergency nurse to understand the implications for discharge advice for the patient who is obese; mobility may be reduced or skin integrity compromised. Any patient who has a BMI >30 should have this noted in the patient discharge letter as the GP should follow up the patient before the issue becomes worse.

Box 21.3

Health concerns of obesity

- Type II diabetes
- Renal failure
- Cardiovascular disease
- Stroke
- Joint injury, degeneration
- Respiratory problems
- Skin rashes
- Vascular problems
- Ineffective wound healing
- Depression
- Cancer and stomach problems

Box 21.4

Working out a body mass index

1. Height in metres × by height in metres
2. Weight in kilograms
3. Divide (2) by (1).

For example, a patient weighing 60 kg who is 1.2 metres tall would have a BMI of 41.6

$1.2 \times 1.2 = 1.44$. $60/1.44 = 41.6$

Epigastric pain

Gastritis is a common condition that relates to an inflammation of the stomach lining and involves the symptoms of vomiting. The term gastroenteritis refers to an inflammation of both the gastric and intestinal mucosa. Gastritis is usually associated with dietary indiscretions due to overindulgence of alcohol or food, but it may also be a result of stress, NSAIDs or uraemia.

The inflammation is usually self-limiting and without sequelae, but patients presenting with gastritis may require antacids to alleviate vomiting and nausea. Advice to patients includes taking clear liquids only until 8–12 hours have passed without vomiting, and then starting with bland foods before gradually resuming a normal diet.

The term 'peptic ulcer' refers to an ulcer in the lower oesophagus, the stomach, the duodenum or the jejunum after surgical anastomosis to the stomach. It is a common condition and has its highest incidence in males aged 40–55 years, with perforation occurring in approximately 5–10% of affected individuals. While epigastric pain resolves with antacids and is self-limiting and short-lived, ulcers are repetitive and are worse after specific foods or drinks. Although peptic ulcer disease is commonly suspected in dyspeptic patients, it is found much less often than suspected when patients undergo endoscopic investigation (Vakil 2005, Aro et al. 2006).

Ulceration of the gastric mucosa leads to excoriation and mucous membrane sloughing. An imbalance between pepsin, hydrochloric acid secretion and bicarbonate causes gastric erosion. Bacterial invasion from *Helicobacter pylori* has been implicated as an important aetiological factor in peptic ulcer disease, accounting for 90% of duodenal ulcers and 70% of gastric ulcers (Lassen et al. 2004). *H. pylori* causes acute inflammation of the mucosa by causing degeneration, detachment and necrosis of the epithelial cells. Chronic ingestion of medications that irritate the gastric mucosa, such as aspirin or NSAIDs, can also lead to the development of ulcers (Butcher 2004). While duodenal and gastric ulcers are different conditions, they share common symptoms and will be considered together.

The most common presentation is that of recent abdominal pain that has three notable characteristics: localization to the epigastrium, relationship to food and episodic occurrence. The pain is probably caused by acid coming into contact with the ulcer. Occasional vomiting may occur in about 40% of patients with peptic ulcer. In some patients the ulcer is completely 'silent', presenting for the first time with anaemia from chronic undetected blood loss, or as an abrupt haematemesis or acute perforation; in others there is recurrent acute bleeding without ulcer pain between attacks.

Peptic ulceration is an umbrella term used to describe areas in the gastrointestinal tract that have been exposed to, and damaged by, acid and pepsin-containing secretions. The most common sites for peptic ulcers are the stomach (gastric ulcers) and the duodenum (duodenal ulcers) (Elliot 2002). A peptic ulcer may progressively erode the submucosal, muscular and serous layers of the gastrointestinal wall. When perforation occurs, the contents of the stomach escape into the peritoneal cavity; this occurs more commonly in duodenal than in gastric ulcers. The most striking symptom is sudden, severe pain; its distribution follows the spread of gastric contents over the peritoneum. Initially, the pain may be referred to the upper abdomen, but it quickly becomes generalized; shoulder tip pain may occur as a result of irritation of the diaphragm. The pain is accompanied by shallow respirations due to epigastric pain and limitation of diaphragmatic movements. A rapid pulse and reduction in blood pressure indicate shock. Pyrexia may also be present as a result of peritonitis. Pallor, a cold clammy skin, nausea and vomiting may be also evident. The abdomen is held immobile and has 'board-like' rigidity.

Non-operative treatment includes i.v. morphine for pain relief, aspiration of the stomach contents using a nasogastric tube and continuous gastric suctioning, i.v. electrolytes and fluids, and antibiotic therapy. After initial treatment for shock, emergency surgery may be performed to close the perforation or resect the affected area; however, perforation carries a mortality rate of approximately 10%. The nurse should monitor the patient's vital signs closely for signs of deterioration and offer reassurance to the patient and his family.

Where there is no indication of perforation, the patient is usually managed with a range of anti-ulcer medications such as omeprazole and/or metronidazole, which have antibacterial effects on *H. pylori*, and referred back to his GP for ongoing treatment and review that may include endoscopy. A patient should be encouraged to follow up any gastro-intestinal disturbance as it can lead to further complications and reattendance at hospital.

Joint injury

For some who have had a history of undertaking sport and continue to do so at an aggressive level, there may be injury due to overuse. This is addressed in further detail in the skeletal injuries chapter (Chapter 6).

Depression and life-changing events

During this phase of life, many people experience life-changing events, including job loss, house moves, children leaving home and bereavement. For many it can be a traumatic time and depression can occur. For some this can manifest itself slowly through a sequence of multiple presentations to the ED with psychosomatic presentations of minor illness, and for others it can be manifested as a suicide attempt or through a violent outburst.

For the nurse assessing it is advisable to be aware of the patient with frequent attendance and to ask for a fuller social history. In acute presentations it is essential that a full psychiatric assessment is undertaken by a specialist in mental health as follow-up treatment may be needed. For the partners and relatives of those who have died suddenly, a referral to a chaplain or a bereavement service may help limit the ongoing development of depression and mental illness. These issues are addressed more fully in Chapters 14 and 15.

Homelessness

Homelessness is the term used to describe a range of situations associated with insecure and inadequate shelter, including rough sleepers, persons staying in homeless shelters and people with nowhere to go following release from institutions such as prisons, psychiatric institutions or from foster care (Wright & Tompkins 2006, Hamden et al. 2011, Cross et al. 2012). Few would need convincing that the extreme conditions of homelessness and sleeping rough are bound to affect health (Joseph Rowntree Foundation 2000, Morrison 2009). The homeless are disproportionately white, male and middle-aged, although there are increasing numbers of young men and women and black and Asian people (Homeless Link 2002, Pleace & Quilgars 1996). In a study of the records of 1873 homeless users of an ED compared with 28 420 housed people, a disturbing health profile emerged (North et al. 1996):

- homeless people's accidents and injuries were four times more likely to be the result of an assault than those of housed people
- homeless people had twice the rate of infected wounds compared with housed people. These infections were twice as likely to be severe enough to warrant an admission to hospital for further treatment
- a substantial proportion (10%) of homeless people attending EDs did so for mental health reasons. This was the second largest presenting category for homeless people to ED, but only ranked tenth for housed attenders
- homeless people were five times more likely to attend EDs due to deliberate self-harm than were housed people. Depression was very common among people of no fixed abode and hostel residents
- asthma was twice as common among homeless as among housed attenders
- epilepsy was four times as common among homeless as among housed users of the ED.

More recent research by Griffiths (2002) has identified that:
- 30–50% of homeless people experience mental health problems
- about 70% of homeless people misuse drugs
- about 50% of homeless people are dependent on alcohol
- rough sleepers are 35 times more likely to kill themselves than the general population.

The average age of death for homeless patients in the UK is between 40 and 44 (Office of the Chief Analyst 2010) and the literature on homelessness reveals the almost universal acceptance that there is a close link between ill health and homelessness (Morrison 2009, Hewett & Halligan 2010, Cross et al. 2012). Difficulties in obtaining access to primary healthcare services have meant that EDs have been an important source of healthcare provision for some homeless men and women. The Scottish Executive Health Department (2001) notes that while EDs are often the first point of contact for homeless people, staff may not have received training on homelessness issues and may not be in a position to respond appropriately to homelessness. Minor, acute illnesses pose particular problems for homeless people, who lack the facilities to look after themselves when well, and who are at risk of particular infections and infestations precisely because of their circumstances. Respiratory illness has been found to be a major health problem associated with being homeless. Other common conditions are chronic obstructive airways disease, tuberculosis, foot problems, infestations and epilepsy. Homeless people attending EDs also exhibit a disproportionate prevalence of infections, scabies and lice (Scott 1993).

One study found that homeless people attended ED six times as often as the housed population, are admitted four times as often and stay in hospital twice as long (Leicester Homeless Primary Heath Care Service 2008). Comparison of duration of stay in Hospital Episode Statistics data shows that the lengths of stay are generally appropriate for the admitting condition (Office of the Chief Analyst 2010). As Hewett & Halligan (2010) note, this means homeless people stay twice as long in hospital because they are twice as sick. Low temperature is an important cause of morbidity and mortality among the homeless. In Britain, for each degree Celsius that the winter is colder than average, there are an extra 8000 deaths (Balazs 1993), although a study by Brown et al. (2010) found no evidence that more homeless people would attend ED in colder weather.

Emergency nurses may offer the only social contact for some homeless people. A novel Canadian study found that compassionate care of homeless people who present to EDs significantly lowered their repeat visits. The researchers identified 133 consecutive homeless adults visiting one inner-city ED who were not acutely psychotic, extremely intoxicated, unable to speak English or medically unstable. Half were randomly assigned to receive compassionate care from trained volunteers. All patients otherwise had the usual care and were followed for repeat visits to EDs. The researchers found that the attendance by homeless people who received compassionate care was significantly lower. While acknowledging that compassionate care is not necessarily cost-effective if staff costs are taken into account, the authors argued that the basic justification for compassion is decency not economics (Redelmeier et al. 1995). At University College Hospital, London, people with an experience of homelessness join a GP and nurse team on regular ward rounds to visit homeless patients throughout the hospital, advocate for their treatment in hospital, plan for their discharge and support them in the community. Early indications are that this approach improves care and discharge planning, while offering overall savings by reducing the small numbers of patients with very prolonged durations of stay (Hewett 2010, Hewett & Halligan 2010).

Conclusion

The middle years is a pivotal timeframe when things can start to go wrong as the adult moves from being almost always healthy to almost always having a health concern. Through this continuum it is essential that the patient is fully assessed and treated with consideration. It may well be that there is nothing wrong and the concerns are psychological, but now is a good time to begin health promotion, ensuring the middle years adult remains healthy for as long as they can.

References

Adam, S.K., Osborne, S., 1997. Critical Care Nursing: Science & Practice. Oxford Medical, Oxford.

Allender, S., Peto, V., Scarborough, P., et al., 2008. Coronary Heart Disease Statistics. British Heart Foundation and Stroke Association, Oxford.

American College of Emergency Physicians, 2000. Clinical Policy: Critical Issues in the Evaluation and Management of Adult Patients Presenting with Suspected Acute Myocardial Infarction or Unstable Angina. ACEP, Dallas.

Aro, P., Storskrubb, T., Ronkainen, J., et al., 2006. Peptic ulcer disease in a general adult population. American Journal of Epidemiology 163 (11), 1025–1034.

Balazs, J., 1993. Health care for single homeless people. In: Fisher, K., Collins, J. (Eds.), Homelessness, Health Care and Welfare Provision. Routledge, London.

Brown, A.J., Goodacre, S.W., Cross, S., 2010. Do emergency department attendances by homeless people increase during cold weather? Emergency Medicine Journal 27, 526–529.

Butcher, D., 2004. Pharmacological techniques for managing acute pain in emergency departments. Emergency Nurse 12 (1), 26–36.

Cross, W., Hayter, M., Jackson, D., et al., 2012. Editorial: Meeting the health care needs associated with poverty, homelessness and social exclusion: the need for an interprofessional approach. Journal of Clinical Nursing 21 (4), 907–908.

Elliot, S., 2002. The treatment of peptic ulcers. Nursing Standard 16 (22), 37–42.

Garner, M., 2012. Chest Pain. In: Wood, I., Garner, M. (Eds.), Initial Management of Acute Medical Patients: A Guide for Nurses and Healthcare Practitioners, second ed. John Wiley & Sons, London.

Gerber, T.C., 2010. Emergency department assessment of acute-onset chest pain: Contemporary approaches and their consequences. Mayo Clinic Proceedings 85 (4), 309–313.

Griffith, S., 2002. Assessing the Health Needs of Rough Sleepers. Office of the Deputy Prime Minister Homelessness Directorate, London.

Hamden, A., Newton, R., McCauley-Elsom, K., et al., 2011. Is deinstitutionalization working in our community? International Journal of Mental Health Nursing 20, 274–283.

Harvey, S., 2004. The nursing assessment and management of patients with angina. British Journal of Nursing 13 (10), 598–601.

Hewett, N., 2010. Evaluation of the London Pathway for Homeless Patients. UCH, London.

Hewett, N., Halligan, A., 2010. Homelessness is a healthcare issue. Journal of The Royal Society of Medicine 103 (8), 306–307.

Homeless Link, 2002. An Overview of Homelessness in London. Homeless Link, London.

Jaffe, A.S. The World Health Organization, The European Society of Cardiology, The American College of Cardiology, 2001. New standard for the diagnosis of acute myocardial infarction. Cardiology in Review 9 (6), 318–322.

Jeremias, A., Gibson, C.M., 2005. Narrative review: Alternative causes for elevated cardiac troponin levels when acute coronary syndromes are excluded. Annals of Internal Medicine 142 (9), 786–791.

Jerlock, M., Welin, C., Rosengren, A., et al., 2007. Pain characteristics in patients with unexplained chest pain with ischaemic heart disease. Journal of Cardiovascular Nursing 6 (2), 130–136.

Joseph Rowntree Foundation, 2000. Research on Single Homelessness in Britain. Joseph Rowntree Foundation, London.

Jowett, N.I., Thompson, D., 1995. Comprehensive Coronary Care, second ed. Scutari, London.

Lassen, A.T., Hallas, J., Schaffalitzky de Muck-adell, O.B., 2004. Helicobacter pylori test and eradicate versus prompt endoscopy for management of dyspeptic patients: 6.7 year follow up of a randomised trial. Gut 53 (12), 1758–1763.

Leicester Homeless Primary Health Care Service, 2008. Annual Report 2007/2008. Leicester, Leicester Community Health Service.

Morrison, D.S., 2009. Homelessness as an independent risk factor for mortality: results from a retrospective cohort study. International Journal of Epidemiology 38 (3), 877–883.

National Clinical Guideline Centre, 2010. Unstable Angina and NSTEMI: The Early Management of Unstable Angina and Non-ST-segment-elevation Myocardial Infarction. Royal College of Physicians, London.

Nicholson, C., 2004. A systematic review of the effectiveness of oxygen in reducing acute myocardial ischaemia. Journal of Clinical Nursing 13, 996–1007.

Nilsson, S., Scheike, M., Engblom, D., et al., 2003. Chest pain and ischaemic disease in primary care. British Journal of General Practice 53, 378–382.

North, C., Moore, H., Owens, C., 1996. Go Home and Rest? The Use of an Accident and Emergency Department by Homeless People. Shelter, London.

Novotny-Dinsdale, V., Andrews, L.S., 1995. Gastrointestinal emergencies. In: Thomas, J., Proeh, J.A., Kaiser (Eds.), Emergency Nursing: A Physiologic and Clinical Perspective, second ed. Saunders, Philadelphia.

Office of the Chief Analyst, 2010. Healthcare for Single Homeless People. Department of Health, London.

Pleace, N., Quilgars, D., 1996. Health and Homelessness in London: A Review. King's Fund, London.

Pride, Y.B., Applebaum, E., Lord, E.E., et al., 2009. Relation between myocardial infarct size and ventricular tachyarrhythmia among patients with preserved left ventricular ejection fraction following fibrinolytic therapy for ST-segment elevation myocardial infarction. The American Journal of Cardiology 104 (4), 475–479.

Redelmeier, D.A., Molin, J.P., Tibshini, R.J., 1995. A randomized trial of compassionate care for the homeless in an emergency department. The Lancet 345, 1131–1134.

Scott, J., 1993. Homelessness and mental health. British Journal of Psychiatry 162, 314–324.

Scottish Executive Health Department, 2001. Health and Homelessness Guidance. Scottish Executive Health Department, Edinburgh.

Shan, Y., 2008. Tackling the obesity crisis in the UK. Primary Health Care 18 (8), 25–30.

Stewart, S., Murphy, N., Walker, A., et al., 2003. The current cost of angina pectoris to the National Health Service in the UK. Heart 89, 848–853.

Vakil, N., 2005. Commentary: toward a simplified strategy for managing dyspepsia. Postgraduate Medicine 1176, 13.

Woodall, N.M., Benger, J.R., Harper, J.S., et al., 2012. Airway management complications during anaesthesia, in intensive care units and in emergency departments in the UK. Trends in Anaesthesia and Critical Care 2 (2), 58–64.

Wright, N., Tompkins, C., 2006. How can health services effectively meet the health needs of homeless people? British Journal of General Practice 56, 286–293.

Older people

Brian Dolan

Introduction

Older people constitute a growing proportion of attendances to the Emergency Department (ED). This chapter addresses the changing UK demographics, and the physiology of ageing, before considering the assessment of common acute older adult presentations, such as hypothermia, confusion and falls.

The effects of polypharmacy and elder abuse will also be described and discussed.

In demographic terms, the UK has an ageing population. From 1971 to 2021 the number of people in the UK aged 65 and over is expected to increase by nearly 70% from 7.3 million to 12.2 million (Office for National Statistics 2006), because average life expectancy in the UK has doubled in the last 200 years. By 2021, there will be more people over 80 than under the age of 5; over a quarter of the population will be over 60. The number of people aged over 65 years is escalating, with the fastest-growing group being those aged over 80 years. In England and Wales, the numbers in this age group increased by >1.2 million between 1981 and 2007 (from 1.5 to 2.7 million), from 2.8% to 4.5% of the population. It is suggested that by 2021 there are expected to be 601 000 people aged 90 and over (Office for National Statistics 2009).

More older people are likely to be admitted to hospital as the population ages; often this is via the ED as the gateway to hospital care. Older peoples' health problems are also often complex clinically and managerially, thus time consuming and challenging for clinical staff (Bridges et al. 2005, Beynon et al. 2011).

Background

There is evidence from the UK, North America and Europe that people who live in areas of socio-economic deprivation have higher rates of emergency admissions, after adjusting for other risk factors. In the UK, admission rates are significantly correlated with measures of social deprivation (Majeed et al. 2000). Socio-demographic variables explain around 45% of the variation in emergency admissions between GP practices, with deprivation more strongly linked to emergency than to elective admission (Duffy et al. 2002). Practices serving the most deprived populations have emergency admission rates that are around 60–90% higher than those serving the least deprived populations (Purdy 2010, Purdy et al. 2011).

http://dx.doi.org/10.1016/B978-0-7020-4315-4.00022-X

There have been concerns about the quality of care delivered to older people for many years. The Health Advisory Service 2000 (1998) identified eight major issues affecting the care of older people (Box 22.1). It was reported that older people waited longer in the ED than any other patient group (Association of Community Health Councils for England and Wales 2001); however, it was also acknowledged that older people present with more complex needs and take longer to process (Clark & Fitzgerald 1999). Meyer & Bridges (1998) found evidence of negative attitudes amongst nurses towards older people in the ED. Spilsbury et al. (1999) interviewed ED patients about their experiences. They reported concerns about lack of assessment, long waiting times, and staff not taking into account their sensory or physical problems while not giving consideration to their privacy, safety and comfort. They also stated that staff did not appear to understand their pre-admission circumstances. Meyer & Bridges (1998) concur, stating that ED nurses perceive their role as primarily providing biomedical care rather than nursing care. This prompted the Royal College of Nursing A&E Nursing Association to release a mission statement on the care of older people in the ED, which highlights the need to:

> 'Provide an environment appropriate to meeting the needs of older people, by creating a culture and supporting practice that is respectful of the complex needs, rights, desires, dignity and life experience' (Sowney 1999).

Higgins et al. (2007) describe the persistent negative attitudes of nurses towards older people in acute clinical settings and the *National Service Framework for Older People* creates a benchmark to underpin the care of older people (Department of Health 2001a). The aim of this document is to address their needs, by promoting knowledge-based practice and partnership working between those who use and those who provide a service (Department of Health 2001a). This highlights the need for emergency nurses to have expert understanding of the ageing process, specialist assessment whilst also developing practice through leadership, teaching and mentoring. Nikki et al. (2012) argue that more attention should also be paid to empathic encounters with family members, who will know the patient's previous functional capacity and medication, which is decisive information when planning further care and thinking about the patient coping at home.

Physiology of ageing

There is no single unifying theory of ageing and it has recently been investigated as a complex, multifactorial process. Death and ageing are distinct entities, but ageing is associated with numerous gradual declines in physiological function that will inevitably lead to death. In broad terms there are two categories of theories to ageing (Maguire & Slater 2010). Ageing is genetically programmed and influenced by the environment, so the rate of ageing among people varies widely (Cheitlin 2003). Ageing is characterized by a general deterioration of bodily function. Although ageing is considered to be inevitable, the reality is that the rate of deterioration in organ function can be reduced by factors such as regular exercise and accelerated by habits such as cigarette smoking and heavy alcohol consumption. Indeed, there is considerable variability in individuals' susceptibility to ageing. Table 22.1 outlines some of the organ and tissue changes associated with ageing, which will underpin patient assessment.

Assessment

An older person presenting to the ED requires a thorough physical, psychological and social assessment. Good communication is vital and the emergency nurse must have the ability to listen effectively. As older people's hearing and vision may be impaired and their responses slow, it is important to give the patient time to express themselves freely. It is also important to remember that the history-taking process may take longer than the physical examination, and studies indicate that over 80% of diagnoses are based on the interview alone (Epstein et al. 2003). Patients have previously expressed concerns about lack of assessment and information-giving (Considine et al. 2010). Older people can present with multiple pathologies and the presenting complaint may not be the only condition that needs to be considered.

The emergency nurse needs to elicit why the person has attended the ED. The assessment can begin with a general question that allows full freedom to respond; for example, 'What brings you here?' or 'What can we do for you?' After the patient answers, probe further by asking 'Is there anything else?' It is imperative to remember that patients may also have complex psychological and social causes and may have complicated feelings about themselves, their illnesses or potential treatments. To gain a thorough history, which fulfils the patient expectations, the interviewing technique must allow patients time to recount their own stories spontaneously (Bickley & Szilagyi 2003). An example of how to structure history taking is provided in Table 22.2.

When first meeting the patient, the nurse should introduce themselves, both as a courtesy and as an opportunity to establish a rapport. If the patient has walked into the department, the nurse should accompany the patient to the cubicle and observe features such as gait, balance and pace.

Box 22.1

Concerns about the quality of care for older people

- Admission delays
- Poor physical environment
- Shortage of medical, nursing and therapy staff
- Lack of expertise and education in the care of older people
- Lack of fundamental care, dignity, respect and assistance with eating and bathing
- Low expectations of recovery, lack of awareness of rehabilitation
- Poor communication with older people and their families
- Poor discharge planning

(After Health Advisory Service 2000 (1998) Not Because They are Old: An Independent Inquiry into the Care of Older People on Acute Wards in General Hospitals. London: HAS (2000).)

Table 22.1 Physiological changes associated with ageing

System	Pre-existing conditions	Physiological changes	Signs and symptoms	Potential traumatic injuries
Cardiovascular	Coronary artery disease Hypertension Congestive heart failure Myocardial infarction Medications (esp. beta blockers, calcium-channel blockers, anticoagulants)	Fat and fibrous tissue replaces conductive pathways Heart valves thicken reducing compliance Reduced coronary artery flow Lower maximum heart rate Reduced cardiac output	Dysrhythmias Hypertension Inability to meet increased myocardial oxygen demands Heart rate may not rise due to stressors	Aortic arch disruption Myocardial contusion Aneurysm
Respiratory	Chronic obstructive pulmonary disease Asthma Pneumonia Pulmonary oedema Pulmonary embolism Congestive heart failure History of smoking	Non-elastic fibrous tissue Fixed expiratory volume Reduced compliance Reduced vital capacity Reduced alveoli in number and size Reduced peak expiratory flow Increased residual volume Under-ventilation despite normal perfusion Reduced baseline PO_2 Reduced cough reflexes Chest wall stiffness Reduced response to foreign antigen Reduced response to hypoxia or hypercarbia	Increased diaphragmatic breathing Shortness of breath	Increased risk of rib fractures Increased risk of pulmonary contusion Air trapping Atelectasis Increased risk of pneumonia Increased risk of aspiration Increased risk of adult respiratory distress syndrome (ARDS)
Renal	Renal insufficiency	Reduced number of glomeruli Reduced number of nephrons Reduced renal flow Reduced glomerular filtration rate Reduced bladder capacity Reduced drug metabolism	Reduced urinary output	Acute renal failure Increased risk of fluid/electrolyte imbalance and fluid overload
Central nervous system	Stroke Dementia Alzheimer's Impaired gait		Confusion Altered mental status	Increased risk of subdural haematoma Brain infarct Closed head injury
Gastrointestinal	Reduced calorie intake Reduced glucose tolerance Diabetes	Reduced calorie requirement Reduced body mass Reduced drug metabolism by liver Reduced gastric emptying Reduced gastric motility Reduced oesophageal sphincter	Oesophageal reflux Bowel dysfunction	Increased risk of bowel injuries Mesenteric infarction
Skin and musculoskeletal	Nutritional deficiency Joint disease Arthritis	Loss of skin tone Reduced sensation Loss of resilient connective tissue Reduced mobility Osteoporosis Spondylosis Kyphosis	Bruising Contusions Skin/wound infections	Tetanus Distal radius fractures Fractured hip C1–C2 fractures from falls at ground level Spinal fractures Rib fractures
Immunological	Autoimmune dysfunction	Altered cellular response	Sepsis without pyrexia	
Hepatic	Coagulopathies		Bruising Bleeding	Contusions Bleeding
Endocrine	Diabetes mellitus Diabetes insipidus Thyroid dysfunction			

Adapted from Stevenson J (2004) When the trauma patient is elderly. Journal of Peri Anaesthesia Nursing, 19(6), 392–400.

Table 22.2 Structured history-taking

Location	Where is the pain/problem?
Timing/onset	When did it start? When did you last feel well? Did it start suddenly or gradually?
Quality	How does the patient describe the pain? Is it constant or intermittent?
Quantity or severity	How does this problem affect their daily living, e.g., shortness of breath, can they walk as far as normal, can they do the stairs?
Aggravating factors	Does anything make it worse?
Relieving factors	Does anything make it better?
Associated manifestations	Are there any other symptoms, e.g., if they are short of breath do they also have a cough?

If the patient needs to get undressed, they should do so themselves if they are able, as it is important for the patient to feel in control as much as possible. Offering the patient a seat while undressing will allow them to remove their clothes more easily. It also enables the nurse to assess the patient's balance and ability to self-care. It is not essential for patients to remove all their clothing when getting undressed, and undergarments should only be removed if necessary. If the patient is wearing pyjamas or a nightdress on presentation, there is rarely a need to change into a hospital gown; however, the patient will usually require a full examination, and clothing should not inhibit this. The patient may require steps to climb onto the trolley where they are able.

Careful attention should be given to the condition of the patient's skin; inspect the patient for old wounds, unhealed ulcers or bruises. The latter may give an indication of elder abuse (considered later in this chapter). An initial nutritional assessment should be completed.

Not all patients attending the ED require a full set of vital signs and the older person must be assessed individually. For many patients, vital signs will form an integral part of the patient assessment. Older people may have altered vital signs that are normal for them; however, it is imperative to establish their normal baseline. This can be gained from the patient or relative, the computer record system or the patient's Single Assessment Process document (Department of Health 2001a). For example, the heart rate of an older person is likely to be slower, with arrhythmias being relatively common in otherwise asymptomatic patients. Similarly, the older person's blood pressure is likely to be elevated, usually as a consequence of atherosclerosis. This predisposes the patient to the development of cardiovascular diseases, such as congestive cardiac failure, stroke, transient ischaemic attacks and dementia. If a normally hypertensive patient appears to have a normal blood pressure they may actually be hypotensive. Similarly, if the patient is prescribed and taking beta-blockers they will fail to have a tachycardic response to shock, so the emergency nurse must apply knowledge of pharmacology and altered physiology when analyzing vital signs.

A baseline temperature should be recorded. In older people, the temperature is usually recorded as 36.5°C or above, due to the reduction in basal metabolic rate. The patient's respiration rate may be increased due to underlying conditions such as chronic obstructive pulmonary disease or asthma. Poor personal hygiene may reflect difficult socio-economic circumstances of the patient rather than an inability to cope, and the nurse should take this into account when assessing the patient. The patient's pre-existing medical and drug history should be assessed and recorded during the assessment.

As with patients of all ages, the nurse needs to use language the patient will understand and provide frequent orienting information about the time, place and person, including explanations of equipment, procedures and routines. Older people may process information more slowly; the nurse should develop comfortable and natural ways of talking to the patient, bearing in mind normal deterioration in hearing and other special senses that are associated with ageing. Others involved in the care of the patient, such as relatives or ambulance crew, should be consulted about the patient's condition. However, the patient's view should be sought as much as possible, with others used to supplement the information provided by the patient.

Elder abuse

Elder abuse, although increasingly recognized as a violation of human rights, remains one of the most hidden forms of inter-family conflict within many societies (Podnieks et al. 2010, Naughton et al. 2012).

The prevalence of elder abuse in the UK is estimated to be 2.6% (Biggs et al. 2009) although international studies range from 2.1% in Ireland (Naughton 2011), to 9–11.4% in the US (Lauman et al. 2009, Lowenstein et al. 2009), which raises several questions. Are the differences related to cultural/societal factors or study design factors or in the risk factors for elder abuse? Nurses should have a high index of suspicion when assessing older people, as with non-accidental injury in children. Clinicians must assess whether the mechanism is consistent with the injury or illness presented (Crouch 2003) as cognitive impairment limits older adults' abilities to advocate for themselves and possibly heightens their risk for abuse (Ziminski et al. 2012). If emergency nurses know the red flags of abuse (Box 22.2), the right questions to ask (Boxes 22.3 and 22.4) and the appropriate action to take in cases of suspected abuse, they can make a critical difference to the welfare of an older person (Gray-Vickery 2005). As Phelan (2012) notes nurses in the ED should be cognizant of interviewing the older person on their own when collecting information, as he may be hugely compromised with the presence of a family member who may be the perpetrator. It is also useful to interview the accompanying relative separately to elicit the cause of attendance, which may deviate from the older person's account. In the context of a relative refusing to leave, it should be noted and the older person should be facilitated to answer the questions rather than being dominated by the relative/other person. This is also why it is essential to build up rapport with the patient to enable to older person to disclose. If nurses suspect abuse, attention to detail when documenting is of paramount importance. Document the person's account in their own words (Community and District Nursing Association 2003) and signs of abuse clearly, and consider the use of illustration through medical photography; this requires specialist consent

Box 22.2

Red flags for identifying elder abuse

For all forms of abuse have a high index of suspicion if the history is inconsistent with the injury or illness

Physical signs of abuse
- Multiple bruising, e.g., inner thigh or bruising at different stages of healing
- Finger marks
- Burns, especially in unusual places
- An injury similar to the shape of an object
- Unexplained fractures
- Pressure ulcers or untreated wounds
- Attempts to hide part of the body on examination
- Inappropriate use of medications, e.g., overdosing

Signs of sexual abuse
- Pain, itching or injury to the anal, genital or abdominal area
- Difficulty in walking or sitting because of genital pain
- Bruising and/or bleeding of external genitalia
- Torn, stained or bloody underclothes
- Sexually transmitted disease or recurrent episodes of cystitis
- An uncharacteristic change in the patient's attitude to sex
- Unexplained problems with catheters

Signs of psychological abuse
- Appears depressed, frightened, withdrawn, apathetic, anxious or aggressive

- Makes a great effort to please
- Appears afraid of being treated by specific staff, carer or relative
- Displays reluctance to be discharged
- Demonstrates sudden mood or behaviour change

Signs of financial abuse
The patient may confide in the emergency nurse:
- Unexplained savings account withdrawals
- Inability to explain what is happening to his/her income
- Unpaid bills
- The disappearance of bank statements and valuables, e.g., jewellery, clothes, personal possessions and money

Signs of neglect
- Weight loss
- Unkempt appearance, dirty clothes and poor hygiene
- Pressure ulcers or uncharacteristic problems with continence
- Inadequate nutrition and hydration
- Inadequate or inappropriate medical treatment or withholding treatment
- A patient who is left in a wet or soiled bed

(Adapted from Klein Schmidt KC (1997) Elder abuse: a review. *Annals of Emergency Medicine*, 30(4), 463–472; Action on Elder Abuse (2005) *Indicators of Abuse*. London: Action on Elder Abuse; Banerjee, J., Conroy, S., O'Leary, V., et al. (2012) Quality care for older people with urgent or emergency care needs ('Silver Book'). London, British Geriatrics Society.)

Box 22.3

Screen for physical abuse with these questions
Has anyone hurt you?
Has anyone touched you without your consent?
Has anyone ever made you do things you didn't want to do?
Has anyone ever threatened you?
Who cares for you at home?
Are you frightened of your care-giver?

Box 22.4

Screen for neglect and financial exploitation with these questions
Are you satisfied with your living situation?
What is a typical day like for you?
Who gives you your medications?
Who helps you with dressing, bathing and/or preparing meals?
Has anyone ever failed to help you when you needed help?

(Adapted from Gray-Vickery P (2005) Elder abuse: are you prepared to intervene? LPN, 1(2), 38–42.)

and adherence to local protocols. Upon detection of abuse local guidelines and policies should be adhered to.

The questions act as a guide; enquiries must be made sensitively in a private and safe environment, allowing the person time to speak. It is important to find out what the person wants to happen.

Polypharmacy

The use of multiple medications (polypharmacy) is common among older people (Linton et al. 2007, Zarowitz 2011). This is caused by many factors, such as co-existing chronic conditions, use of more than one pharmacy, increase in the availability of over-the-counter medicines and multiple prescribing providers. Indeed, interviews carried out with multi-professionals reported that participants admitted that prescribing was sometimes inappropriate and prescribing for chronic diseases was poorly understood (Spinewine et al. 2005). A US study indicated that 23 % of women and 19 % of men take at least five prescription drugs (Kaufmann et al. 2002). These figures, however, do not take into account medication purchased over the counter.

The effects of polypharmacy may have precipitated the patient's attendance at the ED. Falls and dehydration are common risk factors associated with multiple medications (Department of Health 2001b). Emergency nurses need to be aware of medicine-related features, which are known to be associated with problems in older people. These are:

- taking four or more medications
- specific medications, e.g., warfarin, non-steroidal anti-inflammatory drugs (NSAIDs), diuretics and digoxin
- recent discharge from hospital.

Social and personal factors associated with medication-related problems are:

- social support – minimal support available
- physical condition – poor hearing, vision and dexterity
- mental state – delirium/dementia (Department of Health 2001a).

Patients presenting with polypharmacy should have a detailed drug history recorded; it is good practice to have a pharmacist review medications during the patient's ED episode. However, if this service is unavailable, careful attention should be given to taking and documenting the drug history. In addition to the drug name, dose and frequency, the source of the history, compliance and concordance should be noted. The key to ensuring safety is appropriate prescribing and monitoring of the patient's condition; 5–17% of preventable admissions are associated with adverse reactions to medications (Department of Health 2001a). Prescribing should take into account the physiology of ageing, drug interactions, cautions, side-effects and the recommended dose for older people.

Effective communication between the ED and primary care provider is essential to ensure appropriate and effective monitoring is carried out. General practitioners and patients should be provided with information about medications on discharge; this information must include an explanation of why any changes were made.

Hypothermia

Hypothermia is classified as a core temperature below 35°C; it is associated with a high mortality rate among older people. Three types of accidental hypothermia are recognized. Acute hypothermia (often called immersion hypothermia) is caused by sudden exposure to cold such as immersion in cold water or a person caught in a snow avalanche. Exhaustion hypothermia is caused by exposure to cold in association with lack of food and exhaustion such that heat can no longer be generated. Chronic hypothermia comes on over days or weeks and mainly affects the elderly (Guly 2010). It is important to ascertain whether hypothermia is caused by environmental exposure or is a consequence of unknown pathology. Common precipitants include immobility (Parkinson's disease, hypothyroidism), reduced cold awareness (dementia), unsatisfactory housing, poverty, drugs, alcohol, acute confusion and infections (Wyatt et al. 2005). Malnutrition may also be a leading factor associated with hypothermia. A well-balanced diet is essential to provide the calories needed to generate and maintain adequate heat. A decrease in calorie intake can have a profound effect on the ability to produce heat by shivering (Neno 2005).

Physiology

Body temperature is regulated in the anterior hypothalamus. In cold weather, when the body needs to conserve heat, the hypothalamic heat production centres respond to impulses from the thermoreceptors by causing peripheral vasoconstriction via the sympathetic nervous system. This vasoconstriction enhances the insulating properties of the skin, reducing blood flow to the superficial vessels; the result is less heat being lost from the skin (Pocock & Richards 2004).

The ability of people to respond appropriately to changes in the ambient temperature decreases with age. There is a reduction in the awareness of temperature variances and of thermoregulatory responses. Many older people are unable to discriminate a difference between 2.5 and 5°C (Pocock & Richards 2004). When vasoconstriction fails to raise the body temperature, heat is produced by shivering. However, this response is reduced in older people (Box 22.5).

Box 22.5

Clinical features of hypothermia

Mild hypothermia: 32°C–35°C

Cold skin, pallor

Intensive shivering; loss of shiver response at 34°C

Uncoordinated, slow gait

Confusion, disorientation

Apathy or irritability

Bradypnoea, increased heart rate and blood pressure

May not complain of being cold

Moderate hypothermia: 30°C–32°C

Loss of consciousness

Very cold skin and increased pallor

Shivering stops, muscle rigidity develops

Slowed reflexes

Hypertonic muscles

Bradycardia and hypotension

Atrial and ventricular arrhythmias

Severe hypothermia: below 30°C

Extremely cold skin, extreme pallor, cyanosed

Muscle rigidity may become flaccid below 27°C

Unresponsive

Severe respiratory depression

Atrial and ventricular arrhythmias, ventricular fibrillation and finally asystole

(Adapted from Wyatt JP, Illingworth RN, Clancy MJ et al. (2005) Oxford Handbook of Accident and Emergency Medicine. Oxford: Oxford University Press.)

Assessment

Assessment should begin with airway, breathing, circulation and disability; immediate intervention is required if the patient is not breathing or has an absent pulse, when advanced life support should be commenced (Nolan et al. 2010).

Recording of accurate vital signs is essential. The heart rate may be slow or irregular; atrial fibrillation is common due to metabolic disturbances. Similarly the respiration rate may be slower and will be deep or shallow depending on the degree of metabolic acidosis, which is common due to reduced tissue perfusion.

A 12-lead ECG should be recorded and patients with a core temperature <35°C should have continuous cardiac monitoring because of the risk of dysrhythmia or ischaemic changes. The ECG may show a bradycardia or atrial fibrillation: however, in severe hypothermia the ECG may show J waves that occur at the junction of the QRS complex and the ST segment (Haslett et al. 2002). The J wave is a specific finding in hypothermia that disappears when the temperature begins to return to normal (Manning & Stolerman 1993).

Blood screens for full blood count, clotting and U&Es should be taken to detect specific metabolic causes, such as hypoglycaemia or hypothyroidism. Arterial blood gas values are useful in determining respiratory status and acid–base balance. Both hyponatraemia and hypokalaemia are frequently found in hypothermia; however, older people who are severely dehydrated or volume-depleted may present with hypernatraemia.

Management

Re-warming may be passive external, active external or active internal (core re-warming). Patients should be re-warmed at a rate that corresponds with the rate of onset of hypothermia (Nolan et al. 2010). In reality this is difficult to gauge. Re-warming should not exceed increases of 0.3–1.2°C per hour in mild hypothermia; however, in severe cases rapid re-warming of 3°C per hour is essential (Carson 1999). Hypothermic patients should be handled carefully; vigorous procedures such as tracheal intubation can precipitate VF (Nolan et al. 2010).

In mild cases it is sufficient to remove the patient from the cold environment, and prevent further heat loss by wrapping the patient up warmly and providing hot drinks in a warm environment (passive warming). In all cases of hypothermia the removal of wet/soiled clothing should be undertaken as soon as possible, and the patient should be dried and covered with blankets. The patient's head should also be covered, as up to 40% of body heat is lost through the scalp. In moderate cases active external methods should be used which include heated pads that lie beneath the patient, or warm air-filled blankets (Holtzclaw 2004). In severe cases active external methods may include the use of warm humidified gases, and gastric, peritoneal, pleural and bladder lavage with warm fluids at 40°C (Nolan et al. 2010).

In hypothermic cardiac arrest the patient requires circulation, oxygenation and ventilation while the core body temperature is gradually raised; this is best achieved by active internal re-warming using cardiopulmonary bypass. Where this facility is unavailable, continuous veno-venous haemofiltration and warming replacement fluids can be used. Death should not be confirmed until the patient has been rewarmed, or until warming attempts have failed to raise the core temperature (Resuscitation Council (UK) 2005).

During the re-warming phase the emergency nurse must be aware that:

- the patient may become hypotensive as the vascular space expands due to vasodilatation. Patients are therefore likely to require large volumes of fluid. Older people are at greater risk of pulmonary oedema; patients therefore require careful haemodynamic monitoring via arterial blood pressure and central venous pressure and should be transferred to a critical-care environment following the ED episode
- peripheral vasodilatation may cause the core body temperature to drop

- arrhythmias may occur but tend to revert spontaneously (other than VF) and do not require treatment
- rapid metabolic changes can occur and should be monitored closely; hyperkalaemia may occur (Nolan et al. 2010).

Following an episode of hypothermia, it will be essential to prevent a recurrence. An in-depth multi-professional assessment, including occupational therapist, nutritionist and social worker, which addresses the predisposing factors that led to the admission is required. Only patients who have had a mild case of hypothermia, i.e., above 34°C, may be discharged following preventive advice. Those with lower core temperatures will require admission. Although increasing severity of hypothermia does worsen prognosis, the major determinant of outcome is the precipitating illness or injury. Reported mortality rates vary from 0–85% (Rogers 2004).

Delirium

Confusion in older people is a catchall term that covers both dementia and delirium, but may also be a consequence of depression. They are, however, quite different. Dementia is a long-term, non-reversible loss of both short- and long-term memory. Delirium (sometimes called 'acute confusional state') is a common clinical syndrome characterized by disturbed consciousness, cognitive function or perception, which has an acute onset and fluctuating course. It usually develops over 1–2 days. It is a serious condition that is associated with poor outcomes. However, it can be prevented and treated if dealt with urgently (National Institute for Health and Clinical Excellence 2010). The prevalence of older people attending the ED with delirium is 10–12% (Hustey & Meldon 2002).

The ED nurse has an important role in the detection and management of patients with acute delirium. A study by Hustey & Meldon (2002) found that the mental impairment detection rate by emergency doctors was between 28 and 35% and those discharged with delirium had very little discharge advice or follow-up arranged. Information received from the ambulance crew, relatives, home wardens and neighbours can also be crucial in determining the onset and degree of delirium in the patient. This information will be helpful in determining the patient's health and mental status prior to their arrival in the ED.

The aetiology of delirium has to be determined from the history, physical examination and special investigations. This creates a real challenge for emergency nurses, as the history and symptoms can be atypical (Table 22.3); however, linked to knowledge of the altered physiology of ageing, the underlying cause will be found through appropriate investigations.

Assessment

Delirium can result from a pathological lesion within the brain or acting on the brain from a focus elsewhere in the body such as a urine or chest infection. Rapid onset indicates an acute problem. It is therefore important to elicit the timeframe for the development of delirium; information can be gleaned unobtrusively from observing and interacting with the patient. The nurse should note the following:

- is the patient alert?
- does the patient respond appropriately to questions?
- how is the patient groomed?
- are the patient's clothes soiled?
- orientation to time, place and person and situation should also be assessed.

Physical examination will provide clues to the cause of the confusional state. Mental function may be impaired in varying degrees; impaired conscious level is a hallmark symptom of delirium. It is important to exclude hypoxia at this point. Observe the patient's work of breathing; checks for cyanosis and vital signs should include a respiratory rate and oxygen saturation monitoring. Temperature, blood pressure, pulse and respirations should be taken to assess for signs of infection, such as urinary tract and chest infections, which are common causes of delirium in older people (Box 22.6). Simple diagnostic tests such as urinalysis will help to identify potential causes. Evidence of dehydration will often be present in the confused, older person. The nurse should observe mucous membranes, skin turgidity and vital signs, as significant dehydration may be the cause of the confusional state. In addition, hypothermia, myocardial infarction, stroke and metabolic disorders such as diabetes mellitus (Table 22.3) may also present

Box 22.6

Causes of acute confusion

Infection
- Chest
- Urinary

Metabolic disturbances
- Uraemia
- Hyponatraemia
- Hypoglycaemia
- Hypo/hyperthyroidism
- Hypo/hyperthyroidism
- Hepatic failure
- Hypothermia
- B12 deficiency

Hypoxia
- Pneumonia
- Exacerbation of chronic obstructive pulmonary disease
- Pulmonary oedema
- Pulmonary embolism

Hypotension
- Acute myocardial infarction
- Hypovolaemia, e.g., gastrointestinal bleed or diarrhoea

Toxicity
- Drug, e.g., digoxin or opiates
- Drug withdrawal
- Alcohol withdrawal

Cerebral pathology
- Stroke/transient ischaemic attack
- Subarachnoid haemorrhage
- Subdural haematoma
- Tumour
- Epilepsy – postictal state
- Encephalitis

Table 22.3 Disorders presenting with atypical features in older people	
Disorder	**Atypical presentation**
Myocardial infarction or pulmonary embolism	Confusion, collapse, breathlessness and palpitations without chest pain
Bronchopneumonia	Confusion, tachypnoea, minimal chest signs, no pyrexia
Appendicitis	Confusion and constipation or diarrhoea, few localizing signs and no pyrexia
Peptic ulcer	Anaemia, haematemesis or melaena without symptoms of dyspepsia
Urinary tract infection	Confusion and urinary incontinence without pyrexia, dysuria or frequency
Dehydration	No thirst, skin changes indistinguishable from those of ageing
Diabetes mellitus	Asymptomatic until onset of complications, nephropathy, neuropathy or retinopathy
Hypothyroidism	Lethargy and general deterioration with no other characteristic signs and symptoms
Thyrotoxicosis	Apathy, weight loss and cardiac signs without anxiety, excess sweating or heat tolerance
Brain tumour	Confusion, drowsiness and focal neurological signs without headache or papilloedema

(Adapted from Edwards CRW, Bouchier IAD, Haslett C (1995) Davidson's Principles and Practice of Medicine. London: Churchill Livingstone.)

as acute confusion; it is therefore necessary to check the patient's blood sugar, record and analyse a 12-lead ECG and monitor oxygen saturation levels. Blood screening for infections or metabolic causes should also be undertaken. A chest X-ray may confirm a chest infection.

Any of these disorders may lead to delirium and all will require medical management. A history of psychiatric illness should alert the emergency nurse to the possibility of a concurrent mental illness, which could potentiate the confusion. This confusion could be a result of the illness itself or a side-effect of medication the patient is receiving.

Management

There are two key elements to the management of delirium:

- eliminate or correct the underlying aetiological disturbance
- provide symptomatic and supportive care.

Intravenous therapy may be required to correct fluid and electrolyte imbalance. Sedative drugs should not be given unless the patient is at risk of causing harm to themselves. The nurse must ensure environmental risk is assessed; the patient should be nursed in a visible cubicle. Where possible, frequent changes of nurses should be avoided to enable a rapport to be built up with the patient and to facilitate orientation. Effective communication includes ensuring that the patient's hearing aid and spectacles are present and working as necessary.

Stroke

Stroke mostly occurs in elderly people; patient outcomes after stroke are highly influenced by age, with over 80% of strokes occurring in people over 65 years of age (Chen et al. 2010). Stroke is ranked as the second most common single cause of death in the developed world after ischaemic heart disease (Di Carlo 2009). It is also the largest cause of adult disability with up to half of all patients who survive a stroke failing to regain independence and needing long-term healthcare (Sturm et al. 2004).

A stroke is defined as a focal neurological deficit due to a vascular lesion that has a rapid onset and lasts longer than 24 hours (Kumar & Clark 2002). Approximately 150 000 people in England have a stroke every year and a further 20 000 people have a transient ischaemic attack (TIA), which is defined as stroke symptoms and signs that resolve within 24 hours (NICE 2008).

Physiology

Brain tissue is particularly sensitive to the effects of oxygen deprivation, and the effect of occlusion of any part of the vasculature depends on the vessel involved, the collateral blood supply and the duration of occlusion. There are two mechanisms of cerebral injury: cerebral infarction (80%) and intracerebral haemorrhage (20%) (Wyatt et al. 2005). Cerebral infarction is most likely to occur from a thromboembolism secondary to atherosclerosis in the carotid artery and aortic arch (Pocock & Richards 2004). However, this can also be caused by an embolism from atrial fibrillation, valve disease or following a myocardial infarction. Intracerebral haemorrhage is caused by an entry of blood into the brain, which immediately stops function in the area as the neurones are disrupted (Pocock & Richards 2004). This may be caused by hypertension, bleeding disorders and intracranial tumours (Wyatt et al. 2005). Older people who have a stroke are more likely to have an other underlying pathology such as COPD, ischaemic heart disease, visual impairments and renal failure; these co-morbidities must be considered at the time of assessment.

Assessment

The correct diagnosis must be made through careful history-taking, physical examination and investigations. An acute focal stroke is characterized by a sudden appearance of a focal deficit, most commonly a hemiplegia, with or without aphasia, hemi-sensory loss or visual field defect (Haslett et al. 2002).

Classifications of a focal stroke:

- transient if the deficit disappears in 24 hours; however, 20% of these patients will have a stroke within the first month; they are most at risk within the first 72 hours (Royal College of Physicians 2004)
- completed if the deficit persists but does not worsen
- evolving if the deficit continues to worsen after 6 hours (Haslett et al. 2002).

The nursing assessment must commence with airway, breathing, circulation and disability. If the patient is unconscious, resuscitate as per guidelines, otherwise assess the airway for patency as the patient may have difficulty protecting their own airway (Haslett et al. 2002). Open the patient's airway using manual manoeuvres and inspect for foreign bodies, vomit and suction as necessary. If this is successful insert an oropharyngeal or nasopharyngeal adjunct and administer oxygen. If the patient tolerates an airway, the patient will require a definitive airway and the nurse must call for a senior clinician and anaesthetic support.

Assess breathing by observing the rate, rhythm, depth and effort of breathing and monitor oxygen saturation levels. People who have had a stroke should receive supplemental oxygen only if their oxygen saturation drops below 95%. The routine use of supplemental oxygen is not recommended in people with acute stroke who are not hypoxic (National Institute for Health and Clinical Excellence 2008). Chest auscultation may detect underlying pathology and the patient may require a chest X-ray.

To assess circulation record the patient's temperature, heart rate, blood pressure, blood sugar level and an ECG, particularly looking for atrial fibrillation. Hypertension is commonly noted following a stroke; the only indication for lowering blood pressure in the acute phase is if the patient is at risk of complications of hypertension, e.g., hypertensive encephalopathy, aortic aneurysm and renal involvement (Royal College of Physicians 2004, Peters 2009). Blood pressure should return to normal within 24–48 hours spontaneously (Haslett et al. 2002). Intravenous access should be gained and bloods taken for full blood count, U&E and a clotting screen if the stroke is suspected to be caused by a bleeding disorder. Patients should have their gag reflex assessed by a trained professional; until this is completed the patient should receive intravenous fluids. Extent of any disability is assessed by recording a full Glasgow Coma Scale.

Management

The patient and their relatives will require an explanation about what is happening and what they can expect to happen during their stay in the ED. It is important to inform family and friends that the patient may be able to understand even if they are unable to communicate verbally; this can be extremely frightening and frustrating for the patient and their family. The emergency nurse needs to be calming and reassuring whilst supporting the patient and their family.

The emergency nurse must possess knowledge of the medical treatment options to influence care and to support the patient and relatives. The nurse must monitor the patient closely to observe for signs of an evolving stroke and this must be communicated to the medical staff. The neurological assessment should include documentation of the localized signs and brain imaging should be carried out as soon as possible or within 24 hours of the onset. If the pathology or the diagnosis of a stroke is uncertain, an MRI scan should be considered (Royal College of Physicians 2004).

The fundamental approaches to acute ischaemic stroke therapy are reperfusion and neuroprotection, with early reperfusion being the most effective therapy. Early clot lysis with recombinant tissue plasminogen activator (rtPA) up to three hours after ischaemic stroke improves patients' outcomes (Green 2008, Chen et al. 2010). A haemorrhagic stroke must be excluded, and the patient must not be hypertensive. This procedure must be carried out by specialist staff.

Antithrombolytic treatment can be started when a primary haemorrhage has been excluded. Aspirin 300 mg should be given rectally if the patient is dysphagic. Anticoagulation is only necessary if the embolism is from the heart caused by atrial fibrillation; these patients will require oral anticoagulation with warfarin (Haslett et al. 2002).

The Royal College of Physicians (2004) report that surgical evacuation of a primary intracerebral haemorrhage is not supported by evidence. However, they suggest cases of supratentorial haemorrhage with mass effect should be considered for surgical intervention. They recommend that urgent neurosurgical opinion be sought.

Consideration must be given to pressure area care in the ED, a risk assessment should be performed and this communicated to the ward to ensure the patient has appropriate pressure-relieving aids. The patient's acuity will dictate where they are nursed in the ED; however, as patients can deteriorate rapidly they should be cared for where they can have appropriate monitoring, nursing observation and intervention if required. If the patient is nil by mouth in the ED the patient will require oral care and a nutritional assessment when on the ward.

Falls

Falls are the commonest cause of accidental injury in older people, the commonest cause of presentation to urgent care (Kenny et al. 2013, Banerjee et al. 2012) and the commonest cause of accidental death in the 75-plus population. About 6% of falls in those over 65 result in a fracture, including 1% being of the hip. Having fallen is the commonest reason for older people to attend the ED and for being admitted to hospital. Injury occurs more commonly in frailer persons and the nature of the fall affects injury risk and type. Falls due to syncope are particularly likely to result in injury including facial bruising. In more active and younger people, wrist fractures are more common whereas from 75 plus, hip fractures predominate (British Geriatric Society 2007). Traumatic injury caused by falls is the most common surgical reason for presentation to the ED by an older person (Aminzadeh & Dalziel 2002).

Falls can have a profound physical, psychological and social consequence on the patient and their family. Fear of falling or

a loss of confidence occurs in approximately half of all older people who fall. This is associated with functional decline, increasing depression, decreased quality of life and further falls. Sensitivity is required at this point as it can be embarrassing for an adult who has fallen. If it is not the first time they may feel depressed as they chart their own change in physical state associated with ageing. Sensitive history-taking is more likely to elicit a thorough assessment of both the incident and the patient's ability to cope at home.

Falls can result from the interaction of multiple intrinsic and extrinsic factors. Common intrinsic factors include a history of a previous fall, visual disorders, arthritis, confusion, balance impairment, muscle weakness, sensory impairment and polypharmacy (Tideiksaar 2003, Sudip et al. 2004). Extrinsic factors include environmental hazards such as poor lighting, slippery floors and lack of bathroom rails (Tideiksaar 2003). As a consequence, older people are more likely to sustain falls than younger individuals. Illnesses such as cardiac disease, diabetes and sepsis also contribute to the incidence of falls in older people, as do medications such as diuretics, hypnotics and antihypertensive drugs, due to their hypotensive side-effects (Department of Health 2001a).

The emergency nurse must again assess the older person systematically; airway, breathing, circulation, disability and exposure must be assessed. It is important to ensure that the presentation is caused by a mechanical fall and not by a collapse caused by syncope, postural hypotension, visual problems, polypharmacy or carotid sinus syndrome (British Geriatric Society 2003). Physical examination should include an assessment of standing balance and gait; vital signs should include lying and standing blood pressure, blood sugar monitoring, urinalysis and a 12-lead ECG. Any subsequent investigations may be required dependent on clinical findings.

If a mechanical fall is confirmed it is good practice to have a multi-professional approach to the patient assessment. Occupational therapy and physiotherapy should be involved in the ED to assess and promote independence. Their assessment may extend to the patient's home if required. As mentioned earlier, the patient may have a loss of confidence and this should form an important part of the discharge decision.

The emergency nurses' role is pivotal to ensuring that the ED assessment is comprehensive and includes a full social history. A study by Bentley & Meyer (2004) found that the most likely reason for re-attendance at the ED after direct discharge was a fall. In those identified cases, adequate assessment of the patients' social and functional needs was not done and the impact of illness or injury underestimated when considering their ability to cope on discharge.

A risk assessment of the older person prior to discharge should include:

- medical conditions – a thorough history and examination to exclude underlying pathology and problems associated with polypharmacy which may have caused the fall. If an underlying medical condition is the cause of the fall the patient is likely to require admission to hospital. A full social history must be documented as part of this process

- mobility – their ability to walk unaided, with a stick or Zimmer frame, but without carer support, is an important determinant of fitness for discharge. Assessment should be carried out with a multi-professional team
- social support – it is important to establish whether the older person lives alone or has formal or informal support available or whether the ED nurse needs to start coordinating these services in collaboration with primary care
- lifestyle – consider whether the injury incurred will enable the older person to function: for example, in a patient who lives alone but has a fractured wrist, an OT assessment should be considered
- external influences – those living alone in a tower block without working lifts will find it more difficult to mobilize than someone living in sheltered accommodation. The handover ambulance crew can often provide useful information about the environment to which the patient may be returning.

The greatest risk indicator for a future fall is a history of a fall; therefore the assessment and discharge process must be rigorous. There are several tools available; most agree that two predictive risk indicators are a history of falls and polypharmacy (Tideiksaar 2003, Sudip et al. 2004) (Box 22.7). However, remember that seemingly minor infections can cause a fall in older people.

Box 22.7

Falls risk assessment tool

Potential risk factors for a fall:
- History of a fall in the last year
- Four or more prescribed medications
- Diagnosis of stroke or Parkinson's disease
- Reported problems with balance, inability to rise from a chair without using arms

(After Sudip N, Parsons S, Cryer C et al. (2004) Development and preliminary examination of the predictive validity of the falls risk assessment tool for use in primary care. Journal of Public Health, 26(2), 138–143.)

Fractured neck of femur

Fractured neck of femur (hip) is the most serious consequence of falls among older people, with a post-operative mortality rate of 5–10% at 30 days and 19–30% one year after a fall (Roche et al. 2005, Braur et al. 2009, Wiles et al. 2011). Around 20% of patients require institutional care at discharge (Roberts et al. 2004). Recurrent falls are associated with increased mortality, increased rates of hospitalization, curtailment of daily activities and higher rates of institutionalization. Osteoporosis affects 1 in 3 women and 1 in 12 men over the age of 50 years and almost half of all women experience an osteoporotic hip fracture by the age of 70 years (Department of Health 2001a). Over 300 000 patients present to hospitals in the UK with fragility fractures each year, with medical and social care costs - most of which related to hip fracture care - at around £2bn. Current projections in the UK suggest that hip fracture incidence will rise from 70 000 per year in 2007 to 91 500 in 2015 and 101 000 in 2020 (British Orthopaedic Association 2007).

A full assessment of airway, breathing, circulation and disability must be made to ascertain whether the fracture is an isolated injury. This information can be assembled from the history and physical examination. Vital signs need to include a 12-lead ECG to exclude an underlying cardiac cause, which may have precipitated the fall.

Classical features associated with a fractured neck of femur are:

- history of a fall or collapse
- shortened and rotated limb
- groin pain ± radiating to the knee
- inability to mobilize – some patients can mobilize on a fractured hip; if a patient has difficulty mobilizing associated with hip pain, a fracture needs to be excluded.

Management

Emergency nurses should utilize an integrated care pathway where it exists: this will facilitate a seamless assessment, treatment and referral process for the patient. Ninety per cent of patients should be admitted in two hours and 100% within four hours (Department of Health 2006). Patients will require pressure-area care in the ED and consideration should be given to ordering a pressure-relieving mattress.

Analgesia is extremely important in the treatment of hip fractures as pain is likely to be the patient's main problem. Patients with dementia/delirium or cognitive impairment receive less analgesia than those who do not have any cognitive impairment (Heyburn et al. 2000). It is therefore imperative that the emergency nurse is sensitive to subtle non-verbal signs of pain. It must also be remembered that the patient may be pain-free at rest but will have to move for the X-ray and ultimate transfer to a ward or theatre. Analgesia should be administered in accordance with local policy within 20 minutes of arrival; however, greatest efficacy is usually achieved by intravenous opiates titrated to pain; an anti-emetic drug should also be administered.

The patient will require intravenous access via a cannula; blood should be taken for full blood count, U&E along with a group and save as the patient may require blood peri-operatively. The patient may need to be nil by mouth immediately and should receive intravenous fluids as per local policy to avoid dehydration.

A fractured neck of femur is associated with significant morbidity and mortality; it is likely to be anxiety-provoking for the patient and their family, and therefore a sensitive explanation of care is required.

Conclusion

Crouch (2012) has astutely described the elderly as 'the most complex, challenging and rewarding to care for within the emergency department'. This chapter has covered the physiological effects of ageing, and some of the common presenting complaints associated with older people.

As demographic changes in the population continue to evolve, emergency nurses are required to ensure they have the appropriate knowledge and skills to provide older people with the highest standard of care. The assessment of older people, because of their social, psychological and physical vulnerability, is a critically important dimension of care in the ED; however, older people should not be seen as a homogeneous group who are all victims or who are automatically infirm because of their age. The ED nurse has an opportunity to challenge stereotypes, provide health promotion and offer guidance on services available to older patients, as well as acting as an advocate for those unable to communicate for themselves. It presents a challenge which ED nurses should embrace as part of their role as health professionals.

References

Action on Elder Abuse, 2005. Indicators of Abuse. Action on Elder Abuse, London.

Aminzadeh, F., Dalziel, W.B., 2002. Older adults in the emergency department: a systematic review of patterns of use, adverse outcomes and effective interventions. Annals of Emergency Medicine 39, 238–247.

Association of Community Health Councils of England and Wales, 2001. Nationwide Casualty Watch. ACHEW, London.

Banerjee, J., Conroy, S., O'Leary, V., et al., 2012. Quality care for older people with urgent or emergency care needs ('Silver Book'). British Geriatrics Society, London.

Bentley, J., Meyer, J., 2004. Repeat attendance by older people at accident and emergency departments. Journal of Advanced Nursing 48 (2), 149–156.

Beynon, T., Gomes, B., Murtagh, F.E.M., et al., 2011. How common are palliative care needs among older people who die in the emergency department. Emergency Medicine Journal 28, 491–495.

Bickley, L.S., Szilagyi, P.G., 2003. Bates' Guide to Physical Examination and History Taking, eighth ed. JB Lippincott Company, Philadelphia.

Biggs, S., Manthorpe, J., Tinker, A., et al., 2009. Mistreatment of older people in the United Kingdom: Findings from the First National Prevalence Study. Journal of Elder Abuse & Neglect 21, 1–14.

Brauer, C.A., Coca-Perraillon, M., Cutler, D.M., et al., 2009. Incidence and mortality of hip fractures in the United States. Journal of the American Medical Association 302, 1573–1579.

Bridges, J., Meyer, J., Dethick, L., Griffiths, P., 2005. Older people in accident and emergency: implications for UK policy and practice. Reviews in Clinical Gerontology 14, 15–24.

British Geriatric Society, 2003. Standards of Medical Care for Older People: Expectations and Recommendations. British Geriatric Society, London.

British Geriatric Society, 2007. Falls. British Geriatric Society, London.

British Orthopaedic Association, 2007. The care of patients with fragility fracture. BOA, London.

Carson, B., 1999. Successful resuscitation of a 44 year old man with hypothermia. Journal of Emergency Nursing 25 (5), 356–360.

Cheitlin, M.D., 2003. Cardiovascular physiology: Changes with ageing. American Journal of Geriatric Cardiology 12 (1), 9–13.

Chen, R.L., Balami, J.S., Esiri, M.M., et al., 2010. Ischemic stroke in the elderly: a review of the evidence. Nature Reviews Neurology 6, 256–265.

Clark, M.J., Fitzgerald, G., 1999. Older people's use of the ambulance service, a population based analysis. Journal of Accident and Emergency Medicine 16, 108–111.

Community and District Nursing Association, 2003. Responding to Elder Abuse. CDNA, London.

Considine, J., Smith, R., Hill, K., et al., 2010. Older peoples' experience of accessing care. International Emergency Nursing 13, 61–69.

Crouch, R., 2003. Emergency care of the older person. In: Jones, G., Endacott, R., Crouch, R. (Eds.), Emergency Nursing Care, Principles and Practice. GMM, London.

Crouch, R., 2012. The older person in the emergency department: seeing beyond the frailty. International Emergency Nursing 20 (4), 191–192.

Department of Health, 2001a. National Service Framework for Older People. Department of Health, London.

Department of Health, 2001b. National Service Framework for Older People. Medicines and Older People, Implementing Medicines-related Aspects of the NSF for Older People. Department of Health, London.

Department of Health, 2006. Delivering Quality and Value. Department of Health, London.

Di Carlo, A., 2009. Human and economic burden of stroke. Age and Ageing 38, 4–5.

Duffy, R., Neville, R., Staines, H., 2002. Variance in practice emergency medical admission rates: can it be explained? British Journal of General Practice 52 (474), 14–17.

Edwards, C.R.W., Bouchier, I.A.D., Haslett, C., 1995. Davidson's Principles and Practice of Medicine. Churchill Livingstone, London.

Epstein, O., Perkins, D.G., Cookson, J., De Bono, D.P., 2003. Clinical Examination, third ed. Mosby, London.

Gray-Vickery, P., 2005. Elder abuse: are you prepared to intervene? LPN 1 (2), 38–42.

Green, A.R., 2008. Pharmacological approaches to acute ischaemic stroke: reperfusion certainly, neuroprotection possibly. British Journal of Pharmacology. 153 (Suppl 1), S325–S338.

Guly, H., 2010. History of accidental hypothermia. Resuscitation 82 (1), 122–125.

Haslett, C., Chilvers, E.R., Boon, N.A., Colledge, N.R., 2002. Davidson's Principles and Practice of Medicine, nineteenth ed. Churchill Livingstone, London.

Health Advisory Service, 2000. (1998) Not because they are old: An independent inquiry into the care of older people on acute wards in general hospitals. HAS (2000), London.

Heyburn, G., Jenkinson, M., Beringer, T., et al., 2000. The efficiency of analgesia in the elderly hip fracture patient. Age Ageing 29 (Suppl 1), 26.

Higgins, I., Slater, L., Van der Riet, P., et al., 2007. The negative attitudes of nurses towards older patients in the acute hospital setting: a qualitative descriptive study. Contemporary Nurse 26 (2), 225–238.

Holtzclaw, B., 2004. Shivering in acutely ill vulnerable populations. Advanced Practice in Acute Clinical Care 15 (2), 267–279.

Hustey, F.M., Meldon, S.W., 2002. The prevalence and documentation of impaired mental status in elderly emergency department patients. Annals of Emergency Medicine 39, 248–253.

Kaufman, D.W., Kelly, J.P., Rosenberg, L., et al., 2002. Recent patterns of medication use in the ambulatory adult population of the United States: The Slone survey. Journal of the American Medical Association 287 (3), 337–344.

Kenny, R.A. Romero-Ortuno, R., Cogan, L., 2013. Falls. Medicine in Older Adults 41 (1), 24–28.

Klein Schmidt, K.C., 1997. Elder abuse: a review. Annals of Emergency Medicine 30 (4), 463–472.

Kumar, P., Clark, M., 2002. Clinical Medicine, fifth ed. WB Saunders Co, London.

Laumann, E.O., Leitsch, S.A., Waite, L.J., 2009. Elder mistreatment in the United States: Prevalence Estimates From a Nationally Representative Study. Journal of Gerontology, Series B: Psychological Sciences and Social Sciences 63B, S248–S254.

Linton, A., Garber, M., Fagan, N.K., et al., 2007. Examination of multiple medication use among TRICARE beneficiaries aged 65 years and older. Journal of Managed Care Pharmacy 13 (2), 155–162.

Lowenstein, A., Eisikovits, Z., Band-Winterstein, T., et al., 2009. Is elder abuse and neglect a social phenomenon: Data from the First National Prevalence Survey in Israel. Journal of Elder Abuse & Neglect 21, 253–277.

Maguire, S.L., Slater, B.M.J., 2010. Physiology of ageing. Anaesthesia and Intensive Care Medicine 11 (7), 290–291.

Majeed, A., Bardsley, M., Morgan, D., et al., 2000. Cross-sectional study of primary care groups in London: association of measures of socioeconomic and health status with hospital admission rates. British Medical Journal 321 (7268), 1057–1060.

Manning, B., Stolerman, D.F., 1993. Hypothermia in the elderly. Hospital Practice 28 (5), 53–70.

Meyer, J., Bridges, J., 1998. An Action Research Study into People in the A&E Department. City University, London.

National Institute for Health and Clinical Excellence, 2008. Stroke: Diagnosis and initial management of acute stroke and transient ischaemic attack (TIA). NICE, London.

National Institute for Health and Clinical Excellence, 2010. Delirium: Diagnosis, prevention and management. NICE, London.

Naughton, C., Drennan, J., Treacy, P., et al., 2011. The role of health and non-health-related factors in repeat emergency department visits in an elderly population. Emergency Medicine Journal 27, 683–687.

Naughton, C., Drennan, J., Lyons, I., et al., 2012. Elder abuse and neglect in Ireland: results from a national prevalence study. Age and Ageing 48 (1), 98–103.

Neno, R., 2005. Hypothermia: assessment, treatment and prevention. Nursing Standard 19 (20), 47–52.

Nikki, L., Lepistö, S., Paavilainen, E., 2012. Experiences of family members of elderly patients in the emergency department: A qualitative study. International Emergency Nursing 20 (4), 193–200.

Nolan, J.P., Hazinski, M.F., Billi, J.E., et al., 2010. International Consensus on Cardiopulmonary Resuscitation and Emergency Cardiovascular Care Science with Treatment Recommendations. Part 1: Executive Summary. Resuscitation 81, 1219–1276.

Office of National Statistics, 2006. Population Trends. ONS, London.

Office of National Statistics, 2009. Population Figures. ONS, London.

Peters, M.L., 2009. The older person in the emergency department: Aging and atypical illness presentation. Journal of Emergency Nursing 36 (1), 29–34.

Phelan, A., 2012. Elder abuse in the emergency department. International Emergency Nursing 20 (4), 214–220.

Pocock, G., Richards, C.D., 2004. Human Physiology. The Basis of Medicine, second ed. Oxford University Press, Oxford.

Podnieks, E., Anetzberger, G.J., Wilson, S.J., et al., 2010. World view environment scan on elder abuse. Journal of Elder Abuse & Neglect 22, 164–179.

Purdy, S., 2010. Avoiding hospital admissions: What does the research evidence say? The King's Fund, London.

Purdy, S., Griffin, T., Salisbury, C., et al., 2011. Emergency admissions for chest pain and coronary heart disease – A cross-sectional study of general practice, population and hospital factors in England. Public Health 125, 46–54.

Resuscitation Council (UK), 2005. Resuscitation Guidelines. Resuscitation Council (UK), London.

Roberts, H.C., Pickering, R.M., Onslow, E., et al., 2004. The effectiveness of implementing a care pathway for femoral neck fracture in older people: a prospective controlled before and after study. Age and Ageing 33, 178–184.

Roche, J.J.W., Wenn, R.T., Sahota, O., et al., 2005. Effect of comorbidities and postoperative complications on mortality after hip fracture in elderly people: prospective observational cohort study. British Medical Journal 33, 1374.

Rogers, I., 2004. Hypothermia. In: Cameron, P., Jelinek, G., Kelly, A.M. (Eds.), Textbook of Adult Emergency Medicine, second ed. Churchill Livingstone, Edinburgh.

Royal College of Physicians, 2004. National Clinical Guidelines for Stroke, second ed. Royal College of Physicians, London Prepared by the Intercollegiate Stroke Working Party.

Sowney, R., 1999. Older People in Accident and Emergency, a position statement. Emergency Nurse 7 (6), 6–7.

Spilsbury, K., Meyer, J., Bridges, J., et al., 1999. The little things count. Emergency Nurse 7 (6), 24–31.

Spinewine, A., Swine, C., Dhillon, S., et al., 2005. Appropriateness of use of medications in elderly inpatients: qualitative study. British Medical Journal 331, 935–940.

Stevenson, J., 2004. When the trauma patient is elderly. Journal of Peri Anaesthesia Nursing 19 (6), 392–400.

Sturm, J.W., Donnan, G.A., Helen, M., et al., 2004. Quality of life after stroke: the North East Melbourne Stroke Incidence Study (NEMESIS). Stroke 35, 2340–2345.

Sudip, N., Parsons, S., Cryer, C., et al., 2004. Development and preliminary examination of the predictive validity of the Falls Risk Assessment Tool for use in primary care. Journal of Public Health 26 (2), 138–143.

Tideiksaar, R., 2003. Best practice approach to fall prevention in community-living elders. Topics in Geriatric Rehabilitation 19 (3), 199–205.

Wiles, M.D., Moran, C.G., Sahota, O., et al., 2011. Nottingham Hip Fracture Score as a predictor of one year mortality in patients undergoing surgical repair of fractured neck of femur. British Journal of Anaesthesia 106 (4), 501–504.

Wyatt, J.P., Illingworth, R.N., Clancy, M.J., et al., 2005. Oxford Handbook of Accident and Emergency Medicine. Oxford University Press, Oxford.

Zarowitz, B.J., 2011. Polypharmacy: When is enough, enough? Geriatric Nursing 32 (6), 447–449.

Ziminski, C.E., Phillips, L.R., Woods, D.L., 2012. Raising the index of suspicion of elder abuse: Cognitive impairment, falls, and injury patterns in the emergency department. Geriatric Nursing 33 (2), 105–112.

PART 5

Physiology for ED practice

Physiology for ED practice

23

David Corkill

CHAPTER CONTENTS

http://dx.doi.org/10.1016/B978-0-7020-4315-4.00023-1

Introduction

This chapter explores some of the physiological mechanisms that support normal body function, the failure of which may necessitate nursing intervention in the ED patient. The basic physiological concepts of homeostasis are examined and a number of homeostatic mechanisms described. The importance of temperature regulation is discussed and the homeostatic mechanisms that maintain normal levels of fluids and electrolytes, glucose, blood pressure and haemostasis are outlined. The mechanisms of oxygen and carbon dioxide transport to and from the cells are discussed. Finally, the breakdown of homeostatic mechanisms is considered in a discussion of physiological shock.

Homeostasis

A single-celled organism, such as an amoeba, requires warmth, oxygen, nutrients and fluids in order to survive and must be able to rid itself of waste products. It interacts directly with the outside world in order to achieve this (Fig. 23.1). The human body is a highly complex collection of millions of cells, very few of which are in direct contact with the outside world, and yet each individual cell has the same survival requirements as the amoeba – a constant supply of fluids, nutrients, oxygen and warmth in order to live and the ability to remove waste products. The external environment (the 'outside world') of the cells in the body is the interstitial fluid that surrounds them (see Fig. 23.2 for body fluid compartments) and this fluid must be kept supplied with all the components that the cells might need. Individual cells need to maintain a constant environment within relatively narrow limits in order to function optimally and this constant state must be maintained whatever is happening to the body as a whole. The term 'homeostasis', first used by an American physiologist, Walter

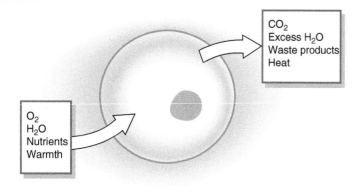

Figure 23.1 ● Cell homeostasis.

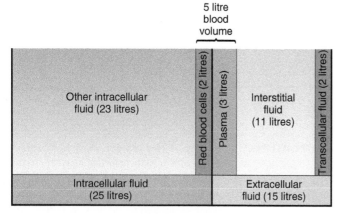

Figure 23.2 ● Body fluid compartments.

Cannon, in 1932, refers to the physiological mechanisms that maintain the body in a relatively constant state despite changes in the environment. The word comes from the Greek and means 'standing the same', something of a misnomer since physiological function is never static but constantly fluctuating. Homeostasis is essential if the metabolic activities that occur constantly in all cells are to continue.

Throughout the body there are many self-regulating homeostatic mechanisms that aim to maintain an internal 'steady state'. Most homeostatic mechanisms within the body work by 'negative feedback', where a deviation from normal will cause a response to restore the steady state – thus too little of something will cause more to be produced, too much of something will trigger mechanisms to reduce the amount. Once steady state is reached, the homeostatic mechanisms are switched off. An example of a see-saw is commonly used to illustrate this concept (Fig. 23.3). In order to function, homeostatic mechanisms require specialized receptors to detect deviations from the 'steady state'; they also require a control centre to receive and process the information and the ability to stimulate appropriate body organs and structures to redress the imbalance.

The homeostatic mechanisms involved in temperature regulation, fluid and electrolyte balance, oxygen and carbon dioxide transport and maintenance of blood glucose and blood pressure will be examined in more detail.

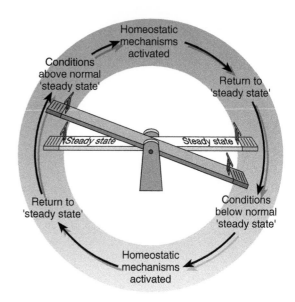

Figure 23.3 ● Homeostasis: maintaining a steady state.

Temperature control

Maintenance of a constant core body temperature, within the internal organs, is essential for optimal functioning of cellular enzymes. Humans are homeothermic and normally maintain a constant core temperature of 37 C regardless of the external temperature. The skin temperature may be several degrees different from the core temperature and varies between areas of the body, as those who always seem to have cold feet and hands will know. Body temperature is usually lower, by about 0.5°C at night and is 0.5–1°C higher in women during the second half of the menstrual cycle as a result of normal circadian rhythms. Children have higher core temperatures than neonates and the elderly, and core temperature can rise by up to 2°C during strenuous exercise. Despite all these normal variations, the body must maintain a careful balance between heat gained and heat lost. A summary of factors influencing heat gain and loss is given in Box 23.1.

Temperature homeostasis

Temperature-sensitive receptors, thermoreceptors, are found peripherally in the skin (sensitive to external temperature changes) and centrally in the hypothalamus in the brain (sensitive to changes in temperature of blood bathing them and thus to core temperature). When stimulated, the thermoreceptors initiate impulses via afferent nerves to the control centre, the temperature-regulating area in the anterior hypothalamus.

When core temperature falls below normal, the hypothalamus acts to conserve heat in the following ways:

● peripheral vasoconstriction mediated via the sympathetic nervous system closes down the surface blood vessels, ensuring that blood is kept closer to the warm core and heat loss through the skin is minimized

Box 23.1

Factors influencing heat gain and loss

Heat gain

- External temperature
- Metabolism
- Food and drink
- Shivering
- Hormones
- Behaviour (put on clothes)
- Drugs/overdose

Heat loss

- External temperature
- Evaporation
- Conduction
- Convection
- Radiation
- Body excretions
  - air
  - urine
  - faeces
- Behaviour (take off clothes)

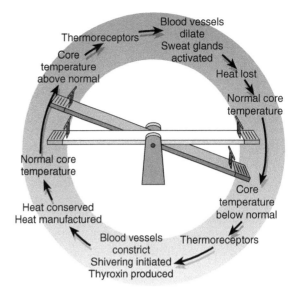

Figure 23.4 • Thermoregulation.

- shivering is initiated by the posterior hypothalamus and results in uncoordinated muscle activity that generates heat
- the thyroid gland is stimulated to produce the hormone thyroxin, which raises the basal metabolic rate of cells, thus increasing heat production
- information is relayed to the cerebral cortex and we become conscious of the cold and will take steps to warm ourselves such as putting on extra clothes, turning on the fire, exercising or having a warm drink.

A rise in core temperature above 37°C will stimulate responses aimed at losing heat:

- peripheral blood vessels are dilated under the influence of the sympathetic nervous system and heat is lost through the skin by radiation, conduction and convection
- sweat glands are stimulated, again via the sympathetic nervous system, to increase secretion, and heat is lost by evaporation. Evaporation of sweat is reduced when humidity is high and this is consequently a less effective means of reducing temperature in hot climates
- again the cerebral cortex receives information and we take steps to cool down – removing clothes, taking a cold shower, drinking iced drinks.

Once temperature returns to normal levels, the physiological mechanisms are switched off. A diagrammatic representation of thermoregulatory mechanisms is given in Fig. 23.4.

Hypothermia, a core temperature below 35°C, is dangerous and, if not treated, will result in failure of the negative-feedback mechanisms that maintain temperature homeostasis, and damage or death may ensue. The ability to shiver decreases when the core temperature falls below

34°C and consequently the core temperature will fall further. Hypothermia slows the chemical reactions of metabolism and reduces blood flow to all organs. The resultant hypoxia will cause drowsiness and loss of consciousness as a result of cerebral ischaemia. Cardiac arrhythmias can occur below 30°C and the heart will cease to beat at about 20°C.

The O_2 requirements of the tissues are substantially reduced at low temperatures, and gradual warming of the patient combined with controlled oxygen therapy may result in full recovery provided no physiological damage has occurred. The elderly and neonates are particularly prone to hypothermia because of less efficient thermoregulatory mechanisms, as are those who misuse drugs and alcohol or who live 'rough' and who are not always able to take voluntary measures to regain heat.

Pyrexia or fever occurs when body temperature rises above normal as a result of pyrogens produced by bacteria, viruses or necrotic tissue, which affect the temperature-regulating centre. Head injury and brain damage may have a similar effect. The temperature-regulating centre is 'reset' at a higher level by the pyrogens and the body will continue to produce heat to maintain the higher level until the pyrogens are removed from the body.

Hyperpyrexia, i.e., a core temperature above 40°C, is a dangerous condition. Cellular metabolism is greatly increased and the body is unable to lose the heat produced sufficiently to reduce the temperature. Cells throughout the body are destroyed by literally burning themselves out and irreversible brain damage can occur at about 42°C.

Fluid and electrolyte balance

Water is the basis of all body fluids, e.g., plasma, tissue fluids and lymph, and accounts for approximately 60% of total body weight. Body water contains many electrolytes, substances that dissolve and dissociate into ions (develop electrical charges). The main electrolytes in the body are sodium (Na⁺),

Figure 23.5 • Electrolytes in fluid compartments.

potassium (K^+), calcium (Ca^{2+}) and magnesium (Mg^{2+}), all of which are positively charged *anions*, and the negatively charged *cations* chloride (Cl^-), bicarbonate (HCO_3^-), protein (Pr^-) and phosphate (PO_4^{2-}).

Fluid is either inside the cells (intracellular) or outside the cells (extracellular). Extracellular fluid includes blood plasma, interstitial or tissue fluid that bathes the cells (see above), and small amounts of transcellular fluid, found in body cavities such as intraocular, peritoneal and pleural fluid, cerebrospinal fluid and digestive juices. Figure 23.2 shows how these fluid compartments compare.

Intracellular fluid contains more positively charged potassium and magnesium and negatively charged protein and phosphate than extracellular fluid (which contains more positively charged sodium ions and negatively charged chloride ions) (Fig. 23.5). The ions are prevented from diffusing into other compartments by the selective permeability of the cell membranes and by the presence of a pumping mechanism within cell walls which actively pumps out sodium and exchanges it for potassium. This difference between intra- and extracellular fluids is essential in nerve and muscle cells (excitable tissues), since nerves would be unable to relay messages and muscles unable to contract without it.

The interstitial fluid which bathes cells throughout the body must be maintained in a stable state as it provides the cells with nutrients and maintains the correct temperature for them to function effectively and receives their waste products. Disturbances in the electrolyte content and the concentration, osmolality and osmolarity of the extracellular fluid will affect the intracellular fluid and will impair cell and body function as a result. Normal cell function relies on fluid and electrolyte homeostasis.

Fluids normally enter the body only through the mouth. Thirst is a stimulus triggered when osmoreceptors in the hypothalamus detect a fall in the osmotic pressure of plasma passing over them. Fluid and electrolyte balance by intake alone would be inefficient, since either too much or too little may be ingested for any number of reasons. The body regulates levels of both water and electrolytes at the point of exit, mainly by the action of hormones on the distal tubules of the kidney.

Water balance is coordinated by the thirst centre in the hypothalamus, which controls the release of antidiuretic hormone (ADH). When the concentration of extracellular fluid rises as a result of a fluid intake below body requirements, osmoreceptors in the anterior hypothalamus sense the change and trigger impulses to allow the release of ADH from the posterior pituitary gland. ADH acts on the distal tubules of the kidney so that water is reabsorbed into the circulation. The

mechanism is switched off once extracellular osmolarity returns to normal. This is another good example of negative feedback.

The hormone aldosterone, secreted from the adrenal cortex, is responsible for maintaining sodium levels in the body. A fall in blood sodium levels or a rise in serum potassium is detected by specialized cells in the adrenal cortex and increases the release of aldosterone, which acts to reabsorb sodium from the renal tubules and to reduce its excretion in saliva, gastric juices and the skin. Aldosterone production is also stimulated by a fall in the extracellular fluid volume via the renin-angiotensin system activated within the kidney. Potassium balance is closely linked with sodium and when sodium is reabsorbed, potassium is generally excreted. The body is inefficient at conserving potassium and blood levels are not indicative of total body potassium as most of this electrolyte is intracellular.

Optimal kidney function is vital for maintaining fluid and electrolyte homeostasis, and damage through whatever causes (trauma, disease, old age, etc.) will reduce the efficiency of the homeostatic system.

Fluid and sodium balance are closely linked and hormonal responses are triggered by both changes in extracellular fluid volumes and changes in plasma osmolality. A diagrammatic representation is given in Fig. 23.6.

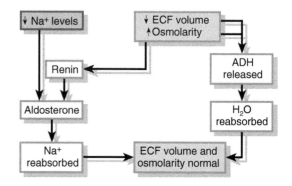

Figure 23.6 • Water and sodium balance.

Calcium levels in the body are regulated by the secretion of parathyroid hormone from the four parathyroid glands. The hormone is released directly in response to low extracellular fluid concentrations of calcium and stimulates the release of calcium from bone and its reabsorption from the kidney tubules. In addition, vitamin D is activated and increases the amount of calcium absorbed in the gut from food. When calcium is reabsorbed, phosphate is lost. High calcium levels stimulate the release of calcitonin from the thyroid gland. Calcitonin inhibits the release of calcium from bone and increases its excretion through the kidney until levels return to normal and the mechanism is switched off (Fig. 23.7).

Oxygen and carbon dioxide homeostasis

All cells require oxygen in order to function, and produce carbon dioxide as a result of metabolic activity. These gases are carried to and from the cells in the blood and their values can be measured as partial pressures (PO_2 and PCO_2). Variations

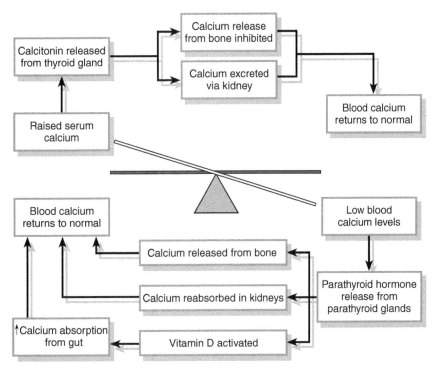

Figure 23.7 • Calcium homeostasis.

in arterial PO_2 and PCO_2 are sensed by chemoreceptors. Peripheral chemoreceptors in the aortic arch and at the bifurcation of the common carotid artery are particularly sensitive to falls in arterial oxygen levels (PaO_2), and rises in arterial carbon dioxide ($PaCO_2$). Once altered levels are sensed, the respiratory centre in the medulla of the brain is stimulated, via the vagal and glossopharyngeal nerves, and stimulates the phrenic and intercostal nerves to the diaphragm and intercostal muscles. The result is that the rate and depth of respiration are increased and more oxygen is inhaled and delivered to the blood. Once arterial blood oxygen levels are restored to normal, the mechanism is switched off.

Central chemoreceptors on the ventral surface of the medulla monitor the acidity of cerebrospinal fluid and are particularly sensitive to rises in $PaCO_2$. Inspiratory neurones in the respiratory centre of the medulla are again stimulated to increase both the rate and depth of respiration until the CO_2 is removed and blown off at the lungs and levels within the blood return to normal. The homeostatic mechanism is switched off once arterial CO_2 levels are normal again.

These homeostatic mechanisms are diagrammatically represented in Fig. 23.8.

In order to understand some common blood gas estimations, the means by which oxygen and carbon dioxide enter and are carried in the blood will be considered.

Oxygen transport

The atmosphere is composed of a mixture of gases of which the most important physiologically is oxygen. Inspired air consists of approximately 21 % oxygen, 79 % nitrogen and small amounts of carbon dioxide (0.04 %) and other gases, including

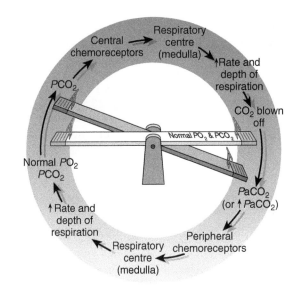

Figure 23.8 • Respiratory homeostasis.

water vapour. Each gas within this mixture exerts its own pressure, known as the *partial pressure*, and the total pressure of the mixture is equal to the sum of the pressures of all the gases within it (Dalton's law of partial pressures). Atmospheric air pressure at sea level is known to be 101.3 kPa or 760 mmHg, and since oxygen comprises 21 % of the mixture, its partial pressure, usually written as PO_2, can be calculated thus:

$$(21 / 100) \times 101.3 = 21.2 \text{ kPa}$$

or

$$(21 / 100) \times 760 = 159.0 \text{ mmHg}$$

The PN_2 and PCO_2 can be similarly calculated.

As atmospheric air passes through the respiratory tract, it becomes humidified with more water vapour, which reduces the partial pressure of the other gases as the pressure exerted by the water accounts for a larger proportion of the total pressure. The partial pressures are further modified as the gases combine with the air in the physiological 'dead space' in the respiratory tract before finally meeting and mixing with gases in the alveoli. As a result, the alveolar PO_2 is considerably less than atmospheric PO_2, and alveolar PCO_2 and water vapour pressure are measurably higher, although the total pressure remains the same as atmospheric pressure. Alveolar PO_2 is 13.3 kPa (100 mmHg) and alveolar PCO_2 is 5.3 kPa, (40 mmHg) and it is these amounts of gas that are available at the alveolar capillary membrane in the lungs where gaseous exchange takes place. Blood within the alveolar capillaries contains less oxygen and more carbon dioxide than alveolar air as a result of cellular metabolism, which removes oxygen from arterial blood and replaces it with carbon dioxide produced as a result of metabolic activity. Blood arriving at the lungs has a PO_2 of 5.3 kPa (40 mmHg) and a PCO_2 of 6.1 kPa (45 mmHg).

In the alveoli, gaseous exchange is possible because of the very thin pulmonary membrane between the alveoli and capillaries and the vast network of capillaries surrounding them. The existence of a pressure gradient, i.e., different pressures on either side of the membrane, results in movement of oxygen into the blood and carbon dioxide out of the blood and into the alveoli ready to be expired. Blood leaving the lungs for the heart contains oxygen and carbon dioxide at virtually the same partial pressures as those contained within the alveoli, so that the normal pulmonary vein and systemic arterial partial pressure of oxygen (PaO_2) is 13.3 kPa (100 mmHg) and $PaCO_2$ is 5.3 kPa (40 mmHg) (Figs 23.9 and 23.10); these quantities of gas are carried within the blood to the tissues.

At the tissues, gases diffuse in the opposite direction across pressure gradients and thin membranes. Oxygen is given up to the tissues and replaced with carbon dioxide produced by the tissues. Partial pressures of oxygen and carbon dioxide within the cells are the same as those in blood arriving at the lungs (Fig. 23.10), since the gases cannot cross the thicker membranes of blood vessels in the rest of the circulation.

Oxygen is not simply carried around the circulation dissolved in blood, as a blood volume in excess of 80 L would be required to supply the 250 mL of oxygen required every minute when the body is at rest. Oxygen carried by this means accounts for only 1 % of the total oxygen transported in the blood, but it is an important 1 % as this is the only oxygen that exerts a pressure: not only does it maintain the pressure gradients necessary for diffusion, but it is this that is recorded when arterial blood gases are measured. Normal PaO_2 and $PaCO_2$ are the same as the pressures within alveolar air. This PO_2 governs the far greater amount of oxygen that can be transported in the blood bound to haemoglobin. Normally, 99% of oxygen is carried bound to haemoglobin (Hb) and, once bound, is no longer free to exert a pressure or to be measured in blood analysis. As the O_2 in solution is used, some of the bound O_2 will be released so that the ratio of 1% in solution:99% bound to Hb is always maintained.

Haemoglobin is a conjugated protein found in red blood cells and consists of four haem groups containing iron and four polypeptide chains. Each of these haem groups can combine with one molecule of oxygen to form oxyhaemoglobin, which is bright red and gives arterial blood its distinctive colour. This process is known as oxygenation. Normal Hb is approximately 15 g/dL and each gram of Hb can carry 1.34 mL O_2, so that the total oxygen capacity of the blood, i.e., the total amount that could be carried, is 15 × 1.34 = 20.1 mL/dL. This equation is simpler if SI units are used – normal Hb is 2.2 mmol/L blood and each molecule of Hb can combine with four molecules of O_2, so the oxygen capacity is 8.8 mmol/L (1 mmol O_2 = 23.4 mL). Amounts of oxygen carried bound to Hb can thus be far in

Figure 23.10 • Oxygen and carbon dioxide exchange throughout the body.

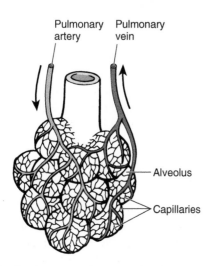

Figure 23.9 • Capillary network surrounding the alveolus.

excess of the normal requirements of the body. A simple sum will allow us to see that the body, which needs 250 mL of O_2 each minute at rest, actually has theoretically available 8.8 × 23.4 (= 197.12 mL per litre) × 5 L pumped out of the heart each minute, i.e., 986 mL per minute.

In normal physiological circumstances, not quite all the available haemoglobin binding sites become bound with oxygen but about 97–98% do; this is the 'oxygen saturation' that is recorded by pulse oximetry. There are many reasons why pulse oximetry may give misleading information, but an important physiological reason is that while Hb may be fully bound with O_2, Hb levels may be very low. In this case pulse oximetry readings will be within normal limits but the blood is unable to carry sufficient oxygen to supply the needs of the cells throughout the body; examples are severe anaemia or in hypovolaemia (see the section on shock below).

Oxygen does not bind to each haem molecule with the same ease, and a graph plotting Hb saturation against PO_2 is not linear. The rate at which they bind is dependent on the PO_2. The first haem group combines with O_2 with relative difficulty, the second and third groups combine more readily and the fourth combines with the greatest difficulty of all. It will be seen from Fig. 23.10 that at a PO_2 of 5.3 kPa, (40 mmHg) as in blood arriving at the lungs, almost 70% of the Hb sites are bound with oxygen and exposure to a PO_2 of 13.3 kPa (100 mmHg) at the alveoli will allow up to 98% of the Hb to become saturated with O_2. At the tissues, O_2 is unloaded from the haem molecules in response to the fall in PO_2, so that a tissue PO_2 of 5.3 kPa (40 mmHg) will mean that oxygen from the 70–97% range can be removed for use.

The 's' shape of the oxygen–haemoglobin dissociation curve is important physiologically for a number of reasons. Normal physiological function occurs over only a small part of this curve (Fig. 23.11) and a large reserve is available in the event of a fall in arterial PO_2, such as in lung disease, during exercise or at altitude. Even at a PO_2 of only 8 kPa (60 mmHg), 90% saturation of Hb with oxygen will be achieved in blood leaving the lungs (point I in Fig. 23.11). During strenuous exercise, it is possible to achieve a PO_2 at the tissues of as little as 2 kPa (15 mmHg) and this will allow 80% of the bound oxygen to be released (point II in Fig. 23.11), thus supplying the increased amount of oxygen required by the tissues.

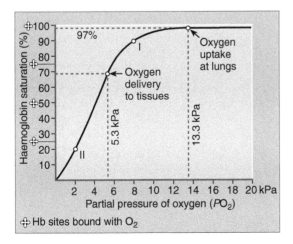

Figure 23.11 • The oxygen dissociation curve.

Several factors affect the ease with which O_2 binds with Hb and will influence the position of the oxygen–haemoglobin dissociation curve. The factors influencing 'shifts' in the curve are summarized in Fig. 23.12. The result of a shift to the left is that loading of Hb with O_2 occurs more readily, i.e., at a lower PO_2, while a shift to the right facilitates release of the O_2 at the tissues.

Figure 23.12 • Factors influencing a shift in the dissociation curve.

Carbon dioxide transport

Carbon dioxide is transported around the body in three ways:

- 7% in simple solution
- 23% bound to the globin portion of haemoglobin and influenced by PCO_2
- 70% as bicarbonate (hydrogen carbonate) ions.

Tissue cells constantly produce CO_2 and this diffuses across a pressure gradient into the capillaries supplying the tissue. Some remains dissolved in the plasma or binds to Hb but most crosses into the red blood cells (erythrocytes), where the presence of an enzyme, carbonic anhydrase, promotes the conversion of CO_2 and water within the cells to carbonic acid. The carbonic acid then dissociates into hydrogen and bicarbonate according to the equation

$$H_2O + CO_2 \leftrightarrow H_2CO_3 \leftrightarrow H^+ + HCO3^-$$

HCO_3^- is then removed to the plasma where it is transported combined with sodium found in the plasma as sodium bicarbonate $NaHCO_3$.

CO_2 carried in this way does not exert a pressure within the blood and the equation reverses readily when blood arrives at the lungs so that CO_2 is readily released to be blown off. Fig. 23.8 shows this process diagrammatically.

Oxygen therapy

The aim of oxygen therapy is to raise the PO_2 in the lungs, thus increasing the pressure gradient across the alveolar capillary membrane and allowing more oxygen to enter the blood for transport to the tissues. There are, however, potential hazards that should be considered when oxygen therapy is indicated.

Patients with long-term respiratory disease may rely on low PO_2 levels to stimulate the respiratory centre (hypoxic drive) rather than rises in PCO_2 levels. High levels of oxygen administered to these patients will cause respiratory depression and possibly apnoea.

High concentrations of O_2 over prolonged periods may cause lung damage with oedema. Concentrations of administered O_2 should be kept as low as possible whilst maintaining adequate blood gas levels.

Compressed O_2 is very drying and should be humidified prior to administration. Patients receiving O_2 will require regular mouth rinses.

In neonates, particularly premature infants, blindness caused by retrolental fibroplasia, i.e., fibrosis behind the lens of the eye, may develop as a result of high-level O_2 administration.

More recently there has been recognition of the harmful effects of hyperoxaemia. It is recommended that critically ill patients, except neonates, be resuscitated in 100% oxygen. After the patient has been successfully resuscitated, the oxygen concentration is rapidly titrated down to ensure an oxygen saturation of 94–98%.

Variations at altitude and depth

As altitude increases, for example, during flight or when ascending mountains, barometric pressure falls. At 10 000 ft (300 m) total atmospheric pressure is 70 kPa or 523 mmHg and the PO_2 will be 21% of this, i.e., 15 kPa. Alveolar PO_2 at this height will be reduced to approximately 9 kPa, causing a marked reduction in the pressure gradient across the alveolar capillary membrane. Hypoxic hypoxia (a deficiency of O_2 at the tissues caused by low PaO_2 levels) may become apparent in anyone above 10 000 ft unless supplementary oxygen is administered. Normal blood oxygen saturation of 98% at sea level will be reduced to 87% at 10 000 ft and to only 60% at 20 000 ft. In pressurized aircraft cabins, pressure is usually maintained at about 8000 ft and the fit adult can readily adjust to cope with the resultant physiological alterations.

The symptoms of hypoxia include increases in heart and respiratory rate, headache, fatigue, nausea and dizziness. Perhaps the most threatening factor is that the onset is insidious and may occur in the carer as well as the patient. Prevention of hypoxia should always be the primary concern.

Pressures within body cavities alter with changes in barometric pressure. At altitude, gases within the cavities expand and then contract again during descent. These effects are particularly noticeable in the smaller body cavities, such as the middle ear and sinuses. Normally expanding and contracting gases will pass through the Eustachian tubes or the sinus cavities so that the pressure changes are equalized. In individuals with allergies, a cold or sinus infection, this movement of gases is limited or obstructed and painful otitis media or sinusitis may result. Those patients in whom respiration is compromised require careful monitoring and any pneumothorax must be treated prior to air transport as it will be likely to collapse further at altitude. Endotracheal tube balloons, intravenous fluid bags, anti-shock trousers and pneumatic splints are also subject to pressure changes and need close observation to ensure accurate functioning.

Gas pressures increase below sea level and at as little as 10 m deep in sea water (10.4 m in fresh water) atmospheric pressure is doubled (i.e., 202.6 kPa) and consequently all the partial pressures of the constituent gases are doubled. Divers and underwater tunnel workers breathe air at high pressure to equalize the pressures on the chest wall and abdomen. Nitrogen dissolves in plasma and interstitial fluid at these pressures but as long as ascent to the surface is slow and controlled, the dissolved N_2 will diffuse at the lungs and be breathed off. If ascent is too rapid, however, the N_2 forms bubbles in the tissues and decompression sickness results. With the current popularity of scuba diving, it is important to be aware of the symptoms of this sickness (joint pain, especially in the limbs, dizziness and fatigue, shortness of breath) as patients may present in departments a day or more after their dive and far from the coast.

Blood glucose homeostasis

Cells need a constant supply of nutrients from which to extract energy for cell work and glucose plays an important role in this as it is a major substrate for the manufacture of adenosine triphosphate (ATP) within the cells. This is particularly true in the brain, where 90% of the cellular energy required for metabolism is derived from glucose. Glucose is obtained from food and food substrates and the body has efficient glucose storage mechanisms for use in times of plentiful supply (for example, following a meal) and equally efficient means of releasing the stores during fasting states. Two hormones – insulin and glucagon – are responsible for maintaining blood glucose within relatively narrow limits so that cells throughout the body receive a constant and adequate supply (Fig. 23.13).

Following a meal, glucose crosses from the gut into the bloodstream and the high levels are detected in the pancreas where the specialized beta cells in the islets of Langerhans are stimulated to secrete insulin. Insulin has a number of ways of reducing blood sugar (by negative feedback):

- encourages the entry of glucose into cells throughout the body, especially the cells of skeletal muscle, to be used to manufacture ATP
- turns glucose into the storage form glycogen (this process is known as glycogenesis) for storage in cells and in the liver
- slows down the processes which turn fats and proteins into glucose.

If blood sugar is low, the alpha cells of the islets of Langerhans are stimulated and secrete the hormone glucagon. This leads to a number of physiological alterations aimed at raising the blood glucose levels:

- acts on liver cells to convert stored glycogen back to glucose (glycogenolysis) and release it back into the blood
- encourages the liver to manufacture glucose from lactic acid and from some amino acids (gluconeogenesis) and release it into the blood
- when blood levels have returned to normal, the mechanism is switched off.

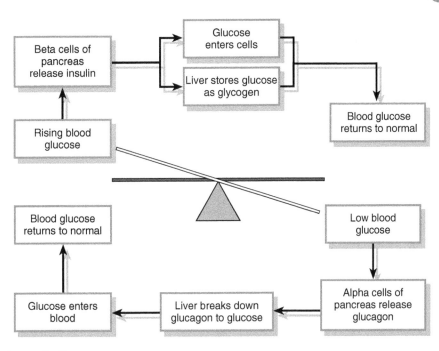

Figure 23.13 • Glucose homeostasis.

Blood pressure homeostasis – a more complex mechanism

The maintenance of blood pressure is essential to life and the body initiates a number of mechanisms to restore pressure to normal resting state. A fall in blood pressure is detected by baroreceptors (pressure receptors) in the aortic arch and carotid arteries and information is relayed to the cardiovascular control centre in the medulla. The sympathetic nervous system is stimulated here and acts to bring about peripheral vasoconstriction so that blood pressure is increased in vessels supplying the vital organs.

The fall in blood pressure is also detected in the kidney where the juxtaglomerular cells release the enzyme renin. Renin converts a plasma protein, angiotensinogen, into angiotensin I and this, in turn, is converted into angiotensin II when it meets angiotensin-converting enzyme (ACE) in the blood vessels. Angiotensin II stimulates the release from the adrenal glands of aldosterone, which increases the amount of sodium and water reabsorbed into the blood as it passes through the kidneys. Angiotensin II also stimulates the release of adrenaline from the adrenal glands and this enhances and maintains the vasoconstrictor effect of sympathetic nervous stimulation described above. Two distinct negative-feedback mechanisms – vasoconstriction and fluid retention – can be seen acting together to increase venous return to the heart and maintain normal blood pressure.

A number of homeostatic mechanisms using negative feedback to maintain a relatively constant internal environment within which cells can function optimally have been examined. There are examples of physiological positive-feedback mechanisms, where too much produces more and too little produces even less, in the body and two of these will now be explored. In the first, the positive-feedback loop is broken once the desired effect has been achieved. In the second, the desired effect is unachievable and the positive feedback continues until the patient's death unless appropriate interventions are made to break the loop.

Haemostasis – an example of positive feedback with a cut-off mechanism

Haemostasis, the arrest of bleeding, is a homeostatic process designed to maintain the body's blood volume. Haemostasis takes place only where blood vessels are damaged as it is essential that blood in the rest of the circulation remains fluid. Normally the haemostatic process will control bleeding in all but large arteries and veins; intervention will be needed if bleeding is to be arrested in these large vessels.

The process of haemostasis can be divided into stages, although physiologically it occurs as a continuous process:

1. *Myogenic reflex* – damaged vessels will normally dilate immediately after injury under the influence of histamine released by mast cells in response to the trauma. Within seconds the vessels constrict and the cut ends retract as platelets within the vessels begin to clump together and release powerful vasoconstrictors, serotonin (also called 5-hydroxytryptamine or 5HT) and thromboxane A. This so-called 'myogenic reflex' occurs even in large vessels and lasts for approximately 20 minutes, enough time for stages two and three to commence.

2. *Platelet plug formation* – when blood vessels are cut, filaments of collagen and elastin are exposed and attract passing platelets which adhere to them. This adherence

causes the release of adenosine diphosphate (ADP) from the platelets, red blood cells and vessel walls. ADP triggers a change in the shape of the platelets which encourages them to clump together. Other substances, including serotonin, also encourage platelet clumping until a plug of platelets is formed which is large enough to close the wounded vessel. A platelet plug is formed within a few seconds of injury and is sufficiently strong to stop bleeding in smaller vessels. The plug must then be stabilized by fibrin fibres or it will break down after about 20 minutes and bleeding will start again.

3. *Fibrin clot* – fibrin is an insoluble protein that is laid down as a mesh of fine threads which adhere to one another and to blood cells and platelets. They become entangled in the platelet plug, attract more cells to plug the damaged area and gradually make the clot firmer and more stable. Fibrin is formed by a complex process initiated when tissues are damaged. The complexity of the process is important since clotting within undamaged vessels would be highly undesirable. The early stages of fibrin formation also trigger the complicated clotting cascade involving 13 different factors, mostly blood constituents, which ultimately results in a blood clot. Blood is prevented from clotting, or the process is prolonged, if any of the factors are absent (as in haemophilia) or by the use of anticoagulants (such as heparin or aspirin), which prevent their production. The positive feedback of this clotting mechanism stops once the cascade is complete.

4. *Fibrinolysis* – during this stage fibrin is broken down and removed by phagocytes. The enzyme plasmin, which is responsible for this process, may be activated by streptokinase and other fibrinolytic agents.

Shock – where homeostasis fails and uncontrolled positive feedback ensues

Shock is a complex clinical syndrome characterized by a lack of adequate tissue and organ perfusion to such an extent that the oxygen and nutritional needs of the cells cannot be met. Cells and organs throughout the body are unable to function adequately and will fail and die unless both the cause and the symptoms of shock are treated.

Shock is commonly classified according to its pathophysiological cause, but any condition, physical or psychological, which reduces the blood supply to the tissues, is a potential cause of shock.

Classification of shock

There are three distinct mechanisms that may lead to hypoperfusion of the tissues:

* hypovolaemia – there is insufficient blood to carry the oxygen and nutrients needed
* pump failure (cardiogenic) – the heart is unable to pump the blood around the body effectively

* distribution problems – blood volume and cardiac output are essentially adequate but widespread vasoconstriction leads to pooling of blood and reduces venous return to the heart. Neurogenic, septic and anaphylactic shock all fall into this category.

Hypovolaemic shock

The causes of hypovolaemia are:

* loss of blood through haemorrhage
* loss of plasma as in severe burns and peritonitis
* loss of body fluids through diarrhoea, vomiting or sweating
* failure to drink sufficient fluids.

Fifteen per cent or more of total blood volume may be lost before signs of hypovolaemic shock are noted in an adult.

Cardiogenic shock ('pump failure')

Events which reduce the ability of the heart to pump efficiently result in cardiogenic shock. These include:

* myocardial infarction
* cardiac arrhythmias
* cardiac tamponade
* disorders in the lungs, e.g., tension pneumothorax or pulmonary embolus.

Neurogenic shock

In neurogenic shock, sympathetic and parasympathetic nervous control is lost. The venous 'tone' essential to the maintenance of normal blood pressure and venous return is lost and blood pools in the venules and capillaries. Common causes include:

* severe head injury
* spinal injury
* drug reaction and anaesthetics
* neurological illness, e.g., Guillain-Barreé syndrome.

Intense pain and severe fright may also result in neurogenic shock.

Septic shock

Damage is caused by overwhelming bacterial infection, usually by Gram-negative bacilli such as *Escherichia coli*, *Pseudomonas* and *Klebsiella*. The bacteria cause damage by releasing endotoxins that cause vasodilatation and increased capillary permeability. Fluid leaks out of the capillaries, causing hypotension and ultimately hypovolaemia. Septic shock often has an insidious rather than a sudden onset and is sometimes referred to as 'hot shock' because sufferers are pyrexial as a result of the precipitating infection. 'Toxic shock' is a type of septic shock and is generally associated with menstruation and prolonged use of tampons. The causative organism in this instance is *Staphylococcus aureus*.

Anaphylactic shock

Anaphylaxis occurs as the result of an antigen–antibody response in sensitive individuals. Antigens combine with immunoglobulin E (IgE) antibodies on the surface of mast cells throughout the body and these cells degranulate and release histamine and prostaglandins into the circulation. Under their influence, capillaries become more permeable, and widespread oedema results, including laryngeal oedema, which can rapidly cause death if not treated with adrenaline (epinephrine). Antigens may be introduced by the following routes:

- by injection, e.g., animal or insect bites and stings, drug therapy and mismatched blood transfusion
- by ingestion – food (shellfish, cheese, egg, nuts are some common causes of allergic reaction) or orally administered drugs
- by inhalation, e.g., dust and chemicals.

It will be noted that, whatever the initial cause of shock, venous return will be increasingly reduced and the cardiac output will continue to fall – a clear example of positive feedback at work.

Physiology of shock

Whatever the initial cause of shock, the pathophysiological response is the same (Fig. 23.14). Cells throughout the body are deprived of oxygen, resulting in cell membrane damage.

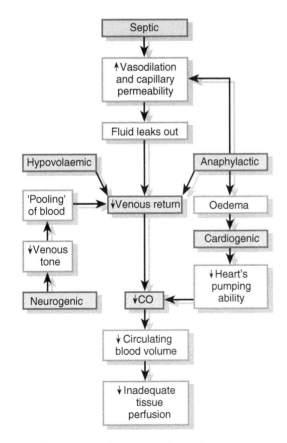

Figure 23.14 • The causative mechanisms of shock.

Histamines and kinins are released in response to the damage and cause vasodilation and increased capillary permeability. White blood cells leak out of the capillaries and proteins pass into the extracellular fluid. Oedema occurs within the cells and the interstitial fluid volume increases as the fluid compartments break down. The result is a decrease in the circulating blood volume and a consequent reduction in venous return, in the amount of blood available for oxygenation and in cardiac output. Metabolism continues within the cells despite the lack of oxygen, and lactic acid, produced as a result of cellular metabolism, builds up causing metabolic acidosis.

Compensatory mechanisms – the early stage

In the initial stages of shock, the body's homeostatic mechanisms are triggered and attempt to return the body to 'steady state'.

Sympathetic nerves are stimulated by the fall in arterial blood pressure and a fall in PO_2. They act to preserve blood supply to the vital organs, i.e., the heart and the brain, by vasoconstriction and by increasing heart rate, although stroke volume, the volume pumped by each contraction, diminishes. This may be felt as a rapid, weak pulse.

The skin becomes cold as blood is diverted to the vital organs and patients may become confused and disoriented as blood supply to the brain is reduced.

The fall in PO_2 levels triggers deep and rapid breathing ('air hunger') but this will only rectify the situation if sufficient blood is passing through the system for adequate oxygenation to occur.

The fall in PO_2 at the tissues means that more O_2 can be released from Hb, but demand will exceed supply unless intervention occurs. Administered O_2 will only partially rectify the situation.

In the early stages of shock, interstitial fluid is returned to the circulation through the capillary walls in an attempt to raise the circulating blood volume, but once cell damage begins this mechanism also fails. Sodium and water are preserved in the body by the production of ADH and aldosterone and this further helps to raise blood volume. Urine output falls as a result.

Progressive shock – when compensatory mechanisms are not enough

Without intervention, these compensatory mechanisms ultimately fail and cells throughout the body begin to malfunction. Some of the resulting effects are:

- metabolic acidosis causes hyperventilation and this causes respiratory acidosis in addition as too much CO_2 is blown off
- PCO_2 falls, causing a reduction in blood flow to the brain and a reduced level of consciousness
- adrenaline (epinephrine) and noradrenaline (norepinephrine) are produced in response to sympathetic nervous stimulation and cause vasoconstriction, which causes further hypoxia by decreasing blood flow through the lungs. Surfactant production in the lungs starts to fail and the lungs begin to collapse, making breathing more difficult. Fluid leaks from the pulmonary capillaries and pulmonary oedema results

- reduced blood volume and flow result in poor renal perfusion with resultant oliguria
- in the liver, cells can eventually no longer conjugate bilirubin; it is returned to the circulation and jaundice becomes apparent
- poor blood flow through the gut leads to breakdown of the gut lumen. Gut contents cross into the circulation and blood passes into the gut – haematemesis and melaena are indications that this is happening
- disseminated intravascular coagulation occurs when the clotting system is activated by enzymes released from the breakdown of cells and this further reduces blood flow
- the heart's pumping ability is so reduced that it is unable to supply even the needs of the cardiac muscle and it becomes weaker and weaker.

Irreversible shock – the final stage

The vicious circle described above, with its many positive-feedback mechanisms, is illustrated in Fig. 23.15. Early intervention may mean that homeostasis can be restored but once cell breakdown and acidosis reach a critical level, the damage is irreversible and death will ensue despite all intervention.

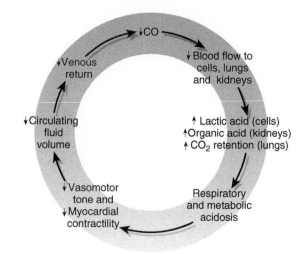

Figure 23.15 • The vicious circle of irreversible shock.

Conclusion

A basic understanding of physiological mechanisms employed to maintain homeostasis is vital if the ED nurse is competently to manage the complex assaults on normal body systems that are regularly witnessed in patients attending ED.

Further Reading

Godfrey, H., 2004. Understanding the Human Body: Biological Perspectives for Healthcare. Churchill Livingstone, Edinburgh.

Montague, S.E., Watson, R., Herbert, R.A., 2005. Physiology for Nursing Practice, third ed. Baillière Tindall, London.

Silverthorn, D.U., 2009. Human Physiology: An Integrated Approach, fourth ed. Prentice Hall, New Jersey.

Sole, M.L., Goldenberg-Klein, D., Moseley, M.J., 2009. Introduction to Critical Care Nursing, fifth ed. WB Saunders, Philadelphia.

Thibodeau, G.A., Paton, K.T., 2009. The Human Body in Health and Disease, fifth ed. Elsevier Mosby, Missouri.

Urden, L.D., Stacey, K.M., Lough, M.E., 2009. Critical Care Nursing: Diagnosis and Management, sixth ed. Elsevier Mosby, Missouri.

Wingerd, B., 2013. The Human Body: Concepts of Anatomy and Physiology, third ed. Lippincott Wilkins & Williams, Philadelphia.

Wound care

Jo-Anne Timms and Kate Gilmour

24

CHAPTER CONTENTS

http://dx.doi.org/10.1016/B978-0-7020-4315-4.00024-3

Introduction

Wound management forms a large percentage of the Emergency Department (ED) nurse's workload, with some 8.5% of the almost 12 million patients attending EDs in the UK in 2008/09 given a primary diagnosis of laceration (>600 000) and/or contusions or abrasions (>400 000) (NHS Information Centre for Health and Social Care 2011).

With changes in working patterns, the ED nurse may be the only health professional involved in a patient's care. It is important that traumatic wound care in the ED is seen as more than the best way to achieve technical closure. Wound care is about an extensive knowledge of skin anatomy, the physiological processes of healing, the causes and impact of wound infection and empowerment of patients to manage their own wounds. This chapter aims to provide the knowledge base needed for safe and effective wound management in the acute setting.

Anatomy of the skin

The skin is the largest external organ, and in adults weighs between 2.7 and 3.6 kg. It covers the whole of the body and its thickness varies around the body, with areas of greatest friction, such as the soles of the feet, being thickest and areas of low friction, like eyelids, being the thinnest (Tortora & Grabowski 2003). It also receives one-third of the body's circulating blood volume – an oversupply compared to its metabolic needs (Baronski & Ayello 2008). The skin has five primary functions (Box 24.1):

- protection
- sensation
- thermoregulation
- vitamin D synthesis
- excretion and reserve.

The skin is made up of two main parts, the epidermis and the dermis, which cover the subcutaneous fat layer and deep structures (Fig. 24.1) (Seidel et al. 2006).

Epidermis

This is subdivided into five distinct layers. Working from the surface, they are listed below.

Stratum corneum

This outer layer consists of keratinized cells that assist with resisting thermal, chemical and mechanical stress and restricts water loss, making the skin susceptible to maceration if constantly exposed to water. These cells shed continuously at a rate of 1 500 000 per hour. The primary function of this layer is to act as a barrier (Seidel et al. 2006).

Stratum lucidum

This layer of dead cells is found in areas needing extra protection, such as the soles of the feet and the palms of the hands (Carville 2007).

Box 24.1

Functions of the skin

Protection
- Bacteria and viruses
- Heat and cold
- Dehydration
- Some chemical substances
- Mechanical damage

Sensation
- Largest sensory organ
- Contains nerve endings – most concentrated in fingertips and lips
- Sensitive to touch, pain, heat, cold, vibration and pressure
- Skin hairs are also sensitive to touch, reducing risk of injury to the skin

Thermoregulation
The skin is responsible for maintaining the body's core temperature. It is controlled by the hypothalamus. The skin stabilizes heat generated by metabolism. This is done by heat conduction, convection and radiation from the skin surface. Heat loss is also influenced by vasodilation and constriction, varying the amount of blood flowing beneath the skin surface. This mechanism also prevents excessive heat loss in cold weather. Sweat production and evaporation have a cooling effect. The body is insulated from the environment by a layer of subcutaneous fatty adipose tissue

Vitamin D synthesis
Vitamin D is synthesized from ultraviolet light falling on the skin. Vitamin D is necessary for calcium absorption. Vitamin D can also be synthesized from dietary intake

Excretion and reserve
Some gaseous exchange takes place through skin. Sodium and urea are excreted via sweat. The skin provides a water reserve which is drawn into the circulating blood volume in cases of sudden fluid loss, such as haemorrhage or chronic dehydration. The fat layer can also be converted into energy

Stratum granulosum

This middle layer contains granular cells containing cytoplasmic granules which are the precursor to keratin. As they migrate from the lower level to this level the cells flatten out and the nuclei die (Carville 2007).

Stratum spinosum

These form a layer of living cells that act as intracellular bridges preventing cell separation. Several different cell types exist in this layer including Langerhans' cells which are dendritic cells involved with antigen processes (Murphy et al. 2005).

Stratum basale (or stratum germinativum)

This layer lies next to the dermis. These cells are responsible for germination of new epithelial cells and are reliant on the dermis for nutrients from the blood supply. Melanocytes are found in this layer and produce melanin which is mainly responsible for skin tones (Murphy et al. 2005).

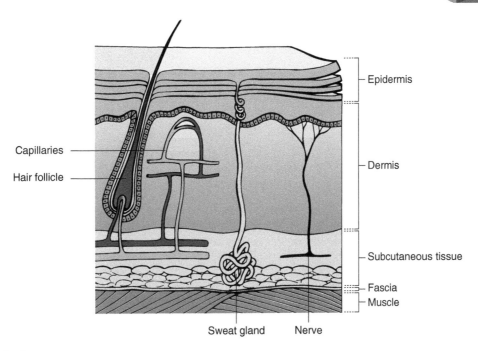

Figure 24.1 • Skin structure.

Dermis

The dermis contains blood vessels, nerves, sebaceous glands and hair follicles and is made up primarily of collagen and elastin. This gives strength and elasticity to the skin (Copstead & Banasik 2005). Sensory nerves located in the dermis provide sensations of touch, temperature and pain. Cells in the dermis include:

- fibroblasts – used in wound healing; they lie between bundles of collagen and act to synthesize elastin and collagen
- tissue macrophages – these phagocytic cells engulf debris and matter during healing
- tissue mast cells – found near hair follicles and blood vessels, these cells produce histamine and heparin.

Between the epidermis and dermis is the basement layer that is an acellular, non-vascular and non-innervated membrane separating the two layers of skin. This membrane provides support to the skin and plays a role in the movement of nutrients between layers (Carville 2007).

The hypodermis is found under the dermis and is composed of adipose tissue, connective tissue and blood vessels. It provides insulation, shock absorption and is responsible for temperature regulation and storage of lipids (Seidel et al. 2006).

Wound healing

Terminology and the number of stages in the healing process vary between texts, however, the general consensus is that four phases of healing occur. They usually follow a set pattern (Clark 2002), but can occur concurrently, and different parts of the same wound can heal at different rates

Table 24.1 Phases of wound healing

Duration	Phase	Signs
First hour	Haemostasis	Initial vasoconstriction Coagulation of wound
10 minutes–5 days	Inflammatory	Vasodilation, pain, heat, swelling
3 days–1 month	Proliferation	Wound size diminishing
		Surrounding skin of normal colour
		Less pain
3 weeks–1 year	Maturation	Wound healed Scarring fades

(Table 24.1). Wound healing can be complex and is affected by the mechanism of injury and the general health of the patient (Gantweker & Hom 2012).

The wound healing process occurs from the time of injury and may last days to years. The phases can be divided into haemostasis, inflammatory stage, the proliferative or maturation stage and the remodeling stage.

Haemostasis

The body's initial response to a cut in the skin is bleeding. This extravasation initiates platelet activity and coagulation of blood. It also results in vasoconstriction and release of histamines and ATP, which also attract leucocytes. Platelets begin to aggregate and the coagulation cascade results in the development of a fibrin mesh and clot, or beginnings of a scab, which temporarily seals the wound. Once the clot is formed, fibrinolysis commences as part of the body's defence mechanism. This ensures the clot does not extend and allows better migration of cells into the wound bed (Baranoski & Ayello 2008).

Inflammatory stage

As well as a haemostatic response, the body also responds to tissue trauma by releasing prostaglandins and activated proteins which initiate vasodilation in the area. This has two main functions:

- it increases blood supply to the area
- it increases capillary permeability.

This is to enable plasma to leak into tissues around the area of injury. This creates wound exudate. Neutrophils are the first leucocytes that usually arrive within 6–12 hours at the injury site (Lewis et al. 2011a), leak into the area of the wound and offer initial protection from infection by engulfing and digesting bacteria. Neutrophils have a short life span, and so are replaced by monocytes that are capable of phagocytosis. These promote new tissue formation and angiogenesis, and continue to engulf and destroy bacteria and debris from the wound, including old neutrophils (Baranoski & Ayello, 2008).

The signs of an inflammatory response are often confused with infection, so it is important to establish a clear history of the duration since injury. Inflammatory responses usually occur before infection has had time to develop. The signs of the inflammatory response include:

- redness – because of local vasodilatation
- heat – because of increased blood supply and metabolic activity
- oedema – because increased capillary permeability allows fluid to leak into the extracellular space
- pain – due to pressure of fluid in tissues and chemical irritation from enzymes such as prostaglandin.

This inflammation is vital to the natural healing. If it is suppressed by drugs or illness, healing will be delayed. Macrophages are essential for transition into the proliferation stage of healing, as they begin to produce transforming growth factor (TGF), which promotes angiogenesis and the formation of new tissues. Macrophages also produce fibroblast growth factor (FGF), which stimulates fibroblast production (Bale & Jones 2006).

Proliferation stage

This starts 3–5 days post-injury and can last up to three weeks (Lewis et al. 2011b). As its name suggests, this part of the healing process is about growth and reproduction of tissue to replace that lost in injury. By day five, the wound surface will only be 7% of its pre-injury tensile strength (Waller & Tan 2009). In order to produce new tissue, the wound needs a good oxygen supply and essential nutrients such as vitamin C, protein and zinc (Kumar et al. 2005, Bishop

2008). As angiogenesis occurs in response to wound hypoxia and TGF, new capillary loops develop and the wound is oxygenated. Three distinct processes occur during the proliferation phase.

Granulation

This is the formation of new tissue up from the base and in from the sides of a wound. It is dependent on the division of endothelial cells forming new capillary loops, until eventually they meet up with existing undamaged blood vessels. At the same time, fibroblasts begin to produce a network of collagen and ground substance that fills tissue spaces and begins to bind fibres together. Collagen synthesis depends on adequate nutrients, i.e., vitamin C, copper and iron (Kumar et al. 2005). These can usually be obtained from a healthy diet. Collagen forms in a haphazard and jelly-like structure, and with adequate vitamin C matures into a strong cross-linked structure which gives the tissue its tensile strength.

Contraction

This occurs at the same time as epithelialization. In wounds where tissue loss has occurred, once the wound bed has filled with healthy granulation tissue, myofibroblasts develop which contract and pull the wound edges together, therefore decreasing the overall size of the wound. Keratinocytes are responsible for the re-epithelialization from the wound edges (Naude 2010).

Epithelialization

This is the resurfacing of the wound by regeneration of epithelial cells. This will only occur where basal cells are in contact with the dermal layer, and therefore in deep wounds regeneration will only occur around wound margins until granulation has taken place. In wounds of varying depth, small islands of epithelialization will occur in superficial parts of the wound. This gradually migrates across wound surfaces until epithelialization is complete. The attachment of this layer to dermal connective tissue is fragile and easily displaced. Regeneration therefore continues until the epidermis has regained its usual thickness. Epithelial regeneration requires a warm, moist environment. If a wound surface has dry scabs or necrotic areas, these will form a barrier to migration of new cells. Cells eventually burrow under scabs.

As the wound cavity is filled with granulation tissue and the surface is regenerated with epithelial cells, the proliferation stops. If this does not happen, e.g., if overgranulation occurs due to continued hypoxic stimulation, perhaps as a result of local ischaemia, then excessive scar tissue is formed (Kumar et al. 2005).

Maturation or remodeling stage

This begins around three weeks after injury, and is a process of returning the area to its usual functional structure. The process is twofold.

Firstly, collagen is remodelled, sometimes over a period of years. The aim of this is to gradually replace newly formed type III collagen, laid down in the proliferation phase, with stronger, more organized collagen fibres. The amount of collagen does not change; its bundles become thicker and shorter and hold the wound together more tightly. Although the skin and wound scar become stronger, the area only usually regains about 80 % of the pre-injury tensile strength (Kumar et al. 2005). This takes a long time; at thee months post-injury 50 % of tensile strength is considered good healing (Baranoski & Ayello 2008).

The second part of the process is the rationalization of blood vessels bringing extra nutrients to the area. This process occurs gradually, and its progression can be monitored by the gradual fading of the scar. It will become paler and flatter as blood vessels diminish. Once maturation is achieved the scar will appear white; it is avascular, has no sebaceous glands and no hairs (Baranoski & Ayello 2008).

Scarring

Dermal damage results in an abnormal formation of connective tissue. This is permanent and manifests as a scar on the skin surface. Scarring follows three phases, although the time span increases with age, skin pigmentation and as a result of poor general health (Table 24.2). Certain areas of the body are notorious for poor scarring – the shoulder, knee, and sternal areas, which are areas under a lot of tension and motion (Bayat et al. 2003, Capellan & Hollander 2003).

Keloid scarring is usually a genetic phenomenon where collagen type I is produced in a tumor-like fashion with uncontrolled growth of scar tissue (Widgerow 2011). Keloid scarring results from the formation of large amounts of scar tissue in the proliferation stage of healing. It results from an increase in collagen synthesis and lysis to an extent where tissue formation exceeds cell breakdown (Bryant & Nix 2006). Keloid scarring is also considered to be related to the melanocyte-stimulating hormone as it is much more common in people with heavily pigmented skin, predominantly those aged 10–30 years (Bayat et al. 2003, Mustoe 2004). Tissue growth is persistent, with scarring often being much larger than the original wound. Early effective wound management can reduce the risk of keloid scarring.

Hypertrophic scarring forms in a similar fashion to tissue growth, but follows the line of incision. This type of scarring is more common in the young and in fair-skinned people and typically occurs after burn injury on the trunk and extremities. In these scars, there is an imbalance in collagen synthesis versus collagen degradation. The resulting wounds are red and raised and can be itchy. In the majority of cases, this is temporary and resolves without treatment although it may take a year or more.

Tattoo scarring results from gravel or foreign bodies being left in a wound. It forms unsightly purple or blue blotches in the scar and is difficult to remedy after initial wound healing. Generally, scars that lie parallel to the body's natural tension lines have a better cosmetic prognosis.

Factors affecting wound healing

Although patients with sudden traumatic wounds do not have the same physiological and educational preparation as patients undergoing surgery, many of the influences on wound healing can be optimized by effective education and empowerment during their initial visit for wound management. Clinical factors affecting healing potential can also be identified at this early stage, and the patient's care can be designed to accommodate them. The main influences on wound healing are listed in Box 24.2.

Nutrition

Nutrition deserves more elaborate exploration, as it is fundamental to adequate healing and is often overlooked both in discharge information and in promoting well-being in hospital inpatients. Malnutrition affects healing in several ways:

- poor healing with reduced tensile strength and an increased risk of wound dehiscence (Scholl & Langkamp-Henken 2001)
- an increased likelihood of infection (Lansdown 2004)
- poor-quality scarring.

Protein and calorie intake need to be above normal recommended levels to support additional collagen synthesis and metabolic activity (Table 24.3).

Table 24.2 Scar formation	
No. of weeks post-injury	**Scar characteristics**
0–4 weeks	Soft, weak scar line
4–12 weeks	Scar contracts, becomes harder and stronger
12–52 weeks	Scar line flattens and becomes soft and supple, moving easily with surrounding skin. Gradually whitens as vascularity decreases. Skin does not regain pre-injury elasticity

Table 24.3 Calorie and protein intake in wound healing		
	Energy (kcal)	**Protein (g)**
Men	2150–2510	54–63
Women	1680–2150	42–45

Vitamin deficiency

Vitamin C is essential for the synthesis of collagen; a deficiency reduces wound tensile strength, increases the fragility of capillaries and impairs angiogenesis. Vitamin A

Box 24.2

Factors affecting wound healing

Age

With age, all metabolic processes slow down and collagen production is lower; therefore wounds heal more slowly and have less tensile strength

Tissue perfusion

Many diseases cause hypoxia and reduced tissue perfusion. Those with a significant effect on wound healing include:

- Anaemia
- Peripheral vascular disease
- Respiratory disease
- Arteriosclerosis
- Dehydration

The result of this is reduced fibroblast activity and collagen synthesis, reduced epithelial regeneration and greater susceptibility to infection because of decreased leucocyte activity

Other diseases

These include diabetes, immune disorders and cancer, because of dampened inflammatory response and susceptibility to infection. Also, inflammatory conditions, liver failure and uraemia

Psychological factors and body image

Stress and anxiety suppress the immune system and are linked with sleep disturbance. This has been shown to delay healing. Anabolic healing is enhanced by sleep. Altered body image can occur from seemingly minor wounds and this can adversely affect healing in terms of stress and compliance with wound care strategies

Poor wound care

Inadequate wound cleansing or inappropriate wound dressing is an avoidable factor in healing

Nutrition

Protein, vitamins and trace elements are vital for prompt, adequate wound healing. These include:

- Iron
- Copper
- Zinc
- Vitamin A
- Vitamin C

Vitamins B, E and K also influence healing, and adequate protein and calorie intake is also necessary

Hydration

To maintain metabolism, between 2 and 2.5 L of fluid in 24 hours is needed. Less than this will result in fluid being drawn from interstitial spaces. Patients who are already clinically dehydrated will have delayed healing

Smoking

Both carbon monoxide and nicotine, as end-products of smoking, have an adverse effect on peripheral tissue perfusion, therefore increasing hypoxia risk. There is also an increased risk of thrombus formation in smokers

Drug therapy

Anti-inflammatory agents, immunosuppressive drugs, cytotoxic agents and corticosteroids all impinge on the healing process

---

supplement improves healing in patients on corticosteroids (Scholl & Langkamp-Henken 2001). It can help to restore inflammatory response and reduces the risk of wound infection. Similarly, a vitamin A deficiency increases infection risk. Vitamin B complex is necessary for wound strength as it contributes to cross-linking of collagen fibres. Vitamin K is essential for the clotting process in early wound healing (Lansdown 2004).

Trace element deficiency

Iron deficiency has two significant impacts on wound healing: first, in patients with anaemia, oxygen transportation is reduced and therefore tissue perfusion is inhibited; and second, iron is a necessary co-factor in collagen synthesis. Copper deficiency is rare but where it occurs, enzyme activity is restricted and collagen cross-linkage is impaired. Zinc deficiency delays wound healing because it slows collagen synthesis, reduces wound strength and decreases speed of epithelialization (Baranoski & Ayello, 2008). The use of a dietician may be of benefit to patients with nutritional issues.

Body type

Body type may also affect wound healing. An obese patient, for example, may experience a compromise in wound healing due to poor blood supply to adipose tissue. In addition, some obese patients have protein malnutrition, which further impedes the healing. Conversely, when a patient is emaciated, the lack of oxygen and nutritional stores may interfere with wound healing (Thomas Hess 2011).

Wound assessment

It is essential that an accurate history is elicited from the patient to ensure systematic assessment and appropriate management of the wound. As with all patients attending the ED, the immediate history of events leading up to ED attendance is imperative. Assessment should consider when, where and how the injury occurred. The mechanism of injury gives important clues to the type of wound being dealt with as well as any materials involved in the injury, such as wood splinters, glass, metal, etc. (Flarity & Hoyt 2010). Table 24.4 relates the mechanism of injury to wound type. The type of skin damage of injury is usually related to the mechanism of injury (Fig. 24.2).

The size, shape, wound depth and anatomical site of the wound should be assessed and documented. Diagrams in the patient's notes, or a photograph with a measurement scale, are useful if the wound is likely to need follow-up care.

Table 24.5 demonstrates the essential principles of wound assessment.

Table 24.4 Mechanism of injury: wound classifications

Mechanism of injury	Type of wound	Appearance	Special considerations
Blunt force such as a direct blow to the skin causing tearing or splitting of the skin (Cole 2003)	Laceration	Irregular break of the skin	
Caused by a sharp cutting implement such as a knife, broken glass or a metal edge	Incision	Straight, clean cut	
Caused by an object penetrating the skin and possibly underlying structures	Penetrating	Appearance may be deceptive; this type of wound needs careful exploration	There may be underlying injury or a foreign body present
Tissue is crushed by the force of the injury, causing skin and underlying structures to split open (Walsh & Kent 2001)	Crush	Jagged with skin loss	This type of wound may be unsuitable for suturing and may need closure using adhesive tissue strips
Skin is forced against a resistant surface in a rubbing or scraping fashion	Abrasion	Superficial skin loss, friction burn	
Blunt trauma	Contusion	Damage to vessels beneath surface with or without lacerations	
Trapped between shearing forces	De-gloving injury	Full-thickness skin loss	There may be damage to underlying structures (Dandy & Edwards 2003)
Thermal sources – caused by intense heat or cold or substances, steam, flame, sun exposure, friction, radiation	Burn	Classified as superficial, partial thickness and full thickness. See wound assessment	
Chemical sources – acids or alkalis. Specialist advice should be sought for chemical burns, an antidote may be needed			There is a risk of underlying tissue damage
Electrical currents			

Figure 24.2 • Mechanism of injury and skin damage.

Table 24.5 Wound assessment

Assessment question	Rationale
How did the wound occur?	To establish mechanism of injury and classification of wound To exclude serious or other injuries To assess potential contamination risk (Clark 2004)
When did the injury occur?	To ensure it is appropriate for primary closure To assess for infection risk (wounds >6 hours old are more prone to infection)
Size, site and depth of wound	To ascertain the most appropriate method of wound closure (e.g., wounds over joints or requiring high tensile strength usually require sutures) (Autio & Olson 2002) To ensure base of wound can be visualized
Past medical history	To detect pathology that may delay or influence healing
Medication history	To detect medication that may delay or influence healing To avoid prescribing contraindicated medications as part of wound management
Allergies	To avoid allergic reactions during the wound management process and during subsequent treatment
Tetanus status	To ensure the patient has tetanus immunity
Occupation and dominant hand	To assess the effect of the injury on the patient's lifestyle To ensure treatment is appropriate for the patient's lifestyle

Wound examination

Extensive wounds may often distract the novice emergency clinician, however it is paramount that the clinician completes the primary survey to rule out life-threatening problems. Please refer to previous chapters for a review of primary survey.

Effective wound examination should reveal the extent of tissue damage, the degree of contamination and specifically the integrity of the nerves, tendons and vascular supply (Autio & Olson 2002, Clark 2004). It should also exclude the presence of foreign bodies (FBs). All findings should be documented, including the normal ones.

Most traumatic wounds occur in unsterile conditions, and therefore all carry a risk of infection. A number of factors affect infection potential, such as mechanism of injury, degree of tissue loss, age of the wound prior to cleansing and anatomical location. All traumatic wounds should be considered contaminated; some of these will appear clean on initial examination, while others will be obviously contaminated. Potential for infection due to all the above reasons may assist with the method of wound closure, i.e., primary or delayed primary closure.

Excessive bleeding and macerated or badly damaged tissue can detract from a thorough examination. Bleeding should be controlled to allow an accurate examination to be carried out

(Clark 2004). Assessment of vascular integrity should include the patient's estimation of blood loss, together with objective evidence of haemorrhage. The wound should be carefully inspected for continuous oozing of blood (suggestive of venous bleeding), spurting of bright-red blood (indicative of arterial injury) and haematoma formation, which could pose a risk to healing in the form of potential infection. Haemostasis is usually achieved through direct pressure and elevation of the injured area. Where bleeding cannot be controlled specialist input should be sought. Vascular integrity distal to the wound can be assessed by observing skin colour distally to the wound, feeling skin temperature, and checking distal pulses and the speed of capillary refill (McKenna 2006).

Nerves have both a sensory and a motor function and therefore both can be checked to eliminate injury. This assessment should occur before local anaesthetic is used. Sensory function distal to the wound should be assessed either by use of a cotton wool wisp to detect the absence or presence of sensation, or by gentle pinprick tests to assess sharp and dull sensation. Motor function should be assessed, particularly in hand or wrist injuries, and this can be done by assessing a variety of movements of the patient's hand and wrist (McKenna 2006).

Tendon injury should also be identified and eliminated as part of the examination stage of wound management. Tendons can often be partially severed and still retain their function, so elimination of this type of injury should be done in two ways. An initial systematic examination of the patient's function in the affected limb may demonstrate reduced power or function. This should be followed by direct visualization of the wound to discover any structural damage (Waller & Tan 2009). This is particularly important in hand injuries where extensor tendon injuries are common, e.g., mallet finger. Flexor tendon injuries following injury to the palmar aspect of the hand are less common, but have a high incidence of disability when missed, as they leave the patient unable to bend the injured digit. Flexor tendon injury is difficult to detect as tendons contract when cut and are therefore not always visible at the wound edges. If the mechanism of injury and initial examination suggest tendon injury, the wound should be explored until tendon edges or intact tendon are visualized. Specialist referral is necessary for wounds such as flexor tendon injuries or wounds involving cosmetic challenges such as the vermillion border or the cartilage of the ear (Reynolds 2004).

During examination and cleansing, FBs should be excluded. Likely FBs include glass, metal, plastic or grit, all of which could lead to infection or tattooing if left in situ. If the history suggests that glass or any other radio-opaque FB may be present in the wound, medical imaging such as ultrasound or X-ray is a useful way of locating or excluding this (Waller & Tan 2009).

Wounds with potential underlying fracture will need referral to a specialist for management. In the ED, the injured area is elevated, splinted and gross debris removed. The treating doctor will decide the need for antibiotics.

Wound pain

Wound pain is initiated by the inflammatory response and is a normal part of the healing process. It is caused by a

Box 24.3

Pain triggers

- Inflammatory response
- Atmospheric exposure – drying to wound
- Tissue tension – due to oedema and angiogenesis
- Irritation from cleaning solutions
- Dressings too tight
- Wound complications, e.g., infection

combination of noxious stimuli, including histamine and peptides such as substance P (a pain transmitter) and prostaglandin (a chemical stimulus for pain) (Kumar et al. 2005). Box 24.3 highlights some of the pain triggers. Part of the pain response is to protect the wound from further injury. The impact of wound pain should not be underestimated and analgesia suitable for the stage of wound healing should be used.

Non-steroidal anti-inflammatory drugs (NSAIDs) modulate pain pathways in multiple ways (Sinatra 2002). NSAIDs reduce inflammatory hyperalgesia and allodynia by reducing prostaglandin synthesis; they can decrease the recruitment of leukocytes and consequently their derived inflammatory mediators; and they cross the blood–brain barrier to prevent prostaglandins (i.e., pain-producing neuromodulators) in the spinal cord (Golan 2008). In this manner, NSAIDs reduce local inflammation and may prevent both peripheral and central sensitization.

NSAIDs are thought to have the potential to affect platelet activity by inhibiting clumping and coagulation, as well as the potential interference with the inflammatory phase of healing where mediators and white cell activity are so important. While analgesia for burns (and wounds) should be a top priority, the potential inhibition of inflammation tends to indicate that other analgesia, such as paracetamol and codeine-based drugs, may be preferable. Opiates should be avoided for ED patients who will invariably be discharged and have no support person able to provide supervision.

Non-pharmacological methods of pain relief should also be considered. If ongoing wound care will be needed, e.g., in management of burns, patients should be prescribed analgesia to take prior to dressing changes. Appropriate explanations of interventions and psychological support will help to alleviate pain (see also Chapter 25).

Distraction techniques are a vital component in managing wounds in children. Activity centres, books, computer games and simple toys that are all age-related assist in distracting the child and reduce the intensity of the intervention. Significantly complex wounds in children may need to be managed under general anaesthetic or sedation. The senior ED medical officer in consultation with the appropriate specialty medical officer and the child's parents should all be included in this decision.

Wound cleansing

There are two important considerations in wound cleansing:

- the way it is carried out
- the solution used.

Wound cleansing is essential for the prevention of infection, tattoo scarring and exclusion of foreign bodies. The practitioner carrying out this cleansing prior to wound closure has a responsibility to ensure that the wound is decontaminated and if any doubt exists the wound should not be closed (Joanna Briggs Institute 2006).

Cleansing solutions

Wound cleansing solutions have been the subject of much debate over recent years. In many emergency departments, normal saline is the cleanser of choice because of its safety and cost-effectiveness (Dulecki & Pieper 2005). Like tap water, it is most effective when warmed to body temperature. Studies have demonstrated that both normal saline and tap water are comparable for wound irrigation in terms of infection rates and healing (Bansal et al. 2002, Valente et al. 2003). A systematic review by the Cochrane Group (Fernandez et al. 2003) suggests that clean, drinkable water is a safe, cheaper alternative to normal saline. Nevertheless water quality may influence outcomes (Betts 2003) and therefore it should be drawn from a tap that is frequently used, from a direct water supply with a nozzle that is regularly swabbed for contamination. Both water and normal saline are less likely to impede the natural healing process compared with other commercial irrigants or detergents such as povidone iodine (Dulecki & Pieper 2005).

Antiseptic solutions include cetrimide and chlorhexidine. It has an immediate and lasting residual action on skin bacteria, including Gram-positive bacteria. It is useful as a hand cleaner and for surgical scrubs (Lee & Bishop 2006).

Povidone-iodine is a broad-spectrum antiseptic agent and is the cleansing agent of choice for contaminated wounds. Iodine is more effective than other antibacterial agents, particularly against Gram-negative bacteria (Lee & Bishop 2006). It has a slow-release capacity where povidone acts as a carrier gradually releasing iodine into the tissues. It has been suggested that this reduces tissue toxicity and irritation but preserves antibacterial properties (Lee & Bishop 2006). There is continued concern over the use of povidone-iodine (Cole 2003) partly because the concentration of iodine in commercial preparations remains cytotoxic to the fibroblasts needed for wound healing and therefore reduces the tensile strength of the wound and slows the epithelialization process. Rabenberg et al. (2002), in a study using human skin samples, found that diluting povidone-iodine solution 1 part solution to 9 parts water provides a safe, antibacterial yet non-toxic compromise.

Desloughing solutions such as hydrogen peroxide are not effective as a routine treatment (Rees 2003). Their ability to destroy bacteria is considerably reduced once in contact with blood or pus. While the oxidizing activity does remove slough, it also breaks down granulating wound tissue and inhibits neo-dermal formation. If diluted to a strength that is non-toxic to tissues, the hydrogen peroxide is no longer effective on bacteria. Hydrogen peroxide should only be used as a one-off treatment for extremely sloughy wounds and the area should be irrigated with saline afterwards. This makes its use in traumatic wound management very limited. There is some evidence that using hydrogen peroxide to irrigate cavity wounds can cause emboli (Haller et al. 2002, Henley et al. 2004) so care should be taken when doing this. The National Institute for Health and Clinical Excellence recommends considering other agents, and suggests that using hydrocolloids or hydrogels, among others, would be more acceptable to patients in terms of comfort and acceptability (National Institute for Health and Clinical Excellence 2005).

Eusol (Edinburgh University Solution Of Lime) type preparations are rarely used and there is no clinical indication for their use in any circumstances. Considerable evidence exists to highlight the limited antibacterial effects of sodium hypochlorite and their devastating degree of tissue damage is well documented (Atiyeh et al. 2009). Table 24.6 lists cleaning solutions and their properties.

Cleansing methods

It is now accepted practice that swabbing a wound with cotton wool or gauze is not the most effective method of cleaning a wound. Fibres can be left in situ and bacteria can be distributed around the wound (Cole 2003). Acute, traumatic wounds should be irrigated with a degree of pressure (using a Steripod™; a pressurized canister of solution or a syringe with or without a blunt needle) to clean the wound and remove debris (Towler 2001). To be effective, the mechanical force used must exceed that of the adhesive forces of the contaminant (Dulecki & Pieper 2005). The amount of pressure needed for adequate irrigation with minimal damage to tissue is approximately 13 psi (Fernandez et al. 2004). Wound irrigation should continue until all obvious contamination has been removed.

In some cases, such as dirty abrasions and gritty wounds of varying depths, surgical scrubbing of the wound may be indicated. If this is necessary adequate anaesthesia or analgesia will be required and often these patients may go to operating theatre for this procedure. More recently, some hydrocolloid dressing or wound irrigation solutions such as Prontostan® can be used to more gently clean contaminated wounds such as abrasions.

Chronic wounds

Chronic wounds are usually the result of poor healing due to a number of underlying issues. As such it is beyond the scope of this chapter to address all of the components of this specialized area, however the important things to consider are:

* how long has the patient had the wound?
* patient dynamics including age, diet, mobility, co-morbidities particularly those affecting wound healing such as circulatory problems
* presence of infection
* compliance with wound management.

It is suggested that chronic wounds need to be assessed and managed by the patient's GP with referral to appropriate specialist medical intervention as needed, e.g., vascular outpatients department. The wound clinical nurse consultant or nurse specialist at most major hospitals can be an excellent resource in management techniques of chronic wounds.

Staff in smaller emergency care centres without a wound care specialist should establish links and establish a referral system that enables staff to confidentially send smart phone photographs of complex chronic wounds for advice regarding the most appropriate treatments.

Chronic wounds should be managed as a potential symptom of underlying disease and therefore management needs to reflect the requirements necessary to address the disease as well as the wound.

Table 24.6 Properties of cleaning solutions

Solution	Antibacterial activity	Tissue toxicity	Advantages	Disadvantages
Tap water	None	None	Cheap. Easily accessible in large volumes	Potential for environmental contamination
Normal saline	None	None	Isotonic. Gentle	Cost (compared with tap water)
Povidone-iodine	Gram negative and Gram positive	Toxic at >5% (sold in 7.5 and 10% solutions only)	Highly antibacterial	Potentially delays healing at strengths commonly used
Chlorhexidine	Strong Gram positive, slight Gram negative	Low toxicity	No clinical advantages	Antibacterial action reduced when in contact with blood or pus
Cetrimide	Low activity	Irritant	Good detergent	Antibacterial properties inactivated by blood and pus. Easily contaminated by infection
Hydrogen peroxide	Weak action on anaerobic surface	Very toxic to cells	No clinical advantages	Inactivated by pus

Local anaesthesia

Local anaesthesia (LA) is used to ensure that wound cleansing or closure using sutures or staples is a painless procedure. Local infiltration of lignocaine or topical application of gel is usually adequate. Some patients find the administration of LA uncomfortable; therefore, careful explanation, expectations of procedure, encouragement and reassurance are helpful in reducing the anxiety and pain of LA administration (Quaba et al. 2005). For further information see Chapter 26.

Wound closure

The closure of traumatic wounds in the ED can be categorized into three types:

- primary wound closure – where edges of wounds are brought together preferably within the first 6 hours after injury
- delayed primary closure – performed 4–5 days after injury provided there is no evidence of infection
- secondary closure – where the wound heals by granulation and epithelialization.

Purposeful delay allows an intervention, such as the use of antibiotics, before the wound is closed. This may happen following debridement of the wound edges.

Primary wound closure

Primary closure should only be carried out once the wound is thoroughly cleaned, foreign bodies have been eliminated and there is minimal or no tissue loss. While it is not suitable for all wound types, primary closure does improve healing and cosmetic appearance. Primary closure occurs when the wound has been brought together by sutures, adhesive tissue strips, staples, tissue adhesive, and hair ties (Fig. 24.3). Primary

closure entails aligning skin layers and underlying structures, eliminating any dead space and so reducing the risk of haematoma, infection and a depressed scar due to precise eversion of skin edges (Lees 2007, Flarity & Hoyt 2010).

The time *elapsed* since initial injury must be considered when undertaking primary closure. Wounds are normally closed up to 6–12 hours post injury, but this may differ according to the site of the wound. A face, for example, should be considered for primary closure up to 24 hours post-injury (Holt 2000). Similarly, if a wound is heavily contaminated or in an anatomical site prone to infection, such as the hand, safe primary closure times are considerably shorter.

Delayed primary closure is usually reserved for those wounds that are heavily contaminated. Secondary closure is more common with chronic wounds (Baranoski & Ayello 2008).

Suturing

Sutures are appropriate for the management of specific wounds, such as deep, large or jagged wounds, those under tension, mobile areas or wounds in awkward places (Autio & Olson 2002). Wound closure using sutures can be more painful than other techniques, usually due to the need to infiltrate the area with local anaesthesia prior to suture insertion.

The wound depth is partial or full dermal depth, and neurovascular damage and functional capacity should be assessed before wound closure and infiltration with local anaesthetic. Healing occurs across wound layers, so it is important to accurately match each skin layer. It is important to eliminate the dead space below the superficial layer of the wound as this provides an ideal location for bacterial colonization (Atiyeh et al. 2002, Richardson 2004a). In addition, because scars contract during the maturation phase of healing, everted wound lines will flatten to the normal plane of the skin. Achieving proper wound edge eversion lies with suturing technique (Flarity & Hoyt 2010).

The most commonly used technique in the ED is an interrupted suture (Waller & Tan 2009). This is basically a square suture, with width and depth of suture equal. This helps to evert wound edges. If suture width is greater than its depth then the wound edges will roll or invert (Fig. 24.4). After thorough wound cleansing the initial suture should be placed centrally, to divide the lesion into two smaller wounds.

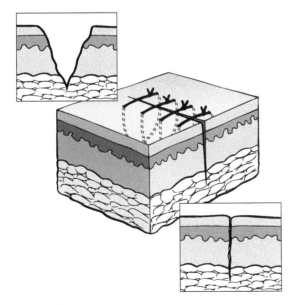

Figure 24.3 • Primary closure.

Figure 24.4 • Everting wound edges with square sutures.

Table 24.7 Suture material

Type	Description	Ease of use	Tensile strength	Inflammatory reaction risk	Infection risk
Silk	Organic, non-absorbable	Easy	Low	High	High
Nylon	Synthetic, non-absorbable monofilament	Moderate	High	Low	High
Polypropylene	Synthetic, non-absorbable monofilament	Difficult	High	Low	High
Catgut (plain or chrome)	Organic from sheep, absorbable	Moderate	Moderate	High	High
Polyglycolic acid	Synthetic braided, absorbable	Moderate	High	Low	Medium
Polydioxanone	Synthetic monofilament, absorbable	Easy	High	Low	Low

Further sutures should then be placed strategically along the wound so that the tension remains constant throughout (Cole 2003). This can be achieved by having all of the knots on the same side.

Suture types

Suture products vary greatly, but general principles for use can be adapted. Sutures are designed to be absorbed or removed (Table 24.7).

Sutures are either absorbable or non-absorbable, with the latter being commonly used for wounds where only the skin requires closure. Where there are deeper structures exposed, such as subcutaneous fat and muscle, then absorbable sutures may be used. These will dissolve over a longer period.

Non-absorbable sutures are used for dermis and epidermal skin closure. They are either monofilament or multifilament. Monofilament nylons and polypropylene are the most commonly used because they carry a low infection risk and are of a high tensile strength as they are made from single strands and not braided. Because they are synthetic, they are far less likely to cause an inflammatory response, which is common with silk and other organic sutures (Cole 2003, Bonham 2011). These sutures need removing.

Absorbable sutures, such as catgut or synthetic polymers, are used for deeper tissue structures as well as the inside of the mouth and perineum. They are broken down by protein synthesis over about 3–4 weeks and therefore do not need removal. Monofilament synthetic polymers are most commonly used as they have a lower infection and inflammation risk than catgut, but they do take longer to reabsorb.

Sutures are measured by gauge, and choice of suture size will be influenced by the extent and site of the wound. The common range of suture sizes found in an ED will be from 3/0 to 6/0, with the lower number indicating the thicker gauge and the higher indicating the finer. A general guide for sutures sizes and wounds can be seen in Table 24.8.

It is usual to utilize a reverse cutting needle for suturing (Clark 2004). This type of needle is manufactured to facilitate ease of use on tissue such as skin. The type and size of needle is depicted on the suture packet. Suture packs usually contain forceps, suture holder and scissors. Forceps may be toothed or non-toothed but regardless of the type used care should be taken not to crush the wound edges (Richardson 2004b).

Table 24.8 A guide to suture size

Area	Size of suture	Suggested removal
Face	5/0–6/0 nylon	5 days (in some circumstances removal after 3 days may be appropriate)
Scalp	3/0 or 4/0 nylon	7 days
Arms, upper legs, torso	3/0, 4/0–5/0 nylon	5–7 days
Hands, lower legs, feet, back	3/0–4/0 nylon	7–10 days

Complications of suturing

Sutured wounds do not need a dressing unless there is associated skin loss or the sutures are in need of protection, e.g., where the patient is a young child or a person working in a dirty environment. Dressings should provide a warm environment and be permeable to allow the wound to breathe. Some patients prefer sutured wounds to be dressed, however, and this should also be taken into consideration. (see Table 24.9).

Staples

Staples are usually associated with surgical wounds, but they also have a place in the closure of acute traumatic wounds, particularly those in the scalp. Staples have the same tensile strength as sutures and can be used for linear wounds of moderate tension. Evidence suggests that overall, staples are quicker and cheaper than sutures for closing scalp wounds (Hogg & Carley 2002) and are associated with good cosmesis (Autio & Olson 2002). Advantages of using staples are the speed of closure and minimal tissue reaction, and low risk of infection when compared with other suture materials (Hoyt et al. 2011). Skill is required to insert staples, and failure to align tissue edges correctly can cause scar deformity (Richardson 2004b). In common with sutures, local anaesthesia should be used prior to insertion of staples. Staples require special equipment for removal and they should be removed in 5–7 days.

Table 24.9 Complications of suturing

Complication	Comment	Solution
Patient fainting	Patient inadequately prepared	Lie patients down while suturing
Sutures too tight	Can result in split sutures and/or devitalized tissue. Can also increase scarring	Tie sutures tight enough to ensure edges are everted. If suture appears too tight remove and replace it
Sutures too loose	Will not hold tissue in apposition and may delay healing or cause a scar	Tie sutures tight enough to ensure edges are everted. If suture appears too loose remove and replace it
Wound edges overlapping	Will not heal optimally and will leave a poor cosmetic finish	Ensure wound edges are apposed and everted
Wound edges inverted	Can result in a depressed scar and delay healing	Ensure wound edges are apposed and everted
Sutures too near to wound edge	May tear skin	Ensure sutures are 4–5 mm from wound edge. Do not suture thin, friable skin: consider other wound closure methods
Sutures too far from wound edge	May cause increased tension and 'cross hatch' scarring	Ensure sutures are 4–5 mm from wound edge
Infection	May cause delayed wound healing, scarring and systemic illness	Scrupulous cleansing and aseptic technique

(Adapted from Clark A (2004) Understanding the principles of suturing minor skin lesions. Nursing Times, 100(29), 32–34; Richardson M (2004b) Wound care: procedures for cleansing, closing and covering acute wounds. Nursing Times, 100(4), 54–58.)

Tissue adhesive

Tissue adhesives (TA) are a useful method of closing simple traumatic wounds. TA is usually supplied in sterile units, which can be disposed after single use. It is easy and quick to use, non-invasive and presents less risk of tissue trauma and needlestick injuries, does not require secondary dressings or the patient to return for removal. They are less painful than other methods and achieves good cosmetic results (Cayton-Richards 2011, Lewis et al. 2011a). TA contains octyl-2-cyanoacrylate, which is also an effective barrier against common bacterial microbes including certain staphylococci, *Pseudomonas* spp., and *Escherichia coli* (Hoyt et al. 2011). The risk of needlestick injuries is eliminated as no sharps are used (Richardson 2004b). TA is particularly useful in the management of acute wounds in children due to its ease and rapidity of use.

When applying TA it is essential that bleeding has been stopped, or the adhesive will not work. Application of TA is normally a two-person technique, and should not be attempted by a lone practitioner, unless the wound is very small and the edges well apposed and the practitioner is skilled in its application.

The wound edges should be apposed as closely as possible, while the adhesive is applied either in a continuous line or dotted along the wound edges (Cole 2003). The wound edges should be held together for at least 30 seconds to allow polymerization to occur (Richardson 2004b), although individual manufacturers' instructions should be followed. TA should never be instilled into the wound and then the wound edges pushed together, as this will cause pain and risk excessive scarring. It will also increase the risk of infection.

Care should be taken when using adhesive on the face to avoid it running into the eyes. This can be avoided by always having the patient lying down and covering the eyes with a damp gauze pad during application.

Following application the patient should be instructed to start washing the affected area with soap and water after five days and the adhesive will start to gently dissolve.

Adhesive tissue strips

Adhesive strips are available in different widths, can be elasticized to allow ease of movement (Richardson 2004b) and have several advantages over suturing. They are usually less traumatic and less painful for the patient, tissue trauma is decreased and there is little risk of reaction to the material being used.

Adhesive tissue strips are useful for wounds that are superficial, straight and where skin edges can be aligned and there is minimal wound tension (Autio & Olson 2002). They are not recommended for patients with frail skin, such as the elderly or patients on steroid therapy, or those with a pre-tibial laceration, these patients are best treated with a zinc-impregnated dressing and light compression for up to six days provided no infection is evident. Adhesive strips should be used with caution in flap injuries, particularly with the elderly as these wounds are fragile and vulnerable and removal of the strips may cause further injury such as shearing (Ireland 2007).

Adhesive tissue strips are unsuitable for wounds where bleeding cannot be stopped and for hirsute areas such as the scalp (Cole 2003). Care should be taken when using them on confused or non-compliant patients, as they can be easily removed.

When applying adhesive tissue strips, ensure that the surrounding skin is clean and dry to allow adequate adhesion (Richardson 2004b). Following the same principles as suturing, and after the wound edges have been apposed, either with forceps or gloved fingers, the first closure should be made in the centre of the wound. Subsequent strips should be placed to bisect the resulting smaller wounds until closure is complete (Richardson 2004b). Tension should be even across the wound and small gaps should be left between the strips to allow exudate to escape (Cole 2003) (Fig. 24.5). Adhesive tissue strips can be used in conjunction with other wound-closure techniques for support.

Adhesive tissue strips require minimal follow-up after application (Autio & Olson 2002), allowing the patient to care for the wound themselves, if they have been given appropriate advice.

A dressing is not strictly necessary over these wounds, but may be used if the wound needs extra protection. Adhesive strips should be removed after 3–4 days from the face, and 5–7 days in most other areas. Patients with friable skin or pre-tibial lacerations should have adhesive strips in place for at least 10 days.

Patients can remove adhesive strips themselves without the need to return to a healthcare professional. Specifying to the patient how long, removal should take place after 5–7 days by gently peeling back both ends of the strip, while supporting the skin, towards the centre of the wound.

Hair apposition technique (HAT)

This is an underused technique, which can be used for superficial wounds on the scalp that are not actively bleeding (Cole 2003). Ong et al. (2002) suggest that this should be the first choice for scalp wounds; however, the patient's hair needs to be long enough to tie. It may be used in situations when other more conventional methods of wound closure may be inappropriate, such as with children or adults who refuse sutures due to needle phobia. However, this method is only suitable for superficial scalp wounds (Richardson 2004b).

HAT is a quick and relatively painless method of wound closure which compares with suturing for wound healing, risk of infection and wound breakdown, but is superior in terms of scarring, overall complications and procedure-related pain (Ong et al. 2002).

The wound edges are pulled together by the hair on either side, which is then tied in a knot. Alternatively, the hair can be twisted rather than tied, and secured with a drop of tissue adhesive (Hock et al. 2002). The patient needs to be advised not to pull on the hair tie with a brush or a comb. After five days the patient should treat the wound as for tissue adhesive.

Secondary closure

This occurs by granulation when primary closure is contraindicated (Fig. 24.6). Wounds healing by secondary closure usually require a dressing. The purpose of a wound dressing is to create the optimal healing environment for that particular wound (Russell 2000) (Box 24.4).

Figure 24.6 • Wound granulation.

Figure 24.5 • Application of adhesive tapes.

Box 24.4

The optimum wound dressing

- High humidity between wound surface and dressing
- Allows gaseous exchange
- Provides thermal insulation
- Impermeable to bacteria
- Removes excess exudate
- Free of particles and toxic wound contaminants
- Can be removed without causing further tissue trauma

See Table 24.10 for an overview of common types of dressings.

Wound humidity

Epithelialization of a wound is faster when the wound surface is covered with a film dressing or hydrocolloid as it allows more rapid movement of epithelial cells to migrate across the surface of the wound. Wound pain is also reduced in a moist healing environment (Baranoski & Ayello 2008). In simple terms, the film dressing acts a little like a scab and can be used on a variety of wounds including pressure ulcers (stage one and two), minor burns and lacerations.

Gaseous exchange

The benefit of wound oxygenation depends on the depth and stage of healing.

For superficial regenerating wounds involving the epidermis, semi-permeable film dressings are advantageous (Baranoski & Ayello, 2008). However, gaseous exchange from the wound surface is inhibited by excessive exudate, making atmospheric oxygen through permeable dressings an unreliable source of oxygenation.

For wounds that heal by granulation, some degree of tissue hypoxia is necessary to stimulate angiogenesis and fibroblastic activity (Broussard 2004). Where healing is by granulation, hydrocolloid dressings are effective.

Thermal insulation

If the thermal environment is kept stable under a dressing, cellular activity is enhanced and wound healing improved. If that wound becomes exposed, perhaps for a dressing change, its surface temperature drops and cellular activity is inhibited. It can take up to 3 hours for this activity to return to normal (Myers 1982). Dressings should therefore only be removed when clinically indicated, as removing dressings has the potential to delay healing.

Permeability to bacteria

Dressings should provide the wound with protection from microorganisms. They should also contain any existing bacteria within the dressing. Any dressing which becomes wet, or where wound exudate soaks through, becomes a passage for infection both in and out of the wound and should be changed.

Table 24.10 Wound dressings[†]

Wound	Dressing classification	Product example	Indications	Contraindications	Application
Abrasion	Non-stick silicone dressing Silver sulphadiazine cream Hydrocolloid dressing	Mepitel SSD cream, Acticoat Duoderm	Superficial wounds, granulating wounds, minor burns or those areas where a non-stick dressing is required	Infected, heavily exuding wounds	Follow manufacturer's guidelines
Epithelializing wounds	Semi-permeable film	Opsite	Superficial regenerating wounds, sites of primary closure	Infected wounds, exuding wounds	Apply to dry skin if it becomes loose or exudate builds up, the wound will need review with potential for a new dressing type
Infected	Impregnated tulle Solugel Silver-based products	Inadine Solugel, SSD Iodosorb	Infected or potentially infected wounds	Non-infected wounds	Follow manufacturer's guidelines
Sloughy	Hydrogel Impregnated tulle Solugel Silver-based products	Intrasyte gel Inadine Solugel SSD Curasalt, Iodosorb	Slough, small areas of necrosis	Non-infected or dry wound	Follow manufacturer's guidelines
Exudating	Hydrophilic/hydrophobic foam	Alginate	Heavily exuding wounds	Dry wounds	Follow manufacturer's guidelines
Granulating	Hydrocolloid	Granuflex, Duoderm	Granulating wounds and burns. Can also be used to deslough wounds	Infected wounds	Follow manufacturer's guidelines
Bleeding	Haemostatic	Kaltostat	Bleeding wounds	Dry or infected wounds	Follow manufacturer's guidelines

[†]It is paramount to ensure all patients receive advice in home wound management and are informed of the indications to return for review at their local primary care service or emergency department. Priorities of home wound management are presence of infection, pain and loss of dressing. Maintenance of the dressing is also important.

Removal of excess exudate

Although the wound surface should be moist, excessive exudate causes skin maceration around the wound. For this reason, the dressing chosen should be of an absorbency level suitable for the amount of exudate. Many commercial dressings are made in a variety of absorbencies. Absorbent pads may be necessary but should only be used over a primary dressing (Holt 2000).

Removal without causing tissue trauma

Dressings that stick to the wound surface should be avoided, particularly dry dressings on open wounds. Exudate can also cause a dressing to stick if it dries, which is why dressings with adequate absorbency are essential. Newly granulating tissue is fragile and easily destroyed in dressing removal. Dressings should be removed slowly while supporting the wound surface in order to reduce the risk of tissue trauma.

Types of dressing

Many wound dressing products are available for hospital use, either for general use or by medical prescription. These can be broadly grouped into seven categories (Table 24.10).

Wound dressings most commonly used in ED warrant further consideration.

Dressings that promote regeneration

These are used for grazes, abrasions, minor burns and other superficial wounds involving the epidermis. The most effective dressings for this are semi-permeable films or membranes. They provide the moist environments needed and some thermal protection; however, membranes have limited absorbency for light exudate. Neither should be used on infected wounds.

Non-adherent dressings also tend to be used for superficial wounds; however, not only do they have little absorbency, but they cannot provide a moist environment for regeneration and are therefore not recommended. They can be useful for the dressing over sutures.

Dressings that promote granulation

These are used for wounds involving the dermal layer where tissue loss has occurred. Occlusive hydrocolloid dressings provide a warm, moist environment and promote granulation. They are designed to absorb moderate amounts of exudate and can be left in place for several days. As exudate is absorbed into the dressing, a distinctive odour is produced, which although not offensive can cause some concern for patients if it is not expected. Hydrocolloid dressings should not be used on infected wounds.

Impregnated tulle

Tulle dressings were commonly used for treating superficial wounds with moderate infection; however, this practice is on the decline with the advent of newer products such as silver-impregnated dressings.

Silver-impregnated dressings

These dressings are useful for treatment of both abrasions and minor burns. They have specific requirements according to the manufacturer and directions of use must be followed. Silver has been found to be an excellent antimicrobial (Ip et al. 2006).

Wound infection

Most traumatic wounds occur in unsterile conditions, and therefore all carry a risk of infection. But just because contaminants can get in does not mean that all wounds become infected. A number of factors affect the infection potential, such as mechanism of injury, degree of tissue loss, age of the wound prior to cleansing and anatomical location.

It is important to recognize infection and differentiate it from the normal inflammatory response. Accurate history-taking and the duration of the injury are important factors in differentiation (Hoyt et al. 2011). Signs of infection include:

* redness
* swelling
* increased pain
* skin warm to touch
* purulent discharge
* odour
* breakdown of the wound
* systemic symptoms
* pyrexia
* tachycardia
* tachypnoea.

Patients with a suspected wound infection may need a wound swab taken for culture and sensitivity prior to considering antibiotic therapy. Antibiotics are generally only considered for those infections that are not responding to local dressing techniques or the patient demonstrates local or systemic inflammatory markers such as cellulitis, fever, tachycardia, etc. In the initial injury, the use of antibiotics remains controversial with Goodson & Simmons (2012) noting that routine use of prophylactic antibiotics in traumatic injuries has not been shown to significantly reduce infection rates. Antibiotics are generally only prescribed for certain injuries such as some bites (see bite section) and those patients with complex, contaminated wounds often involving a fracture and potentially requiring surgery. Patients who suffer unexpected traumatic wounds are at greater risk of infection if they are malnourished, immunosuppressed or taking steroids. Tetanus status must be considered early in the management of wounds (Denke 2009).

Wounds that require special consideration

Bite wounds

Bite wounds make up a small but significant proportion of injuries seen in the ED and warrant special consideration because of their potential for infection. About 1 in 5 people bitten by a dog seek medical attention. It has been estimated that dog bites account for 60–90 % of bites; cat bites for 5–18 %, and human bites for 4–23 % (Smith et al. 2000, Richardson 2006). Between a third and half of all mammalian bites occur in children, who are often bitten by a household pet.

Bite wounds most commonly occur on the hands and are potentially at high risk for infection. The reasons for this are twofold; first, because of the number of pathogens found in the perpetrator's mouth, both human and animal; second, because of the way the pathogens are transferred – usually by deep, penetrating puncture wounds, which means that bite wounds, especially those from animals, tend to be heavily contaminated. Crush injury, lacerations and abrasions are common in dog bites, as dogs' teeth and jaws are designed to crush and tear their prey. These wounds, on top of being inoculated with bacteria, will have devitalized tissue that requires surgical excision. Cats, in contrast, usually inflict puncture wounds, as they have long, slender incisors that can penetrate deeply into tendon, bone and joints. These wounds tend to be underestimated because they are small and seal off early. In fact, deep abscesses and osteomyelitis are more common in cat than dog bites, as is infection (Cheah & Chong 2011). All these factors mean that a bite wound can lead to complications such as local wound infection, lymphangitis, abscess formation, septic arthritis and potentially rarer complications such as meningitis (Brook 2003, 2005). Bites to the hand also have a 30–40 % infection rate so thorough irrigation of lavage of the wound is necessary to reduce the bacterial load (Morgan & Palmer 2007, Cheah & Chong 2011).

Human bite wounds to the hand, particularly from clenched-fist injuries, may not present initially as a bite-injury, and may accompany other co-existing injuries, such as fractures to metacarpals. Nonetheless, these should be treated as bite injuries (Cole 2003). Where a human bite is sustained, consideration should be given to the possibility of transmission of other diseases, such as hepatitis B (HBV) and human immunodeficiency virus (HIV). The greater risk is with potential HBV transmission and so the opinion of an infectious disease physician or virologist should be sought, with a view to the patient commencing an accelerated course of HBV vaccine. HIV levels are low in saliva and so the risk of transmission via human bites is thought to be negligible (Eckerline et al. 1999). Rigorous wound management can go some way to reducing the infection risk (Bower 2002).

The closure of bite wounds is a subject of ongoing debate, with some authors advocating delaying closure of hand wounds (Dearden et al. 2001, Bower 2002) for 24–48 hours. Suturing may be appropriate where cosmetic appearance is of a primary concern, such as on the face (Chen et al. 2000, Correira 2003).

There is general agreement that prophylactic antibiotics should be given when the bite is sustained on the hand, head, neck or groin (Taplitz 2004) or if the wound is considered to be high-risk, such as very deep wounds (Brook 2005). Amoxicillin-clavulanic acid is the mainstay of prophylaxis, as it provides excellent coverage against the usual organisms that are inoculated. Doxycycline with metronidazole is a good alternative in individuals who are allergic to penicillin (Oehler et al. 2009, Chea & Chong 2011).

Insect bites and stings

Insect bites and stings are seen commonly in this country throughout the summer and early autumn months although they can occur at other times. Most commonly, people attend the ED following a sting from an insect of the classification Hymenoptera such as a wasp or bee, which has not resolved or from which they are suffering ill-effects (Klotz et al. 2009).

Reactions to an insect sting range from local to systemic. The majority will be local and will consist of symptoms such as localized pain, redness and itching. For these reactions, the treatment is symptomatic and the use of antihistamines and simple analgesics will usually result in a resolution of symptoms. Where cellulitis has developed, the patient should be treated with antibiotics and reviewed within 24 hours to ensure the infection is resolving. It is helpful to mark the outer border of the erythema with a marker pen so that the patient, and also the practitioner who reviews the patient, can see if there is an improvement of symptoms.

Where patients have a systemic reaction due to anaphylaxis, treatment must be prompt and should follow the resuscitation guidelines of their country, e.g., *Resuscitation Guidelines* (Resuscitation Council (UK) 2010).

Abrasions

Abrasions are caused by shearing trauma to the epidermis and dermis, resulting in the variable loss of these two layers of skin and potentially deeper layers of tissue such as fat and muscle. These injuries can be small or can potentially cover a large surface area of the body, such as in the case of the cyclist who comes off a bike at speed and slides along a road.

Due to the nature of these injuries, they are often contaminated with dirt, debris and sometimes tar from road surfaces. This debris, if not removed at initial presentation, can become trapped under the skin and lead to unsightly tattooing, which is very difficult to remove later (Richardson 2004b).

Analgesia should be given some time prior to cleansing to make the patient more comfortable. Large pieces of grit or dirt can be removed using forceps or by gentle scrubbing with a surgical sponge. The patient may require additional pain relief such as inhaled nitrous oxide, local anaesthetic infiltration or even intravenous opiates, if the area is particularly large or painful. More recently, utilization of dressings to assist with debridement of these wounds has become more popular. Some hydrocolloid dressing or wound irrigation solutions such as Prontostan® can be used to more gently clean contaminated wounds such as abrasions.

A non-adherent dressing can be applied (see Table 24.10).

Minor burns

Most minor burns are dealt with in EDs and in the community. Minor burns are usually considered to be where the surface area of the burn is less than 5% with only superficial or partial-thickness involvement. Minor burn injuries will heal in the same manner as a minor wound, with epithelialization complete within 7–14 days.

If the burn has occurred within the previous three hours, initial treatment should start with cooling the burned area in running water for 20 minutes and giving the patient analgesia (Cuttle & Kimble 2010). Before considering an appropriate wound dressing, the site and extent of a burn need to be assessed in accordance with the burns unit referral criteria. Intact reddened skin can be treated with non-perfumed emollients such as Vaseline® or E45 cream®. As burn wound infection is the main source of bacteraemia, silver sulphadiazine cream or silver-impregnated dressings are the first-line treatment for burns in the ED. The effectiveness of silver dressings is due to the bacteriostatic effect of the sulphadiazine and the bactericidal effect of silver (Leaper 2006); however, in a systematic review of the literature, Aziz et al. (2011) found that silver-containing dressings and topical silver were either no better or worse than control dressings in preventing wound infection and promoting healing of burn wounds.

Once dressed, the patient should be encouraged to keep flexion surfaces such as the hands and fingers, for example, mobile and the patient referred to a physiotherapist and/or hand therapist where appropriate.

Partial-thickness burns need to be protected against infection and encouraged to heal. Individual gauze and pad dressings for hand and finger burns should be avoided as the mobility of the hand will be impeded (Cole 2003). A burn bag or glove filled with silver sulphadiazine (SSD), silicone or paraffin is an effective alternative as a method of allowing movement, moisture and collection of exudate. Non-flexure surfaces may be dressed with a semi-permeable film dressing (DuKamp 2000); however, there may be leakage in cases of large amounts of exudate. Multiple layers of sterile paraffin tulle dressing (*at least 4*) or a non-stick silicone dressing (e.g. Mepitel©) may be useful alternatives. Silver-based dressings which need to be kept moist are applied for three to seven days, depending on the product. These dressings require a secondary dressing with light compression bandages.

The management of partial-thickness burn blisters is contentious (Rennekampff & Tennenhaus 2010). It is suggested that a blister should be deroofed as not doing so could increase the size of the lesion (Collier 2000); however, this is contradicted by Flanagan & Graham (2001), who describe the detrimental and deepening effects of exposing a burn injury to air. Furthermore, calmodulin, a protein found in burn blisters, has been shown to have a positive effect on healing (Flanagan & Graham 2001), indicating the need to leave the blister intact during the inflammatory phase. Many patients find it very painful to have a blister deroofed in the first day or two following a burn injury; therefore the blister may be left intact and covered with a protective dressing. When the devitalized tissue has become loose and grey it is ready for debridement (Cole 2003).

Major burns are resuscitated as per usual ED procedures and referred for specialist treatment. Burns to functional areas, although often small, are usually referred to burns centres for opinion and ongoing management.

Burns requiring transfer to a specialist centre are often covered with cling wrap to enable the receiving centre to assess the burns prior to dressing. Advice should be sought from the accepting specialist centre.

Skin tears

Skin tears most commonly occur in the elderly and the incidence is expected to increase due to the ageing population (Morey 2007, Baranoski & Ayello 2008). Skin tears are seen in the older population due to the ageing effects on skin from normal ageing processes, disease, mediation and sensory loss leaving the skin more likely to be injured by shearing and friction. These forces are most commonly caused by poor manual handling techniques, wheelchairs and falls. This definition still holds well for today:

> A skin tear is a traumatic wound that occurs principally on the extremities of older adults, as a result of friction alone, or shearing and friction forces, which separate the epidermis from the dermis (partial thickness wound) or which separates both the epidermis and dermis from the underlying structures (full thickness wound) (Payne & Martin 1990).

Classification, descriptions and management of skin tears are variable.

Assessment, management and documentation include identifying other injuries, a thorough assessment and description of the wound, distal neurovascular assessment and comparison between injured and non-injured limb. Given these injuries occur predominantly in the elderly, observation of the patient's general state of health is paramount and plays a role in the ongoing management of the patient for prevention strategies (Ireland 2007, Hoyt et al. 2011).

Treatment of skin tears depends on the category of tear identified. Analgesia should be provided prior to wound cleansing with consideration of the patient's co-morbidities. An anaesthetic cream such as EMLA™ may be placed on the wound with a film dressing for up to 30 minutes provided the wound is not too large as this may lead to toxicity of the local anaesthetic. Wounds require gentle cleansing with saline or tap water ensuring all debris and haematoma are removed from the wound. The viable flap should then be gently realigned to approximate skin edge location and a dressing applied (Stephen-Haynes & Carville 2011).

The choice of dressing is variable and the practitioner must consider the likely amount of exudate and choose the most effective dressing. A compression bandage is then usually applied as per the manufacturer's instructions. Reassessment of the wound may not be needed for 5–7 days provided there is no evidence of infection.

Some centres recommend securing the flap with adhesive strips, but care must be taken when removing the dressing. The outer dressing can be marked with an arrow to designate the direction of the flap and therefore which way the dressing and tapes should be removed. Obviously the dressings must be removed with extreme care and gentleness.

Table 24.11 Classification of skin tears

Category	Depth	Loss of tissue	Management
1A	Lineal tear – partial to full thickness No necrosis, heamatoma or oedema	Occurs in a wrinkle of furrow of skin similar to incision Nil loss of tissue	Gentle cleansing Adhesive strips Cover with non-adherent dressing and review in 5–7 days if no signs of infection
2A	Partial-thickness skin flap No necrosis, no haematoma, mild oedema	Less than 25% loss of epidermal flap and 75% of dermis is covered Limb is warm and well perfused	Gentle cleansing Spread flap gently to approximate edges without tension, Non-adherent dressing Double-layer tubular bandage from tips of fingers or toes to elbow or knee Review in 5–7 days if no signs of infection
2B	Partial-thickness skin flap	Greater than 25% of flap is lost and greater than 25% of dermis is exposed Edges of skin flap may be necrosed, no haematoma, some bruising and oedema Limb is warm and well perfused	Gentle cleansing Spread flap gently to approximate edges without tension Non-adherent dressing for exudating wound, e.g., hydrogel Double-layer tubular bandage from tips of fingers or toes to elbow or knee Review in 5–7 days if no signs of infection
2C	Partial thickness	Greater that 50% of dermis is exposed Edges of flap necrosed, no haematoma, moderate bruising and oedema Limb is warm and well perfused	Gentle cleansing Spread flap gently to approximate edges without tension Non-adherent dressing that abdorbs exudate, e.g. hydrogel Double-layer tubular bandage from tips of fingers or toes to elbow or knee Review in 5–7 days if no signs of infection
3A	Full-thickness dermal skin flap	Fat and potential for fascia exposure in <5 cm² Moderate bruising, no necrosis, minimal haematoma, moderate oedema Limb feels cooler than other limb	Gentle cleansing Spread flap gently to approximate edges without tension, Non-adherent dressing such as hydrogel Double-layer tubular bandage from tips of fingers or toes to elbow or knee Review in 5–7 days if no signs of infection
3B	Full-thickness dermal skin flap	Fat and potential for fascia exposure in less that 5–10 cm² Moderate bruising, up to 50% of flap is necrosed, moderate haematoma, moderate oedema Limb feels cooler than other limb	Gentle cleansing Cover with moist saline dressing pending surgical review

The patient should also be assessed for potential of further skin tears with consideration of adjuncts that will minimize the patient's risk, e.g., manual handling techniques, pressure mattresses, care with types of adhesive tapes for dressings – consider non-adherent stockings to assist and so on. Table 24.11 lists the classification of skin tears as described by Battersby (2009).

Tetanus prophylaxis

Clostridium tetani are Gram-positive, spore-forming anaerobic bacteria found in the soil and animal and human faeces that cause tetanus. Once activated, the bacillus is extremely resistant to almost anything, including sterilization. The incubation period for tetanus is four days to three weeks or more post-injury. Spores may contaminate wounds but remain dormant in tissue for years. After C. *tetani* enters the circulatory system, bacilli attach to cells

in the CNS, causing depression of the respiratory centre in the medulla. Symptoms may be mild or severe and include local joint stiffness and mild trismus or inability to open the jaw, which is where the term 'lockjaw' came from. Severe tetanus is characterized by severe trismus, back pain, penile pain, tachycardia, hypertension, dysrhythmias, hyperpyrexia, opisthotonos, and seizures and can be fatal (Denke 2009). Immediate life-saving treatment involves sedation, airway and respiratory support, active and passive immunization and neutralizing of the tetanus toxin in the body with intravenous antibiotics (Scott 2012).

The Health Protection Agency (2003) states that lifelong immunity to tetanus is achieved after five doses of a vaccine such as Revaxis® (Adsorbed Diphtheria, Tetanus and inactivated Poliomyelitis vaccine 0.5 mL), delivered in three doses as a primary course, followed by a booster 10 years later and a final booster again 10 years later (Reynolds & Cole 2006). Lifelong immunity may not protect against tetanus-prone wounds. These may include wounds that have been

Table 24.12 Anti-tetanus prophylaxis

Immunization status	Clean minor wounds	All other wounds	
Previous doses of tetanus toxoid	Tetanus toxoid-containing vaccine	Tetanus toxoid-containing vaccine	Human tetanus immunoglobulin
< 3 doses or unknown	Yes	Yes	Yes
> 3 or more doses	Only if last dose given greater than 10 years ago	Only if last dose given greater than 5 years ago	No

(Adapted from Department of Health (England) (2011) Tetanus. London: Department of Health.)

crushed, devitalized or contaminated by dirt (Rhee et al. 2005), wounds that are more than six hours old or wounds that have been in contact with soil or manure. Patients with tetanus-prone wounds may need human tetanus immuno-globulin 250 IU intramuscular injection for further protection. See Table 24.12 for Department of Health (England) recommendations.

Wound care and nursing documentation

The Nursing and Midwifery Council has guidelines on record-keeping and state that it is an integral part of nursing practice which should be factual, consistent and accurate. Clinical documentation can be pivotal in cases of negligence and the Nursing and Midwifery Council describes record keeping as an integral part of nursing and midwifery (Nursing and Midwifery Council 2009). Documentation must be clear, legible, timed and dated, signed for, unambiguous and fully completed (Table 24.5).

When assessing and describing a wound it is essential that the correct terminology is used. This is important for two reasons. First, from a medico-legal perspective, a patient's notes are sometimes called in evidence during a coroner's or criminal investigation. Therefore an accurate record of how the wound occurred and the subsequent treatment undertaken is mandatory. Second, poor descriptions of injuries are common and therefore, if in doubt about the causation of the wound, it is preferable to describe it as a wound. Photography can be used to record the initial wound and its subsequent progress during treatment and provides a useful objective record of the injury (Bianco & Williams 2002).

Discharging patients

It is important that patients fully understand what has happened to them during their time in the ED and what to expect in terms of wound healing and wound management. Patient education and applicable fact sheets explaining the wound management will ensure compliance with treatment regimens. Flanagan (1997) highlighted the importance of a number of factors influencing a patient's ability to manage an injury at home (Box 24.5). Patients should have access to

---

Box 24.5

Personal influences on wound healing

- Knowledge and understanding – the patient's and carer's level of knowledge will affect their ability to promote wound healing. The nurse needs to ensure the patient understands wound care guidance and any dieting changes necessary
- Compliance – this is complex and is influenced by the success of treatment so far, the duration of injury, previous experience and the degree of trust in the healthcare professional
- Motivation – this may be influenced by the carer's fear, guilt and how the patient sees the injury in relation to the rest of her life
- Attitude – a positive attitude to recovery will enhance motivation and compliance, particularly if supported with appropriate education
- Body image – this may impact on how the patient cares for the wound
- Financial status – this affects the patient's ability to comply with healthcare advice

---

wound-care materials if appropriate, and access to advice and support from the ED staff.

If the patient has a co-existing illness or condition that may influence their wound healing status, they should be given the appropriate advice related to their condition. For example, patients taking anticoagulants may need sutures or tissue strips left in situ for longer periods. All information should be given in both written and verbal format (using health advocates as required).

If the patient is referred to another healthcare provider for follow-up, it is good practice to give the patient a discharge letter summarizing care to date and the materials for the next dressing. If ongoing wound care will be needed, e.g., in management of burns, patients should be prescribed analgesia to take prior to dressing changes.

Conclusion

Wound care is an important part of the ED nurse's work and is an area of practice where nurses have a great deal of experience and influence. It is imperative that, in addition to good wound-management skills, the nurse also has an in-depth knowledge of wound healing, the threats to healing and the range of wound care methods available.

References

Atiyeh, B.S., Ioannovich, J., Al-Amm, C.A., et al., 2002. Management of acute and chronic open wounds: the importance of moist environment: I optimal wound healing. Current Pharmacological Biotechnology 3, 179–195.

Atiyeh, B.S., Dibo, S.A., Hayek, S.N., 2009. Wound cleansing topical anaesthetics and wound healing. International Wound Journal 6 (6), 20–30, 4.

Autio, L., Olson, K.K., 2002. The four S's of wound management: staples, sutures, steri-strips and sticky stuff. Holistic Nursing Practice 16 (2), 80–88.

Aziz, Z., Abu, S.F., Chong, N.J., 2011. A systematic review of silver-containing dressings and topical silver agents (used with dressings) for burn wounds. Burns 37 (8), 307–318.

Bale, S., Jones, V., 2006. Wound Care Nursing. Mosby Elsevier, Philadelphia.

Bansal, B.C., Wiebe, R.A., Perkins, S.D., et al., 2002. Tap water for irrigation of lacerations. American Journal of Emergency Medicine 20, 469–472.

Baranoski, S., Ayello, E., 2008. Wound Care Essentials: Practice Principles, second ed. Lippincott Williams & Wilkins, Philadelphia.

Battersby, L., 2009. Exploring best practice in the management of skin tears in older people. Nursing Times 105 (16), 22–26.

Bayat, A., McGrouther, D.A., Ferguson, M.W.J., 2003. Skin scarring. British Medical Journal 326, 88–92.

Betts, J., 2003. Wound cleansing with water does not differ from no cleansing or cleansing with other solutions for rates of wound infection or healing. Evidence Based Nursing 6 (3), 81.

Bianco, M., Williams, C., 2002. Using photography in wound assessment. Practice Nursing 13 (11), 505–508.

Bishop, A., 2008. Role of oxygen in wound healing. Journal of Wound Care 17 (9), 399–402.

Bonham, J., 2011. Comparison on suture types in the closure of scalp wounds. Emergency Nurse 19 (3), 34–39.

Bower, M., 2002. Evaluating and managing bite wounds. Advances in Skin and Wound Care 15 (2), 88–90.

Brook, I., 2003. Microbiology and management of human and animal bite wound infections. Primary Care Clinics in Office Practice 30 (1), 25–39.

Brook, I., 2005. Management of human and animal bite wounds: an overview. Advances in Skin & Wound Care 18 (4), 197–203.

Broussard, C.L., 2004. Hyperbaric oxygenation and wound healing. Journal of Vascular Nursing 22 (2), 42–48.

Bryant, R.A., Nix, D., 2006. Acute and Chronic Wound Current Management Concepts, fourth ed. Mosby Year Book, Elsevier, St Louis.

Capellan, O., Hollander, J.E., 2003. Management of lacerations in the emergency department. Emergency Medicine Clinics of North America 21 (1), 205–231.

Carville, K., 2007. Wound Care Manual, fifth ed. Silver Chain Foundation, Western Australia.

Cayton-Richards, M., 2011. Closure of minor wounds with tissue adhesive. Emergency Nurse 18 (9), 18–20.

Chea, A.E.J., Chong, A.K.S., 2011. Bites to the hand: are they more than we can chew? Singapore Medical Journal 52 (10), 715–719.

Chen, E., Hornig, S., Shepherd, S.M., et al., 2000. Primary closure of mammalian bites. Academic Emergency Medicine 7 (2), 157–161.

Clark, A., 2004. Understanding the principles of suturing minor skin lesions. Nursing Times 100 (29), 32–34.

Clark, J.J., 2002. Wound repair and factors influencing healing. Critical Care Nursing Quarterly 25 (1), 1–12.

Cole, E., 2003. Wound management in the A&E department. Nursing Standard 17 (46), 45–52.

Collier, M., 2000. Expert comment on managing burn blisters. NT Plus 96 (4), 20.

Copstead, L., Banasik, J., 2005. Pathophysiology, third ed. Elsevier, Philadelphia.

Correira, K., 2003. Managing dog, cat and human bite wounds. Journal of American Academy of Physicians Assistants 16 (4), 28–37.

Cuttle, L., Kimble, R.M., 2010. First aid treatment of burn injuries. Wound Practice & Research 18 (1), 6–13.

Dandy, D.J., Edwards, D., 2003. Essential Orthopaedics and Trauma, fourth ed. Churchill Livingstone, London.

Dearden, C., Donnelly, J., Dunlop, M., et al., 2001. Traumatic wounds: local wound management. NT Plus 97 (35), 55–57.

Denke, N., 2009. Wound management. In: Sheehy, S. (Ed.), Sheehy's Emergency Nursing, sixth ed. Elsevier, St Louis.

Department of Health (England), 2011. Tetanus. Department of Health, London.

DuKamp, A., 2000. Managing burn blisters. NT Plus 96 (4), 19–20.

Dulecki, M., Pieper, B., 2005. Irrigating simple acute traumatic wounds: a review of the current literature. Journal of Emergency Nursing 31 (2), 156–160.

Eckerline, C., Blake, J., Koury, R., 1999. Puncture wounds and bites in: Topics in Emergency Medicine: A Comprehensive Study Guide, fifth ed. McGraw-Hill, New York.

Fernandez, R., Griffiths, R., Ussia, C., 2003. Water for Wound Cleansing (Cochrane Review). The Cochrane Library. Issue 4. John Wiley & Sons, Chichester.

Fernandez, R., Griffiths, R., Ussia, C., 2004. Effectiveness of solutions, techniques and pressure in wound cleansing. Joanna Briggs Institute, Adelaide.

Flanagan, M., 1997. Wound Healing. Churchill Livingstone, Edinburgh.

Flanagan, M., Graham, J., 2001. Should burn blisters be left intact or debrided? Journal of Wound Care 10 (1), 41–45.

Flarity, K., Hoyt, K.S., 2010. Wound Care and Laceration Repair for Nurse Practitioners in Emergency Care: Part I. Advanced Emergency Nursing Journal 32 (4), 360–372.

Gantwerker, E.A., Hom, D.B., 2012. Skin: histology and physiology of wound healing. Clinics in Plastic Surgery 39 (1), 85–97.

Golan, D.E., 2008. Principles of Pharmacology: The Pathophysiologic Basis of Drug Therapy, second ed. Lippincott Williams & Wilkins, Baltimore, MD.

Goodson, A.M.C., Simmons, J., 2012. Suturing Part 3: Suturing traumatic facial wounds; special areas and tips for tricky closures. Face, Mouth and Jaw Surgery 2 (1), 3–11.

Haller, G., Faltin-Traub, E., Kern, C., 2002. Oxygen embolism after hydrogen peroxide irrigation of a vulval abscess. British Journal of Anaesthesia 88 (4), 597–599.

Health Protection Agency, 2003. Tetanus: Information for Health Professionals. HPA, London.

Henley, N., Carlson, D.A., Kaehr, D.M., et al., 2004. Air embolism associated with irrigation of external fixator pin sites with hydrogen peroxide: A report of two cases. Journal of Bone and Joint Surgery (American) 86 (4), 821–822.

Hock, M., Ong, E., Ooi, S.B.S., et al., 2002. A randomized controlled trial comparing the hair apposition technique with tissue glue to standard suturing in scalp lacerations. Annals of Emergency Medicine 40 (1), 19–26.

Hogg, K., Carley, S., 2002. Staples or sutures for repair of scalp laceration in adults. Emergency Medicine Journal 19 (4), 327–328.

Holt, L., 2000. Wound care. In: Dolan, B., Holt, L. (Eds.), Accident and Emergency: Theory into Practice. Baillière Tindall, Edinburgh.

Hoyt, K.S., Flarity, K., Sanning Shea, S., 2011. Wound care and laceration repair for nurse practitioners in emergency care: Part II. Advanced Emergency Nursing Journal 33 (1), 84–99.

Ip, M., Poon, V., Lung, I., et al., 2006. Antimicrobial activities of silver dressings: An in vitro comparison. Journal of Medical Microbiology 55, 59–63.

Ireland, C., 2007. Pretibial lacerations: management and treatment in the emergency department. Emergency Nurse 14 (9), 18–25.

Joanna Briggs Institute, 2006. Solutions, Techniques and Pressure in Wound Cleansing: A Systematic Review. JBI Reports 10 (2), 1–4.

Klotz, J.H., Klotz, S.A., Pinnas, J.L., 2009. Animal bites and stings with anaphylactic potential. The Journal of Emergency Medicine 36 (2), 148–156.

Kumar, V., Abbas, A., Fausto, N., 2005. Robbins and Cotran Pathologic Basis of Disease, seventh ed. Elsevier, Philadelphia.

Lansdown, A.B.G., 2004. Nutrition 2: A vital consideration in the management of wounds. British Journal of Nursing 13 (20), 1199–1208.

Leaper, D.J., 2006. Silver dressings: their role in wound management. International Wound Journal 3, 282–294.

Lee, G., Bishop, P., 2006. Microbiology and Infection Control for Health Professionals, third ed. Pearson Prentice Hall, Sydney.

Lees, S., 2007. The removal of sutures. Nursing Times 103 (17), 26–27.

Lewis, S., Styles, J., Hamer, J., et al., 2011a. Wound healing outcomes after laceration repair with adhesive. Emergency Nurse 18 (10), 18–21.

Lewis, S.L., Ruff Dirsksen, S., Heitkemper, M.M. (Eds.), 2011b. Medical-Surgical Nursing, Assessment & Management of Clinical Problems, eighth ed. Mosby, St Louis.

McKenna, D., 2006. Hand assessment. Emergency Nurse 14 (6), 26–37.

Morey, P., 2007. Skin tears: A literature review. Primary Intention 15 (3), 122–129.

Morgan, M., Palmer, J., 2007. Dog bites. British Medical Journal 334, 413–417.

Murphy, G., Sellheyer, K., Mihm, M., 2005. In: Kumar, V., Abbas, A., Fausto, N. (Eds.), Robbins and Cotran Pathologic Basis Of Disease, seventh ed. Elsevier, St Louis.

Mustoe, T.A., 2004. Scars and keloids. British Medical Journal, 1329–1330.

Myers, J., 1982. Modern plastic surgery dressings. Health and Social Services Journal 92, 336–337.

National Institute for Health and Clinical Excellence, 2005. Skin Disorders and Wounds. NIHCE, London.

Naude, L., 2010. The practice and science of wound healing. Professional Nurse Today 14 (3), 17–21.

NHS Information Centre for Health and Social Care, 2011. Hospital Episode Statistics Online: Accident and Emergency Attendances in England (Experimental Statistics) 2008-09. NHS Information Centre, London.

Nursing and Midwifery Council, 2009. Record Keeping: Guidance for Nurses and Midwives. Nursing and Midwifery Council, London.

Oehler, R.L., Velez, A.P., Mizrachi, M., et al., 2009. Bite-related and septic syndromes caused by cats and dogs. The Lancet Infectious Diseases 9, 439–447.

Ong, M.E.H., Hock, M., Ooi, S.M., et al., 2002. A randomized controlled trial comparing the hair apposition technique with tissue glue to standard suturing in scalp lacerations (HAT study). Annals of Emergency Medicine 40, 19–26.

Payne, R., Martin, M., 1990. The epidemiology and management of skin tears in older adults. Ostomy/Wound Management 26, 26–37.

Quaba, O., Huntley, J.S., Bahia, H., et al., 2005. A users guide for reducing the pain of local anaesthetic administration. Emergency Medicine Journal 22, 188–189.

Rabenberg, V.S., Ingersoll, C.D., Sandrey, M.A., et al., 2002. The bacterial and cytotoxic effects of antimicrobial wound cleansers. Journal of Athletic Training 37 (1), 51–54.

Rees, J., 2003. Where have all the bubbles gone? An ode to hydrogen peroxide, the champagne of all wound cleaners. Accident & Emergency Nursing 11, 82–84.

Rennekampff, H.O., Tennenhaus, M., 2010. Debridement of the burn wound. Color Atlas of Burn Reconstructive Surgery 1, 10–14.

Resuscitation Council (UK), 2010. Resuscitation Guidelines. Resuscitation Council (UK), London.

Reynolds, T., 2004. Ear, nose and throat problems in accident and emergency. Nursing Standard 20 (1), 55–64.

Reynolds, T., Cole, E., 2006. Techniques for acute wound closure. Nursing Standard 20 (21), 55–64.

Rhee, P., Reynolds, T., Nunley, M.K., et al., 2005. Tetanus and trauma: a review and recommendations. Journal of Trauma, Injury, Infection and Critical Care 58 (5), 1082–1088.

Richardson, M., 2004a. Acute wounds: an overview of the physiological healing process. Nursing Times 100 (4), 50–53.

Richardson, M., 2004b. Wound care: procedures for cleansing, closing and covering acute wounds. Nursing Times 100 (4), 54–58.

Richardson, M., 2006. The management of animal and human bite wounds. Nursing Times 102 (3), 34–36.

Russell, L., 2000. Understanding Physiology of Wound Healing and how dressings help. British Journal of Nursing 9 (1), 10–12.

Scholl, D., Langkamp-Henken, B., 2001. Nutrient Recommendations for Wound Healing. Journal of Intravenous Nursing 24 (2), 124–132.

Scott, T., 2012. Point-of-care tetanus immunoassay: An audit of tetanus prophylaxis. International Journal of Orthopaedic and Trauma Nursing 16 (2), 97–103.

Seidel, H., Ball, J., Dains, J., et al., 2006. Mosby's Guide to Physical Examination, sixth ed. Elsevier, St Louis.

Sinatra, R., 2002. Role of COX-2 inhibitors in the evolution of acute pain management. Journal of Pain Symptom Management 24(Suppl 1), S18–S27.

Smith, P.F., Meadowcroft, A.M., May, D.B., 2000. Treating mammalian bite wounds. Journal of Clinical Pharmacy & Therapeutics 25 (2), 85–99.

Stephen-Haynes, J., Carville, K., 2011. Skin tears made easy. Wounds International 2 (4), 3–5.

Taplitz, R.A., 2004. Managing bite wounds. Postgraduate Medicine 116 (2), 49.

Thomas Hess, C., 2011. Checklist for factors affecting wound health. Advances in Skin & Wound Care 24 (4), 192.

Tortora, G.J., Grabowski, S.R., 2003. Principles of Anatomy and Physiology, tenth ed. John Wiley & Sons, New Jersey.

Towler, J., 2001. Cleansing traumatic wounds with swabs, water or saline. Journal of Wound Care 10 (6), 231–234.

Valente, J.H., Forti, R.J., Freundlich, L.F., et al., 2003. Wound irrigation in children: saline solution or tap water? Annals of Emergency Medicine 41, 609–616.

Waller, R., Tan, G., 2009. Wound care and repair. In: Cameron, P., Jelinek, G., Kelly, A.M., Murray, L., Brown, A.F.T., Heyworth, J. (Eds.), Textbook of Adult Emergency Medicine (eds), third ed. Churchill Livingstone Elsevier, Sydney.

Walsh, M., Kent, A. (Eds.), 2001. Soft tissue injury. In: Accident & Emergency Nursing, fourth ed. Butterworth Heinemann, Oxford.

Widgerow, A.D., 2011. Current concepts in scar evolution and control. Aesthetic Plastic Surgery 35, 628–635.

Pain and pain management

Paula Grainger

Introduction

Pain is a primitive, multi-dimensional experience with physiological, psychological, social and emotional components. The International Association for the Study of Pain (IASP) Subcommittee on Taxonomy (Merskey & Bogduk 1994) describes pain as 'an unpleasant sensory and emotional experience associated with actual or potential tissue damage or described in terms of such damage'. Pain is also a valuable and necessary part of the body's defence mechanism and usually indicates that something is wrong, for example, physical damage or disease (Scholz & Woolf 2002). Pain management meanwhile is a fundamental feature of healthcare with the aim to achieve comfort through some form of analgesia – taken from the Greek word for painlessness.

This chapter will consider the physiological and psychological elements of pain and will identify assessment tools that may be used in the Emergency Department (ED). Pharmacological and non-pharmacological analgesic methods will be considered and the nurse's role in relieving pain and suffering will be explored.

Feeling pain – transmission anatomy and physiology

Pain is felt when sensory nerve endings are stimulated and neurones relay information to the brain. Specialized pain receptors, known as nociceptors, are found in free nerve endings close to mast cells and small blood vessels that all work together to respond to pain (McHugh & McHugh 2000). Nociceptors are found in large numbers in the skin, arterial walls, periosteum and joint surfaces and in smaller numbers in all of the deep tissues of the body (Marieb & Hoehn 2007).

There appear to be two distinct types of nociceptors: high-threshold mechanoreceptors that respond to strong mechanical stimuli, and polymodal nociceptors that respond to mechanical, thermal and chemical stimuli (McHugh & McHugh 2000). Mechanical stimuli, e.g., compressing or stretching tissues and thermal stimuli, e.g., excess heat or cold, appear to stimulate the nociceptors through chemical mediator release (Allan 2005). Chemical stimuli occur as a result of the substances that are released from damaged tissues, e.g., prostaglandins, serotonin, bradykinin and histamine (McHugh & McHugh 2000). Examples of tissue damage when such chemicals are released are infection, ischaemia, inflammation, ulceration and nerve damage (Godfrey 2005).

Once nociceptors are stimulated, the sensory or afferent nerve fibres of which they are formed carry the impulses to the spinal column. Two types of sensory (afferent) fibre are involved in this transmission:

- A-delta fibres respond to stimulation of the high-threshold mechanoreceptors. The fibres are large diameter and thinly myelinated. They transmit pain impulses rapidly (about 5–30 m/s) and are known as 'first' or 'fast' fibres. Pain sensation is usually sharp pricking, well-localized or stinging (Hudspith et al. 2006).
- C fibres connect to the polymodal receptors. They are smaller, unmyelinated fibres that conduct at 0.5–2 m/s and are known as 'second' or 'slow' pain fibres. Pain sensation may be burning, dull and poorly localized or aching.

Other fibres and receptors involved are:

- A-beta fibres are thicker and heavily myelinated, conducting information such as touch, pressure and temperature very rapidly (30–100 m/s) but not pain.
- opioid receptors are found throughout the brain and spinal cord and respond to naturally occurring endogenous opioids and to synthetic exogenous opioids.

A-delta fibres, C fibres and T (transmitter) neurones in the spinal cord

Information carried by the A-delta fibres and C fibres is relayed to the substantia gelatinosa in the dorsal horn of the spine where the neurones terminate and synapse with T (transmitter) neurones (Fig. 25.1). For the transfer of this information between the A-delta and C fibres to the T neurones excitatory neurochemical transmitters need to be released, since there is a synaptic cleft between the two (Strøma et al. 2012). These transmitters include adenosine triphosphate, glutamate, calcitonin gene-related peptide, bradykinin, nitrous oxide and substance P. The T neurones cross the spinal cord and ascend on the opposite side of the spino-thalmic tract carrying pain information to the medulla where they re-cross to the original side and synapse with secondary sensory neurones that transmit the sensation onto the thalamus in the brain. It is at this point that the sensation is experienced in a general manner without detail. From the thalmus a third group of neurones relay the information to the cerebral cortex and the somatosensory cortex to allow pain localization and stimulus interpretation. This perception of pain in the brain is vital as it allows us to act to

relieve or alleviate the situation. Fibres from the thalamus also connect with the hypothalamus and reticular system, accounting for the changes in the autonomic nervous system outlined below and the motor response, and to the limbic system where emotional and behavioural responses are generated (Godfrey 2005).

A-beta nerve fibres

A-beta fibres do not carry pain information, but do attach to low-threshold mechanoreceptors. They enter the spine at the dorsal horn but do not synapse with other neurones or cross the spine; instead they ascend to the brain in the ipsilateral column of nerve fibres and relay information to the lower medulla where they synapse with connecting neurones to the thalamus and cerebral cortex.

Opioids and opioid receptors

While substance P and glutamate have been implicated in the transmission of pain, other neurochemicals appear to possess analgesic properties. These include endorphins, enkephalins and dynorphins, which are produced by the body and have an analgesic action similar to that of morphine. Further research is required, but the existence and action of these chemicals help to explain phenomena such as the placebo response, where an individual perceives pain relief even though no analgesic agent has been given. It appears that, in such cases, the mere expectation of pain relief is sufficient to release psychogenically the endogenous opiates, which would then cause a genuine analgesia even without the administration of an analgesic drug (Allan 2005).

Pain theories

Pain was originally thought to be due to the activities of demons and evil spirits or to be the penalty for wrongdoings. A number of theories have been proposed and developed in order to understand and explain the process of pain. Two will be considered here: the specificity theory and the gate control theory.

Specificity theory

The traditional specificity theory was developed by Descartes in 1644 (Godfrey 2005). Descartes thought there was a direct link from the point of pain to the brain, suggesting that pain is a specific sensation and that pain intensity is proportional to the extent of the tissue damage (Watt-Watson & Ivers Donovan 1992). According to this theory, pain associated with a minor cut gives minimal discomfort, whereas pain associated with major trauma hurts far more. It is now known that pain is not simply a function of the amount of bodily damage, but is influenced by attention, anxiety, suggestion, experience and other psychological variables (Melzack & Wall 1982). However, current research indicates that conduction

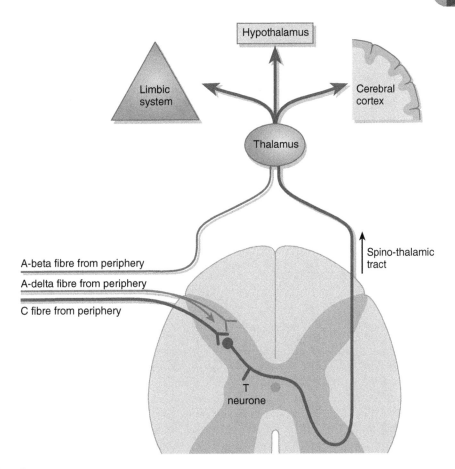

Figure 25.1 • The pain pathway.

of pain impulses is more complex than was originally proposed. The recognition of the pain pathways inherent in the specificity theory provides the basis for surgery of intractable pain where the pain pathway is interrupted so impulses cannot reach consciousness (Hallet 1992).

Gate control theory

The gate control theory of pain proposed by Melzack & Wall (1965) revolutionized the understanding of pain. They proposed the idea of a 'gate' in the substantia gelatinosa in the dorsal (or posterior) horn of the spinal cord through which pain information must pass on its way to the brain. The substantia gelatinosa is an area of special neurones located close to each posterior column of grey matter and extending the length of the spinal cord. A number of factors can block or close the 'gate' to pain messages, but equally other factors will open the gate and allow pain to be experienced by the individual. When nerve impulses from the nociceptors are brought to the dorsal horn by A-delta and C fibres and relayed to the T neurones, the gate is opened.

The T neurones can be inhibited by neurochemical transmitters released by tiny interneurones in the substantia gelatinosa. The A-beta fibres synapse with these interneurones and inhibit transmission of information to the T neurone (Fig. 25.2).

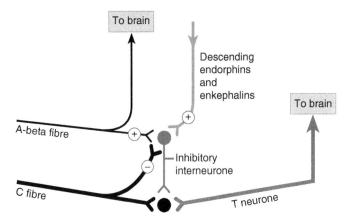

Figure 25.2 • Inhibitory interneurone and pain transmission.

Inhibition of the T neurone reduces the flow of pain information to the brain, effectively 'closing' the pain gate. Increasing activity in the A-beta fibres (touch, pressure, temperature) lessens the pain felt, while an increase in activity in the small-diameter A-delta and C fibres means that more pain is perceived (Barasi 1991). This is the basis for many of the non-pharmacological pain-relieving measures, including 'rubbing it better', the application of heat or cold, electrical stimulation and countercurrent irritation, all of which stimulate the A-beta fibres and so reduce the pain messages being relayed to the brain.

The gating mechanism is affected by information flowing from the brain through the descending inhibitory pathways. These pathways originate in a number of areas of the brain (i.e., reticular formation, periaqueductal grey matter, raphe nuclei) and synapse with the inhibitory neurones in the substantia gelatinosa, releasing the neurotransmitters serotonin and noradrenaline norepinephrine (Barasi 1991). These inhibitory neurotransmitters excite the interneurones in the dorsal horn of the spine secreting the body's natural endogenous opioids (endorphins, enkephalins and dynorphins) that inhibit the T neurones suppressing pain transmission. They also block the release of substance P from the A-delta and C fibres and block the receptors for substance P on the T neurones (Sherwood 2010). Allowing the brain to release endogenous opiates is a key factor in pain relief and several methods can be employed in emergency settings to try to achieve this:

- use of sensory input, such as distraction, guided imagery and hypnotism
- reducing fear and lowering the level of anxiety
- patient education about the cause and relief of pain.

If the inhibitory interneurones are stimulated, either by the A-beta fibres or by input from descending brain pathways, fewer pain impulses will be relayed to the T fibres and so less pain information will be carried to the brain. Melzack & Wall (1965) felt that this theory explains why the relationship between pain and injury is so variable and why the location of pain can differ from the site of injury. It also explains how pain can persist in the absence of injury or after healing and why the nature and location of pain can change over time. Hallet (1992) suggested that the gate control theory expands the role of the spinal cord; it is not just a relay station, but a centre for filtering and integrating incoming sensory information.

Effects of pain

Physiological effects

The physiological responses that occur when the nociceptors are stimulated are similar to those of the acute stress ('flight-or-fight') response as first described by Cannon (1915) also known as the freeze, fight, or flight response (Bracha et al. 2004). The sympathetic nervous system is activated causing general vasoconstriction, while dilating the arteries supplying vital organs such as the muscles (McArdle et al. 2006). This results in tachycardia, tachypnoea, hypertension, sweating and pallor. Tidal volume and alveolar ventilation may be reduced, as is gastric motility. Skeletal muscle spasm may occur and hormonal changes may cause electrolyte imbalances and hyperglycaemia (Sutcliffe 1993).

Non-physiological effects

There is evidence that everyone has the same pain threshold, i.e., they perceive pain at the same stimulus intensity. Sternback & Tursky (1965) found that there was no difference among four different ethnic groups in the level of electric shock that was first reported as producing a detectable sensation.

Box 25.1

Pain thresholds

- Sensation threshold – the lowest stimulus value at which a sensation, such as tingling or warmth, is first reported
- Pain perception threshold – the lowest stimulus value at which the person reports that the stimulation feels painful
- Pain tolerance (or upper threshold) – the lowest stimulus level at which the subject withdraws or asks to have the stimulation stopped
- Encouraged threshold – the highest stimulus level the subject will tolerate after being encouraged to tolerate higher levels than identified in the pain tolerance threshold

---

Heat, for example, is perceived as painful by everyone at the 44–46°C range when it begins to damage tissues (Marieb & Hoehn 2007). The sensory conducting apparatus, in other words, appears to be essentially similar in all people so that a given level of input always elicits a sensation. However, an individual's tolerance of and response to pain will be affected by a number of factors other than those described above. The different thresholds associated with pain are identified in Box 25.1.

Although there is evidence that everyone, regardless of cultural background, has a uniform threshold, cultural background does have a powerful effect on the pain tolerance levels. Sternback & Tursky (1965) reported that the levels at which subjects refused to tolerate electric shocks, even when they were encouraged by experimenters, depended in part on the ethnic origin of the subject. For the emergency nurse, this may explain the differing reactions to pain of individuals from different cultural backgrounds.

Anxiety and the experience of pain have also been linked (Hayward 1975, Cave 1994). Hayward (1975) demonstrated that if patients were given information regarding their post-operative pain, they experienced less pain and required less analgesia. Walsh (1993) found in a study of patients with relatively minor problems that of the 90% with pain, many were anxious. He suggested that this might be due to a variety of reasons:

- the sudden and unexpected disruption of the illness or injury
- fear of treatment
- fear of the possible long-term effects of the illness or injury
- fear of the unknown hospital treatment.

Pain is not simply a physiological response; rather it is a psycho-physiological phenomenon, explaining why the experience of pain is unique for each person (Sofaer 1992). As McCaffery (1983) noted, 'pain is always a subjective experience and pain is what the patient says it is and exists when the patient says it does'.

Assessing pain

Uncontrolled acute pain is known to cause psychological distress, and it may also lead to adverse physiological changes in some organs and systems (Green & McGhie 2010). As a consequence, it needs to be assessed and addressed early and effectively.

Individuals not only feel and react differently to pain, but describe it differently as well (Sofaer 1998). It is difficult to measure pain as it is a subjective phenomenon especially in relation to the cultural values and norms regarding the expression of pain as well as a result of the psychological response. This is further complicated where patients are unable to describe their pain because of the location or severity of their injury, their age or cognitive ability or because they are unconscious or intubated. In part, this may explain why pain levels are often poorly documented in emergency settings (Chisolm et al. 2008, Easton et al. 2012). The aim of pain assessment is to take the patient's subjective experience and transform it into objective data which health professionals can understand and use to plan relevant pain-relieving measures and monitor their effect.

In some situations it will be immediately obvious that the patient is profoundly distressed and requires urgent intervention, e.g., the patient suddenly presenting to the ED with severe crushing chest pain. Intervention in these circumstances should be immediate and only a brief assessment of the situation is required. In other circumstances, however, a more thorough assessment is required and should be ongoing in the light of the patient's current and in some cases their already known clinical condition. Hallet (1992) identified the range of information that should be included when making pain assessments (Box 25.2).

Pain assessment tools

A number of pain assessment tools are available (Green & McGhie 2010) that are potentially useful in the ED. Scales can be used to measure pain, treatment effectiveness and satisfaction. Three scores are the Verbal Rating Scale (VRS) scoring from 'no pain' to 'severe pain'; the Visual Analogue Scale (VAS) consisting of a line that ranges from 'no pain' to 'worst pain imaginable' where the patient points to a position on the line; and the Numeric Rating Scale (NRS), using a scoring 0-10 or 0-5. Williamson & Hoggart (2005) argue that the VAS and NRS are not interchangeable; however, they continue to be used in combination. The VRS has the benefit of simplicity but is less sensitive than either the VAS or the NRS (Green & McGhie 2010). The advantages of the VAS combined with a NRS are as follows:

- it is sensitive to small changes
- it can be used to measure pain intensity
- it can be used to measure pain relief
- it is easy for the patient to use
- the numerical interpretation that facilitates documentation.

The disadvantages of VAS are that:

- pain is scored on a single dimension only
- some patient groups, such as the visually impaired, cognitively impaired, children or the elderly, may find it difficult to use.

Box 25.2

Detailed pain assessment (after Hallet 1992)

Location

The location should be identified as specifically as possible. For instance, abdominal pain may be localized to the lower or upper left or right quadrant, epigastrium or mid-abdomen. The site may be well defined or diffuse or the pain may radiate, involving a wide area. Observing the pain's location(s) on the patient's body can help to localize the sites of pain, as well as identifying physical changes at the site, such as swelling or discoloration.

Intensity

The intensity or severity of pain experienced should be translated into words or numbers that can provide objective data for ongoing assessment. Visual analogue scales and numerical scales, with or without written descriptions, are often used.

Quality

A description of pain, using the patient's own words, is helpful in determining the origin of pain, its cause and possible pain relief measures. For instance, patients with cardiac-related chest pain may describe it as 'crushing', whereas patients with non-cardiac-related chest pain may describe a 'sharp' pain, usually related to inspiration. Other words used to describe pain are throbbing, stabbing, cramping, squeezing, hot or burning, heavy, dull, tearing, stretching and aching.

Onset and duration

When the pain first began and how the pain has changed over time should be determined. If the pain varies over the course of a day, this variation and the circumstances surrounding the variation should be noted. The pattern may be constant, intermittent, variable, etc.

Relief measures

The efficacy of measures used by the patient to relieve pain should be identified. Any medications, including analgesia, taken by the patient prior to attendance at ED should be recorded.

Exacerbating factors

Often patients may be comfortable at rest, but have difficulty moving due to pain. For instance, patients with abdominal pain may be more comfortable sitting upright than lying flat on the ED trolley. In most instances, the ED nurse should support patients by making them as comfortable as possible, except where this may compromise their safety such as lying over the end of the trolley.

Associated symptoms

Associated symptoms can include nausea and vomiting, profuse perspiration, fainting, inability to perform usual functions, dulling of senses, apathy, clouding of consciousness, disorientation and inability to rest and sleep.

For children under three years old the observational FLACC scale (Merkel et al. 1997) is available. This includes five categories: face, legs, activity, cry and consolability with each category scoring 0–2 with a maximum of 10 points awarded overall.

For children over the age of three years and those unable to grasp the concept of linear scales, pain rating scales using pictures of faces have become popular, e.g., Wong-Baker

FACES™ (Hockenberry & Wilson 2009). The faces, which are in increasing degrees of distress, are shown to patients who are then asked to point to the one that depicts the amount of pain they are feeling. Each face has a numeric link to it making it easily recordable. However, concern about these pain scales has been expressed by Mather & Mackie (1983), who noted that children sometimes played down their pain because they did not want to be given an injection. They found that pain reporting has the potential to be inaccurate where the consequences were known or expected to be unpleasant, e.g., administration of an injection.

Similarly, adult patients, particularly those who are elderly, may minimize their pain reports and will suffer in silence because they do not want to be seen as a 'nuisance' to nursing staff or to their families. The emergency nurse should therefore reassure patients that their needs are being taken seriously and evaluate pain requirements and relief at regular intervals. As none of these assessment tools is of use in the semi-conscious patient or in infants, the nurse must use her observational skills and knowledge of physiological responses to pain to estimate its severity. The most important observations include facial expression, grimacing, movement, posture and interaction with others. In severe pain, the patient's blood pressure, pulse rate and respiration may increase and therefore should be recorded.

Pharmacological pain management

Most acute pain is managed solely with drugs. Analgesic drugs work in several ways: by altering the pain sensation, depressing pain perception or modifying the patient's response to pain. As a general principle, drugs are used most effectively if their selection is based on the cause and intensity of pain. They can be delivered in a variety of routes (Box 25.3).

Analgesics act in the brain, spinal cord, nerve endings and at the site of tissue damage to reduce the amount of pain being felt. They are selective as they are able to diminish pain without affecting other sensations (O'Hara & Campling 1996). Moreover, analgesics do not 'mask pain', particularly that of abdominal pain hindering assessment (Helfand & Freeman 2009). Analgesics can be divided into two groups: opiates and non-opiates.

Box 25.3

Routes of analgesia administration

- Oral (p.o.)
- Rectal (p.r.)
- Topical
- Transmucosal/Intra-nasal (i.n.)
- Inhalation (Inh)
- Subcutaneous (s.c.)
- Intramuscular (i.m.)
- Intravenous (i.v.)
- Epidural

Opiates

Opiates are used in the treatment of moderate to severe pain and work by binding to the opiate receptors in the CNS and thus modulate the transmission of nociceptive pain messages via the 'gate' in the spinal cord. Opiate analgesics may also initially produce sedation, reduce fear and anxiety and promote sleep. Drawbacks of opiate use is that they stimulate the chemoreceptor trigger zone (CTZ) in the brain stem, causing nausea and vomiting in about 30% of patients and can produce respiratory depression by acting on respiratory centres in the brain. The antidote naloxone can reverse this effect. Four opiates used as analgesics are morphine, diamorphine, fentanyl and pethidine.

Morphine

Morphine is a derivative of the opium poppy and is extremely effective. In the ED it is usually administered intravenously or orally. It alleviates pain and anxiety; however, the nurse should note the following (Greenstein & Gould 2004):

- the pupils of the eye are constricted due to an effect on the nucleus of the third facial nerve
- morphine stimulates the vagus nerve, which may present difficulties when morphine is used for the pain of coronary thrombosis as it may further reduce the pulse rate and blood pressure
- morphine causes spasms of the sphincters, including the sphincter of Oddi, and therefore should not be used in pancreatitis.

In trauma cases, oral or intramuscular morphine should not be given as the shocked patient will have poor perfusion leading to limited initial drug absorption and bolus absorption following resuscitation (Driscoll et al. 1994).

Diamorphine

The actions of diamorphine are similar to those of morphine, but it is 2.5 times more potent as an analgesic agent (Thompson & Webster 1992) with a similar rise in side effects. It is the drug of choice in the management of severe central chest pain in many countries. Intravenous (i.v.) administration should be accompanied with anti-emetics, and the depressant effects on the respiratory centre need to be monitored, particularly in patients with chronic chest disease. Diamorphine is usually administered in a dose of 2.5–5 mg i.v., repeated as necessary. Diamorphine, a class A controlled drug, is also known as heroin and the antidote naloxone 0.4 mg i.v. should always be available.

Fentanyl

The actions of fentanyl are similar to those of morphine although it has a faster peak, shorter duration of action, and a non-histamine release that can reduce adverse effects experienced by the patient, particularly hypotension (Braude & Richards 2004). Fentanyl lends itself well to situations where establishing i.v. access may be difficult, e.g., in young children, but where significant pain needs to be addressed. This is because it may be administered intranasally for absorption by the mucosa (Borland et al. 2007), or nebulized and inhaled for absorption across alveoli (Furyk et al. 2009).

Pethidine

Pethidine is a synthetically derived analgesic that has similar actions to diamorphine and is chemically related to atropine. It is less powerful than morphine but has a lower risk of respiratory depression and does not cause constriction of the pupils; it is therefore used in head injuries where observation of the pupil size may be important (Goldstein & Gould 2004). Unlike morphine, it does not cause spasms of the sphincters and is the analgesic of choice in pancreatitis. It is worthy of note that pethidine can react with monoamine oxidase inhibitor (MAOI) drugs and cause severe hypertension (Carr & Mann 2000).

Non-opiates

Effective relief can be achieved with oral non-opioids and NSAIDs. These drugs are appropriate for treating much pain after minor surgery, such as incision and drainage, or on discharge home, for instance, following musculoskeletal injury. Two examples of non-opiates are Entonox, paracetamol/acetaminophen and non-steroidal anti-inflammatory drugs (NSAIDs).

Entonox

This gaseous mixture of 50 % oxygen and 50 % nitrous oxide can be effective as a short-term analgesic agent. Its primary use is to provide pain relief to conscious patients who are able to use the demand valve system of delivery for analgesia during unpleasant procedures, e.g., during splinting (Adam & Osborne 1997). It is contraindicated when there is a pneumothorax or a fracture to the base of the skull (Driscoll et al. 1994) or in a prolonged manner for potential bowel obstruction (McKinnon 1980).

Paracetamol/Acetophinomen

This is most suitable for mild to moderate pain. Its mechanism of action remains in debate. It is thought to act by inhibiting the cycloxygenase (Cox-I, Cox-II, Cox-III) enzymes, therefore increasing the patient's pain threshold. It has no impact on the inflammatory response nor on platelet function or gastric mucosa. It can be used in combination with other analgesia but caution needs to be used as many patients self-administer this pre-hospital which can lead to the unintentional self-poisoning (Bronstein et al. 2010).

NSAIDs

These are the most widely used analgesics. Commonly used NSAIDs include aspirin, indometacin and ibuprofen. They are effective particularly in relieving pain associated with inflammation, such as musculoskeletal disorders, trauma to peripheral tissues and headache. Some studies have shown that NSAIDs provided pain relief equal to or better than 10 mg intramuscular morphine (McQuay & Moore 1998). NSAIDs also act on the hypothalamus to reset the body's thermostat during febrile episodes, reducing the temperature.

NSAIDs inhibit the enzyme cyclo-oxygenase and thus affect the body's production of prostaglandins (Carr & Mann 2000), which cause pain and inflammation. However, prostaglandins are also responsible for maintaining the mucous lining of the gastric mucosa. As a consequence, the use of NSAIDs can lead to gastric damage, which may range from nausea or 'heartburn' to gastrointestinal bleeding. This can be ameliorated by recommending the patient to take the NSAIDs with meals and/or milk. NSAIDs can also trigger asthmatic reactions, and patients should be asked if they suffer from asthma before NSAIDs are prescribed or dispensed. In the past five years, selective cyclo-oxygenase II specific inhibitors (COX-II) have been developed which produce analgesia with fewer side effects.

Non-pharmacological pain management

In addition to pharmacological interventions, there is a wide range of pain-relieving strategies that can be employed by the nurse to relieve patient pain and suffering. These include information, positioning, thermal, mechanical and/or electrical stimuli and distraction and the placebo effect. McCaffery (1990) has suggested that a combination of pharmacological and non-pharmacological methods probably yields the most effective relief for the patient.

Information

Attention to factors identified by the patient and, for example, to his level of anxiety regarding pain is essential. Hayward's classic study showed that patients who were kept informed about the level of discomfort and pain they could expect reported lower levels of pain (Hayward 1975). It is both unwise and unethical for the nurse to state that a patient will not feel pain before a painful procedure. This is especially true for children, who may subsequently lose trust in their health carers. Honesty with reassurance can do much to alleviate the mental suffering associated with current or impending pain from nursing and medical procedures.

Positioning

Immobilization and elevation are simple but effective measures can do much to alleviate pain and suffering and are particularly useful for patients who have sustained musculoskeletal injuries. The nurse can use slings, splints, pillows or blankets to place the injured limb in a comfortable position and should advise the patient to move it as little as possible. Swelling and pain, particularly when associated with soft tissue injury, can also be reduced by elevation of an injured limb (Walsh 1996).

Thermal and mechanical stimulation and electroanalgesia

For patients who have sustained musculoskeletal injuries, superficial burns or other injuries, the use of cold compresses can reduce swelling and alleviate pain. They act by reducing the release of pain-causing chemicals, such as lactic acid, potassium ions, serotonin and histamine (Lee & Warren 1978). The nurse should ensure that the cold compress does not cause further injury, such as frostbite, and therefore ice should be placed in a plastic bag and covered with a paper or cloth towel. The use of gel packs which can be kept cool in the fridge or warmed in hot water can reduce this risk.

Warm compresses may also be used to reduce pain by triggering pain-inhibiting reflexes through temperature receptors. They are particularly effective for muscle and joint pain. However, because warmth increases swelling and the tendency to bleed, it is contraindicated after trauma. Because heat can burn, it should be used with particular caution over areas with impaired sensation or in patients with limited or no ability to communicate. These types of stimulation reduce the pain message relayed to the brain through the stimulation of A-beta nerve fibres. Examples are massage, stretching and transcutaneous electrical nerve stimulation (TENS).

Distraction

McCaffery (1990) defined distraction as simply focusing attention on stimuli other than the pain sensation. One of the most frequently used distraction techniques in the ED involves breathing exercises. Patients are directed to focus their breathing by concentrating on inhalations and exhalations. Appropriate use of humour is also a successful distraction strategy that has been shown to improve the release of the body's natural endorphins (Watt-Watson & Ivers Donovan, 1992). More recent distractions include use of audio-visual media, such as artwork, music, movies and electronic games.

Conclusion

The emergency nurse has a key role in the assessment and management of pain. This chapter has outlined the physiological and psychological effects of pain as well as a number of assessment tools the nurse may employ in the ED. Pharmacological and non-pharmacological means of delivering pain relief have also been considered. Non-pharmacological methods in particular are usually effective, simple to apply and easy to learn.

The emergency nurse has a responsibility to obtain a working knowledge of the range of strategies available to decrease pain and to use them to alleviate patient suffering and improve the quality of care.

References

Adam, S.K., Osborne, S., 1997. Critical Care Nursing: Science and Practice. Oxford Medical, Oxford.

Allan, D., 2005. Sensory receptors and sense organs. In: Montague, S.E., Watson, R., Herbert, R.A. (Eds.), Physiology for Nursing Practice, third ed. Elsevier, London.

Barasi, S., 1991. The physiology of pain. Surgical Nurse 4 (5), 14–20.

Borland, M., Jacobs, I., King, B., et al., 2007. A randomized controlled trial comparing intranasal fentanyl to intravenous morphine for managing acute pain in children in the emergency department. Annals of Emergency Medicine 49 (3), 335–340.

Bracha, H.S., Ralston, T.C., Matsukawa, J.M., 2004. Does 'fight or flight' need updating? Psychomatics 45 (5), 448–449.

Braude, D., Richards, M., 2004. Appeal for fentanyl prehospital use. Prehospital Emergency Care. 8, 441–442.

Bronstein, A. C., Spyker, D. A., Cantilena, L. R., et al. 2009. Annual Report of the American Association of Poison Control Centres (NPDS) 27th Annual Report Clinical Toxicology 48, 979–1178.

Cannon, W.B., 1915. Bodily Changes in Pain, Hunger, Fear and Rage: An Account of Recent Researches into the Function of Emotional Excitement. Appleton-Century-Crofts, New York.

Carr, E.C.J., Mann, E.M., 2000. Pain: Creative Approaches to Effective Management. Macmillan Press, Basingstoke.

Cave, I., 1994. Pain in A&E: the patient's view. Emergency Nurse 2 (2), 19–20.

Chisholm, C.D., Weaver, C.S., Whenmouth, L.F., et al., 2008. A comparison of observed versus documented physician assessment and treatment of pain: the physician record does not reflect the reality. Annals of Emergency Medicine 52, 383–389.

Driscoll, P., Gwinnutt, C., Brook, S., 1994. Extremity trauma. In: Driscoll, P.A., Gwinnutt, C.L., LeDuc Jimmerson, C., Goodall, A. (Eds.), Trauma Resuscitation: The Team Approach. Macmillan, Basingstoke.

Easton, R.M., Bendinelli, C., Sisak, K., et al., 2012. Recalled pain scores are not reliable after acute trauma. Injury 43 (7), 1029–1032.

Furyk, J.S., Grabowski, W.J., Black, L.H., 2009. Nebulized fentanyl versus intravenous morphine in children with suspected limb fractures in the emergency department: A randomized controlled trial. Emergency Medicine Australasia 21 (3), 203–209.

Godfrey, H., 2005. Understanding the Human Body: Biological Perspectives for Healthcare. Churchill Livingstone, Edinburgh.

Green, L., McGhie, J., 2010. Assessment of acute and chronic pain. Anaesthesia and Intensive Care Medicine 12 (1), 911.

Greenstein, B., Gould, D., 2004. Trounce's Clinical Pharmacology for Nurses, seventeenth ed. Elsevier, Edinburgh.

Hallet, N., 1992. Pain: prevention and cure. In: Royle, J.A., Walsh, M. (Eds.), Watson's Medical-Surgical Nursing and Related Physiology. Baillière Tindall, London.

Hayward, J., 1975. Information: A Prescription Against Pain. RCN, London.

Helfand, M., Freeman, M., 2009. Assessment and management of acute pain in adult medical inpatients: A systematic review. Pain Medicine 10 (7), 1183–1199.

Hockenberry, M.J., Wilson, D., 2009. Wong's Essentials Of Pediatric Nursing, eighth ed. Mosby, St. Louis.

Hudspith, M.J., Siddall, P.J., Munglani, R., 2006. Physiology of pain. In: Hemming, H.C., Hopkins, P.M. (Eds.), Foundations of Anesthesia, second ed. Mosby, London.

Lee, J.M., Warren, M.P., 1978. Clinical applications of cold for the musculoskeletal system. Cold Therapy in Rehabilitation. Bell & Hyman, London.

Marieb, E.N., Hoehn, K., 2007. Human Anatomy and Physiology, seventh ed. Pearson Benjamin Cummings, San Francisco.

Mather, L., Mackie, J., 1983. The incidence of post-operative pain in children. Pain 15, 271–282.

McArdle, W.D., Katch, F.I., Katch, V.L., 2006. Essentials of Exercise Physiology Volume 1, third ed. Lippincott Williams & Wilkins, Baltimore, MD.

McCaffrey, M., 1983. Nursing the Patient in Pain. Chapman & Hall, London.

McCaffrey, M., 1990. Nursing approaches to non-pharmacological pain control. International Journal of Nursing Studies 27 (1), 1–5.

McHugh, J.M., McHugh, W.B., 2000. Pain: neuroanatomy, chemical mediators and clinical applications. AACN Clinical Issues 11 (2), 168–178.

McKinnon, K.D.L., 1980. Dr McKinnon replies. Canadian Family Physician 26, 639–643.

McQuay, H., Moore, A., 1998. An Evidence-Based Resource for Pain Relief. Oxford University Press, Oxford.

Melzack, R., Wall, P.D., 1965. Pain mechanisms: a new theory. Science 150, 971–979.

Melzack, R., Wall, P.D., 1982. The Challenge of Pain. Basic Books, New York.

Merkel, S.I., Voepel-Lewis, T., Shayevitz, J.R., et al., 1997. The FLACC: A behavioral scale for scoring postoperative pain in young children. Pediatric Nurse 23 (3), 293–297.

Merskey, H., Bogduk, N., 1994. Classification of chronic pain. In: Merskey, H., Bogduk, N. (Eds.), Part III: Pain Terms, A Current List with Definitions and Notes on Usage. IASP Task Force On Taxonomy. IASP Press, Seattle.

O'Hara, P., Campling, J., 1996. Pain Management for Health Professionals. Chapman and Hall, London.

Scholz, J., Woolf, C.J., 2002. Can we conquer pain? Nature Neuroscience 5 (Suppl), 1062–1067.

Sherwood, L., 2010. Human Physiology: From Cells to Systems. Peripheral nervous system, afferent division, special senses, seventh ed. Cengage Learning, Sydney.

Sofaer, B., 1992. Pain – A Handbook for Nurses, second ed. Chapman & Hall, London.

Sofaer, B., 1998. Pain – Principles, Practice and Patients. Stanley Thorne, Cheltenham.

Sternback, R.A., Tursky, B., 1965. Ethnic differences among housewives in psychophysical and skin potential responses to electrical shock. Psychophysiology 1, 241–246.

Strøma, V., Røeb, C., Matrea, D., et al., 2012. Deep tissue hyperalgesia after computer work. Scandinavian Journal of Pain 3 (1), 53–60.

Sutcliffe, A.J., 1993. Pain relief for acutely ill and injured patients. Care of the Critically Ill 9 (6), 266–269.

Thompson, D.R., Webster, R., 1992. Caring for the Coronary Patient. Butterworth Heinemann, Oxford.

Walsh, M., 1993. Pain and anxiety in A&E attenders. Nursing Standard 17 (7), 40–42.

Walsh, M., 1996. Accident and Emergency Nursing: A New Approach, third ed. Butterworth Heinemann, Oxford.

Watt-Watson, J.H., Ivers Donovan, M., 1992. Pain Management: Nursing Perspectives. Mosby Year Book, St Louis.

Williamson, A., Hoggart, B., 2005. Pain: A review of three commonly used pain rating scales. Journal of Clinical Nursing. 14, 798–804.

Local and regional anaesthesia

Paula Grainger

26

CHAPTER CONTENTS

Introduction

Local and regional anaesthesia is a method of rendering surgical interventions painless to a conscious patient while also being spontaneously reversible, enabling the complete recovery of function following the treatment. Local and regional anaesthetics are suitable for the management of the nociceptive pain that many patients present with to the emergency department (ED). They can be used either as an adjunct to treatment or as definitive treatment in itself. Local anaesthesia is limited to a discrete field, while regional anaesthesia is the use of the same or similar chemicals applied so that the effect is experienced over a larger area, such as a finger distal from the point of administration.

This chapter will describe local and regional anaesthetics, the applicable aspects of the physiology of the conduction of the pain signal, and the pharmacology of the drugs used. (Other aspects of pain and pain management in the ED situation are discussed in Chapter 25.) This will be followed by the consideration of the advantages and disadvantages associated with local anaesthetics, a review of the various methods of use, and an outline of the principles of managing patients undergoing these procedures in the ED.

Note: Except where explicitly stated in this chapter, the term local anaesthetic also includes regional anaesthetics.

Conduction of the nociceptive pain signal

Local anaesthetics address the nociceptive pain signal in the first two of stages of nociception, which is the normal method of processing the sensation along the neuron. Nociceptive pain has been classified as tissue damage that triggers the release of inflammatory mediators that bathe and sensitize the nociceptors (Butcher 2004). The neuron has a range of receptors including the nociceptors for the sensation of pain, named from the Latin 'noci' to injure or harm. The process of nociception contains four stages, the first of which is transduction followed by transmission or conduction, perception, and modulation (National Pharmaceutical Council and Joint Commission on Accreditation of Healthcare Organizations 2001).

Before the process of transmitting the nerve impulse begins, the neuron is in the resting phase in which all the active ion channels and almost all voltage-gated sodium (Na^+) and potassium (K^+) gates are closed, with the exception of the leakage channels allowing some potassium ions to diffuse

http://dx.doi.org/10.1016/B978-0-7020-4315-4.00026-7

out and smaller quantities of sodium ions to diffuse in (the movement ratio is 3 Na$^+$ out of the neuron to every 2 K$^+$ in; Clark 2008). In this phase the neuron interior is negatively charged at −70 mV.

Transduction (conduction) occurs when a noxious stimulus (e.g., excessive mechanical energy, thermal energy, or chemical interaction) is converted into electrical energy by the release of chemical mediators from the damaged cells. These mediators include: prostaglandin, bradykinin, serotonin, substance P, potassium and histamine. The chemical mediators sensitize the nociceptors in the neuron causing a rise in the action potential of approximately 15 mV to −55 mV that triggers cell depolarization. This depolarization takes place by the opening of the voltage-gated sodium channels to increase the neuron membrane's permeability to sodium ions, thus allowing more sodium to enter. Ultimately the neuron allows in enough positively charged sodium ions that the cell interior is positively charged.

Transmission happens when this depolarization travels the length of the nociception fibres in milliseconds, causing the impulse to be experienced as a conscious sensation in the brain (McCaffery & Passero 1999). For this to transpire, a critical level of depolarization of the neuron membrane must be reached; this is known as the threshold potential. This is reached when the ion flow becomes self-generating and the membrane potential alters from −70 mV to a maximum +30 mV, with the process slowing at 0 mV as the membrane becomes less permeable to sodium ions and the electrical gradient begins to prevent the sodium ions from entering freely.

Repolarization commences when the transmission process has passed from each nociception fibre. In the repolarization phase the voltage-gated potassium channels open, allowing positively charged potassium ions to flow out of the neuron. This decreases the excess internal positive charge and brings the membrane potential closer to the resting potential leading to the cell interior becoming negatively charged once more.

Pharmacology of local anaesthetics

Local anaesthetics act by blocking the conduction of the nerve impulses when applied either locally to the nerve fibre endings or regionally to the nerve trunks that convey the impulses from the affected area. They do this by binding to the sodium channels in the membrane to prevent changes to membrane permeability, creating a membrane-stabilizing effect that blocks the depolarization of the membrane (Fatovich & Brown 2004). The smaller the diameter of the neuron, the more sensitive it is to the effects of local anaesthetic. The clinical consequences following injection of a local anaesthetic are initial loss of autonomic function, followed by loss of pain sensation, then touch and pressure sensation, and finally motor function; recovery occurs in the reverse order (Rosenberg 2000).

All local anaesthetics, with the exception of cocaine, interfere with autonomic function, which means that they cause local or regional vasodilatation depending on the technique used. This vasodilatation can lead to rapid dispersal, thereby minimizing the duration of the local anaesthetic. To address this effect a vasoconstrictor such as adrenaline (epinephrine)

can be added, which can delay absorption, prolonging anaesthesia and preventing flooding of the circulation (Fatovich & Brown 2004). For example, the normal duration of action for lignocaine of 15–45 minutes when infiltrated subcutaneously can be increased by 50% by the addition of adrenaline (De Jong 2001). If adrenaline is used, the total dose should not exceed 0.5 mg/ml or the concentration 1:200 000 (British National Formulary 2011). The duration of anaesthetic action is dependent upon:

- the drug used
- the concentration and dose of local anaesthetic
- the mode of drug administration
- the rate of diffusion from the injection site to the axon.

This latter point is important as it emphasizes the need to allow sufficient time for the local anaesthetics to work before commencing the procedure.

Classification of local anaesthetics

History

The oldest recorded method for local or regional analgesia for medical interventions is the use of cooling or freezing by Hippocrates (460–377 BC) (Trescot 2003). Ether spray was introduced for topical anaesthesia (Richardson 1866) followed by ethylchloride spray in 1891 which is still in use today alongside other variations (Trescot 2003). The first chemical local anaesthetic agent to be isolated was cocaine, isolated from the coco leaf by German chemist Albert Nieman in 1860; the first recorded clinical use was topically on a cornea by Köller in 1884 (Brown & Allen 2009, Walsh & Walsh 2011). Since then, the field of local and regional anaesthesia has advanced with the synthesis of other agents, particularly procaine in 1904 and lignocaine in 1947. These agents and the establishment of increasingly sophisticated techniques have led to a growth in the use of local anaesthetics to achieve pain-free procedures. Brown & Allen (2009) provide a detailed chronology of the development of local and regional anaesthesia and agents (Table 26.1).

Types of anaesthesia

There are two commonly used types of anaesthetic in the average emergency department: coolant and non-coolant. Coolant anaesthesia (known as cryoanaesthesia or cryoanalgesia) is a technique that produces prolonged analgesia by applying cold to nerves. This causes an injury to the myelin sheath that temporarily impairs the nerve's ability to conduct signals while leaving the sheath structure of the nerve intact that enables the regeneration of the nerve.

Non-coolant local anaesthetics can be divided into two chemical groupings: ester caines and amide caines. Esters are readily metabolized in the plasma by pseudocholinesterase, and then by the liver to para-aminobenzoic acid. Amides are slowly metabolized by the liver and can therefore only be

Table 26.1 Development of local anaesthetic agents by date and type

	Synthesized by	Year of synthesis	Clinical introduction where documented
Esters			
Cocaine	Niemann	1860	1884
Benzocaine	Salkowski	1895	
Procaine	Einhorn	1904	1905
Amylocaine	Fourneau	1904	
Cinchocaine	Meischer	1925	
Tetracaine	Eisler	1928	1932
Chloroprocaine	Marks & Rubin	1949	1952
Amides			
Dibucaine	Meischer	1925	1930
Lidocaine	Løfgren and Lundqvist	1943	1947
Mepivacaine	Ekenstam & Egner	1956	1957
Bupivacaine	Ekenstam	1957	1963
Prilocaine	Løfgren & Tegnér	1959	1959
Articaine	Rusching	1969	
Etidocaine	Takman	1971	1972
Ropivacaine	Ekenstam	1957	1997
Levobupivacaine	Chiroscience, Mather & Tucker	1972	1999

(Sources: Cartwright & Fyhr 1988; Horlocker & Wedel 2002; Johansen 2004; Mather & Tucker 2009; Brown & Allen 2009.)

Table 26.2 Categories of nerve blocks

Category	Method	Region
Local		
Topical	Surface application	Within wound
Field (infiltration) block	Injection into area around a wound/injury	Within injection sites
Regional		
Haematoma block	Injection into haematoma	Site of injection
Peripheral nerve block	Injection into nerves proximal to a wound/injury	Dermatonal pattern distal to injection site
Intravenous regional block (Bier's block)	Injection intravenously proximal to a wound/injury	Limb distal to tourniquet site
Epidural (extradural) block (caudal block)	Injection into the epidural space of the spine cord	Below the injection site
Spinal (subarachnoid) block	Injection into the subarachnoid space around the spinal cord	

Categories of anaesthesia

Local anaesthesia is categorized according to the method of administration or the site of injection, and these are broadly divided into local or regional with seven subcategories of nerve block (Table 26.2).

Local anaesthesia is used for relatively minor procedures, whereas regional anaesthesia is reserved for those that are more complex or requiring a longer duration of action. The last two techniques are not usually seen in ED and are therefore beyond the scope of this chapter.

Uses of local anaesthetics

The pharmacological properties of four commonly used local anaesthetic agents for field blocks, haematoma blocks and peripheral nerve blocks are outlined in Table 26.2. Note: both generic and some brand names have been used, including those related to the combination preparations known by acronyms and based upon their contents.

Topical or surface application

This involves direct application of the local anaesthetic to mucous membranes, intact skin, or open wounds, such as grazes. Suitable sites for topical anaesthesia include the cornea, conjunctiva, upper airway, epidermal and dermal layers of the skin, and urethra. Local anaesthetics for this purpose come in various forms, including refrigerant sprays, aerosol sprays, liquid solutions, creams, jellies, balms and ointments. One local anaesthetic used as a topical agent is cocaine. The initial formulation of tetracaine, adrenaline and cocaine (TAC)

used in those patients whose liver function is uncompromised. The esters are less stable and more readily metabolized than the amides (Titcomb 2003). Table 26.1 lists some of these agents according to their chemical group.

The ideal local anaesthetic should be non-irritant, non-toxic, have a rapid onset of effect, have an action duration that is appropriate to the procedure, and leave no local after-effects. Butterworth (2009) lists three classifications for local anaesthetic agents for humans as:

- low potency and short action duration, e.g., procaine and chloroprocaine
- intermediate potency and action duration, e.g., lignocaine, mepivacaine and prilocaine
- high potency and prolonged action duration, e.g., tetracaine, bupivacaine, ropivacaine and etidocaine.

Table 26.3 Topical anaesthetics

Type	Agent	Onset	Duration (minutes)	Skin condition
TAC	Tetracaine (amethocaine) 4%, epinephrine (adrenaline) 1:2000–1:4000, and cocaine 4%	20 minutes	30–45 After solution /gel removal	Intact only
EMLA cream	Prilocaine 2.5% and lignocaine 2.5%	60 minutes for venepuncture 120 minutes for cannulation (maximum effect after 2–3 hours)	60–120 After cream removal	Intact only
Ametop gel	Tetracaine (amethocaine) 4%	30 minutes for venepuncture 45 minutes for cannulation (maximum effect after 45 minutes)	120–180 After cream removal	Intact only
ALA, LET, LAT or XAP	Tetracaine (amethocaine) 0.5%, lignocaine (lidocaine/xylocaine) 4%, and adrenaline (epinephrine) 0.05%	10 minutes (up to a maximum of 30 minutes)	15–60 After solution /gel removal	Intact or into/onto wounds
Refrigerant spray	Ethylchloride, fluroethyl or dichlorotetrafluoroethane (Frigiderm)	Cools <10°C within 10–15 seconds	N/A	Intact only
Ophthalmic use	Tetracaine 0.5–1%, oxybuprocaine, proxymetacaine	<1 minute	20–40	N/A

(Sources: McCaffery & Passero 1999, Lander & Weltman 2002, Butcher 2004, Dunn et al. 2003.)

gained widespread acceptance in North America and largely supplanted infiltration anaesthesia (Grant & Hoffman 1992). Unlike other local anaesthetics, cocaine potentiates the action of the sympathetic nervous system, thus causing local vasoconstriction. It is highly effective on very vascular areas, such as the nasal membranes. It also causes dilatation of the pupil when used on the cornea. Cocaine, however, has powerful central effects, making it too dangerous to inject. It also has complex administrative and financial issues resulting from it being a drug of addiction, which has led to the development of cocaine-free alternatives in the last decade as seen in Table 26.3 (Eidelman et al. 2005).

These alternatives include creams and jellies containing a combination of lignocaine and prilocaine that can be used prior to venepuncture or cannulation in children. One example of such a topical anaesthetic is the Eutectic Mixture of Local Anesthetics (EMLA©) cream. The 'eutectic' property refers to the liquefaction of the constituents (McCaffery & Passero 1999). EMLA cream is applied only to intact skin (British National Formulary 2011) for cutaneous anaesthesia. To do this a thick layer is applied under an occlusive dressing and left for 60–120 minutes, dependent on the indication for its use. Numbing of the skin should occur one hour after application, reaching a maximum at two to three hours, and one hour for children less than three months old. The effect lasts for one to two hours after removal of the cream (Lander & Weltman 2002). However, this time lag sometimes makes it impractical for use in the ED especially when a painful

activity needs to be performed before that time. An alternative option is amethocaine gel (Ametop©), which is similarly indicated for local topical anaesthesia prior to venepuncture or venous cannulation. As with EMLA, this gel is applied to the site required and sealed with an occlusive dressing; however, it is ready for the procedure to occur after 30 minutes for venepuncture and after 45 minutes for venous cannulation as it has a faster action. Like EMLA, it should only be applied to intact skin as it is rapidly absorbed and it should not be applied to inflamed, traumatized, highly vascular surfaces, or mucous membranes (British National Formulary 2011).

A further option is a solution or gel containing tetracaine (amethocaine/pontacaine), lignocaine (lidocaine/xylocaine) and adrenaline (epinephrine), known as ALA, LET, LAT or XAP (according to country of use), which can be made by the hospital pharmacy (McCaffery & Passero 1999). It is a faster-acting option and can be applied directly into or onto a wound in conjunction with the application of a piece of gauze soaked in the solution and left on the wound with a clear non-absorbent dressing used to hold it in place for 10 minutes (up to a maximum of 30 minutes). This can provide sufficient anaesthesia lasting up to 15 minutes to enable wound cleansing and closure with sutures if required (McCaffery & Passero 1999). Care should be taken to avoid the mucous membranes to avoid systemic absorption and possible toxicity, and the eyes should be avoided also due to the risk of causing corneal abrasions (McCaffery & Passero 1999). The benefit of these topical treatments is that they are painless to use.

Other uses of anaesthesia include those for ophthalmic procedures in the ED such as irrigation or examination, in which case tetracaine is often chosen due to its profound effect although oxybuprocaine and proxymetacaine are options recommended by the College of Optometrists since they are less irritating than tetracaine (Titcomb 2003). Tetracaine, oxybuprocaine and proxymetacaine have a similar duration of action, approximately 30 minutes, that of lignocaine is somewhat longer (45 minutes).

Lignocaine can be used alone in a 4% solution or a 1–2% jelly form for relief from the discomfort of procedures such as urinary catheterization. Chronic long-term use of topical preparations can lead to sensitization and local allergic reactions.

An alternative to chemical topical agents is the use of cryo-anaesthesia via a refrigerant spray, in which the rapid cooling of the skin causes superficial anaesthesia suitable for immediate pinpoint pain relief (Brown 2004). Examples of these sprays are ethylchloride, fluroethyl and dichlorotetrafluoroethane (Frigiderm®). Refrigerant sprays work by extremely rapid cooling of the skin (<10°C within 10–15 seconds of application); however, their duration of action is briefer than that provided by EMLA, amethocaine gel or ALA/LET/LAT/XAP and this sudden cooling can be distressing and children particularly may object to it (McCaffery & Passero 1999). Refrigerant sprays should be used with caution as prolonged application can cause frostbite.

Local infiltration and field block

Local infiltration and field block are ideal methods of anaesthesia for the suturing and extensive cleansing of minor wounds or small abscesses (although local anaesthetic may be less effective when used for infiltrating an abscess due to the altered pH of the infected tissue/fluid). It is recommended that infiltration is not used for inflamed or infected tissues (British National Formulary 2011). It is also imperative to avoid introducing lignocaine directly into a vein due to its cardiac arrhythmia properties.

The difference between these two methods of drug administration is that local infiltration involves the injection of the anaesthetic drug directly into the subcutaneous tissue involved, while a field block involves injecting the chosen drug into the surrounding area for treatment (Chan et al. 2002). The latter has the advantage of avoiding distortion of the wound edges. Care needs to be exercised to avoid injection of large volumes of local anaesthetic as this can lead to localized oedema, causing distortion of wound edges and tissue hypoxia, which makes the apposition and healing of the wound edges difficult.

While these methods provide excellent levels of pain relief, the act of infiltration or injection can be painful. Warming the vial between the hands prior to drawing up and use can relieve this discomfort to some extent. Buffering the lignocaine with sodium bicarbonate 8.4% has been seen to significantly decrease the pain perceived by the patient on infiltration by raising the pH of the solution (Achar & Kundu 2002, Chan et al. 2002). However, this latter option significantly decreases the solution's shelf-life, limiting the efficacy of the anaesthetic to one week post combination with the sodium bicarbonate, and it is recommended to only mix the two drugs together immediately prior to the procedure. Lignocaine 1% or 2% with or without adrenaline (dependent on the wound location) is the drug of choice for these methods of administration due to its rapid onset. Toxicity can be avoided if the dose of lignocaine does not exceed 3 mg/kg body weight, which is approximately 20 ml of a 1% solution in an adult, increased to a maximum of 500 mg if the lignocaine solution contains adrenaline. Table 26.4 details the pharmacological properties of the drugs involved in these blocks.

Haematoma blocks

Haematoma blocks are principally used for the reduction of wrist fractures. They involve injecting the anaesthetic drug directly into the haematoma surrounding the fracture (Chan et al. 2002). The benefit of this type of block is that it is

Table 26.4 The pharmacological properties of common anaesthetics used for infiltration, field blocks or regional blocks

Category	Concentration	Max. single dose without adrenaline	Onset of action for infiltration	Duration of action for infiltration	Onset of action for nerve block	Duration of action for nerve block
Lignocaine	1–4%	4.5 mg/kg, maximum 200 mg	Fast	60–120 minutes	4–10 minutes	60–120 minutes
Prilocaine	1%	6 mg/kg, maximum 400 mg	Slow	60–120 minutes	Fast	30–90 minutes
Bupivacaine	0.25–0.5%	2–2.5 mg/kg maximum 150 mg	Moderate	240–480 minutes	8–12 minutes (up to 30 for full effect)	240–480 minutes
Ropivacaine	7.5–10 mg/ml	30–40 ml of 7.5 mg/ml maximum 300 mg	Not indicated	N/A	8–12 minutes long	

(Sources: British National Formulary 2011, Rayner-Klein & Rowe 2005, Fatovich & Brown 2004, Chan et al. 2002.)

easy and quick to give, and is sufficiently effective to enable the reduction and immobilization of the fracture; however, a peripheral nerve block is more selective in that the local anaesthetic drug is injected around nerve trunks supplying the injury/operation site.

Peripheral nerve blocks

Peripheral nerve blocks are occasionally mistakenly referred to as haematoma blocks; however, a peripheral nerve block affects a larger area and in a dermatonal pattern (McCaffery & Passero 1999). Various peripheral nerve blocks using local anaesthetic agents have been described in order to reduce pain and facilitate treatments; these nerve blocks are used to administer an anaesthetic agent locally to nerves serving particular parts of the body. The techniques for administering peripheral nerve blocks are also more difficult than that of haematoma blocks. They provide excellent analgesia over limited fields with minimal systemic effects, and are generally easy to perform, inexpensive and safe (Summers 2011). They also act as muscle relaxants since the motor fibres are also blocked. Care should be taken not to exceed maximum local anaesthetic doses (shown in Table 26.4).

The most frequent uses of regional nerve blocks in the ED setting are ring blocks to achieve anaesthesia of a digit and femoral blocks for pain relief of a hip or femur fracture, although others are used according to the skill of the clinician. A ring block involves injection into the base of the finger via the interdigital web; bilateral infiltration is required to ensure blockage of all four digital nerves. Brachial plexus or axillary blocks can be used to achieve anaesthesia of the forearm and hand, for which the local anaesthetic is injected into the neurovascular sheath surrounding the axillary artery and the median, radial and ulnar nerves. A number of options are available for femoral blocks, which differ according to the experience and skill of the practitioner and include the lateral cutaneous nerve of thigh, subcostal nerve, femoral nerve, sciatic nerve, triple nerve block (femoral, obturator and sciatic nerves), psoas (lumbar plexus) block, or continuous epidural block (Parker et al. 2002). The triple nerve femoral block using a three-in-one injection method has been found to effectively reduce pain and the need for opiates, and can be given by all grades of medical staff trained in the procedure (Fletcher et al. 2003). The main advantage of the triple nerve block is it requires fewer injections and avoids the pain involved in injection directly into already sensitive tissue.

Potential complications, as with all nerve blocks, relate to the possibility of damage to surrounding structures (Rivellini 1993). It is imperative that adrenaline is not added to the local anaesthetic solution for any procedure where it may compromise the flow of blood to an area that has an end-arteriole blood supply, as the adrenaline leads to vasoconstriction and can cause the occlusion of the supplying arteries: these include fingers or toes, skin flaps with marginal viability, penis and tips of the ears, or the nose-tip (McCaffery & Passero 1999, Achar & Kundu 2002). It should also be noted that the onset and duration of action of the various drugs differ according to the site of injection: for example, there has been seen a difference of up to 25 minutes for onset time and 6 hours difference of duration time of bupivacaine when comparing an intercostal nerve block with a brachial plexus block (Chan et al. 2002) (see Table 26.4).

Intravenous regional anaesthesia (Bier's block)

The technique of intravenous regional anaesthesia (IVRA) was first described by Karl Bier in 1908 and the technique later became known as a Bier's block (Checketts 2010). It is used primarily to achieve anaesthesia below the elbow, although it can also be used for procedures below the knee and in ED the main uses of this technique are for the manipulation of Colles' and Smith fractures. The use of IVRA has been found to provide better relief from pain and it facilitates better limb reduction with a reduced risk of re-dislocation or the need for re-plastering in comparison to the use of haematoma blocks (Handoll 2005).

IVRA can be a useful option in the ED, although it requires training for safe use. Contraindications for the use of IVRA are outlined in Box 26.1.

In preparation for an IVRA procedure, the patient's blood pressure, ECG and weight must be recorded. A cuffed tourniquet underlaid by wool is placed around the proximal limb – a double-cuffed tourniquet is recommended. Two points of intravenous access are required; the first for the IVRA should ideally be placed distal to the injury (Dunn et al. 2003) or at the antecubital fossa (ACF) (Blyth et al. 1995), although there is a greater risk of leakage under the inflated tourniquet with the latter location (Kamming 2010). The second is to enable the administration of other drugs as required. The injured limb needs to

---

Box 26.1

Contraindications to the use of intravenous regional anaesthesia

- Patient refusal
- Peripheral vascular disease including
  - Sickle cell disease
  - Raynaud's disease
- Severe atheroma
- Unstable epilepsy
- Heart failure
- Heart block
- Systolic blood pressure >200 mmHg
- Severe liver disease
- Anticoagulant therapy
- Confusion/uncooperative patient
- Compromised limb circulation
- Compartment syndrome in the injured limb
- Injuries at the tourniquet site including fractures or soft tissue injuries
- Local infection, e.g., cellulitis

be elevated for between 30 seconds and 2 minutes following insertion of the intravenous cannula to drain some of the blood from the veins in order to reduce the dilatation of the local anaesthetic (Dunn et al. 2003). When the procedure is ready to begin, the proximal cuff is inflated to a pressure at least 100 mmHg above the patient's systolic blood pressure and the anaesthetic, e.g., 40 ml prilocaine 0.5%, can then be injected into the collapsed veins of the limb, which will cause the limb to develop a blue, mottled appearance. If a single-cuff tourniquet is used the pain from the direct compression of nerve and muscle tissue will be evident after 30 minutes and may be unbearable after an hour. Where a double-cuff is used, once the anaesthetic has taken effect the distal cuff is inflated to the same pressure and the proximal cuff is then deflated reducing the patient's discomfort as the inflated cuff is now over an anaesthetized area.

The maximum length of time for which the cuff can remain inflated is 1½ hours as the tourniquet is preventing blood from entering the limb and extended use can lead to ischaemia of the area. The minimum time for constant inflation is at least 30 minutes to permit fixation of the local anaesthetic to the tissues of the limb (Rivellini 1993). Release or leakage of the anaesthetic into the systemic circulation prior to this time can lead to cardiovascular and CNS depression and therefore the presence of resuscitation facilities and circulatory access are mandatory for this procedure. It is recommended that lipid therapy is always available wherever IVRA is undertaken. (For signs of toxicity, see Box 26.2.)

Box 26.2

Potential toxic effect of local anaesthetics (in order of increasing plasma levels)

Central nervous system
- Paraesthesia of mouth and tongue
- Dizziness and light-headedness
- Tinnitus
- Visual disturbance
- Talkativeness
- Feelings of disorientation
- Confusion
- Agitation or tremor
- Drowsiness
- Convulsion
- Coma

Cardiovascular system
- Myocardial conduction
- Sinus bradycardia
- AV block
- Reduced cardiac output
- Hypotension
- Resistant ventricular arrhythmias
- Apnoea
- Cardiac arrest (highest plasma levels)

Benefits of local anaesthetics

In the ED setting local and regional anaesthesia either enables otherwise painful procedures to occur, leading to the patient's discharge from ED rather than admission to an inpatient bed, or it can ensure a patient's comfort while waiting for surgical intervention after their transfer from the ED.

The principal benefit of local anaesthesia is the absence of complications that may arise from the use of general anaesthetics and intubation. These include: the laryngeal and cough reflexes remain unimpaired, reducing the risk of respiratory obstruction and respiratory function is not automatically depressed, making them ideal for patients with poor lung function. Also the patient does not experience the discomforts associated with general anaesthetic, such as nausea, vomiting, dizziness, and/or a sore throat. The associated shorter recovery time facilitates an earlier discharge. In addition, many, though not all, minor procedures can still be performed even if the patient has eaten.

The numbing effect of local anaesthetics on the surgical site usually lasts beyond the operative period, providing highly specific, temporary postoperative pain relief. Because the patient remains conscious, they are able to cooperate if required, and report any abnormalities, making the early detection of complications more likely.

Disadvantages and limitations of local anaesthesia

The first major disadvantage with local anaesthesia is that, while patients may not feel pain, they will often experience other sensations associated with the procedure, such as pressure and movement. Because they are conscious they will be able to see, hear and smell all that is going on. There will be many patients who simply do not wish to be awake because they would rather not know anything; they may find the feelings of numbness, paraesthesia, paralysis and the sense of being detached from the affected part of the body disconcerting (Rivellini 1993). For this reason, many, although not all, children and adults with learning difficulties are not suitable candidates for treatment under local or regional anaesthesia. The use of local anaesthetic requires the active cooperation of the patient and so may not be suitable for confused, aggressive and agitated people. Children and patients with learning difficulties may pose a challenge for the nurse, but they should by no means automatically be excluded from the use of local anaesthesia.

A second disadvantage is that the use of local anaesthetic may be limited by the suitability of the surgical site. In addition, some of the procedures involved for regional anaesthesia may be perceived as technically difficult and require a high level of expertise beyond that of the majority of ED medical and nursing staff. However, standardized training in the use of each technique could and should be available and local anaesthesia has been recommended as a practical alternative to general anaesthesia (Graham et al. 1997).

It is important to remember that while the term 'local' is used, local anaesthetics are only minimally metabolized at the site of injection; most pass ultimately into the bloodstream and, potentially, may produce systemic toxic effects. These result from the membrane-stabilizing effects on other cells, notably those of the cardiovascular and central nervous systems.

Allergic reactions to local anaesthetic drugs are uncommon; those seen are generally caused by the preservative added (e.g., methylparaben) rather than by the anaesthetic drug (Chan et al. 2002). Also allergic reactions have been confused with systemic toxicity; however, the amino-ester drugs have a higher frequency of allergic reactions than the amino-amide group (Fatovich & Brown 2004) and adverse side-effects have been reported (British National Formulary 2011). The potential effects of toxicity are listed in Box 26.2.

Other potential toxic effects include hypotension due to loss of vascular tone, respiratory depression, and allergic reactions (British National Formulary 2011), although the latter two are uncommon.

Nursing implications of procedures involving local anaesthetics

Pre-operatively

The patient's past and current medical history should be assessed and factors that might contraindicate the use of local anaesthetics should be noted, in particular previous allergic reactions. A baseline of the current neurovascular status of the proposed surgical site should be established. When intravenous regional anaesthesia is proposed, the patient's baseline cardiovascular status in the form of their haemodynamic observations and their weight is necessary. The nurse needs to be familiar with the technique to be used, the length of time the block will last, and whether any vasoconstrictive agent has been added (Rivellini 1993).

Thorough preparation of the patient includes the provision of information about both the nature of the procedure and the feelings the patient may experience during it. Explanation of sights and sensations that may result from the procedure need to be given before they occur, e.g., that local anaesthesia will remove the sensation of pain but not the sensation of pressure or that during intravenous regional anaesthesia a change of limb colour associated with the infiltration of local anaesthetic is expected.

Informed consent will need to be obtained. For minor procedures such as suturing this can be obtained verbally, but for techniques involving intravenous regional anaesthesia formal written consent will be required.

Intra-operatively

Special consideration should be given to the fact that patients are awake. Careless remarks should be avoided and technical terms, when used, even between staff, need to be explained. The focus of conversation should be the patient rather than the procedure. Where conscious awareness of the procedure causes distress, social conversation can be used to distract the patient (Edwards 1994).

Constant vigilance is required to assess for signs of toxicity and allergic reaction. Should there be a risk of systemic absorption, it is recommended that a reversal agent, i.e., an intravenous lipid emulsion, is available for use. The administration of such a reversal agent can restore haemodynamic stability after local anaesthetic-induced cardiac arrest (Clark 2008) and may be used to pre-empt complete cardiovascular collapse when toxicity has been identified. Examples of lipid emulsions are Intralipid® and Liposyn®.

The neurovascular function of the affected area should be continuously observed and compared with that of equivalent unaffected areas. This is particularly pertinent with procedures involving manipulation of a limb or the application of a plaster cast, as the complications of either are mimicked by the action of local anaesthetic. The tourniquet time, where appropriate, should be noted. The patient should be encouraged to report any discomfort experienced during the procedure.

Post-operatively and advice for discharge

Pain provides a protective function both as an initiator of reflex mechanisms and by alerting the person when a body part has sustained trauma. In eliminating pain, local anaesthetics eliminate these protective mechanisms. Nurses will need to consider measures to ensure the safety of the patient and the body part involved; for example, the patient's limb should not be allowed to rest on or become trapped in cot sides. The transient loss of motor function necessitates that affected extremities will need to be supported in anatomically neutral positions. A sling will serve both to protect and to support the weight of an arm. Any attempt at using the affected area until full sensation has returned should be discouraged. The post-anaesthesia levels of sensory and motor function should be continually assessed and delays in expected dissipation times reported. It is vital that care is taken to differentiate between paraesthesiae related to dissipation of the block and those of neurovascular compromise (Jasinski & Snyder 1996). These observations should be documented at least once prior to discharge.

The residual effect of the local anaesthetic will provide immediate pain relief. However, as this is only temporary, post-operative analgesia will need to be prescribed and administered before the effect dissipates. As far as possible, it is helpful to give some indication as to the possible levels of discomfort the patient may experience once the local anaesthetic has worn off. This will help the patient to determine whether this is normal or an indicator of residual or developing complications.

Conclusion

This chapter has highlighted both the rationale for the use of local anaesthetics and the nursing implications. Local anaesthetics are a valuable tool in the options available in ED care. Used with vigilance they can provide an alternative to the torture of the 'one quick pull' or the fear of 'being put to sleep', and improve the experiences of the patients and their supporters while in ED.

References

Achar, S., Kundu, S., 2002. Principles of office anesthesia: Part 1. Infiltrative anesthesia. American Family Physician 66 (1), 91–95.

Blyth, M.J.G., Kinninmonth, A.W.G., Asante, D.K., 1995. Biers block: a change of injection site. Journal of Trauma-Injury & Critical Care 39 (4), 726–728.

British National Formulary, 2011. British National Formulary No. 62. British Medical Association and the Royal Pharmaceutical Society of Great Britain, London.

Brown, A., 2004. Pain relief. In: Cameron, P., Jelinick, G., Kelly, A.-M., Murray, L., Brown, A., Heyworth, J. (Eds.), Textbook of Adult Emergency Medicine, second ed. Churchill Livingstone, Edinburgh.

Brown, D.L., Allen, R.F., 2009. The history of regional anesthesia. In: Cousins, M.J., Carr, D.B., Horlocker, T.T., Bridenbaugh, P.O. (Eds.), Cousins & Bridenhaugh's Neural Blockade in Clinical Anesthesia and Pain Medicine, fourth ed. Kluwer/Lippincott Williams and Wilkins, Wolters Philadelphia.

Butcher, D., 2004. Pharmacological techniques in managing acute pain in emergency departments. Emergency Nurse 12 (1), 26–36.

Butterworth, J.F., 2009. Clinical pharmacology of local anesthetics. In: Cousins, M.J., Carr, D.B., Horlocker, T.T., Bridenbaugh, P.O. (Eds.), Cousins & Bridenhaugh's Neural Blockade in Clinical Anesthesia and Pain Medicine, fourth ed. Wolters Kluwer/ Lippincott Williams and Wilkins, Philadelphia.

Cartwright, P.D., Fyhr, P., 1988. The manufacture and storage of local anesthetics. Regional Anesthesia & Pain Medicine 13 (1), 1–12.

Chan, S.K., Karmakar, M.K., Chui, P.T., 2002. Local anesthesia outside the operating room. Hong Kong Medical Journal 8 (2), 106–113.

Checketts, M.R., 2010. Intravenous regional anaesthesia. Anaesthesia and Intensive Care Medicine 11 (3), 111–112.

Clark, M.K., 2008. Lipid emulsion as rescue for local anesthetic-related cardiotoxicity. Journal of PeriAnesthesia Nursing 23 (2), 111–121.

De Jong, R.H., 2001. Local anesthetics in clinical practice. In: Waldman, S.D. (Ed.), Interventional Pain Management, second ed. WB Saunders Company, Philadelphia.

Dunn, R., Dilley, S., Brookes, J., et al., 2003. The Emergency Medicine Manual, third ed. Venom Publishing, Adelaide.

Edwards, B., 1994. Local and regional anesthesia. Emergency Nurse 2 (2), 10–15.

Eidelman, A., Weiss, J.M., Enu, I.K., McNicol, E., Lau, J., Carr, D.B., 2005. Topical anesthetics for repair of dermal lacerations (Protocol). The Cochrane Database of Systematic Reviews, John Wiley & Sons, London.

Fatovich, D.M., Brown, A.F.T., 2004. Pain relief in emergency medicine. In: Cameron, P., Jelinick, G., Kelly, A.-M., Murray, L., Brown, A., Heyworth, J. (Eds.), Textbook of Adult Emergency Medicine, second ed. Churchill Livingstone, Edinburgh.

Fletcher, A.K., Rigby, A.S., Heyes, F.L., 2003. Three-in-one femoral nerve block as analgesia for fractured neck of femur in the emergency department: a randomized control trial. Annals of Emergency Medicine 42 (4), 596–597.

Graham, C.A., Gibson, A.J., Goutcher, C.M., et al., 1997. Anesthesia for the management of distal radius fracture in adults in Scottish hospitals. European Journal of Emergency Medicine 4 (4), 210–212.

Grant, S., Hoffman, R., 1992. Use of tetracaine, epinephrine, and cocaine as a topical anesthetic in the emergency department. Annals of Emergency Medicine 21, 987–997.

Handoll, H.H.G., 2005. Anesthesia for treating distal radial fracture in adults. Cochrane Review, Cochrane Collaboration. John Wiley & Sons, London.

Horlocker, T.T., Wedel, D.J., 2002. Local anesthetic toxicity - does product labeling reflect actual risk? Regional Anesthesia and Pain Medicine 27 (6) 562–267.

Jasinski, D., Snyder, C., 1996. Invasive interventions. In: Sallerno, E., Williams, J. (Eds.), Pain Management Handbook: An Interdisciplinary Approach. Mosby, St Louis.

Johansen Ø, 2004. Comparison of articaine and lidocaine used as dental local anaesthetics. Thesis paper. University of Oslo.

Kamming, D., 2010. Day Surgery Analgesia. In: Bromley, L., Brander, B. (Eds.), Acute Pain. Oxford University Press, Oxford.

Lander, J.A., Weltman, B.J., 2002. Topical anesthetics (EMLA and AMETOP creams) for reduction of pain during needle insertion in children (Protocol). The Cochrane Database of Systematic Reviews, Issue 4. John Wiley & Sons, London.

Mather, L.E., Tucker, G.T., 2009. Properties, absorbtion and disposition of local anesthetic agents. In: Cousins, M.J., Carr, D.B., Horlocker, T.T., Bridenbaugh, P.O. (Eds.), Cousins & Bridenhaugh's Neural Blockade in Clinical Anesthesia and Pain Medicine, fourth ed. Wolters Kluwer/Lippincott Williams and Wilkins, Philadelphia.

McCaffery, M., Passero, C., 1999. Pain: Clinical Manual, second ed. Mosby, St Louis.

National Pharmaceutical Council and Joint Commission on Accreditation of Healthcare Organizations, 2001. Pain: Current Understanding of Assessment, Management, and Treatments. National Pharmaceutical Council, Reston, VA.

Parker, M.J., Griffths, R., Appadu, B.N., 2002. Nerve blocks (subcostal, lateral cutaneous, femoral, triple, psoas) for hip fractures. The Cochrane Database of Systematic Reviews, Issue 4. John Wiley & Sons, London.

Rayner-Klein, J., Rowe, C.A., 2005. Analgesia and anesthesia. In: O'Shea, R.A. (Ed.), Principles and Practice of Trauma Nursing. Elsevier Churchill Livingstone, Edinburgh.

Richardson, B.W., 1866. On a new and ready mode of producing local anesthesia. Medical Times and Gazette, 1–115.

Rivellini, D., 1993. Local and regional anesthesia. Nursing Clinics of North America 28 (3), 547–572.

Rosenberg, P.H., 2000. Local and Regional Anesthesia. Blackwell Publishing, Oxford.

Summers, A., 2011. Use of digital nerve blocks to provide anaesthetic relief. Emergency Nursing 19 (5), 25–29.

Titcomb, L.C., 2003. Drugs used in optometric practice. Optometry Today 46 (13), 26–33.

Trescot, A.M., 2003. Cryoanalgesia in Interventional Pain Management. Pain Physician 6 (3), 345–360.

Walsh, A., Walsh, S., 2011. Local anaesthesia and the dermatologist. Clinical and Experimental Dermatology 36 (4), 337–343.

PART 6

Emergency care

Cardiac emergencies

27

Chris Morrow-Frost

CHAPTER CONTENTS

http://dx.doi.org/10.1016/B978-0-7020-4315-4.00027-9

Introduction

Cardiovascular disease accounts for approximately 40% of all deaths under the age of 75 years in Europe (Resuscitation Council (UK) 2011). One-third of all people suffering from myocardial infarction (MI) will die prior to reaching hospital, with a high proportion of these dying within one hour from the onset of symptoms (Resuscitation Council (UK) 2011) and approximately 15% of those admitted will die within the first 30 days (British Heart Foundation 2010). Ischaemic heart disease is the leading cause of death in the world (Fuhrmann et al. 2008) and 50% of men and 64% of women who die suddenly of chronic heart disease do so without having had or recognizing any early warning signs (Williams 2009). More than 1.4 million people suffer from angina and 300 000 have MIs every year (Department of Health 2000) with up to 28 000 new cases of angina reported in the UK each year (British Heart Foundation 2010). Thus, Emergency Departments (EDs) will see a high proportion of patients suffering from a cardiovascular disorder.

The aim of this chapter is to give a systematic approach to the multiple problems that may be encountered by cardiac patients. A general overview of anatomy and physiology has been included to enable the disease process to be more accurately defined. The management of the particular cardiac problems described in this chapter is set out as a suggested guideline and is not a definitive directive for all cardiac patients, as each problem should be judged on an individual basis.

Related anatomy and physiology

The heart can be described as a muscular pump containing four chambers, situated at an oblique angle in the mediastinal cavity (Tortora & Grabowski 2000) (Figs 27.1 and 27.2).

As the heart beats it expels blood into two closed circuits. The first circuit is fed from the left side of the heart. This supplies oxygenated blood from the lungs to the systemic circulation. The second circuit is the pulmonary circuit. This enables the right side of the heart to receive deoxygenated blood which is then pumped back to the lungs via the pulmonary artery (Marieb 2000).

The heart is composed of a triple layer, which enables the protection of the inner components (Tortora & Grabowski 2000):

* the pericardium – the outer layer is composed of thick fibrous tissue that surrounds and protects the heart
* the myocardium – this is the muscular layer that forms the basis of the pumping action of the heart. It is present within both the atria and the ventricles, with the ventricles having the greater ratio of muscle
* the endocardium – this is composed of a thin layer of endothelial and connective tissue covering the inside of the heart, including the valves, which enables a smooth flow of blood through the heart, with little resistance.

Cardiac valves (Fig. 27.3)

The atrioventricular (AV) valves refer to the mitral and tricuspid valves, which lie between the atria and the ventricles, the mitral on the left and the tricuspid on the right. The valves are supported by a network of strands called chordae tendineae. The passive movement of blood from the atria to the ventricles, across the AV valves, occurs in the cardiac cycle in the phase known as ventricular filling. As the pressure in the ventricles increases, the valves are forced to close, preventing a back-flow of blood.

At the origin of the aorta and the pulmonary artery sit the semilunar valves. These consist of three cusps, and prevent the back-flow of blood into the heart. During ventricular diastole (relaxation), these valves are closed, but as ventricular systole (contraction) occurs the valves are forced to open and blood is ejected out into either the aorta or the pulmonary artery. Should these valves be diseased or damaged, stenosis or regurgitation may occur. More often than not this precludes the need for the surgical intervention.

Coronary circulation

To maintain oxygenation and the supply of nutrients, the heart derives its own blood supply via the coronary arteries (Fig. 27.4). The left and right coronary arteries originate from the aorta. As suggested, they branch into a network of arteries supplying both the right and left sides of the heart.

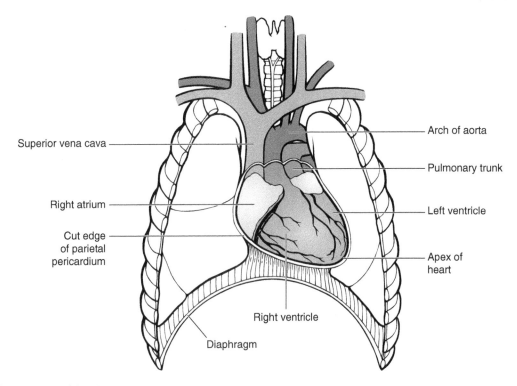

Figure 27.1 • Anterior view of the chest.

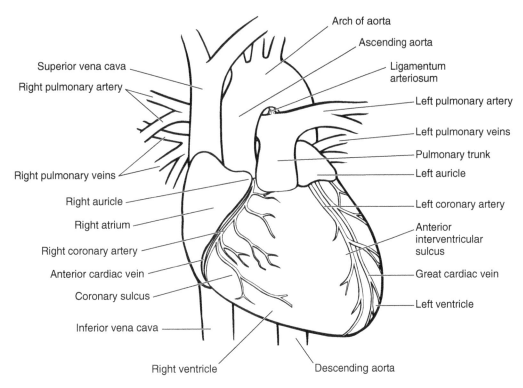

Figure 27.2 • Anterior view of the heart.

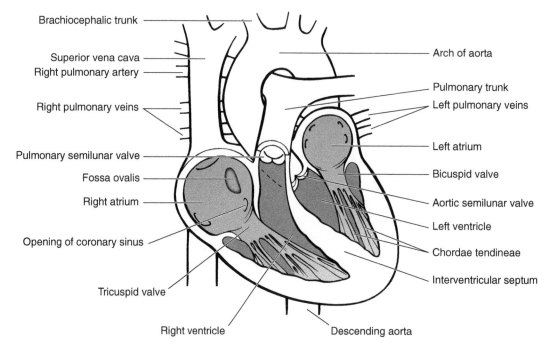

Brachiocephalic trunk

Superior vena cava
Right pulmonary artery

Right pulmonary veins

Pulmonary semilunar valve

Fossa ovalis

Right atrium

Opening of coronary sinus

Tricuspid valve

Right ventricle

Arch of aorta

Pulmonary trunk
Left pulmonary veins

Left atrium

Bicuspid valve

Aortic semilunar valve

Left ventricle

Chordae tendineae

Interventricular septum

Descending aorta

Figure 27.3 • Valves of the heart.

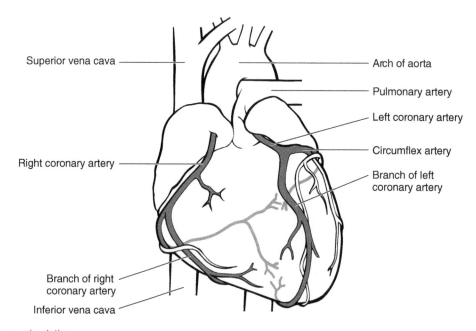

Superior vena cava

Right coronary artery

Branch of right
coronary artery

Inferior vena cava

Arch of aorta

Pulmonary artery

Left coronary artery

Circumflex artery

Branch of left
coronary artery

Figure 27.4 • Coronary circulation.

The cardiac cycle

The cardiac cycle is divided into three main phases (Tortora & Grabowski 2000):

- ventricular relaxation (diastole)
- ventricular filling
- ventricular contraction (systole).

For simplification only the left side of the heart will be explained.

Ventricular relaxation

This follows ventricular contraction (systole). The ventricles relax, resulting in pressure within the left ventricle falling below that of the aorta, and thus the aortic valve closes. As Tortora & Grabowski (2000) indicate, all valves within the heart are now closed. At the same time, blood is passively flowing into the left atrium via the pulmonary system. As pressure and volume within the left atrium increase, the mitral valve opens and the second phase of the cardiac cycle is now entered.

Ventricular filling

Tortora & Grabowski (2000) identified that the ventricular filling phase of the cardiac cycle is divided into three stages. The first stage is referred to as rapid ventricular filling and involves passive filling of the left ventricle from the left atrium. The second stage of ventricular filling is known as diastasis and refers to slow ventricular filling. At the end of diastasis, the pressures in the left atrium and the left ventricle are now equal. The third stage of ventricular filling is due to the contraction of the atrium, with blood being forced into the left ventricle.

Ventricular contraction

As the left ventricle starts to contract the mitral valve closes. The left ventricle is now a closed chamber. The muscles within the left ventricle start to contract and there is a resultant increase in pressure. Once the pressure in the left ventricle is greater than that of the aorta, the aortic valve opens and blood is ejected out (the stroke volume). As the pressure in the left ventricle drops with the expulsion of blood, the aortic valve closes and the cardiac cycle starts again.

Assessment

The presenting history when a patient attends the ED with a cardiac event remains one of the most crucial aspects in aiding diagnosis. The history provides subjective information about the presenting complaint, symptoms, past medical history and any other relevant information (Castle 2009). During initial assessment, the patient's need for immediate care must be paramount. Hence, the use of the ABC principle should be initiated automatically (Box 27.1).

The remainder of the assessment should include:

- assessment of patient's appearance – this should include pallor, posture and any non-verbal signs
- pain assessment – location, type, site and severity of pain, including any measures taken to relieve the pain
- baseline observations – these should include blood pressure, pulse, temperature, respiration and oxygen saturation. Often temperature is forgotten, but the incidence of a mild pyrexia is a common response to muscle damage (Alexander et al. 2000)

Box 27.1

ABCs

A – check the patency of the **airway**

B – check the adequacy of the **breathing**

C – **circulation**: check the adequacy of the pulse (centrally and peripherally), signs of shock, pallor, etc.

- Electrocardiograph (ECG) – note any arrhythmia and use of cardiac monitor. (Note that it may be necessary to perform repeat ECGs on a patient whose condition changes, experiences further chest pain, or whom may have an evolving cardiac event.)

Clinical investigations

Clinical investigations to support assessment should include blood analysis (Box 27.2) and chest X-ray to determine heart size and detect oedema (Jowett & Thompson 2007). These blood tests, specifically the troponin/cardiac enzymes, may be repeated at defined times; normally between 6 and 12 hours past the initial onset of chest pain (Baliga & Eagle 2008).

Box 27.2

Blood analysis in cardiac patients

- *Cardiac enzymes* – these indicate muscular damage which may suggest cardiac ischaemia
- *White cell count* – a raised white cell count in the cardiac patient is usually indicative of myocardial damage
- *Erythrocyte sedimentation rate (ESR)* – a raised ESR may indicate an increase in fibrinogen due to myocardial necrosis
- *Urea and electrolytes (U&E)* – any change in the sodium or potassium should be noted as these ions are related to cardiac cells and their function
- *Glucose* – the appearance of hyperglycaemia can be stress-related and linked to any acute changes in the myocardium, e.g. myocardial infarction (Woods et al. 2000)
- *Lipids* – these will give an indication as to the risk factors incorporated with ischaemic heart disease; they include cholesterol and triglycerides
- *Clotting screen* – this is useful when the patient may be anticoagulated

Basic ECG interpretation

It is important for ED nurses to accurately record and interpret an ECG of a patient presenting with a cardiac condition. An inherent and rhythmical electrical activity is the reason for the heart's continuous beating (Tortora & Grabowski 2000). The cardiac cells (myocardial cells) located within the myocardium undergo chemical changes, which in turn trigger electrical impulses (action potentials) and result in myocardial contraction.

The normal heartbeat is known as sinus rhythm. In essence, this means that the impulses have been generated by the normal heart conductive system (Fig. 27.5). These electrical impulses can be recorded via an ECG. To obtain a 12-lead ECG, electrodes are placed across the chest and each limb (Fig. 27.6).

Having positioned the ECG electrodes, it is important to understand the representation being made by each electrode. The heart's electrical impulses start at the SA node and

Figure 27.5 • Cardiac conduction.

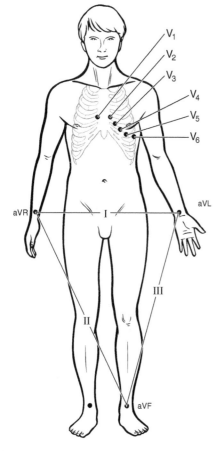

Figure 27.6 • Lead placements for 12-lead ECGs.

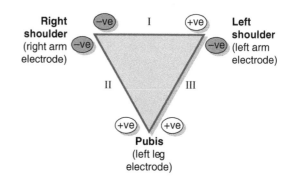

Figure 27.7 • Einthoven triangle.

Box 27.3

Areas of heart shown in specific leads

I – Left lateral surface
II – Left lateral and inferior surface
III – Inferior surface
AVR – Right atrium
AVL – Left lateral surface
AVF – Inferior surface
V_1 – Right anterior
V_2 – Right anterior surface and some of left anterior surface
V_3 – Septal area
V_4 – Anterior surface of left ventricle
V_5 – Left anterior/lateral surfaces
V_6 – Lateral aspect of left ventricle

depolarize down the conductive system as far as the apex of the heart. This directional flow is known as the cardiac vector. The four limb leads attached as shown in Figure 27.7 form what is known as the Einthoven triangle. The fourth lead not shown within the triangle acts as an earth and helps to standardize

recordings. Leads I, II and III are known as bipolar leads, because each lead represents the electrical activity between two poles:

• lead I represents electrical activity from the right arm to the left arm

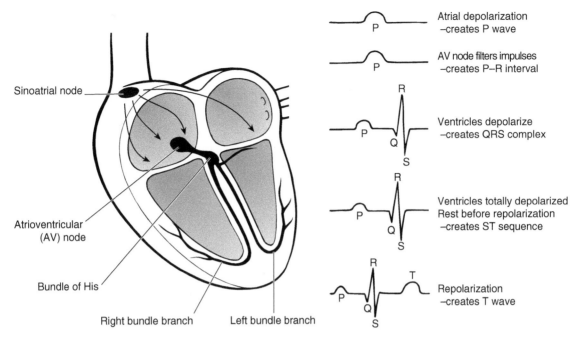

Atrial depolarization
–creates P wave

AV node filters impulses
–creates P–R interval

Ventricles depolarize
–creates QRS complex

Ventricles totally depolarized
Rest before repolarization
–creates ST sequence

Repolarization
–creates T wave

Figure 27.8 • Electrical activity of the heart in relation to the ECG recording.

- lead II represents electrical activity from the right arm to the left leg
- lead III represents electrical activity from the left arm to the left leg.

Leads AVR, AVL and AVF are known as unipolar leads. They read electrical impulses from one electrode, with the ECG machine calculating the effect of the other limb leads to give an average reading between the points of the triangle formed by the bipolar leads.

The abbreviations for the unipolar leads are as follows:

- A – augmented (amplified)
- V – vector (force of direction of impulse)
- R, L, F – the direction being viewed, i.e., right, left or foot.

Thus, AVR looks at the right atrium (although in practice this is of little consequence), AVL looks at the lateral aspect of the heart, and AVF looks at the inferior aspect (Box 27.3). The chest leads are a much more simplified version for looking at the frontal plane of the heart. These are unipolar leads that pick up electrical activity from the point at which they are placed (Box 27.3):

- V_1 is placed over the 4th intercostal space to the right of the sternum
- V_2 is placed over the 4th intercostal space to the left of the sternum
- V_1 and V_2 thus view the anterior surfaces of the right and part of the left ventricles
- V_3 is placed on the chest midway between V_2 and V_4; hence it is useful to apply V_4 before V_3. V_3 looks at the septum
- V_4 is placed on the fifth intercostal space, midway along the clavicular line, and views the septum and the anterior wall of the left ventricle

- V_5 is placed along the same line as V_4, but anteriorly to the midaxillary line
- V_6 is again placed along the same line as V_4 and V_5, but rests on the midaxillary line
- V_5 and V_6 view predominately the lateral wall of the left ventricles.

Components of a normal ECG

The ECG complex is made up of a sequence of electrical events occurring in the heart. The activity starts with impulses being transmitted from the sinoatrial node across the atria. As the atria depolarize, the P wave is created. The AV node filters and holds atrial impulses to allow significant ventricular filling time prior to contraction. This is represented as a straight line (isoelectric line) on the ECG and is called the P–R interval. As depolarization occurs through the bundle branches, and a wave of depolarization spreads across, the QRS complex is created on the ECG. This is followed by a short resting period, depicted again as an isoelectric line called the ST segment, before the T wave is created by ventricular repolarization (Fig. 27.8).

When this is all put together, a single heartbeat is represented in the ECG trace as shown in Figure 27.9.

Basic rhythm recognition

To make an accurate analysis of cardiac activity it is necessary to obtain a 12-lead ECG trace as opposed to a rhythm strip. The rhythm strip only shows one view of the heart that is dependent on the electrode positioning. As a result, myocardial damage or stress can easily be missed.

Once the 12-lead ECG has been obtained (Fig. 27.10), it is necessary to work through each lead methodically, looking at each waveform to ensure that any changes/abnormalities are recognized. To interpret an ECG, the ED nurse should start by looking at the rhythm strip to determine whether a basic rhythm is present. If a rhythm exists, complexes will be repetitive and components of those complexes will form the same pattern. It is also necessary to determine whether this pattern is occurring at regular intervals or not. Once an underlying rhythm is established, the rate of the rhythm should be determined (Evans 2007).

ECG tracings are standardized so that heart rate can be calculated from the tracing. Most ECG machines are set to pass paper through at 25 mm/s. As graph paper is standardized, one small square represents 0.04 s (1 mm of paper), one large square represents 0.2 s (5 mm of paper) and five large squares represent 1 s (25 mm of paper). Therefore, if there is one QRS complex per five large squares, the heart rate would be approximately 60 beats/min. Once an approximate rate is established, the nurse should look at the make-up of the repetitive complexes, checking whether the P waves are followed by the right length of interval and the QRS complex is followed by a T wave (Box 27.4).

Once a basic rhythm has been established from the rhythm strip, attention should be focused on the various

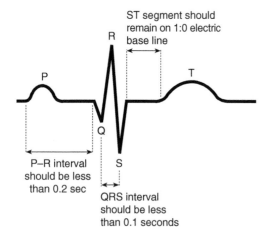

Figure 27.9 • Normal ECG complex from a single heartbeat.

Box 27.4

ECG analysis

- *Rhythm* – is it regular? Are the R–R intervals equal? To check this, place a piece of paper on the trace and mark off three R waves, moving the paper alone to see if other R waves match this pattern
- *Rate* – sinus, tachycardic or bradycardic?
- *P waves* – are P waves present? Are they of a uniform shape? Do they precede the QRS complex? These represent atrial activity or abnormality
- *QRS complex* – normal width/shape? These represent ventricular activity or abnormality
- *T waves*– are the ST segments above or below the isoelectric line? Uniform shape and size?
- *Intervals* – are all the intervals normal?
  - P–R 0.12–0.2 s
  - QRS 0.07–0.1 s
  - Q–T 0.33–0.43 s
  - P–R and Q–T intervals vary with heart rate

leads to determine whether any area of the heart is damaged or ischaemic. ECG interpretation grows with experience, time and practice utilizing learning opportunities within the ED. However, it is important that ECG interpretation does not take precedence over the patient's clinical condition. The clinical picture and condition of the patient are by far the best indicators of overall well-being. For this reason there is no substitute for the ED nurse's fundamental assessment skills.

Cardiac arrest

Cardiorespiratory arrest can be defined as the sudden or acute cessation of the heartbeat and subsequently cardiac function, resulting in loss of effective circulation and respiration and therefore, incompatible with life (Evans 2007). There are numerous causes of cardiorespiratory arrest but there are only four cardiac rhythms an arrested patient will be in, they are:

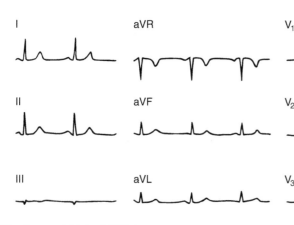

Figure 27.10 • A normal 12-lead ECG trace.

* or national emergency number

Figure 27.11 • Adult basic life support. (*, or call national emergency number) • (Copyright European Resuscitation Council – www.erc.edu – 2012/027)

* ventricular fibrillation (VF)
* pulseless ventricular tachycardia (VT)
* asystole
* pulseless electrical activity (PEA).

It is identified by:

* loss of consciousness
* absence of a central pulse (carotid/femoral)
* absence of spontaneous respiration.

Systemic management

In EDs, cardiac arrests in most instances are anticipated. Therefore, the ED nurse is responsible for (Alexander et al. 2000):

* recognizing cardiac arrest
* correct procedure for summoning help
* commencing basic life support (Fig. 27.11).

Ventricular fibrillation and pulseless ventricular tachycardia

The most common cause of cardiac arrest is usually VF or VT, which has an 80% mortality rate for patients outside the hospital environment (Nolan et al. 2010) although women have a higher survival rate (Teodorescu et al. 2012). In VF, the cardiac cycle is disrupted and the cardiac cells behave chaotically, depolarizing in a disoriented and disorderly fashion or fibrillation (Fig. 27.12). As a result, cardiac output is compromised to the extent that blood circulation stops. This results in hypoxia, loss of consciousness within 10–20 seconds and absence of respiration. The physiology of VT is discussed later in this chapter. Simply put, the ventricular contractions occur at such a rate that ventricular filling time is inadequate and cardiac output is compromised. In severe cases, circulation ceases as in VF.

Immediate management

Cardiac arrest management has been standardized by the development of advanced life support (ALS) protocols (International Liaison Committee on Resuscitation 2005a, Resuscitation Council (UK) 2011). If the VF arrest is witnessed and monitored, a precordial thump may be of benefit in an attempt to 'shock' the heart and restore normal electrical activity; however it has a very low success rate for cardioversion of a shockable rhythm and is only likely to succeed if given within the first few seconds of the onset of a shockable rhythm (Haman et al. 2009, Pellis et al. 2009). It should never lead to a delay in getting a patient on to a defibrillator or being shocked (Resuscitation Council (UK) 2011). Potential complications of the precordial thump include rhythm deteriorations, such as rate acceleration of VT and asystole (Krijne 1984). A precordial thump is most likely to

Figure 27.12 • Ventricular fibrillation.

be successful in converting VT into sinus rhythm. Successful treatment of VT by precordial thump is much less likely (Resuscitation Council (UK) 2011). Having reviewed the evidence, the International Liaison Committee on Resuscitation (2005b) recommends one immediate thump may be considered after a monitored cardiac arrest if an electrical defibrillator is not immediately available.

The optimum first-line treatment for VF and pulseless VT is early defibrillation. The aim of defibrillation is to depolarize the myocardium simultaneously, to allow normal cardiac cell function to resume (Colquhoun et al. 1999). A key factor in reducing mortality lies with the speed of defibrillation, which should be given, safely, without delay (International Liaison Committee on Resuscitation 2005b). For this reason, ED nurses should be appropriately skilled in performing defibrillation as they are likely to be the first personnel in attendance. The resuscitation training officer for the ED should provide or ensure this training is given and updated yearly.

Defibrillation

Defibrillators used to require someone holding onto paddles and placing them on the chest; these have now all but been withdrawn, replaced by hands-free pad systems. Most EDs will have hands-free defibrillator systems. The pads or paddles of the defibrillator are positioned to enclose as much myocardium as possible (Fig. 27.13). A conductive medium, such as jelly pads, should always be used if older-style paddle defibrillators are used, both to enhance contact and to reduce skin damage. However, the widely used hands-free systems in most EDs have this gel component included already in the pads provided. Good contact with the chest is vital to maximize conduction and prevent 'arcing' of electrical current. If using the paddles, then they should be placed firmly over the jelly pads and perpendicular pressure should be applied (approximately 8 kg). If using the hands-free pads then the pads should be firmly pressed against the skin without kinks or folds and care should be taken to ensure nothing has become stuck between the pad and the patient. One pad/paddle should be placed to the right of the sternum, below the right clavicle in the mid-clavicular line, and the other vertically in the mid-axillary line, approximately level with the V$_6$ electrode position or the female breast. This position should be clear of any breast tissue (Resuscitation Council (UK) 2011).

Prior to defibrillation, glyceryl trinitrate (GTN) patches and external pacing generators should be removed and the bare chest should be dried. Excessive hair should be shaved off quickly to allow for pad/paddle contact to the skin. Jewellry should be moved to one side so as not to touch the pads/paddles. Nothing should delay in providing a patient with a safe defibrillation. Any internal pacers or defibrillating systems do not preclude the need for external DC shock in the case of VF or pulseless VT; however, the electrode should be placed away from the device.

In very rare occasions a patient may have internal defibrillation performed where small paddles are placed either side of the heart inside the open chest cavity. The ED nurse would never be expected to perform this role.

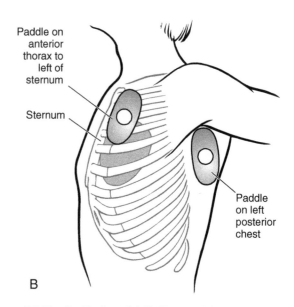

Figure 27.13 • Positioning of defibrillator paddles.

As even short interruptions to perform rhythm analysis causes significant interruptions in CPR and thus survival, the Resuscitation Council (UK) (2011) now recommends a single-shock strategy. The rationale is that with the first wave of biphasic waveforms exceeding 90%, failure to terminate VF/VT successfully implies the need for a period of CPR to improve myocardial oxygenation, rather than a further shock. The Resuscitation Council (UK) (2011) notes that even if defibrillation is successful in restoring a perfusing rhythm, it is very rare for a pulse to be palpable immediately afterwards, and the delay in trying to palpate a pulse will further compromise the myocardium if a perfusing rhythm has not been restored (van Alem 2003). The SOS-Kanto study group (2007) found in witnessed out-of-hospital cardiac arrest, cardiac-only resuscitation improved survival rate.

The safety of the resuscitation team is paramount and it is the responsibility of the person administering DC shocks to ensure that other team members are clear of the patient. This should be ascertained verbally and visually before proceeding with defibrillation. ALS courses provide a standardized approach to training for all team members and should be a priority for ED nurses. These courses and updates are usually attained through a hospital's resuscitation training department. The defibrillation regime should follow the algorithm shown in Figure 27.14.

Asystole

This is total cessation of circulation, brought about by the lack of cardiac pacemaker activity, either natural or artificial (Colquhoun et al. 1999). Asystole accounts for 25% of all cardiac arrests within the hospital environment (Jowett & Thompson 2007). The treatment is continued cardiac compression with ventilation. Adrenaline (epinephrine) and atropine are used to stimulate cardiac activity, but the prognosis for a successful

Figure 27.14 • Universal algorithm • (Copyright European Resuscitation Council – www.erc.edu – 2012/027)

Figure 27.15 • Asystole.

resuscitation remains poor, with the overall survival rate being about 20–22% of the survival rate compared with VF/VT rhythms (Resuscitation Council (UK) 2011) (Fig. 27.15).

Pulseless electrical activity (PEA)

This presents as a full QRS complex on the heart trace, but with the absence of any palpable pulse, hence the lack of systemic circulation. The causes are divided into the categories primary and secondary (Box 27.5).

 Box 27.5

Causes of electromechanical disassociation

Primary causes
- Myocardial infarction (particularly inferior wall)
- Drugs (beta-blockers or calcium antagonists) or toxins
- Electrolyte abnormalities (such as hypocalcaemia, hyperkalaemia)
- Atrial thrombus or tumour (myxoma)

Secondary causes
- Tension pneumothorax
- Pericardial tamponade
- Cardiac rupture
- Pulmonary embolism
- Prosthetic heart valve occlusion
- Hypovolaemia

For the resuscitation attempt to be of any success, the cause must be isolated and the appropriate treatment initiated, namely the non-VF/VT side of the algorithm shown in Figure 27.14.

Drug therapy

Pharmacological intervention may be used during cardiac arrest to (Jowett & Thompson 2007, Resuscitation Council (UK) 2011):

- correct hypoxia and acidosis
- accelerate or reduce the heart rate
- suppress ectopic activity
- stimulate the strength of myocardial contraction.

Adrenaline

Adrenaline (epinephrine) is the first drug used in cardiac arrest. Its therapeutic action is to improve coronary and cerebral perfusion. To date, substantial clinical evidence that adrenaline improves survival or neurological recovery in humans is absent (International Liaison Committee on Resuscitation 2005a), but some clinical findings have ensured that it has been continually used in arrests for the last 40 years (Resuscitation Council (UK) 2011). Adrenaline is an alpha- and beta-agonist and acts upon receptor sites to increase circulation to vital sites (Opie 2000). Its action in cardiac arrest is to cause vasoconstriction, increasing cerebral and coronary perfusion. Arrich et al. (2012) found, however, that an increasing cumulative dose of adrenaline during resuscitation of patients with asystole and pulseless electric activity is an independent risk factor for unfavourable functional outcome and in-hospital mortality.

Atropine

Atropine used to be recommended in the first-line treatment of arrests. However, the Resuscitation Council (UK) Resuscitation Guidelines (2010) no longer recommend its use for this purpose.

Amiodarone

Amiodarone is used to increase the duration of the action potential in both the atrial and ventricular myocardium, thus prolonging the QT interval. Amiodarone 300 mg is considered for use in treating shock-refractory cardiac arrest due to VF or pulseless VT after the third shock. A further dose of 150 mg can be given if VF/pulseless VT persists. Lidocaine may be given as an alternative if amiodarone is not available; however, both should not be given at the same time.

Calcium salts

In cardiac cell activity, calcium ions play a vital role in contraction, as well as during the cell's action potential. Calcium is indicated during resuscitation from PEA when the cause is:

- hypocalcaemia
- hyperkalaemia
- overdose of calcium-channel-blocking drugs
- overdose of magnesium (e.g., during treatment of pre-eclampsia (Resuscitation Council (UK) 2011).

Sodium bicarbonate

Controversy continues as to the efficacy of this drug and its routine use is not recommended. It may be considered for the reversal of life-threatening hyperkalaemia, pre-existing metabolic acidosis or tricyclic antidepressant overdose (Resuscitation Council (UK) 2011).

Normal sinus beat   Ventricular ectopic beat

Figure 27.16 • Ventricular ectopic beat.

Ethical considerations

Whether the resuscitation is successful or not, thought and consideration for family or relatives must be a priority. Clear lines of communication must exist between medical and nursing staff and any family/friends. If the need to break bad news arises, ideally the doctor and the ED nurse should perform this, with one or the other actually breaking the news. More often than not these simple communication skills are forgotten (Box 27.6). A detailed discussion of this subject is given in Chapter 14.

Box 27.6

Communicating with relatives/friends
- Prepare yourself. Compose your thoughts
- Enter the room/area with another person, e.g., a doctor or nurse
- Confirm that you are talking to the correct relatives/friends
- Spend time with the relatives. Avoid appearing harassed or impatient
- Maintain eye contact when talking
- Be prepared to emphasize and repeat any information
- Avoid using the wrong terms, i.e., 'slipped away' or 'passed on'. Be honest, say the person has died
- Don't be afraid of silences
- Be prepared for a wide variety of reactions

Occasionally the subject of 'do not attempt resuscitation' orders (DNAR) will present itself. In a joint statement from the British Medical Association and Royal College of Nursing (Resuscitation Council (UK) 2007), it was determined that the overall responsibility for decisions about CPR and DNAR rests with the consultant in charge of the patient's care. This decision should involve the medical and nursing staff, the patient, if possible, and the family and must be clearly documented, including the date, decision and the reasons for it (Resuscitation Council (UK) 2007, Nolan et al 2011). It is also discussed in Chapter 14.

Rhythm disturbances

It is important when caring for a patient with a presenting cardiac condition that the recognition of any abnormalities is accurate and prompt. Reference to the UK treatment algorithms

for tachycardias and bradycardias may prove useful to the ED nurse when considering the management of arrhythmias (Resuscitation Council (UK) 2011). Rhythm disturbances can be divided into two groups: ventricular and atrial arrhythmias. Those commonly treated in ED are discussed below.

Ventricular ectopics (VEs)

This is due to premature discharge of an ectopic ventricular focus (Schamroth 2001) (Fig. 27.16). The impulse avoids travelling through conducting tissue, but travels through ordinary muscle structure. Causes of VEs include:

- hypoxia
- myocardial ischaemia
- hypokalaemia
- hypercalcaemia
- acidosis
- caffeine
- digoxin toxicity.

Assessment

The aim of assessment is to determine both causative factors and level of systemic compromise. This should include pulse speed, regularity and pressure, respiration and blood pressure. Repeated VEs reduce ventricular filling time and can result in a reduction of circulatory volume. A 12-lead ECG should be obtained to confirm diagnosis. ECG characteristics are shown in Table 27.1.

Table 27.1 ECG characteristics of ventricular ectopics

Component	Finding
Rhythm	Irregular, due to premature beats
Rate	60–100 beats/min
P wave	Not related to QRS complex of the VE
QRS	Wide and bizarre complex of a VE

Management

The patient may present with palpitations, nausea, diaphoresis or shortness of breath. Immediate treatment of VEs can

Figure 27.17 • Ventricular tachycardia.

include the use of anti-arrhythmic drugs, such as intravenous amiodarone. For long-term control, oral preparations such as beta-blockers, calcium-channel blockers or amiodarone can be used. Correction of the urea and electrolyte imbalance can lead to the resolution of VEs.

Ventricular tachycardia (VT)

Ventricular contraction is stimulated from within as ventricular myocardium and does not follow normal electrical conductivity (Fig. 27.17). The causes of VT are the same as those of VEs, but it is considered more dangerous due to its capacity to significantly decrease cardiac output. The cardiac output is compromised due to the shortening of the cardiac cycle, and thus there is a reduced amount of blood available for ejection (Woods et al. 2000). The ventricular myocardium is not able to sustain rapid contraction over prolonged periods and there is therefore a tendency for VF to follow untreated VT.

Assessment

This is the same as assessing a patient with multiple VEs. VT is usually caused by ischaemic or structural heart disease or electrolyte disturbances. The important factor is determining the degree of systemic compromise through levels of consciousness, pulse, respirations and blood pressure (McDonough 2009). ECG characteristics are shown in Table 27.2.

Table 27.2 ECG characteristics of ventricular tachycardia

Component	Finding
Rhythm	Either regular or slightly irregular
Rate	Faster than 100 beats/min
P waves	Dissociated from QRS complexes
QRS	Wide and bizarre

Management

Presenting symptoms may include shortness of breath, palpitations, dizziness, nausea and diaphoresis. Treatment may incorporate the use of 300 mg amiodarone i.v. over 20–60 minutes, followed by an infusion of 900 mg over 24 hours (Resuscitation Council (UK) 2011). If initial drug therapy is not successful and the patient is showing signs of cardiovascular compromise, cardioversion with synchronized DC shock should be carried out. The patient should be sedated for this procedure, unless his clinical condition is deteriorating too rapidly to facilitate this. If VT becomes pulseless at any time, emergency defibrillation should be carried out, and the algorithm in Figure 27.14 should be followed.

Supraventricular tachycardia (SVT)

This does not always stem from atrial activity, but it does originate from above the ventricles and it is difficult to pinpoint the exact causative factor from the ECG (Fig. 27.18). The atria can depolarize in a retrograde fashion or a circular fashion depending on the causative factors.

Causes include:

- atrial tachycardia
- atrial flutter/fibrillation
- stimulants, e.g., caffeine or nicotine
- idiopathic.

Assessment

This should concentrate on determining the patient's capacity to compensate for the rapid heart rate. Pulse, respirations and blood pressure are vital indicators. The patient will probably be aware of palpitations or 'pounding' in his chest and may complain of pain, dizziness and shortness of breath. The ECG characteristics are shown in Table 27.3.

Management

Depending on the patient's tolerance of the SVT, vagal stimulation can be attempted to slow down the heart rate. This can be achieved by carotid sinus massage and is sufficient to control SVT in about 20% of cases (International Liaison Committee on Resuscitation 2005a); however, over-zealous treatment can result in profound bradycardia or VF. Drug therapy of choice is adenosine, with the initial dose of 6 mg

Figure 27.18 • Supraventricular tachycardia.

Sinus beat   Atrial ectopic beat

Figure 27.19 • Atrial ectopic beats.

Table 27.3 ECG characteristics of supraventricular tachycardia	
Component	**Finding**
Rhythm	Regular
Rate	>100 and up to 280 beats/min
P wave	Not usually visible
QRS	Usually narrow

given by rapid bolus injection. If required, two further doses of 12 mg can be administered. Adenosine works by depressing AV node conduction and therefore prevents re-entry rhythms from sustaining SVT, allowing sinus rhythm to return. Side-effects of adenosine are common, and the nurse should expect the patient to be flushed, nauseous, have some chest discomfort and 'a sense of impending doom'. These effects are short-lived and should have passed in a matter of minutes (Opie 2000). If the patient's condition continues to deteriorate, a synchronized DC shock is indicated.

Atrial ectopics

This is a premature discharge of an ectopic atrial focus from a point other than the sinoatrial node (Fig. 27.19). Causes include:

* alcohol
* mitral valve disease
* coronary artery disease
* hyperthyroidism
* heart failure
* viral infections.

It can also occur in healthy individuals.

Assessment

Diagnosis is made on ECG tracing as the patient is usually unaware of the occurrence of atrial ectopics. Pulse rate should be checked for irregularity and respiration may be slightly increased. ECG findings are shown in Table 27.4.

Table 27.4 ECG characteristics of atrial ectopic beats	
Component	**Finding**
Rhythm	Slightly irregular
Rate	Usually within normal limits
P wave	Precede every QRS
QRS	Normally no change is seen

Management

The patient is usually unaware, but can present with shortness of breath. The treatment of atrial ectopics is not usually required unless the patient shows signs of compromise. Drugs used include disopyramide.

Atrial fibrillation

Atrial fibrillation (AF), is the most common cardiac arrhythmia, and is associated with an increased risk of embolus-related stroke, heart failure due to reduced cardiac output and premature death (Bilal Iqbal et al. 2005, Evans 2007, von Besser & Mills 2011). It affects 5–10% of older people (Houghton & Gray 1997), and is a rapid and disorganized depolarization occurring throughout the atrial myocardium, replacing normal rhythmic activity by the SA node (Hand 2002). Every minute 400–600 impulses reach the AV node

Irregular QRS complexes   No discernible P waves

Figure 27.20 • Atrial fibrillation.

Figure 27.21 • Atrial flutter.

Table 27.5 ECG characteristics of atrial fibrillation	
Component	**Finding**
Rhythm	Irregular
Rate	Variable, but usually >100 beats/min
P waves	Not present
QRS	Normal

from different atrial foci rather than the SA node, but only 120–180 of these reach the ventricles to produce QRS complexes (Fig. 27.20). Causes include:

- hypertension
- ischaemic heart disease
- binge alcohol drinking
- atrial septal defect
- pulmonary embolus
- pneumonia
- cardiomyopathy
- idiopathic
- rheumatic heart disease
- myocardial infarction
- mitral valve disease.

Assessment

The fast pace at which the atria depolarize leads to failure of the atria to contract effectively, causing them to quiver. This means that the ventricles do not fill adequately, which can lead to a 10–15% fall in cardiac output (Houghton & Gray 1997). Patients with AF often present with palpitations or symptoms of an underlying cause. Respirations, pulse and blood pressure should be ascertained. The patient may complain of weakness, dizziness or shortness of breath. ECG changes are listed in Table 27.5.

Management

The aim of treatment of AF is usually to eliminate the cause in order to control the ventricular rate, thereby optimizing cardiac function, reducing the risk of embolism and restoring sinus rhythm (Hand 2002, Neumar et al. 2010). If the duration is less than 48 hours, and rhythm control is considered appropriate, this may be attempted using amiodarone 300 mg i.v. over 20–60 minutes followed by 900 mg over 24 hours (Resuscitation Council (UK) 2011). If the patient is severely compromised, cardioversion may be necessary. Other symptoms can include an increased risk of thrombus formation, and hence the need for anticoagulants.

Atrial flutter

Atrial flutter occurs when there is rapid atrial excitement and is much less common than atrial fibrillation. The term flutter is used as the P waves appear 'saw-toothed' (Fig. 27.21). It is almost always associated with significant cardiac abnormalities (Hand 2002). The atrial rate can be anything between 250 and 350 beats/min, but the ventricular rate is much lower because of AV filtering which acts as a 'gatekeeper'. In contrast to atrial fibrillation, the rate is regular.

The causes include:

- ischaemic heart disease with left ventricular dysfunction
- mitral valve disease
- acute MI
- hypertension.

Prolonged P–R interval

Figure 27.22 • First-degree heart block.

Assessment

Assessment is the same as for AF (Table 27.6).

Table 27.6 ECG characteristics of atrial flutter

Component	Finding
Rhythm	Usually regular
Rate	Variable, but usually >100 beats/min
P waves	Usually obscured by flutter waves
QRS	Normal, may be widened by bundle branch block

Management

Hudak et al. (1998) suggest that slowing down the rhythm using adenosine or vagal manoeuvres should increase the degree of AV block and make the rhythm more apparent. Although drugs can be used to control the ventricular rate, the aim should be to restore sinus rhythm. If the patient is compromised, oxygen will be required. Treatment comprises digoxin or verapamil, or in severe cases cardioversion may be required. Other drugs that may aid treatment include amiodarone, beta-blockers or disopyramide.

Heart block

Heart block occurs when the impulses from the atria to the ventricles are delayed at the AV node (Hampton 2003). There are, for the purpose of this chapter, three types of heart block:

* first-degree heart block
* second-degree heart block
* third-degree (complete) heart block.

These can be a complication of a myocardial infarction.

First-degree heart block (Fig. 27.22)

As can be seen from the rhythm strip, the P–R interval is prolonged. This is due to the delay at the AV node, where impulses conduct to the ventricles but with delayed conduction times (Jacobson 2000, Jowett & Thompson 2007). The ECG characteristics are given in Table 27.7.

Table 27.7 ECG characteristics of first-degree heart block

Component	Finding
Rhythm	Regular
Rate	Sinus, between 60 and 100 beats/min
P wave	Normal
P–R interval	Prolonged, i.e. >0.20 s
QRS	Normal

Management

In most instances the patient remains asymptomatic and does not require any further treatment, but for the reasons of safety should be re-evaluated at regular intervals.

Second-degree heart block (Fig. 27.23)

There are two types of second-degree block: type I (Wenckebach) and type II (Mobitz) (see Table 27.8 for ECG characteristics). In type I second-degree AV block a gradual lengthening of the P–R interval occurs because of lengthening AV conduction time, until an atrial pulse is non-conducted, so a P wave is not followed by a QRS. Then the sequence begins again. The blocked P wave may occur occasionally or frequently, regularly or irregularly. Of the second-degree heart blocks, type I is the most common, is usually transitory and rarely progresses to complete heart block. It produces few or no clinical symptoms although a 2:1 type block may develop with haemodynamic instability. In type II second-degree AV heart block, a P wave is blocked without progressive antecedent P–R elongation and occurs almost always in a setting of bundle branch block. Type II second-degree block is often caused by irreversible damage and frequently progresses to complete heart block. Clinical symptoms such as dizziness or faintness may occur with frequent non-conducted P waves (Wyatt et al. 2012).

Management

Depending on the patient's tolerance to the rhythm, there may or may not be a need for treatment. If the patient is compromised, i.v. atropine is the first-line drug for bradycardias. Then consider adrenaline (epinephrine) and seek expert help. The patient may need temporary pacing to avert the

Figure 27.23 • Second-degree heart block. (A) Wenckebach type I. (B) Mobitz type II.

Figure 27.24 • Complete (third-degree) heart block.

Table 27.8 ECG characteristics of second-degree heart block	
Component	**Finding**
Rhythm	Regular
Rate	Sinus or atrial beats
P waves	Normal
P–R interval	Can lengthen or can be normal
QRS	Normal

need for pacemaker insertion in a compromised patient if sudden complete heart block develops (Hand 2002).

Third-degree (complete) heart block (Fig. 27.24)

This type of heart block is characterized by the unrelated impulses sent between the atria and the ventricles. When this occurs there is no correlation of the electrical activity and a disassociation develops between the atria and ventricles. This in turn means that the cardiac output is reduced to the point where the patient usually becomes symptomatic.

Assessment

A nodal rhythm gives a rate of around 40–60 beats, while a ventricular rhythm gives a rate of 30–40 beats/min. If this so-called 'escape' rhythm does not develop, ventricular standstill will occur and this is fatal if not treated (Hand 2002). It is important to assess the level of circulatory compromise as a treatment guideline. Some patients will present profoundly, with a history of collapse. This is due to severe circulatory collapse as a result of poor cardiac output due to decreased atrial and ventricular synchronicity. The ECG characteristics are given in Table 27.9.

Table 27.9 ECG characteristics of third-degree heart block	
Component	**Finding**
Rhythm	Regular
Rate	Normal atrial rate, but the ventricular rate can be less than 45 beats/min
P wave	Normal, but shows no relation to the QRS complexes
P–R interval	No consistent P–R interval exists
QRS	Normal, although sometimes wide

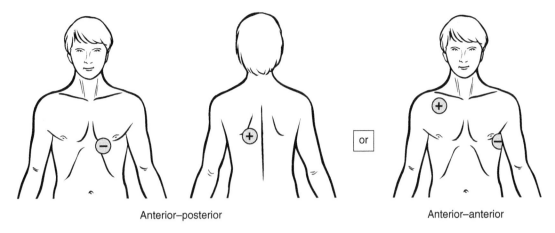

Anterior–posterior   or   Anterior–anterior

Figure 27.25 • Positioning of pacing pads for non-invasive temporary pacing.

Pacing spike

Broad QRS complexes

Figure 27.26 • Non-invasive temporary pacing.

Management

Treatment ultimately depends on the symptoms encountered. If the cause is acute inferior MI, drug toxicity, acute pericarditis or myocarditis, total AV block is usually a passing phenomenon. Drug therapy includes atropine and isoprenaline, but in most instances requires the insertion of either a temporary or a permanent pacing system to maintain the patient's cardiac equilibrium. In cases of profound collapse, external pacing is necessary to maintain circulatory volume. Nolan et al. (1998) estimate that up to 89 % of patients who develop complete heart block following anterior MI die, often from pump failure due to ventricular damage.

Pacing

It is sometimes necessary to support a patient's conductive system by means of a pacing system. The purpose of pacemakers is to control the electrical activity of the heart. Both temporary and permanent pacing systems contain two components:

- pulse generator (pacing box) – this forms the electrical supply source for pacing; the box usually contains batteries as its power source
- pacing catheter – this conductive wire has either one or two electrodes to provide an electrical stimulus to the heart, once the pacing catheter electrodes are in direct contact with the myocardium.

There are currently three types of pacemaker available:

- non-invasive temporary pacing
- temporary (transvenous) pacing
- permanent pacing.

Non-invasive temporary pacing (NTP)

This system of pacing is used predominately by EDs to treat symptomatic bradycardias and ventricular asystole. Most EDs in the UK have access to a defibrillator with pacing facilities, e.g., the Physio Control Lifepak 20. The advantages of NTP include its ability to be initiated rapidly, its ease of use and the fact that CPR can be continued without risk to the user. To use NTP, two large electrodes are placed on the chest as shown in Figure 27.25.

Once NTP has been commenced it is important to look for signs of electrical and mechanical capture. When looking for signs of electrical capture, a heart trace can provide the evidence required. A pacing spike should be followed by a wide QRS and a tall broad T wave (Fig. 27.26). Mechanical capture is seen by the improvements in the patient's condition. Compared with other forms of pacing, NTP is, on the surface, a more favourable approach to emergency pacing. Pacing can be painful for the patient so analgesia and sedation should be considered and given appropriately (Resuscitation Council (UK) 2011).

Temporary pacing (transvenous)

The indications for the insertion of a temporary transvenous pacing wire include (Harrigan et al. 2007):

- extreme bradycardia
- complete heart block
- asystole
- very occasionally for tachycardias.

A bipolar pacing catheter is inserted through a central or peripheral vein (subclavian, external jugular or antecubital fossa) under sterile conditions, using ECG monitoring and fluoroscopy equipment. A local anaesthetic is used prior to insertion. Once the pacing catheter has been sited, the electrodes are then connected to the external pulse generator (pacing box). Complications include:

- pneumothorax
- infection
- cardiac perforation
- arrhythmias.

Permanent pacing

The decision to use an implantable pacing system remains dependent on the patient's symptoms. Symptomatic patients are fitted with a permanent pacemaker by inserting the power source (lithium-driven) with a subcutaneous pocket under the clavicle or axilla. The procedure is performed under a local anaesthetic. The majority of permanent pacemakers fitted today have an approximate life span of up to 15 years.

Acute chest pain

Acute coronary syndromes

These consist of:

- Q wave myocardial infarction (full-thickness myocardial necrosis) known as ST segment elevation MI (STEMI)
- non-Q wave myocardial infarction, now better known as non-ST elevation MI or non-STEMI (subendocardial or intramural wall damage)
- unstable angina (myocardial ischaemia without necrosis).

Non-ST segment elevation myocardial infarction can occur with partial or transient blocking of the coronary artery. This can produce less extensive damage to the surrounding muscle. However, testing serum troponin levels will show that necrosis has occurred. With Q wave myocardial infarction, sometimes the typical ST changes are not seen; however, if ischaemia persists, typical Q waves will appear on the ECG.

Unstable angina is a symptom, not a disease, brought on by inadequate coronary blood flow to the myocardium (Jowett & Thompson 2007). Castle (2003) notes that while the myocardium has no 'pain fibres', ischaemic hearts do produce lactic acid, bradykinin, adenosine, prostaglandins, potassium and carbon dioxide. Each of these has been linked with the stimulation of pain fibres in coronary arteries or the transmission of pain as a noxious stimulus (International Liaison Committee on Resuscitation 2005c). It usually presents as central chest pain with either a rapid or gradual onset over several minutes, with possible radiation to the jaw, back and arms. Pain is frequently described as crushing, burning, sharp, or heavy (Williams 2009). It can occur at rest or on exertion. When chest pain has been unremitting for 20 minutes at rest, myocardial infarction should be considered (Braunwald et al. 2000). Other associated symptoms include breathlessness, dizziness, belching and epigastric discomfort after eating.

Assessment

When a patient presents to the ED with chest pain secondary to unstable angina it is usually because previous attempts to relieve the pain have failed. On average patients delay seeking medical care for acute MI symptoms for two or more hours (Zerwic 1999); however, prompt assessment of the patient with acute coronary syndromes is critical as the incidence of ventricular fibrillation is greater during the first hour after the onset of acute MI symptoms (Barnason 2003).

It is very often difficult to distinguish between unstable angina and acute MI during the initial assessment of the patient, thus the management in the first few hours will often be similar to that for an MI. When assessing the patient it is important to gain a detailed history. This should include: the type (e.g., crushing, burning, sharp), severity and duration of the pain, what the patient was doing when the pain started, and whether anything has been taken to relieve it. Any radiation of pain should be noted because it helps to confirm a clinical picture of cardiac pain. Any symptoms associated with the onset of pain or still present are also important as they act as an indication of the level of systemic compromise resulting from myocardial hypoxia. The patient's medical and drug history should also be noted.

Physical assessment should include baseline observations of pulse rate, regularity and pressure, respirations and blood pressure. These should enable the ED nurse to determine the impact of the angina on the patient's overall condition. Temperature should also be checked, as a rise in temperature can be indicative of tissue breakdown, consistent with a myocardial infarction. Cardiac monitoring, 12-lead ECG recording and X-ray help complete the clinical picture. The ECG may show any associated rhythm disturbance and most importantly any ischaemic changes to the myocardium as a result of hypoxia. ECG changes may show as ST-segment depression in the area affected by hypoxia (Fig. 27.27, Table 27.10).

Clinical investigations include blood analysis to detect electrolyte imbalance, cardiac enzymes or cardiac troponins consistent with myocardial infarction. Blood should be taken for full blood count (FBC), urea and electrolyte (U&E) levels, glucose (which can rise after acute infection) and cardiac enzymes and troponins. Detection of raised troponin levels indicates a diagnosis of non-ST-elevated MI, and absence of detectable troponin is indicative of unstable

| I II III | aVR aVL aVF | V₁ V₂ V₃ | V₄ V₅ V₆ |

Figure 27.27 • Inferior/lateral ST depression.

Table 27.10 Classification of angina

Classification	Characteristics
Stable angina	Condition in which the frequency and severity of angina remain well controlled and unchanged over months
Angina decubitus	Pain occurring when lying down
Unstable angina	Condition in which the pain is increasing in frequency, severity and duration. Occurs with less activity or at rest
Prinzmetal's angina	Unusual form where pain occurs at rest or long after activity has ceased. Accompanied by transient ST-segment elevation. Coronary artery spasm without underlying disease is often the cause
Crescendo angina	Form of angina where chance of an MI occurring within a few days is high
Intractable angina	Continued pain with increasing frequency, despite treatment

angina (Fox 2004). Troponin reaches detectably raised levels hours after a cardiac event, and so may not be abnormal at initial presentation. Raised levels can be detected three to four hours after the event and remain elevated for up to two weeks. Coady (2006) argues this is important if the patient re-presents within this timeframe. French & White (2004) recommend that troponin levels should be measured at presentation, at 6 to 9 hours and at 12 hours to ensure correct diagnosis, although the optimum time to measure troponin (I or T) for diagnosis or prognostic risk stratification is 12 hours from the onset of symptoms (Scottish Intercollegiate Guidelines Network 2007, National Institute for Health and Clinical Excellence 2010). In patients with an acute coronary syndrome who present to the ED within six hours of pain onset, around half will have an elevated troponin I on admission (Hamm et al. 1997). Edwards et al. (2011) found that for patients who present to the ED with potential acute coronary syndrome, severe pain is not related to likelihood of acute myocardial infarction at presentation or death, acute myocardial infarction or revascularization within 30 days.

It is important to note that troponins are specific to myocardial injury rather than to myocardial infarction so other causes of cardiac damage should be excluded through the patient history and clinical examination. In addition, elevated troponin levels may be present in other conditions, such as renal failure, sepsis and heart failure, so it is important this test is used as part of an overall clinical assessment (Coady 2006). A chest X-ray is useful to detect any cardiac failure or enlargement. Isoenzymes may also be useful if other trauma, such as cardiac massage, has taken place.

Management

It is useful to obtain i.v. access early in the patient's management in order to administer pain relief or supportive drugs if necessary. The aim is to restore a normal blood flow through the coronary arteries, so that myocardial oxygen supply and demand is met. It is important that oxygen therapy is commenced at the earliest opportunity. This both acts as a pain-relieving agent and reduces the likelihood of tissue damage. It is necessary to reduce the workload of the heart, which relieves the symptoms experienced by the patient. Sublingual GTN is an effective first-line treatment. It works by causing venous and coronary artery dilatation. This in turn causes a reduction in preload and consequently a reduction in afterload (Khan 2000), therefore allowing blood to flow with less effort from the myocardium, increasing the amount of oxygen to the heart and subsequently decreasing chest pain. Diamorphine is the preferred agent for the treatment of patients with ongoing chest pain. It relieves chest pain and anxiety, which decreases myocardial oxygen consumption. Opiate and GTN substances should also be given as an i.v. infusion titrated to the patient's pain and blood pressure, to ensure that vasodilatation is not excessive. Aspirin should be given as a general measure.

Other drugs that can be used include:

- beta-blockers
- calcium antagonists.

Other aspects in the management of unstable angina include a reduction in activity and adjustments in lifestyle, if risks to the patient's health have been noted. If symptoms do not settle with analgesia, or if ECG changes persist after pain subsides, the patient should be admitted for observation and specialist management.

Myocardial infarction

Myocardial infarction is defined as the death or necrosis of part of the myocardium due to the reduction or cessation of blood flow (Alexander et al. 2000). The universal definition of MI criteria for the diagnosis of MI is pivotally centred on elevated troponins, in an ischemic setting, with either ischaemic symptoms or ischaemic electrocardiographic changes, and a rise and/or fall in troponin levels (Thygesen et al. 2007, White 2010).

The treatment of acute MI remains a major medical challenge, with over 300 000 patients presenting annually in the UK (Department of Health 2000). The major cause of the final event leading to acute MI is thrombosis formation in a narrowed coronary artery from ruptured or fissured atherosclerotic plaque. Subsequent vessel occlusion and thrombosis cause myocardial hypoxia and necrosis. Myocardial hypoxia may also be caused by coronary artery spasm and dissecting aortic aneurysm. Complete necrosis occurs in 4 to 6 hours and the area surrounding the zone of necrosis is ischaemic. Damage of the myocardium predisposes the patient to pump failure and various dysrhythmias secondary to conduction defects and irritability of myocardial tissue. The location and size of the infarct depend on the coronary artery affected and where the occlusion occurs. Most acute MIs are caused by a blockage of the left anterior descending coronary artery, which causes involvement of the anterior wall of the myocardium (Barnason 2003) (Fig. 27.28).

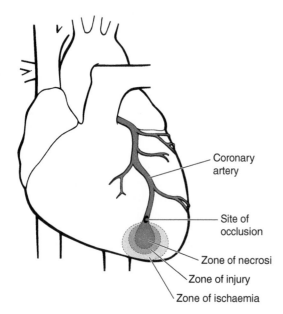

Figure 27.28 • Post-myocardial infarction damage.

The crucial aspect in the management of MIs is rapid commencement of treatment as soon as possible after the onset of symptoms. In ED, rapid treatment relies on accurate and thorough assessment by ED nurses.

Assessment

Assessment of patients having an MI should follow the same structure as a patient with acute coronary syndrome. In addition, the patient is likely to appear:

- pale
- sweating or clammy
- short of breath
- possibly cyanosed
- nauseous and vomiting
- anxious.

The 12-lead ECG is an important tool in the diagnosis of an MI, but should be taken in context with the overall clinical picture. The ECG usually demonstrates specific changes in the areas of myocardial damage. These are linked to the time span of injury and duration of pain. During the first hour of pain there is little change to the ECG; however, T waves may flatten. After this, the ST segment may elevate and during the next 12–24 hours Q waves begin to develop as myocardium becomes necrotic and electrical conduction ceases. In general, ST segment elevation myocardial infarctions are associated with a larger region of myocardial necrosis, higher enzyme levels, fresh coronary thrombosis, frequent vomiting, congestive heart failure, conduction defects, dysrhythmias and less collateral circulation (Barnason 2003). T waves become inverted because repolarization changes. In some instances, the ECG trace will remain with Q waves and inverted T waves in damaged areas. In other instances, T waves will turn upright after a period of time (Fig. 27.29).

In addition to the progress of the MI, the ECG will also depict the areas of the myocardium affected by the infarct (Box 27.3, p380).

Blood pressure

In the majority of cases the blood pressure appears low. This is due to poor ventricular function and a reduced cardiac output. The frequency of BP recordings should be of an optimum level to detect any further changes in the patient's condition. Note that use of nitrates may keep the blood pressure low or even drop it further.

Pulse

Predominately the patient will be tachycardic as a response to the decreased cardiac output, but the anxiety levels should also be taken into account as these can also induce a tachycardia due to the sympathetic response. Specific side-effects of infarction should also be considered. Bradycardia is frequently associated with inferior infarction.

Respiration

Tachypnoea or dyspnoea will usually be evident. These can indicate levels of hypoxia and the onset of pulmonary oedema. Oxygen therapy is vital in MIs to ensure that the myocardium is receiving as much oxygen as possible. Note the relevance of keeping the patient calm and reassured so as to attempt to relieve symptoms caused by anxiety or fear.

Temperature

Temperature is sometimes forgotten, but in the instance of an MI a mild pyrexia can be indicative of muscle damage due to an inflammatory response (Woods et al. 2000).

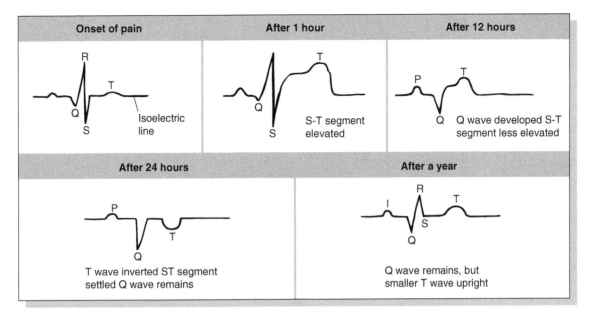

Onset of pain	After 1 hour	After 12 hours
Isoelectric line	S-T segment elevated	Q wave developed S-T segment less elevated

After 24 hours	After a year
T wave inverted ST segment settled Q wave remains	Q wave remains, but smaller T wave upright

Figure 27.29 • ECG changes following myocardial infarction.

Blood analysis

Similar to chest pain from unstable angina, blood analysis should include cardiac enzymes and cardiac troponins (troponin I and troponin T). Following an MI there is a rise in the levels of myocardial enzymes present. Assessment of troponins, which are highly sensitive and more specific than creatinine kinase, can now identify smaller areas of myocardial necrosis than previously (Coady 2006). It is these enzymes that aid in the diagnosis of an MI (Jowett & Thompson 2007) and they include (see also Table 27.11):

- creatinine kinase (CK)
- lactic dehydrogenase (LDH)
- aspartate aminotransferase (AST)
- cardiac troponins (troponin I and troponin T).

CK, LDH and AST are released in the first 24 hours after the onset of a myocardial infarct. These enzymes may provide retrospective confirmation of infarction rather than a guide to immediate management (analgesia, aspirin, thrombolysis). While troponin is a sensitive biomarker to 'rule out' non-ST-segment elevation myocardial infarction, it is less useful to 'rule in' this event because it may lack specificity for acute coronary syndromes (Jaffe et al. 2001).

Changes to other levels are as follows:

- FBC – a rise in both the white blood count and ESR is indicative of muscle necrosis
- U&Es – sodium and potassium ions are important in cardiac function due to their involvement within the action potential; this analysis is also important as it helps to determine if there is any renal function impairment present
- glucose – as previously stated, a rise in the blood glucose can be indicative of stress-related hyper glycaemia;

Table 27.11 Cardiac enzyme changes following a myocardial infarction

Enzyme	Released into circulation		Range (normal)
	Initially	Peaks	
Creatinine phosphokinase (CPK)	6 h	18–36 h	200–1000 u/mL (100 u/mL)
Serum aspartate transferase (formerly glutamic oxalo-acetic transaminase, SGOT)	12–24 h	36–48 h	>100 u/mL (50 u/mL)
Lactic dehydrogenase (LDH)	2–3 days	7 days	
Troponin	4–6 h	10–24 h	< 0.5 ng/mL

however, 5 % of cardiac patients admitted to hospital have previously undiagnosed diabetes (Alexander et al. 2000)
- lipids – raised cholesterol and triglycerides are common in ischaemic heart disease.

Chest X-ray

Chest X-rays may show fluid levels associated with oedema or an enlarged heart.

Management

The aim of care is to (Alexander et al. 2000):

- limit the infarction size
- re-establish an optimal cardiac output
- relieve pain
- detect and prevent any life-threatening complications.

Oxygen therapy should be commenced as early as possible in an attempt to limit myocardial damage and relieve pain. Pain control in patients with an MI should be achieved by using i.v. opiates, such as diamorphine or cyclomorph. These provide pain relief but also have a mild diuretic effect, hence enabling a better ventricular function (Opie 2000). An anti-emetic, such as cyclizine or metoclopramide, is also indicated as it reduces any previous nausea and counteracts the nauseated feelings associated with opiates.

Reperfusion therapy

The two most frequently used ways of treating patients with acute myocardial infarctions are thrombolysis and percutaneous coronary interventions (PCIs). Reperfusion therapy is vital if the integrity of the myocardium is to be preserved. Thrombolysis is a chemical intravenous method of treatment whereas PCI is an invasive procedure that artificially widens the coronary arteries potentially through balloon angioplasty or stenting. Thrombolysis is almost always administered in EDs due to ease of use after quick diagnosis. However, PCI requires specialist staffing and equipment and, as such, will require the patient to be transferred to an appropriate laboratory within a hospital or transferred to another which has these facilities.

These two methods and their use are discussed below.

Percutaneous coronary intervention (PCI)

PCI has become the preferred reperfusion therapy choice if it can be performed within 90 minutes and by an experienced team with the correct equipment (Castle 2006, Leahy 2006). A review of 23 trials comparing PCI with thrombolytic therapy showed more positive long-term outcomes in a reduction of further infarction, stroke and death (Tough 2006).

PCI is defined as balloon angioplasty and/or stenting where an artery is artificially widened and kept patent (Leahy 2006). These stents ensure that the lumen does not recoil or narrow again (Kern 2003). In the procedure, which is carried out in a cardiac laboratory, a catheter is inserted into an artery through a small puncture hole – usually above the femoral or radial arteries. Local anaesthetic is applied before inserting diagnostic and interventional catheters, coupled with a guiding catheter, up into the aorta and on to where the blockage has occurred. Contrast solution is injected into the artery and, with X-ray guidance, the source of the problem can be identified. A wire is then passed into the narrowed area and a balloon within a stent is inflated to re-open the artery and consequently restore normal blood flow (Leahy 2006).

Some regions in the UK may have centralized services headed by a local coordinator and will triage the patients based on their ECGs and clinical condition over the phone. Local ambulance services may even perform an ECG on transit and electronically send it to a PCI centre for assessment in order to decide whether the patient should be sent to them directly. If the transfer, whether from another hospital or the community, is performed in a timely fashion, the benefits to the patient have been shown to exist (Castle 2006).

Before transfer to the PCI unit, the ED nurse should ensure initial anticoagulation and pain management treatment has been started as prescribed and the patient is fully informed and comfortable. Whether performing an intra- or inter-hospital transfer, the ED nurse must ensure that they have the appropriate skills to ensure this can be done safely. These patients are at high risk of cardiac arrest or arrhythmias (Leahy 2006, Tough 2006) and nursing staff should be able to function as an integral member of the team; therefore the nurse should ideally be Adult Life Support (Resuscitation Council (UK)) qualified.

Thrombolytic therapy

Thrombolysis is the lesser preferred option for STEMIs but may be chosen in unstable patients who are not suitable to be transferred to a PCI unit. Rapid administration of thrombolytic therapy reverses the effects of ischaemia and injury before necrosis can occur, therefore dramatically changing the outcome for the patient (Quinn & Thompson 1995).

Thrombolytic therapy has been a well-established reperfusion treatment that reduces mortality (Fibrinolytic Therapy Trialists' Collaborative Group 1994) after STEMI, but its use has reduced in favour of PCI treatment instead. The amount of time that passes from onset of symptoms to myocardial salvage relates directly to patient mortality. There is a decrease in lives saved from 65 per 1000 patients treated with thrombolytic therapy within an hour of onset of symptoms to 29 per 1000 patients treated at between three and six hours (Castle 2006). Thrombolytic therapy retains a clinical benefit for up to 12 hours after onset of symptoms and, under specific conditions, benefit may be evident for up to 24 hours (Late Assessment of Thrombolytic Efficacy Steering Committee 1993).

Thrombolytic therapy dissolves the thrombus/clot occluding a coronary artery and restores blood flow to the myocardium, therefore limiting damage. Therapy is administered via an intravenous route, usually prepared as an infusion.

There are four thrombolytic agents available for use in the management of STEMI: streptokinase, and three fibrin-specific agents, alteplase, reteplase and tenecteplase. Streptokinase is a bacterial protein that reduces circulatory fibrinogen and clotting factors V and VIII (Alexander et al. 2000); however, it is also associated with significant incidence of hypotension, bradycardia and allergic reaction when compared with third-generation thrombolytic agents such as alteplase, reteplase and tenecteplase (Castle 2006). Recombinant tissue-type plasminogen activator (tPA) (alteplase) is a single bolus, fibrin-specific and works mainly on dispersement of the clot, therefore reducing the risk of systemic effects (Box 27.7).

During therapy, the ED nurse should be vigilant for signs of reperfusion (Box 27.8) and complications. Along with continual cardiac monitoring, blood pressure and 12-lead ECG monitoring should be frequent, and the patient should not be left unattended. Complications include reperfusion arrhythmias, including VF, allergic reactions and hypotension. The patient may feel flushed, generally unwell and have a headache. Bleeding episodes can also occur.

Other drugs of benefit include aspirin, which inhibits platelet aggregation and reduces blood viscosity, therefore reducing

Box 27.7

Contraindications of thrombolytic therapy

Absolute

- Previous haemorrhagic stroke
- Ischaemic stroke during the past 6 months
- Central nervous system damage or neoplasm
- Recent (within 3 weeks) major surgery, head injury or other major trauma
- Active internal bleeding (menses excluded) or gastro intestinal bleeding within the past month
- Known or suspected aortic dissection
- Known bleeding disorder

Relative

- Refractory hypertension (blood pressure > 180 mmHg)
- Transient ischaemic attack in preceding 6 months
- Oral anticoagulant treatment
- Pregnancy or less than 1 week post-partum
- Traumatic CPR
- Non-compressible vascular puncture
- Active peptic ulcer disease
- Advanced liver disease
- Infective endocarditis
- Previous allergic reaction to the thrombolytic drug to be used
- If streptokinase has been given more than four days previously, use a different thrombolytic agent as antibodies reduce effectiveness

Box 27.8

Signs of reperfusion

- Abrupt end to chest pain
- ECG change to ST segment – ST elevation rapidly returns to normal and Q waves do not develop
- Improved left ventricular function
- Early peak in cardiac enzyme excretion because of renewed blood flow
- Reperfusion arrhythmias or conduction defects

the risks of further thrombus activity. For the appropriate management of patients suffering from an MI, ED staff must be aware of current trends and treatments in cardiac care in order to understand more fully, and care more competently for, this group of patients. For optimal care, patients with an acute MI should be 'fast-tracked' to either a PCI unit for PCI treatment or to a coronary care unit, otherwise, at the earliest opportunity.

Acute cardiac failure

In 1995, the New York Heart Association renamed and reclassified all types of heart failure under the heading of 'heart failure'. There are now four classifications of heart failure, but for the purposes of this chapter the term is used to depict the clinical manifestations that relate to this condition. Heart failure is characterized as the heart's inability to provide an adequate cardiac output for the body's metabolic requirements (Alexander et al. 2000).

Acute left ventricular failure

Left ventricular failure (LVF) often presents suddenly and is usually associated with pulmonary oedema. LVF is also a frequent complication of MI. Common causes include:

- myocardial infarction
- coronary artery disease
- diabetes mellitus
- cardiac drugs – beta-blockers or calcium antagonists
- alcohol
- hypertension
- cardiomyopathy
- valvular disease
- arrhythmias
- hypertension
- pericarditis
- pericardial effusion
- pregnancy
- severe anaemia
- ventricular or atrial septal defect.

The mechanics of LVF mean that the heart is regarded as a failing pump, with more blood remaining in the ventricle at the end of each cardiac cycle (Tortora & Grabowski 2000). Often, this build-up of pressure results in blood being forced to seep back into the lungs, causing an increase in pressure and resulting in pulmonary oedema. In response to the pump mechanism failing, blood can also back up from the right ventricle into the systemic circulation, causing peripheral oedema due to the increase in capillary pressure causing fluid to seep into the tissues. This is most noticeable in the ankles and feet.

Assessment

Typically, LVF and pulmonary oedema occur in the night or early hours of the morning due to an increase in venous return when lying down. The usual presentation in ED includes:

- cold/clammy appearance
- severe dyspnoea
- cyanotic appearance
- tachycardia
- raised jugular venous pressure (JVP).

The assessment findings are summarized in Box 27.9.
Immediate priorities for care include:

- airway assessment
- oxygen therapy
- baseline observations

Box 27.9

Assessment findings in left ventricular failure

- *Respirations* – airway is of paramount importance, as the presence of pulmonary oedema exacerbates any shortness of breath and causes hypoxia. Depending on the severity of the hypoxia, airway adjuncts such as oropharyngeal or nasopharyngeal airways may be required. Extreme cases may require intubation and ventilation
- *Pulse* – tachycardias are prominent in LVF with the heart beating faster in an attempt to compensate for the reduced cardiac output
- *Blood pressure* – hypotension is usually present due to the failure of the pumping mechanism and hence a reduced cardiac output
- *Temperature* – possible occurrence of pyrexias
- *Urine output* – with the use of diuretics, it is vital to keep an accurate hourly record of the output to monitor the effectiveness of the diuretics
- *Cardiac monitoring* – this should be maintained throughout the stay in the emergency department and on transfer. Rhythm changes, such as increasing ventricular ectopics, or left bundle branch block should be considered. Profuse sweating may make electrode placement difficult to achieve
- *Central venous pressure monitoring* – this measurement is important in monitoring and maintaining the haemodynamic status of the patient

---

- cardiac monitoring
- intravenous or central line access
- diuretics
- catheterization for urine output measurement.

Clinical investigations should include:

- blood chemistry analysis – both to monitor renal function and to maintain adequate potassium levels if loop diuretics, such as frusemide, are being administered
- cardiac enzymes/cardiac troponins – to check for muscular damage
- full blood count – a low haemoglobin would show any evidence of anaemia
- arterial blood gases – monitor frequently to assess respiratory function
- chest X-ray – useful in determining the degree of pulmonary oedema and any evidence of heart enlargement.

Management

The aims of first-line management are:

- to relieve symptoms
- to treat the underlying cause.

Oxygen therapy is vital to counteract the effects of hypoxia. Positioning is also important in LVF, as sitting patients in an upright position reduces venous return. LVF is highly treatable and good nursing and medical care should provide symptomatic relief very quickly for the patient. Symptomatic relief comes in the form of i.v. diuretics, namely frusemide, due to its rapid onset of action. This type of diuretic is a potent 'loop diuretic' causing almost immediate diuresis. In severe cases, inotropic drugs may be required, such as dobutamine, dopamine or adrenaline to increase the contractility of the myocardium and thus to assist the left ventricular function. Other drugs of note include vasodilatation agents such as angiotensin-converting enzyme (ACE) inhibitors, nitrates and calcium-channel blockers. These reduce preload and thus enable an increase in the cardiac output (Nicholas 2004).

Cardiogenic shock

Shock is a systemic clinical syndrome that can be said to exist when perfusion is insufficient to meet the metabolic demands of body tissues (Hunt & Hunt 2011). If left uncorrected it will lead to irreversible cell damage and multiple organ failure and death. In the case of cardiogenic shock, the degree of heart failure is so severe that the extreme reduction in cardiac output leads to inadequate organ perfusion. It can occur because of one significant or multiple smaller infarcts in which over 40% of the myocardium becomes necrotic, a ruptured ventricle, significant valvular dysfunction or at the end stage of heart failure. It can also result from cardiac tamponade, cardiomyopathy, pulmonary embolism or dysrhythmias (Smeltzer & Bare 2000). Kinney & Packa (1996) suggest a mortality rate of at least 80% during the course of MI, with the incidence of cardiogenic shock among survivors of MI likely to be 6–20%, indicating the seriousness of the condition (Hand 2002).

Assessment

Patients presenting with cardiogenic shock require urgent attention as they are acutely ill. The patient will appear clinically shocked and hence consideration must be given to the following symptoms:

- acute dyspnoea
- profound hypotension
- pale/cyanotic
- cold/clammy
- arrhythmias.

The assessment findings are summarized in Box 27.10.

Priorities for care

Ideally the patients should be cared for in the resuscitation environment with:

- cardiac monitoring
- i.v. access and CVP access
- oxygen therapy
- baseline observations
- catheterization.

Clinical investigations include:
- renal care – urine measurement is vital to measure the effectiveness of drug therapy and U&Es to monitor potassium levels

Box 27.10

Assessment findings in cardiogenic shock

- *Blood pressure* – severe hypotension, due to a radically reduced cardiac output
- *Pulse* – tachycardia; the heart rate increases to compensate for the reduced cardiac output, but in profound stages the rate may become weaker and arrhythmias may occur
- *Respirations* – oxygen therapy is vital if hypoxia is to be restricted. An upright posture will help to reduce venous return. Again, in extreme cases intubation and ventilation may be required. Arterial blood gases must be performed on a regular basis to monitor levels of hypoxaemia and any rise in the carbon dioxide levels

- blood analysis – for routine FBC and cardiac enzymes/cardiac troponins
- ECG – may show multifocal ventricular ectopics indicative of an irritable ventricle, or ischaemic changes suggestive of an acute MI
- chest X-ray – evidence of pulmonary oedema and cardiac enlargement may be present.

Management

Close, frequent observations and cardiac monitoring are vital if life-threatening abnormalities are to be detected. Adequate i.v. access is essential if the haemodynamic status of the patient is to be stabilized. Aggressive i.v. diuretic therapy should be administered to this end and its effectiveness monitored. Volume replacement is sometimes necessary, but should be titrated to CVP and pump functioning. Vasodilators (i.v. nitrates) and inotropic agents (dobutamine, dopamine or adrenaline) may be used to support the cardiovascular system. Rapid administration of alteplase to dissolve thrombi has been shown to increase aortic pressure and survival significantly (Hand 2002). On occasions an intra-aortic balloon pump may be required to support the left ventricle. Thought and consideration must be given to the family and/or friends as this undoubtedly will be a very stressful experience for them.

Viral/inflammatory conditions

Pericarditis

Acute pericarditis is an acute inflammation of the pericardial sac. The presence of a respiratory tract infection may indicate a viral infection. Causes of pericarditis include:

- idiopathic (non-specific)
- bacterial infection
- viral infection
- pregnancy
- uraemia

- connective tissue disease, e.g., systemic lupus erythematosus (SLE), arthritis
- following an acute MI
- hypothyroidism
- neoplasm, e.g., breast, lung, etc.
- radiation.

Assessment

The patient with pericarditis presents in ED with sharp chest pain localized to the retrosternal area and left precordium. It is typically pleuritic and positional, worsening on deep inspiration, coughing or movement. Other symptoms include:

- dyspnoea
- fever
- production of sputum
- weight loss
- on auscultation of the chest, the sound of a friction rub confirms the diagnosis of pericarditis.

Immediate priorities for care

- baseline observations
- cardiac monitor
- intravenous access
- oxygen therapy.

Specific investigations should include:

- ECG – the classical sign seen on the ECG, of which 90% are abnormal in patients with acute pericarditis, is the presence of widespread concave ST elevation, often referred to as saddleback. Late presentations of pericarditis can include generalized T wave inversion on most leads (Humphreys 2006)
- blood analysis – U&Es due to the possibility of uraemically induced pericarditis as a result of decreased renal function
- FBC – a raised white cell count would be indicative of bacterial infections
- blood culture – to investigate for infections
- chest X-ray – this is usually normal, unless the presence of a pericardial effusion shows cardiac enlargement.

Management

The immediate management is pain relief. In the initial stages the use of opiates may be required, e.g., diamorphine, or if the pain is less acute, NSAIDs are given, particularly ibuprofen due to its rare side-effects, favourable impact on coronary flow and large dose range (300–800 mg every 6–8 hours).

With viral pericarditis no further treatment is required. For bacterial pericarditis, antibiotic therapy should be initiated. If pericarditis is left uncorrected, it can become potentially life-threatening, leading to pericardial effusion and cardiac tamponade.

Endocarditis

Endocarditis is caused by either bacterial or fungal infiltration of the heart valves or endocardium and should be considered a multisystem disease (Lee 2004). It is prevalent in a heart already damaged by congenital or acquired heart abnormalities. The main characteristic of endocarditis is a vegetative growth on the leaflets of the valves, causing dysfunctional or incompetent valvular action.

Assessment

The symptoms of endocarditis include:

- anaemia
- rigors
- heart murmur
- night sweats
- fever (present in 80–85% of cases) (Karchmer 1997)
- haematuria
- chills.

Immediate priorities for care

A major complication of endocarditis is heart failure. Hence, on presentation in the ED, the patient, along with the symptoms listed above, may be acutely short of breath, dyspnoeic and pale. Thus, immediate priorities are:

- oxygen therapy where required
- baseline observations – check temperature for recurrent pyrexias
- i.v. access.

Specific investigations include:

- ECG – to detect damage or stress to the heart
- blood analysis – FBC for possible raised white cell count in response to an infection
- U&E – imbalance may occur if heart failure is present
- blood cultures – these are performed to enable isolation of the causative pathogen, so that the correct antibiotics are used to target the source of the infection.

Management

This is dependent upon the causative factor for endocarditis. There are three approaches:

- bacterial endocarditis – suggested antibiotics include benzylpenicillin and gentamicin
- fungal endocarditis – amphotericin is the drug of choice
- surgical intervention – to replace the diseased valve.

Antibiotic prophylaxis is required when undertaking any dental work. This is necessary to reduce the risk of reinfection.

Despite refinements in diagnostic techniques and advances in antibiotic and surgical therapy, infective endocarditis (IE) remains a serious condition (Tleyjeh 2007). The overall mortality for endocarditis is 20–25% and up to 50% in patients with concomitant diabetes mellitus (Chu et al. 2004). Primary treatment failure can occur even with combined medical and surgical treatment if the organism is *Staphylococcus aureus*, Enterobacteriacae or fungi (Lee 2004).

Cardiomyopathy

Cardiomyopathy is a broad term that includes subacute or chronic disorders of the myocardium. Heart failure often results from cardiomyopathy and not from coronary artery disease as previously thought (Laurent-Bopp 2000). The definition and diagnosis of cardiomyopathy are ambiguous due to the fact that it is a disease of the heart muscle of an unknown cause.

There are four classifications of cardiomyopathy:

- dilated cardiomyopathy (DCM)
- hypertrophic cardiomyopathy
- arrhythmogenic right ventricular cardiomyopathy
- restrictive cardiomyopathy.

Assessment

The majority of patients in the acute phase will be suffering from heart failure due to their cardiomyopathy. Other symptoms include:

- dyspnoea, because of heart failure
- fatigue, because of hypoxia due to inadequate cardiac output
- chest pain related to a decreased cardiac output (mainly with hypertrophic cardiomyopathy)
- syncope
- palpitations
- anxiety
- depression.

Immediate priorities for care

In the presence of heart failure or an acute episode, the priorities should be:

- cardiac monitoring for ventricular arrhythmias, suggestive of a stressed heart
- oxygen therapy
- i.v. access
- baseline observations
- ECG
- routine FBC and U&Es
- chest X-ray – this will show cardiac hypertrophy and may show pulmonary oedema.

During non-acute phases, patients with cardiomyopathy are usually asymptomatic.

Management

A fundamental goal of treatment in cardiomyopathy is the alleviation of symptoms and the prevention of sudden cardiac death (Cruickshank 2004). The only true treatment to offer a cure is heart transplantation. During the interim period, the use of ACE inhibitors such as captopril may be of benefit. Other drugs used in the treatment of cardiomyopathy include:

- diuretics
- amiodarone to control ventricular arrhythmias
- prophylactic anticoagulants, e.g., warfarin – these are indicated as the risk of thrombus formation and subsequent pulmonary embolus is great.

Conclusion

The diversity of cardiac conditions presenting in ED is vast. It is therefore essential for ED nurses to understand the principles of a systematic approach to the elements of cardiac care. This chapter has explored one of the most exciting aspects of ED nursing by identifying distinct aspects of patient care and subsequent management.

References

Alexander, M.F., Fawcett, J.N., Runciman, P.J., 2000. Nursing Practice: Hospital and Home: The Adult, second ed. Churchill Livingstone, Edinburgh.

Arrich, J., Stertz, F., Herkner, H., et al., 2012. Total epinephrine dose during asystole and pulseless electrical activity cardiac arrests is associated with unfavourable functional outcome and increased in-hospital mortality. Resuscitation 83 (3), 333–337.

Baliga, R., Eagle, K., 2008. Cardiology: Evaluation and Treatment of Common Cardiovascular Disorders. Lippincott Williams & Wilkins, Philadelphia.

Barnason, S., 2003. Cardiovascular emergencies. In: Newberry, L. (Ed.), Sheehy's Emergency Nursing: Principles and Practice, fifth ed. Mosby, St Louis.

Bilal Iqbal, M., Taneja, A.K., Lip, G.Y.H., 2005. Recent developments in atrial fibrillation. British Medical Journal 330, 238–243.

Braunwald, E., Antman, E.M., Beasley, J.W., et al., 2000. ACC/AHA guidelines for the management of patients with unstable angina and non-ST-segment elevation myocardial infarction: executive summary and recommendations. A report of the American College of Cardiology/American Heart Association task force on practice guidelines (Committee on the Management of Patients with Unstable Angina). Circulation 102 (10), 1193–1209.

British Heart Foundation, 2010. Coronary Heart Disease Statistics: 2010 edition. British Heart Foundation, London.

Castle, N., 2003. Effective relief of acute coronary syndrome. Emergency Nurse 10 (9), 15–19.

Castle, N., 2006. Reperfusion therapy. Emergency Nurse 13 (9), 25–35.

Castle, N., 2009. Cardiovascular Emergencies. In: Crouch, R., Charters, A., Dawood, M., Bennett, P. (Eds.), Oxford Handbook of Emergency Nursing. Oxford University Press, Oxford.

Chu, V.H., Cabell, C.H., Benjamin, D.K., et al., 2004. Early predictors of in-hospital death in infective endocarditis. Circulation 109, 1745–1749.

Coady, E., 2006. Managing patients with non-ST-segment elevation in acute coronary syndrome. Nursing Standard 20 (37), 49–56.

Colquhoun, M.C., Handley, A.J., Evans, T.R., 1999. ABC of Resuscitation, fourth ed. BMJ, London.

Cruickshank, S., 2004. Cardiomyopathy. Nursing Standard 18 (23), 46–52.

Department of Health, 2000. National Service Framework for Coronary Heart Disease. HMSO, London.

Edwards, M., Chang, A.M., Matsuura, A.C., et al., 2011. Relationship between pain severity and outcomes in patients presenting with potential acute coronary syndromes. Annals of Emergency Medicine 58 (6), 501–507.

Evans, C., 2007. Acute Cardiac Emergencies. In: Evans, C., Tippins, E. (Eds.), The Foundations of Emergency Care, Open University Press, Maidenhead.

Fibrinolytic Therapy Trialists' Collaborative Group, 1994. Indications for fibrinolytic therapy in suspected acute myocardial infarction: collaborative overview of early mortality and major morbidity results from all randomized trials of more than 1,000 patients. The Lancet 343 (8893), 311–322.

Fox, K.A., 2004. Management of acute coronary syndromes: an update. Heart 90 (6), 698–706.

French, J.K., White, H.D., 2004. Clinical implications of the new definition of myocardial infarction. Heart 90 (1), 99–106.

Fuhrmann, L., Lippert, A., Perner, A., et al., 2008. Incidence, staff awareness and mortality of patients at risk on general wards. Resuscitation 77, 325–330.

Haman, L., Parizek, P., Vojacek, J., 2009. Precordial thump efficacy in termination of induced ventricular arrhythmias. Resuscitation 80, 14–16.

Hamm, C.W., Bu, Goldmann, Heeschen, C., et al., 1997. Emergency room triage of patients with acute chest pain by means of rapid testing for cardiac troponin T or troponin I. New England Journal of Medicine 337 (23), 648–653.

Hampton, J., 2003. The ECG Made Easy, sixth ed. Churchill Livingstone, Edinburgh.

Hand, H., 2002. Common cardiac arrhythmias. Emergency Nurse 10 (3), 29–38.

Harrigan, R.A., Chan, T.C., Moonblatt, S., et al., 2007. Temporary transvenous pacemaker placement in the emergency department. The Journal of Emergency Medicine 32 (1), 105–111.

Houghton, A., Gray, D., 1997. Making Sense of the ECG: A Hands-on Guide. Arnold, London.

Hudack, C., et al., 1998. Critical Care Nursing: A Holistic Approach. Lippincott, Philadelphia.

Humphreys, M., 2006. Pericardial conditions: signs, symptoms and electrocardiogram changes. Emergency Nurse 14 (1), 30–36.

Hunt, P., Hunt, F., 2011. Shock. In: Smith, J., Greaves, I., Porter, K. (Eds.), Oxford Desk Reference: Major Trauma. Oxford Medical Publications, Oxford.

International Liaison Committee on Resuscitation, 2005a. Part 4: Advanced life support. Resuscitation 67, 213–217.

International Liaison Committee on Resuscitation, 2005b. Part 3: Defibrillation. Resuscitation 67, 203–211.

International Liaison Committee on Resuscitation, 2005c. Part 5: Acute coronary syndromes. Resuscitation 67, 249–269.

Jacobson, C., 2000. Arrhythmias and conduction defects. In: Woods, S.L., Froelicher, E.S.S., Motzer, S.U. (Eds.), Cardiac Nursing, fourth ed. Lippincott, Williams and Wilkins, Philadelphia.

Jaffe, A.S., The World Health Organization, The European Society of Cardiology, The American College of Cardiology, 2001. New standard for the diagnosis of acute myocardial infarction. Cardiology in Review 9 (6), 318–322.

Jowett, N.I., Thompson, D.R., 2007. Comprehensive Coronary Care, fourth ed. Bailliére Tindall, London.

Karchmar, A.W., 1997. Infective endocarditis. In: Braunwald, E. (Ed.), Heart Disease: A Textbook of Cardiovascular Medicine, fifth ed. WB Saunders, Philadelphia.

Kern, M., 2003. The Cardiac Catheterization Handbook, fourth ed. Mosby, Philadelphia PA.

Khan, M.G., 2000. Manual of Cardiac Drug Therapy, sixth ed. WB Saunders, London.

Kinney, M.R., Packa, D.R., 1996. Comprehensive Cardiac Care. Mosby, St Louis.

Krijne, R., 1984. Rate acceleration of ventricular tachycardia after a precordial chest thump. American Journal of Cardiology 53, 964–965.

Laurent-Bopp, D., 2000. Cardiomyopathies and myocarditis. In: Woods, S.L., Froelicher, E.S.S., Motzer, S.U. (Eds.), Cardiac Nursing, fourth ed.. Lippincott, Williams and Wilkins, Philadelphia.

Late Assessment of Thrombolytic Efficacy Steering Committee, 1993. Late assessment of thrombolytic efficacy (LATE) study with alteplase 6–24 hours after onset of acute myocardial infarction. The Lancet 342 (8874), 759–766.

Leahy, H., 2006. Primary angioplasty for acute ST-elevation myocardial infarction. Nursing Standard 21 (12), 48–56.

Lee, M., 2004. Heart valve emergencies. In: Cameron, P., Jelinek, G., Kelly, A.M., Murray, L., Brown, A.F.T., Heyworth, J. (Eds.), Textbook of Emergency Medicine, second ed.. Churchill Livingstone, Edinburgh.

Marieb, E., 2000. Human Anatomy and Physiology, fifth ed.. Benjamin Cummings, California.

McDonough, M., 2009. Treating ventricular tachycardia. The Journal of Continuing Education in Nursing 40 (8), 342–343.

National Institute for Health and Clinical Excellence, 2010. Chest Pain of Recent Onset: Assessment and Diagnosis of Recent Onset Chest Pain or Discomfort of Suspected Cardiac Origin. NICE, London.

Neumar, R.W., Otto, C.W., Link, M.S., et al., 2010. Part 8: Adult Advanced Cardiovascular Life Support: 2010 American Heart Association Guidelines for Cardiopulmonary Resuscitation and Emergency Cardiovascular Care. Circulation 122 (Suppl. 3), S729–s767.

Nicholas, M., 2004. Heart failure: pathophysiology, treatment and nursing care. Nursing Standard 19 (11), 46–51.

Nolan, J.P., Greenwood, J., MacKintosh, A., 1998. Cardiac Emergencies: A Pocket Guide. Butterworth Heinemann, Oxford.

Nolan, J.P., Soar, J., Zideman, D.A., et al., 2010. European Resuscitation Council Guidelines for Resuscitation 2010 Section 1: Executive summary. Resuscitation 81, 1219–1276.

Nolan, J.P., Ornato, J.P., Parr, M.J.A., et al., 2011. Resuscitation highlights in 2011. Resuscitation 83, 1–6.

Opie, L., 2000. Drugs and the Heart, fifth ed. WB Saunders, London.

Pellis, T., Kette, F., Lovisa, D., et al., 2009. Utility of pre-cordial thump for treatment of out of hospital cardiac arrest: a prospective study. Resuscitation 80, 17–23.

Quinn, T., Thompson, D.R., 1995. Administration of thrombolytic therapy to patients with acute myocardial infarction. Accident and Emergency Nursing 3, 208–214.

Resuscitation Council (UK), 2007. Decisions Relating to Cardiopulmonary Resuscitation: A Joint Statement from the British Medical Association and the Royal College of Nursing. Resuscitation Council, London.

Resuscitation Council (UK), 2010. Resuscitation Guidelines. Resuscitation Council, London.

Resuscitation Council (UK), 2011. Advanced Life Support Course Provider Manual, sixth ed. Resuscitation Council, London.

Schamroth, L., 2001. An Introduction to Electrocardiography, eighth ed. Blackwell Scientific, Oxford.

Scottish Intercollegiate Guidelines Network, 2007. Acute coronary Syndromes: A National Clinical Guideline. NHS Scotland, Edinburgh.

Smeltzer, S., Bare, B., 2000. Brunner and Suddarth's Textbook of Medical and Surgical Nursing. Lippincott, Philadelphia.

SOS–Kanto study group, 2007. Cardiopulmonary resuscitation by bystanders with chest compression only (SOS–Kanto): an observational study. Lancet 369, 920–926.

Teodorescu, C., Reinier, K., Uy-Evanado, A., et al., 2012. Survival advantage from ventricular fibrillation and pulseless electrical activity in women compared to men: the Oregon Sudden Unexpected Death Study. Journal of Interventional Cardiac Electrophysiology 34 (3), 219–255.

Thygesen, K., Alpert, J.S., White, H.D., et al., 2007. Universal definition of myocardial infarction. Journal of American College of Cardiology 50, 2173–2195.

Tleyjeh, I.M., Abdel-Latif, A., Rahbi, H., et al., 2007. A systematic review of population-based studies of infective endocarditis. Chest 132, 1025–1035.

Tortora, G.J., Grabowski, S., 2000. Principles of Anatomy and Physiology, ninth ed. Harper Collins, New York.

Tough, J., 2006. Primary percutaneous coronary intervention in patients with acute myocardial infarction. Nursing Standard 21 (2), 47–56.

van Alem, A.P., Sanou, B.T., Koster, R.W., 2003. Interruption of cardiopulmonary resuscitation with the use of the automated external defibrillator in out-of-hospital cardiac arrest. Annals of Emergency Medicine 42, 449–457.

von Besser, K., Mills, A.M., 2011. Is discharge to home after emergency department cardioversion safe for the treatment of recent-onset atrial fibrillation? Annals of Emergency Medicine 58 (6), 517–520.

White, H.D., 2010. Higher sensitivity troponin levels in the community: What do they mean and how will the diagnosis of myocardial infarction be made? American Heart Journal 159 (6), 933–936.

Williams, D., 2009. Cardiovascular Emergencies. In: Kunz Howard, P., Steinmann, R.A. (Eds.), Sheehy's Emergency Nursing: Principles and Practice, sixth ed. Mosby Elsevier, St Louis.

Woods, S.L., Sivarajan-Froelicher, E.S., Halpenny, C.J., et al., 2000. Cardiac Nursing, fourth ed. Lippincott, Williams and Wilkins, Philadelphia.

Wyatt, J.P., Illingworth, R.N., Graham, C.A., et al., 2012. Oxford Handbook of Accident & Emergency Medicine, fourth ed. Oxford University Press, Oxford.

Zerwic, J.J., 1999. Patient delay in seeking treatment for acute myocardial infarction symptoms. Journal of Cardiovascular Nursing 13 (3), 21–32.

Medical emergencies

28

Barry McCarthy

CHAPTER CONTENTS

http://dx.doi.org/10.1016/B978-0-7020-4315-4.00028-0

Introduction

A substantial proportion of the Emergency Department (ED) nurse's workload involves dealing with patients who present with medical emergencies. Medical emergencies are many and varied, and it is beyond the scope of this chapter to consider them all. The main conditions are identified and the assessment and management detailed. It is, however, possible to provide initial management of any life-threatening medical emergency by making an assessment of, and interventions to support, the airway, breathing, circulation, and other aspects of the Primary Survey.

Knowledge of the early signs of a deteriorating patient, and the 'Emergency Nurses Intuition' are essential skills to possess in recognizing the medical emergency. Following these, and providing the initial aspects of the presenting illness are stable, are secondary investigations, which are baseline observations of temperature, pulse, respiration and blood pressure. When coupled with effective communication, these 'routine' actions form the basis of care for the patient with a potentially life-threatening medical condition.

Respiration

Respiration is a process that is fundamental to life itself. In the absence of external respiration, oxygen is not absorbed into the circulation and carbon dioxide is not removed from it. Such a state is clearly incompatible with life and is of an importance few would fail to acknowledge. The process of respiration is considerably more complex than external respiration alone (Fig. 28.1). Respiration also takes place at a cellular level, known as internal respiration, where oxygen plays a fundamental part in cell energy production, or metabolism,

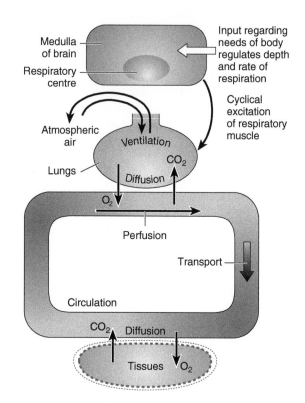

Figure 28.1 • Process involved in respiration. • (After Hinchliff S, Montague S, Watson R (1996) Physiology for Nursing Practice, 2nd edn. London: Bailliére Tindall.)

with one of the by-products of this process being carbon dioxide. Internal and external respiration cannot sustain life without the existence of an adequate transport system that enables the oxygen absorbed by external respiration to be delivered to the cells to support internal respiration, and the removal of carbon dioxide produced by internal respiration to the lungs for excretion by means of external respiration.

It is essential that assessment of the respiratory system takes into account *all* of these processes, as the presence of one process does not ensure that other processes are functioning. It is equally important that an assessment evaluates the adequacy of these processes and not just their presence or absence. For example, readings of the patients' respiratory rate, as well as assessment of depth of breathing, increased or decreased work of breathing, anxiety and skin colour and hydration are all markers that gas exchange is occurring and the patient is adequately respiring.

The mechanics of respiration

Inspiration occurs when intrathoracic pressure falls below atmospheric pressure. This fall in intrathoracic pressure is caused by an increase in the intrathoracic volume, which occurs when muscle contraction causes the rib cage to move upwards and outwards at the same time as the diaphragm is flattening. During normal inspiration it is the movement of the diaphragm that accounts for the greatest change in intrathoracic volume and not the expansion of the rib cage (Ganong 2003). The fall in intrathoracic pressure causes air to be drawn into the lungs. This generally occurs at approximately −4 to −8 mmHg.

Expiration occurs when the lungs recoil, at the end of inspiration, bringing the chest wall back to its pre-inspiratory position. The diaphragm domes, returning to its pre-inspiratory state. Air leaves the lungs by this passive process. Movement of gas is proportional to changes in volume. Therefore, small changes in volume will result in small movements of gas, with the risk that inspired air may only be moving in and out of the anatomical dead space, never reaching the site of gas exchange at the alveoli.

Assessment of the mechanics of respiration

For external respiration to be adequate, the chest wall must be intact, the thorax and diaphragm must be able to rise and fall and that movement must be sufficient to create a negative pressure which will draw air beyond the anatomical dead space and to the alveoli. Patient assessment should reflect this and at least include an assessment of the adequacy of respiratory volume by observing the extent and symmetry of chest expansion and recoil. Observation must also be made to ascertain whether the chest is moving symmetrically and to note if movement is in any way paradoxical.

Neural control of respiration

The rate, rhythm and volume of respiration are governed by the central nervous system, with the involuntary or automatic component being controlled by the respiratory centre in the medulla of the brain. There is a degree of voluntary control over respiration, for instance when an individual intentionally takes a deep breath, which is controlled by the cortex of the brain.

Chemoreceptors in the carotid and aortic body sense changes in blood pH. As the levels of carbon dioxide rise in the blood, the blood becomes more acid and impulses from the chemoreceptors to the respiratory centre increase. In response to this, the respiratory centre increases the respiratory rate. A similar process occurs in the brain where chemoreceptors in the medulla respond to changes in the pH of cerebrospinal fluid. Chemoreceptors are also responsive to a fall in blood oxygen concentrations, increasing impulses to the respiratory centre as the levels of oxygen fall.

In those individuals with chronic respiratory disease, the respiratory centre becomes unresponsive to the changes in carbon dioxide concentration. In these circumstances the falling oxygen concentrations become the main stimuli for respiration. Consequently the administration of high concentrations of inspired oxygen may lead to an increase in carbon dioxide retention, a decrease in respiratory rate and ultimately respiratory arrest. Administration of oxygen to those patients who may have chronic respiratory disease should be done with great care and weaned down to a lower flow rate earlier. This is considered further in respect of chronic obstructive pulmonary disease later in the chapter.

Assessment of respiratory control

Assessment should be made of the rate, rhythm and volume of respiration, as this may give an early indication of the increased carbon dioxide or decreased levels of oxygen in the blood. A further and often more striking indication of these physiological processes is the use of the accessory muscles of respiration in the neck, shoulders and abdomen. This is often associated with tracheal tug and recession of the sternum and intercostal muscles.

Bronchial tone

The tone of the bronchi and bronchioles is maintained by the smooth muscle contained within their walls.

Hypoxia

Hypoxia is regarded as being one of the leading causes of preventable death in the trauma patient, but it is often overlooked as a potential threat to life in the many patients who attend ED for reasons other than having sustained an injury. Hypoxia, or inadequate tissue oxygenation, falls broadly into four broad groups (Box 28.1):

- hypoxic hypoxia
- anaemic hypoxia
- stagnant hypoxia
- histotoxic hypoxia.

Assessment of gas exchange

In recent years there has been an increased reliance upon pulse oximetry in respiratory assessment. In many cases, this technology is helpful in identifying hypoxia. However, pulse oximetry must be used with caution as it has the potential to mislead (Moyle 2002). Pulse oximetry gives an indication of the degree to which the available haemoglobin is saturated with oxygen. However, oximetry must only be trusted in situations where a correlation can be made to other assessments of hypoxia and it is strongly recommended to use an oximeter device that has 'photoplethysmograph' (PPG) capability (or 'pleth' as it is more commonly known). It can measure the change in the volume of arterial blood with each pulse beat and therefore can be useful in comparing to a peripheral pulse rate, and watching for signs of cardiac insufficiency (especially when ectopics occur) and, of course, prove that you have a strong enough signal and can trust the percentage reading. The relationship between oxygen saturation and the amount of oxygen within the circulation is illustrated in graphical format as the oxygen dissociation–haemoglobin dissociation curve. Assuming that the relationship on this curve is normal for a given patient, Gibson (2003) suggests that an oxygen saturation of 90% represents a blood oxygen tension of 8 kPa. The normal range for arterial blood gases is shown in Box 28.2.

Box 28.1

Types of hypoxia

Hypoxic hypoxia

Oxygen is not available to haemoglobin in the red blood cells. This may occur when the patient is in an atmosphere which has a reduced oxygen content, although it is most likely to occur as a result of a decrease in respiratory rate and/or volume. If untreated, conditions such as pulmonary oedema or pneumonia lead to hypoxic hypoxia by preventing the diffusion of oxygen at the alveolar/capillary interface in the lungs.

Anaemic hypoxia

The oxygen-carrying capacity of the blood is reduced because of a lack of available haemoglobin. In the acute episode, this is likely to be due to hypovolaemia where haemoglobin is lost in proportion to the number of red cells lost. This type of hypoxia may also occur following chronic conditions where the number of red cells is normal but the haemoglobin is either reduced or not readily available, e.g., in iron deficiency anaemia and sickle cell anaemia. Following carbon monoxide poisoning, the carbon monoxide preferentially binds to the haemoglobin, preventing oxygen binding with the haemoglobin and thus resulting in anaemic hypoxia.

Stagnant hypoxia

This occurs as a result of failure of the circulatory system to transport oxygenated blood to the tissues. Normal diffusion occurs at the alveolar/capillary interface in the lungs, but inadequate circulation prevents the oxygen from being delivered to the tissues. This type of hypoxia is classically associated with physiological shock, be that cardiogenic, neurogenic, anaphylactic, etc. This type of hypoxia may also occur at a local level where vascular obstruction causes a reduction in blood flow distal to the obstruction.

Histotoxic hypoxia

In this case, adequate concentrations of oxygen are transported to the tissues, but the cells are unable to utilize the oxygen. This type of hypoxia usually results from certain types of poisoning, classically cyanide poisoning.

Box 28.2

Normal arterial blood gas values

- pH – 7.35–7.45
- PCO_2 – 4.6–6.0 kPa
- PO_2 – 10.0–13.3 kPa
- Bicarbonate – 22–26 mmol/L
- Base excess – −2.4 to +2.2

A patient with carbon monoxide poisoning may well have an anaemic hypoxia whilst still presenting what appears to be a normal oxygen saturation on the pulse oximeter. Similarly, patients with other forms of hypoxic anaemia may have normal pulse oximetry readings because the pulse oximeter is a reflection of the degree of saturation of each red blood cell and not of the total oxygen content of the blood. Again pulse oximetry must be used with caution when there is probe

movement or when peripheral perfusion is low, as recorded saturation may be inaccurate (Levine & Fromm 1995).

It must be remembered that pulse oximetry only provides information about the patient's oxygen saturation; it is not able to offer information regarding carbon dioxide in the blood. Consider the patient who is having an acute asthma attack and who has been given oxygen therapy by facemask. They may well have what may be regarded as satisfactory oxygen saturation, yet have inadequate ventilation with high and increasing levels of blood carbon dioxide. The most accurate way to assess the gaseous content of the circulating volume is by arterial blood gas analysis. Not only does this investigation provide information regarding respiratory gases in the circulation, but it is also a vital tool in the assessment of acid–base balance.

Asthma

Asthma is a complex disorder characterized by variable and recurring symptoms, airflow obstruction, bronchial hyper-responsiveness, and an underlying inflammation (National Institutes of Health 2007). While many of the 10% of children and 5% of adults in the population who have asthma are asymptomatic or are well controlled with medication, approximately 1500 people per year die from asthma (Newman-Taylor 2003). Acute asthma is characterized by an acute attack of bronchospasm in which the airways become swollen, constricted and plugged with mucus. The airflow obstruction, which characteristically fluctuates markedly, causes a mismatch of alveolar ventilation and perfusion and increases the work of breathing. Being more marked during expiration it also causes air to be 'trapped' in the lungs.

Respiratory arrest may occur within a few minutes of the onset of a severe episode or death may occur from alveolar hypoventilation and severe arterial hypoxaemia in the patient exhausted by a prolonged attack. Severe airflow obstruction is manifested in the symptoms of shortness of breath, wheezing, chest tightness and a cough. Acute severe asthma may arise from absence of treatment or from inadequate or unsuccessful treatment and is life-threatening and should be considered a medical emergency.

In the non-asthmatic individual, there is a minimal reaction of the smooth muscle in the bronchial wall to stimulation by inhaled allergens such as the house dust mite, animal hair or pollen. Non-allergenic stimulants such as cold weather, cigarette smoke, anxiety and exercise also have a minimal effect on the reactivity of the smooth muscle. In the individual with asthma, reaction to such stimulation is exaggerated, a response termed bronchial hyperreactivity, which is thought to be associated with an inflammatory process.

Asthma can be broadly divided into two main types: allergic and non-allergic. Allergic asthma, as the name suggests, is triggered by allergens such as the house dust mite and others previously identified. This condition generally appears in childhood and may improve as the child reaches adolescence. Conversely, non-allergic asthma is triggered by factors such as anxiety or cold weather, first presenting in middle age. The symptoms of non-allergic asthma tend to intensify in both severity and frequency as the individual becomes older (Axford 1996).

Attendance at the ED is usually precipitated by one of two events:

1. an acute event in the individual who has episodic asthma, i.e., symptom-free between distinct acute episodes; or

2. an acute increase in the severity of symptoms in the individual who has chronic asthma, where tightness and wheezing are present most of the time, if not controlled by regular medication.

Initially, the most obvious sign of asthma may be noisy respiration in the form of a wheeze, which is generally expiratory but can also be inspiratory. One must be cautious not to make false assumptions based upon this symptom, for, as Axford (1996) notes, 'all that wheezes is not asthma'. Wheezing is a sign of airway obstruction that may or may not be asthmatic in origin.

Assessment

A full and objective assessment is essential and should include a full history. It may not be possible to obtain this from the patient, if breathless. In cases of severe and life-threatening asthma, treatment should not be delayed in order to obtain a full history. The assessment should include the following:

- full history
  - onset of symptoms
  - duration
  - exacerbation
  - medication history; beta blockers, aspirin and non-steroidal anti-inflammatory drugs (NSAIDs) may precipitate a severe asthma attack in some patients with asthma
  - previous admissions, especially to intensive care units (British Thoracic Society 2012)
- observation
  - respiratory effort
  - use of accessory muscles
  - chest movement and symmetry
  - skin colour and appearance, such as sweating
  - respiratory rate, rhythm and depth
  - pulse
  - blood pressure
  - temperature (episode may have been precipitated by a chest infection)
  - anxiety
- Palpation
  - degree of chest expansion
  - temperature of the skin
- percussion – resonance of the chest
- auscultation
  - quality of breath sound
  - degree of air entry
  - silence

- peak expiratory flow rate
  - measured against predicted and actual normal for that individual
  - should not be done if the patient has signs of severe or life-threatening asthma (i.e., is unable to speak a complete sentence)
- pulse oximetry – use with caution; remember it will not tell you the amount of carbon dioxide the patient is retaining
- arterial blood gas analysis
- chest X-ray.

From the assessment it will be possible to identify those patients with severe and life-threatening asthma who need immediate intervention (Tables 28.1 and 28.2).

Table 28.1 Features of severe asthma

Adult	Child
Cannot complete sentences	Cannot talk or feed
Pulse >110 beats/min	Pulse >140 beats/min
Respiratory rate >25 min	Respiratory rate >50 min
Peak flow rate <50% of predicted	

(After Greaves I, Hodgetts T, Porter K (2005) Emergency Care: A Textbook for Paramedics, 2nd edn. London: WB Saunders.)

Table 28.2 Features of life-threatening asthma

Adult	Child
Exhaustion	Reduced conscious level
Cyanosis	Agitation
Bradycardia	Cyanosis
Hypotension	Silent chest
Silent chest	Coma
Peak flow <33% of predicted	
Coma	

(After Greaves I, Hodgetts T, Porter K (2005) Emergency Care: A Textbook for Paramedics, 2nd edn. London: WB Saunders.)

Management

Position the patient to sit upright to maximize ventilation. Patients may need high concentrations of oxygen or medication nebulized by an oxygen-driven system. The drug regimen recommended by the British Thoracic Society and Scottish Intercollegiate Guidelines Network (British Thoracic Society 2012) includes nebulized or i.v. salbutamol, and oral or i.v. steroids depending upon the mechanism and severity of the attack. In life-threatening asthma, ipratropium should be added to the nebulizer and expert advice must be sought, which may include progression to non-invasive intermittent positive pressure ventilation (IPPV) with pressure support (PS) and positive end expiratory pressure (PEEP) (such as CPAP or BiPap). This can be done on the spontaneously breathing patient, via a face mask and a ventilator that is capable of delivering the non-invasive positive support safely, but is a skill that requires extra knowledge and training as there is risk of barotrauma. For children with moderate to severe exacerbation, bronchodilators can be given by inhaler using a spacer device. ED nurses must be familiar with the current British Thoracic Society and Scottish Intercollegiate Guidelines Network guidelines on asthma (British Thoracic Society 2012) and in particular the flow charts relating to the management of acute asthma in adults in ED and the management of acute asthma in children in ED. In addition to continued reassessment based upon the initial assessment, monitor the cardiac rhythm. Provide psychological care for patient and family in dealing with their stress and anxiety. The use of spacers for adult asthma patients as well as children is currently being evaluated.

In the less severe episodes, it is important to check out the patient's understanding of the illness and management. It is not uncommon for some individuals with asthma to have a poor understanding of the purpose of their medication, when it should be taken and how to take it correctly. This can lead to poor compliance and leave the patient in a brittle state, with decreased reserve to cope with any triggering episodes. It is important to make use of such opportunities to provide some preventive care. It is also essential that appropriate follow-up is arranged to continue patient education and monitoring in the primary healthcare setting. Patients with little understanding of their condition and medication regimen will continue to attend EDs where their symptoms will be treated without resolving the underlying issues.

It is important to differentiate asthma from hyperventilation, as the presenting symptoms of both are dramatic and can easily be confused by the inexperienced nurse (Yeh & Schwartzstein 2010). A hyperventilating patient will be tachypnoeic but not tachycardic and will usually have oxygen saturation levels of 100%. Hyperventilation is associated with anxiety and responds quickly to rebreathing through a paper bag. Hyperventilating patients generally do not have a history of asthma.

Chronic obstructive pulmonary disease

Chronic obstructive pulmonary disease (COPD) is a collective term for a number of chronic respiratory diseases, the most common of which are chronic bronchitis and emphysema and is characterized by airflow obstruction that is not fully reversible (National Institute for Health and Clinical Excellence 2010). Airflow obstruction has profound effects on cardiac function and gas exchange with systemic consequences (Barnes & Celli 2009, MacNee 2011).

Chronic bronchitis

Chronic bronchitis is most frequently seen in adults of middle age and beyond. It is characterized by a productive cough resulting from increased mucus secretion from hypertrophied mucus-secreting glands in the bronchi. The patency of the smaller bronchi is further compromised by inflammation of the mucosa. The cough and associated inflammation last for several months each year and occur on consecutive years.

Assessment

When the individual with chronic bronchitis attends the ED, it is usually because of an acute exacerbation of symptoms associated with a superimposed upper respiratory tract infection. Assessment of the individual will include:

- a full history, including past history as well as the history of the current episode
  - onset of symptoms
  - duration
  - exacerbation
- observation
  - signs of chronic respiratory disease, e.g., clubbing of the fingers, barrel chest
  - respiratory effort
  - use of accessory muscles
  - chest movement and symmetry
  - skin colour
  - respiratory rate, rhythm and depth
  - pulse
  - blood pressure
  - temperature
  - anxiety
- palpation
  - degree of chest expansion
  - temperature of the skin
- percussion – resonance of the chest
- auscultation
  - quality of breath sound
  - degree of air entry
- pulse oximetry – use with caution; remember many of these patients retain carbon dioxide which can result in fatal respiratory acidosis, even in the presence of adequate oxygen saturation. Pulse oximetry will not provide any information about elevated levels of carbon dioxide
- arterial blood gas analysis – will be abnormal given the chronic respiratory disease and should be viewed in the light of the individual's actual or predicted normal
- sputum sample – for microbiological examination (microscopy, culture and sensitivity)
- chest X-ray.

Assessment of the patient is likely to reveal the following clinical features:

- purulent productive cough
- increased sputum volume
- dyspnoea
- tachypnoea
- wheezing

- respiratory distress and use of accessory muscles
- poor chest expansion
- cyanosis.

Management

Position the patient sitting upright to maximize ventilation. Oxygen should be given at a low concentration, initially no more than 28%; increased concentrations may be necessary if improvement does not occur, but this should be based on the results of arterial blood gas analysis. Whilst on oxygen the patient must be closely monitored for signs of respiratory depression. Antibiotics, bronchodilators and steroids should be given if asthma is an element in the acute episode. Where nebulized medication is indicated the British Thoracic Society (2012) recommend that a compressed air nebulizer should be used and the patient given supplemental oxygen by nasal prongs. In addition to continued reassessment based upon the initial assessment, the cardiac rhythm should be monitored. Arterial blood gas analysis must be carried out within the first hour of admission to the ED and results used to inform on-going management of the patient. Psychological care for patient and family should be provided in dealing with their stress and anxiety. Progression to invasive, or non-invasive positive pressure ventilation may also be needed if the condition deteriorates and there is a clinical need, however the medical staff will need to take into consideration all aspects of the individual's medical history including their normal functioning state and any advanced health directives. Discussions with family members will also be valuable in deciding the next appropriate step in resuscitation.

Emphysema

Dilatation of the alveoli reduces the functional surface area of the lung available for gas exchange. The mechanics of respiration are also compromised by the reduction of elasticity and recoil of the lung. As with other chronic respiratory conditions, emphysema is commonly seen in adults beyond middle age. The individual attends the ED with an increase in the severity of the symptoms, often associated with additional respiratory disease or infection.

Assessment should follow the format as for the patient with chronic bronchitis. Such assessment will reveal:

- dyspnoea
- quiet breath sounds
- over inflation of the chest
- forced expiration through pursed lips.

Management of the patient is much the same as that for chronic bronchitis.

Pulmonary oedema

Although pulmonary oedema for many patients has its origins in the cardiac system, it is a manifest problem in the respiratory system.

Cardiac-related pulmonary oedema

The most common presentation of pulmonary oedema of cardiac origin seen in the ED is as a result of left ventricular failure that may or may not be secondary to acute myocardial infarction. Failure of the left ventricle leads to back-pressure in the pulmonary circulation. As the pressure builds, fluid is forced from the circulation first into the pulmonary interstitial spaces and then, with further increases in pressure, into the alveoli. This fluid within the interstitial spaces and the alveoli reduces the efficacy of gas exchange at the alveolar−capillary interface.

Other possible causes of pulmonary oedema

It is important to remember that pulmonary oedema is not a disease in itself but is merely a symptom of some other underlying pathology, for example:

- opiate overdose
- inhalation of toxic or irritant substances
- allergic reactions
- airway burns/inhalation injury
- circulatory volume overload (overinfusion)
- pulmonary embolism
- hypoalbuminaemia
- near drowning.

Assessment

Onset is usually sudden with the individual attending the ED as symptoms worsen and respiratory function deteriorates. Assessment must focus upon the presenting symptoms, but must also aim to consider the possible underlying causes:

- a full history (past history as well as the history of the current episode)
  - onset of symptoms
  - duration
  - exacerbation
- observation
  - airway
  - signs of possible underlying mechanisms, e.g., inhalation injury, substance misuse
  - respiratory effort
  - use of accessory muscles
  - chest movement
  - skin colour
  - respiratory rate, rhythm and depth
  - pulse
  - blood pressure
  - temperature
  - level of consciousness
  - anxiety

- palpation
  - degree of chest expansion
  - temperature of the skin
- percussion – resonance of the chest
- auscultation
  - quality of breath sound
  - degree of air entry
- pulse oximetry – with caution
- arterial blood gas analysis
- chest X-ray.

Assessment is likely to reveal:

- dyspnoea
- orthopnoea
- tachypnoea
- exhaustion
- respiratory distress
- noisy respiration
- expectoration of frothy sputum, sometimes blood-stained in the later, more severe stages.

Management

Management of the patient is dependent upon the underlying pathology, but will include securing the airway and positioning the patient upright to maximize ventilation. Provide high-concentration oxygen through a Hudson mask with reservoir bag at a flow rate of 10–15 L/min. Diuretics may reduce the fluid load from the circulation. Morphine/diamorphine, if not contraindicated, causes venous pooling, thus reducing venous return on loading on the heart. Opiates will also help in the reduction of anxiety, but one must be vigilant for signs of respiratory depression. Vasodilators in the form of nitrates, if indicated, sublingual or i.v. infusion also cause venous pooling. Catheterization should be considered and the patient's fluid output should be carefully monitored. A 12-lead ECG should be performed to monitor any cardiac changes. Progression to non-invasive IPPV with PS and PEEP (such as CPAP or BiPap). This can be done on the spontaneously breathing patient, via a face mask and a ventilator that is capable of delivering the non-invasive positive support safely, but is a skill that requires extra knowledge and training as there is a risk of barotrauma. In addition to continued reassessment based upon the initial assessment, monitor the cardiac rhythm and raise the back of the trolley to sit the patient up and support with pillows if necessary (Wyatt et al. 2012). Psychological care should be provided for patient and family in dealing with their stress and anxiety.

Pulmonary embolism

Venous thromboembolism (VTE) is a common cause of death in Europe. The total estimated number of VTE-related deaths for 2004 across six EU countries (UK, France, Germany, Italy, Spain and Sweden) was 370 012. Of these deaths, 7 % (26 473) were expected to have resulted from diagnosed

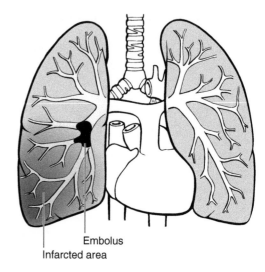

Figure 28.2 • Pulmonary embolism.

(and presumably treated) VTE, 34 % (126 145) from sudden fatal pulmonary embolism (PE), and 59 % (217 394) from PE-related deaths following undiagnosed (untreated) VTE (Cohen et al. 2007). Pulmonary embolism is a common cause of respiratory-related death in the UK, with an estimated 60 000 deaths each year (Cohen et al. 2007). It is a commonly associated complication of deep vein thrombosis (DVT), where a fragment detaches from the thrombus to form an embolus (Fig. 28.2). The embolus flows through the circulation until it wedges in narrow branches of the arterial system, classically branches of the pulmonary artery. The pulmonary circulation becomes obstructed, which consequently reduces the efficacy of gas exchange and ventilation–perfusion mismatch occurs.

Predisposition to pulmonary embolism, generally speaking, is determined by a predisposition to DVT:

- sluggish circulation due to
  - bed rest
  - limb immobilization
  - heart failure/reduced cardiac output
- venous injury
  - trauma
  - venous cannulation
- increased coagulability
  - drugs, such as oral contraceptives
  - dehydration
  - polycythaemia
- increased age.

Emboli may arise from other mechanisms such as air, fat or amniotic fluid entering the circulatory system, but these are less common. Symptoms are related to the size of the area of lung affected, the rate of onset and the severity of the symptoms being determined by the size and number of emboli:

- small emboli – these wedge in smaller vessels, close to the alveolar–capillary interface, and affect only a small area of lung

- medium emboli – these wedge in the larger branches of the pulmonary artery some distance from the alveolar–capillary interface; they affect a larger area of lung than do smaller emboli and result in a greater ventilation–perfusion mismatch
- large emboli – these wedge in the largest branches of the pulmonary artery, furthest away from the alveolar–capillary interface; they affect very large areas of the lung and result in a massive ventilation–perfusion mismatch.

Assessment

A good assessment is vital, as the symptoms of pulmonary embolism are often confused with those of acute myocardial infarction:

- a full history, considering predisposition to and evidence of DVT, as well as the history of the current episode
  - onset of symptoms
  - duration
  - exacerbation
- observation
  - signs of possible underlying mechanisms, in particular DVT
  - respiratory effort
  - use of accessory muscles
  - chest movement
  - skin colour
  - respiratory rate, rhythm and depth
  - pulse
  - blood pressure
  - sputum
  - level of consciousness
- palpation
  - degree of chest expansion
  - temperature of the skin
- percussion – resonance of the chest
- auscultation
  - quality of breath sound
  - degree of air entry
- pulse oximetry – with caution
- arterial blood gas analysis
- chest X-ray
- 12–lead ECG.

Table 28.3 outlines the features of emboli of different sizes. An ECG may reveal an S wave in lead I, a Q wave in lead II and an inverted T wave in lead III. The ECG may also be useful in excluding other diagnoses such as myocardial infarction and pericardial disease.

Management

Position the patient sitting upright to maximize ventilation. Administer high-concentration oxygen using a Hudson mask with reservoir bag at a flow rate of 10–15 L/min.

Table 28.3 Features of pulmonary emboli

Small emboli	Medium emboli	Large emboli
Slow onset	Rapid onset	Sudden onset
Mild to moderate dyspnoea	Pleuritic chest pain	Dyspnoea
Fatigue	Dyspnoea	Chest pain
	Haemoptysis	Haemoptysis
		Tachycardia
		Compromised circulation
		Hypotension
		Cyanosis
		Reduced level of consciousness
		Unconsciousness

Bloods should be taken for clotting screen. Anticoagulants, such as heparin, are often the only form of treatment given for massive pulmonary embolism. A thrombolytic, such as alteplase, may be indicated primarily in patients who are haemodynamically unstable (British Thoracic Society 2003). Silent pulmonary embolisms have also been found to be present in 1665 of 5233 patients (32%) with deep venous thrombosis so routine screening may be advantageous (Stein et al. 2010).

Anaphylaxis

Anaphylaxis is an acute, life-threatening systemic reaction with varied mechanisms, clinical presentations, and severity that results from the sudden systemic release of mediators from mast cells and basophils. The more rapidly anaphylaxis develops, the more likely the reaction is to be severe and potentially life-threatening. The prevalence of anaphylaxis is increasing and the number of cases of fatal anaphylaxis appears to be rising (Nasser 2012). Prompt recognition of signs and symptoms of anaphylaxis is crucial (Lieberman et al. 2010). Symptoms will usually occur rapidly within minutes of exposure to the causative allergen, especially if given parenterally. Repeated administration of parenteral or oral therapeutic agents may also precipitate an anaphylactic reaction.

Commonly cited riggers include:

- antibiotics, e.g., penicillin or other penicillin derivatives
- bee or wasp stings
- insect or snake venom
- foodstuffs, e.g., nuts or shellfish.

Clinical features

The clinical features of anaphylactic shock may occur singly or in combination and may include respiratory distress, cyanosis, bronchospasm, laryngeal obstruction, circulatory collapse, hypotension, tachycardia, generalized erythema, urticaria, nausea, vomiting, abdominal pain and diarrhoea. Generally, the faster the onset of symptoms, the more life-threatening is the reaction.

Management

The priority is to secure and maintain the airway; intubation may be required especially if laryngeal oedema is present. If the patient is able to maintain an open airway, she/he should be administered supplemental oxygen by a face mask at a high flow rate of 10–15 L/min. Adrenaline (epinephrine) slows the release of cellular chemical mediators and, additionally, causes vasoconstriction. It also has beneficial effects on myocardial contractility, peripheral vascular tone and bronchial smooth muscle. Adrenaline should be administered via the intramuscular route and NOT the intravenous route.

The ED nurse should be alert to the dangers of anaphylactic reactions and have knowledge of any relevant patient history. The nurse should avoid giving medication to patients with a known allergic disorder, such as hayfever or asthma, unless absolutely necessary. Ensure that prescribed medication is given by the most appropriate route; anaphylactic reactions are more likely to occur when drugs are given via the parenteral route.

Near drowning

There are about 700 drowning deaths in the UK each year and many times that number of near drowning (Joint Royal Colleges Ambulance Liaison Committee 2006). Worldwide, over 175 000 children under 20 years of age died from drowning in 2004. For each fatal event it is estimated that there are 1–4 non-fatal submersions (Taneja et al. 2008).

Near drowning following submersion in water results from one of two main mechanisms: 'dry' drowning and 'wet' drowning. Dry drowning occurs in 10–20 % of cases following immersion in cold water, where the cold water causes intense and persistent laryngospasm and vagal stimulation leading to asphyxiation, hypoxia and cardiac arrest. Little or no water enters the lower airways or lungs and death is secondary to airway obstruction rather than pulmonary oedema (Morris 2003). More commonly, drowning and near drowning occur as a result of wet drowning. After a period of breath-holding following immersion, the individual is forced to inhale by reflex mechanism. Water is aspirated into the lungs along with the large volumes of water which have been swallowed. This causes pulmonary vasoconstriction and hypertension with ventilation/perfusion mismatch, aggravated by surfactant destruction and washout and atelectasis. Consequently, the individual rapidly becomes hypoxic, which leads to unconsciousness and cardiac arrest (Wyatt et al. 2012).

Near drowning is often associated with other factors which complicate the individual's condition. In adults, as much as 25 % of cases have been documented as being associated with alcohol use (Mills et al. 1995). Hypothermia is common in UK waters. This is inevitable when the water is below 10°C as body heat is lost despite the individual actively exercising (Greaves et al. 2005). Near drowning is frequently associated with head and neck injury, when individuals dive into shallow water or water that contains submerged objects.

Occasionally, near-drowning victims can be asymptomatic; however, most present with mild dyspnoea, a deathlike appearance with blue or grey colouring, apnoea or tachypnoea, hypotension, heart rate as slow as 4 to 5 beats per minute or pulselessness, cold skin, dilated pupils known as fish eyes, hypothermia and vomiting (Morris 2003). Significant neurological impairment occurs in up to 25 % of near-drowning patients. Neurological injury results from hypoxia and can lead to cerebral oedema and brain stem herniation. Approximately 20 % of comatose patients recover completely. Secondary drowning, which is a deterioration in a previously apparently well patient following successful resuscitation after submersion, may occur in 5–10 % of initial survivors (Wyatt et al. 2012). Hypothermia is an important clinical feature in determining outcome as it decreases the metabolic demands of the body, and severe cerebral hypoxia may be prevented or delayed. Acidosis is a common finding in near-drowning patients. Metabolic acidosis is primarily due to tissue hypoxia, but a respiratory component may be present following aspiration. Hypoxia and acidosis act as myocardial depressants and precipitate circulatory collapse.

Assessment

There are some physiological differences between near drowning in fresh water and that in salt water. These differences are functionally irrelevant in the early management of the individual in the ED. Assessment of the individual must ensure that due consideration is given to the mechanism of injury in respect of potential head and neck trauma. This should include:

- a full history
  - onset of symptoms
  - duration
  - exacerbation
- observation
  - airway
  - signs of possible underlying factors; head and neck trauma, alcohol use
  - respiratory effort
  - use of accessory muscles
  - chest movement
  - skin colour
  - respiratory rate, rhythm and depth
  - pulse
  - blood pressure
  - temperature
  - level of consciousness
- palpation
  - degree of chest expansion
  - temperature of the skin

- percussion – resonance of the chest
- auscultation
  - quality of breath sound
  - degree of air entry
- pulse oximetry – with caution
- arterial blood gas analysis
- chest X-ray.

The presentation of the individual following near drowning may be diverse, but is likely to include at least some of the following:

- head and neck trauma
- reduced level of consciousness – unconscious
- apnoea
- tachypnoea
- shallow respiration
- pulmonary oedema
- hypothermia arrhythmias
- asystole.

Symptoms may be delayed. Apparently well patients must be observed and reviewed over the subsequent 48 hours due to the risk of secondary drowning.

Management

- airway management with cervical spine control
- high-concentration oxygen, with intermittent positive pressure ventilation if indicated
- rewarming if indicated (see hypothermia)
- management of arrhythmias
- management of injuries
- cardiac monitoring
- continued reassessment based upon the initial assessment
- psychological care for the patient and family in dealing with their stress and anxiety.

Good prognostic factors include patients who are alert on admission, hypothermia, older children adults, brief submersion time, and those who receive rapid on-scene basic life support and respond to initial resuscitation measures (Wyatt et al. 2012).

Carbon monoxide poisoning

Carbon monoxide poisoning is the most common cause of poisoning in the UK, and is thought to cause approximately 50 deaths per year. Carbon monoxide is a colourless, odourless, tasteless gas produced by incomplete combustion of organic material. Poisoning is usually associated with inhalation of smoke from fires in confined spaces, engine exhausts and faulty heating systems. Because its earliest symptoms are vague and mimic a viral illness, carbon monoxide has been coined 'the great masquerader' (Sivilotti & Abu-Laban 2012). It is often referred to as the silent killer as victims of accidental exposure often have no idea they are being poisoned, even when they develop severe symptoms. Consequently, victims are likely to remain in a life-threatening environment without realizing the dangers. Carbon monoxide combines more readily with haemoglobin than oxygen does – its affinity is more than 200 times that of oxygen. Once combined with carbon monoxide, haemoglobin is unable to bind with oxygen, resulting in a fall in PO_2 and an anaemic hypoxia.

Assessment

Assessment is largely dependent upon a clear history and a high index of suspicion, as symptoms in themselves may not be self-evident:

- a full history
  - has the individual been in a confined space in which carbon monoxide may be present?
  - onset of symptoms
  - duration
  - exacerbation
- observation
  - airway – soot, carbonaceous sputum as evidence of an inhalation injury
  - respiratory effort
  - use of accessory muscles
  - chest movement
  - skin colour – may look pink or flushed in the later stages (cherry red appearance may not be evident)
  - respiratory rate, rhythm and depth
  - pulse
  - blood pressure
  - temperature
  - level of consciousness
- auscultation
  - quality of breath sound
  - degree of air entry
- pulse oximetry – can be extremely misleading, giving high readings even though the patient is hypoxic
- arterial blood gas analysis
- bloods for carboxyhaemoglobin.

Presentation will depend upon the percentage of carboxyhaemoglobin present (Table 28.4).

Management

A carboxyhaemoglobin level greater than 3 % in non-smokers or greater than 10 % in smokers confirms exposure to carbon monoxide, but the level does not correlate with the presence or absence of initial symptoms (Weaver 2009). The patient should be given high-concentration oxygen, with intermittent positive pressure ventilation if indicated. In the presence of 100 % oxygen there is a 50 % reduction of carboxyhaemoglobin in the first 20 minutes. Consider hyperbaric oxygen, which forces oxygen onto the haemoglobin and reduces the half-life of carbon monoxide as well as decreasing intercranial

Table 28.4 Presentation of carbon monoxide poisoning

Carboxyhaemoglobin	Symptoms
<10%	No symptoms
10–20%	Headache Nausea Vomiting Loss of manual dexterity
21–40%	Confusion Lethargy ST depression on ECG Apathy – loss of interest in leaving dangerous environment, and therefore may be fatal
41–60%	Ataxia Convulsions Apnoea Coma
>60%	Usually fatal

pressure and cerebral oedema. The indications for hyperbaric oxygen (Axford 1996) are:

- conscious patients with levels of carboxyhaemoglobin of >20%
- neurological symptoms other than headache at any time since exposure
- pregnancy
- cardiac arrhythmias.

Renal disorders

The renal system is an important system as it influences a large number of physiological processes, e.g., the control and maintenance of blood pressure, fluid and electrolyte balance, acid–base balance and excretion of by-products of metabolism.

Maintenance of blood pressure

Baroreceptors in the renal arterial system respond to a fall in blood pressure by stimulating the release of renin from the juxta-glomerular apparatus. The renin enters the bloodstream and acts upon angiotensinogen, produced in the liver to form angiotensin I. Angiotensin I is then converted to angiotensin II by angiotensin-converting enzyme (ACE) found mainly in the lungs and kidney. Angiotensin has a number of effects which raise blood pressure:

- acts directly on arterioles to cause vasoconstriction
- stimulates the circulation centre in the central nervous system resulting in vasoconstriction

- stimulates the thirst mechanism in the hypothalamus
- influences renal blood flow and the glomerular filtration rate by renal vasoconstriction
- stimulates the adrenal cortex to secrete aldosterone, which increases sodium reabsorption by the kidney and so causes water retention.

Fluid and electrolyte balance

A fluid deficit in the circulating blood volume is detected by the osmoreceptors, located in the hypothalamus. This causes the secretion of antidiuretic hormone from the posterior pituitary. This hormone stimulates increased water absorption in the kidney and this is supported by the effects of the renin-angiotensin pathway (described above).

Acid–base balance

In cases where the blood is acidotic the lungs play a major part in the reduction of the acidosis by the excretion of the acid-producing hydrogen ions in the form of carbon dioxide. However, the kidney provides a valuable additional role in the reduction of the hydrogen ion concentration. The kidney provides a back-up in the case of inadequate respiration; it removes acid produced by fat and protein metabolism which cannot be removed by the lungs and it allows bicarbonate to be reabsorbed to supplement that being used in buffering processes. Acid is excreted by the kidney in a buffered form.

Excretion of by-products of metabolism

Carbohydrates and fats are broken down to carbon dioxide and water and are excreted by means of processes as detailed previously. Many substances such as protein and amino acids contain nitrogen, which relies upon the kidney to excrete nitrogenous by-products in the form of urea, uric acid and creatinine.

Assessment of the renal system

The renal system gives an insight into many physiological processes and should not be underestimated when making a patient assessment. Likewise, an assessment of the renal system should not be restricted to those patients with renal conditions. The assessment of these processes and of renal function is via the urine output in terms of volume, frequency and content. This may be achieved by accurate fluid balance measurement and recording at intervals appropriate to the patient's condition. Routine urine testing using reagent strips offers a wealth of information, as does a visual inspection of the urine, which is frequently undervalued in assessment.

Urinary tract infection

Of the many conditions which are of renal or urinary tract origin, few are seen in the ED. Where the patient does attend with an underlying renal or urinary tract pathology, it is generally because of pain rather than any other symptom, the most common conditions being urinary tract infection (UTI) and renal colic. *Escherichia coli* is associated with 80–90% of UTIs (Ejernæs 2011). Other organism groups that cause UTI include *Proteus*, *Pseudomonas*, *Streptococcus*, *Staphylococcus epidermidis* and *Klebsiella* (Cetti & Venn 2012). Following inoculation, organisms rapidly multiply in the ideal culture material of the urine. The individual will generally present at the ED complaining of pain on micturition. Recurrent UTIs (RUTIs) are reported in 25% of women within six months of an acute UTI episode and pose a major problem (Ejernæs 2011).

Assessment

- a full history
  - ○ onset of symptoms
  - ○ duration
  - ○ exacerbation
- observation
  - ○ skin colour
  - ○ temperature
  - ○ urine – colour, opacity, odour
- midstream specimen of urine – for microscopy, culture and sensitivity.

Symptoms of UTIs include:

- dysuria
- frequency of micturition
- haematuria.

In its advanced stages UTI may lead to infection of the kidney or kidneys in the form of pyelonephritis, which may present as:

- signs of UTI
- fever
- loin pain
- nausea
- vomiting.

Management

Management of the condition is based upon:

- antibiotics
- increased oral fluid intake
- patient education.

Renal colic

Renal colic is the most common presentation of renal calculi. It occurs most frequently between 20 and 50 years of age with a male:female ratio of 3:1. About 50% of patients have a single episode but the remaining 50% have recurrences within 5 years (Nicholson 2004). Renal calculi are predominantly calcium in origin, although they may be calcium/ammonium phosphate, urate or cysteine. The calculi form in the kidney when the urine is saturated with the given solute and the kidney is unable to excrete it. The solute, in its crystalline form, deposits in the kidney causing pain. Pain is at its most intense when the calculi pass through the urinary tract.

Assessment

- a full history and pain assessment
  - ○ onset of symptoms
  - ○ duration
  - ○ exacerbation
  - ○ skin colour
  - ○ temperature
  - ○ urine – colour, opacity, odour, laboratory stick test; urine should be filtered through filter paper to identify evidence of grit from the calculi
- observation
- midstream specimen of urine – for microscopy, culture and sensitivity.

The main feature identified by the assessment is likely to be pain; however, other features may be present:

- pain – unilateral pain radiates from the loin to left or right lower quadrants. Suprapubic pain may also be present. Pain may be sudden or intermittent in onset
- restlessness
- dysuria urgency
- frequency
- haematuria
- proteinuria
- UTI.

Management

- Antispasmodics – atropine
- Anti-emetics
- Increase fluid intake – orally or i.v.
- Patient education – advise patient to increase fluid intake especially at night when urine normally concentrates.

NSAIDs provide excellent analgesia in renal colic, but should be used with care in patients at risk of renal impairment, cardiac failure and gastric ulceration (Davenport & Waine 2010).

Dehydration – fluid volume deficit

The mechanisms leading to dehydration are many and varied. It is likely that the patient will attend the ED with a condition resulting in dehydration rather than with dehydration perse.

Table 28.5 Dehydration: fluid deficit

	Hypertonic deficit	Isotonic deficit
Mechanism	Occurs when fluid is lost without the loss of electrolytes Extracellular fluid becomes concentrated and fluid moves from the intracellular compartment to the extracellular compartment	Occurs when fluid and electrolytes are in normal physiological proportions Extracellular and intracellular fluid remains unchanged
Possible causes	Severe GI infections, causing fluid loss and sodium concentration Increased insensible loss Low-volume, concentrated feeds (infants or nasogastric) Inability to access water (environmental isolation/entrapment loss of consciousness)	Diarrhoea and vomiting Increased urine output (renal disease, diuretics) Increased sweating Burns Haemorrhage Lack of fluid and electrolyte intake
Symptoms	Decreased skin elasticity Dry mucous membranes Hypotension Tachycardia Increased respiratory rate and volume Increased thirst Pitting oedema	Acute weight loss Dry mucous membranes Hypotension Tachycardia Increased respiratory rate and volume Decreased and concentrated urine output Sunken eyes Pleural effusion Pulmonary oedema Dependent oedema
Management	Water replacement Hypotonic i.v. fluids	i.v. replacement of isotonic fluids Blood and blood products Anti-emetics

(After Paradiso C (1995) Fluids and Electrolytes. Philadelphia: JB Lippincott.)

It is important to consider the processes involved in the underlying illness to identify the potential for dehydration. There are two main types of dehydration, depending on the type of fluid deficit, i.e., hypertonic, isotonic (Table 28.5).

In an effort to correct dehydration, patients may inadvertently overhydrate, leading to subsequent physiological disturbance. This is covered in Table 28.6.

Assessment

This should include:

- a full history, including past history as well as the history of the current episode
  - onset of symptoms
  - duration
  - exacerbation
- observation
  - respiratory effort
  - use of accessory muscles
  - chest movement
  - skin colour
  - respiratory rate, rhythm and depth
  - pulse
  - blood pressure
  - temperature
  - level of consciousness
  - urine – volume, colour and concentration
- palpation
  - degree of chest expansion
  - skin temperature and elasticity
- auscultation
  - quality of breath sound
  - degree of air entry
- pulse oximetry (depending upon respiratory symptoms) – with caution
- arterial blood gas analysis
- chest X-ray.

Thermoregulation

The control of body temperature takes place in the hypothalamus in response to changes in core temperature, detected by thermoreceptors in the hypothalamus, skin and spinal cord. When the body temperature rises, the hypothalamus responds by increasing sweating, respiration and blood flow to the skin, via the autonomic nervous system. Normal human body temperature displays a circadian rhythm, ranging from 35.8°C (96.4°F) in the predawn hours to 37.3°C (99.1°F) in the late afternoon (Bickley & Szilagyi 2009) and body temperatures that exceed the norm

Table 28.6 Overhydration: fluid excess

	Hypertonic excess	Isotonic excess
Mechanism	Increased sodium concentrations with fluid volume remaining normal Extracellular fluid becomes concentrated with intracellular fluid moving into the extracellular compartment	Increase in fluid and electrolyte concentrations of normal physiological concentrations No movement of fluid across the compartments
Possible causes	Intake of relatively large volumes of salt water	Excessive intake of isotonic fluids either orally or i.v. Abnormal fluid and electrolyte retention following renal disease Corticosteroid therapy
Symptoms	Circulatory overload Oedema Increased cardiac output Congestive cardiac failure Pulmonary oedema Increased BP Full bounding pulse Decreased level of consciousness Muscle twitching Fitting Coma Hypernatraemia	Circulatory overload Oedema Increased cardiac output Congestive cardiac failure Pulmonary oedema Increased BP Full bounding pulse
Management	Management of underlying disease Removal of sodium with diuretics Replacement of fluid lost by drug-induced diuresis	Diuretics Treatment of underlying disease, e.g., CCF i.v. replacement of hypertonic fluids with caution

(After Paradiso C (1995) Fluids and Electrolytes. Philadelphia: JB Lippincott.)

of 37.0°C (98.6°F) are often observed in healthy people. Abnormal elevation of temperature (pyrexia) is categorized as hyperthermia or fever. Hyperthermia is the result of a failure of thermal control mechanisms. In fever, the thermal control mechanisms are intact.

When the temperature falls, the body aims to raise the body temperature by heat conservation and increased heat production. Heat is conserved by reducing the activity of the sweat glands, erection of the body hair and diverting the blood flow from the periphery to the core. Heat is produced by involuntary muscle activity in the form of shivering and by voluntary muscle activity such as stamping the feet.

Assessment of body temperature

Assessment of the body temperature is reliant upon thermometry, which has traditionally been by means of the clinical thermometer either orally, axillary or rectally. These methods often yield inaccuracies in temperature measurement as thermometers are often removed before an accurate temperature has been recorded. With the advent of electronic tympanic thermometers, this has become less of a problem. However, inaccuracies do occur if the ear canal is occluded by either wax or other debris. Again it is important not to discount the value of patient observation as a means of assessment.

Heat illness

Heat illness is inextricably linked to fluid and electrolyte balance. An increase in body temperature is controlled by an increase in sweating as a means of dissipating heat by evaporation. Increased sweating, although a relatively efficient way of reducing temperature, results in the loss of considerable amounts of fluid. Consequently, electrolyte concentrations, especially sodium, become deranged.

A number of factors predispose heat illness. These are rarely of significance individually, but pose a great risk in combination:

- high ambient temperature
- high humidity (humidity reduces effective evaporation through sweating)
- exercise
- clothing which reduces the skin surface area available for evaporation.

Assessment

Good assessment is important to establish the type of heat illness that has occurred and to guide management:

- a full history, including past history as well as the history of the current episode
  - onset of symptoms

○ duration
○ exacerbation
- observation
  ○ airway
  ○ respiratory effort
  ○ use of accessory muscles
  ○ chest movement
  ○ skin colour
  ○ respiratory rate, rhythm and depth
  ○ pulse
  ○ blood pressure
  ○ temperature
  ○ level of consciousness
- palpation
  ○ degree of chest expansion
  ○ temperature and elasticity of the skin
- blood for urea and electrolytes.
- pulse oximetry – with caution.

From the assessment, two conditions may be identified. These are heat exhaustion and heat stroke.

Heat exhaustion

The signs and symptoms are:

- loss of fluid and electrolytes
- slight increase in core temperature
- tachycardia
- headache
- dizziness
- sweating.

Heat stroke (life-threatening)

Signs and symptoms are:

- core temperature above 41°C
- heat increases beyond the body's ability to lose heat (beyond 42°C hypothalamic control of temperature is lost)
- sweating may be absent
- hot dry skin
- nausea and vomiting
- hypovolaemia
- hypokalaemia
- decreased level of consciousness – unconsciousness.

Management

Heat exhaustion

- place in a cool environment, with gentle air flow
- remove clothing preventing heat loss
- replace isotonic fluid – orally if conscious and oriented and not vomiting; otherwise by the intravenous route
- tepid sponging and the use of a fan is not advocated as this causes peripheral vasoconstriction, pooling the blood to the core with a consequential rise in core temperature.

Heat stroke

- secure the airway if indicated
- administer high-concentration oxygen and assisted ventilation if required
- remove clothing
- carry out active cooling – consider immersion in cool water, taking into account potential airway and breathing problems. Spraying the skin with cool water in the presence of air flow may be a more practical intervention to reduce body temperature through evaporation
- carry out intravenous fluid replacement and correction of electrolyte imbalance.

Nervous system

The brain is highly intolerant to a fall in oxygen and glucose levels and is therefore highly sensitive to changes in its blood flow. This sensitivity is manifest in changes in the level of consciousness and subtle signs such as confusion or disorientation. As the brain is responsible for the control and regulation of many vital functions, such as respiration, cardiac output or movement, by means of the somatic or autonomic nervous system, symptoms may be manifest in these systems or processes.

Neurological assessment

As with all assessment, neurological assessment is about the interpretation of trends in clinical signs and not single observations viewed in isolation. One of the most important and informative signs is the level of consciousness. The accepted tool for this assessment is the Glasgow Coma Score (GSC).

Headaches

Headaches of non-traumatic origin account for approximately 0.5% of ED attendances and 10–15% have serious underlying pathology (Wyatt et al. 2012). Headaches with no other neurological signs fall broadly into three main groups: tension, migraine and cluster. In order to differentiate between the three and to identify any serious underlying conditions, a full assessment is essential, with great emphasis being placed upon the history:

- a full history, including past history as well as the history of the current episode
  ○ location of pain
  ○ type of pain
  ○ severity/intensity of pain
  ○ onset of pain
  ○ duration of pain
  ○ frequency of pain
  ○ context in which pain occurs
  ○ what exacerbates or relieves pain
  ○ other associated neurological symptoms

○ health history – has the individual experienced these headaches previously?

○ current medication – especially over-the-counter medications taken for symptom relief, vasodilators or caffeine-containing drugs

○ allergies

○ diet – including intake of caffeine

○ alcohol and substance use

○ smoking

• observation

○ signs of possible underlying mechanisms, substance misuse for example

○ skin colour

○ respiratory rate, rhythm and depth

○ pulse

○ blood pressure

○ temperature

○ level of consciousness (GCS)

○ photophobia

○ neck stiffness.

Tension headaches

These are associated with stress and can often be associated with identifiable causes, such as increase in workload, financial pressures and bereavement. Pain is usually slow in onset, often increasing in intensity over a number of hours and is described as a dull or nagging ache. Generally the pain is generalized and described as a band around the head, rather than focused in a specific area. Tension headaches are frequently chronic as the underlying stress may be chronic.

Management is based upon managing the stress through relaxation techniques and addressing underlying problems where possible. In the immediate term, pain relief may be achieved with simple over-the-counter analgesics as appropriate in the light of current medication history. Ensure that analgesics do not contain caffeine.

Migraine

Migraine may be described as a headache with associated symptoms such as photophobia or sensitivity to movement. However, visual disturbances and aura only occur in about 15% of sufferers. At the onset the pain is unilateral and is accompanied by nausea, vomiting, numbness of hands, face and tongue, weakness and clumsiness. The pain is described as throbbing or pounding and is often intensified by light. Common migraine has similar clinical features, but without the aura, individuals often being awoken from sleep by the pounding headache.

Individuals often find the symptoms less intense if they are able to lie down in a quiet darkened room. Analgesia, especially containing codeine, may help in symptom relief but should be preceded by an anti-emetic. Analgesia alone is of little benefit, as reduced gastric motility prevents its absorption. If vomiting is severe, consideration should be given to administering the anti-emetic per rectum.

The majority of migraine sufferers experience their first episode before the age of 30 and so any individual who presents with a first attack over the age of 40 should be viewed with suspicion and carefully investigated.

Cluster headaches

Cluster headaches refer to repeated episodes of headaches occurring several times a day and lasting between 30 minutes and 2 hours, clusters lasting from 1 to 4 months followed by a period of remission. Pain can occur at any time, but often follows a pattern and frequently occurs an hour after falling asleep. The pain is described as a stabbing, boring pain, which causes the individual to be restless, pacing the floor rather than going to bed. Vomiting is not common. Trigger factors have been linked with alcohol and vasodilators in particular. Treatment is based on analgesia, which is best taken prophylactically prior to expected episodes.

Headaches with associated neurological symptoms

Serious neurological illness may manifest in the form of headaches, but is likely to be accompanied by other neurological signs. Brain tumours, for example, are often associated with fitting and focal neurological signs. The form of the focal signs is dependent upon the site of the tumour, but may include changes in mood, memory, balance, motor function, gait and coordination. The most serious indication of underlying pathology is failing vision and/or reducing levels of consciousness. Again, a thorough history is important in order to establish trends; single occurrences are open to misinterpretation.

Any headache associated with other neurological symptoms must be treated with suspicion and the patient referred immediately.

Subarachnoid haemorrhage

Spontaneous subarachnoid haemorrhage (SAH) generally results from the rupture of an intercranial aneurysm on a major artery in the circle of Willis. The occurrence of SAH is 3% of all strokes and one third of haemorrhagic strokes and has a mortality ranging between 32–67% (Taqi & Torbey 2012). The patient generally presents with sudden onset of an intense headache which may initially be frontal or occipital, but eventually becomes generalized. The blood in the subarachnoid space leads to irritation and neurological signs such as drowsiness, confusion, neck stiffness, photophobia, convulsions and loss of consciousness. Depending upon the location of the bleed, the individual may have aphasia, hemiparesis or hemiplegia.

Management is focused on supporting the vital functions in terms of airway, breathing and circulation. Particular attention should be given to the monitoring of the blood pressure, as a raised blood pressure may increase the degree of bleeding. Preventing and managing the secondary insults on the brain are also important, e.g., hypo-/hyperglycaemia, seizures, hypo-/hyperthermia, hypoxia, irregular respiratory patterns.

Cerebrovascular accident and transient ischaemic attacks

Ischaemic brain injury

The most frequently observed types of brain ischaemia seen in the ED are transient ischaemic attacks and ischaemic stroke. In both cases, ischaemia leads to focal loss of cerebral function. As the name suggests, the symptoms of the ischaemia are short-lived, lasting less than 24 hours, the actual ischaemia being shorter in duration than this. When symptoms last more than 24 hours, death occurs from what is thought to be a cerebral vascular event alone. A person who has had one or more transient ischaemic attacks is almost ten times more likely to have a stroke than someone of the same age and gender who has not had one. Those who have had a myocardial infarct are also at increased risk for having a stroke (Bergman et al. 2012).

More than 85 % of strokes are ischaemic in origin leading to infarction; haemorrhagic brain injuries account for the remaining cases (Wang et al. 2009). These mainly result from either a primary intercerebral bleed or a subarachnoid haemorrhage. A quick way to triage stroke is to use the FAST acronym, based on the Cincinnati Stroke Scale that was developed to raise public recognition of stroke. FAST stands for Face, Arm, Speech, and Time, and *time is brain* is a key concept in the management of those who have had a stroke (Arto et al. 2012, Bergman et al. 2012).

Assessment

- a full history
  - onset of symptoms
  - duration
  - exacerbation
- observation
  - skin colour, appearance
  - respiratory rate, rhythm and depth
  - pulse
  - blood pressure
  - temperature
  - GCS.

The modes of presentation of both transient ischaemia and stroke differ little other than in the duration of the symptoms. Symptoms vary depending upon the area of brain affected:

- hemiparesis
- hemiplegia
- dizziness
- dysarthria
- dysphagia
- dysphasia
- ataxia
- visual disturbances
- confusion
- reduced level of consciousness
- unconsciousness.

Management

As with subarachnoid haemorrhage, management is focused upon supporting the vital functions in terms of airway, breathing and circulation. Particular attention should be given to monitoring of the blood pressure, as a raised blood pressure may increase the degree of bleeding. Patients should be screened for intravenous thrombolytic drugs such as Alteplase/recombinant tissue plasminogen activator which should be given within 3–4.5 hours after acute ischaemic stroke. Exclusion criteria include >80 years of age, taking oral anticoagulant drugs, and/or combined history of diabetes and stroke (ECASS III 2008, Bergman et al. 2012).

Epilepsy

Epilepsy in itself is not a medical emergency; however, there are a number of mechanisms that may make it so, the most common being injury sustained during a convulsion and several seizures following on from the previous in quick succession – status epilepticus. This is more common at the extremes of age, with over 50 % of all cases occurring in children and a disproportionately high incidence in those over 60 years of age. It also occurs most commonly in patients with no previous history of epilepsy (Wilkes 2004).

Neurones within the brain communicate in a systematic way. During a seizure, discharge from the neurones is chaotic, often manifesting in a tonic–clonic fit, but it may manifest in many other ways. During the tonic phase, the individual loses consciousness, this being accompanied by muscle contraction causing the body to become stiff, jaw to be clenched, air to be forced out of the lungs and possibly incontinence. The tonic phase is followed by the clonic phase that is characterized by rhythmic contractions of the limbs and trunk – convulsions.

Normally when convulsions cease, the individual is drowsy, confused and may have a headache. The main danger for the individual in such circumstances is from injury when falling to the ground or colliding with objects or from having objects forced into the mouth by unwitting 'helpers'. It is important to establish if the fit is related to epilepsy or if it is a symptom of some other condition such as head injury or subarachnoid haemorrhage. Status epilepticus, where one seizure ends and another immediately commences, is a potentially life-threatening condition requiring immediate intervention to break the cycle. Status epilepticus has a significant mortality (2–4 %) and morbidity (10 %) with irreversible neurological damage (Appleton 1994). The mainstay of management is securing the airway, administration of oxygen, assessment of respiratory and cardiac function and the administration of either lorazepam or diazepam intravenously (Scottish Intercollegiate Guidelines Network 2003).

Glucose regulation

Two of the hormones secreted by the pancreas, insulin and glucagon, have an important function in the maintenance of blood glucose levels. Insulin is secreted in response to elevated blood glucose levels, its function being to promote the storage of glucose by facilitating its uptake by the cells and by the synthesis of glycogen in the liver, renal cortex and the muscles. Consequently, these actions reduce blood glucose.

Unlike insulin, the stimuli for glucagon release are hunger and a low blood sugar level, the net effect of its release being to raise the blood sugar level. This is achieved by glycogenolysis, the conversion of stored glycogen into glucose. In addition, glucose is synthesized from lactate, amino acids and glycerol.

Assessment of blood sugar

Patient observation and a nursing history may provide an indication that the patient has an altered blood sugar. The use of single drop of blood laboratory sticks is a rapid and accurate method of providing objective confirmation of your observations. This should always be followed up with a laboratory test of a larger sample of blood drawn by venepuncture. Such assessments should also be considered for those patients who have an altered level of consciousness and where a raised or lowered blood sugar cannot be excluded.

Diabetes mellitus

Diabetes mellitus is a condition whereby the cells are unable to access and utilize glucose taken in through the diet, due to either a lack of insulin or ineffective insulin. A lack of naturally occurring insulin is referred to as type 1, commonly known as insulin-dependent diabetes mellitus (IDDM), which generally first appears in childhood. Where naturally occurring insulin is present but is ineffective, the condition is termed type 2, commonly known as non-insulin-dependent diabetes mellitus (NIDDM). This often first appears in later life. As a consequence of the cells' inability to access the glucose, it remains in the circulation, with some being excreted by the kidneys. In the absence of effective glucose metabolism, the body begins to metabolize fats.

Three main conditions occur in diabetes which may present a threat to life: hypoglycaemia, diabetic ketoacidosis (DKA) and hyperglycaemic hyperosmolar state (HHS) also known as hyperosmolar non-ketotic state (HONK). HHS replaces the older terms, 'HONK coma' and 'HONK', because mild to moderate ketosis is commonly present in this state and alterations of sensoria may be present without coma (English & Williams 2004).

Hypoglycaemia occurs in all types of diabetics and non-diabetics and occurs when there is a lowered plasma level of glucose. DKA almost only ever occurs in type 1 diabetes. In the presence of uncontrolled hyperglycaemia metabolism of lipids occurs, resulting in the production of large amounts of ketones and an associated metabolic acidosis. Hyperglycaemic hyperosmolar state most commonly occurs among type 2 diabetics and is associated with often very high blood glucose levels, frequently without the production of ketones and the associated acidosis.

Assessment

Assessment of the neurologically impaired patient is important regardless of the suspected mechanism:

- a full history
  - onset of symptoms
  - duration
  - exacerbation
- observation
  - skin colour, appearance
  - respiratory rate, rhythm and depth
  - pulse
  - blood pressure
  - temperature
  - odour on the breath
- reagent strip blood test for glucose
- formal blood sample for laboratory blood glucose measurement
- assessment for dehydration.

Hypoglycaemia

Symptoms and signs of hypoglycaemia include:

- blood glucose of less than 3.0 mmol/L
- rapid in onset in IDDM, where synthetic insulin intake oversupplies glucose intake or where there is an increased glucose demand
- slower in onset in NIDDM.

Early signs:

- weakness
- sweating
- tachycardia
- palpitations
- tremor
- irritability
- confusion
- amnesia
- visual disturbance.

Later signs:

- unconsciousness
- fitting.

All individuals with a reduced level of consciousness, especially if associated with alcohol, should routinely have blood glucose measured by use of a reagent lab stick.

Management

The conscious individual

- fast-acting sugar in the form of a drink, e.g., sugar in tea or coffee, soft drink – not diet/low calorie. It is important to note that metformin is a sucrose inhibitor therefore sugar in the form of glucose is required for patients on this medication
- longer-acting sugar, e.g., a sandwich or biscuits.

The unconscious individual

- maintain the airway
- support breathing
- glucagon by injection – converted into glucose by the body; benefits are temporary and so it must be followed up with oral long-acting sugar when consciousness returns and the individual is able to protect his own airway
- 50% glucose intravenous infusion – must be into a large vein as hypertonic fluids are highly irritant.

Diabetic ketoacidosis

Symptoms and signs include:

- blood glucose persistently above 15 mmol/L
- usually type 1, but can occasionally be type 2
- osmotic diuresis – water following glucose excreted by the kidney
- thirst
- polyuria
- oliguria
- fatigue
- warm dry skin
- nausea
- vomiting
- electrolyte imbalance
- loss of consciousness.

Management

- airway management as required
- support of breathing
- rehydration with i.v. isotonic fluids
- insulin – guided by measured blood glucose
- correction of electrolyte imbalance.

Haematology

The blood has a number of important functions, many of which impinge on other systems and processes. It plays a vital role in the transportation of respiratory gases, maintenance of body temperature, acid–base balance, fluid and electrolyte balance and immunity. Blood, by volume, is predominantly plasma, in which are suspended red blood cells, white blood cells and platelets. Red blood cells are predominantly involved in the transportation of oxygen by means of the haemoglobin. The red cells are produced in the bone marrow and remain in the circulation for about 120 days. Changes in blood concentration, infection and some drugs are known to easily damage the relatively fragile red blood cells.

White cells are produced in the bone marrow and are considerably less numerous than the red blood cells. The white cells are of three main types: granulocytes (neutrophils, eosinophils and basophils), lymphocytes and monocytes.

Collectively these cells form the basis of the body's defence system. Platelet formation also takes place in the bone marrow; 60–75% of platelets stay in the circulation and the bulk of the remainder are found in the spleen (Waugh & Grant 2010). Platelets are predominantly involved in clotting processes.

The plasma, as well as being a transport medium for the red cells, white cells and platelets, contains a number of salts and proteins. The proteins have a wide range of functions, including maintaining the osmotic pressure of the blood, clotting and immunity.

Haematological assessment

Much of the assessment may be based upon patient observation and the nursing history. However, much information may be gained from the appropriate haematological and biochemical tests and the interpretation of the results.

Sickle cell disease

While 70% of those with sickle cell disease are of African ethnic origin, it is also seen in Mediterranean, Middle Eastern and Indian communities (Rees et al 2010). Sickle cell disease is thought to have evolved over a considerable time in malaria-endemic areas, as a defence against malaria. The evolutionary changes have resulted in a change in the structure of the haemoglobin, which in sickle cell disease can lead to a change in the shape of the red blood cell to form the classically sickle-shaped blood cell, and these changes are at a genetic level, accounting for the hereditary element of sickle cell disease.

The most commonly occurring crisis experienced by sufferers of sickle cell disease is painful crisis and this accounts for over 90% of hospital admissions for patients with sickle cell disease. Sickle cells can cluster together causing occlusion of small blood vessels. Such obstruction reduces the blood flow to the distal tissues and causes the acute pain. It is the acute pain which precipitates the attendance at the ED, but it is essential that an adequate assessment is made to identify factors which may have triggered the episode, such as:

- reduced oxygenation – often following exercise
- cold or excessive heat
- dehydration
- fever
- infections
- stress.

Assessment

Assessment will include:

- a full history, including past history as well as the history of the current episode
  - onset of symptoms
  - duration
  - exacerbation
- observation
  - respiratory effort
  - use of accessory muscles
  - chest movement and symmetry
  - skin colour
  - respiratory rate, rhythm and depth (respiration may be compromised if sickling occurs in the pulmonary circulation)
  - pulse
  - blood pressure
  - temperature
  - GCS as sickling in cerebral vessels can lead to ischaemic stroke
- palpation
  - degree of chest expansion
  - temperature of the skin
- auscultation
  - quality of breath sound
  - degree of air entry
- pulse oximetry – with caution
- chest X-ray.

Clinical features

These include severe pain which commonly starts in the limbs, but may occur in the back and chest. Other clinical features may be associated with the precipitating factors, such as dehydration.

Management

This includes rapid and adequate analgesia, usually requiring opiate analgesics. These should not be delayed by undertaking a detailed examination. Intravenous fluids are particularly important for patients with renal involvement and the aim should be to generate urine output in excess of 100 mL/h (McLaren 2004). Seek specialist advice from the haematologist. As well as pain relief, ensure the patient is warm and able to rest. Oxygen therapy should be given if indicated; however, oxygen will be of little or no benefit to most individuals in sickle cell crisis as the problem is associated with obstructed blood flow and not oxygenation of that blood. Sickle cell disease is associated with an increased risk of cerebral infarction (Verduzco & Nathan 2009). It is highly recommended that each department has a policy for managing individuals with sickle cell disease and information on where to access specialist advice and support locally.

Neutropaenic pyrexia

One of the major causes of fevers in cancer patients is infection, especially in relation to neutropaenia. Fever in the neutropaenic cancer patient represents an absolute emergency, since undetected and untreated infections in neutropaenic patients can progress quickly (Bosnjak 2004). Fever in a neutropaenic cancer patient may signify a life-threatening infection and in a cancer patient should be considered indicative of infection until proven otherwise and appropriate assessments should be instituted immediately.

Assessment

Clinical evaluation of an infection-related fever includes a complete history and physical examination with careful attention to inspection of the skin, all body orifices, fingerstick and venepuncture sites, biopsy sites, and skin folds (e.g., breasts, axilla, groin). The perirectal area should also be assessed, since a history of haemorrhoids places neutropaenic patients (especially those with leukaemia) at particular risk for infection. Assessment should include the respiratory, gastrointestinal, urinary and neurological systems. Patients should be checked for abdominal distension and tenderness. Cultures should be obtained from each port and lumen, as well as from a peripheral vein.

Management

All neutropaenic cancer patients should be considered to be at risk for infection and, once febrile, should be treated immediately with antimicrobials, without waiting for clinical and/ or microbiological documentation of infection (Bosnjak 2004): this is known as empirical antibiotic therapy. Empirical antibiotic treatment of all neutropaenic patients at the onset of fever continues to be controversial. However, it also remains the key aspect of infection management. The specific composition of the empirical antibiotic regimen also remains subject to change, which is due to the changing pattern of pathogens, the emergence of antibiotic-resistant organisms, the appearance of the new clinical entities, the availability of new drugs and the improved models for patient's infection risk categorization (Bosnjak 2004). While there is a general consensus that empirical therapy is appropriate, there is no consensus as to which antibiotics or combinations of antibiotics should be used.

Conclusion

In the modern ED, a 'medical emergency' can range from a full cardiac arrest to a GP referral patient with an exacerbation of a chronic condition. This chapter has considered the more common medical conditions which may result in ED attendances. The ED nurse plays an important role in identifying and alleviating symptoms and conditions which can be debilitating for the patient. While many medical conditions are chronic, the exacerbation of these conditions may require the patient to attend ED for subsequent admission. The provision of supportive care can alleviate the suffering and disruption caused by these medical emergencies.

References

Appleton, R., 1994. The Nursing Times Guide to Epilepsy. Macmillan, Basingstoke.

Arto, V., Putaala, J., Strbian, D., et al., 2012. Stroke mimics and intravenous thrombolysis. Annals of Emergency Medicine 59 (1), 27–32.

Axford, J., 1996. Medicine. Blackwell Science, Oxford.

Barnes, P.J., Celli, B.R., 2009. Systemic manifestations and comorbidities of COPD. European Respiratory Journal 33 (5), 1165–1185.

Bergman, K., Kindler, D., Pfau, L., 2012. Assessment of stroke: A review for ED nurses. Journal of Emergency Nursing 38 (1), 36–42.

Bickley, L.S., Szilagyi, P.G., 2009. Bates' Pocket Guide to Physical Examination and History Taking, sixth ed. Lippincott, Williams & Wilkins, Philadelphia.

Bosnjak, S., 2004. Treatment of a febrile neutropenic patient. Archives of Oncology 12 (3), 179–181.

British Thoracic Society, 2003. British guidelines on the management of suspected acute pulmonary embolism. Thorax 58, 470–484.

British Thoracic Society, 2012. The British Guideline on the Management of Asthma: A National Clinical Guideline. BTS & SIGN, Edinburgh.

Cetti, R., Venn, S., 2012. The management of acute urinary tract infection. In: Dawson, C., Nethercliffe, J. (Eds.), ABC of Urology, third ed. John Wiley & Sons, London.

Cohen, A.T., Agnelli, G., Anderson, F.A., et al., 2007. Venous thromboembolism (VTE) in Europe: The number of events and associated morbidity and mortality. Thrombosis and Haemostasis 98, 756–764.

Davenport, K., Waine, E., 2010. The role of nonsteroidal anti-inflammatory drugs in renal colic. Pharmaceuticals 3, 1304–1310.

ECASS III, , 2008. Thrombolysis with Alteplase 3 to 4.5 hours after acute ischaemic stroke. New England Journal of Medicine 359, 1317–1329.

Ejernæs, K., 2011. Bacterial characteristics of importance for recurrent urinary tract infections caused by *Escherichia coli*. Danish Medical Bulletin 58 (4), B4187.

English, P., Williams, G., 2004. Hyperglycaemic crises and lactic acidosis in diabetes mellitus. Postgraduate Medical Journal 80, 253–261.

Ganong, W.F., 2003. Review of Medical Physiology, twenty-first ed. Appleton & Lange, Connecticut.

Gibson, G.J., 2003. Respiratory function tests. In: Warrel, D.A., Cox, T.M., Firth, J.D. (Eds.), Oxford Textbook of Medicine. Oxford University Press, Oxford.

Greaves, I., Hodgetts, T., Porter, K., 2005. Emergency Care: A Textbook for Paramedics, second ed. WB Saunders, London.

Hinchliff, S., Montague, S., Watson, R., 1996. Physiology for Nursing Practice, second ed. Bailliere Tindall, London.

Joint Royal Colleges Ambulance Liaison Committee, 2006. The Immersion Incident. JRCALC, Warwick.

Lieberman, P., Nicklas, R.A., Oppenheimer, J., et al., 2010. The diagnosis and management of anaphylaxis practice parameter: 2010 update. The Journal of Allergy and Clinical Immunology 126 (3), 477–480.

Levine, R.L., Fromm, R.E., 1995. Critical Care Monitoring: From Pre-hospital to the ICU. Mosby, St Louis.

MacNee, W., 2011. Pathology and pathogenesis. In: Currie, G.P. (Ed.), ABC of COPD, second ed. Wiley-Blackwell, Oxford.

McLaren, H., 2004. Anaemia. In: Cameron, P., Jelinek, G., Kelly, A.M., Murray, L., Brown, A.F.T., Heyworth, J. (Eds.), Textbook of Emergency Medicine, second ed. Churchill Livingstone, Edinburgh.

Mills, K., Morton, R., Page, G., 1995. Colour Atlas and Text of Emergencies, second ed. Mosby-Wolfe, London.

Morris, J., 2003. Environmental emergencies. In: Newberry, L. (Ed.), Sheehy's Emergency Nursing: Principles and Practice, fifth ed. Mosby, St Louis.

Moyle, J., 2002. Pulse Oximetry, second ed.. British Medical Journal Publishing Group, London.

Nasser, S., 2012. Anaphylaxis: current state of knowledge for the modern physician. Postgraduate Medical Journal 88, 458–464.

National Institute for Health and Clinical Excellence, 2010. Chronic Obstructive Pulmonary Disease: Management of Chronic Obstructive Pulmonary Disease in Adults in Primary and Secondary Care. NICE, London.

National Institutes of Health, 2007. Guidelines for the Diagnosis and Management of Asthma: National Asthma Education and Prevention Program Expert Panel Report 3. NIH, Bethseda, MD.

Newman Taylor, A.J., 2003. Endocrine disorders. In: Warrel, D.A., Cox, T.M., Firth, J.D. (Eds.), Oxford Textbook of Medicine. Oxford University Press, Oxford.

Nicholson, P., 2004. Renal colic. In: Cameron, P., Jelinek, G., Kelly, A.M., Murray, L., Brown, A.F.T., Heyworth, J. (Eds.), Textbook of Emergency Medicine, second ed. Churchill Livingstone, Edinburgh.

Paradiso, C., 1995. Fluids and Electrolytes. JB Lippincott, Philadelphia.

Rees, D.C., Williams, T.N., Gladwin, M.T., 2010. Sickle-cell disease. The Lancet 376 (9757), 2018–2031.

Scottish Intercollegiate Guidelines Network, 2003. Diagnosis and Management of Epilepsy in Adults: A National Clinical Guideline. Scottish Intercollegiate Guidelines Network, Edinburgh.

Sivilotti, M.L.A., Abu-Laban, R.B., 2012. Inhaling smoke causes smoke inhalation: put that in your hookah pipe! Canadian Journal of Emergency Medicine 14 (1), 3.

Stein, P.D., Matta, F., Muzammil, H.M., et al., 2010. Silent pulmonary embolism in patients with deep vein thrombosis: A systematic review. The American Journal of Medicine 123 (5), 426–431.

Taqi, M.A., Torbey, M.T., 2012. Subarachnoid haemorrhage. In: Manno, E. (Ed.), Emergency Management in Neurocritical Care. John Wiley & Sons, London.

Taneja, G., Van Beeck, E., Brenner, R., 2008. Drowning. In: Peden, M., Oyebgite, K., Ozanne-Smith, J. (Eds.), World Report on Child Injury Prevention. World Health Organization, Geneva.

Verduzco, L.A., Nathan, D.G., 2009. Sickle cell disease and stroke. Blood 114, 5117–5125.

Waugh, A., Grant, A., 2010. Ross and Wilson's Anatomy and Physiology in Health and Illness, eleventh ed. Churchill Livingstone, Edinburgh.

Wang, C.X., Stroink, A., Casto, J.M., et al., 2009. Hyperthermia exacerbates ischaemic brain injury. International Journal of Stroke 4, 274–284.

Weaver, L.K., 2009. Carbon monoxide poisoning. New England Journal of Medicine 360, 1217–1225.

Wilkes, G.J., 2004. Seizures. In: Cameron, P., Jelinek, G., Kelly, A.M., Murray, L., Brown, A.F.T., Heyworth, J. (Eds.), Textbook of Emergency Medicine, second ed. Churchill Livingstone, Edinburgh.

Wyatt, J.P., Illingworth, R.N., Graham, C.A., et al., 2012. Oxford Handbook of Accident & Emergency Medicine, fourth ed. Oxford University Press, Oxford.

Yeh, S.Y., Schwartzstein, R., 2010. Asthma: Pathophysiology and diagnosis. In: Harver, A., Kotses, H. (Eds.), Asthma, Health and Society: A Public Health Perspective. Springer, New York.

Surgical emergencies

29

Valerie Small

CHAPTER CONTENTS

http://dx.doi.org/10.1016/B978-0-7020-4315-4.00029-2

Introduction

The management of patients presenting with surgical emergencies relies upon rapid assessment, the formulation of an accurate working diagnosis and timely appropriate management to reduce overall morbidity and mortality. The emergency nurse may be the first person to assess the patient, and therefore finely tuned assessment skills are vital. To ensure patient assessment is safe and thorough, the skills of inspection, auscultation, palpation and percussion should be utilized appropriately during patient consultations. Some of the physical examination skills described in this chapter will require both instructions in the technique and repeated practice to achieve a proficient level of competence. This chapter will describe non-traumatic surgical emergencies of the abdominal and pelvic regions in adults, according to the following classification: acute abdomen, vascular and genitourinary emergencies.

Anatomy and physiology of the abdomen

A comprehensive knowledge of the anatomy and physiology of the abdomen is vitally important for the emergency nurse to assist in the rapid assessment and initiation of treatment for patients who present with a surgical emergency. The external and internal anatomy of the abdomen is broadly described in Chapter 9. The anatomy and physiology of specific abdominal organs are outlined throughout this chapter.

Oesophagus

This muscular tube extends from the pharynx to the stomach. It is about 25 cm long and lies in front of the vertebral column and behind the trachea within the mediastinum. The oesophagus transports food from the pharynx, and upper and lower oesophageal sphincters regulate the movement of food into

and out of the oesophagus. Lubrication of the food is provided by mucous glands coating the inner surface of the oesophagus (Moore et al. 2009).

Stomach

The stomach is a J-shaped organ lying under the diaphragm in the epigastric, umbilical and left hypochondrial regions of the abdomen. The most superior part of the stomach is called the fundus. The largest part is the body, which has a convex area laterally called the greater curvature and a concave area medially called the lesser curvature. The final part of the stomach is the pylorus, which provides the opening into the first part of the small intestine. The muscular coats of the stomach consist of three layers: a longitudinal outer layer, a middle circular layer and an inner oblique layer of muscle fibres. The lining mucosa of the stomach is arranged into folds called rugae. These folds allow the stomach to stretch, and they disappear as the stomach is filled. The stomach acts as a food blender and reservoir, its chief function is enzymatic digestion. The cells in the stomach produce mucus, hydrochloric acid, intrinsic factor, regulatory hormones and pepsinogen, which is involved in protein digestion. The gastric juice gradually converts a mass of food into a liquid mixture – chyme – that passes fairly quickly into the duodenum (Moore et al. 2009).

The small intestine

The small intestine is about 6 m in length and is composed of three parts: the duodenum, the jejunum and the ileum. The duodenum is about 25 cm long, the jejunum is 2.5 m long and the ileum is 3.5 m long. The duodenum nearly completes a 180° arc that contains the head of the pancreas. The common bile duct from the liver and the pancreatic duct both empty into the duodenum. The surface area of the duodenum is greatly increased by tiny projections called villi, which are covered by columnar epithelium. The villi are about 1 mm high, and with around 10–40 mm^2 the surface area is greatly increased for absorption of nutrients. About 9 L of water enter the small intestine each day, most of which is reabsorbed, with only about 1 L reaching the large intestine. The jejunum and the ileum are similar in structure to the duodenum. The junction between the ileum and the large intestine is the ileocaecal sphincter which has a one-way valve.

The large intestine

The large intestine is responsible for the elimination of food residue and the maintenance of water and electrolyte balance. It consists of the caecum, the appendix, the ascending, transverse, descending colon, the sigmoid colon, the rectum and anal canal. The caecum – the first part of the large intestine that is continuous with the ascending colon – is a blind interstitial pouch. The vermiform (wormlike) appendix, a blind intestinal diverticulum (6–10 cm in length), arises from the caecum. The colon is about 1.8 m long, consisting of ascending, transverse, descending and sigmoid colons. The lining of the large intestine contains many mucus-producing goblet cells and columnar cells which reabsorb water. About 1 L of water enters the large intestine each day, but only about 100 mL is lost in the faeces – the rest is reabsorbed. The circular muscle layer is complete, with an incomplete longitudinal layer of muscle. Contraction of this longitudinal layer gives the colon a pouched appearance called haustra. The rectum is a straight muscular tube running from the sigmoid colon to the anal canal. This canal is about 3 cm long and is the final part of the digestive tract (Moore et al. 2009).

Peritoneum

The abdominal cavity is lined by a serous membrane called the parietal peritoneum, with the organs being covered by the visceral layer of the peritoneum. There is a potential space between these two layers called the peritoneal cavity, which contains serous fluid. A small amount of fluid in the peritoneal cavity allows the abdominal organs to move freely. The intestines are supported in the abdominal cavity by a fan-like structure of connective tissue called the mesentery. The mesentery connecting the lesser curvature of the stomach to the liver and diaphragm is called the lesser omentum. The greater omentum connects the greater curvature of the stomach to the transverse colon and the posterior abdominal wall. The greater omentum also covers the front of the abdominal organs. It contains a lot of adipose tissue and looks like a fatty apron hanging over the organs. If infection occurs in the peritoneum, the greater omentum tries to wall off the infection by surrounding it, to prevent its spread. The mesenteries contain blood and lymphatic vessels and nerves that supply the abdominal organs.

Abdominal organs that lie against the posterior abdominal wall have their anterior surface covered by peritoneum and are described as retroperitoneal organs. These are the duodenum, pancreas, ascending colon, rectum, kidneys, adrenal glands and the bladder.

Abdominal wall

The abdominal wall is composed of skin, fascia and four pairs of flat, sheet-like muscles called rectus abdominis, external and internal oblique and transverse abdominis. The linea alba is a tough, fibrous band of tissue that stretches from the sternum to the symphysis pubis and is made up of the aponeurosis of the abdominal muscles. Part of the external oblique muscle forms the inguinal ligament, which runs from the anterior superior iliac pubic tubercle. Just superior to the medial end of this ligament is the superficial inguinal ring which is the outer opening of the inguinal canal. This canal contains the spermatic cord and the ilio-inguinal nerve in males and the round ligament of the uterus and the ilio-inguinal nerve in females. The posterior abdominal wall is composed of the bones of the lumbar spine and the hip bones, along with the psoas, quadratus lumborum and iliacus muscles (Moore et al. 2009).

Nursing assessment of the acute abdomen

The clinical approach to patients with surgical emergencies is the same as that of any emergency presentation. An initial overview is accomplished rapidly to evaluate that the airway is patent and protected, that air exchange is adequate, and that the patient has adequate systemic perfusion. The tools for evaluating abdominal complaints are: patient history, physical examination, imaging studies and laboratory tests. Once airway, breathing and circulation have been assessed and appropriate interventions to correct any abnormalities have been performed, the emergency nurse may proceed to gather the history of the presenting complaint. According to the literature the most common pitfall in evaluating abdominal pain is the failure to obtain a sufficiently detailed and accurate history (Bickley 2007).

History

The essential elements of the history are to determine:

- the nature, onset, location and radiation of the abdominal pain
- the presence and sequence of onset of associated symptoms such as fever, nausea, vomiting, urinary symptoms, and pelvic symptoms (in women)
- pertinent history related to bowel movements, appetite, weight changes, and menstrual history
- previous medical history of similar episodes, prior medical and surgical history, and current medication use. Alcohol intake, tobacco use and known allergies should also be ascertained
- social history related to occupation, family history, activity level, and recent foreign travel.

To establish a full clinical picture, the emergency nurse may further ascertain the following:

- *appetite:* has there been a recent alteration in dietary habits? Does the patient avoid certain foods for any reason? Is there any difficulty in swallowing; is there any sensation of food sticking in the throat or chest? Has there been any change in the patient's weight? Do the patient's clothes still fit? Is the abdomen bloated?
- *tongue:* the state of the tongue gives some indication of the state of hydration of the body. Patients who have been ill for some time with a gastrointestinal problem frequently have a fluid and electrolyte deficit. A dry brown tongue may be found in any severe illness, uraemia or acute intestinal obstruction. Additional longitudinal furrows may indicate dehydration
- *skin:* any change in skin colour, bruising or itching may be as a result of liver disease
- *bowel habits:* is there any constipation, diarrhoea, blood or mucus in the stool?
- *energy:* are there any feelings of lethargy or changes in mental status?

Pain assessment

Abdominal pain is due to:

- contraction of muscle tissue
- irritation of the mucosa
- stretching of an organ
- inflammation of the peritoneum
- irritation of nerves in the area.

The body is programmed to appreciate pain from areas under voluntary control and the skin. We are therefore not able to appreciate the precise location of the source of visceral pain. In pain originating in the heart, for example, impulses pass along the dermatomes of T1–T4, so the patient experiences pain across the chest and down the arms. Pain may therefore be referred to a site far from its origin; for instance, pain from the spleen may be referred to the left shoulder due to irritation of the phrenic nerve. There are several aspects to consider when assessing a patient's pain, which can be usefully remembered by the mnemonic TROCARS (Box 29.1).

Box 29.1

Assessing abdominal pain using mnemonic TROCARS

Timing – duration of the pain
Radiation – does the pain go anywhere else?
Occurrence – when does the pain start?
Characteristics – colicky, sharp, dull
Aggravating factors – food, exercise
Relieving factors – rest, medicines
Site and severity – location and pain score

General principles of patient assessment and abdominal examination

Begin the assessment of the gastrointestinal tract by examining the patient's hands to discover signs of disease (Table 29.1). Next examine the patient's eyes for pale conjunctiva as this is indicative of anaemia. Enlarged lymph nodes may be found in the supra-clavicular fossa, suggestive of secondaries from a gastric carcinoma.

For the purposes of specific examination the abdomen can be divided into four quadrants (Fig. 29.1). To divide the abdomen into quadrants draw an imaginary line from the xiphoid process of the sternum through the umbilicus to the symphysis pubis, draw a second perpendicular line across the abdomen through the umbilicus. This divides the abdomen into quadrants: right upper quadrant, right lower quadrant, left upper quadrant and left lower quadrant and is the most common method of mapping the contents of the abdomen (Douglas et al. 2009).

In order to perform the abdominal examination satisfactorily it is essential to have a good light source and the patient should be made as relaxed as possible. Patient privacy and a full explanation of the procedure will assist in making

Table 29.1 Hand examination

Clinical finding	Cause
Pallor	Anaemia
Clubbing	Cirrhosis
	Crohn's disease
	Ulcerative colitis
Palmar erythema	Liver disease
Spoon-shaped nails	Iron deficiency

the patient comfortable. The patient should be placed in a supine position with the head resting on a small pillow and the arms resting by the sides. In some cases the patient may be more comfortable with a small pillow under the knees, to help relax the abdominal muscles. Although it is necessary to expose the area from the sternum to the pelvis, the patient should be kept as warm as possible during the procedure, which should be performed quickly and efficiently. The patient should be examined from his right side, in a gentle manner, with warm hands and short fingernails (McGrath 2004, Bickley 2007).

Inspection

Inspection can reveal important information, including the presence of distension, masses, surgical scars, discoloration by ecchymosis (Cullen's and Grey-Turner's signs), and skin abnormalities such as spider angiomata, petechiae, jaundice and rashes. Look for any visible peristalsis and pulsations. Pulsation of the abdominal aorta may be observed in thin patients or in those with an aortic aneurysm. The location of operation scars may give clues as to the type of surgery previously performed. The abdomen is normally symmetrical, and may be asymmetrical due to bowel obstruction, hernia or spinal deformity. It is useful to try to visualize the underlying organs during the examination. For example, asymmetry of the lower abdomen may be due to a distended bladder, masses of the ovary, uterus or colon. Distended veins around the umbilicus signify portal hypertension. Generalized distension of the abdomen may be due to one of the five Fs:

- fat
- fluid
- faeces
- flatus
- foetus.

The abdomen should move freely with respiration, but this will be diminished or absent in generalized peritonitis (McGrath 2004, Epstein et al. 2008, Turner et al. 2009).

Auscultation

Auscultation should precede palpation as the latter can induce peristalsis artificially. Bowel sounds are regarded as the least

Right upper quadrant

Right lobe of liver
Gallbladder
Pylorus
Duodenum
Head of pancreas
Upper right kidney

Left upper quadrant

Left lobe of liver
Spleen
Stomach
Left kidney
Body of pancreas
Splenic flexure of colon

Right lower quadrant

Lower right kidney
Cecum
Appendix
Ascending colon
Right fallopian tube (female)
Right ovary (female)
Right ureter
Bladder (distended)

Left lower quadrant

Descending colon
Sigmoid colon
Left fallopian tube (female)
Left ovary (female)
Left ureter
Bladder (distended)

Figure 29.1 • Abdominal contents.

helpful element of the abdominal examination because reflex ileus can occur with virtually any painful abdominal condition and might persist for some time, even with intra-abdominal catastrophes (Epstein et al. 2008, Turner et al. 2009). The emergency nurse may gain valuable experience from listening to many normal abdomens to establish a baseline. Initially, it is best to listen using the diaphragm of the stethoscope to the right of the umbilicus. Bowel sounds should be checked for at least 1 minute in all four quadrants, before declaring that they are absent. Absent bowel sounds are a feature of paralytic ileus, late obstruction and generalized peritonitis.

In an obstructed patient, the absence of bowel sounds suggests strangulation or ischaemia. In small bowel obstruction the bowel sounds are exaggerated initially, with frequent low-pitched gurgles, rising to become high-pitched tinkling sounds as peristalsis increases above the obstruction. The presence of these sounds coincides with the peristalsis and the colicky abdominal pain suffered by the patient. In between these painful episodes, the bowel is quiet. The bowel is also hyperactive in gastroenteritis and severe diarrhoea.

Normally, blood flow along arteries cannot be heard using a stethoscope. However, when the vessel becomes diseased the resultant turbulence, as the blood flows over atheromatous plaques, produces soft high-pitched sounds called bruits. These bruits may be heard using the bell of the stethoscope over a diseased aorta and renal, hepatic, splenic or femoral vessels. Check the aorta by listening in the mid-epigastric region above the umbilicus. Renal bruits may be heard in this area, and additionally in the flanks or posteriorly over the kidneys. Femoral bruits may be heard in the groin. Bruits are heard even if the patient changes position.

Percussion

Light percussion is performed to determine the presence of masses, enlargement of an organ or abdominal distension. The middle finger of the left hand is placed on the area to be percussed, and the back of its middle phalanx is struck with the tip of the middle finger of the right hand. The percussing finger should be bent, so that when the blow is delivered its terminal phalanx is at right angles to the metacarpal bone it is striking. Tympany is the normal percussion note and is a hollow resonant sound heard over the abdomen, apart from over the solid organs. Dull percussion notes will be heard over dense organs such as the liver and spleen, tumours or over a fluid-filled bladder (Epstein et al. 2008, Turner et al. 2009).

Palpation

Palpation is saved for last and should be performed gently, beginning with the quadrant most remote from the patient's pain, moving towards the painful area. Deep palpation and the classically described test for rebound tenderness have limited utility and might be misleading (McGrath 2004, Turner et al. 2009). If the patient is not relaxed, the abdominal muscles will tense, making examination impossible. Using a warm hand flat on the abdominal wall, gently palpate all four quadrants. Palpation of specific organs requires practice, and further description is beyond the scope of this chapter. Check for the presence and equality of the femoral pulses, and assess the femoral and inguinal lymph nodes for tenderness or enlargement.

Vomit

The strongest stimuli for vomiting are irritation and distension of the stomach. Nerve impulses are transmitted to the medulla, and returning impulses to the upper gastrointestinal organs, diaphragm and abdominal muscles. The stomach is then squeezed between the diaphragm and the abdominal muscles. Prolonged vomiting will lead to loss of gastric juice and fluid. This can lead to disturbance in fluid and acid–base balance. If bleeding is severe, the vomit may look like pure blood or it may be dark with clots. Bleeding may be altered to a dark brown or black colour by gastric juice. The dark colour is due to the conversion of haemoglobin into haematin. The altered blood is sometimes compared to 'coffee grounds'. Blood in vomit may have been swallowed from mouth injuries or epistaxis. Vomit may have a faecal odour in advanced intestinal obstruction.

Faeces

Black stools may be due to the presence of blood or iron. Bleeding high in the intestinal tract produces offensive 'tarry' stools. If bleeding is from the large intestine, the blood may be less mixed with the faeces and may be seen as streaks. Stools may be pale in obstructive jaundice, diarrhoea or malabsorption.

Shock

Shock is a condition which results from inadequate blood supply to the tissues, leading to a decreased supply of oxygen and other nutrients, which are essential to maintain the metabolic needs of the body. Without oxygen, the cells shift from aerobic to anaerobic metabolism. Anaerobic metabolism is a less efficient method of extracting energy, and the cells begin to use up their stores of adenosine triphosphate (ATP) faster than they can be replaced. This disturbs the cell electrolyte balance, causing sodium to be retained and potassium lost. Excessive sodium in the cell means that it becomes waterlogged. This immediately affects the cells of the nervous system and myocardium leading to depression of their function. The water that leaks into the cells is coming from the interstitial space and will be replaced from the intravascular space, causing further hypovolaemia. Anaerobic metabolism produces large quantities of acid. This increase is detected by the brain, which increases the respiratory rate to reduce the carbon dioxide level and correct the imbalance.

As the supply of oxygen and nutrients fails to meet the demand, the body responds by activating compensatory mechanisms to improve perfusion to the vital organs. As the blood volume decreases, the peripheral blood vessels constrict due to sympathetic stimulation, which increases peripheral resistance and raises the blood pressure. As a result the patient looks pale and has cold clammy skin. As perfusion of the vital centres in the brain is reduced, the patient becomes anxious and restless.

The increase in peripheral resistance may be detected clinically by a rise in the diastolic blood pressure. Eventually as the body loses the battle, the systolic pressure will begin to fall. Reduced blood flow to the kidney, because it is not a vital organ as far as the body is concerned, causes the release of certain chemicals which increase sodium retention, increase water retention and increase vasoconstriction. The release of adrenaline causes glycogen to be broken down to supply the additional glucose needed and as a result an increased blood sugar level will occur.

The management of the patient who has lost blood or body fluids is the most important aspect of dealing with surgical emergencies. It is vital that the condition is recognized and treated promptly to reduce both morbidity and mortality. Rapid volume repletion is indicated in patients with severe hypovolaemia or hypovolaemic shock; delayed therapy can lead to ischaemic injury and possibly to irreversible shock and multiorgan failure (American College of Surgeons 2008, Smeltzer et al. 2009). The management of the patient with haemorrhage may be surgical, or in certain cases conservative. Clinical symptoms include tachycardia, hypotension, peripheral vasoconstriction, oliguria and a narrowed pulse pressure in the absence of jugular venous distension or pulmonary oedema. Monitoring of vital signs and nursing observations are of vital importance and should be carried out at least quarter-hourly. Accurate measurement of intake and all output including vomiting will assist in assessing adequate tissue perfusion. Hourly urinary output of approximately 1 mL/kg per hour is indicative of effective circulating volume (American College of Surgeons 2008, Smeltzer et al. 2009).

Management principles

It is important to provide emotional support for the patient, since fear and anxiety can aggravate the condition:

- administer supplementary oxygen to maintain oxygen saturation at greater than 95 % on pulse oximetry. Oxygen can be administered through a tight-fitting oxygen reservoir face mask with a flow rate of at least 11 L/min. Other methods, such as nasal cannula, nasal catheter and non-rebreather mask can improve inspired oxygen concentration (American College of Surgeons 2008)
- initiate intravenous fluid replacement by inserting two large-bore cannulas, 14 or 16 gauge (as a minimum). Cannula should be placed in the antecubital fossa and well secured to provide an adequate flow rate. If circumstances prevent the use of peripheral veins, large-caliber, central venous access or cut-down is indicated (American College of Surgeons 2008). As intravenous lines are inserted blood is drawn for baseline laboratory investigations including blood group and cross-match and other appropriate analyses. Arterial blood gas (ABG) analysis is also performed at this time (American College of Surgeons 2008). The choice of replacement fluid depends in part upon the type of fluid that has been lost: as an obvious example blood components are indicated in patients who are bleeding (Scott 2009). In general an initial bolus of 1–2 L of warmed isotonic saline is recommended and is the preferred solution in managing patients with severe volume depletion not due to haemorrhage. Both isotonic saline solutions (crystalloid) and colloid-containing solutions are used to replace extracellular fluid deficit, but research has shown that saline solutions are as safe and effective in expanding the plasma volume as colloid and are much less expensive (American College of Surgeons 2008, Scott 2009). Following the administration of a fluid bolus it is important to assess the patient's response by rechecking vital signs and assessing the patient's general condition. The rate of flow is usually slowed as the blood pressure increases: too rapid an increase in blood pressure can cause further bleeding.

In extreme cases of haemorrhage or haemorrhagic shock it may be necessary to give the patient O-negative blood (universal donor), while awaiting type-specific blood. Fluids should be given rapidly using a pressure device, but should be warmed to prevent inducing hypothermia. Hypothermia results in decreased tissue extraction of oxygen from haemoglobin and impaired cardiac contraction. Hypothermia also causes problems with blood clotting due to disruption of cellular enzymes and platelets, and increased fibrinolysis. An arterial line should be placed in all patients who fail to respond promptly to initial fluid resuscitation

- administer prescribed analgesia
- gastric distension can lead to vomiting, therefore inserting a gastric tube will allow decompression of the stomach and provide a sample for testing
- inserting a urinary catheter will allow accurate fluid balance and provide evidence of successful fluid volume replacement
- monitor the temperature to determine hypothermia, or pyrexia due to infection
- prepare the patient physically and psychologically for surgery where indicated.

Acute abdominal emergencies

Bowel obstruction

Obstruction to the passage of contents may occur in the small or large bowel and is a serious life-threatening condition. Obstruction is one of the most common disorders afflicting the small bowel (Sarraf-Yazdi & Shapiro 2010) and is more common because the ileum is the narrowest segment, and therefore more easily obstructed. Obstruction of the large bowel tends to develop more slowly and is associated with a high mortality rate (Biondo et al. 2004). The most common cause of small bowel obstruction is post-operative adhesions, with hernias being the second most common cause (Baker et al. 2009). Adhesions are bands of scar tissue following inflammation which can constrict the intestine. Other causes of bowel obstruction are:

- volvulus – twisting of bowel more common in the elderly
- intussusception – segment of intestine prolapsed into an adjacent part, usually in infants
- mesenteric embolus – interferes with blood supply, foreign bodies (e.g., drug smugglers swallowing packages), faecal impaction, tumours
- paralytic ileus – peristalsis may be interrupted by disturbance of the nerve supply following peritonitis, pancreatitis, shock, spinal cord lesions, or after abdominal surgery
- inflammatory bowel disease (Crohn's disease).

Pathophysiology

Obstruction of the bowel causes fluid, gas and air to collect near the obstruction site. The bowel tries to force its contents past the obstruction by increasing peristalsis. This causes damage to the intestinal mucosa, which results in further swelling at the site. This increased pressure exceeds venous and capillary pressure, causing reduced blood supply to the bowel. As the bowel wall swells, instead of performing its normal function in this area, it starts to secrete water, sodium and potassium, leading to dehydration. Gas-forming bacteria collect in the area and aggravate distension by fermentation, which produces more gas. If untreated, the interruption of the blood supply to the bowel will lead to gangrene, perforation of the bowel and peritonitis. Patients who develop septicaemia in these cases have a 70% mortality rate (Herrington 2009).

Assessment

Obstruction of the small bowel is commonly associated with sudden onset of colicky abdominal pain radiating over the whole abdomen. Appendicitis is characterized by a dull pain in the right lower quadrant, accompanied by an elevated temperature. The pain of pancreatitis is constant, not colicky, and the pain of diverticulitis usually occurs in the left lower quadrant and may be accompanied by blood in the faeces (Herrington 2009). In large bowel obstruction, the pain has a more gradual onset. In small bowel obstruction there is vomiting of gastric juice, mucus and bile in high obstructions. If the obstruction is in the ileum or large bowel, the patient may vomit faecal contents. This loss of fluid by vomiting and increased intestinal secretion leads to severe dehydration and electrolyte imbalance. The extravasation of plasma from the capillaries adds to the accumulation of fluid in the intestines, which compresses the veins, reducing venous return and contributing to the shock.

The patient will display the classic features of shock as previously described; rapid weak pulse, restlessness, low blood pressure and cold, clammy skin. There is constipation and no flatus is passed. The patient suffers abdominal distension due to the accumulation of gas and fluids, with active tinkling bowel sounds initially, progressing to absent bowel sounds as peristalsis diminishes. The stretched weakened intestinal wall becomes permeable to organisms and perforation of the bowel may lead to peritonitis. Obstruction of the large bowel is less acute, with complete constipation (obstipation) and slowly developing distension; diarrhoea may be present with partial obstruction. The pain is described as colicky, with vomiting and dehydration occurring later.

Clinical, laboratory, and radiographic factors should all be considered when making a decision about treatment of small bowel obstruction. The four clinical features, intraperitoneal free fluid, mesenteric oedema, lack of the 'small bowel faeces sign' and history of vomiting are predictive of requiring operative intervention (Zielinski et al. 2010). The small bowel faeces sign is a finding that can be observed on CT scan and is defined by the presence of particulate feculent matter mingled with gas bubbles in the lumen of dilated loops of the small intestine.

Investigations

Blood should be sent for full blood count, electrolytes, amylase, glucose and cross-match. A raised white cell count can be an indicator of infection, which can suggest perforation or even ensuing sepsis and possible bacterial translocation as the gut becomes so distended that the bowel contents are able to pass through its membranes. Abdominal radiographs in both the supine and upright positions may reveal bowel distortion and distension, with air or fluid levels, however during the past two decades, computed tomography has become a mainstay in the evaluation of patients with known or suspected small bowel obstruction. Computed tomography scans should be performed and interpreted with attention to establishing the diagnosis of small bowel obstruction, locating the transition point indicating the site of obstruction, and determining the cause of the obstruction (Desser & Gross 2008, Zielinski et al. 2010).

Management

Strategies for the management of small bowel obstructions have changed significantly over the years. Non-operative medical management has become the mainstay of treatment of many small bowel obstructions. However, the key to the management of small bowel obstructions is identifying those patients who need surgical intervention (Trevino 2010). The most life-threatening problem for the patient is fluid volume deficit and therefore the initial priorities are to treat the shock due to the hypovolaemia and to prevent further complications (Diaz et al. 2008). Administer 100% oxygen via a non-rebreather mask at 12–15 L/min. Initiate large-bore intravenous infusions, using crystalloids such as normal saline. A nasogastric tube should be inserted to decompress the stomach, as fluid shifts can be more severe as the bowel becomes decompressed. Accurate recording of fluid balance and vital signs is essential. Assist the patient into a comfortable position, and give prescribed analgesia and antibiotics, which reduce the risk of sepsis if the bowel perforates (Diaz et al 2008).

In less urgent cases of large bowel obstruction, the patient may be given an enema to attempt to clear the obstruction. Intestinal obstruction other than paralytic ileus is treated surgically. In some cases, it may be possible to delay surgery to improve the patient's general condition, but if there is evidence of compromised blood supply to the intestines, emergency surgery is indicated. If the bowel is strangulated or if there is gross distension, surgery should take place within one hour to avoid perforation.

The extent of the surgery required will depend upon the cause of the obstruction. Simple adhesions may be divided, but if the blood supply to the bowel has been interrupted, the bowel is checked for viability and, if gangrenous, will require resection with anastomosis or a stoma. Stomas may be temporary or permanent.

Ileus is most often associated with intraperitoneal or retroperitoneal infection; it may be produced by mesenteric ischaemia, arterial or venous injury or after intra-abdominal surgery. Gastric and colonic motility disturbances after abdominal surgery result from abdominal manipulation. The small bowel is rarely affected, with motility and absorption returning to normal within a few hours of operation. The large bowel may remain inert for 48 to 72 hours. Symptoms include abdominal distension, vomiting, obstipation and cramp.

Treatment is usually conservative and involves nasogastric suction to reduce distension. Intravenous fluids to correct electrolyte deficiencies are essential; the condition usually resolves gradually (Trevino 2010).

Peritonitis

This is a life-threatening condition due to inflammation of the visceral and parietal peritoneum (Smeltzer et al. 2009). The most serious causes of peritonitis are perforation of a viscus into the peritoneal cavity, trauma, infected peritoneal blood, foreign bodies, strangulating intestinal obstruction, pelvic inflammatory disease, mesenteric thrombosis or embolism. This chemical and bacterial invasion causes an inflammatory response, with depressed intestinal motility and distension of the bowel with gas and fluid.

Pathophysiology

The peritoneal cavity is a closed sac, which normally contains a little fluid to allow the abdominal organs to move freely. The great omentum is a sheet of peritoneum which is reflected off the stomach and hangs down in front of the intestines like a curtain. If peritonitis occurs, the great omentum tries to wall off the infection by surrounding it, to prevent spread of infection. The peritoneum is remarkably resistant to infection and unless contamination continues from an uncontrolled source, tends to heal with treatment.

Assessment

The symptoms of peritonitis depend on the virulence and extent of the infection. In a previously well patient the sudden onset of abdominal pain is either localized if the process is confined by viscera or omentum, or generalized if the entire peritoneal cavity is involved. The patient usually lies very still, reluctant to breathe deeply or cough and looks unwell. The abdomen is distended, rigid like a board and there is rebound tenderness, with absent bowel sounds. Signs of shock may be present (tachycardia, pallor, sweating, low blood pressure), along with pyrexia, nausea and vomiting. Respirations may be shallow due to interference by extreme abdominal distension. The peritoneal membrane becomes oedematous, with loss of protein and electrolyte fluid into the peritoneal cavity aggravating the shock.

Investigations

Blood should be sent for full blood count, glucose, electrolytes, amylase (to exclude pancreatitis), arterial blood gas and group and cross-match.

Plain abdominal radiographs in both supine and upright positions may show distension of both small bowel and colon, or air under the diaphragm. As little as 20 mL of air will produce a gas shadow between the liver and the diaphragm. Abdominal ultrasonography may be helpful in the evaluation of right upper quadrant (e.g., perihepatic abscess, cholecystitis, biloma, pancreatitis, pancreatic pseudocyst), right lower quadrant, and pelvic pathology (e.g., appendicitis, tubo-ovarian abscess, Douglas pouch abscess), but the examination is sometimes limited because of patient discomfort, abdominal distension, and bowel gas interference (Cameron et al. 2009). If the diagnosis of peritonitis is made clinically, a CT scan is not necessary and generally delays surgical intervention without offering clinical advantage. CT scans of the abdomen and pelvis remain the diagnostic study of choice for peritoneal abscess and related visceral pathology. CT scanning is indicated in all cases in which the diagnosis cannot be established on clinical grounds and findings on abdominal plain films. Whenever possible, the CT scan should be performed with enteral and intravenous contrast. CT scans can detect small quantities of fluid, areas of inflammation, and other GI tract pathology, with sensitivities that approach 100% (Cameron et al. 2009, Herrington 2009).

Management

The treatment of peritonitis primarily involves treatment of the underlying disease; therefore early diagnosis is imperative. Two large-bore intravenous cannulas should be inserted and intravenous crystalloid fluids (either normal saline 0.9% or Hartmann's solution) should be commenced to treat hypovolaemia; blood transfusion may be commenced to treat shock and replace the protein lost in the inflammatory response in the peritoneum. One hundred per cent oxygen should be administered via a non-rebreather mask, at 12–15 L/min. A nasogastric tube should be passed to decompress the stomach and relieve distension. The use of antibiotics is advocated prior to results of cultures being available, with third-generation cephalosporins being regarded as the most safe and effective treatment. Immediate surgery is nearly always indicated for patients with peritonitis arising from appendicitis, perforated peptic ulcer, or diverticulitis. Acute pancreatitis and pelvic inflammatory disease (PID) are exceptions.

Appendicitis

This is a common cause of acute abdominal pain and is the commonest surgical emergency. The overall lifetime occurrence is approximately 9% for males and 6% for females (Petroianu 2012). It is more common in children, adolescents and young adults. Accurate and early diagnosis is essential to minimize morbidity. Prompt surgical treatment may reduce the risk of appendix perforation. The case fatality rate is reported to be >1% in non-perforated cases, which rises to 5% or higher when perforation occurs (Old et al. 2005).

Several factors are claimed to predispose the patient to appendicitis, including:

- faecoliths – hard pellets of faeces
- food residues
- enlargement of lymphoid tissue in response to a viral infection in children.

All of these causes will lead to blockage of the appendix, allowing secretions to collect.

Pathophysiology

The appendix is a narrow blind tube which is attached to the inferior part of the caecum. It has no known physiological function, and if diseased it can be removed. Inflammation begins in the mucosa after a breach in the epithelium, allowing the entry of bowel bacteria. The appendix is a blind tube, and if secretions cannot pass the obstruction they will accumulate, causing enlargement and pain. The resulting infection leads to ulceration of the mucosa, which eventually spreads, causing peritonitis. Inflammation can cause the greater omentum to become adherent to the appendix in an attempt to wall off the infection. If the area has time to be walled off and the appendix then ruptures, an abscess will form. However, the build-up of pressure within the wall can lead to the distal part of the appendix becoming gangrenous and perforating, before it has time to be walled off, causing generalized peritonitis.

Assessment

Typical signs and symptoms of acute appendicitis appear in >50% of patients: they complain of sudden onset of epigastric or peri-umbilical pain followed by brief nausea and vomiting after a few hours. The pain is described as steady, persistent or constant by the patient. As the inflammation spreads through the walls of the appendix, involving the parietal peritoneum, it becomes confined to the right lower quadrant (Smeltzer et al. 2009). Pain is aggravated by coughing, and on rectal examination there is increased pain on the right side. There may be rebound tenderness in the right lower quadrant, although rebound tenderness in other areas suggests that the appendix has perforated and caused peritonitis. The patient may also exhibit low-grade pyrexia of 38–39°C. The patient will try to avoid sudden movements, which increase the pain, and may keep the right thigh flexed to provide pain relief.

The following signs may demonstrate the pain of appendicitis:

- McBurney sign – tenderness on palpation in an area about 2 inches from the anterior superior iliac spine on a line with the umbilicus (the single most important sign)
- Aaron's sign – pain or distress in the area of the heart or stomach when McBurney's point is palpated
- Rovsing sign – pain in the right lower quadrant with palpation of the left lower quadrant
- Psoas sign – pain in the abdomen on hyperextension of the right thigh (often indicates retroperitoneal retrocaecal appendix)
- Obturator sign – pain on internal rotation of the right thigh (pelvic appendix)
- Dunphy's sign – increased pain in right lower quadrant with coughing.

It is worth noting that all of the above occur in <40% of patients with appendicitis and even their absence should not prevent the clinician from establishing an accurate diagnosis. Plain abdominal X-rays are abnormal in 95% of patients with appendicitis (Petroianu 2012).

Investigations

If the diagnosis of appendicitis is clear from the history and physical examination no further testing is required and prompt surgical referral is warranted (Yeh 2008, Smeltzer et al. 2009). When diagnosis is not clear, options include observation and limited diagnostic tests. Blood should be sent for full blood count which may reveal a leucocytosis. Leucocyte count is raised above 10 000 in 90 % of cases. Other blood tests may include glucose, amylase (to exclude pancreatitis) and electrolytes. Females with lower abdominal pain should always have their beta human chorionic gonadotropin (beta-hCG) checked, to help exclude ectopic pregnancy. A urine specimen may help to exclude urinary tract infection or urinary calculi as a cause of the pain. Imaging studies are cost-effective if a definitive diagnosis can be made and observation in a hospital can be avoided; however, outcome studies to date suggest that imaging has a small part to play in assessing atypical presentations of appendicitis (Old et al. 2005).

Differential diagnosis

- right-sided lobar pneumonia or pleurisy
- perforated ulcer
- acute cholecystitis
- intestinal obstruction
- gastroenteritis
- acute salpingitis.

Management

Initiate intravenous fluids to re-hydrate the patient. Keep the patient fasting. Administer prescribed analgesia. Pre-operative intramuscular or intravenous antibiotics should be commenced, with third-generation cephalosporins the preferred choice. If the condition is still located within the appendix, and it has not perforated, an appendectomy is performed. If it has progressed to peritonitis, the patient may be managed conservatively with antibiotics and intravenous fluids and surgery arranged at a later stage to remove the appendix.

The appendix may be removed by open appendectomy or laparoscopic appendectomy. The laparoscope is particularly useful in young women to allow widespread visualization of the abdomen and pelvis. This allows differentiation of appendicitis from gynaecological disease with minimally invasive surgery. The laparoscope also reduces hospital stay by decreasing post-operative ileus because the tissues are handled less. There are fewer adhesions and there is less scarring from smaller incisions.

Acute pancreatitis

Acute pancreatitis has become increasingly common in Western countries in recent years, particularly in the middle aged and elderly (Wyatt et al. 2012). It is a protean disease capable of wide clinical variation and may be classified as mild, involving minimal organ dysfunction with uneventful recovery, or severe, leading to necrosis and multisystemic organ failure and death (UK Working Party on Acute Pancreatitis 2005, Lankisch et al. 2009).

Pancreatitis is an inflammatory process in which pancreatic enzymes autodigest the gland (Goldacre & Roberts 2004). Recurrent attacks are referred to as chronic pancreatitis, and both forms of disease present in the Emergency Department (ED) with acute clinical findings. Studies report that acute pancreatitis remains a disease with a high mortality rate. It is reported that death rates in the first month after admission are 30 times higher than in the general population of the same age; there have been no significant improvements in fatality rates since the 1970s (Goldacre & Roberts 2004).

Pathophysiology

The pancreas is located in the retroperitoneal space but as it does not have a capsule inflammation can spread easily. In acute pancreatitis, parenchymal oedema and peripancreatic fat necrosis occur first, leading to a process known as acute oedematous pancreatitis. The inflammatory process may remain localized in the pancreas, spread to regional tissues, or involve remote organ systems. Local complications of severe disease include pseudocyst, abscess and pseudoaneurysm formation (Mitchell et al. 2003).

Acute pancreatitis has numerous causes; however, two of the common causes are biliary tract obstruction related to cholelithiasis and alcohol abuse (Goldacre & Roberts 2004). Attacks of acute pancreatitis in biliary disease are the result of temporary impaction of a gallstone in the sphincter of Oddi. Although the precise pathogenic mechanism is unclear, the literature suggests that the obstruction of the pancreatic duct in the absence of biliary reflux can increase ductal pressure, triggering extravasation of enzymes into the parenchyma, leading to acute pancreatitis.

Long-term alcohol abuse or alcohol intake >100 g/day over several years cause the protein of pancreatic enzymes to precipitate within small pancreatic ductules. In time, protein plugs accumulate, inducing additional histological abnormalities. At the ductal level ethanol increases the permeability of ductules which allow enzymes to reach the parenchyma, resulting in organ damage. On the cellular level ethanol leads to intracellular accumulation of digestive enzymes; the premature activation of pancreatic enzymes results in leaks out of the ducts into the pancreatic acinar cells, causing auto-digestion of the gland.

Oedema or necrosis and haemorrhage are prominent gross pathological changes. Tissue necrosis is caused by activation of several pancreatic enzymes, including trypsin and phospholipase A2. Haemorrhage is caused by extensive activation of pancreatic enzymes, including pancreatic elastase, which dissolves elastic fibres of blood vessels. In oedematous pancreatitis inflammation is usually confined to the pancreas, resulting in a mortality rate >5 %. Where there is severe necrosis and haemorrhage, inflammation is not confined to the pancreas and the mortality rate ranges from 10 % to 50 %.

Pancreatic exudate containing toxins and activated pancreatic enzymes permeates the retroperitoneum and sometimes the peritoneal cavity, inducing a chemical burn and increasing the permeability of blood vessels. This causes extravasation of large amounts of protein-rich fluid from the systemic circulation into 'third spaces', producing hypovolaemia and shock. On entering the systemic circulation these activated enzymes and toxins increase capillary permeability throughout the body and may reduce peripheral vascular tone, thereby intensifying hypotension. Circulating activated enzymes may also damage tissue directly, e.g., phospholipase A2 is thought to injure alveolar membranes of the lungs, leading to acute respiratory distress syndrome (ARDS).

Incidence and causes of acute pancreatitis

The incidence of acute pancreatitis per 100 000 of population ranges from 5 to 80-years-old. Patients suffering from haemorrhagic-necrotizing pancreatitis die in 10–24% of cases; 80% of all cases of acute pancreatitis are aetiologically linked to gallstone disease and/or immoderate alcohol consumption (Mayerle et al. 2012). About 25% of patients develop severe or life-threatening complications and require support in high-dependency or intensive-care units. Biliary tract disease and alcoholism account for 80% of hospital admissions for acute pancreatitis; the remaining 20% are attributed to other conditions (Box 29.2) (Munoz & Katerndahl 2000).

Assessment

Acute pancreatitis may be difficult to diagnose as the signs and symptoms are common to many illnesses (Lankisch et al. 2009). In acute pancreatitis abdominal pain may develop

Box 29.2

Minor causes of acute pancreatitis

- Medications (e.g., azathioprine, corticosteroids, sulfonamides, thiazides, frusemides, non-steroidal anti-inflammatory, methyldopa and tetracyclines)
- Viral infections (e.g., mumps, cytomegalovirus, hepatitis virus, Epstein-Barr virus and rubella)
- Structural abnormalities of the pancreatic duct (e.g., stricture, cancer)
- Structural abnormalities of the common bile duct (e.g., choledochal cyst, sphincter of Oddi stenosis)
- Peptic ulcer disease
- Abdominal or cardiopulmonary surgery which may insult the gland by ischaemia
- Endoscopic retrograde cholangiopancreatography (ERCP)
- Vascular disease (especially severe hypotension)
- Trauma to the abdomen or back resulting in sudden compression of the gland
- Hypercalcaemia (almost always due to hyperparathyroidism)
- Hyperlipidaemia
- Renal transplantation
- Hereditary pancreatitis
- Intestinal parasites such as *Ascaris* that can block pancreatic outflow
- Idiopathic

quickly, is frequently devastating in severity, fluctuates very little in intensity and usually persists for at least several days. Abdominal pain is located in the epigastric region or in the right upper quadrant radiating to the back or flank. The pain is classically described as constant, dull and boring and is worse when the patient is supine. The discomfort may lessen when the patient assumes a sitting or foetal position; however, coughing, vigorous movement and deep breathing may accentuate or aggravate pain. A heavy meal or drinking binge may trigger the pain and onset of symptoms. Nausea and vomiting are present in 75–90% of patients (Smeltzer et al. 2009). The patient will appear acutely ill and diaphoretic, and pulse rate will be elevated usually between 100–140 beats/min. Respirations may be shallow and rapid and blood pressure may be transiently high or low, with significant postural hypotension. Temperature may be normal or even subnormal in the first instance but may increase to 37.7–38.3°C within a few hours. The patient may also present with jaundice and dehydration. Examination of the lungs may reveal limited diaphragmatic excursion and evidence of atelectasis. About 20% of patients experience upper abdominal distension caused by gastric distension or a large pancreatic inflammatory mass displacing the stomach anteriorly. Abdominal tenderness always occurs and is usually isolated to the upper abdomen; it may be associated with mild to moderate muscular rigidity in that region. The entire abdomen rarely exhibits severe peritoneal irritation in the form of a rigid board-like abdomen. Bowel sounds may be hypoactive. Rectal examination usually discloses no tenderness and stool usually tests negative for occult blood. The literature suggests that acute pancreatitis should be considered in the differential diagnosis of every acute abdomen (Epstein et al. 2008, Smeltzer et al. 2009).

The differential diagnosis of acute pancreatitis includes perforated gastric and duodenal ulcer, mesenteric infarction, intestinal obstruction, ectopic pregnancy, dissecting aneurysm, biliary colic, appendicitis, diverticulitis haematoma of abdominal muscles or spleen. In comparison the abdominal pain associated with choledocholithiasis tends to last for several hours rather than days. Pain associated with a perforated ulcer or mesenteric ischaemia may also develop quickly and is characteristically very severe, but nausea and vomiting are usually mild and disappear soon after the onset of pain. Pain associated with intestinal obstruction tends to increase and recede in a pattern similar to labour pains.

Investigations

Laboratory tests alone cannot confirm a diagnosis of acute pancreatitis but can support the clinical impression (UK Working Party 2005, Lankisch et al. 2009). Laboratory tests include full blood count, in particular white cell count, blood for group and cross-match, serum amylase, serum lipase, blood glucose, urea and electrolyte and liver function tests. The literature suggests that the expected rise in serum amylase levels in patients with pancreatitis may not always be seen as in cases of coexisting conditions such as hypertriglyceridaemia; conversely a rise in serum amylase can occur as a result of numerous non-pancreatic conditions (Mitchell et al. 2003, Lankisch 2009). Serum lipase concentration rises within 4–8 hours of an episode of acute pancreatitis, peaks at 24 hours and returns to normal after 8–14 days. As the pancreas is the only source of lipase, estimation of plasma lipase has a slightly superior sensitivity and specificity and greater overall accuracy than amylase, making it a useful diagnostic method in patients presenting late, e.g., >24 hours after the onset of pain (UK Working Party 2005, Banks & Freeman 2006). An elevated trypsin level has a better likelihood ratio for detecting pancreatitis than the amylase level and is reported as the most accurate serum indicator for acute pancreatitis; however, this test is not widely available and is therefore not routinely used (Banks & Freeman 2006). Imaging studies such as chest X-ray may be indicated if pleural effusion is suspected. Plain abdominal radiograph and ultrasound may reveal the presence of air under the diaphragm, or gas shadows secondary to bowel distension, but the most reliable imaging modality in the diagnosis of acute pancreatitis is computed tomography (Banks & Freeman 2006, Lankisch et al. 2009).

Prediction of the severity of the attack at the time of admission can prove difficult; however, several scoring systems with clinical, laboratory and radiological criteria have been developed and are recommended for use in assessing patients with clinical features of acute pancreatitis (UK Working Party 2005, Lankisch et al. 2009).

The Apache II system (Knaus et al. 1985) has the advantage of being available at the time of admission as opposed to 48 hours later as is the case for the Glasgow criteria and Ranson criteria systems.

The Ranson scoring system aims to estimate the severity of acute pancreatitis but has limitations in that it is recorded over two days and therefore the score is only valid after 48 hours post admission (Table 29.2). A Ranson score of 0–2 has a minimal mortality rate; a Ranson score of 3–5 has a 10–20% mortality rate, with scores higher than 5 having a mortality rate of more than 50% and being associated with more system complications. The UK Working Party on Acute Pancreatitis (2005) revised the recommendations of the British Society of Gastroenterology (1998) published guidelines and outlines key prognostic features which predict complications in acute pancreatitis. Features that may predict a severe attack incorporate clinical evaluation, body mass index >30, pleural

effusion on chest X-ray and APACHE II score >8 on immediate assessment. After 24 hours, a repeat of initial assessment along with Glasgow Criteria (Table 29.3) plus persistent organ failure and C reactive protein > 150 mg/L. By 48 hours after admission, the patient's clinical state, the Glasgow score, and C reactive protein all contribute to the assessment of severity, in addition to the features noted earlier (UK Working Party on Acute Pancreatitis 2005).

An imaging grading system was developed by Balthazar (2002) to evaluate abdominal computerized tomography scan results (Box 29.3). The chance of infection or death in grades A or B is almost nil, but this increases in C and D and in patients graded E there is a 50% increased incidence of infection with a mortality of 15%. Although there is a multitude of predictive models for identifying which patients will develop severe pancreatitis no perfect system exists, future developments may depend upon new factors such as biomarkers and new methods of analysis to develop more accurate predictive models (Chauhan & Forsmark 2010).

Table 29.3 Glasgow scoring system for the initial prediction of severity in acute pancreatitis

Age	>55 years
White blood cell count	>15 × 10⁹/L
Glucose	>10 mmol/L
Urea	>16 mmol/L
PaO₂	<60 mmHg
Calcium	<2 mmol/L
Albumin	<32 g/L
Lactate dehydrogenase	>600 units/L
Asparate/alanmeammotransferase	>100 units/L

Box 29.3

Balthazar CT grading system for staging acute pancreatitis

Grade A – normal pancreas
Grade B – focal of diffuse gland enlargement
Grade C – peripancreatic inflammatory changes
Grade D – fluid collections in a single location
Grade E – multiple fluid collections, gas in or near pancreas

Management

The majority of patients presenting to the ED are treated conservatively and approximately 80% respond to such treatment. The patient should have baseline observation of vital signs and a pain score recorded by the emergency nurse. Supplemental oxygen should be administered to maintain an arterial saturation greater than 95%. A large-bore 14 gauge

Table 29.2 Ranson's (1982) criteria of severity in acute pancreatitis

At admission	Age > 55 years WBC>16 000/mm³ Glucose > 200 mg/dL LDH > 350 IU/L AST >250 U/L
During initial 48 hours	HCT decrease of >10% BUN increase of > 5 mg/dL Ca <8 mg/dL PaO₂ <60 mmHg Base deficit >4 mEq/L Fluid sequestration >6 L

cannula should be inserted for rapid infusion of crystalloid or colloid solution for fluid resuscitation to maintain urine output >0.5 mL/kg body weight (UK Working Party on Acute Pancreatitis 2005). A urinary catheter should be inserted in order to record and closely monitor fluid intake and output. Laboratory and radiological investigations should be initiated immediately to assist with establishing a diagnosis. A nasogastric tube is indicated where vomiting is protracted or if obstruction is seen on the abdominal radiograph; studies have shown that the use of a nasogastric tube with suction is no longer advocated as routine therapeutic measure as it has not demonstrated a decrease in symptom mortality or hospital stay (UK Working Party on Acute Pancreatitis 2005, Banks et al. 2006). There is conflicting evidence in the literature regarding the use of narcotic analgesics such as pethidine or meperidine. Morphine would appear to be the recommended drug of choice for pain management initially in the ED (Banks et al. 2006, Chaudhari et al. 2007). The role of antibiotics in the management of early acute pancreatitis remains controversial (UK Working Party on Acute Pancreatitis 2005) but antibiotic therapy may be commenced in severe cases associated with septic shock, in other conditions such as cholangitis or when CT scan indicates that there are fluid collections in the pancreas. The preferred antibiotics are those secreted by the biliary system such as ampicillin and third-generation cephalosporin.

Vascular disorders

Oesophageal varices

These refer to the localized dilatation of veins in the lower oesophagus, due to the impairment of portal blood flow through the liver.

Pathophysiology

In patients suffering from cirrhosis of the liver, the blood flow from the portal vein meets resistance in the damaged organ. This increased resistance causes back pressure into the veins that normally empty into the portal system. The veins most affected are those at the lower end of the oesophagus. The veins become weak and varicosed, lifting the mucosa so that they protrude into the oesophagus, where they can be damaged by passing food, coughing, vomiting or straining. Patients with liver disease may also have abnormal blood clotting, which exacerbates the problem. Bleeding from these veins can be both dramatic and fatal; because of the high pressure within the vascular bed, hypovolaemia occurs quickly. The mortality rate for each bleeding episode is 30%; if underlying conditions remain untreated 70% of patients who develop haemorrhage die within one year of the initial bleeding episode (Gow & Chapman 2001).

Assessment

The patient may have a history of alcohol abuse and ascites, without abdominal pain. Painless haematemesis is suggestive of varices. Haematemesis following peptic ulceration may cause significant vomiting of bright-red blood, but is usually accompanied by abdominal pain. In bleeding, there may be a dramatic haematemesis, occasionally preceded by a feeling of dizziness, as the bleeding into the stomach causes the blood pressure to fall. There may be a history of previous episodes. Features of portal hypertension are splenomegaly and ascites. Some of the blood will pass through the intestinal tract and will appear later as melaena. Patients with portal hypertension may be asymptomatic until they suddenly suffer catastrophic haemorrhage.

Investigations

Full blood count, group and cross-match, electrolytes, glucose, arterial blood gas, clotting factors and liver function tests should be requested.

Management

This life-threatening condition is one of the most complex emergency conditions to manage as the patient requires prompt aggressive resuscitation. The patient and relatives will require significant emotional and psychological support also as haemorrhage is generally profuse and is extremely frightening for all concerned.

In massive haemorrhage, the patient may lose consciousness and therefore airway clearance will be a priority. Ensure that there are adequate receivers and working suction to hand, as bleeding can be sudden and profuse. Supplemental oxygen should be administered to maintain an arterial saturation greater than 95%. Establish at least two large-bore intravenous lines and be prepared to give large quantities of 5% dextrose. Saline should be avoided as this may worsen ascites. Blood should be drawn for immediate group and cross-match for six units of blood (O-negative can be used initially). A central line should be inserted to monitor the central venous pressure as a guide to fluid replacement along with a urinary catheter to monitor output and maintain accurate fluid balance records. Prevention of encephalopathy and aspiration are important measures during resuscitation; therefore obtunded and actively bleeding patients should have endotracheal intubation to prevent aspiration. Urgent endoscopy is essential to confirm the presence of oesophageal varices but should only take place in a well-equipped specialist centre after the patient has been adequately resuscitated.

Balloon tamponade

Endoscopic therapy probably has replaced balloon tamponade as the initial therapy for variceal bleeding. Balloon tamponade is now rarely necessary, and, when it is used, it must be performed by experienced personnel because the procedure is potentially dangerous.

A Sengstaken triple-lumen or a Minnesota quadruple-lumen tube may be inserted orally to apply pressure to the bleeding veins and to allow aspiration from the stomach and upper oesophagus (Fig. 29.2). Applied by an experienced team, balloon tamponade can achieve control of variceal bleeding in

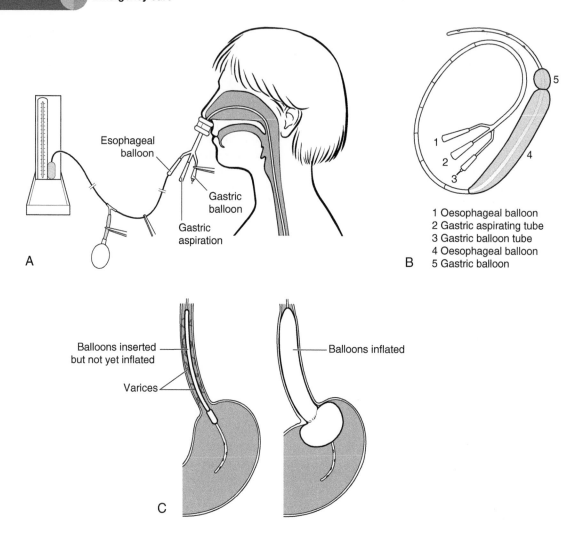

A

Esophageal
balloon

Gastric
balloon

Gastric
aspiration

B

1 Oesophageal balloon
2 Gastric aspirating tube
3 Gastric balloon tube
4 Oesophageal balloon
5 Gastric balloon

Balloons inserted
but not yet inflated

Varices

Balloons inflated

C

Figure 29.2 ● Use of Sengstaken tube.

up to 90% of cases, with acceptably low morbidity (Habib & Sanyal 2007). If time permits, the tube may be chilled prior to insertion as this makes the tube more rigid and aids insertion. Insertion of the tube is a fairly unpleasant procedure for the patient, but many patients will be sedated and intubated to allow the clinician to have more control over the airway. The patient will need to be placed in the left lateral decubitus position to allow for tube placement although the tube can be placed while the patient is supine. The tube can remain in position for up to 12 hours. Leaving the tube in excess of 12–24 hours carries a significant risk of oesophageal necrosis, oedema, ulceration and perforation. Inflation of the oesophageal balloon will make swallowing difficult for the patient, and suction may be required (Christensen & Christensen 2007). Suction should be available before, during and after removal of the tube.

The emergency nurse should maintain a vigilant assessment of the patient's respiratory status after the tube has been inserted. If signs of respiratory distress or obstruction develop, the nurse should immediately cut away the valves from the end of the tube and remove it (Smith & Fawcett 2004). Care should be taken to ensure that the correct balloons are inflated and deflated. Inadequate inflation will be ineffective

at controlling bleeding, while excessive pressures will cause tissue damage. As soon as the tube is placed the balloons are inflated and a portable chest X-ray is carried out to confirm the position of the tube. X-ray should be repeated every four hours as long as the tube is inflated to assess position and balloon size; progressive decline in balloon size indicates a leak and the balloon must be re-inflated. Inflation of the oesophageal balloon should always be done under pressure control with a manometer. Manometer pressure should read between 25 and 40 mmHg and the balloon should be deflated every two hours for ten minutes and then re-inflated. Regular monitoring of the patient's vital signs and fluid balance should be maintained to assess the effectiveness of the tube at achieving haemorrhage control (Christiansen & Christiansen 2007).

Pharmacological control

Vasoactive drugs to control variceal bleeding have been used for 40 years. Vasopressin is still the most widely used agent and is best administered by continuous intravenous infusion at a rate of 0.4 U/min. This may be given to produce arterial vasoconstriction, which will reduce the amount of blood entering the portal system. Potentially serious cardiac complications (which occur in 15% of patients) and plasminogen activator and factor VIII release (which may aggravate coagulopathy) are important factors limiting the use of vasopressin alone (Gow & Chapman 2001, Habib & Sanyal 2007). Terlipressin, the triglycyl synthetic analogue of vasopressin, given in a bolus injection has a longer therapeutic action (4 hours vs 40 minutes) and there are no cardiac side-effects.

Somatostatin does not cause systemic vasoconstriction: its action is on the smooth muscle of splanchnic vessels, resulting in a reduction in splanchnic and hepatic blood flow. The efficacy of somatostatin to control variceal bleeding has been tested in studies against vasopressin and proved in some studies to be more effective at reducing bleeding and transfusion requirements (Habib & Sanyal 2007).

Endoscopic sclerotherapy

In this technique a coagulating substance is injected into the varices, which seals the bleeding veins by coagulation and is the primary method of treatment (Smith & Fawcett 2004). The patient will require repeated treatments at regular intervals for a few years. Severe complications of injection sclerotherapy include:

- haemorrhage
- aspiration
- oesophageal perforation
- portal vein thrombosis.

Percutaneous transhepatic portal vein embolization

This may be done under X-ray control to insert embolic material directly into the blood vessels. Emergency surgery carries considerable risk and it is preferable to stabilize the patient's condition and undertake surgery when bleeding is controlled. Various options are available:

- a portacaval shunt – this makes an anastomosis between the portal vein and the inferior vena cava
- a splenorenal shunt
- a mesocaval shunt between the superior mesenteric vein and the inferior vena cava
- a transoesophageal ligation of the bleeding vessels.

Surgery will reduce the risk of further ruptured varices, but will not resolve the underlying liver disease. Other procedures involve oesophageal transection and anastomosis, or ligation of bleeding veins. In patients with oesophageal varices, there is a 60–80% recurrence over 2 years, with 20% mortality during each further episode of bleeding.

Abdominal aortic aneurysm

An aneurysm is a focal dilatation of a blood vessel that has been weakened by atheroma. The normal aorta is approximately 2 cm in diameter: aneurysm is diagnosed in cases where dilation is in excess of 3 cm. The commonest site for aneurysms is the aorta, although they can occur elsewhere, such as the common iliac vessels.

Pathophysiology

The largest-diameter arteries, such as the aorta, have a greater proportion of elastic tissue and a smaller proportion of smooth muscle compared with other arteries. Elastic arteries are stretched when the ventricles of the heart pump blood into them. The elastic recoil prevents blood pressure from falling rapidly and maintains blood flow while the ventricles are relaxed. As the arteries become smaller, they undergo a gradual transition from having walls containing more elastic tissue than smooth muscle to having walls with more smooth muscle than elastic tissue. This allows these arteries (radial, brachial, etc.) to have a greater degree of vasoconstriction and vasodilatation, allowing them to alter blood flow according to local demands.

Arteries are composed of three layers. From the inside to the outer wall the layers are:

- tunica intima – an endothelium composed of simple squamous cells and a small amount of connective tissue
- tunica media – the middle layer consists of smooth muscle arranged circularly around the blood vessel
- tunica adventitia – composed of connective tissue.

The walls of the arteries undergo changes as they age, mainly in the large elastic arteries such as the aorta, coronary arteries serving the heart and carotid arteries serving the brain. Atherosclerosis refers to the deposition of material in the walls of arteries to form plaques. This fatty material contains cholesterol and may be replaced by connective tissue and calcium deposits. Atherosclerosis increases resistance to blood flow, as the deposits reduce the internal diameter of the arteries. The rough plaques attract passing platelets, which adhere to them, increasing the chances of thrombus formation. As the tunica media becomes weakened, the wall of the aorta begins to bulge.

The aneurysm may form a sac or it may separate through the layers of the vessel, called a dissecting aneurysm, without a visible dilatation (Fig. 29.3). Dissecting aneurysms can spread for some distance along the aorta and affect other organs, such as the kidneys. Aneurysms can also send off emboli to distant sites. Risk factors for rupture relate to the size of the dilatation and range from 4–5 cm = 0.5–5% to >8 cm = 30–50%. Contributing factors for rupture include hypertension, chronic obstructive airway disease, diabetes, smoking, family history, ratio to adjacent normal aorta, rapid expansion. Fatal rupture is commoner among women than men, although there is a higher instance of aneurysm in men, of the order of 5:1. Abdominal aortic aneurysm (AAA) is one of the most common killers of men >65 years, causing approximately 6000 premature deaths a year in England and Wales (Earnshaw 2011). They noted that there has been a significant decline in overall AAA incidence since 2001, the reasons for which may be complex but almost certainly include the decline in smoking rates (Choke et al. 2012). Mortality following rupture of an AAA is more than 90%, with many people dying before reaching hospital. In comparison,

Figure 29.3 • Dissecting aortic aneurysm.

mortality rates following emergency repair are approximately 50%, and following elective AAA repair are between 5 and 10% (Bick 2000, Irwin & Rippe 2008).

Assessment

Abdominal aortic aneurysms tend to affect middle-aged to elderly people. There may be a history of atherosclerosis and the patient may have suffered a previous myocardial infarction or stroke or may have peripheral vascular disease or chronic obstructive pulmonary disease (Bick 2000). If the aneurysm is pressing on other structures, there may be abdominal pain radiating to the back or groin. There may be few initial indications that the patient has an aneurysm, until it is large and causes pressure on other structures, or it starts to leak. The immediate problem is of sudden abdominal pain and collapse. Patients with a dissecting aneurysm may complain of a sudden tearing or ripping pain. There is no history of haematemesis, which tends to exclude oesophageal varices or perforated ulcer.

The patient has signs of hypovolaemic shock, pale, cold, clammy skin and rapid respirations. The blood pressure may be low with an accompanying tachycardia. Physical examination may reveal a pulsatile mass in the centre of the abdomen, and in extreme cases pulsation may be visible. A pulsatile mass can be found in 80–90% of patients (Drake 1993, Irwin & Rippe 2008). The patient's femoral pulses may be weak or absent. Impaired blood supply to a limb may lead to 'blue toe syndrome', which is a classical manifestation of AAA in 5% of patients. This presentation may cause an ischaemic, painful extremity or cyanotic toes due to atheroembolism. Emboli may also involve the mesenteric and renal arteries, leading to intestinal ischaemia, haematuria and renal failure (Irwin & Rippe 2008).

Differential diagnosis

- pancreatitis
- renal colic
- biliary disease
- musculoskeletal back pain.

The classic triad of AAA therefore is abdominal or back pain, hypotension, and a pulsatile abdominal mass.

Investigations

Blood should be cross-matched urgently – initially at least 10 units in anticipation of surgery. Also request full blood count, amylase, glucose, gases and clotting studies. Further investigations should be tailored to the clinical condition of the patient. Chest and abdominal X-rays waste time in unstable patients who need urgent intervention. Ultrasound can be performed in the ED, allowing continual monitoring of the patient in a controlled environment. CT scan is time-consuming and involves moving the patient to the X-ray department. Angiography provides very detailed information and is best reserved for stable patients.

Management

A senior surgeon should be involved early in the care of these patients, and in unstable patients limited investigations should be undertaken prior to surgery. Supplemental oxygen should be administered to maintain an arterial saturation greater than 95%. Initiating large-bore intravenous access with two 14 gauge cannulas and controlled fluid resuscitation are critical for a patient with an aneurysm.

The patient's systolic blood pressure should be maintained <90 mmHg to decrease the pressure of ventricular systole against the fragile aorta. Attempting to increase blood pressure beyond this range may rupture the aneurysm, with fatal consequences for the patient. Fluids should be warmed to prevent hypothermia and coagulopathy. Frequent monitoring of the patient's vital signs and fluid balance are essential to detect subtle changes in the patient's condition. Analgesia can be administered intravenously and titrated according to the patient's response. The analgesia of choice is morphine, as non-steroidal anti-inflammatories may induce renal failure. Antibiotics may be prescribed to reduce post-operative infection. Surgery may involve an endovascular repair which involves an endograft being inserted to replace the diseased aorta. Timely surgery is crucial: operative mortality for unruptured aneurysm is less than 5%, whereas emergency surgery after rupture is greater than 50%. Morbidity rates are between 15 and 30%, with a five-year survival rate of 60%. The mortality rate in untreated patients is 100% (Bick 2000, Rogers & McCormack 2004, Irwin & Rippe 2008).

Arterial embolism

Occlusion of an artery may follow external compression, thrombosis or embolism. This deprives the tissues of vital blood supply. An arterial embolus is a fragment of thrombus, fat, atherosclerotic plaque, bacterial vegetation or air that mobilizes within the arterial vessels and obstructs the lumen of the vessel disrupting blood flow distal to the embolus. The arterial thrombus is a dry, friable mass composed of layers of platelets and fibrin (Walsh & Young 2007). Diagnosis is usually made on the basis of the sudden nature of the onset of symptoms and an apparent source for the embolus (Smeltzer et al. 2009).

Pathophysiology

Emboli travel along blood vessels until they reach a point where the vessel diameter stops them from going any further. The effect on the tissue supplied by that vessel depends upon the presence of collateral circulation to that area. The most common emboli are derived from thrombi in the circulatory system. Thrombi can develop in peripheral blood vessels due to atheroma, aortic aneurysms or trauma. Thrombi in the arterial system can form within the heart on areas of dead myocardium, where the circulating platelets are exposed to the rough collagen, thus encouraging clot formation. Atrial fibrillation causes blood to stagnate in the heart, allowing thrombi to form. Emboli from the right side of the heart or the veins cause pulmonary embolism, while emboli from the left side can travel to the brain, viscera or limbs.

If the occlusion has been gradual, collateral circulation will have developed, so that blood is able to flow around the occlusion. However, if the occlusion is sudden, there will be no collateral vessels and blood flow will stop at the occlusion. The resulting ischaemia may cause necrosis, gangrene and loss of a limb if circulation is not restored quickly. In the case of the abdominal organs, death of a small part of the kidney will leave a scar, whereas death of a small area of the bowel will lead to perforation and peritonitis. Thromboses tend to occur in association with atheroma at areas of turbulent blood flow, such as at the bifurcation of arteries.

Assessment

The limb may feel cold to the touch compared with the other limb, and the skin may appear pale or cyanosed. Peripheral pulses below the obstruction disappear. In the lower limb, the following peripheral pulse sites may be assessed: femoral popliteal, posterior tibial and dorsalis pedis.

The likely findings can be remembered as the six Ps:

- pain – this may be sudden and severe in embolic episodes, or occur over several hours in the case of thrombosis; it is aggravated by flexion and extension of the limb
- pulseless – with decreased or absent capillary refill – this is a very late sign
- pallor – the limb will look pale when compared to the non-affected limb
- paraesthesia – the patient may complain of tingling sensations in the limb
- perishing cold – the limb feels cold to the touch
- paralysis – there is loss of function due to the decreased blood supply to the nerves and muscles

Investigations

Blood should be sent for full blood count, electrolytes, glucose and coagulation studies as a baseline prior to treatment. Blood flow to the limb can be assessed using noninvasive duplex and Doppler ultrasonography or arteriography. ECG and chest X-ray are also required as baseline investigations.

Management

Supplemental oxygen should be administered to maintain an arterial saturation greater than 95%. Intravenous access should be established in the unaffected limb and prescribed analgesia administered. The limb should be kept warm and in a dependent position to encourage vasodilatation. Regular monitoring of vital signs and distal pulses in the affected limb as well as cardiac monitoring and pulse oximetry in the normal limb should be carried out as standard practice. Heparin therapy is initiated quickly to prevent further development of emboli or extension of existing thrombi. An initial intravenous bolus of 5000 units of heparin or 60 mL/kg body weight is typically the loading dose followed by an intravenous infusion of 12 units/kg/hour until the patient undergoes appropriate management.

Management is usually dependent on the cause of the embolus. Acute embolic occlusion usually requires surgery (Smeltzer et al. 2009). Catheter-directed thrombolysis (CDT) is the treatment of choice for patients with relatively mild acute limb ischemia with no contraindications to thrombolytic therapy (Morrison 2006).

Surgical embolectomy is the simple surgical removal of a clot following incision into a vessel by open surgery on the artery. Surgery should be undertaken as soon as possible, and is most effective within 6–12 hours of occlusion. Embolectomy may be carried out under local or general anaesthesia. In some cases, more advanced surgery requiring patch grafting of the blood vessels may be required. In the case of arterial reconstruction, the percentages of limbs saved in survivors are 80% in femoropopliteal bypass grafts and 60% in femorotibial bypass grafts.

Genitourinary disorders

Retention of urine

Pathophysiology

The urethra exits the bladder inferiorly and anteriorly near the entrance of the two ureters. The ureters and bladder are lined with transitional epithelium which is specialized to stretch as the volume of urine increases. The walls of the ureter and bladder have smooth muscle, and waves of muscle contraction propel the urine along from the kidneys to the bladder. Contraction of muscle in the bladder will force urine to flow along the urethra to exit the body.

At the junction of the urethra and bladder, the smooth muscle of the bladder forms the internal sphincter. The external sphincter is skeletal muscle surrounding the urethra as it extends through the pelvic floor. These sphincters regulate the flow of urine through the urethra. Enlargement of the gland causes stretching and distortion of the urethra, which obstructs the bladder outflow. The bladder muscle enlarges in an attempt to overcome the obstruction, causing high pressures to be generated. Eventually the bladder becomes dilated and the muscle hypotonic.

Assessment

Urinary retention in younger men is relatively rare, occurring in 7 in every 1000 patients aged 40–59 years. The risk rises dramatically in men aged 70–79 years with moderate to severe lower urinary tract symptoms; they have a five-year cumulative incidence of more than 13.8%. Urinary retention may be acute or chronic (Wareing 2004, Gosling 2005). Urinary retention may develop in males with previous symptoms of prostatic obstruction (hesitancy, poor stream, dribbling). Benign prostatic enlargement occurs most often in men over the age of 60 years. Retention may be precipitated by constipation, 'holding on too long', infection, neurological disease or post-operatively. Chronic retention is relatively painless, and although the bladder is distended it is not tender because the distension is more gradual. There may be a history of frequency, with overflow incontinence usually at night. The patient may present with severe lower abdominal pain or discomfort, a palpable distended bladder, and feeling the need to pass urine but unable to do so. The nurse should consider the last time of voiding, intake and output and relevant history. In addition, vital signs to establish a baseline should be checked.

Investigations

Urine, when available, should be taken for culture and routine analysis. Blood should be sent for full blood count, renal profile and acid phosphatase – a marker of disease activity. Further investigations will be arranged at a later time, such as ultrasound, urine flow rates, etc.

Management

Patients with retention of urine can be quite distressed and will need reassurance. It may be possible to overcome the retention by ensuring privacy for the patient and altering his position if possible. Warm baths and letting the patient listen to running water may help; however, in a number of cases the patient will require catheterization, by either the transurethral or suprapubic method.

If retention has been acute, not more than 1000 mL of urine should be drained initially, and then 300 mL each hour until the bladder is empty (Wareing 2004, Gosling 2005). Sudden decompression of the bladder can result in an inflow of blood to the area and some capillary bleeding. The sudden emptying of an over-distended bladder can result in an atonic bladder wall. The suprapubic route may be chosen when there is trauma to the urethra or when it has proved impossible to pass a urethral catheter. It is a surgical procedure and, in common with urethral catheterization, requires aseptic technique. It may be performed under local or general anaesthesia. The catheter is sutured in place and taped to the abdomen to reduce traction on the tube.

Urinary catheters

Although urinary catheterization is seen as a last resort for urinary retention, it remains a common procedure for short-, medium- and long-term management. National Occupational Standards (NOS) to guide practice in catheter care have been developed in partnership with the Royal College of Nursing and Skills for Health (SFH). These guidelines were published in 2008 for use across the NHS and independent healthcare sectors and provide a comprehensive resource and framework for practice (Royal College of Nursing 2008).

Torsion of the testis

Torsion of the spermatic cord involves twisting of the testis and epididymis on their axis. It is a urological emergency and must be differentiated from other complaints of testicular pain, because delay in diagnosis can lead to loss of the testicle. It is most commonly seen in children and young adults (Wyatt et al. 2012).

Pathophysiology

The scrotum is divided into two by a connective tissue septum which separates the testes. Beneath the skin of the scrotum there is a layer of loose connective tissue and a layer of smooth muscle called the dartos muscle. In cold temperatures the dartos muscle contracts, causing the skin of the scrotum to become firm and wrinkled and thus reducing its overall size. At the same time, extensions of the abdominal muscles, called cremaster muscles, which extend into the scrotum, contract. The testes are then pulled nearer to the body and their temperature is raised. During warm weather the process is reversed and the testicles descend away from the body, which lowers their temperature. If the testes become too cold or too warm, normal sperm production does not occur.

The outer part is a white connective tissue capsule. Part of the capsule extends to the interior of the testis, dividing it into about 250 lobules with tubules in which sperm cells develop. Interstitial cells secrete the hormone testosterone. Sperm cells move from these tubules to the epididymis, where they mature in a few days and develop their capacity to function as sex cells. The vas deferens passes from the epididymis via the inguinal canal through the abdominal wall to the prostate gland. The urethra is a passage for both urine and male reproductive fluids. While semen is passing through the urethra, a reflex causes the urinary sphincter muscles to contract, stopping urine from passing from the bladder to the urethra.

Torsion of the testis is due to an anatomic abnormality in which the testicle is not attached to the scrotum (Fig. 29.4). The congenital anomaly is present in approximately 12% of males, 40% of whom have the abnormality in the contralateral testicle. Torsion produces an initial occlusion of the venous return from the testis, although the arterial supply continues for some time. There follows congestion of the testis, with haemorrhagic infarction as the arterial system becomes impaired. The infarction produces a shrunken,

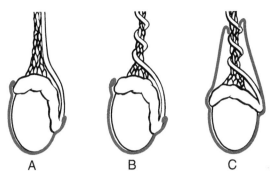

Figure 29.4 • Testicular torsion.

fibrotic testis. Toncich (2009) notes that the extent and rapidity of the damage depends on the degree of torsion, i.e., the number of turns:

• incomplete torsion (<360°) may not completely obstruct arterial flow
• one turn (360°) causes necrosis in 12–24 hours
• two or more (>720°) causes necrosis in less than 2 hours because arterial flow is completely obstructed (Herbener 1996).

Assessment

Torsion is often precipitated by exertion which causes contraction of the cremaster muscle producing the torsion. The patient is usually 15–30 years old, with sudden onset of pain in one testis. Pain may radiate up to the abdomen, the original site of the testicles in the embryo. Nausea and vomiting are common, and on examination the patient is found to have a hot swollen testis.

Differential diagnosis

• epididymitis
• testicular tumour
• trauma
• hydrocele.

Investigations

Use of a Doppler ultrasound on the spermatic cord is an attempt to measure arterial blood flow to the involved testis. While absence of blood flow obviously supports the diagnosis, the presence of blood flow does not exclude torsion. Ultrasound may be helpful, although most would agree that if there is doubt it is best to perform surgical exploration.

Management

The patient may be in considerable pain and will require both emotional support and prescribed analgesia. Surgery should be performed as soon as possible, and viability depends on the number of twists and the time taken to untwist the testis (Toncich 2009). A salvage rate of 100% is found in patients if the testis is untwisted within four hours; after six to eight

hours the salvage rate markedly decreases. Informed consent will include an explanation by the surgeon that the testis may have to be removed if it is found to be non-viable at operation, as well as an explanation that both testes will be fixed by suturing. As torsion is a bilateral phenomenon in 40% of individuals, the uninvolved testis will be fixed to the scrotum during the operation to prevent subsequent torsion. If the testis is viable at operation, it is sutured to the scrotal wall, and if it is deemed unsalvageable it is removed.

Pre-operative preparation

The length of time available for the preparation of the patient for surgery will depend upon the patient's clinical condition. The chief objective is to ensure that the patient goes to surgery in the best physical and psychological condition. There will be some overlap between the medical and nursing input in the preparation of the patient.

Psychological

While surgical procedures and their preparation may be relatively routine for staff in the ED, the need for surgery may come as quite a shock to patients and their relatives, with little time for psychological preparation. Jaworski & Wirtz (1995) noted that during an acute crisis the patient may seem to understand, but information and instructions may have to be repeated. It has been shown that providing patients with information pre-operatively leads to more favourable post-operative outcomes (Hayward 1975, Royal College of Anesthetists 2003). It has also been demonstrated that informing patients about anticipated pain and giving them some control over the pain experience decreased apprehension, increased pain tolerance and resulted in earlier discharges (Hayward 1975, Royal College of Anesthetists 2003). Even where the patient's condition is grave and surgery is being undertaken as a desperate last measure, it remains important to be truthful to both patients and their relatives without unduly frightening them.

Consent

The word consent literally means 'to feel together' that something should be done (Curtin 1993). In today's legal and ethical climate, patient involvement is so important that treating a patient without adequately informing him/her about the treatment is considered negligence, and treatment without consent is considered battery. When signing the consent form, the patient should be rational and not under the influence of drugs or alcohol that may impair comprehension. As far as the law is concerned there is no specific requirement that consent should be given in a particular way; however, consent in writing is by far the best method for all procedures involving risk. Besides explaining treatments and alternatives in terms the patient understands and specifying who will perform the procedure, the provider must invite and answer his/her questions (Dunn 2000, Sims 2008). It is important that the nurse is present during the surgeon's explanation to the patient to allow for continuity. It is, however, not the nurse's responsibility to explain the procedure: the nurse's role in obtaining informed consent is to advocate for the patient: protect his/her rights, preserve their dignity, identify fears, and determine the level of understanding and approval of the care to be given (Sims 2008). Keep in mind that each patient's response is unique and based on personality, education level, emotional make-up, and intellectual capacity. To verify that your patient has received enough necessary information to give consent, ask him/her to state in his/her own words what information has been given. If any doubts exist about the level of patient understanding or decision-making capacity the surgeon or healthcare provider should be notified (Nursing and Midwifery Council 2008, Sims 2008).

In an emergency, where the patient's life is in danger and the patient is not able to consent, the doctor may proceed and do what is required without formal consent (Nursing and Midwifery Council 2008). This is rarely necessary, and even in the unconscious patient consent should be sought where possible from the next of kin.

Skin preparation

Kjonniksen et al. (2002) conducted a systematic literature review and found there was strong evidence to recommend that when hair removal is considered necessary, shaving should not be performed. Instead a depilatory or electric clipping, preferably immediately before surgery, should be performed.

Nursing issues in pre-operative preparation

In emergencies, preparation is limited to the essentials but there are many opportunities for the emergency nurse to ensure that the patient has adequate physical and psychological support prior to urgent operative intervention.

The following list identifies some important nursing considerations, both practical and psychological, that may be tailored to the individual patient:

- patient privacy and confidentiality
- family issues such as young or aged dependants addressed
- notification of relatives
- informed consent – patient has reached age of consent (16 years)

- spiritual needs addressed (minister of religion or appropriate other)
- psychological preparation (post-operative anxieties, altered body image, phobias)
- non-pharmacological pain control (warm packs, positioning)
- prescribed pharmacological pain control
- allergy status established
- identification and removal, where appropriate, of prosthetics, cosmetics and jewellery, including body piercing
- adequate intravenous access
- oral hygiene and gastric decompression using nasogastric tube where appropriate
- appropriate laboratory tests such as blood for group and cross-match, full blood count and biochemistry
- urine testing to detect diabetes, impaired renal function or pregnancy
- catheterization when strict fluid monitoring is required
- patient identification bracelet to correspond with clinical record
- clinical records should include recent vital signs, fluid balance, drug history, allergy history, property list and any other relevant information such as contact telephone number for next of kin.

In more controlled circumstances additional information may be gathered on the patient's condition through

- radiological investigations
- electrocardiograph
- special investigations specific to the patient's condition.

Conclusion

An emergency is defined as a serious condition requiring immediate treatment. The management of surgical emergencies in this chapter covers the full spectrum of patients, from those suffering the discomfort of urinary retention to life-threatening conditions such as aortic aneurysm. With the exception of trauma very few conditions warrant immediate surgery, and a period of resuscitation and stabilization is of considerable benefit to the patient and remains the key to ensuring the best outcome for the patient (American College of Surgeons 2008, McQuillan et al 2008, Smeltzer et al. 2009, Sedlack 2010).

References

American College of Surgeons, 2008. Advanced Trauma Life Support, eighth ed. American College of Surgeons, Chicago.

Baker, Q.F., Devalia, H., Sulliaman, T., 2009. Management of surgery in elderly patients. In: Baker, Q., Aldoori, M. (Eds.), Clinical Surgery: A Practical Guide. Edward Arnold, London.

Balthazar, E.J., 2002. Staging of acute pancreatitis. Radiological Clinics of North America 40 (96), 1199–1209.

Banks, P.A., Freeman, M.L., 2006. The Practice Parameters Committee of the America College of Gastroenterology: Practice Guidelines in Acute Pancreatitis. American Journal of Gastroenterology 101, 2379–2400.

Bick, C., 2000. Abdominal aortic aneurysm repair. Nursing Standard 15 (3), 47–52.

Bickley, L.S., 2007. Bates' Guide to Physical EXamination and History Taking, ninth ed. Lippincott, Williams & Wilkins, Philadelphia.

Biondo, S., Pares, D., Frago, R., et al., 2004. Large bowel obstruction: predictive factors for postoperative mortality. Diseases of the Colon and Rectum 47 (11), 1889–1897.

British Society of Gastroenterology, 1998. UK Guidelines for the management of acute pancreatitis. GUT 42 (Suppl. 2), S1–S13.

Cameron, P., Jelinek, G., Kelly, A.M., et al., 2009. Textbook of Adult Emergency Medicine, third ed. Churchill Livingstone Elsevier, Edinburgh.

Chaudhari, M., Chaudhari, S., Mather, S., 2007. Ketamine for pain relief in acute pancreatitis. Acute Pain 9 (2), 83–86.

Chauhan, S., Forsmark, C.E., 2010. The difficulty in predicting outcome in acute pancreatitis. American Journal of Gastroenterology 105 (2), 435–441.

Choke, E., Vijaynager, B., Thompson, J., et al., 2012. Changing epidemiology of abdominal aorti aneurysm in England and Wales: Older and more benign? Circulation 125 (13), 1617–1625.

Christensen, T., Christensen, M., 2007. The implementation of a guideline of care for patients with a Sengstaken-Blackmore tube in situ in a general intensive care unit using transitional change theory. Intensive Critical Care Nursing 23 (4), 234–242.

Curtin, L.L., 1993. Informed consent: cautious, calculated candor. Nursing Management 24 (4), 18–20.

Desser, T.S., Gross, M., 2008. Multidetector row computed tomography of small bowel obstruction. Seminars in Ultrasound MR and CT 28 (5), 308–321.

Diaz J.J, Jr, Bokheri, F., Mowry, W.T., et al., 2008. Guidelines for management of small bowel obstruction. Journal of Trauma 64 (6), 1651–1664.

Douglas, G., Nicol, F.E., Robertson, C., 2009. MacLeod's Clinical Examination, twelveth ed. Churchill Livingstone-Elsevier, Edinburgh.

Drake, T., 1993. Aortic aneurysm and aortic dissection. In: Pons, P.T., Wolfe, R.E. (Eds.), Emergency Medicine Secrets, third ed. Hanley & Belfus, Philadelphia.

Dunn, D., 2000. Exploring the grey areas of informed consent. Nursing Management 31 (7), 20–25.

Earnshaw, J.J., 2011. Doubts and dilemmas over abdominal aortic aneurysm. British Journal of Surgery 98, 607–608.

Epstein, O., Perkin, G.D., Cookson, J., et al., 2008. Clinical Examination. In: Mosby (Ed.), fourth ed. Elsevier, Edinburgh.

Goldacre, M.J., Roberts, S.E., 2004. Hospital admission for acute pancreatitis in an English population, 1963–98: database study of incidence and mortality. British Medical Journal 328, 1466–1469.

Gosling, J., 2005. Management of urinary retention. Nursing Times 101 (18), 61.

Gow, P.J., Chapman, R.W., 2001. Modern management of oesophageal varices. Postgraduate Medicine Journal 77 (904), 75–81.

Habib, A., Sanyal, A.J., 2007. Acute variceal hemorrhage. Gastrointestinal Endoscopy Clinics of North America 17 (2), 223–252.

Hayward, J., 1975. Information: A Prescription Against Pain. Royal College of Nursing, London.

Herbener, T.E., 1996. Ultrasound in the assessment of the acute scrotum. Journal of Clinical Ultrasound 24, 405–421.

Herrington, A., 2009. Gastrointestinal Emergencies. In: Howard, P.K., Steinmann, R.A. (Eds.), Sheehy's Emergency Nursing: Principles and Practice, sixth ed. Mosby Elsevier, St Louis.

Irwin, R.S., Rippe, J.M., 2008. Intensive Care Medicine, sixth ed. Wolters Kluwer/Lippincott Williams & Wilkins, Philadelphia.

Jaworski, M.A., Wirtz, K.M., 1995. Spinal trauma. In: Kitt, S., Selfridge-Thomas, J., Proehl, J., Kaiser, J. (Eds.), Emergency Nursing: A Physiological and Clinical Perspective. WB Saunders, Philadelphia.

Kjonniksen, I., Andersen, B.M., Sondenaa, V., et al., 2002. Preoperative hair removal – a systematic literature review. AORN (Association of Perioperative Registered Nurses) 75 (5), 928–939.

Knaus, W.A., Draper, E.A., Wagner, D.P., et al., 1985. APACHE II: a severity of disease classification system. Critical Care Medicine 13 (10), 818–829.

Lankisch, P.G., Weber-Dany, B., Hebel, K., et al., 2009. The Harmless Acute Pancreatitis Score: A clinical algorithm for rapid initial stratification of non-severe disease. Clinical Gastroenterology and Hepatology 7 (6), 702–705.

Mayerle, J., Dummer, A., Sendler, M., et al., 2012. Differential roles of inflammatory cells in pancreatitis. Journal of Gastroenterology and Hepatology 27 (S2), 47–51.

McGrath, A., 2004. Examination of the Abdomen. In: Cox, C.L. (Ed.), Physical Assessment for Nurses. Blackwell Science, Oxford.

McQuillan, K.A., Flynn Makic, B.A., Whalen, E., 2008. Trauma Nursing: From Resuscitation through Rehabilitation, fourth ed. WB Saunders, Edinburgh.

Mitchell, R.M.S., Byrne, M.F., Baillie, J., 2003. Pancreatitis. The Lancet 361 (9367), 1447.

Moore, K., Dalley, A.F., Agur, A.M.R., 2009. Clinically Oriented Anatomy, sixth ed. Wolters Kluwer/Lippincott, Williams & Wilkins, Philidelphia.

Morrison, H.L., 2006. Catheter-directed thrombolysis for acute limb ischaemia. Seminars in Interventional Radiology 23 (3), 258–269.

Munoz, A., Katerndahl, D.A., 2000. Diagnosis and management of acute pancreatitis. American Family Physician 62 (1), 164–174.

Nursing and Midwifery Council, 2008. The Code: Standards of conduct, Performance and Ethics for Nurses and Midwives. Nursing and Midwifery Council, London.

Old, J.L., Dusing, R.W., Yap, W., et al., 2005. Imaging for suspected appendicitis. American Family Physician 71 (1), 71–78.

Petroianu, A., 2012. Diagnosis of acute appendicitis. International Journal of Surgery 10, 115–119.

Ranson, J.H., 1982. Etiological and prognostic factors in human acute pancreatitis: a review. American Journal of gastroenterology 77 (9), 633–638.

Rogers, R.L., McCormack, R., 2004. Aortic disasters. Emergency Medicine Clinics of North America 22 (4), 887–908.

Royal College of Anaesthetists, 2003. Raising the Standard: Information for Patients. Royal College of Anaesthetists, London.

Royal College of Nursing, 2008. Catheter Care: RCN Guidelines for Nurses. Royal College of Nursing, London.

Sarraf-Yazdi, S., Shapiro, M.L., 2010. Small bowel obstruction: The eternal dilemma of when to intervene. Scandanavian Journal of Surgery 99, 78–80.

Sedlack, K., 2010. Vascular access and fluid replacement. In: Howard, P.K., Steinmann, R.A. (Eds.), Sheehy's Emergency Nursing:Principles and Practice, sixth ed. Mosby-Elsevier, St Louis.

Scott, R.A., 2009. Shock. In: Cameron, P., Jelinek, G., Kelly, A.M., Murray, L., Brown, A.F.T., Murray, L. (Eds.), Textbook of Adult Emergency Medicine, third ed. Churchill Livingstone, London.

Sims, J.M., 2008. Your role in informed consent: Part 1. Dimensions of Critical Care Nursing 27 (2), 70–73.

Smeltzer, S.C., Bare, B.G., Hinkle, J.L., et al., 2009. Brunner and Suddarths Textbook of Medical-Surgical Nursing, twelfth ed. Wolters Kluwer/Lippincott, Williams & Wilkins, Philadelphia.

Smith, G.D., Fawcett, T., 2004. Oesophageal varices. Gastrointestinal Nursing 2 (5), 33–39.

Toncich, G., 2009. The acute scrotum. In: Cameron, Jelinek, G., Kelly, A.M., Murray, L., Brown, A.F.T. (Eds.), Textbook of Adult Emergency Medicine, third ed. Churchill Livingstone, Edinburgh.

Trevino, C., 2010. Small bowel obstruction: The art of management. Advanced Critical Care 21 (2), 187–194.

Turner, R., Angus, B., Hatton, C., et al., 2009. Clinical Skills and Examination: The Core Curriculum, fifth ed. Wiley Blackwell, Oxford.

UK Working Party on Acute Pancreatitis, 2005. UK guidelines for the management of acute pancreatitis. Gut 54, 1–9.

Walsh, T., Young, M.E., 2007. Disorders of the Peripheral Vascular System. In: Swearingen, P.L. (Ed.), Manual of Medical – Surgical Nursing Care: Nursing Interventions and Collaborative Management, sixth ed. Mosby Elsevier, Edinburgh.

Wareing, M., 2004. Urinary retention: Issues of management and care. Emergency Nurse 11 (8), 24–27.

Wyatt, J., Illingworth, R., Graham, C., et al., 2012. Oxford Handbook of Emergency Medicine, fourth ed. Oxford University Press, Oxford.

Yeh, B., 2008. Evidence-based emergency medicine/rational clinical examination abstract. Does this adult patient have appendicitis? Annals of Emergency Medicine 52 (3), 301–303.

Zielinski, M.D., Eiken, P.W., Bannon, M., et al., 2010. Small Bowel Obstruction – Who needs an operation? Multivariate prediction model. World Journal of Surgery 34 (5), 910–919.

Gynaecological and obstetric emergencies

30

Orla Devereux

CHAPTER CONTENTS

Introduction

This chapter considers women's health in both pregnant and non-pregnant patients. Although many of the principles of management are similar, significant anatomical differences exist, and many of the signs and symptoms have different implications. Conditions relating to female reproduction form a relatively small part of Emergency Department (ED) work; however, many women actively choose the ED for both emergency care and preventative intervention. As well as its physical implications, for many patients an obstetric or gynaecological condition can be distressing and value-laden. This chapter seeks to equip the ED nurse to rapidly assess the patient's condition and intervene appropriately. It will provide an outline of relevant anatomy and physiology before identifying conditions commonly treated in ED.

Anatomy and physiology

The female reproductive organs consist of:

* uterus
* ovaries
* fallopian tubes
* vagina
* external genitalia.

http://dx.doi.org/10.1016/B978-0-7020-4315-4.00030-9

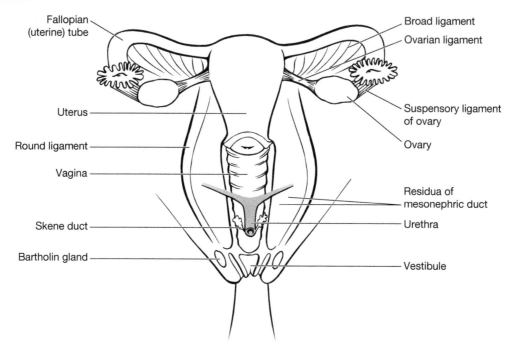

Figure 30.1 • The female reproductive system.

They are situated outside the peritoneal cavity (Fig. 30.1).

The uterus is located in the anterior pelvis above the bladder. It is a pear-shaped organ with thick walls, made up of three layers: an outer serous membrane, a middle layer of smooth muscle, and the mucosal inner layer of endometrium, which is extremely vascular. The top of the uterus is called the fundus; it is the height of this that is measured to determine the gestation of pregnancy (Fig. 30.2).

The neck of the uterus is called the cervix. This opens into the vagina, the opening of which is called the os. The status of the os is an important consideration in assessing bleeding in early pregnancy. The ovaries sit bilaterally to the uterus, on the lateral pelvic wall, and are connected to the uterus by fallopian tubes. The fallopian tubes have a funnel-like opening below the ovaries, which collects the ova and transports them by peristalsis to the uterus. The tubes are made up of smooth muscle and mucous membrane. The vagina is an elastic tube leading to the external genitalia. There are two small glands either side of the vaginal opening called Bartholin's glands which can be prone to cyst formation in some women (Bickley & Szilagyi 2003).

During child-bearing years, each ovary is 2.5–5 cm long, 1.5–3 cm wide, and 0.6–1.5 cm thick. Size diminishes significantly after menopause. The number of ova present in the ovaries also decreases with age, from approximately 2 million at birth to 300 000–400 000 by puberty (Sanders Jordan 2009). The female reproductive cycle varies in length between 21 and 35 days, but for most the average cycle is 28 days. The cycle consists of ovulation and menstruation, and is governed by changes in hormone levels. The first 5–7 days of the cycle represent menstruation. This is followed by a 7–8-day follicular phase preparing the endometrium for implantation of a fertilized egg. At around days 14–15 of the cycle, ovulation occurs. Once the ovum is released from the follicle, the luteal phase then commences: the collapsed

Figure 30.2 • Change in fundal height during gestation.

follicle becomes an endocrine gland called the corpus luteum. It secretes oestrogen and progesterone to support the egg if it is fertilized. If the egg is not fertilized the luteal phase is responsible for the degeneration of the corpus luteum, after which the thickened lining of the endometrium sheds and the cycle begins again. If the egg is fertilized, the corpus luteum continues to secrete hormones until about three months into the pregnancy when the placenta takes over.

Fertilization of the ovum takes place in the fallopian tube, and during the first few days it passes slowly towards the uterus while a series of cell divisions take place forming a mass of embryotic cells. The embryo reaches the uterus between 3 and 5 days after fertilization. It then begins to implant into the uterine wall by about 6–7 days after fertilization. The placenta forms around where the embryo is embedded and, after a few weeks, begins to provide oxygen and nutrients to support fetal growth for the rest of the pregnancy. By five weeks after implantation the fetal heart is pumping well, and nutrients pass from the maternal blood supply across the placental membrane to nourish the fetus.

The pregnancy is divided into trimesters of growth: in the first the internal organs develop; in the second the fetus grows in length and systems begin to mature; and in the last trimester the fetus fattens out and builds up reserves for birth. Physiological changes in pregnancy are plentiful, and an overview of key changes is given in Box 30.1; however,

a detailed description is beyond the scope of this text and only those changes related to emergency care in ED will be discussed.

Emergency care of the non-pregnant woman

History

Obtaining an accurate history is vital to establish the severity of a patient's condition. Because of the personal nature of gynaecological complaints, the nurse should ensure that assessment is carried out in private and in a sensitive and non-judgemental manner. Box 30.2 highlights the information that should be obtained.

Assessment

General assessment of the woman with a gynaecological condition should include baseline observations of pulse, respiration, blood pressure and temperature to detect signs of shock or infection. The level of pain should be determined, together with the exact location. Gentle abdominal examination will assist in this. If clinically indicated, a vaginal examination should be carried out once, either by the nurse or, more commonly, by the doctor. Assessment should include urinalysis to detect a urinary tract infection as a primary cause of pain. Initially this can be diagnosed by the presence of leucocytes, protein and blood in urine, but culture and sensitivity should follow to ensure appropriate antibiotic therapy. A pregnancy test should also be carried out routinely to exclude unknown pregnancy. Abdominal pain is often the primary reason women with gynaecological complaints attend ED. Conditions causing acute abdominal pain are shown in Box 30.3.

Box 30.1

Physiological changes in pregnancy

Cardiovascular

- Blood vascularity increases by 30 %
- Red cell mass rises by 20 %
- Plasma increases by up to 50 %
- Peripheral resistance decreases, reducing diastolic BP in the first and second trimesters
- Heart rate increases by up to 20 beats/min
- CVP falls by 65 % by term
- Cardiac output increases by up to 30 %

Respiratory

- Oxygen consumption increases by 20 %
- Respiratory rate increases
- Pulmonary function alters, residual capacity decreases, minute volume increases by 40–50 % and tidal volume increases

Renal

- Renal plasma flow and glomerular filtration rate increase steadily throughout pregnancy to a 50 % greater capacity by term
- Speed of urine formation increases
- Water and sodium reabsorption rates are increased

Gastrointestinal

- Smooth muscle relaxes, and therefore gastric emptying is faster
- Intestines are relocated into the upper abdomen
- Acid regurgitation is common

Endocrine

- Base metabolic rate increases by up to 25 %
- Anterior pituitary hypertrophy occurs
- Thyroid hypertrophy occurs

Other

- Anaemia develops because of rapid increase in iron requirements
- Cell-mediated immunity is depressed
- Autoimmunity disease eases during pregnancy

Box 30.2

History related to gynaecological assessment

- Duration of symptoms
- Type and location of any pain
- Is there any redness or itching?
- Date of last menstrual period, and duration
- Was menstrual period normal?
- Is there any possibility of pregnancy?
- Is the patient sexually active? What (if any) contraception is being used?
- Is there any abnormal vaginal discharge or bleeding? If so, what is the discharge like?
- How heavy is bleeding, i.e., how often are pads or tampons being changed?
- Past history of pregnancy
- Coexisting medical problems/drug therapy
- Is there a history of assaults?

Causes of acute abdominal pain in gynaecology

- Menstrual cycle
  - mid-cycle pain
  - menstruation
- Ovarian cyst
- Pelvic inflammatory disease (PID)

Menstrual pain

Mid-cycle pain

This is known as Mittelschmerz disease and is a benign, transient mid-cycle pain occurring at or after ovulation. Pain is usually unilateral and lasts 24–48 hours. Some women experience this every month as part of their usual cycle; for others it is an unexpected pain sometimes associated with per vaginal (PV) bleeding that causes enough discomfort and anxiety for the patient to seek emergency healthcare. Mittelschmerz pain is thought to be caused by a combination of local irritation due to blood, follicular fluid and prostaglandins released after ovulation, and increased peristalsis in the fallopian tubes. At this time, most women experience microscopic PV bleeding, a few regularly have overt bleeding and most women will have an occasional mid-cycle PV bleed. This is due to a temporary fall in hormone levels between the follicular and luteal phases of the menstrual cycle. Bleeding usually lasts only a few hours.

Mittelschmerz, from the German 'middle pain', is a periodic pain at mid-cycle due to irritation of the peritoneum by follicular fluid at the time of its rupture (Salhan 2011). It should only be diagnosed once other causes, such as ovarian cyst and pelvic inflammatory disease (PID), have been ruled out (Reedy & Brucker 1995). The condition is self-limiting, and therefore treatment involves symptom control and education. Non-steroidal anti-inflammatory drugs (NSAIDs), such as ibuprofen, are usually the most effective analgesia. The patient should be made aware of the cyclical nature of the condition, and the possibility of recurrence.

Dysmenorrhoea

In most cases, dysmenorrhoea (period pain) is self-diagnosed and treated at home; however, when symptoms are unusually severe, some women seek emergency care. Two types of dysmenorrhoea exist: primary and secondary dysmenorrhoea. In the former, uterine spasm involves A nerve fibres, responsible for acute pain, and C nerve fibres responsible for chronic and referred pain (see also Chapter 25). Primary dysmenorrhoea is most common in adolescents and young women who have not had children (Horne & Critchley 2012).

Secondary dysmenorrhoea is more common in women over 30 with gynaecological problems such as endometriosis or PID. Other causes include intrauterine devices, adhesions and benign tumours of the uterus. In both types of dysmenorrhoea, the patient will have crampy, low abdominal pain either at onset of menses or 24 hours prior to onset. The woman may have referred pain in the back and legs. Associated symptoms include breast tenderness, nausea/vomiting, diarrhoea and headache, all due to rapid hormonal changes.

Diagnosis should be made only after other causes of pain and bleeding have been excluded. Management revolves around symptom control and the condition is self-limiting. NSAIDs are the analgesia of choice because they inhibit intra-uterine synthesis of prostaglandin as well as decreasing pain. Small quantities of alcohol are effective in the treatment of dysmenorrhoea because it reduces oxytocin and vasopressor activity, therefore reducing uterine spasm. Ethically, however, this method of pain control should only be advocated for women who understand the potential dangers of alcohol ingestion and are legally old enough to use it (Reedy & Brucker 1995). Discharge information should include the commonality of dysmenorrhoea and, in the case of secondary dysmenorrhoea, information and advice about the predisposing condition.

Ovarian cyst

These usually result from a dysfunction in the menstrual cycle, when a collection of fluid forms around the corpus luteum. Cyst formation is more common in endometriosis and most are benign, self-limiting and asymptomatic. In some instances, the cyst increases in size and becomes symptomatic causing pelvic discomfort at about 8–10 cm diameter due to the stretching of the capsule, although most regress spontaneously over a period of 1–3 months (Sanders-Jordan 2009). Eventually, if growth persists, bleeding, rupture or torsion can occur. Ovarian cysts are uncommon in women using oral contraception.

Assessment

The patient will have abdominal pain, worse on the affected side, with possible guarding on examination. Onset of pain is usually during the latter half of the menstrual cycle or the week prior to menses where the cycle is regular. The patient will experience prolonged menstruation. If a small cyst ruptures, the fluid collected in it is reabsorbed without any clinical evidence. Rupture of a large cyst can cause potentially life-threatening hypovolaemia.

Assessment of vital signs should be ongoing, as a mild tachycardia can quickly deteriorate into severe hypotension and shock in ovarian cyst rupture. Prior to rupture, a large cyst can twist around the vascular pedicle, causing ovarian torsion. This is identified by a sudden onset of intermittent but sharp pain. Nausea or vomiting is an early sign of ovarian torsion.

Management

Cysts not causing haemodynamic compromise tend to be managed conservatively with follow-up investigation from a GP or gynaecological clinic. If adequate pain control cannot be achieved, hospital admission should be considered. If the patient has mild to moderate signs of hypovolaemia, intravenous fluid support should be established, and laparoscopic surgical decompression of the cyst should be considered. In cases of severe hypotension or torsion, fluid resuscitation and urgent surgical intervention are necessary. These women will need both information and psychological support during a time which potentially threatens their fertility.

Pelvic inflammatory disease

Pelvic inflammatory disease comprises a range of upper genital tract inflammatory disorders in women that usually result from microorganisms ascending from the cervix to the upper genital tract (French et al. 2011). Recurrent PID is associated with an increased risk for infertility and chronic pelvic pain (Trent et al. 2011). It is also linked to an increase in ectopic pregnancy. PID is a generic term used to describe infection of the pelvic peritoneum, connective tissue and reproductive organs – most commonly the fallopian tubes (also termed salpingitis). PID results from:

- sexually transmitted infections (STIs), particularly gonorrhoea and chlamydia
- termination of pregnancy
- childbirth with assisted delivery
- gynaecological surgery.

For most women, intrauterine contraceptive devices (IUCD) are a safe option. Upper genital tract infections occur when pathogenic microorganisms ascend from the cervix and invade the endometrium and the fallopian tubes, causing an inflammatory reaction (Martinez & Lopez-Arregui 2009). Sexually transmitted infections are the most common cause of PID, especially caused by *Chlamydia trachomatis* and *Neisseria gonorrhoeae*. The infection occurs in the genital area and spreads along mucosal surfaces, causing transient bouts of inflammation. Infection tends to settle in fallopian tubes, causing scar tissue and adhesions. This makes ovum passage more difficult and increases the likelihood of ectopic pregnancy because the fertilized egg is unable to pass to the uterus and implants in the tube. PID is most common in young women with multiple sexual partners, women who experienced their first sexual intercourse at a young age, or women with a high frequency of sexual intercourse, and within that group PID has a higher incidence in women from lower socio-economic groups (Bryan 2004). The most common age group is 20–24 years of age (French et al. 2011), which has considerable implications for future healthcare and fertility therapy, as women with PID are at increased risk of chronic pelvic pain, ectopic pregnancy and infertility.

A patient with PID will present with moderate to severe abdominal pain, worse with urination, bowel action and intercourse. Because the pain increases with movement, patients characteristically shuffle, the 'PID shuffle'. She may be tachycardic and will be pyrexic. If STI is the cause, the patient will have a thick vaginal discharge. If pelvic abscess or peritonitis is developing, the patient will also have nausea or vomiting. Lichtman & Parera (1990) highlighted three grades of PID (Box 30.4).

Management

Pain relief is a priority for management of all types of PID. The strength of analgesia needed will vary depending on the severity of infection and the patient's individual perceptions of her condition. Grade I infection can be treated with broad-spectrum antibiotics, usually cefotaxime or tetracycline, and the patient can be discharged and followed up in the STI clinic. Grade II conditions warrant hospital admission for i.v. antibiotics. Grade III PID is uncommon, but necessitates hospitalization and surgical intervention as well as antibiotic therapy.

If the woman is pregnant or has not responded to, or complied with, oral antibiotics, hospital admission should be considered. If the patient is discharged from the ED, it is essential that she has appropriate health education to enable her to recognize a recurrence and get treatment. This is important in reducing potential long-term health problems, including chronic pelvic pain, dyspareunia and infertility. If the PID originates from an STI, the patient's partner should be encouraged to attend an STI clinic and advice should be given about the use of barrier methods of contraception during intercourse. Patients with PID, gonorrhoea, or chlamydial infection should also have serological testing and be offered confidential counselling and testing for HIV infection (Sacchetti 2009).

Bartholin's cyst

The Bartholin's glands lie on either side of the vagina and secrete fluid onto the surface of the labia. In normal health these cannot be seen or palpated. If the duct becomes blocked, a small cyst forms; these are usually benign and self-limiting. They can, however, become infected with *Escherichia coli* or STIs such as gonorrhoea. Bartholin's cyst/abscess affects 2% of women (Haider et al. 2007). If infection occurs, the labium becomes inflamed and oedematous to the extent that the patient may have difficulty walking. This is a painful and distressing condition, which is resolved by early excision and drainage of the cyst. This is usually performed as an inpatient procedure. Antibiotic therapy is also indicated (Wechter et al. 2009).

Sexually transmitted infections

Patients may present to ED because of its relative anonymity compared with GP attendance. Many people are still unaware of the existence and accessibility of STI clinics. Broadly,

Table 30.1 Sexually transmitted infections

Organism	Incubation	Symptoms	Discharge	Treatment
Neisseria gonorrhoea	3–5 days	Dysuria	Yellow	Cefotaxime
Chlamydia trochomatis	5–10 days	Urethral itching	Mucopurulent vaginal discharge	Tetracycline
Trichomonas vaginalis	1 week	Vaginal itching	Thin, frothy, greenish, foul-smelling	Metronidazole
Gardnerella vaginalis	5–10 days	Itching	Thin, white, fishy odour	Metronidazole
Candida albicans	Variable	Inflammatory itching	Thick white discharge	Clotrimazole
Herpes simplex II	2–12 days	Painful, genital lesions	–	Acyclovir
Genital warts	1–6 months	Wart-type lesions on genitals spreading up genital tract	–	Paint with 5 % acetic acid

common symptoms of STI are genital irritation or pain, infection, discharge and sometimes bleeding. Specific symptoms and management are shown in Table 30.1.

The role of the ED nurse in caring for patients with STIs is twofold: first, to provide immediate therapy to resolve the acute episode with appropriate STI clinic follow-up; and second, to provide non-judgemental health education aimed at preventing the spread of STIs. All direct sexual contacts of the patient should be advised to have a health check. It is not possible for the ED nurse to personally follow up patient contacts, but the nurse can support the patient in informing a current partner, and information can then be cascaded to anyone else who may be involved. Patients should refrain from sexual activity until the infection is clear. Advice about barrier contraception should also be given and where appropriate, opportunities for serological testing, confidential counseling and testing for HIV infection (Sacchetti 2009).

Emergency contraception

Emergency contraception is available in the form of oral progesterone-based pills taken within 72 hours of intercourse or an IUCD that needs to be inserted within 5 days of intercourse.

Progesterone-based pills

The most widely used emergency contraception is that containing levonorgestrel. While it was initially prescribed in two divided doses, a single dose is now the preferred method of administration (Black 2009). Administration of the drug which should be taken within 72 hours of unprotected intercourse. Nausea and vomiting are significant side-effects of oral postcoital contraception and some doctors prefer to prescribe prophylactic anti-emetic drugs with the pill. Follow-up care should be sought around three weeks after postcoital contraception. It is because these facilities are not available in ED that some consultants choose not to offer emergency postcoital contraception. Most women will commence menses within 21 days of the postcoital pill. If this does not happen, a

pregnancy test should be performed; however, the failure rate of the postcoital pill is less than 2 % if taken within 72 hours of coitus (Task Force on Postovulatory Method of Fertility Regulation 1998).

The patient should be advised about contraception in the short term while still in the ED. The patient must also be advised to use barrier methods of contraception for the rest of this cycle as the postcoital pill alters the timing of ovulation. Longer-term contraception will be discussed in the follow-up check. It should also be noted that, because the postcoital contraceptive pill prevents uterine implantation, it does not preclude ectopic pregnancy. The patient should be advised of the symptoms of ectopic pregnancy and advised to seek medical care should these be experienced.

Intrauterine contraceptive device

The IUCD may be used up to five days after ovulation, or after unprotected intercourse if the date of ovulation is not known. It also works by preventing implantation, and failure is rare at 0–0.2 % (Black 2009). There are disadvantages to its use in nulligravida women because of pain associated with insertion. It is not ideal for women with existing pelvic infection as it could exacerbate this. Irregular vaginal bleeding is also common after IUCD insertion. The advantage of this method is that it provides longer-term contraception. The use of prophylactic antibiotics may be considered for women who are at increased risk of sexually transmitted infection if an IUCD is to be inserted before results of tests are available (French et al. 2004).

Rape and sexual assault

In England and Wales, under the Sexual Offences Act 2003 (Home Office 2003), the definition of rape is the non-consensual penetration of vagina, mouth or anus by a penis. Sexual assault by penetration is the non-consensual, intentional insertion of an object other than the penis into the vagina or anus. The Act also treats any sexual intercourse with a child under the age of 13 as rape and defines the age of consent as 16 (College of Emergency Medicine 2011).

Rape and sexual assault are violent crimes. Police forces are increasingly caring for physically injured survivors of rape in dedicated rape suites equipped for the privacy and comfort of women who have been assaulted. In the UK and Ireland, Sexual Assault Referral Centres (SARCs)/Sexual Assault Treatment Units (SATUs) are located at most major hospitals providing an integrated response to adult survivors of rape and sexual assault. The services provided include forensic and medical examination, one-to-one counselling, screening for sexually transmitted diseases, postcoital contraception and 24-hour information and support (Lovett et al. 2004, Lovett & Kelly 2009). Specialist Forensic Nurses trained in the collection of forensic evidence, photo documentation and legal testimony ensure high standards of practice are maintained. Thorough, compassionate assessment and treatment of survivors, as well as the meticulous collection and documentation of forensic evidence, are vital for successful prosecution (Fitzpatrick et al. 2012).

These clinicians are dedicated to the care of survivors of sexual and domestic violence, liaising with medical and nursing staff, police social services and support agencies (Markowitz et al. 2005).

EDs should have a rape protocol that has been discussed with the local police force and rape support groups. This should ensure that the patient's best interests are served in terms of both immediate healthcare and her subsequent ability to produce evidence to prosecute the assailant. ED nurses should attempt to reinstate the patient's perception of control over what happens to her. Unless associated injuries prevent it, the patient should be encouraged to give explicit consent, either written or verbal, for any investigations or examination she, or he in the case of male survivors, undergoes.

There were 54 509 sexual offences recorded by the police in England and Wales in 2009/10; however, police-recorded statistics on sexual offences are likely to be more heavily influenced by under-reporting than the British Crime Survey (BCS) and therefore should be interpreted with caution (Flately et al. 2010). Analysis of the 2007/08 BCS self-completion module showed that 11 % of victims of serious sexual assault told the police about the incident (Povey et al. 2009).

The decision to report sexual assault is entirely that of the patient, and ED staff must support that decision and plan care around it. Box 30.5 shows care paths for reporting and non-reporting of sexual assault. If the patient does not have significant physical injury, it may be appropriate to obtain a full history jointly with the police if the patient wishes to report the attack. This is simply to prevent the patient having to describe the incident several times, which can be unnecessarily distressing. The decision to take a joint history should be the patient's. Box 30.6 highlights the essential information needed.

It is important that any potential forensic evidence is preserved. This is equally important in a patient who is unconscious or who has significant physical injury; however, treatment of associated immediate life-threatening injuries takes priority over forensic examination. A paper sheet should be placed under the patient to collect debris if possible; otherwise linen used should be saved. A mobile patient should be asked to stand on a paper sheet while undressing so that debris can be saved. If unconscious, the paper couch liner should be retained also. Wet or blood-stained garments should

Box 30.5

Reporting/non-reporting sexual assault care paths

Incident reported to police

- Police officer allocated to support patient
- Examination carried out by forensic medical examiner (FME)
- Entrance to victim support scheme
- Police statements obtained
- Police officer support throughout court case

Incident not reported

- Medical examination by senior A&E doctor
- Support agency contacted
- Follow-up at STI clinic
- Nurse support throughout
- Retain option of police involvement

(After Holloway M (1994) Care of the sexually assaulted woman. Emergency Nurse, 2(3), 18–20.)

Box 30.6

Obtaining a history from a survivor of sexual assault

- Establish the date, time and location of the attack
- Circumstances of assault
  - where injured, i.e., in mouth, skin, breast, anus, vagina
  - was a condom used?
  - removal or damage to clothing by assailant
  - number of assailants
  - drugs/alcohol used
  - any associated physical injuries
- Action taken after assault
  - cleaned teeth, mouthwash gargled
  - wash/shower/bath
  - changed clothes
  - urinated/bowels opened
  - changed tampon/pad
  - subsequent sexual intercourse
- Alcohol/drugs (prescribed or recreational) taken prior to the attack or since
- Previous sexual intercourse, if within 2 weeks
- Menstrual stage, date of last period and usual method of birth control if of child-bearing age
- Medical and obstetric history

not be put into a plastic bag as this will lead to decomposition rendering forensic analysis very difficult. The responsibility to collect evidence and maintain the chain of evidence resides with the police and a forensic medical examiner (College of Emergency Medicine 2011). Physical examination should be carried out at once by a forensic medical examiner (FME).

In some areas, the FME will take on this role whether or not the patient intends to prosecute, although Kelly (2002) notes that the vast majority of survivors, both female and male, express a preference for a female forensic examiner. The first priority must lie in protecting the patient from further

Box 30.7

Forensic evidence from survivors of sexual assault

- Observe and document the condition of clothing, i.e., damaged, stained, debris attachment to it. Clothing should be placed in a paper bag for dry storage
- Full medical examination, documenting injuries in detail; provide photographs if possible
- Obtain following samples

Sample	Collect in	Store in
Blood group/DNA profile	EDTA bottles	Fridge
Blood alcohol	Fluoride oxadate bottle	Fridge
Saliva/sperm group	Universal container	Fridge
Urine/drugs/alcohol screen	Sodium fluoride	Fridge
Skin swabs	Plastic tube	Freezer
Vaginal/cervical swabs	Plastic tube	Freezer
Anal swabs	Plastic tube	Freezer
Loose hairs/debris	Plastic bag	Dry storage
Fingernail clippings	Plastic bag	Dry storage
Tampon/sanitary towel	Plastic bag	Freeze

(After Stevens L, Kenney A (1994) Emergencies in Obstetrics and Gynaecology. Oxford: Oxford University Press; Schofield S (2006) Body of Evidence. Emergency Nurse 13(9), 9–11.)

Box 30.8

Rape trauma syndrome

Acute phase (during the attack and the period afterwards)

- Shock
- Disbelief and terror
- Anxiety
- Vulnerability
- Guilt
- Physical pain
- Suppressed/controlled emotions

Adjustment phase (during weeks and months following)

- Sleep disturbance
- Flashbacks disturbance
- Phobias
- Eating disorders
- Voluntary isolation and rejection of close friends/relatives
- Denial of incident
- Insecurity

Long-term implications

Most women carry emotional scars for the rest of their lives. Some common problems include:
- Depression
- Inability to trust others
- Inability to maintain intimate relationships
- Constant reminders triggered by smells, sounds, etc.
- Some women have persistent flashbacks

(After Holloway M (1994) Care of the sexually assaulted woman. Emergency Nurse, 2(3), 18–20.)

humiliation and distress and, on those grounds alone, one examination is good practice. For evidence to be submissible in court, the examination, evidence collection and documentation should follow local police policy. The primary role of the ED nurse is in supporting the patient and ensuring her privacy and safety until examination can take place. Box 30.7 shows what evidence should be collected and how it should be preserved.

Once the medical examination has been carried out, the patient needs to be advised about pregnancy risk and offered emergency contraception if appropriate. The patient should also be offered follow-up STI screening and it is imperative she has either actual contact with a rape survivors' support counsellor or contact telephone numbers for later use should she wish to do so. Rape trauma syndrome (RTS) is experienced by most sexual assault survivors in some form (Burgess & Holmstrom 1974, McGrath 2010). Good, sensitive, non-judgemental care immediately following the attack can help to reduce the impact of RTS. It is important that ED nurses understand the progression of this syndrome, both for immediate care of attack survivors and to help recognize and rationalize associated symptoms of patients sometime after the assault. Box 30.8 outlines the stages of RTS.

Domestic violence refers to the use or threat of physical, sexual or emotional force by spouses, partners, relatives or anyone else with a close relationship with their victims. It occurs among people of all social classes, age groups, ethnic groups and cultures; among disabled and able-bodied people; and in homosexual and heterosexual relationships (Kearns et al. 2008, Gibbons 2011). Domestic violence can involve slapping, kicking, hitting, punching, burning or scalding, use of weapons or destruction of property; it often results in injury and can lead to death

(Boursnell & Prosser 2010). There are a number of tell-tale signs of domestic abuse of which emergency nurses should be aware (Health Service Executive 2007, Gibbons 2011) (see Box 30.9).

Based on findings of the BCS of 22 643 women and men aged 16–59 years, Walby & Allan (2004) found that interpersonal violence is both widely dispersed and it is concentrated. It is widely dispersed in that some experience of domestic violence (abuse, threats or force), sexual victimization or stalking is reported by over one-third (36%) of people. It is concentrated in that a minority, largely women, suffer multiple attacks, severe injuries, and experience more than one form of inter-personal violence and serious disruption to their lives.

The practice of efficient patient processing in EDs may obscure subtle signs of abuse, which may not be picked up until the woman presents with more serious physical injuries (Olshansky 2002). The confidential enquiry into maternal deaths (Confidential Enquiry into Maternal and Child Health 2004) found that 14% of the women whose deaths were assessed had a history of domestic violence which was either self-reported to healthcare professionals or was known to health and social services. This is believed to be a conservative estimate of the true prevalence of violence among these women, and ED nurses should be vigilant to the signs of abuse and the local services available to these patients.

Box 30.9

Signs of domestic violence (Health Service Executive 2007, Gibbons 2011)

- Patients presenting with choking or attempted strangulation injuries; these are 'red flag' indicators of high-risk abusive situations
- Patients making light of their injuries
- Patients exhibiting extreme panic, fear and apprehension
- The constant presence of overly attentive spouses or partners
- Patients giving inaccurate or incomplete explanations for injuries
- Frequent presentations to EDs. These may not be injury-related but involve substance or alcohol abuse, para-suicide, anxiety, chronic pain, deterioration of or poor compliance with long-term medical problems
- Delays between when patients sustained injuries and when they present to EDs. These delays can be calculated by assessing bruises, which change from a red or purple colour to blue, green and yellow
- Signs of sexual violence
- X-rays showing old, healed fractures and fractures at various stages of healing
- The presence of injuries to sites such as the head, face and neck, chest, breasts or abdomen that are associated with domestic violence
- The presence of injuries, such as forearm fractures, bruising, marks to the back of shoulders or neck, or those of a defensive nature

(After Health Service Executive (2007) Domestic Abuse Guidelines for Hospital Staff. Dublin, HSE; Gibbons L (2011) Dealing with the effects of domestic violence. Emergency Nurse 19(4), 12–17)

Emergency care of the pregnant woman

History

As with other aspects of healthcare, an accurate history of events leading to ED attendance is imperative. In the case of a pregnant patient, a full obstetric history should be obtained as well as the history of the presenting complaint. Box 30.10 highlights the information needed for an obstetric history.

Assessment

General assessment should include baseline observations of pulse, blood pressure, respirations and temperature to detect signs of shock, infection or preeclampsia. Routine urinalysis should also be carried out for glucose and protein. The progress of the pregnancy should be assessed in terms of the height of the fundus compared with estimated gestation, and after about 14–16 weeks fetal heartbeat should be assessed. Any vaginal discharge or bleeding should only be assessed in terms of type, quality and odour. Vaginal examination should only be carried out if it is necessary to determine the state of the cervical os or to identify causes of fresh vaginal bleeding.

Box 30.10

Obtaining an obstetric history

- Number of previous pregnancies
  - terminations
  - miscarriages
  - live births – combinations in pregnancy, delivery, postnatal care
- This pregnancy
  - gestation
  - antenatal care
  - PV bleeding to date
  - other complications
  - ultrasound scans
  - fetal abnormality tests

Most patients receiving antenatal care in the UK have patient-held notes which contain a detailed account of their obstetric history.

During assessment and care, maternal health should be paramount whatever the gestation of the fetus.

Miscarriage

Miscarriage is also termed 'spontaneous abortion' and describes the delivery of a non-viable fetus before 24 weeks' gestation. There are six types of miscarriage and these are listed in Table 30.2.

Marquardt (2011) notes that women with threatened miscarriage can present at any point during the first 24 weeks of pregnancy and half of them will progress to actual miscarriage (Dighe et al. 2008). Patients may or may not report pain that is similar to period pain or cramps. This is due to the contraction of the uterus in response to irritation caused by the bleeding. In women with threatened miscarriage, the cervix is likely to be closed. In inevitable miscarriages, the os is usually open, due to dilation and there has been a partial loss of products of conception, which can be seen or felt through the os. Inevitable miscarriages present as complete miscarriages, in which all products of conception are passed, or as incomplete miscarriages, in which some products are retained (Wyatt et al. 2012). Where there is complete miscarriage the cervical os is closed and the uterus is small and contracted.

Where a cause is investigated, pathological abnormalities with the fetus or placenta are commonly found. Immunological incompatibility with the father, maternal infection, substance misuse and malnutrition have also been linked with spontaneous abortion (Reedy & Brucker 1995).

Despite the relative commonness of miscarriage, it can be devastating for the woman and her partner. Apart from the physical pain associated with miscarriage, the woman and her family are grieving for the loss of a baby, the dreams and plans they will have had for that baby, and their identity as a family. It is essential that ED nurses recognize the enormity of this loss and do not attempt to trivialize it with comments like 'you can have another', or by functional care avoiding conversation about the miscarriage. Parents want

Table 30.2 Categorization of miscarriage

Type	Bleeding	Passed tissue	Cervical os	Pain	Size of uterus
Threatened	Slight	No	Closed	Mild	Normal for gestation
Inevitable	Moderate-heavy	No	Open	Moderate-severe	Normal for gestation
Incomplete	Heavy	Yes	Open with tissue present	Severe	Smaller than expected for gestation
Complete	Slight	Yes	Closed	Mild	Smaller than expected for gestation
Missed	None	No	Closed	Nil	Smaller than expected for gestation
Septic	Varies, foul odour often accompanies loss	Sometimes	Open	Moderate-severe High temperature	Normal or small for dates

their loss acknowledged and it is much better for the nurse to express condolences for the loss of their baby (Olga & van den Akker 2011).

Assessment

This should revolve around maintaining maternal health, as little can be done to alter fetal prognosis. The patient's haemodynamic stability should be assessed, in terms of heart rate, respirations and blood pressure, as well as blood loss. When enquiring about blood loss, the nurse should seek to establish quantity in terms of the number of pads used per hour. The type of loss should also be noted, whether it is fresh or dark blood, and whether clots or tissue have been passed. This will help to determine the category of miscarriage occurring.

The amount and location of pain should be established, and appropriate analgesia given. A urine sample should be obtained to confirm pregnancy and to rule out urine infection as a cause of bleeding. Blood should also be taken to confirm rhesus status in case the patient is rhesus negative and anti-D serum is required. A vaginal examination will confirm the status of the cervical os, rule out a vaginal source for bleeding and identify any products of conception in the cervix or vagina. An ultrasound scan should be organized to confirm clinical findings, i.e., to identify a potentially viable pregnancy or retained products of conception. For humanitarian reasons, this should be done as soon as possible, as most patients and their partners need confirmation of a visible heartbeat to believe that everything is all right or, more commonly, they need the reinforcement that their baby is dead, or has been miscarried, in order to come to terms with their loss.

Management

In most cases of miscarriage, ED care revolves around symptomatic management and psychological support. If the patient shows signs of hypovolaemia, intravenous fluid replacement should be commenced. Adequate analgesia should be given, particularly if the pregnancy is not viable. If the miscarriage has been an incomplete or missed abortion, the patient should be prepared physically and emotionally for an evacuation of retained products of conception (ERPC) in theatre. Psychological support for both the woman and her partner is important throughout their stay in ED, as the initial handling of

their loss will impact on the grieving process they must work through (see also Chapter 14).

The use of the term 'spontaneous abortion' should be avoided at this time, as many people associate abortion with voluntary termination of pregnancy. Miscarriage, on the other hand, is seen as involuntary. Using the term abortion can therefore cause unnecessary distress (Olga & van den Akker 2011).

The length of the gestation may alter physical symptoms, but it does not alter emotional ones. All patients should be offered contact numbers for support groups or specialist counsellors. It is also useful to reinforce their need to grieve, and identify times which may be hard, such as the period around the baby's estimated delivery date. This helps the patient and her partner to legitimize their feelings. Some hospitals offer bereavement counselling and a book of remembrance for babies; others also offer the services of the hospital chaplain.

Ectopic pregnancy

The word ectopic comes from the Greek word for 'out of place'. Ectopic pregnancy (EP) describes any pregnancy implantation outside of the uterine cavity. Classification of EPs can be broadly divided into two main categories, tubal and non-tubal. The vast majority of EPs are tubal (95%). Although non-tubal EPs make up only 5% of all EPs, these disproportionately contribute to the morbidity and mortality associated with EPs (Winder et al. 2011) (Fig. 30.3). It is also an important cause of first trimester morbidity and mortality and accounts for 80% of first trimester maternal deaths (Lewis 2011), and EP currently accounts for 1% of all pregnancies (Winder et al. 2011).

A diagnosis of ectopic pregnancy should be considered in all women of childbearing age presenting with abdominal pain or an unexpected collapse (Moulton & Yates 2004). This ratio has risen over the last decade and indications are that it will continue to rise with the increase in PID and IUCD use (Shennon 2003).

The use of oral postcoital contraceptives and some fertility treatments also appear to increase the risk of ectopic pregnancy. Ectopic implantation appears to occur because of delay in passage of the fertilized egg. This passage is induced by muscular contraction and ciliary activity. If the fallopian tubes are damaged due to adhesions following infection, the ciliary

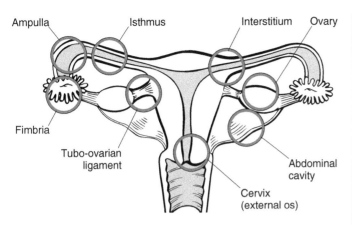

Figure 30.3 • Sites of implantation of ectopic pregnancies.

activity is reduced and the egg cannot pass into the uterus, so it implants in the tube. Hormonal changes of the corpus luteum continue as, physiologically, the pregnancy is still viable at this stage. As a result, the uterus grows and softens as it would with a normal uterine pregnancy. The products of conception continue to expand, causing pain and vaginal bleeding in a 'spotting' form. It is usually at this stage that the woman seeks health intervention. If left unchecked, the products of conception will continue to grow until rupture of the tube occurs and devastating haemorrhage follows (Fig. 30.3).

Assessment

Most patients will give a history of abdominal pain, sometimes unilateral or generalized lower abdomen and pelvic pain. The patient usually has intermittent vaginal bleeding or spotting and, as a result, may or may not be aware that she is pregnant. Most embryos die within 6–12 weeks of gestation due to lack of placental development. For this reason, most women with ectopic pregnancy suffer a lot less nausea than those with a uterine pregnancy with a healthy developing placenta. Once the embryo dies, endometrium is shed and a large PV bleed ensues. This is different to the potentially life-threatening haemorrhage that occurs with a ruptured fallopian tube. The degree of haemodynamic compromise determines the urgency of intervention, and therefore accurate assessment of basic haemostasis is vital. Slight tachycardia would be expected because of the emotion and anxiety attached to ectopic pregnancy, but bradycardia together with an increase in respirations and postural and persistent hypotension should be treated seriously. As part of the assessment, a urine and blood sample should be taken for serum human chorionic gonadotropin (hCG) testing to confirm pregnancy, and a transvaginal ultrasound scan will show the location of pregnancy after about five weeks' gestation. Table 30.3 highlights the clinical differences between a threatened miscarriage and an ectopic pregnancy.

Management

Early management revolves around symptom control and psychological support. Pain relief and routine intravenous access should be established via two large-bore cannulas. Blood samples are sent for group and cross-match, beta hCG, full blood

Table 30.3 Differential diagnosis of ectopic pregnancy vs. threatened miscarriage (after Stevens & Kenney 1994)

Symptom	Ectopic		Threatened miscarriage	
	Nature	Percentage of patients affected	Nature	Percentage of patients affected
Abdominal pain	General or affected side	90	Midline, crampy	10
Shoulder tip pain		26		None
General abdominal tenderness	General	45	Usually non-tender	
	Lower	25		
	Unilateral	30		
Vaginal bleeding	Light/ spotting	64	Light	100
Amenorrhoea		75		90
Uterus size	Normal	80	Right for dates	100
Shock		17		None
Dysuria		11		None
Rectal pain		9		None

(After Stevens L, Kenney A (1994) Emergencies in Obstetrics and Gynaecology. Oxford: Oxford University Press.)

count and coagulation studies. If the woman demonstrates signs of shock, fluid replacement should commence. Once the diagnosis has been made, using transvaginal/abdominal ultrasound and blood/urine hCG levels, treatment is prescribed dependent on the patient's haemodynamic status and gestation of pregnancy. In most instances, both haemodynamically stable and unstable patients can be managed by laparoscopy (Royal College of Obstetricians and Gynaecologists 2004).

Medical management of ectopic pregnancy reduces the need for surgical intervention in women who are haemodynamically stable and at an early stage of the pregnancy. This involves the use of cytotoxic intramuscular methotrexate, two dose regimen (Barnhart 2009), administered using special safety precautions for its preparation, administration and disposal. As the embryo is one of the fastest growing cells in the body the proliferating trophoblastic tissue is very sensitive to the action of methotrexate, causing cell death and dissolution. Close monitoring of beta hCG levels by the gynaecological team is required to ensure this treatment has been successful (Miller & Griffin 2003). Local injections of prostaglandins and laparoscopic injections of hyperosmolar glucose solutions have also been used successfully with fewer side-effects. Conservative surgical management involves the removal of the conceptus via laparoscopic salpingostomy, conserving the fallopian tube. In cases where the conceptus has implanted within the fimbrial region of the fallopian tube, fimbrial evacuation may be considered. These procedures carry an increased risk of future ectopic pregnancies because of scarred tissue. If salpingostomy is not possible, the fallopian tube is removed to prevent tubal rupture, with obvious implications for future fertility.

If ectopic rupture is suspected, the patient should be considered to have a life-threatening condition. Ruptured ectopic pregnancy is the highest single cause of maternal death. Death usually occurs as a result of uncontrolled haemorrhage. This is because occult bleeding into the abdominal cavity can occur as well as PV loss; therefore, blood loss can be underestimated. The patient compensates initially, then becomes rapidly shocked. It is important to commence vigorous fluid resuscitation. Urgent surgical intervention is necessary to preserve maternal life.

The woman and her partner's psychological needs should not be overlooked. As well as the physical distress, they are also coming to terms with the loss of their baby and the threat to future fertility that surgery brings. The nurse needs to acknowledge, not minimize, these feelings. A full description of psychological care and appropriate follow-up is given in the section on miscarriage.

As the mortality rate for deaths from ectopic pregnancy continues to rise, the confidential enquiry into maternal and child health 2000—2002 found that of those who died as a result of ectopic pregnancy, 66% were assessed as having had some form of substandard care. As a result the Royal College of Obstetricians and Gynaecologists (2004) set out recommendations for EDs. They advised that ectopic pregnancy should be excluded in all women of childbearing age with unexplained abdominal pain. Furthermore all clinicians, including undergraduate medical and nursing students, need to be made aware of the typical and atypical presentations of ectopic pregnancy and how it may mimic gastrointestinal disease (Lewis 2011).

Pre-eclampsia/eclampsia

Pre-eclampsia, or pregnancy-induced hypertension, complicates about 10% of all pregnancies and is associated with increased risk of adverse fetal, neonatal and maternal outcomes, including preterm birth, intrauterine growth restriction, perinatal death, acute renal or hepatic failure, antepartum haemorrhage, postpartum haemorrhage and maternal death (Steegers et al. 2010). Worldwide, pre-eclampsia/eclampsia is one of the three leading causes of maternal morbidity and mortality (Ghulmiyyah & Sibai 2012).

Its causes have not been proven, however, pre-eclampsia is known to have hereditary elements (Williams & Broughton Pipkin 2011). Other theories link eclampsia to a possible immunological cause where an antigenic reaction to the fetus causes maternal symptoms. Historic linkage of eclampsia to socioeconomic status has no foundation in research. Women most susceptible to pre-eclampsia/eclampsia are those at either end of the child-bearing age range, i.e., younger than

16 or older than 35 years of age. It is most common in first pregnancies and in those women expecting twins or more, and there appears to be a familial link. Women with pre-existing health problems, such as diabetes and chronic hypertension, are more susceptible to pre-eclampsia.

The disease usually has a gradual onset, the pre-eclampsia phase. Because of good antenatal screening, most patients are identified and treated early. Therefore, the use of ED for care in the pre-eclampsic phase is uncommon, but it is important to understand the disease process in order to treat life-threatening eclampsia in ED. Pre-eclampsia has a multisystem impact (Box 30.11).

Box 30.11

Multisystem impact of pre-eclampsia/eclampsia

Cardiovascular
- Hypertension – increased peripheral resistance
- Damage to blood vessels – vasopression traumatizes vessels and induces coagulopathy
- Haemorrhage – due to reduced platelets

Haematological
- Thrombocytopenia – results from coagulopathy and reduces platelets and fibrinogen activity
- Abnormal clotting
- Disseminating intravascular coagulopathy

Renal
- Impaired glomerular function – glomerular filtration rate (GFR) and renal blood flow are increased in pregnancy; with pre-eclampsia a decrease occurs
- Proteinuria – due to renal impairment
- Sodium/potassium retention – contributes to oedema
- Acute renal failure

Neurological
- Headache – due to cerebral oedema. In severe cases cerebral infarct/haemorrhage may occur
- Hyperreflexia – nerve-end irritation due to vasospasm
- Visual disturbance – due to retinal oedema; can lead to retinal detachment
- Convulsions – late sign of eclampsia

Respiratory
- Pulmonary oedema – due to cardiovascular and renal complications
- Haemorrhage – due to thrombocytopenia

Hepatic
- Abnormal liver enzymes
- Periportal haemorrhage – secondary to other system changes
- Infarction
- Rupture

Placental/fetal
- Placental infarction
- Abruptio placentae
- Fetal intrauterine growth retardation
- Fetal death

Pre-eclampsia

A triad of symptoms exists:

- hypertension – 30 mmHg or more above the woman's usual systolic BP or 15 mmHg above her usual diastolic BP
- proteinuria
- oedema – where this is present in the face or upper limbs it is of greater concern. Lower limb oedema, particularly of the feet or ankles, is usually mechanical in nature.

If any two of these symptoms are present, the woman is considered to have pre-eclampsia. Persistent hypertension should be treated, and initially close maternal and fetal monitoring will necessitate admission.

Eclampsia

This is usually defined as the onset of seizures in pregnancy occurring after 21 weeks' gestation or within 10 days of delivery. It is accompanied by at least two of the following signs: hypertension, proteinuria and oedema. Later signs include thrombocytopenia of raised aspartate amino transferase. Eclampsia is one of the main causes of maternal deaths, occurring in approximately 1 in 2000 pregnancies (Munro 2000). Prior to fitting, most patients complain of headache, visual disturbance, shortness of breath or right hypochondriacal pain. They may also have oliguria and appear confused. These symptoms are all derived from the physiological processes described in Box 30.11. While some women present to the ED at this stage, more appear as emergency admissions once fitting has commenced. Staff should be alert to the possibility of a concealed pregnancy in young women who have no previous history of seizures. Eclampsic fitting is life-threatening to both the mother and fetus. It must be brought under control rapidly using small doses of diazepam, 10 mg i.v. repeated up to five times. It is administered in this manner to prevent fetal depression. Intravenous infusion of chlormethiazole or phenytoin should also be considered. Occasionally, short-term ventilation and paralysis may be necessary. Other presentations of impending eclampsia include severe right hypochondriacal pain and shock as a result of hepatic rupture.

Urgent laparotomy is indicated to control haemorrhage and preserve maternal life. In these circumstances, however, it has a mortality of about 70%. Symptoms of disseminating intravascular coagulopathy (DIC) accompany about 7% of eclampsic conditions (Stevens & Kenney 1994). Once pre-eclampsia reaches this stage, or fitting has occurred, urgent preparation to deliver the fetus should be made. Delivery usually resolves maternal symptoms, although in some cases they may persist for up to 10 days (Reedy & Brucker 1995). The baby has a greater chance of survival even if delivered premature.

Abruptio placentae

This is more commonly treated in obstetric units than in EDs. It occurs as a result of premature separation of the placenta from the uterine wall and is an obstetric emergency and is a major risk factor for foetal and perinatal mortality and morbidity (Jabeen 2010). Haemorrhage and blood usually track between the uterus and placental membranes, causing PV bleeding and pain. Bleeding can be occult in about 10% of cases, and therefore diagnosis should not be made simply by the presence of PV bleeding. A pelvic ultrasound should be used to confirm diagnosis. Predisposing factors include substance misuse, pre-eclampsia, a maternal age of 35 or more, multiple gestation and as a result of trauma.

Emergency childbirth

The majority of births are normal deliveries requiring little assistance and the duration of labour is usually long enough for the woman to seek maternity care. Occasionally, however, it is necessary to deliver a baby in the ED if there is insufficient time to reach the delivery unit. The most common causes of emergency childbirth include multiparous women with precipitous (rapid) deliveries and adolescent girls who successfully conceal their pregnancy until they present with abdominal pains or do not recognize the signs of active labour. Some women in pre-term labour may also have precipitous deliveries. Child protection issues may be raised in cases where a woman whose child may be at risk may choose to avoid traditional routes of maternity care and travel to a hospital outside of their area, presenting to EDs in labour (McLoughlin 2001).

Labour can be described as a process by which the fetus, placenta and membranes are expelled through the birth canal. Normal labour begins spontaneously at approximately 40 weeks' gestation, referred to as 'term', with the fetus presenting by the head or 'vertex'. Box 30.12 outlines the stages of labour.

Box 30.12

The three stages of labour

First stage

This is the longest phase during which the body prepares for delivery. The cervix effaces then dilates. There is usually a pink, mucous 'show' as this begins, and the amniotic membranes rupture as the cervix dilates. If this has not already occurred, contractions gradually increase in frequency and intensity. Transition to second stage occurs once the cervix is fully dilated to 10 cm. This phase usually lasts several hours, however the time reduces with the number of pregnancies.

Second stage

This is from full dilation until after delivery of the baby. During this phase, the baby's head travels down the birth canal. When it reaches the outlet, it flexes to present occiput first. This is a complicated but natural process. The visible occiput is termed 'crowning' and highlights the imminence of delivery. The head is followed by the shoulders, then the trunk and legs. This usually lasts up to one hour.

Third stage

This is from the delivery of the baby until complete delivery of the placenta and membranes and control of haemorrhage.

First-stage labour management

The nurse's role in the care of a woman facing imminent childbirth is to provide physical and emotional support in a calm, relaxed manner (McCormack 2009). The nurse should obtain enough information to assess the woman's immediate circumstances:

- what parity is the woman?
- at what gestation is the pregnancy?
- what signs of onset of labour has she experienced?
- has she a history of precipitous labour?
- what are the frequency and duration of the contractions?

The assistance of a midwife, obstetric and neonatal team should be obtained immediately, and provision for the imminent birth should be made. Signs of imminent childbirth include:

- the mother experiences tension, anxiety and intense contractions
- blood 'show' as a result of rapid dilation of the cervix
- bulging or gaping of the anus as a result of descent of the fetal presenting part
- bulging or fullness of the perineum
- 'crowning' of the fetal head at the introitus, which occurs when the fetal skull escapes under the pubic arch and no longer recedes (Fig. 30.4)
- the mother saying 'the baby is coming'.

In multiparous women, the last sign is symptomatic of imminent birth; however, in primiparous women, birth may take up to 30 minutes. Birth is near when the head stays visible between contractions. The mother should be made to feel in control, protecting her dignity, and should be kept informed of all that is happening. Her partner should be included as a source of constant support and encouragement to the mother at this time. The mother should be encouraged to adopt a position which is most comfortable for her, which is usually sitting on the trolley with her back well supported with pillows or a foam wedge. Nitrous oxide is the preferred method of pain relief when birth is imminent and the mother should be encouraged to inhale the gas while she is feeling the contractions. As well as providing pain relief, it is also an effective means of providing extra oxygen to both the mother and

the fetus. Neither shaving, urinary catheterization nor enema administration are required (Priestly 2004).

Baseline recordings of maternal temperature, pulse, respirations and blood pressure should be obtained. The fetal heartbeat is also recorded and may be auscultated using a fetal stethoscope or fetal Doppler when the head is presenting. The fetal heart sounds are more commonly located close to the midline below the umbilicus. The normal fetal heart rate is between 120 and 160 beats/min. A further assessment of fetal condition includes observation of the amniotic fluid or 'waters'; these are normally straw-coloured, but they may become green as a result of meconium.

Second-stage labour management

The attending nurse/midwife should open a sterile delivery set and wash the woman's vulva with sterile swabs and warmed antiseptic solution. With the next contraction, the woman should be encouraged to inhale deeply and bear down to facilitate the delivery. The nurse should place his/her fingers over the advancing head to prevent expulsive 'crowning', which may result in perineal tearing and a heightened risk of intraventricular haemorrhage to the newborn infant (Fig. 30.5). As the fetal head advances and gradually distends the perineal tissue, the mother should be encouraged to pant to facilitate a controlled delivery and reduce maternal trauma. Once the baby's head emerges, the nurse should slip a finger over the occiput to feel if the cord is round the baby's neck. If this has happened, the cord should be released either by slipping it over the head or, if this is unsuccessful, by applying two artery forceps 2–5 cm apart and cutting the cord between them.

The nurse should continue to support the head, taking care not to put any traction on it (Fig. 30.6). Mucus should be removed with a sterile swab, but the eyes should not be cleansed due to the risk of infection. At the next contraction, the anterior shoulder should be delivered by gentle downward traction of the head. Then the baby should be raised and the posterior shoulder will deliver rapidly, followed by the trunk and legs. The baby should be dried and placed in a warm towel, as a cold baby has an increased oxygen consumption and cold babies more easily become hypoglycaemic and acidotic; they also have an increased mortality (Advanced Life Support Group 2011). The newborn baby should be allowed to lie on the bed or be placed on the mother's abdomen,

Figure 30.4 • Cross-sectional view of crowning.

Figure 30.5 • Hold infant's head gently in both hands.

allowing her to see and touch the baby. The umbilical cord should be clamped and cut if this has not already been done and syntometrine given intramuscularly to the mother. This contains oxytocin and ergometrine. The oxytocin provides marked uterine contraction after approximately three minutes but is short-lived, and as its effects begin to wear off the ergometrine begins to act and provide longer-lasting uterine contractions, reducing the risk of postpartum haemorrhage.

The time of the delivery and those involved in it should be recorded accurately. The Apgar score should also be recorded. This is a numerical scoring system used to assess the newborn baby's condition at one minute after birth and reassessed again after five minutes. The factors assessed are heart rate, respiratory rate, muscle tone, reflex response to stimulus, and colour (Finster & Wood 2005). A score of 0–2 is given to each sign in accordance with the guideline in Table 30.4. A normal infant in good condition at birth will achieve an Apgar score of between 7 and 10. A score below 7 indicates some degree of asphyxia which requires some form of resuscitation.

Third-stage labour management

The third stage of labour is from delivery of the baby to delivery of the placenta and usually takes about 5–20 minutes. A sterile receiver should be placed between the woman's thighs to collect any blood lost, and the umbilical cord is placed in the

Figure 30.6 • Carefully support infant's head as it is born.

receiver. Once the signs of placental separation are observed, i.e., lengthening of the umbilical cord, a fresh gush of blood and contraction of the uterus causing the fundus to rise to the level of the umbilicus, the mother should be asked to bear down as for delivery to expel the placenta and membranes. Once delivered, the placenta should be examined for completeness. The fundus of the uterus may be massaged to promote contractions, expel blood clots and control haemorrhage. The woman's vagina and perineum should be examined for tearing, which may require suturing. The mother's temperature, pulse and blood pressure should be recorded and her lochia, i.e., PV loss, observed. The baby should also be examined, weighed and have a rectal temperature taken. Two identity bands should also be placed on the baby. Both mother and baby should then be transferred to the nearest maternity unit for post-natal care.

Postpartum haemorrhage

Postpartum haemorrhage (PPH) is a major cause of maternal deaths around the world. The incidence of PPH is between 2 and 11% (Oyelese et al. 2007, Lombaard & Pattinson 2009). It can be described as any bleeding from the genital tract that adversely affects the mother's condition following the birth of a baby, up to 6 weeks post-delivery. A blood loss of 500 mL or more at delivery is regarded as PPH, irrespective of maternal condition. There are two types of PPH:

- primary PPH, which occurs within the first 24 hours post-delivery
- secondary PPH, which occurs at any time after the first 24 hours, up to 6 weeks post-delivery, but most commonly occurs between 7 and 14 days postpartum. It can be described as bleeding in excess of the normal lochial loss and may be associated with retained placental tissue or uterine infection.

Assessment

History should include the following information:

- duration of symptoms
- quantity of bleeding in terms of number of pads used per hour
- type of blood loss, i.e., red, brown clots
- type of pain
- location of pain
- date of delivery and any subsequent period/PV bleeding
- any infection
- any trauma
- other related medical history.

The woman will have an enlarged, 'boggy', uterus. On palpation the uterus will feel soft, distended and lacking in tone. The fundal height will rise above the umbilicus as a result of retained blood in the uterus preventing uterine contraction. A low-grade pyrexia, rising pulse and falling blood pressure characterize postpartum haemorrhage, together with lower back and abdominal pain, and general restlessness.

Table 30.4 Apgar scores			
Factor	**Score**		
	0	1	2
A – appearance (colour)	Blue	Blue limbs, pink body	Pink
P – pulse (heart rate)	Absent	<100 beats/min	>100 beats/min
G – grimace (muscle tone)	Limp	Some flexion	Good flexion
A – activity (reflexes irritable)	Absent	Some motion	Good motion
R – respiratory effort	Absent	Weak cry	Strong cry

Sanitary pads should be checked to evaluate the amount of bleeding and note the presence or absence of clots or odour.

Management

The aim of ED management is to control haemorrhage and maintain blood volume. Blood should be taken for group and cross-match, and large-bore i.v. lines for warmed crystalloids and blood should be established. Oxygen should also be administered. An i.v. injection of ergometrine or syntometrine may be given in order to cause uterine contraction, which assists in haemorrhage control. If the uterus is palpable, it may be massaged to enable it to contract and expel any clots. The presence of retained products of conception should be excluded on pelvic ultrasound. If debris is found or haemorrhage is not controlled, urgent ERCP should be performed in theatre.

Conclusion

This chapter has considered the common gynaecological and obstetric reasons for presentation to the ED. Many of these conditions have a life-long impact on the patient and her family, in terms of either physical or, more commonly, psychological well-being. It is imperative that ED staff are sensitive to the needs of the woman and her partner, and can offer privacy and compassionate, non-judgemental care. Inappropriate assessment or intervention can have catastrophic consequences. The information provided in this chapter should enable the nurse to make an informed assessment and plan therapeutic care for this emotionally and physically vulnerable group.

References

Advanced Life Support Group, 2011. Advanced Paediatric Life Support: The Practical Approach. West Sussex, Wiley-Blackwell.

Barnhart, K.T., 2009. Ectopic pregnancy. The New England Journal of Medicine 361 (4), 379–387.

Bickley, L.S., Szilagyi, P.G., 2003. Bates' Guide to Physical Examination and History Taking, eighth ed. Lippincott, Williams & Wilkins, Philadelphia.

Black, K.I., 2009. Developments and challenges in emergency contraception. Best Practice & Research Clinical Obstetrics & Gynaecology 223 (2), 221–231.

Boursnell, M., Prosser, S., 2010. Increasing identification of domestic violence in emergency departments: a collaborative contribution to increasing the quality of practice of emergency nurses. Contemporary Nurse 35 (1), 35–46.

Bryan, S., 2004. Pelvic inflammatory disease. In: Cameron, P., Jelinek, G., Kelly, A.M., Murray, L., Brown, A.F.T., Heyworth, J. (Eds.), Textbook of Adult Emergency Medicine, second ed. Churchill Livingstone, Edinburgh.

Burgess, A., Holmstrom, L., 1974. Rape: Victims of Crisis. RJ Brady, Maryland.

College of Emergency Medicine, 2011. Management of Adult Patients who attend Emergency Departments after Sexual Assault and/or Rape. College of Emergency Medicine, London.

Confidential Enquiry into Maternal, Child Health, 2004. Maternity Services in 2002 for Women with Type 1 and Type 2 Diabetes, England, Wales and Northern Ireland. CEMACH, London.

Dighe, M., Cuevas, C., Moshiri, et al., 2008. Sonography in first trimester bleeding. Journal of Clinical Ultrasound 36 (6), 352–366.

Finster, M., Wood, M., 2005. The Apgar Score has survived the test of time. Anesthesiology 102, 855–857.

Fitzpatrick, M., Ta, A., Lenchus, J., et al., 2012. Sexual assault forensic nurses' training and assessment using simulation technology. Journal of Emergency Nursing 38 (1), 85–90.

Flately, J., Kershaw, C., Smith, K., et al., 2010. Crime in England and Wales 2009/10. Home Office, London.

French, C.E., Hughes, G., Nicholson, A., et al., 2011. Estimation of the rate of pelvic inflammatory disease diagnoses: Trends in England, 2000–2008. Sexual Transmitted Diseases 38 (3), 158–162.

French, K., Ward, S., McRae, J., et al., 2004. Emergency contraception. Nursing Standard 18 (42), 49–53.

Ghulmiyyah, L., Sibai, B., 2012. Maternal mortality from preeclampsia/eclampsia. Seminars in Perinatology 36 (1), 56–59.

Gibbons, L., 2011. Dealing with the effects of domestic violence. Emergency Nurse 19 (4), 12–17.

Haider, Z., Condrus, G., Kirk, E., et al., 2007. The simple outpatient management of Bartholin's abscess using Word catheter: A preliminary study. Australia and New Zealand Journal of Obstetrics and Gynaecology 47 (2), 137–140.

Health Service Executive, 2007. Domestic Abuse Guidelines for Hospital Staff. HSE, Dublin.

Holloway, M., 1994. Care of the sexually assaulted woman. Emergency Nurse 2 (3), 18–20.

Home Office, 2003. Sexual Offences Act. HMSO, London.

Horne, A.W., Critchley, H.O.D., 2012. Menstrual problems: Heavy menstrual bleeding and primary dysmennorrhoea. In: Edmonds, D.K. (Ed.), Dewhurst's Textbook of Obstetrics and Gynaecology, eighth ed. John Wiley and Sons Ltd., London.

Jabeen, M., 2010. Abruptio placentae: Risk factors and perinatal outcome. Journal of Postgraduate Medicine Institute 18 (4), 669–676.

Kearns, N., Coen, L., Canavan, J., 2008. Domestic Violence in Ireland: An Overview of National Strategic Policy and Relevant International Literature on Prevention and Intervention Initiatives in Service Provision. Child and Family Research Centre, Galway.

Kelly, L., 2002. A Research Review on the Reporting, Investigation and Prosecution of Rape Cases. HMCPSI, London.

Lewis G (ed) (2011) Saving Mothers' lives: Reviewing maternal deaths to make motherhood safer - 2006-2008. The Eighth Report of the Confidential Enquiries into Maternal Deaths in the United Kingdom. British Journal of Obstetrics and Gynaecology 118 Supp 1, 1–205

Lichtman, R., Papera, S., 1990. Gynecology: Well Woman Care. Appleton & Lange, Norwalk, CT.

Lombaard, H., Pattinson, R.C., 2009. Common errors and remedies in managing postpartum haemorrhage. Best Practice & Research Clinical Obstetrics and Gynaecology 23, 317–326.

Lovett, J., Kelly, L., 2009. Different Systems, SImilar Outcomes: Tracking Attrition in Reported Rape Cases Across Europe. London Metropolitan University, London.

Lovett, J., Regan, L., Kelly, L., 2004. Sexual Assault Referral Centres. Developing Good Practice and Maximising Potentials: Home Office Research Study 285. Home Office, London.

Markowitz, J.R., Steer, S., Garland, M., 2005. Hospital-based intervention for intimate partner violence victims: a forensic nursing model. Journal of Emergency Nursing 31 (2), 166–170.

Marquardt, U., 2011. Management of miscarriage and ectopic pregnancy. Emergency Nurse 19 (7), 29–35.

Martinez, F., Lopez-Arregui, E., 2009. Infection risk and intrauterine devices. Acta Obstetricia et Gynecologica 88 (3), 246–250.

McCormack, C., 2009. The first stage of labour: physiology and early care. In: Fraser, D.M., Cooper, M.A. (Eds.), Myles Textbook for Midwives, fifteenth ed. Churchill Livingstone, Edinburgh.

McGrath, M., 2010. Rape Trauma Syndrome and the investigation of sexual assault. In: Savino, J.O., Turvey, B.E. (Eds.), Rape Investigation Handbook, second ed. Academic Press, London.

McLoughlin, A.M.P., 2001. Unexpected birth in A&E departments. Accident and Emergency Nursing 9, 242–248.

Miller, J.H., Griffin, E., 2003. Methotrexate administration for ectopic pregnancy in the Emergency Department: one hospital's protocol/competencies. Journal of Emergency Nursing 29 (3), 240–244.

Moulton, C., Yates, D., 2004. Obstetric, Gynaecological Genitourinary and Perinal Problems. Emergency Medicine, second ed. Blackwell Science Ltd., London.

Munro, P.T., 2000. Management of eclampsia in the Accident and Emergency Department. Journal of Accident and Emergency Medicine 17 (1), 7–11.

Olga, B.A., van den Akker, 2011. The psychological and social consequences of miscarriage. Expert Review of Obstetrics & Gynecology 6 (3), 295–304.

Olshansky, E., 2002. Emergency care of women who were abused was driven by the prevailing practice pattern of effective patient processing. Evidence Based Nursing 5 (1), 29.

Oyelese, Y., Scorza, W.E., Mastrolia, R., et al., 2007. Postpartum hemorrhage. Obstetric & Gynecology Clinics of North America 34, 421–441.

Povey, D., Coleman, K., Kaiza, P., et al., 2009. Homicides, Firearm Offences and Intimate Violence 2007/08 (Supplementary Volume 2 to Crime in England and Wales 2007/08). Home Office Statistical Bulletin 02/09. Home Office, London.

Priestly, S., 2004. Emergency delivery. In: Cameron, P., Jelinek, G., Kelly, A.M., Murray, L., Brown, A.F.T., Heyworth, J. (Eds.), Textbook of Adult Emergency Medicine, second ed. Churchill Livingstone, Edinburgh.

Reedy, N., Brucker, M., 1995. Emergencies in gynecology and obstetrics. In: Kitt, S., Selfridge-Thomas, J., Proehl, J.A., Kaiser, J. (Eds.), Emergency Nursing: A Physiologic and Clinical Perspective, second ed. WB Saunders, Philadelphia.

Royal College of Obstetricians and Gynaecologists, 2004. The Management of Tubal Pregnancy (Guideline 21). RCOG, London.

Sacchetti, A., 2009. Pelvic inflammatory disease. In: Wolfson, A.B., Hendey, G.W., Ling, L.J., Rosen, C.L., Schaider, J.J., Sharieff, G.Q. (Eds.), Harwood-Nuss' Clinical Practice of Emergency Medicine, fifth ed. Lipincott Wilkins & Williams, Philadelphia.

Salhan, S., 2011. Dysmenorrhea and chronic pelvic pain. In: Salhan, S. (Ed.), Textbook of Gynaecology. Jaypee Brothers Medical Publishers, New Delhi.

Sanders Jordan, K., 2009. Gynecologic emergencies. In: Howard, P.K., Steinmann, R.A. (Eds.), Sheehy's Emergency Nursing: Principles and Practice, sixth ed. Mosby Elsevier, St Louis.

Schofield, S., 2006. Body of evidence. Emergency Nurse 13 (9), 9–11.

Shennon, A.H., 2003. Recent developments in obstetrics. British Medical Journal 327, 604–608.

Steegers, E.A., von Dadelszen, P., Duvekot, J.J., et al., 2010. Pre-eclampsia. Lancet 376, 631–644.

Stevens, L., Kenney, A., 1994. Emergencies in Obstetrics and Gynaecology. Oxford University Press, Oxford.

Task Force on Postovulatory Method of Fertility Regulation, 1998. Randomized controlled trial of levonorgestrel versus Yupze regimen of combined oral contraceptives of emergency contraception. Lancet 352, 428–433.

Trent, M., Bass, D., Ness, R., et al., 2011. Recurrent PID, Subsequent STI, and reproductive health outcomes: Findings from the PID Evaluation and Clinical Health (PEACH) Study. Sexually Transmitted Diseases 38 (9), 879–881.

Walby, S., Allen, J., 2004. Domestic Violence, Sexual Assault and Stalking: Findings from the British Crime Survey. Home Office, London.

Wechter, M.E., Wu, J., Marzano, D., et al., 2009. Management of Bartholin Duct Cysts and Abscesses: A Systematic Review. Obstetrical & Gynaecological Survey 64 (6), 395–404.

Williams, P.J., Broughton Pipkin, F., 2011. The genetics of pre-eclampsia and others hypertensive disorders of pregnancy. Best Practice & Researach Clinical Obstetrics and Gynaecology 25 (4), 405–417.

Winder, S., Reid, S., Condous, G., 2011. Ultrasound diagnosis of ectopic pregnancy. Australasian Journal of Ultrasound Medicine 14 (2), 29–33.

Wyatt, J., Illingworth, R., Graham, C., et al., 2012. Oxford Handbook of Emergency Medicine, fourth ed. Oxford University Press, Oxford.

Ophthalmic emergencies

31

Janet Marsden

CHAPTER CONTENTS

http://dx.doi.org/10.1016/B978-0-7020-4315-4.00031-0

Introduction

A significant proportion, generally around 6% of the workload of the Emergency Department (ED), is made up of patients with ophthalmic problems (Ezra et al. 2005). Tan et al. (1997) found a lack of basic ophthalmic training for ED Senior House Officers leading to a lack of confidence on their part in the management of eye emergencies. This lack of confidence on the part of junior doctors is reflected in the nursing teams of many EDs, although Ezra et al. (2005) found that nurses were significantly more accurate than junior doctors in their assessment of ED patients, and combined with the apparent health of many ophthalmic patients, can lead to inappropriate management in the ED.

Being able to see and make a visual assessment of surroundings is taken for granted by most people and the sudden decline in or loss of sight is an extremely frightening experience. In the ED, patients attend with acute and chronic ophthalmic conditions of varying degrees of severity. For some, immediate intervention can be sight-saving. This chapter will equip ED nurses to assess, identify and initiate care for patients with common ophthalmic conditions. Knowledge of the anatomy and physiology of the eye and surrounding structures will aid nurses in using mechanism of injury, signs and symptoms to assess the patient's condition.

The chapter will address ophthalmic conditions in terms of assessment findings, which can be broadly categorized into two groups:

- trauma
- non-traumatic red eye.

Anatomy and physiology of the eye (Fig. 31.1)

Orbit

The orbit is a large bony socket that contains the eyeball or globe with its associated muscles, nerves, blood vessels, fat and most of the lacrimal apparatus. Each of the two orbits is roughly pyramidal in shape with the apex lying posteriorly. The orbit is made up of seven individual bones: the maxilla, palatine, zygoma, sphenoid, frontal, ethmoid and lacrimal bones.

Eyelids

The lids are layered structures covered on their outer surfaces by skin and on their inner surfaces by conjunctiva (Fig. 31.2).

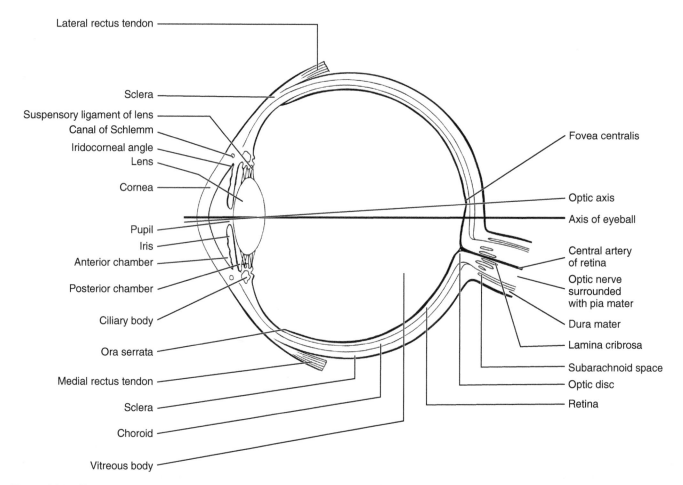

Figure 31.1 • Basic structure of the eye.

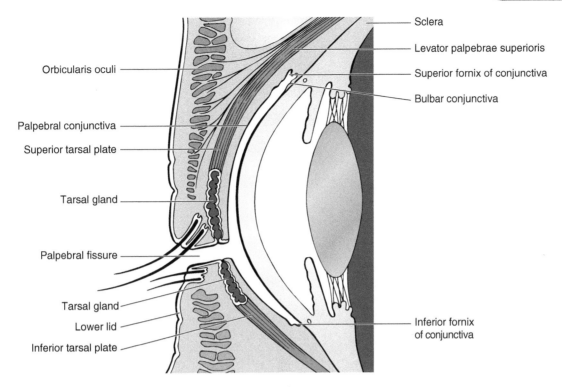

Figure 31.2 • Lids and conjunctival fornices.

In between is subcutaneous tissue, the orbital septum of which thickens within the lids to form fibrous tarsal plates that give structure to the lid. The upper lid contains the levator muscle and the lower contains the inferior tarsal muscle, which retracts it. The lids are maintained in position by the medial and lateral canthal tendons that attach to the periosteum. The lids are closed by the orbicularis muscle.

Within the lid structure are a number of glands. Tarsal or Meibomian glands are arranged perpendicular to the lid margin on the conjunctival surface of the tarsal plate; when blocked and infected, these are known as chalazia (singular, chalazion). The eyelashes are more numerous on the upper lid than on the lower. Sebaceous and modified sweat glands open into each lash follicle – infection produces a hordeolum or stye.

Behind the lashes is the join between the conjunctiva and the skin of the lids. This is known as the grey line because of its relative avascularity. The lids protect the eye by preventing contact with foreign bodies and by preventing drying of the cornea and conjunctiva. Lid closure and blinking help to spread the tear film over the front of the eye and move it into the lacrimal drainage apparatus.

Lacrimal system

The tear film is composed mainly of watery fluid from the lacrimal gland (99%), which is situated in the lacrimal fossa of the frontal bone in the orbit. The other important components of the tear film are mucin from the conjunctival goblet cells and oil from the Meibomian (tarsal) glands and the glands of Möll and Zeiss. The tear film is distributed over the surface of the eye by gravity, capillary action of the puncta and canaliculi and the eyelids. The tears leave the eye by evaporation and by way of the puncta, the upper of which takes around 30% of the unevaporated tears and the lower around 70%. From the puncta, the tears flow into the canaliculi, into the common canaliculus and then into the lacrimal sac and through the nasolacrimal duct (Fig. 31.3).

Conjunctiva

The conjunctiva is a thin, transparent mucous membrane lining the inner surface of the eyelid (palpebral conjunctiva), reflecting back on itself at the upper and lower fornices and covering the sclera as far as the corneoscleral junction (bulbar conjunctiva). The conjunctiva is adherent to the lid and rather less so to the Tenon's capsule overlying the sclera. It is most adherent at the corneoscleral junction (limbus). The conjunctiva is quite mobile in the fornices and over the globe and can absorb a large volume of fluid and become oedematous. The epithelium of the conjunctiva is continuous with the corneal epithelium. It contains goblet cells which secrete mucus. The main body of the conjunctiva is connective tissue housing blood vessels, nerves and other glands.

Cornea

The transparent cornea forms the anterior one-sixth of the globe. Its curvature is higher than that of the rest of the globe and it is the main structure responsible for the refraction of light entering the eye. It is an avascular structure which is

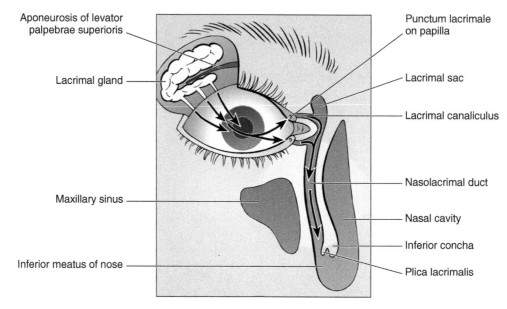

Figure 31.3 • Lacrimal system showing tear production and drainage.

nourished by the aqueous humour, the capillaries at its edge and from the tear film. Microscopically, it consists of five layers:

- the epithelium – consists of five layers of cells centrally, ten or more at the limbus. Running between the cells are the nerve endings of sensory nerve fibres, which are sensitive mainly to pain. The epithelium regenerates by the movement of cells from the periphery towards the middle
- Bowman's layer – is acellular and consists of collagen fibres
- substantia propria or stroma – comprises 90% of the thickness of the cornea. It is transparent and fibrous, and is made up of lamellae of collagen fibres arranged parallel to the surface. This arrangement ensures corneal clarity
- Descemet's membrane – a strong membrane which is the basement membrane of the endothelium
- endothelium – a single layer of flattened cells which plays a major role in controlling the hydration of the cornea by a barrier and active transport method. Loss of endothelial cells leads to corneal oedema and lack of clarity.

Sclera

Sclera forms the posterior five-sixths of the eye. It is 1 mm thick posteriorly and thinnest (0.3 mm) immediately posterior to the insertion of the recti muscles. The sclera forms the 'white' of the eye; its outer surface is smooth, except for where the six orbital muscles are attached. It is perforated posteriorly by the optic nerve at an area known as the lamina cribrosa. In this area, the sclera forms a meshwork rather than a solid structure to allow nerve fibres and the central retinal artery and vein to pass through it. The sclera is weakened at this point. Raised intraocular pressure can make the lamina cribrosa bulge outwards, producing a cupped disc.

The sclera is composed of two main layers: the episclera, a loose connective tissue that provides most of the nutritional support of the sclera via a vascular plexus; and the main body of the sclera, which is a dense fibrous tissue that is relatively avascular. The function of the sclera is to protect the intraocular contents and preserve the shape of the globe, maintaining the placement of the optical system. It provides the insertion for the muscles.

The uveal tract

The uveal tract is composed of the iris, the ciliary body and the choroid. The iris is a thin-pigmented diaphragm with a central aperture or pupil. It is located between the cornea and the lens. The pupil varies in size from 1–8 mm and differs in size on the two sides in 25% of 'normal' people. The iris divides the anterior segment into anterior and posterior chambers. Its periphery is attached to the ciliary body. The colour of the iris is produced by pigment in melanocytes within its structure. The main body of the iris consists of highly vascular connective tissue; it also contains nerve fibres, the muscle of the sphincter pupillae and the dilator pupillae. The sphincter forms a ring of smooth muscle around the pupil. When it contracts in bright light and during accommodation, the pupil constricts. The dilator is a thin layer of muscle extending from the iris root to the sphincter pupillae. When the dilator pupillae contracts in low-intensity light and during sympathetic activity such as fear, the pupil enlarges.

The ciliary body is continuous with the choroid and the margin of the iris. It contains the ciliary muscle used to change the shape of the lens during accommodation. Its outer, pigmented layer is continuous with the retinal pigment epithelium. Its inner, non-pigmented layer produces aqueous humour. The lens attaches to the ciliary body by a suspensory ligament whose fibres are known as zonules.

The choroid is a thin, soft, brown coat covering the inner surface of the sclera. It extends from the optic nerve to the ciliary body at the ora serrata. The inner surface of the choroid is firmly attached to the pigment layer of the retina. The main body of the choroid is a vascular layer, the choriocapillaris, which supplies nutrition to the external half of the retina and the macula. Its outer layer consists of larger vessels and collecting veins.

The angle and aqueous

The anterior segment of the globe is divided into two chambers. The anterior chamber lies between the cornea and the root of the iris. At the periphery of the anterior chamber is a junction between the cornea, sclera, ciliary body and iris, known as the angle. Within this angle is the trabecular meshwork. The posterior chamber is a slit-like cavity between the back of the iris and the ciliary processes and lens.

Aqueous humour is a clear fluid which fills both of these chambers. It is formed by the ciliary processes of the ciliary body. From the ciliary processes, the aqueous flows through the pupil into the anterior chamber and from there through the trabecular mesh-work into a sinus, the canal of Schlemm. From this structure, it drains into the aqueous veins and into the general circulation. There is a continuous dynamic production and drainage of aqueous which supplies the metabolic needs of the lens and cornea. Pathologically high pressure, such as glaucoma, is usually due to reduced outflow of aqueous and causes damage to the retina.

The lens

The lens is a transparent, biconvex structure situated behind the iris and in front of the vitreous. It is flexible and kept in position by suspensory ligaments attached to the ciliary body. The convexity of its anterior surface is less than that of its posterior surface and it contributes to the refractive power of the eye. The lens consists of a capsule, an epithelial layer on its anterior surface and the lens fibres. The capsule is elastic and encloses the whole lens. The lens fibres constitute the main part of the lens. Epithelial cells change to become lens fibres throughout life. No cells are lost and therefore the centre of the lens becomes denser and less pliable over time. With age, the nucleus becomes dense and yellow; if it becomes opaque, it is known as a cataract.

When in its normal state, the lens is designed to focus light onto the retina. In order to focus on a near object, the lens must become more powerful. Contraction of the ciliary muscle moves the ciliary body forwards. This relieves pressure on the fibres of the zonule and allows the lens to relax and become more spherical. At the same time, the sphincter pupillae contracts, allowing light to enter through the thickest part of the lens. Light from a near source is therefore enabled to focus on the retina. This is known as accommodation and the amount of accommodative power possible reduces as the lens becomes less flexible with age, resulting in the need for 'reading glasses' in middle age.

Retina

The retina is the nervous coat of the eye and the internal layer of the globe. It is a thin, transparent membrane, continuous with the optic nerve and extending to the ora serrata behind the choroid. The retina consists of a pigmented layer next to the choroid which absorbs light and releases vitamin A, which is necessary for the functioning of the photoreceptors. The neural retina consists of photoreceptors and then a number of layers of nerve cells which serve to amplify and transmit the impulses from the photoreceptors to the optic nerve and from there to the brain.

Two types of photoreceptor are present within the retina: 'rods', which allow vision in dim light and in black and white; and 'cones', which are adapted to bright light and can resolve fine detail and colour. Rods are absent at the fovea and rise rapidly in numbers towards the periphery of the retina. Cones are most dense at the fovea and reduce in number towards the periphery. Light impinges on the photo-receptors, producing a chemical reaction which results in an electrical impulse. This is amplified by the various nerve cells and synapses in the neural retina and transmitted through the nerve fibre layer to the optic nerve.

Vitreous

The vitreous body fills the posterior segment of the eye. It is a clear, jelly-like substance consisting of a collagen framework with hyaluronic acid. Collagen fibrils attach the vitreous to the retina at the ora serrata and the optic disc. Its function is to transmit light and to contribute slightly to the resolving power of the eye. It supports the posterior surface of the lens and assists in holding the neural part of the retina in place against its pigment layer.

Assessing ophthalmic conditions

History

As in any presentation, establishing the exact history of a patient's condition is fundamental to making an accurate diagnosis. The history of the presenting problem should include:

- how long the patient has had symptoms for and whether they are getting worse
- rapidity and mode of onset (Box 31.1)
- is vision reduced and to what degree?
- degree, type and location of pain

Box 31.1

Determining mechanism of injury
- Chemical involvement – identify type of chemical substance
- Force of injury and size of projectile
- Possibility of penetration – may be small and high speed
- What first aid has taken place?

- is there any discharge, watering or photophobia?
- has the patient had this, or a similar problem before?
- are there any concurrent systemic problems?
- does the patient wear glasses/contact lenses?

Discussion of systemic problems and medication is important as it can point to possible ophthalmic problems. For example, there is a link between ankylosing spondylitis and uveitis, and a link between rheumatoid arthritis and dry eyes, and there are many ophthalmic side-effects of systemic drugs. The assessing nurse needs to investigate any pre-existing ophthalmic or other medical conditions. Of particular importance are conditions such as glaucoma, iritis (uveitis) and blepharitis; systemic conditions such as diabetes and rheumatoid arthritis; and any drug therapy, as all of these may affect the health of the eye.

Visual acuity

Assessment of visual acuity should be undertaken at initial assessment for any ophthalmic patient, before any other investigations or treatment, except irrigation or instillation of topical anaesthetic. The patient's affected or poorer-seeing eye should be tested first, and the other occluded with a card or the patient's hand. Any distance glasses should be worn. He should be asked to read down from the top of the Snellen chart, making an attempt at all possible letters. Visual acuity should be recorded as:

Distance at which the eye is being tested (usually 6 m) /
Last line read by the patient

The number for this line is indicated on the Snellen chart, just above or just below the letters. If part of a line only is read, this may be recorded as the line above plus the extra letters, or the line below minus the missed letters. For example, if the patient reads the '12' line except for one letter, at 6 m, it should be recorded as 6/12 – 1.

If the patient's vision appears poor (less than 6/9), a pinhole (a small hole in a card or a commercial pin-hole) can be held in front of the eye to negate the effects of any refractive error. The visual acuity should be recorded with and without pinholes and a note should be taken of whether distance glasses or contact lenses are worn. If the patient is unable to read the top letter, the distance should be reduced until the patient can see the top letter on the chart, i.e., 5/60, 4/60, etc. to 1/60. If the patient cannot see the top letter at 1 m, it should be ascertained whether he can count fingers (CF), see hand movements (HM) or just perceive light (PL) at 1 m. Lack of light perception is recorded as NPL. Normal visual acuity is 6/6, but normal visual acuity *for the patient* may be less for a variety of reasons.

Problems in accurate visual acuity assessment may occur if the patient does not speak English or is not able to read. Strategies to overcome this may include:

- using a recognition chart so that the patient may match letters or shapes
- obtaining the services of an interpreter or family member to translate for the patient

- with children, using picture tests such as the Kay picture test and making the procedure into a game – this will usually encourage greater cooperation.

Patients who are in pain should have a drop of topical anaesthetic instilled so that any corneal pain is alleviated and the patient can cooperate more fully with the procedure, thus achieving an accurate visual acuity. Patients sometimes feel that this is a test that they have to pass and 'cheat' by looking through their fingers etc. It should be explained that the nurse is attempting to obtain an accurate assessment of their vision and that it is important that they are not tempted to make it seem better than it really is.

Examining the eye

Eye examination must be systematic. It is very easy to assume a diagnosis from the history and, in that way, miss less obvious problems. The eye should be examined from the 'outside' – the eye position and surrounding structures – working 'in' to consider the globe itself. Considerations for a thorough eye examination are given in Box 31.2.

Remember to compare the findings with the normal eye. What appears to be an abnormality may be bilateral and normal for the patient.

Equipment to aid assessment

An adequate eye assessment can be performed with minimal equipment. A bright light source, such as a pen torch or adjustable light, is essential for examination of the eye. Ophthalmoscopes are useful for retinal examination, but not for general examination as they only produce a small spot of light. Magnification is a useful aid, particularly in the hunt for foreign bodies. A hand-held magnifier, head loupe or ring light can be used. Cotton buds are used to evert the eyelids, remove foreign bodies and during irrigation.

Fluorescein drops or strips that stain damaged epithelial tissue are useful in examining abrasions. The stain is inserted and then the eye is viewed through a cobalt blue filter, as a penlight attachment, slit lamp or ophthalmoscope filter. While slit lamps (a binocular microscope for eye examination) offer the optimum provision for examination, they are expensive and not vital to initial assessment. Topical anaesthetic, such as tetracaine 1 % or oxybuprocaine 0.4 %, should be available in single-dose applications for pain relief and to facilitate examination. Proxymetacaine stings less on initial application and may be preferable, especially in children (Andrew 2006).

Contact lenses

If the patient is wearing contact lenses, the lens should be removed from the injured eye or from both eyes if inflammation or swelling is present. If possible, the patient should remove his own lens; each contact lens wearer develops his own way of doing it.

Box 31.2

Systematic eye examination

The eyes

- Are they in their normal position for the patient?
- Is there any enophthalmos/exophthalmos?
- Is movement normal?

The lids

- Position – look for entropion (lid turning inwards) and ectropion (lid turning outwards)
- Integrity – look for lacerations
- Lash line – is it intact; is there any ingrowing lashes/crusting/infestation?
- Swelling – the whole or part of the lid/pointing onto the lid margin/one or both lids

Conjunctiva

- Integrity – look for lacerations
- Structure – is it smooth or are there follicles or papillae?
- Other features – conjunctival cysts, pterygia, pingueculae
- Inflammation – is it generalized or local?
- Subconjunctival haemorrhages
- Discharge – type
- Fornices (both lower and subtarsal area) – concretions or foreign bodies

Cornea

- Integrity – lacerations, abrasions, ulcers
- Clarity
- Foreign bodies

Anterior chamber

- Depth (the distance between the curved cornea and the iris) – generally equal in both eyes
- Contents, e.g., red blood cells – inflammation is difficult to see without a slit lamp

Iris

- Colour – may be dull if there is inflammation in the anterior chamber
- Integrity – iris changes may occur in both blunt and penetrating trauma
- Position – a deviated pupil may indicate a perforated eye
- Size and shape – smaller or larger than the fellow eye; round or oval?
- Reaction – to light and to near objects

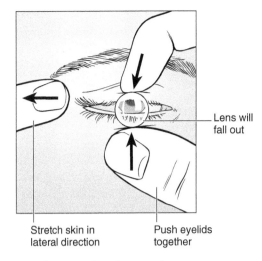

Figure 31.4 • Removal of hard contact lenses.

Lens will fall out

Stretch skin in lateral direction

Push eyelids together

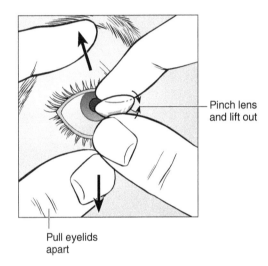

Figure 31.5 • Removal of soft contact lenses.

Pinch lens and lift out

Pull eyelids apart

Removal of lenses

To remove hard lenses, the nurse should stretch the skin of the eyelid by pulling gently in a lateral direction from the outside corner of the patient's eye. Once the skin is stretched, the nurse should push the upper and lower lids together using a finger from each hand. This movement catches the edges of the lens and breaks its suction to the cornea. Once this happens, the lens will fall out (Fig. 31.4). Alternatively, the nurse could put a (washed) index finger on the lens and gently move away from the cornea. The lids can then be used to lever the edge of the lens away from the cornea, and as the adhesion to the cornea breaks, the lens can be gently removed (Shaw et al. 2010).

Hard lenses can also be removed using a specifically designed suction cup. The cup should be soaked in saline and then gently pressed against the contact lens. This forms a stronger suction than that of the lens to the cornea. The lens can then be lifted away from the eye. Other suction extractors must be squeezed before applying to the lens. The lens should be put into a labelled container with normal saline. If any significant corneal infection is present, such as an ulcer or abscess, the lens must be kept for microbiological culture.

Removal of soft lenses is demonstrated in Figure 31.5.

Triage decisions

Similar to other illness and injury, ophthalmic conditions vary considerably in severity and urgency. Using the Manchester Triage Group guidelines (Mackway-Jones et al. 2005) eye complaints can be prioritized as follows:

- priority one (red) – acute chemical eye injury; failure to act to dilute or neutralize chemical agents results in increased tissue damage and can lead to vascular damage and ischaemia and is therefore sight-threatening
- priority two (orange) – severe pain, penetrating eye injury or acute complete loss of vision; these presentations have the potential to be sight-threatening or result in further damage if not treated promptly
- priority three (yellow) – moderate pain, reduced visual acuity or inappropriate (where the history does not explain the findings as this can be an indication of a safeguarding issue)
- priority four (green) – recent mild pain, red eye, foreign body sensation, diplopia, recent problem/injury
- priority five (blue) – chronic complaint without acute exacerbation.

Ocular burns

Ocular burns may be divided most commonly into chemical, thermal and radiation (UV) burns.

Chemical burns

These are the most urgent category of ocular burns and causes may include alkalis, acids or solvents. Alkali burns are caused by substances such as sodium or potassium hydroxide, used as cleaning agents; calcium hydroxide, found in plaster and mortar; and ammonia, which is found in fertilizer and used in liquid form. Alkalis rapidly penetrate corneal tissue, combining with lipids in cell membranes, which results in cell disruption and tissue softening. A rapid rise in the pH in the anterior chamber may damage intraocular structures, and damage to vascular channels leads to ischaemia. Acids are less penetrating, and most damage is done during and soon after exposure. Acid substances combine with tissue, forming barriers against deeper penetration and localizing damage to the point of contact, although they can still be devastating. Acid burns are often due to car battery (sulphuric) acid or more complex organic and inorganic compounds. Solvent burns, although very painful, usually cause only transient irritation and damage. Thermal and/or contusion injuries due to the temperature or pressure of the chemical may be superimposed on the chemical injury (Marsden 1999a).

Primary management

A prompt and effective response to a chemical injury is vital to minimize tissue damage. One of the main determinants of ultimate outcome is duration of contact (Waggoner 1997), and as Glenn (1995) suggested, the initial treatment given by the nurse in the case of chemical eye injury may have more impact on the final vision than any subsequent care by the ophthalmologist.

Irrigation

The initial treatment of acute chemical injury involves copious irrigation to dilute the chemical and remove particulate matter. Irrigation should commence immediately, using whatever source is available and no time should be wasted in trying to find out what chemical was splashed into the eye (Marsden 2009). In a multi-centre trial, Moscati et al. (2007) found no difference in the efficacy of irrigation fluids and therefore, in the ED, the irrigating fluid of choice is normal saline (0.9%) administered via a giving set to provide a directable and controllable jet. Sterile water is also used. The eyelids should be held open and contact lenses removed. A drop of topical anaesthetic should be instilled prior to irrigation to assist in patient compliance and minimize pain. All aspects of the cornea and conjunctiva (exposed by everting the upper lid) should be thoroughly irrigated. All particulate matter should be removed, by wiping with a cotton-tipped applicator if necessary.

Any delay in irrigation adds to the contact time and increases the risk of more severe injury. It is best to assume that any previous irrigation is inadequate and carry out adequate irrigation when the patient presents, unless a significant time has elapsed (hours) between injury and presentation. Specific irrigation time and fluid volume depend on the nature of the chemical and its physical state as well as the patient's condition. Waggoner (1997) suggested that it is impossible to over-irrigate a chemically injured eye and recommended irrigation for 15–30 minutes and one to two litres of saline is generally sufficient.

The use of pH paper to check for adequate irrigation may be debated. In alkaline injury in particular, the chemical leaches out of the eye for a number of hours after injury, thus altering the pH. Delay in therapy of a number of hours until the pH is back to normal will delay healing. It is useful though if used before irrigation to determine the type of chemical involved and again later to check any progress in returning to a normal pH. When measured by sensitive experimental methods, normal pH of the conjunctival sac is 6.5–7.6 (Forrester et al. 1996) but when measured by touching pH measuring paper to the conjunctiva, it is most often near 8 (Adler et al. 1968). It must be remembered that a chemical may have a neutral pH and still cause injury. Ultimately then, indicator paper is no substitute for adequate irrigation. Following irrigation, the patient's visual acuity should be checked.

Acute chemical eye injury is defined by Mackway-Jones et al. (2005) as injury by chemicals occurring in the last 24 hours. While this is true, and places the patient into a red triage category, this should lead to immediate further assessment rather than immediate irrigation. If there is still particulate chemical material in the eye after 24 hours, then it needs irrigation, but small amounts of liquid will have been irrigated by profuse tearing over that period of time and if a period of a few hours has elapsed between chemical exposure and presentation to an ED, and the pH of the conjunctiva is between 7 and 8 at initial assessment, there is little need for irrigation. After irrigation, pH should not be expected to be 7 and is more likely to stabilise around 8 (Sharma et al. 2006).

Ophthalmic management

All but the most trivial chemical injuries should be referred to an ophthalmologist. The eye may look deceptively normal due to tissue blanching and ischaemia, which needs urgent assessment and treatment.

Ophthalmic management usually includes:

- mydriatics, which are used to dilate the pupil, reduce pain due to ciliary spasm and prevent adhesions between the iris and the lens (posterior synechiae)
- topical antibiotics – prophylactic use prevents secondary infection
- topical steroids to reduce and control inflammation
- admission to hospital may be required.

Solvent injury

This may be seen after staining with fluorescein as punctate stains on the cornea. They may be treated with a mydriatic drop to dilate the pupil and chloramphenicol ointment to prevent secondary bacterial infection and aid comfort. They usually resolve very quickly.

Thermal burns

These usually involve damage to the lids and are often associated with facial burns. Treatment is similar to that of thermal burns elsewhere on the body. Thermal burns range from very mild corneal injury which may be treated as an abrasion, with dilatation of the pupil and chloramphenicol ointment, to devastating injury such as that caused by molten metal which may require reconstruction of the globe and surrounding structures. Thermal burns involving the lids should be referred due to the possibility of aberrant healing, leading to lid closure and mobility problems (see also Chapter 11).

Radiation burns

These are likely to be caused by ultraviolet light in the form of sun lamps or from welding equipment. The symptoms are similar, ranging from mild discomfort to severe pain, photophobia and lacrimation. The condition is usually bilateral and symptoms are delayed by 6–10 hours. Topical anaesthetic drops may be used to facilitate examination but should not be given to the patient to use at home. Treatment may include dilatation of the pupil and topical chloramphenicol ointment. The most affected eye may be double padded. The condition resolves spontaneously within 24–36 hours.

Patients who have been using a MIG welder may need a fundal check if there is any residual loss of visual acuity after epithelial healing. The intensity of the light produced by this type of equipment may cause retinal burns (Marsden 1999b).

Penetrating trauma

Intraorbital foreign bodies are frequently the result of high-velocity injuries with varying clinical presentations. Penetrating injuries and intraocular foreign bodies may cause eye damage by:

- disruption of the ocular tissues at the time of injury
- introduction of infection
- scar tissue formation (corneal, disrupting vision, retinal detachment caused by contracting scars inside the eye)
- reaction of the eye to foreign bodies – from organic material introducing infection or inflammation and from the deposition of pigments caused by degrading metal foreign bodies.

Large penetrating eye injuries are very obvious, but small perforations may be easily missed. The eye may look intact if the perforation is small and the wound may be sealed by iris tissue. It is very important, therefore, that a systematic eye examination is carried out and the particular circumstances of the incident are ascertained (Marsden 1996, 2009). Corneal perforations always leave a full-thickness scar, even if it is very small. Scleral perforations may be masked by overlying sub-conjunctival haemorrhage.

The use of Seidel's test may help to identify a full-thickness laceration. This involves instilling a drop of fluorescein into the eye and watching for dilution of it from escaping aqueous. The cobalt blue filter will identify dark tracks in the bright fluorescence, from escaping aqueous.

Patients with penetrating trauma should be referred urgently to an ophthalmologist. Wounds with retained foreign bodies should be protected with a rigid shield such as a cartella shield or a gallipot. Retained foreign objects should not be removed from the eye. In the case of other penetrating injuries, the eye should be covered with a single pad, so no pressure is applied to the eye, and a cartella shield if possible. The patient should be cared for lying flat or sitting at around 30 degrees in order to reduce the possibility of further injury or loss of ocular contents. After consultation with the ophthalmologist, a single drop of unpreserved antibiotic drop (a chloramphenicol minim) instilled in the eye may be useful. Preserved drops or ointments should not be used as both are toxic to intraocular tissues. There should never be an occasion when both eyes are covered. This can lead to extreme distress and disorientation.

Poor prognostic factors associated with globe loss include a wound larger than 10 mm, injuries that involve the retina, initial visual acuity of less than 5/200 at time of injury, no light perception at the time of injury, pellet mechanism of injury, injuries from blunt objects (Ehlers et al. 2008, Lemley et al. 2008, Abrames & Folio 2012).

Lid trauma

The eyelids must be intact, in the correct position and without any disruption to their structure and function in order that the eyes are protected effectively. Repair of lid trauma may be a planned activity rather than an emergency procedure due to the good vascularization of the lids and associated structures. Lid trauma, unless very superficial, should be referred to ophthalmologists, who are best able to achieve the necessary functional and cosmetic results for the patient.

Major closed trauma

A direct blow to the eye from a blunt missile such as a clenched fist, squash ball or champagne cork may produce one or a combination of the following:

- ecchymosis (or black eye)
- hyphaema
- dislocation of the lens
- iridodialysis
- traumatic mydriasis or miosis
- traumatic uveitis
- traumatic angle recession
- posterior segment problems such as retinal oedema (commotio retinae), choroidal rupture and retinal detachment
- blow-out fracture of the orbital floor or nasal wall
- orbital apex trauma and optic nerve injury
- retrobulbar haemorrhage.

Patients with reduced vision following blunt trauma should be referred to an ophthalmologist.

It is important to recognize the possibility of ocular involvement after indirect trauma such as base of skull fractures, as well as from more direct trauma where the eyes themselves do not appear to be involved. Any apparent loss or reduction of vision after trauma should be taken very seriously and the patient should be referred to an ophthalmologist urgently in order to reduce preventable vision loss.

Ecchymosis

Ecchymosis is more commonly known as a 'black eye'. It results from a blow to the orbit that leads to bruising and oedema of the eyelids. In itself, it is a relatively minor injury, treated with ice packs to relieve swelling. The force needed to cause this sort of injury may cause contusion or concussion injuries to any or all of the structures within the eye, as well as orbital rim or floor fractures. It is important, therefore, that the eye and surrounding structures are assessed carefully. The patient may be able to assist in opening the lids enough for the clinician to be able to assess the eye. This kind of injury is common is some sports, such as rugby and squash, however, nearly 90% of all sports-related eye injuries can be prevented with adequate eye protection (Cass 2012).

Hyphaema

Traumatic hyphaema may only be detectable with a slit lamp, when red blood cells may be seen floating in the anterior chamber, or alternatively it may be visible with the naked eye, when blood may fill the whole of the anterior chamber. Its presence usually indicates significant intraocular trauma (Woodcock 2009). The signs and symptoms of hyphaema are:

- history of trauma
- reduced visual acuity

- reddish haze present diffusely through the anterior chamber, a settled layer of blood inferiorly or complete filling of the anterior chamber
- pain – due to raised intraocular pressure and other eye injury
- pupil irregular or poorly reactive
- drowsiness – particularly in children.

Admission may be necessary in the treatment of hyphaema in children, and in the treatment of large hyphaema with raised intraocular pressure in adults, but is rare and generally patients are advised to rest at home. Daily intraocular pressure monitoring by an ophthalmologist is usual, and treatment with agents such as acetazolamide, glycerol or mannitol may be indicated if the intraocular pressure is raised.

Patients who need to be transported to an ophthalmic unit should be transported sitting upright to allow the blood cells to settle and the visual axis to clear as pigment from haemolysed red blood cells may permanently stain the corneal endothelium and reduce vision.

Luxation or subluxation of the lens

A patient with a total dislocation of the lens or a partial dislocation (subluxation) can also present to the ED. It may be the result of trauma, hereditary, or associated with certain syndromes, such as Marfan's syndrome (Shaw et al. 2010). Vision will be disturbed, but the degree of visual disturbance will depend on the degree of dislocation. If 25% or more of the zonules of the lens are ruptured, the lens is no longer held securely behind the iris. The signs and symptoms of luxation or subluxation of the lens are:

- deepening of the anterior chamber due to tilting of the lens posteriorly – the anterior chamber may be shallow if the lens moves anteriorly
- pupil block – this may occur if the lens occludes the pupil
- a tremulous iris (iridodonesis).

The patient should be referred to an ophthalmologist. In general, if no complications occur dislocated lenses are best left untreated. If complications do occur, such as raised intraocular pressure, these are treated before lens extraction is attempted, as surgery in these instances is difficult.

Iridodialysis

This is the disinsertion of the iris base from the ciliary body and it is often associated with hyphaema. No immediate treatment is undertaken. Whether or not surgical intervention is undertaken depends on the effect of iridodialysis on visual acuity after a suitable recovery period.

Traumatic mydriasis or miosis

This may be present after blunt trauma. Additionally, the pupil may react only minimally to light, or not at all, and may have an irregular shape. This deformity is indicative of complete or partial rupture of the iris sphincter. It may be permanent or transient.

Traumatic uveitis

A mild inflammatory reaction of the iris and/or ciliary body is frequently seen after blunt trauma. The patient complains of aching in the eye and cells, and flare may be seen in the anterior chamber. Treatment is as for any uveitis, i.e., dilatation and topical steroids by an ophthalmologist.

Angle recession

Angle recession refers to a separation or posterior displacement of the tissues at the anterior chamber angle at the site of the trabecular meshwork. At least 20% of patients with a hyphaema have some degree of angle recession and are followed up, as secondary glaucoma may eventually follow damage to the trabecular meshwork.

Cataract

A cataract is an opacity of the lens of the eye. It prevents light entering the lens properly and causes dimness of vision. When the structure of the lens is altered, e.g., as a result of a blunt (contusion) injury from a squash ball, aqueous enters the lens substance, causing it to swell and become cloudy. Contusion cataracts may occur as an immediate or long-term consequence of blunt trauma.

Posterior segment problems

A number of posterior segment problems may result from blunt trauma. Their common feature from the patient's perspective is a reduction in visual acuity which may be relatively temporary, usually a matter of weeks, or permanent. It is not possible to give the patient an accurate prognosis for vision initially as this may take some time and early referral to the ophthalmologist is important.

Orbital fractures

The orbits are each composed of seven bones, the thinnest of which are the lamina papyracea over the ethmoid sinuses, along the medial wall, and the maxillary bone on the orbital floor.

Medial orbital fractures

The lacrimal secretory structures, especially the nasolacrimal duct, may be damaged and the medial rectus muscle may be trapped within fractures of the medial wall of the orbit.

Orbital floor fractures

These are often referred to as 'blow-out fractures' and are produced by transmission of forces through the bones and soft tissues of the orbit by an object such as a ball or fist. They typically may be found in young patients in their teens and twenties and may not be clinically obvious. Diplopia, nausea, and vomiting with no subconjunctival haematoma in a young patient requires immediate referral (Lynham et al. 2012). Fractures may be complicated by fat and muscle entrapment which limits ocular motility, causing double vision. They are often found by plain X-rays, but CT scans are used to investigate them further. Symptoms resolve without surgery in almost 85% of patients, as oedematous tissues usually settle, freeing muscles and allowing correct motility (Egging 2009). Visual loss following trauma has a poor prognosis for recovery; however, evolving loss may be indicative of retrobulbar haemorrhage and is potentially treatable (Mackenzie & Gibbons 2011). Signs and symptoms of orbital floor fracture include:

- diplopia
- enophthalmos
- surgical emphysema
- infraorbital anaesthesia.

A sentinel presentation is that the patient attends the ED stating that he has had a blow to the eye and when he blew his nose, his eyelids swelled hugely. This indicates a facture between orbit and sinus and air blown into orbital tissues from the sinus. Antibiotics are indicated to prevent orbital infection from contaminated air from the sinus.

Orbital fractures are not considered an ocular emergency unless visual involvement or globe injury is present. Discharge instructions should include cautions about Valsalva's manoeuvres, such as straining at stool and nose blowing. Antibiotics should be prescribed to prevent orbital cellulitis as air from sinuses contaminates orbital tissue.

Orbital apex trauma and optic nerve injury

Orbital apex fractures may result from both direct, non-penetrating trauma or from penetrating trauma such as large foreign bodies. A number of syndromes have been defined to describe different presentations which depend on the degree of injury to vascular and neural structures within the orbital apex.

Optic nerve injury may occur, often due to traumatic optic neuropathy from indirect trauma (such as fractures of the base of the skull). The nerve may be compressed by haematoma, damaged by foreign body or fracture, resulting in anything from minor trauma to the nerve to transection. Injury to the cranial nerves present in the orbit will present as double vision in injury to the III, IV and VI nerves and as sensory disturbance to the areas supplied by the trigeminal nerve (V). Visual acuity should be checked repeatedly in this group of patients and any reduction should prompt immediate referral to an ophthalmologist (Marsden 2006).

Retrobulbar haemorrhage

This may occur from direct or indirect trauma to the orbit and progress rapidly, resulting in pain, proptosis of the globe, lid and conjunctival swelling and congested conjunctival vessels with subconjunctival haemorrhage. An ophthalmologist should be involved immediately if the globe begins to proptose after trauma and CT or MRI scan may be required urgently. Visual acuity should be checked very frequently as reduction in acuity suggests compression of the optic nerve, and emergency decompression of the haemorrhage by lateral canthotomy (a horizontal incision at the lateral canthus, through skin and conjunctiva and then through the lateral canthal tendon, under topical anaesthetic) will be required to relieve this.

Minor trauma

The vast majority of eye injuries are relatively minor and involve the anterior segment only. It is important, however, to bear in mind the possibility of more major trauma and not to rule it out without a comprehensive examination. If it is assumed that the eye injury is likely to be trivial, sight-threatening injuries may easily be missed. The degree of pain following eye trauma is not a good indication of the severity of the injury. Corneal abrasions can be extremely painful, whereas a sight-threatening perforating injury may be virtually painless.

Traumatic subconjunctival haemorrhage

This is common after a variety of injuries and is, in itself, relatively minor. Fluorescein should be used to rule out a conjunctival laceration. The condition is self-limiting and does not require treatment. A traumatic subconjunctival haemorrhage which extends backwards so that the posterior border is not visible may be an indication of significant orbital trauma and may warrant further investigation if the history and other signs and symptoms are indicative of this. The patient should be reassured that the haemorrhage will resolve, usually over a period of weeks.

Corneal abrasion

Corneal abrasions are very common as the corneal epithelium is easily damaged. The damage to the cornea exposes superficial corneal nerves, causing tearing, eyelid spasms and pain. The degree of pain may be considerable and visual acuity is likely to be reduced. Providing the deeper layers of the cornea are not involved, there should be no visual impairment after the abrasion has healed. Topical anaesthetic may be needed in order to examine the eye effectively. The eye should be stained with fluorescein, and the extent of the abrasion documented.

Eye pain is difficult to control. The pain associated with a breach in the corneal epithelium has a component of ciliary muscle spasm which can be relieved, along with a degree of the patient's pain, by the use of a dilating drop such as cyclopentolate 1%. Topical non-steroidal anti-inflammatory (NSAI) drops provide a significant degree of effective pain relief for patients with corneal pain and are usually prescribed four times daily (Brahma et al. 1996).

Any breach in the corneal epithelium places the eye at risk of infection. A prophylactic antibiotic is necessary and chloramphenicol is usually the antibiotic of choice. Short courses of topical chloramphenicol do not appear to cause systemic side-effects (McGhee & Ananstas 1996) and it is considered to be a very safe drug, widely used throughout ophthalmology in the UK. In the treatment of corneal abrasions, this is often prescribed in ointment form, as this provides a lubricant layer over the eye that enables the lid to slide over the damaged epithelium, and is therefore much more comfortable for the patient. As the antibiotic is for prophylaxis rather than treatment of infection and the ointment base is for comfort, there is no need to prescribe a 'course' of antibiotics. When the abrasion is healed, the patient will know as the pain will have resolved. At that point, the antibiotic treatment may be stopped. Corneal abrasions generally heal within 48–72 hours. Abrasions which appear slow to heal or involve loose epithelium should be referred to an ophthalmologist.

In some instances, the cornea is at particular risk of infection, slow healing or recurrent abrasion. This is particularly the case in human, animal or vegetable material scratches. It is important, therefore, that the patient uses the antibiotic ointment at night for a period of 3–4 weeks to prevent this occurring. Follow-up visits are not usually necessary unless the abrasion is particularly large, involves the deeper layers of the cornea or the patient is a child. The patient should be reassured that a corneal abrasion usually heals and pain relief occurs within 24–48 hours (Kumar et al. 2012).

Conjunctival abrasion and foreign body

Foreign bodies do not often penetrate the conjunctiva and are therefore easily wiped off using a moistened cotton bud after instillation of topical anaesthetic. The resulting (and any concurrent) abrasion may be treated with antibiotic ointment. A pad is not usually necessary and the degree of pain experienced is much less than with corneal trauma.

Subtarsal foreign body

In this case, the patient often presents with a foreign-body sensation and a history of something falling or blowing into the eye. Management involves everting the upper lid using a moistened cotton-tipped swab. Any foreign material trapped underneath the lid may be wiped off with the swab. The eye should then be stained with fluorescein to rule out any corneal abrasion. If corneal abrasions are present, they are often linear, superficial and quite characteristic of this type of injury. If the corneal injury is minimal, a stat dose instillation of antibiotic ointment is usually sufficient. If larger abrasions are present, they should be treated as corneal abrasions.

Corneal foreign body

These commonly occur from grinding wheels and other industrial machines, from DIY and even windborne materials. The patient may present with a foreign-body sensation, especially when opening or closing the eye. The final resting place of an intraocular foreign body, and the damage caused by it depend on the size, shape and moment of the object at the time of impact and the momentum of the object at the time of impact, and the site of ocular penetration (Scott 2011). Superficial foreign bodies are often easily removed with a moistened cotton bud after instillation of topical anaesthetic. Dry cotton buds should not be used as they can stick to the corneal epithelium, which is moist, and this may result in a large abrasion, complicating the injury.

Impacted corneal foreign bodies need to be removed using the edge of a hypodermic needle (most commonly 21 gauge) held tangentially to the cornea with the hand supported on the patient's cheek or nose. The needle may be mounted on a cotton bud or syringe for easier manipulation. After the initial removal of the foreign body, a rust ring often remains which must be removed completely. This is easier after 24–48 hours of treatment with antibiotic ointment; referral to an ophthalmic unit is recommended.

Removal of corneal foreign body with a needle is a procedure that must be carried out with extreme care. It is quite possible to penetrate the cornea with a needle and corneal scarring will result if the deeper layers of the cornea are damaged. This can cause visual problems if it involves the visual axis. It is therefore important that if the ED possesses a slit lamp, it is utilized for the removal of corneal foreign bodies so that both a high degree of magnification and support for the patient's head are possible. ED staff may feel most comfortable removing only peripheral foreign bodies and referring on central ones. If in any doubt, the patient should be referred to an ophthalmic unit.

After removal of the foreign body, treatment is as for a corneal abrasion. Many patients have repeat visits for removal of corneal foreign bodies and treat them as something of an occupational hazard, although opportunities should still be taken to reinforce the need for adequate eye protection as it is most unlikely that one foreign body would penetrate the eye while another stayed on the cornea. X-ray examination is only indicated if there is a definite history of a high-speed foreign body hitting the eye, such as a hammer and chisel, and no foreign body can be found.

Eye pads

There is no evidence that padding the eye enhances healing; however, for many patients, padding can make the eye much more comfortable. The decision to pad the eye of a patient with a corneal abrasion should therefore be accompanied by the advice that if the pad makes the eye more comfortable, it can be left in place, without disturbance for 24 hours and then removed and antibiotic treatment commenced. If the pad makes the eye less comfortable, it may be removed and antibiotic ointment commenced immediately. In this way, those patients who can be helped by padding are, and others are not made worse by the indiscriminate application of eye pads (Marsden 2006).

A single pad will not keep the eye closed and further damage to the cornea may be caused by the surface of the pad. If padding is required, the following method should be used. Fold one pad in half and place over the closed eyelids after instilling the necessary medication. Place the second pad, flat, over the first and secure with two or three pieces of tape (Fig. 31.6). It is unnecessary to pad an eye merely because topical anaesthetic has been used. Anaesthetic drops last for only around 20–30 minutes and the risk of the patient sustaining any further injury because of the topical anaesthetic drop is minimal (Cheng et al. 1997).

The ED nurse should not pad the eye of a patient who is driving home. If the patient leaves the eye pad on and drives anyway, he is breaking the law, invalidating his insurance and

Eye closed after instillation of antibiotic ointment

Single folded pad over the closed lid and taped down – ensures the patient cannot open his eye under the pad

Second pad – open (unfolded) over the first and taped firmly to the face

Figure 31.6 • Use of eye pads.

is a danger to other road users. A drop of topical anaesthetic will facilitate driving home safely and the patient may then pad the eye at home.

Eye drops

Topical anaesthetic drops are a valuable tool for examination purposes. They 'magically' remove all the patient's pain and he may be very keen to have some to take home so that this pain-free state may continue. Unfortunately, topical anaesthetic drops also inhibit epithelial healing. The patient will be pain-free, but the epithelial defect will not heal (Andrew 2006).

Topical non-steroidal anti-inflammatory drugs (NSAIDs) have been evaluated for use in corneal pain (Brahma et al. 1996) and found to be extremely useful. Their use does not appear to delay healing and no adverse effects have been found. A number of NSAIDs are available in eye drop form, including diclofenac sodium, flurbiprofen sodium and ketorolac trometamol.

Mydriatic and cycloplegic drops, such as cyclopentolate, dilate the pupil and paralyze accommodation. The patient's near vision is therefore blurred for a period. This does not mean that the patient should not drive. If he feels safe to do so, there is nothing to stop him driving, as the legal standard for driving only includes distance vision and distance vision is not affected by dilatation. Near vision, which is affected, is not used to any great extent for driving. However, he should be warned that, if it is a bright day, he may be quite dazzled by sunlight and should wear sunglasses and take extreme care.

Steroid drops should not be prescribed in the ED as the effects of steroids on the eye in a misdiagnosed condition can be catastrophic.

Red eye

Ophthalmic trauma is fairly easy to recognize with the aid of a history and a brief eye examination. However, ophthalmic medical problems are, on the whole, less easily diagnosed and therefore may be dealt with less well than other problems. The differential diagnosis of the red eye (Marsden 2006) is shown in Table 31.1.

Subconjunctival haemorrhage

Patients may present with a spontaneous subconjunctival haemorrhage. The patient may not have noticed any irritation and is often prompted to attend by others noticing the haemorrhage, which presents as a deep red patch of blood under the conjunctiva. It may be quite small and circumscribed or may be severe enough for the conjunctiva to protrude like a 'bag of blood'. Providing there is no history of trauma, no treatment is needed except reassurance. Patients with clotting disorders or those on anticoagulants may be prone to repeat episodes. Subconjunctival haemorrhages will take up to three weeks to resolve and the blood may spread under the conjunctiva and actually appear worse before it begins to resolve.

Blepharitis

This chronic eyelid condition is very common. The patient is likely to present with gritty, sore eyes and red-rimmed eyelids with crusting, which may be mild to very severe, along the lid margin – the lash line. Treatment involves regular lid cleaning,

Table 31.1 Differential diagnosis of the red eye

	Conjunctivitis	Uveitis	Glaucoma	Corneal ulcers
Lids	? Swollen follicles, papillae if allergic	Normal	Normal	May be swollen
Conjunctiva	Injected	Injected	Injected	Injected
Cornea	? Punctate staining	Normal, bright reaction	Very hazy	Opacity/stains with fluorescein
Anterior chamber	Deep	Deep	Shallow or flat	Deep
Iris	Normal	May look muddy	May be difficult to see	Normal
Pupil	Normal	Slight miosis (compared with fellow) sluggish	Fixed, oval, semi-dilated	Usually normal, may be slightly sluggish
Pain	Gritty	Deep pain in eye	Severe pain in and around eye and head	Gritty
Discharge	Pus/watery/sticky in morning	May water	No	May water
Photophobia	If severe	Yes	No	Not usually
Systemically	? Flu-like symptoms (URTI)	Well	Nausea, vomiting, severe abdominal pain, dehydration	Well

using a cotton bud dipped in a solution of baby shampoo and water to 'scrub' the lid margin along the lash line to remove all the crusts. When the condition is acute, antibiotic ointment should be rubbed into the lid margin after lid hygiene two to four times a day. As this is a chronic condition, lid cleaning should continue even after the symptoms have resolved, or the condition will recur. Occasionally, punctate staining may occur at the corneoscleral junction. This is marginal keratitis, an inflammatory change. The patient should be referred to an ophthalmologist.

Conjunctivitis

Inflammation of the conjunctiva is by far the most common cause of red eyes. Bacterial conjunctivitis in adults is uncommon (Tullo & Donnelly 1995) and most conjunctivitis in adults is viral. Conjunctivitis in children is more likely to be bacterial.

Bacterial conjunctivitis

The patient is likely to present with a red, irritable eye, describing the sensation as 'gritty' rather than painful. Discharge is likely to be purulent and profuse, and the lashes may be coated with it. There will be no corneal staining with fluorescein. Treatment is usually with a broad-spectrum antibiotic such as chloramphenicol or fusidic acid, applied topically in the form of drops. Drops are often prescribed quite frequently during the first 48 hours; for example, in the case of chloramphenicol drops, two-hourly application would not be unreasonable.

Health education information, particularly on how to control the spread of infection, should be given and the nurse must ensure that the patient understands how to use his medication before leaving the ED. Information on how to keep the lids clean and free from discharge may be needed, e.g., using cooled, boiled water and cotton wool or tissues, especially by parents of small children who may also need extra help instilling the prescribed medication effectively. Patient education should also, where appropriate, incorporate discussion of cross-contamination through eye makeup, pillows and towels (Egging 2009).

Viral conjunctivitis

Viruses, often types of adenovirus, are by far the most common cause of conjunctivitis in adults (Kaufman 2011). Once again, the patient is likely to complain of a gritty sensation, but the discharge is much less likely to be purulent than profuse watering, with stickiness often only in the morning when the watery discharge has dried and the lids are stuck together. If the lid is everted, the conjunctiva covering it will appear very bumpy rather than smooth. These 'bumps' are follicles and are inflamed lymphoid tissue. This roughness of the conjunctiva is what makes the eye feel so gritty and irritable. The patient with viral conjunctivitis often complains of dryness, along with a watery eye. The tears, although profuse, are inadequate in quality and dry up very quickly; the eye responds to the irritation and dryness by producing more. There may be punctate erosions on the cornea when stained with fluorescein.

Some types of adenovirus, of which there are about 30, cause upper respiratory tract infection and this, when combined with an eye infection, is known as pharyngoconjunctival fever. The patient may feel generally unwell with flu-like symptoms and the preauricular lymph node may be enlarged. Treatment of viral conjunctivitis is based on controlling the symptoms. Unless the eye is particularly sticky, antibiotics are not indicated. Artificial tears may help to control the feeling of dryness and irritation and these may be used very frequently, e.g., every 30 minutes. A bland ointment such as simple eye ointment may also be helpful. Cold compresses on the lids may ease the irritation of this very distressing condition. The patient should be aware that viral conjunctivitis may persist for 3–6 weeks and the symptoms of dryness may last much longer.

Adenoviral conjunctivitis is a condition with symptoms out of all proportion to its relative clinical importance. Once the symptoms have peaked, however, the patient may be said to be no longer an infection risk. Adenovirus is highly infectious and infection control is of paramount importance, both for the patient and for the department. Hand washing is the first line of defence in infection control and is vital to stop the spread of viral conjunctivitis. Swabs to identify specific organisms are not required. Results do not change treatment and the swab is both painful and costly.

Chlamydial conjunctivitis

A patient presenting with a uniocular, chronic conjunctivitis causing only mild symptoms may have a chlamydial infection. A swab should be taken for culture and chlamydial identification and the patient referred to genito urinary medicine if the swab proves positive.

Allergic conjunctivitis

Allergic conjunctivitis is very common and presents acutely in two distinct ways. Firstly, the patient may have red eyes with itching and watering and an appearance of large bumps (papillae) on the subtarsal conjunctiva. This presentation is particularly common during spring and summer – the 'hay fever' season – and may also be associated with a runny nose, sneezing, etc. Treatment is with systemic antihistamines and/or topical antihistamine treatment such as emedastine or olopatadine. Topical mast cell stabilizing drops such as sodium cromoglycate are of little value in an acute exacerbation but may be useful if used throughout the whole of the 'hay fever' season by patients who are aware that they are likely to develop allergic conjunctivitis.

The second allergic presentation is an acute and frightening atopic reaction that involves massive swelling of the conjunctiva (chemosis) which the patient often describes as 'jelly' on the eye. This is usually due to the patient rubbing the eye with an allergen present on the hand or finger. Common allergens include some plant juices and cat hairs, although it is unlikely that the particular allergen will be identified. This condition is completely self-limiting and requires no treatment unless the chemosis is severe and protruding from the closed lids. In this case, lubricant drops may be helpful to prevent drying. Adequate reassurance is needed and, if the reaction is severe, the patient may need to be monitored for systemic effects of the allergen.

Anterior uveitis (also known as uveitis, iridocyclitis, iritis)

Uveitis is an inflammatory condition of part or all of the uveal tract (iris, ciliary body and choroid) (McDonald et al. 2012). It may be associated with systemic disease such as ankylosing spondylitis but which is often idiopathic. It may also occur secondary to trauma. The most common presentation is anterior uveitis (inflammation of iris and ciliary body, also commonly known as iritis). Common presenting symptoms are photophobia, pain due to iris and ciliary spasm, conjunctival redness (injection), which may be more marked around the corneoscleral junction (limbus), and decreased visual acuity. The reduction in vision is due to protein and white blood cells (part of the inflammatory response) in the anterior chamber. The pupil, because of spasm and inflammation, is likely to be small (miosed) compared with the unaffected eye and may react sluggishly. There will be a clear reflection of light when a light is shone onto the cornea, demonstrating the lack of corneal involvement, and there will be no staining with fluorescein. Prompt referral to an ophthalmologist is required and treatment is with topical corticosteroids, and mydriatics to dilate the pupil to reduce inflammation and prevent adhesions of the iris and lens.

Acute glaucoma

In acute glaucoma, the outflow of aqueous in the eye is obstructed by the peripheral iris covering the trabecular meshwork. The pressure inside the eye increases rapidly as aqueous continues to be produced, resulting in the sudden onset of severe pain, due to the increased intraocular pressure, and blurred vision due to corneal oedema. Haloes may be seen around lights. The pain is not likely to be localized in the eye, but may involve the whole head and may be accompanied by nausea, vomiting and abdominal pain. Patients are usually elderly and are likely to be hypermetropic (long-sighted). On examination, the patient's eye will be red and the reflection of light from the cornea will be very diffuse, demonstrating that the cornea is oedematous. The pupil is likely to be semi-dilated, oval and fixed.

Acute glaucoma is an ophthalmic emergency and the patient should be referred to an ophthalmologist urgently, including emergency ambulance transportation if necessary. Prolonged raised ocular pressure at this level will cause permanent loss of vision, which may be severe and will occur quickly. Treatment involves the use of carbonic anhydrase inhibitors, such as acetazolamide intravenously, constriction of the pupil once the pressure has reduced and, eventually,

laser treatment when the pressure is back to normal. In the ED, analgesia and anti-emetics may be required. Occasionally, patients present having coped with these symptoms for some time and may be dehydrated due to prolonged vomiting, and rehydration may therefore be necessary. A great deal of explanation, reassurance and care are needed by these ill and often terrified patients.

Corneal ulcers

There are three main types of corneal ulcer that are likely to be seen in the ED. All should be referred to an ophthalmic unit because differentiation between the different types of corneal ulcer is sometimes difficult and the treatment is completely different.

Bacterial ulcers occur as 'fluffy' white demarcated areas on the cornea which stain with fluorescein. They are caused by a number of organisms, some of which, e.g., *Pseudomonas*, are very difficult to treat. All need a number of investigations to be carried out, such as Gram stain and culture, which will be done in the ophthalmic unit without delay. Patients may be treated with frequent antibiotic drops on either an outpatient or, if the infection is severe, an in-patient basis. Delay in treatment of infected corneal ulcers can result in devastating intraocular infection.

Marginal ulcers appear as ulcerated areas that stain with fluorescein and are usually close to the limbus. They are part of a hypersensitivity response by the eye to staphylococcal exotoxins and are usually treated with steroid eye drops by an ophthalmologist.

Viral ulcers caused by herpes simplex virus are known as 'dendritic' ulcers because of their branching, tree-like shape when stained with fluorescein. They are treated with acyclovir eye ointment, again only by an ophthalmologist.

Health promotion

Many patients with ophthalmic conditions are only seen for a short period in the ED, before either discharge or referral, and there is therefore limited time to advise patients. It is important, however, that patients leave the department with a basic knowledge of their condition, in order to understand the importance of drug treatment and follow-up requirements and instruction on correct eye drop instillation and side-effects of any drug therapy. Patients with newly diagnosed conditions should also be aware of recurring symptoms which should prompt them to seek early treatment.

Many activities in the home and workplace cause eye injuries, due to equipment, materials, chemicals and radiation. Patients with such injuries should be encouraged to wear eye protection or to check that any equipment already in use is of a suitable standard. All eye protection should conform to British Standard BS 2092 requirements. Children, in particular, are vulnerable to eye injuries. Parents need sympathetic health education to minimize the risks of sight-damaging injury (Kutsche 1994).

Conclusion

While ocular emergencies do not present a threat to the patient's life, sight is precious and the ED nurse can have a critical impact on a patient's vision. Once lost, vision cannot be replaced, and therefore knowledge of the management of the most common ophthalmic conditions will assist the nurse in protecting sight and promoting health.

References

Abrames, F., Folio, L., 2012. CT severity spectrum of penetrating eye injuries from blasts. Military Medicine 177 (2), 169–173.

Adler, I.N., Wlodyga, R.J., Rops, S.J., 1968. the effects of pH on contact lens wearing. Journal of American Optomotrists Association 39, 1000–1001.

Andrew, S., 2006. Pharmacology. In: Marsden, J. (Ed.), Ophthalmic Care. Wiley, Chichester.

Brahma, A.K., Shah, S., Hillier, V.F., et al., 1996. Topical analgesia for superficial corneal injuries. Journal of Accident and Emergency Medicine 13, 186–188.

Cass, S.P., 2012. Ocular injuries in sports. Current Sports Medicine 11 (1), 11–15.

Cheng, H., Burdon, M.A., Buckley, S.A., et al., 1997. Emergency Ophthalmology. BMJ, London.

Egging, D., 2009. Ocular emergencies. In: Newberry, L. (Ed.), Sheehy's Emergency Nursing: Principles and Practice, sixth ed. Mosby, St Louis.

Ehlers, J.P., Kunimoto, D.Y., Ittoop, S., et al., 2008. Metallic intraocular foreign bodies: characteristics, interventions, and prognostic factors for visual outcome and globe survival. American Journal of Ophthalmology 146 (3), 427–433.

Ezra, D.G., Mellington, F., Cugnoni, H., et al., 2005. Reliability of opthalmic accident and emergency referrals: a new role for the emergency nurse practitioner? Emergency Medicine Journal, 696–699.

Forrester, J., Dick, A., McMenamin, P., et al., 1996. The Eye: Basic Sciences in Practice. WB Saunders, London.

Glenn, S., 1995. Care of patients with chemical eye injury. Emergency Nurse 3 (3), 7–9.

Kaufman, H.E., 2011. Adenovirus advances: new diagnostic and therapeutic options. Current Opinion in Ophthalmology 22 (4), 290–293.

Kumar, K., Dodds, C., Gayer, S., 2012. Ophthalmic Anaesthesia. Oxford University Press, Oxford.

Kutsche, P.J., 1994. Ocular trauma in children. Journal of Ophthalmic Nursing and Technology 13 (3), 117–120.

Lemley, C.A., Wirostko, W.J., Mieler, W.F., et al., 2008. Intraocular foreign bodies. In: Albert, D.M. (Ed.), Principles and Practice of Ophthalmology. Saunders, Philadelphia.

Lynham, A., Tuckett, J., Warnke, P., 2012. Maxillofacial trauma. Australian Family Physician 41 (4), 172–180.

Mackenzie, N., Gibbons, A., 2011. Maxillofacial fractures. In: Smith, J., Greaves, I., Porter, K. (Eds.), Oxford Desk Reference: Major Trauma. Oxford Medical Publications, Oxford.

Mackway-Jones, K., Marsden, J., Windle, J., 2005. Emergency Triage, second ed. BMJ, London.

Marsden, J., 1996. Ophthalmic trauma in accident and emergency. Accident and Emergency Nursing 4 (1), 54–58.

Marsden, J., 1999a. Ocular burns. Emergency Nurse 6 (10), 20–24.

Marsden, J., 1999b. Painless loss of vision. Emergency Nurse 6 (9), 13–18.

Marsden, J., 2006. The care of patients presenting with acute problems. In: Marsden, J. (Ed.), Ophthalmic Care. Wiley, Chichester.

Marsden, J., 2009. Ophthalmological emergencies. In: Crouch, R., Charters, A., Dawood, M., Bennett, P. (Eds.), Oxford Handbook of Emergency Nursing. Oxford University Press, Oxford.

McDonald, R.J., Lawlor, M., McCluskey, P.J., 2012. Anteriour uveitis: is the cause of a red eye? Medicine Today 13 (2), 58–60.

McGhee, C.N., Ananstas, C.N., 1996. Widespread ocular use of topical chloramphenicol: is there justifiable concern regarding idiosyncratic aplastic anaemia? British Journal of Ophthalmology 80, 182–184.

Moscati, R.M., Mayrose, J., Reardon, R.F., et al., 2007. A multicentre comparison of tap water versus sterile saline for wound irrigation. Academic Emergency Medicine 14, 404–410.

Scott, R., 2011. Eye trauma. In: Smith, J., Greaves, I., Porter, K. (Eds.), Oxford Desk Reference: Major Trauma. Oxford Medical Publications, Oxford.

Sharma, A., Smilkstein, M.J., Fraunfelder, F.W., 2006. Ophthalmic principles. In: Flomenbaum, N.E., Goldfrank, L.R., Hoffman, R.S. (Eds.), Goldfrank's Toxicologic Emergencies, eighth ed. McGraw Hill, New York.

Shaw, M., Lee, A., Stollery, R., 2010. Ophthalmic Nursing, fourth ed. Wiley Blackwell, Oxford.

Tan, M.M.S., Driscoll, P.A., Marsden, J.E., 1997. Management of eye emergencies in the accident and emergency department by senior house officers: a national survey. Journal of Accident and Emergency Medicine 14, 157–158.

Tullo, A.B., Donnelly, D., 1995. Conjunctiva. In: Perry, J.P., Tullo, A.B. (Eds.), Care of the Ophthalmic Patient, second ed. Chapman and Hall, London.

Waggoner, M.D., 1997. Chemical injuries of the eye: current concepts in pathophysiology and therapy. Survey of Ophthalmology 41 (4), 275–313.

Woodcock, M., 2009. Ophthalmic injuries. In: Greaves, I., Porter, K., Garner, J. (Eds.), Trauma Care Manual, Hodder Arnold, London.

Ear, nose and throat emergencies

32

Tina Roche

CHAPTER CONTENTS

http://dx.doi.org/10.1016/B978-0-7020-4315-4.00032-2

Introduction

Ear, nose or throat (ENT) conditions presenting at the Emergency Department (ED) are often trivialized, even though some can subsequently become life-threatening. For those patients who attend the ED with an ENT disorder, the onset of symptoms is likely to be acute or that the current episode may also be a feature of a chronic condition. It is important to be alert to the danger of viewing the patient only in terms of the presenting symptoms.

It is often the case that such conditions are accompanied by systemic illness precipitated by local infection. Equally important is the fact that the individual may have psychological, social and emotional needs as well as the presenting pathophysiological needs. This may be obvious in the case of an individual who has hearing loss as a direct result of being in close proximity to the seat of an explosion, but may be less apparent in the individual whose hearing loss results from wax impaction, but who is concerned that she may be becoming permanently deaf.

This chapter broadly examines ENT conditions in terms of infection, trauma and foreign bodies. The nursing care of patients is discussed in relation to presenting conditions.

The ear

The attendance at the ED of a patient with an ear-related problem is usually precipitated by one or more of the following symptoms:

- pain
- discharge from the ear
- hearing loss
- foreign bodies in the ear canal
- direct trauma to the external structure of the ear.

Anatomy of the ear

The ear is divided into three sections: external, middle and inner ear (Fig. 32.1). The outer ear funnels sound into the middle ear, which serves to transmit the sound to the auditory apparatus of the inner ear. The external ear consists of the auricle (or pinna), ear canal and tympanic membrane. The S-shaped ear canal is approximately 2.5–3 cm long and terminates at the tympanic membrane. The canal is lined with glands that secrete cerumen, a yellow waxy material that lubricates and protects the ear. Ear wax, sloughed off skin cells and dust may impair sound transmission through the outer ear, especially if a plug of wax attaches to the eardrum. The bone behind and below the ear canal is the mastoid part of the temporal bone. The lowest portion of this, the mastoid process, is palpable behind the lobule (Bickley & Szilagyi 2003).

The tympanic membrane (or eardrum) is a thin, translucent, pearly grey oval disc separating the external ear from the middle ear. It can easily be observed with an otoscope. The tympanic membrane vibrates and moves in and out in response to sound. The middle ear is an air-filled cavity containing three tiny bones, the ossicles, which are individually called the malleus (hammer), the incus (anvil) and the stapes (stirrup), so named because of their appearance. The malleus is attached to the tympanic membrane by a set of ligaments. The incus is attached to the malleus and they move as one. The stapes attaches to the oval window, the membrane separating the middle and inner ear. When the tympanic membrane vibrates in response to sound, the malleus and incus are displaced, and the stapes vibrates against the oval window continuing the transmission of sound. The pharyngotympanic tube, formerly known as the Eustachian tube, which connects the middle ear with the nasopharynx, allows the passage of air to equalize pressure on either side of the tympanic membrane. The inner ear is composed of several fluid-filled chambers encased in a bony labyrinth in the temporal bone. The semicircular canals are also important for balance (Zemlin 2011).

Presentation to the ED may be prompted by a single symptom, such as hearing loss resulting from wax impaction. The patient may alternatively have multiple symptoms, resulting from, for example, an ear infection where pain, discharge and hearing loss may be present in combination with systemic illness.

Infections of the ear

Acute otitis externa

The external auditory meatus is a canal-shaped structure which extends from the external opening of the ear to the tympanic membrane. The integrity of the canal is protected from pathogens by its lining. The lateral one-third is composed of skin that is a continuation from the concha, which is the depression in the centre of the shell-shaped external structure of the ear – the pinna. The lining continues as an epithelial layer, protecting not only the medial two-thirds of the external auditory meatus but also the tympanic membrane.

The protective lining of the external auditory meatus may be easily breached by direct trauma, although pre-existing dermatological conditions, typically eczema and psoriasis, as well as external mediators such as maceration by water, may influence the resilience of the lining.

Clinical evidence and management

Acute otitis externa is essentially a localized or diffuse infection of the lining of the external auditory meatus commonly associated with organisms such as *Pseudomonas aeruginosa*, *Staphylococcus aureus* and occasionally fungi like *Candida* and *Aspergillus* (Sander 2001). Acute otitis externa frequently occurs following bathing or swimming because excessive moisture removes the protective cerumen from the ear canal allowing keratin debris to absorb water to create a nourishing environment for bacteria. For this reason it is often referred to as 'swimmer's ear'. Infection may be diffuse within the

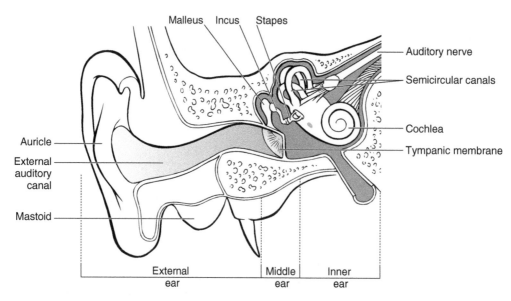

Figure 32.1 • Anatomy of the ear.

external auditory meatus or it may be focal in the form of a local swelling known as a furuncle, which may be extremely painful. Taking swabs for microbiological studies may not be well tolerated by the patient. It is essential that careful preparation of the patient takes place before any attempt is made to take a swab, especially if the individual is a child. Attempts to take a swab from an uncooperative child should be avoided as there is a risk that the tympanic membrane may be perforated by the swab if the child moves her/his head.

As the external auditory meatus contains no mucus-secreting cells, discharge from the ear is minimal; however, any discharge that does occur is usually thick and foul-smelling infected wax. The canal may also contain cell debris, which is unlikely to cause hearing loss, but may contribute to the intense irritation the individual may experience.

Treatment is based upon cleaning and drying the external auditory meatus. This should only be done after examination of the ear canal to determine the integrity of the tympanic membrane. Following cleansing of the external auditory meatus, topical medication containing steroids and antibiotics is necessary (Abelardo et al. 2007). Acute otitis externa largely results from identifiable causes and therefore lends itself to prevention strategies. The focus of much of the nursing care may revolve around educating the patient on keeping ears dry and on how to instill their prescribed medication.

Acute otitis media

An acute infection of the middle ear, that is, medial to the tympanic membrane, may cause pain, a feeling of pressure or fullness in the ear and hearing loss, the symptoms being caused by infective material splinting the tympanic membrane. Discharge from the external ear may be present, but in order for this to occur, the tympanic membrane must have been damaged, usually as a result of the increased pressure causing perforation.

Clinical evidence and management

Acute otitis media is often associated with systemic illness and fever, which may be attributed to the otitis media alone or occur in conjunction with coincidental upper respiratory tract infection (Ludman 2007). Acute otitis media is characterized by rapid onset of ear pain, headache, tinnitus, hearing loss, and nausea or vomiting. Infants and young children may present with irritability, crying, rubbing or pulling the ear, restless sleep and lethargy (Olson 2003). Children are often prone to acute otitis, with up to 30% of those presenting with otitis media being children under three years of age, as the infection frequently results from upper respiratory tract infection of bacterial or viral origin.

Antibiotics are not often necessary in the treatment of uncomplicated otitis media with the mainstay of treatment being analgesia with antipyretic properties. Antibiotics in otitis media provide a modest benefit that must be balanced against the risk of adverse effects (Coker et al. 2010). In most cases involving children, antibiotics only provide symptomatic benefits after the first 24 hours, at which time symptoms are generally resolving. Serious complications, such as meningitis, mastoiditis, intracranial abscess, permanent

hearing loss and neck abscess can develop as a result of otitis media (Olson 2003).

If the tympanic membrane has perforated, it is often the painful result of otitis media, trauma or foreign body insertion and is associated with loss of hearing. The individual should be advised to keep the ear dry and prevent water entering the ear. However, the ear should not be packed, and the patient should be advised not to do this at home, as it may prevent the discharge draining from the ear. More than 90% of tympanic membrane perforations heal spontaneously and management includes antibiotics, analgesia and antipyretics (Olson 2003). In some cases, where the tympanic membrane is intact, the infective material may cause the membrane to bulge, which also causes pain and loss of hearing. In such cases, admission to hospital is required in order that the tympanic membrane may be surgically perforated under general anaesthetic and grommets inserted to allow the discharge to drain out freely.

Mechanical obstruction

Impacted wax

The lateral one-third of the external auditory meatus contains cells that secrete a waxy substance called cerumen, the purpose of which is to act as a defense against dust and other foreign material entering the external auditory meatus.

Clinical evidence and management

Cerumen may build up in the external auditory meatus, causing mechanical obstruction, which may be exacerbated by cleaning the ear with cotton-tipped buds. Such activities often cause cerumen to be pushed deep into the canal, causing impaction against the tympanic membrane. Obstruction in either case may cause a reduction in hearing, but rarely causes complete deafness. Impacted cerumen is often hard and resistant to removal by syringing alone; thus, in the ED the most appropriate management is to initiate a regimen to soften the cerumen using commercially available eardrops.

Patient education involves self-administration with advice to contact their GP in 2–3 weeks to arrange for ear syringing. Ear syringing is rarely indicated in the ED. Poor technique and failure to take adequate precautions may cause the patient serious harm; it is therefore imperative that ear syringing is carried out by a nurse who is suitably trained in the technique.

Foreign bodies

Clinical evidence

Older children and adults may present with a history of having a foreign body in the ear. Young children have a tendency to put foreign bodies in their ears, but as they often do not disclose this information, the nurse should be suspicious of children who present with earache, hearing loss and discharge from the ear. Small insects may also crawl into the ear canal and become trapped, causing a great deal of discomfort if still alive and buzzing.

Management

Foreign bodies may be removed using a variety of techniques including irrigation, suction and instrumentation, by individuals with the appropriate skills (Davies & Benger 2000). Care should be taken to ensure that this process does not impact the foreign body further in the ear, causing trauma to the external auditory meatus and the tympanic membrane.

If the tympanic membrane is intact then syringing the external auditory meatus with warm water may flush the foreign body out. However, this should only be carried out under direct visualization by those skilled in the technique.

Severe pain and distress are caused to patients when live insects enter the ear and they need to be killed in situ by the instillation of oil or lignocaine prior to removal (Davies & Benger 2000). Analgesic and/or antibiotic treatments should be prescribed as necessary.

Safe removal of a foreign body from the external auditory meatus requires a skilled operator and a cooperative patient, which is not always possible to achieve in the ED. If in any doubt, the patient should be referred to the ENT department. If the object is not retrieved at the first attempt, the patient should be referred to the ENT department.

Perforation of the tympanic membrane

Perforation of the tympanic membrane may be caused by two main mechanisms – either direct or indirect trauma. In both cases the symptoms are much the same, i.e., hearing loss, pain and possibly bleeding from the external auditory meatus.

Direct trauma

This is commonly caused by the insertion of objects either to clean the ear or to relieve itching, although any object inserted into the external auditory meatus has the potential to cause tympanic perforation. Objects frequently used are cotton-tipped buds and hair grips. In most cases, the ruptured tympanic membrane will heal spontaneously in 1–3 months (Bluestone 2007); however, ENT opinion should be sought. Pain relief and prophylactic antibiotics may be required, especially if the mechanism of injury includes contamination by water or a foreign body.

This provides the ED nurse with a health education opportunity in terms of prevention of subsequent episodes particularly in relation to aural hygiene. The importance of keeping the ear dry at all times must be stressed. A protective cotton plug coated with petroleum jelly will enable the patient to shower safely; however, swimming and generally getting the ears wet should be avoided.

Indirect trauma

Perforation of the tympanic membrane may be caused by high pressure transmitted along the external auditory meatus to the tympanic membrane. This barotrauma to the tympanic membrane results from significant changes in atmospheric pressure causing air trapped in the external ear canal or behind the tympanic membrane to expand or contract enough to rupture the eardrum. This pressure may be generated by such forces as a slap to the ear, flying, diving or exposure to an explosion. Pressures of as little as 35 kPa on the tympanic membrane may cause it to rupture, although in the explosion scenario some individuals will be protected from these pressures because of the orientation of the external auditory meatus to the blast wave (Garner 2011). As it is unlikely that data will be available regarding blast wave pressure, all individuals who have been in close proximity to an explosion should be carefully assessed and referred to the ENT department if appropriate.

Although tympanic membrane rupture may be seen in isolation from other injuries following an explosion, the nurse should be aware of other injuries that may have occurred, such as lung and gastrointestinal injury, which may be covert in nature. The nurse should also be aware of the emotional and psychological crisis the patient will be experiencing, not only from the incident itself, be it explosion or assault, but also from anxieties about the permanency of hearing loss and the problems associated with communication. As perforation of the tympanic membrane may be caused by a slap to the ear, such injuries in children may be resultant of a non-accidental injury.

External trauma

Wounds to the external ear or pinna in most cases may be closed by conventional wound closure methods. However, if the cartilage of the pinna is involved, scrupulous wound cleansing is required, as any subsequent infection is likely to lead to permanent deformity of the pinna. All wounds require antibiotic cover, such as amoxiclav (Corbridge & Steventon 2010).

Blunt trauma to the pinna, commonly occurring in contact sports, may result in haematoma formation. The haematoma, if untreated, may lead to the necrosis of the underlying cartilaginous skeleton of the pinna. O'Donoghue et al. (1992) advocate early incision and drainage as the most appropriate course of action in order to reduce morbidity. This is likely to require a general anaesthetic, and therefore referral to the ENT department is pertinent.

There is an increasing trend of cosmetic piercings of the upper one third of the pinna that puncture the cartilage. Hanif et al. (2001) report how infections following such piercings can result in auricular perichondritis.

The nose

Anatomy and physiology

The nose is a structure with a bony and cartilaginous skeleton that is attached to the skull via the frontal bone and the maxilla. It is a vascular structure whose prime functions are to interface with the respiratory system, to warm, filter and moisten inhaled air and to act as a sense organ involved in the enjoyment of food and the detection of danger in the case of smoke and gas. The upper third of the nose, where the frontal and maxillary bones form the bridge, is bony (Fig. 32.2).

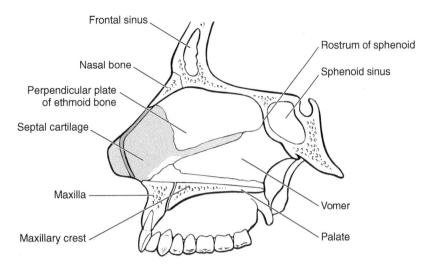

Figure 32.2 • Anatomy of the nose.

Foreign bodies

A foreign body in the nose usually occurs in children and they often will be accompanied by parents who are distressed and anxious about their child's well-being.

Clinical evidence and management

Usually the child will have told the parents that she/he has put something up her/his nose, or the parents will have noticed that the child has a purulent discharge from one nostril. Unilateral discharge is highly suggestive of a foreign body in the nose; however, children are not averse to placing foreign bodies in each nostril, resulting in a bilateral discharge.

The removal of a foreign body in the nose follows the same rules as the removal of a foreign body in the ear. The child should be seated in a dental chair or on a parent's lap in a semi-recumbent position. Initial assessment and history should ascertain the type of foreign body present, how long it has been in the nostril and whether there has been any bleeding or discharge. Careful explanation and instruction regarding the procedure for removal are required and psychological support for both parents and child is essential both for humanitarian reasons and to gain their cooperation during the procedure. Removal can be attempted using some topical anaesthetic spray, a ring curette or alligator forceps (Olson 2003). Care should be taken to prevent damage to the highly vascular nasal septum and mucosa during removal of a nasal foreign body. If the child is too distressed, the foreign body is too far into the nostril or there is any evidence of trauma to the nostril already, then the child should be referred to the ENT surgeon (Reynolds 2004).

Epistaxis

Epistaxis is often seen as a relatively minor problem in the ED. However, something as simple as a nose bleed can quickly turn into a life-threatening condition if it is not treated swiftly and correctly. Epistaxis can occur from either local or systemic causes including direct trauma, nose picking, inflammatory disease involving the nasal mucosa, coagulation deficits (including medication) and hypertension (Castelnuovo et al. 2010).

Clinical evidence and management

The patient will present with active bleeding from the nose, or a recent history of bleeding that may have stopped. The main aim of treatment is to stop the epistaxis. If the bleeding is from the anterior end of the septum (Littles' area), bleeding can usually be alleviated by seating the patient upright and advising her to hold the front soft part of the nose very firmly (Reynolds 2004). The patient's head should be tilted forward over a bowl.

This compression must be applied for at least 30–40 minutes without interruption. The use of ice can be helpful for its vasconstricting action; however, children and the elderly may find it difficult to tolerate. The patient should be encouraged to expectorate blood rather than swallow it, as this can lead to vomiting, which makes measurement of blood loss difficult. Haematemesis is also very anxiety-provoking for the patient.

If the bleeding is from the posterior part of the nose, as indicated by continued bleeding after compression or as seen on examination, the patient may need to have the nose packed. The procedure may be performed in the ED following the application of local anaesthetic spray to the area. Ribbon gauze, haemostatic absorbent nasal tampons or catheters may be used as directed by the clinician. If unsuccessful, the patient may need to be referred to the ENT surgeon.

Once active haemorrhage is controlled, any precipitating medical factors should be identified and corrected if clinically safe to do so. The anticoagulated patient can pose a challenging problem, because they tend to have more severe epistaxis and bleed from several sites. Because of the risk for serious medical complications, reversal or discontinuation of the anticoagulation medication should not be performed unless it is deemed safe by the initiating medical specialty. During warfarin-related epistaxis, 80 % of patients were outside their disease-specific international normalized ratio (INR) range; therefore, in addition to a complete blood count, all patients should have an INR evaluated at the time of presentation (Smith et al. 2011, Rudmik & Smith 2012). If the patient is hypertensive on presentation an antihypertensive agent, such as nifedipine, may need to be administered.

Occasionally, the patient with an epistaxis may need resuscitative care due to blood loss. The siting of a large-bore intravenous line and commencement of replacement fluid, monitoring of vital signs, and taking of blood for a full blood count and cross-match are necessary in this case. All patients with epistaxis have the potential to become shocked if bleeding is not stopped. Initial assessment involves an estimate of the amount of bleeding, the length of time active bleeding has been taking place and any previous relevant medical history. Physical assessment of the patient should always include monitoring of vital signs (Melia & McGarry 2011).

Nasal fracture

This is the most common facial fracture accounting for almost 60% of all facial fractures (Allareddy & Nalliah 2011). It usually caused by blunt trauma and commonly seen in the ED patient who has been assaulted. Clinically, the injury can usually be recognized immediately afterwards by the distortion from normal shape, although this soon becomes obscured by soft tissue swelling.

Clinical evidence and management

There will be a history of trauma to the nose, swelling deformity and occasionally epistaxis. It is important to examine the nose for any evidence of cerebrospinal fluid (CSF), rhinorrhoea and any indication of fractures to the cribiform plate. Normal CSF is clear and slightly yellow, but CSF nasal drainage is frequently mixed with blood. Gisness (2003) describes septal haematoma as a bulging, tense bluish mass that feels doughy when palpated. Septal haematomas should be urgently drained to prevent airway obstruction and necrosis of the septal cartilage. Septal haematoma may strip the septal cartilage of blood supply and progress to abscess formation or later cartilage necrosis, resulting in significant nasal deformity and septal perforation. An overlooked septal haematoma may critically disfigure the patient and it should always be ruled out (Lynham et al. 2012).

Generally, little can be done for patients following a fracture of the nose until 5–10 days after the initial injury, due to soft tissue swelling. The patient should therefore be referred to the ENT outpatients department. Since the nasal bones will become firmly set within 3 weeks of the injury, reduction of a nasal fracture is indicated in any patient with significant cosmetic deformity or functional compromise (Vats et al. 2007). X-rays are often requested for medico-legal reasons, but are not strictly necessary (see also Chapter 10).

Rhinorrhoea

Otherwise known as a 'runny nose', this is caused by excess mucus being produced by an inflamed nasal mucosa.

Clinical evidence and management

The patient presents with a runny nose or the sensation of something dripping down the back of the throat. The discharge may be clear or purulent. The causes are:

- allergy
- infection
- foreign body
- underlying tumour.

The patient may need to have a foreign body removed. If an allergy is suspected, antihistamines may be prescribed, and advice should be given on avoidance of common allergens, i.e., grass/tree pollen, dust and cat or dog fur. The patient may also need to be referred to an allergy clinic. Infective rhinosinusitus may need treatment with antibiotics. If a tumour is suspected, urgent referral to ENT will be necessary.

Advice, explanation and health education regarding the taking of antihistamines (whose main side-effect is drowsiness) and antibiotics should be given to the patient. If the rhinitis is viral in origin, antibiotics will have little or no effect, and they should therefore not be seen as a panacea for this, or any other, condition.

Allergic rhinitis

This can be seasonal or perennial. The symptoms are those of sneezing, nasal obstruction and rhinorrhoea. There is often itching of the nose, eyes and palate, accompanied by loss of smell, rhinorrhoea and episodes of sneezing. Secondary symptoms such as headache and facial pain may also occur due to nasal congestion (Stearn 2005). Evidence of associated allergic diseases, such as asthma and eczema, should also be sought as there is a high correlation between the conditions. Bousquet et al. (2001) note that some 80% of asthma patients also suffer from allergic rhinitis. Patients should be advised to avoid common allergens as much as possible, such as grass/tree pollen, cat or dog fur and house dust, especially in the early morning and later afternoon/early evening when pollen counts are at their highest. Wearing sunglasses, spectacles or contact lenses (if appropriate) may also be beneficial in reducing eye symptoms. Patients should be given antihistamines and advised to see their GP for further prescription of any topical decongestants and for referral to a local allergy clinic.

Sinusitis

Sinusitis is an inflammatory, and usually infective, condition of the paranasal sinus, which is associated with approximately 90% of viral infections of the upper respiratory tract. Complications of untreated or inadequately treated acute sinusitis include chronic sinusitis, orbital abscess, meningitis, brain abscess, cavernous sinus thrombosis and osteomyelitis of the maxillary or frontal bones (Olson 2003, Kumar 2004).

Clinical evidence and management

The main symptoms a patient can present to the ED are sneezing, headache and facial pain which are worse when bending forward, and a recent history of upper respiratory tract infection. Maxillary toothache without obvious dental cause may also occur. The patient may be very worried about the severity of their headache. A set of baseline observations of pulse, blood pressure, temperature and respirations will aid diagnosis. This, along with a clinical history, may help to rule out other diagnoses such as hypertension or subarachnoid haemorrhage.

Treatment usually involves prescription of a broad-spectrum antibiotic. Advice can be given to take analgesia and to use a decongestant spray. The patient should be advised to see their GP if symptoms persist, as referral to the ENT department may be necessary. Complications of sinus disease include meningitis, orbital extension and brain abscess (Kumar 2004).

The throat

Anatomy and physiology

The throat, or pharynx, consists of the nasopharynx, oropharynx and laryngopharynx. It is a funnel-shaped tube that starts at the internal nares (nasal passages) and extends to the level of the cricoid cartilage. Its wall is composed of skeletal muscles and lined with mucous membrane. The central portion (oropharynx) provides a common passage for air, drink and food (Bickley & Szilagyi 2003). Pharyngeal constrictor muscles propel food or liquid into the oesophagus. These muscles are also responsible for the gag reflex, which is controlled by the cranial nerves. The larynx helps to prevent aspiration, assists in coughing and serves as the organ for speech.

Airway obstruction

Many patients who attend the ED with either an apparently trivial throat condition or more severe conditions are potentially at risk of airway obstruction. Thus the potential for a life-threatening condition to be overlooked is ever-present, unless there is a high index of suspicion and a rigorous assessment of these patients takes place (see also Chapter 2).

Airway obstruction can be partial or complete and is dynamic in nature. In the case of oedema, where the airway may initially be partially obstructed, it can progress rapidly to complete obstruction as the oedema progresses. Relatively large foreign bodies inhaled into the airway may well rapidly obstruct it, while oedema of the airway in response to an allergic reaction may obstruct it in a more progressive manner.

Should the airway become compromised, by whatever means, patency must be achieved as a matter of urgency, in order for ventilation to occur. Airway management should initially be in the form of basic techniques, such as positioning the patient and the Heimlich manoeuvre where the obstruction is caused by a foreign body. The Heimlich manoeuvre is not recommended for infants because of poor protection of the upper abdominal organs (International Liaison Committee on Resuscitation 2006).

Circumstances such as complete obstruction by an impacted foreign body or rapidly progressing oedema may dictate the early use of advanced techniques, such as endotracheal intubation, cricothyrotomy and surgical airway. Oxygen should be administered to all patients with actual and potential airway obstruction. Admission must be considered for observation of patients whose airway has been compromised and where deterioration is a possibility.

A number of events can compromise the airway. If these are dealt with effectively, complete obstruction can be prevented. These events will be discussed under the headings traumatic, infective and reactive.

Oral cavity

Trauma

Trauma to the oral cavity can cause a great deal of tissue swelling. Extensive bleeding can occur because of the vascular nature of the region, which is why lacerations to the tongue can bleed dramatically. Teeth can be dislodged or broken and inhalation can occur. Fracture of the mandible may also cause problems and these are dealt with in Chapter 10. Injuries to the oral cavity are common in young children (Zimmermann et al. 2006).

A visual assessment is vital in determining the extent of any injury. Suction may be required to enable visual assessment to take place. Blind suction should be avoided as this can exacerbate trauma and increase the likelihood of additional problems, such as vomiting. X-rays can be of benefit in suspected fractures or in locating lost teeth when inhalation is suspected. Where an assault has occurred, photographs may be of use for medico-legal purposes. Bleeding from tooth sockets can usually be arrested with haemostatic agents and slight pressure. Antibiotics may be prescribed prophylactically.

It is essential that anxiety is reduced by reassuring the patient at the time of initial assessment. In the case of children, injuries frequently appear worse than they really are, especially when bleeding is profuse, and parents require as much reassurance as the children. Not all lacerations in the mouth will require sutures. Small lacerations, particularly to the inside of the lip, will usually heal well without intervention, other than advice on oral hygiene and the use of medicated mouth washes. Similarly, lacerations of the tongue bleed profusely, but they too usually heal well. Sutures inside the oral cavity should be soluble so that removal is not required. Those patients with extensive lacerations in the oral cavity will require appropriate referral. External cold compresses may be helpful in reducing swelling.

Infective

Infections of the oral cavity most commonly involve the teeth and gums and referral to a dentist may be the most appropriate action.

Clinical evidence and management

Abscesses of the teeth may need drainage and/or antibiotic therapy, which is most appropriately carried out by a dental practitioner. Frequently the most appropriate course of action is to refer the patient to their GP, but in the interim the patient may be prescribed antibiotics and analgesia. Patient education may focus upon the safe and efficacious use of prescribed medication and the initiation of oral hygiene measures including saline mouthwashes and tooth brushing.

Reactive

Reactions occur as a result of exposure to foreign substances to which the body has developed an allergy, resulting in a local or systemic allergic reaction which in severe cases may manifest as anaphylactic shock.

Aetiology of anaphylactic shock

Anaphylaxis is a severe, life-threatening, generalized or systemic hypersensitivity reaction. It is characterized by rapidly developing life-threatening airway and/or breathing and/or circulation problems usually associated with skin and/or mucosal changes. The incidence of anaphylaxis appears to be increasing, in part given the possibility of omission of a precise diagnosis for a patient (Simons & Sampson 2008, Younker & Soar 2011). It generally follows from exposure to a foreign protein to which the patient has been previously sensitized. The individual becomes sensitized to the allergen by the production of antibodies in response to this exposure. These bind to basophils in the blood and sensitize the cells. Common sensitizing substances are antibiotic medication, especially penicillin and penicillin derivatives, bee stings, foodstuffs such as peanuts and non-steroidal anti-inflammatory medications. When the allergen re-enters the body, this stimulates the release of mediators of anaphylaxis, e.g., histamine, serotonin, slow-release substances of anaphylaxis (SRS-A) and platelet-activating factors (PAF), which result in cellular damage.

Clinical evidence of anaphylactic shock

Anaphylaxis is likely when *all* of the following three criteria are met:

- sudden onset and rapid progression of symptoms
- life-threatening airway and/or breathing and/or circulation problems
- skin and/or mucosal changes (flushing, urticaria, angio-edema) (Younker & Soar 2011).

Physiological changes include:

- increased blood capillary permeability – causing localized oedema
- smooth muscle contraction (bronchioles)
- increased gastric secretion
- increased mucus secretion
- inhibited coagulation.

These changes may result in some or all of the following symptoms:

- wheezing
- urticaria
- pruritis
- stridor
- respiratory difficulty
- tachypnoea
- hypotension
- collapse.

Symptoms can occur within minutes of ingestion, with the allergen gaining rapid access to the circulatory system through the digestive tract and activating mast cells in the mouth, throat, lungs, skin, abdomen and other tissues and organs (Crusher 2004). Management is based on positioning of the patient in the supine position and the administration of adrenaline (epinephrine) via the intramuscular route. This is supported with high-flow oxygen to combat potential hypoxia. Where adrenaline is administered, the patient should be admitted for a period of observation. If possible, the allergen should be identified to enable the patient to avoid this in the future.

Those patients with mild reactions and who are discharged home require advice on the safe and efficacious use of any prescribed medications, most likely antihistamine tablets. Specifically they should be warned of the sedative effects of this type of medication and thus the implications for driving and operating machinery while taking the medication. Subsequent exposure to an unidentified allergen may cause a more severe reaction which could be potentially fatal. It is crucial that these patients are offered advice on identifying the allergen which caused the reaction. This is perhaps best achieved by referral to their own GP who may arrange appropriate tests and support.

Pharynx

Swelling in this region is more likely to compromise the airway than in the oral cavity because of the smaller diameter of the lumen of the airway. This is highly significant in children, where as little as 1 mm of oedema may cause 75 % occlusion of the airway.

Traumatic

Clinical evidence

External as well as internal trauma may cause oedema in this region. People who have attempted suicide by hanging or strangulation and those involved in accidents involving strictures around the neck account for a proportion of this group of patients. In cases of strangulation and hanging where the patient is unable to self-advocate, for whatever reason, consideration should be given to any medico-legal implications, and where appropriate the police may need to be informed. Victims of road traffic accidents may also suffer trauma to this region of the body which can be easily overlooked in the presence of more obvious injuries, highlighting the importance of thorough primary and secondary surveys. Where neck injuries are apparent, the possibility of trauma to the internal structures should be considered.

Inhalation injury due to hot gases and flames may be present in burn-injured patients. Signs of inhalation injury from hot substances are not always evident, but a useful sign to look for is singed nostril hairs. If the gas was hot enough to damage these hairs then airway damage should be expected. Similarly, the ingestion of corrosive substances may also cause burns and swelling to the pharynx area. Inhalation of small foreign bodies, such as fish bones, rarely causes airway obstruction, but they can be troublesome, causing irritation, increased salivation and coughing because they are lodged in the pharynx. Patients should be advised that fish bones can often scratch the side of the throat on the way down, leaving them with the feeling that the foreign body is still there.

Management

The airway is the number one priority. Careful and accurate assessment of the patient and the extent of injuries must be carried out early. If the patient is conscious, a history of the event and mechanism of injury will give an indication of the stresses involved. Signs of airway obstruction such as noisy breathing should be noted and monitored for deterioration. Admission is essential where there is a degree of swelling which is likely to increase, leading to the airway becoming compromised.

For patients with small foreign bodies in their pharynx, X-ray examination may be helpful and could reveal radioopaque objects. A plain lateral soft-tissue X-ray of the neck can provide valuable information about tissue swelling.

Infective

Clinical evidence

There will be a number of patients attending the ED with simple sore throats. They often only need reassurance and simple advice, possibly with referral to their GP if symptoms persist. There will be some adults among them with a peritonsillar abscess that will require further intervention. Children are less likely to complain of a sore throat but often go off their food and generally feel unwell and are pyrexial. These children may present with dysphagia, a wheeze or stridor and will need careful assessment. The possible cause of these symptoms is epiglottitis, which is a potentially fatal inflammation of the epiglottis and pharynx as a result of infection. McEwan et al. (2003) report an age range of presentation between 6 months and a little over 10 years.

Management

Peritonsillar abscesses in need of drainage will require the attention of the ENT team. The patient should be referred as soon as the diagnosis has been made. As a general anaesthetic may be required, the patient should be kept nil by mouth, and unnecessary examination of the throat should be avoided as this is likely to be very uncomfortable.

Children with epiglottitis will require urgent assessment and admission by the paediatric team. It is essential that the child is kept calm and is not distressed, that examination in the ED is kept to a minimum, and that insertion of instruments, such as thermometers or tongue depressors, should not take place, as this may cause the epiglottis to be pushed onto the larynx, thus occluding the airway completely. Endotracheal intubation should only be carried out by those who are extremely experienced in these techniques. If the airway becomes occluded then patency should be ensured by means of cricothyrotomy.

Conclusion

This chapter has examined the care of the individual who attends the ED with a condition relating to the ear, nose or throat. For practical purposes, care has been artificially described in terms of specific conditions, when in reality many of the identified conditions form only a part of a broader clinical picture. Care should encompass the psychological, emotional and social needs of patients and their families. What may be regarded as a minor condition to the ED nurse is often a terrifying experience for the affected individuals.

The key element in care with these individuals, as with all aspects of ED care, is communication. Patients who attend the emergency department with an acute ENT condition are often regarded as having a trivial condition, yet many of these conditions have the potential to become life-threatening. Patients who have traumatic injuries are rightly given high priority and are treated aggressively, yet the preventable causes of death in both groups of patients are the same, i.e., hypoxia and hypovolaemia – hypoxia resulting from a foreign body impacted in the airway, and hypovolaemia resulting from epistaxis. People die from acute ENT conditions and, in many instances, these deaths are preventable. The ED nurse has a critical role to play in reducing the number of these preventable deaths.

References

Abelardo, E., Pope, L., Rajkumar, K., et al., 2007. A double-blind randomised clinical trial of the treatment of otitis externa using topical steroid alone versus topical steroid–antibiotic therapy. European Archives of Oto-Rhino-Laryngology 266 (1), 41–45.

Allareddy, V., Nalliah, R.P., 2011. Epidemiology of facial fracture injuries. Journal of Oral & Maxillofacial Surgery 69, 2613–2618.

Bickley, L.S., Szilagyi, P.G., 2003. Bates' Guide to Physical Examination and History Taking, eighth ed. Lippincott, Williams & Wilkins, Philadelphia.

Bluestone, C., Klein, J., 2007. Otitis Media in Infants and Children. BC Decker Inc, Hamilton.

Bousquet, J., van Cauwenberge, P., Khaltaev, N., 2001. Allergic rhinitis and its impact on asthma. The Journal of Allergy and Clinical Immunology 108 (5), S147–S333.

Castelnuovo, P., Pistochini, A., Palma, P., 2010. Epistaxis. Otorhinolaryngology, Head and Neck. European Manual of Medicine, Part 2, 205–208.

Coker, R., Chan, L., Newberry, S., et al., 2010. Diagnosis, microbial epidemiology, and antibiotic treatment of acute otitis media in children. The Journal of the American Medical Association 304 (19), 2161–2169.

Corbridge, R., Steventon, N., 2010. Oxford Handbook of ENT and Head and Neck Surgery. Oxford University Press, Oxford.

Crusher, R., 2004. Anaphylaxis. Emergency Nurse 12 (3), 24–31.

Davies, P., Benger, J., 2000. Foreign bodies in the nose and ear: a review of techniques for removal in the emergency department. Journal of Accident and Emergency Medicine 17, 91–94.

Garner, J., 2011. Ballistic and blast injuries. In: Smith, J., Greaves, I., Porter, K. (Eds.), Oxford Desk Reference: Major Trauma. Oxford Medical Publications, Oxford.

Gisness, C., 2003. Maxillofacial trauma. In: Newberry, L. (Ed.), Sheehy's Emergency Nursing: Principles and Practice, fifth ed. Mosby, St Louis.

Hanif, J., Frosh, A., Marnane, C., et al., 2001. High ear piercing and the raising incidence of perichondritis of the pinna. British Medical Journal 322, 906–907.

International Liaison Committee on Resuscitation, 2006. The International Liaison Committee on Resuscitation (ILCOR) consensus on science with treatment recommendations for pediatric and neonatal patients: Pediatric basic and advanced life support. Paediatrics 117 (5), e955–e977.

Kumar, S., 2004. Ear, nose and throat. In: Cameron, P., Jelinek, G., Kelly, A.M., Murray, L., Brown, A.F.T., Heyworth, J. (Eds.), Textbook of Emergency Medicine, second ed. Churchill Livingstone, Edinburgh.

Ludman, H., 2007. Pain in the ear. In: Ludman, H., Bradley, P.J. (Eds.), ABC of Ear, Nose and Throat, fifth ed. Blackwell Publishing/BMJ Books, London.

Lynham, A., Tuckett, J., Warnke, P., 2012. Maxillofacial trauma. Australian Family Physician 41 (4), 172–180.

McEwan, J., Giridaran, W., Clarke, R., et al., 2003. Paediatric acute epiglottitis: not a disappearing entity. International Journal of Pediatric Otorhinolaryngology 67, 317–321.

Melia, L., McGarry, G.W., 2011. Epistaxis: update on management. Current Opinion in Otolaryngology & Head & Neck Surgery 19 (1), 30–35.

O'Donoghue, G.M., Bates, G.J., Narula, A.A., 1992. Clinical ENT: An Illustrated Textbook. Oxford University Press, Oxford.

Olson, C., 2003. Dental, ear, nose and throat emergencies. In: Newberry, L. (Ed.), Sheehy's Emergency Nursing: Principles and Practice, fifth ed. Mosby, St Louis.

Reynolds, T., 2004. Ear, nose and throat problems in Accident and Emergency. Nursing Standard 18 (26), 47–53.

Rudmik, L., Smith, T., 2012. Management of intractable spontaneous epistaxis. American Journal of Rhinology & Allergy 26 (1), 55–60.

Sander, R., 2001. Otitis externa: A practical guide to treatment and prevention. American Family Physician 63 (5), 927–937.

Simons, F.E., Sampson, H.A., 2008. Anaphylaxis epidemic: fact or fiction? Journal of Allergy & Clinical Immunology 122, 1166–1168.

Smith, J., Siddiq, S., Dyer, C., et al., 2011. Epistaxis in patients taking oral anticoagulant and antiplatelet medication: Prospective cohort study. Journal of Laryngology & Otology 125 (1), 38–42.

Stearn, R., 2005. One airway, one disease. Primary Health Care 15 (2), 31–34.

Vats, A., Narula, A., Bradley, P.J., 2007. Trauma, injuries and foreign bodies. In: Ludman, H., Bradley, P.J. (Eds.), ABC of Ear, Nose and Throat, fifth ed. Blackwell Publishing/BMJ Books, London.

Younker, J., Soar, J., 2011. Recognition and treatment of anaphylaxis. Nursing in Critical Care 15 (2), 94–98.

Zemlin, W.R., 2011. Speech and Hearing Science: Anatomy and Physiology, fourth ed. Allan and Bacon, Boston.

Zimmermann, C.E., Troulis, M.J., Kaban, L.B., 2006. Pediatric facial fractures: Recent advances in prevention, diagnosis and management. International Journal of Oral Maxillofacial Surgery 35 (1), 2–13.

PART 7

Practice issues in emergency care

People with learning disabilities

33

Margaret Sowney and Michael Brown

CHAPTER CONTENTS

Introduction

There is an increasing recognition of the need to respond to and meet the health needs of vulnerable groups within society. There are a range of people who may, for a variety of reasons, be vulnerable; this includes people with learning disabilities, children, people with mental health problems, people with acquired brain injury, some older people and those with dementia. Nurses who work in emergency care are often the first point of contact with healthcare services for patients and they are in a good position to ensure that the needs of vulnerable patients are appropriately assessed and responded to in a person-centred way. In order to respond appropriately it is necessary for these nurses to have an understanding and overview of the key health and care needs of vulnerable patients. This knowledge and understanding is important, as needs are often different and distinct, requiring specific responses and actions.

People with learning disability in society

People with learning disabilities are an integral part of society and need to be recognized and valued as equal citizens. It is estimated that as a group they form almost 2 % of the overall population across the UK, totaling some 1.5 million people. It is further estimated that prevalence rates per thousand of the general population indicate that there are 3 to 4 persons with severe learning disabilities and 25 to 30 with milder learning disabilities. The population of people with learning disabilities is ageing and increasing (Tyler et al. 2007). As a consequence, nurses working in emergency care settings will come into contact with more of this group of people in the future; hence the need for core knowledge and skills.

Across the world a range of definitions are used when referring to this population. The term learning disability has been adopted within the UK and refers to people with cognitive impairments that impact significantly upon their development, which in turn may affect the ability of some to live independently. Other terms used across the world include developmental disability, mental handicap and mental retardation. Increasingly the term intellectual disability is being adopted; however, irrespective of the current terminology used it is generally agreed that the term learning disability relates to:

- a significantly reduced ability to understand new or complex information, to learn new skills

- a reduced ability to cope independently
- which started before adulthood, with a lasting effect on development (Department of Health 2001a, 2001b).

A learning disability is a disorder that covers a spectrum of the population and is frequently referred to as mild, moderate, severe or profound. The level of cognitive impairment increases with the severity of learning disability, thereby affecting a person's ability to understand new or complex information, learn and develop skills and use them independently. In order to be considered as a learning disability it is generally accepted that the disorder usually occurs on or around the time of birth and certainly before the age of 18.

There is a wide range of causes that result in the development of a learning disability. These can be conceptualized as occurring in the prenatal (prior to birth), perinatal (during birth), and postnatal (following birth) periods.

Prenatal issues

Some of the causes of learning disability are preventable, highlighting the need for access to genetic counselling and effective nutrition, including vitamin supplements. For example, folic acid taken prior to and up to the 12th week of pregnancy is known to help prevent neural tube defects. The management of pre-existing health conditions such as diabetes is important.

Additionally there is a range of lifestyle issues such as smoking, alcohol and drug misuse that can have an impact on pregnancy and can result in learning disability. Environmental risk factors that can lead to learning disability include exposure during pregnancy to infections such as rubella (German measles), cytomegalovirus and genitourinary infections such as syphilis.

Perinatal issues

Perinatally, there are risk factors that can result in learning disability. There is increasing evidence that premature and low-birth-weight babies are at risk from developmental delay and that some will have a learning disability of a nature that will require ongoing additional support. Trauma during birth can occur and factors such as breech presentations and asphyxia can be causes. Therefore good maternal care is necessary along with access to health education.

Postnatal issues

Postnatally, poor nutrition, social deprivation and abuse are known to intervene in a child's growth and development. In addition there are also a number of infections that are common in childhood that carry a risk of brain damage, such as gastroenteritis, meningitis and encephalitis. Environmental factors, such as trauma and injury resulting from falls and injuries from car accidents, can result in brain damage and learning disability.

Changing policy and legislative directions

The four countries of the UK all have clear policy frameworks regarding the care and support of people with learning disabilities:

- Scotland – *The Same as You?* (Scottish Executive 2000)
- England – *Valuing People* and *Valuing People Now* (Department of Health 2001a, 2009)
- Wales – *Fulfilling the Promises* (Welsh Assembly 2002a)
- Northern Ireland – *Equal Lives* (Department of Health, Social Services and Public Safety 2004).

Collectively these policies are seeking to bring about change and improvement in the lives of children, adults and older people with learning disabilities that support and enable them to contribute as equal and valued members of society. These changes and developments are important, as people with learning disabilities have not always been valued and respected. Today, however, there is a clear shift in focus for the care and support of this group towards community inclusion, which has brought about the closure of long-stay institutions across the country (Scottish Executive 2003).

In addition to the clear policy frameworks that have been developed, there are specific pieces of legislation that are particularly relevant that impact on the lives of people with learning disability. Across the UK, the Disability Discrimination Act (1995) is particularly significant as this legislation makes it explicitly illegal to discriminate against a person with a disability, including those with learning disabilities. The Act requires all public services, including health services, to make a *reasonable adjustment* to enable people with disabilities to access services. In 2006, the Disability Equality Duty came into force in England, Wales and Scotland making it a requirement of public services, such as health and social care services to ensure that all people with disabilities, including those with learning disabilities, are treated equally and fairly. In 2011 the Equality Act (2010) came into force in England, Wales and Scotland to eliminate unlawful discrimination, harassment and victimization and other conduct prohibited by the Act.

Also of significance is the Human Rights Act (1998); it is relevant from a number of perspectives. The Act contains articles that seek to protect the rights of citizens in areas such as the right to life, the right to marriage, the right to freedom of expression and the right to freedom from discriminating and humiliating treatment. It is important that healthcare professionals in emergency care have an understanding of the implications and potential impact on their practice and care. The House of Lords and House of Commons published the findings of their independent inquiry that highlighted that the human rights of people with learning disabilities are not always respected when receiving healthcare (House of Lords & House of Commons 2008).

As a result of cognitive impairment some people with learning disabilities may experience capacity difficulties that impact upon their ability to make decisions about certain aspects of their life. Healthcare procedures and treatments can have important implications for a patient and there may be particular difficulties for some people with learning disabilities regarding their comprehension and understanding and as a result their capacity to give informed consent (Cummings 2012). In Scotland the Adults with Incapacity (Scotland) Act (2000) provides a clear framework to support people with capacity issues, including people with learning disabilities and in England and Wales the Mental Capacity Act (2005) provides a clear statutory framework to protect vulnerable people, including those with learning disabilities, who are not able to make their own decisions. The Act sets out who can make decisions and in what situations and what they need to do to comply. The Act sets out the presumption of capacity and the right of all individuals to make decisions about their care, the right to receive support in making decisions, the right to make decisions, even when they may seem unwise, that all actions must be in the best interest of the patients and that all interventions must be the least restrictive. It is therefore a requirement of their professional practice that all clinicians have a clear understanding of the legal frameworks in place to ensure the rights of people with learning disabilities are protected and their needs addressed.

The health profile of people with learning disabilities

As a group, people with learning disabilities have a differing health profile when compared to the general population and as a result particular responses are required. Additionally they have higher health needs, many of which frequently go unrecognized and unmet. This has a significant impact on their health and well-being and contributes to their need to access healthcare services and to premature death.

The health needs of people with learning disabilities can be complex and bring many into contact with all aspects of the healthcare system. For some their need for ongoing healthcare will be life-long in order to manage and limit the consequences of a range of chronic health conditions found within this population (Jansen et al. 2005, Van Schronjenstein et al. 2008). There are a range of health issues experienced by this group that frequently require them to access emergency care services, and therefore all nurses require an overview and understanding of the care needs, not only those who work in specialist services (Janicki et al. 2002, Scottish Executive 2002, Balogh et al. 2005). Fifty per cent of people with learning disabilities who present at ED are subsequently admitted, a proportion considerably higher than the 31 % of people without such disabilities who are admitted after presentation (Blair 2012, Emerson et al. 2012).

People with learning disabilities have the same everyday health needs as the general population, such as requiring treatment, investigation and management of conditions like asthma and diabetes (NHS Health Scotland 2004). The notion of everyday health needs includes access to emergency care services, as people with learning disabilities experience accidents and trauma as do the general population (Alborz et al. 2005). Collectively therefore nurses in emergency care will encounter people with learning disabilities and need to be able to respond appropriately, yet many report feeling poorly prepared to meet the needs of this group (McConkey &

Truesdale 2000, Iacono & Davis 2003, Sowney & Barr 2006a, Gibbs et al. 2008).

It is relevant to reflect on healthcare education programmes, where it is clear that few health care professionals have received any significant education or clinical experience in assessing and meeting the distinct health needs of this population and as a consequence they lack confidence in providing care. It is therefore apparent that many healthcare professionals, including nurses in emergency care, are not well prepared to respond effectively to this group of patients (Brown 2005). It is not, however, acceptable to fail to respond due to a lack of confidence and experience, and the role of continuing practice development and education programmes is important and all should incorporate a focus on the needs of people with learning disabilities (NHS Education for Scotland 2004a).

An evolving evidence base of health needs

As a result of the overall improvements in health experienced by the general population, people with learning disabilities are living longer and into older age. Previously their life expectancy was significantly shorter. Now there is a new phenomenon, with more living on into older age, meaning there will be more people with learning disability in the future, many with complex care needs (Glasson et al. 2002, Carling-Jenkins et al. 2012). This will mean that nurses in emergency care will see the full spectrum of people with learning disabilities, from those with a mild learning disability through to those with highly complex physical and mental disabilities related to old age.

Communication is the number one ranked problem experienced across the spectrum of the learning disability population. They experience a high prevalence of difficulty with comprehension, expression and pragmatic communication (UK Parliament 2008). Additionally, paid carers frequently overestimate their communication abilities. This overestimation is an important issue that needs to be taken into account when emergency nurses are undertaking patient assessments, where they may rely on a carer for additional information and background about the person with learning disabilities. Merrifield (2011) argues that the assumption should not be made that because a person has poor or limited verbal speech, they are unable to understand what is being said to them.

People with learning disabilities experience higher prevalence rates of sensory impairment when compared with the general population. It is estimated that there is a 4 % prevalence of visual problems experienced by people with a mild learning disability under 50 years old in comparison to 2–7 % in the general population; the level of visual impairment increases with the level of learning disability. There is a 21 % prevalence rate of hearing impairment being experienced by those with mild learning disabilities less than 50 years in comparison with 0.2–1.9 % in the general population (Evenhuis et al. 2001). There is also a higher prevalence of hearing disorders in people with severe learning disability. These issues are particularly prevalent in people who have very severe learning disabilities and are frequently associated with a range of other health needs such as epilepsy, gastric disorders, cerebral palsy, hydrocephalus, respiratory disorders and immobility. Many will require tube feeding, increasingly via PEG tubes, some may need ventilation and routine suctioning, while others may have valves and shunts inserted due to blockage in the circulation of cerebrospinal fluid. Their presence needs to be considered when undertaking assessment in emergency departments.

Respiratory disease is the commonest cause of death in this population and is associated with pneumonia, often secondary to swallowing and aspiration problems (Hollins et al. 1998). In contrast to the general population, cardiovascular disease is the second commonest cause of death within this population. Cardiac abnormalities are a feature of specific syndromes such as Down syndrome, and ongoing investigation, treatment and monitoring are required for such persons (Hollins et al. 1998). People with learning disabilities experience higher rates of gastric problems, including gastric oesophageal reflux disorder (GORD), oesophagitis and *Helicobacter pylori* infection. Complications can result from these problems and investigation and treatment are indicated (Böhmer et al. 2000, Merrifield 2011).

Constipation is an important and frequent problem experienced by a significant number of people with learning disabilities, particularly those with severe learning disabilities, and is an issue that may bring some into contact with emergency services, yet it can be overlooked. Those most at risk are those with mobility problems, poor diets and fluid intake combined with medication for epilepsy and gastric problems (Böhmer et al. 2001). Assessment and diagnosis can prove challenging and patients with learning disabilities who are constipated may exhibit challenging behaviours due to their abdominal pain and discomfort.

People with learning disabilities experience a different pattern of cancer when compared to the general population. Gastric, oesophagus and gall bladder cancer are more prevalent in this population and there are higher levels of leukaemia experienced by people with Down syndrome (Hasle et al. 2000, Patja et al. 2001).

Within the learning disability population there are high rates of tooth and gum disease and an increased use of anaesthetics for examinations and treatment (Cumella et al. 2000). It is important for nurses undertaking assessments with people with learning disabilities to look beyond what may appear to be challenging behaviours, as closer review may indicate pain and distress associated with dental problems and this is an issue that needs to be excluded.

Epilepsy is extremely common in the learning disability population, with some 10–20% of people with mild learning disabilities experiencing seizures, moving to over 50% in those with severe and complex learning disabilities. This is in comparison with some 1% of the general population. The epilepsy presentation within the learning disability population is more complex than that experienced by the general population and there are higher levels of polypharmacy, complex seizure types and sudden unexplained death as a result of seizures (Sillanpaa et al. 1999). As a consequence of seizures, people with learning disabilities may require emergency treatment of status epilepticus, while some will experience injury and trauma that will also require attention from emergency care services.

As with the general population people with learning disabilities experience accidents and orthopaedic problems associated with falls that will bring them into contact with emergency nurses. It is now recognized that women with learning disabilities have higher rates of osteoporosis and associated fractures. Additionally, as a result of mobility, balance and gait problems people with learning disabilities experience accidents and fractures that are linked to their premature death (Center et al. 1998).

While there is an increasing recognition of the sexual health needs of people with learning disabilities, this is in an area requiring a higher focus. People with learning disabilities can be victims of sexual abuse, with an associated impact on their sexual healthcare. Additionally women with learning disabilities have a low uptake of cervical and breast-screening programmes targeted at the general population (Brown et al. 1995, Hollins & Perez 2000).

People with learning disabilities have a higher prevalence of psychiatric ill health and, as with their physical health needs, their mental health pattern differs when compared to the general population. This point is significant when linked with the communication difficulties that may be present and is an important factor that needs to be considered by emergency nurses when undertaking patient assessment. People with learning disabilities have a higher prevalence rate of schizophrenia, 3% compared with 1% in the general adult population (Lund 1985, Doody et al. 1998). Furthermore, depression was found in 22% of people with learning disabilities compared with 5.5% in the general adult population (Richards et al. 2001). Anxiety and panic disorders are common in the general population and are also experienced by people with learning disabilities of all ages, although the disorder may fail to be recognized in this population and be considered to be challenging behaviour, thereby affecting diagnosis and treatment (Patel et al. 1993, Moss et al. 2000).

Emergency nurses will be familiar with patients who self-injure. Self-injury is found in the learning disability population and is associated with autism, IQ, level of immobility and hearing difficulties. Prevalence rates of self-injury have been found to be as high as 17.4% in this population, with some 1.7% being of a severe and sustained nature (Collacott et al. 1998). Dementia is found in higher rates within the learning disability population and occurs at an earlier age. It is particularly common within people with Down syndrome (Patel et al. 1993, Holland 2000).

Autistic spectrum disorder is a life-long disability that affects the way a person communicates and relates to others around them. People with autism also experience problems and difficulties with social interaction as well as having altered capacity to understand emotional expressions. Autism may be associated with learning disabilities; however, it is important to recognize that autism covers a spectrum. Not all people with autism also have a learning disability. It is estimated that there are some 60 per 10000 population of children with autistic spectrum disorder, though data are currently not available for the prevalence within the adult population. People with autistic spectrum disorder present with a range of additional health needs, including mental health, communication, epilepsy and some may experience problem behaviours (Medical Research Council 2001, Public Health Institute of Scotland 2001).

People with learning disabilities as health service users

People with learning disabilities are high users of all aspects of health services. Yet when compared with the general population their care episodes are shorter. Mencap (2004) suggest that on average 14% of the general population will require general hospital services: this is in comparison to 26% of people with learning disabilities. Therefore it becomes evident that all nurses irrespective of the clinical focus of their role will come into contact with people with learning disability as a result of their health needs and the need to access health services. This contact is also likely to increase, as people with learning disabilities are now living longer and into old age, resulting in them also developing health needs associated with older age.

As a result of their health profile people with learning disabilities will come into contact with emergency services. However, their opportunity to access quality healthcare is dependent in part on emergency nurses' ability and willingness to learn and respond appropriately to their communication patterns, the number one ranked problem experienced by this population. The challenge then for nurses within this fast-moving environment is to find ways in which the needs of people with learning disabilities are both identified and met in equity with others who access the service.

Reducing challenges in accessing services

The challenges in accessing health services and the impact of poor-quality care that potentially lead to poor outcomes for individuals was highlighted more recently in the document 'Death by Indifference' following the deaths of six people with learning disability in general hospitals (Mencap 2007). In response to this report an independent inquiry into access to healthcare by this population was undertaken by Sir Jonathan Michael in 2007. The subsequent Michael Report (Department of Health 2008) found that despite clear legislation related to equality of treatment, people with learning disabilities continue to have both unmet health needs and they receive a poorer quality of health treatment. The Joint Committee on Human Rights in their report on the Human Rights of people with learning disabilities highlighted that although the key principles such as human rights, dignity, respect, autonomy, and equality should apply to all, they are often breached in relation to meeting the needs of people with learning disabilities (UK Parliament 2008). The Michael Report also suggests that there is evidence indicating that both morbidity and deaths in this population could be avoided and made a number of recommendations to improve the care of people with learning disabilities (Department of Health 2008).

A follow-up on the progress to improving access to healthcare for people with learning disabilities (Parliamentary and Health Services Ombudsman 2009) recommended that NHS and social care organizations in England urgently review the quality of their service in meeting the needs of people with learning disabilities. In addition the Ombudsman's report placed the onus on the regulators of health and social care services to monitor adherence to both statutory and regulatory requirements. Furthermore the implementation and monitoring of the recommendations should be undertaken by the Department of Health, within 18 months of the report's publication (Parliamentary and Health Services Ombudsman 2009).

Many of the negative experiences outlined by people with learning disabilities and their families of being in general hospitals are associated with poor communication (Gibbs et al 2008). Indeed ineffective communication was a common issue highlighted in the *Death by Indifference* document and failures in communication were highlighted in The Parliamentary and Health Ombudsman's 'Six Lives' Report (Department of Health 2009). Communication is a basic human right and a fundamental principle central to inclusion within society. It is a two-way process and all people use a variety of means to communicate, including both verbal and non-verbal means. Yet within society there is a significant dependence on verbal communication, leaving those with reduced or no verbal skills at a significant disadvantage in interacting in the world around them (Arnold & Boggs 1999).

The Department of Health (1992) estimates that between 40 and 50% of people with learning disabilities experience some degree of difficulty with communication, with sensory impairments being more common in this population. Evidence consistently shows that poor communication is one of the key barriers experienced by people with learning disabilities in accessing quality health and contributes to their poor care (Cumella & Martin 2000, PAMIS 2001, US Public Health Services 2002, Department of Health, Social Services and Public Safety 2004, Department of Health 2008).

For the healthcare professional, poor communication increases the challenges normally encountered in assessing the patient's needs, informing them of their current health status and seeking and gaining valid consent, all of which are prerequisites in providing quality care. As attendance at emergency care is often unplanned, for people with learning disabilities being in an unfamiliar fast-moving environment can increase their feelings of fear and increase distress. Both the environmental and personal factors increase the risk of limited information exchange and as such increase the risk of harm to the patient (Department of Health, Social Services and Public Safety 2004, National Patient Safety Agency 2004).

Thus it is crucial that nurses within the emergency care settings develop a greater understanding of the communication difficulties experienced by people with intellectual disabilities, as a failure to communicate effectively can result in serious consequences. Primarily poor communication impacts on the nurse's ability to conduct an appropriate assessment of the individual's holistic needs, which in turn can have many negative consequences for the patient who has a learning disability, including:

- needs not being assessed and identified, thus not met
- an increased risk of harm due to non-compliance
- a greater risk of diagnostic overshadowing or differential diagnosis
- difficulties informing consent leading to a reluctance of staff to carry out previously identified care
- a reduction of patient involvement in discussions and decisions about healthcare
- reduction in opportunities to exercise the right to give or withhold consent.

Assessing needs

Currently there is little documented evidence available on the experience of people with learning disabilities of the emergency department, although this situation is gradually changing. Houghton (2001) suggests that this dearth of information within the emergency care literature may indicate a lack of awareness of emergency nurses regarding the health needs of people with learning disabilities. What is more concerning is a misconception that the needs of people with learning disability are not associated with emergency care (Sowney & Barr 2006b). This is an issue that requires to be challenged, as it is now accepted that general hospital services can present significant risk to the lives and health of people with learning disabilities. The National Patient Safety Agency state that:

'People with learning disability may be more at risk of things going wrong than the general population, leading to varying degrees of harm being caused whilst in general hospitals' (National Patient Safety Agency 2004, p. 11).

The risk factors identified include a limited knowledge and understanding of the health needs, an increased prevalence and risk of dysphagia and aspiration pneumonia, barriers preventing equal access to healthcare, a lack of education and practice development opportunities, complex communication issues and misdiagnosis or no diagnosis. When these issues are considered in relation to the research evidence of the range of health needs experienced by people with learning disabilities and their communication issues and behavioural challenges, it is vital that nurses in emergency care recognize these risk factors, assess for them and plan and implement individual care; they have a legal and professional duty to do so (NHS Health Scotland 2004, Disability Rights Commission 2006, NHS Quality Improvement Scotland 2009).

Though the number of people with learning disabilities accessing emergency services is increasing, few organizations have systematic mechanisms in place to quantify their attendance. Whilst the absence of these figures may actually be seen as a positive step towards inclusion, nurses within emergency care frequently ask the question 'how do we know if a person has a learning disability if there are no obvious signs?' There is no guaranteed way of gaining this understanding, particularly if the person has a mild learning disability and does not wish anyone to be aware of this. However, there may be a few indicators of the presence of a learning disability, including:

- vagueness providing a history
- difficulties expressing current need
- slowness in answering questions.

It is important that the right of people to withhold this information is respected; however, if the emergency care nurse suspects that a person may have learning disability and may require some further support to aid their assessment, treatment and recovery, this understanding is then justified. During the patient assessment some broad general questions may then help clarify the situation, for example, 'do you have any contact with health or social care professionals?' and 'do you receive visiting support at home?' In addition, following the provision of information throughout the whole process (whether verbal or written) emergency nurses need to continually ask broad questions that will establish the patient's current understanding.

While emergency nurses are skilled at carrying out a rapid assessment of needs, this process is not, however, as straightforward when the patient has a learning disability and communication difficulties and as such some further issues require consideration.

Hospitalization regardless of the time involved is known to cause stress, which is often demonstrated in people with learning disabilities by heightened emotional responses and behaviours. These emotional responses, including fear, insecurity or physical discomfort, can impact on the individual's ability to express needs and understand information regarding their condition and their compliance with treatment. Although compliance is required for many of the interventions associated with examination, treatment and care, ineffective communication and inappropriate timing of interventions, particularly at the heightened emotional stage, can cause harm to the individual (Arnold & Boggs 1999).

People with learning disabilities often need more time to express their needs, particularly when they are ill, yet within emergency departments, where time is considered to be of the essence, affording extra time to encourage interaction is problematic (Walsh & Dolan 1999). In order to conduct the assessment safely the emergency nurse must afford more time to the process of triage (Houghton 2001), which may be up to four times more than that required for a person without such disabilities. The challenge for nurses is to find out how the individual communicates, then investigate ways in which they can best communicate with each other to gain the appropriate information required for the assessment, rather than apportion blame for ineffective communication with people with learning disabilities. In doing so, they can reduce the patient's distress, fear and insecurities, whilst facilitating opportunities for the nurse to inform the patient, thus increasing compliance with examination, treatment or care (Boore 1978, Merrifield 2011).

Many people with learning disabilities who have little or no speech exhibit unusual behaviours as a way of communicating with others. Such behaviours can include rocking; head banging; increased flexion or extension and hypersensitivity to either sound or touch in their response to pain. However, as these messages are sent in a way that is quite different to what emergency nurses experience on a daily basis, there is a greater chance that these messages are misunderstood, being associated with learning disability and not a means of communicating a need. The danger in not understanding behavioural cues is a risk of diagnostic overshadowing and differential diagnoses.

An understanding of these two terms, diagnostic overshadowing and differential diagnosis, is particularly relevant in relation to assessing the health needs of people with learning disabilities. Diagnostic overshadowing occurs when clinicians, due to their limited knowledge and understanding of the differing presentations of illness in people with learning disabilities, assume that all clinical presentations and symptoms are as a result of the person's learning disability, as opposed to considering other possible physical or psychological underlying reasons (Jopp & Keys 2001). Clearly the consequences of diagnostic overshadowing could be potentially fatal for some people with learning disabilities as their true underlying health need will not be identified and treated (Parliamentary and Health Services Ombudsman 2009). Furthermore the term differential diagnosis relates to the range of possible clinical diagnoses that may result from the patient's history and from assessment and investigation (Reiss et al. 1982). In relation to people with learning disabilities where communication can be impaired there is an increased possibility that the range of differential diagnoses is not explored fully, and the potential seriousness of the condition going unrecognized – the problem of misdiagnosis is real and can have fatal consequences for persons with learning disabilities.

Thus, the assessment of healthcare needs, including pain, in people with learning disabilities can be very challenging. There may be the added issue of discriminating between what may be the distress of the patient in being in the emergency care situation and that of pain in emergency care settings. Nurses therefore need to assess levels of distress that may be experienced by patients with learning disability as well as pain and respond accordingly and the Disability Distress Assessment Tool is one example of an assessment that may assist (Regnard et al. 2007, Gates & Barr 2009). Pain presents in many ways and people have varying thresholds of pain; however, this is complicated further if the individual also has communication difficulties. Nonetheless, pain needs to be accurately assessed in people with learning disabilities through a comprehensive holistic approach informed by the use of appropriate pain assessment tools and where possible including information from a carer who is knowledgeable of the patient when well, thereby allowing a comparison with the presenting history. In addition to the knowledge of and skills in using various pain assessment tools the emergency care nurse also requires knowledge of how the perception of pain is verbalized and demonstrated in people with intellectual disabilities (Cumella & Martin 2000, Kerr & Wilkinson 2006, Kerr et al. 2006). Furthermore, the assessment of pain and the provision of adequate pain relief are also associated with the nurse's attitudes. Consequently, if emergency nurses believe that people with learning disabilities experience pain differently to those who do not have learning disabilities, then the opportunity to receive appropriate pain relief is reduced, increasing the patient's experience of stress, anxiety and fear. However, while

pain is a subjective experience, the opportunity to be pain-free must be seen by emergency nurses as a patient's priority.

The role of the families and carers in the assessment process is very important too, as they can provide essential support to the person with a learning disability, assisting them to express needs and make choices known. This is particularly so if the person has severe to profound learning disability with complex needs. Therefore it is both good practice and a duty of care for nurses within emergency care to work collaboratively with family members, demonstrating the value of their contribution, as well as showing a caring, respectful attitude towards the individual. Whilst the role of the carer in assisting with the provision of vital information cannot be underestimated, nurses are, however, responsible for using various skills to gain the information required to carry out a patient assessment, then to analyse the information, judging the value and worth (Sowney & Barr 2006b).

Involving people with learning disabilities

Involving people with learning disabilities in their care when they are acutely ill can be challenging. However, all patients need to be adequately informed of their health status to enable them to make informed decisions regarding their healthcare. Additionally the receipt of information in a format that is understood reduces fears and anxieties experienced by people with learning disabilities in acute general hospitals and increases opportunities for greater compliance and recovery. Evidence shows that informed people are better able to manage and cope with treatment and the effects of hospitalization and this is particularly important when working with vulnerable people.

People with learning disabilities may have difficulty understanding written information provided in general hospitals and frequently require the help of others to gain an understanding of the documents and their significance. Recent research on access to acute general hospitals has highlighted many areas of good practice within the emergency care environment in the development of various means of gaining and providing information to people with learning disabilities (NHS Quality Improvement Scotland 2006, Brown et al. 2010, MacArthur et al. 2010). This includes working guidelines and the development of more appropriate user-friendly leaflets and posters. Emergency nurses have an obligation to be aware of the good practice within their own area to facilitate good communication with people with learning disabilities.

Consent

It is impossible to consider communication difficulties experienced by people with learning disabilities without discussing the connection with the provision of valid consent. Central to the process of gaining valid consent is good communication; however, without the required information in a format that is clearly understood and accessible, people with learning disabilities remain passive in asserting control over their ability to self-determine and their own bodies.

The law recognizes the right of all adults to consent to examination, treatment and care and this includes people with a learning disability. Yet people with learning disabilities are often viewed by healthcare professionals as being incapable of making decisions and as such are frequently excluded from discussions and decisions regarding their healthcare (Mencap 2004, Hutchinson 2005, Sowney et al. 2006). Such false beliefs regarding the capacity to maintain control over their own bodies reduces opportunities for people with learning disabilities to be empowered, increasing their passivity in decision-making. Evidence shows that parents and other relatives are often asked to consent on behalf of an adult who has a learning disability, even though the law states that no one can give valid consent on behalf of another adult. It is therefore important to distinguish between consent and assent from a relative or carer. A relative or carer assenting and agreeing with a course of action is not valid consent.

In order to give valid consent, individuals must first have the ability to understand, maintain and judge information and in addition communicate a choice to others (Wong et al. 1999). The support mechanism of using the relative/carer to assist with explanations is good practice by nurses; however, no decisions should be made by the relatives or carers regarding the treatment or care that has not been the patient's identified choice. Healthcare professionals have both a legal and professional responsibility to obtain valid consent prior to the commencement of any examination, treatment or care and have a responsibility to ensure people with learning disabilities are empowered to make healthcare decisions (Department of Health 2001c, Welsh Assembly 2002b, Department of Health, Social Services and Public Safety 2004, NHS Health Scotland 2004, Mental Capacity Act 2005, Disability Rights Commission 2006, Nursing and Midwifery Council 2008). In addition, many investigations and treatments may be required within the emergency care environment and nurses must appreciate that valid consent for one aspect of care does not cover all other aspects of care. In addition nurses need to remember that consent is ongoing, being context-dependent, in that a person may have capacity to consent at one time and not at another (Dye et al. 2004). If, however, there is concern from the health care professional about an individual's capacity to consent this must be confirmed through a test of capacity.

In the absence of consent to examination, treatment and care within the emergency care environment, there is an increased risk of harm to the person with a learning disability from procedures being carried out by nurses without the full cooperation of the patient. Furthermore treatment without valid consent is unlawful. Similarly nursing staff can inadvertently cause harm through decisions not to act rather than to act, due to difficulties gaining valid consent (Barr 2004).

Emergency nurses need to be familiar with the issue of valid consent, having an understanding that both choice and control over healthcare decisions are key principles for all patients. In addition these aspects are central to the provision of inclusive services for people with learning disabilities (Department of Health 2001c, 2009, Welsh Assembly 2002b, Department of Health, Social Services and Public Safety 2004, NHS Health Scotland 2004, Mental Capacity Act 2005, Scottish Executive 2005). See Box 33.1.

> **Box 33.1**
>
> ## Improving communication and facilitating valid consent
>
> - Take a little extra time to communicate
> - Seek other means of gaining and providing information, verbal and non-verbal. Some people respond better to short phrases and pictures
> - Be aware of good practice elsewhere to enhance communication with people with learning disabilities, such as the development of leaflets and posters more suitable to providing information to people with learning disabilities
> - Always direct questions to and converse with the person with a learning disability first. Being valued and respected increases opportunities for trust
> - Encourage relatives or carers to support the individual in communicating needs or decisions, not to do this for them
> - Understand that behaviour is a means of communicating and expressing a need. It is not a symptom of a learning disability
> - Use the guidelines on consent as a framework to aid decision-making

Additional support models

The main focus of the work of emergency nurses is not with people with learning disabilities. However, they are a group who have significant health needs and have experienced institutional discrimination from healthcare professionals in the past (NHS Health Scotland 2004). While there are actions that can be taken by nurses in emergency care that will have a significant impact on the care experience of this group, there are times when people with learning disabilities require support beyond that which is available. Models of additional support are now being developed that see experienced learning disability nurses taking on liaison roles within general hospitals (Brown et al. 2005, 2010, Gibbs et al. 2008, MacArthur et al. 2010, Royal College of Nursing 2011). These liaison models help to ensure that those with the most complex of care needs receive appropriate care and support and help to create a partnership between patients, their carers, general hospital nurses and specialists in learning disability healthcare as well as providing education and practice development and contributing to strategic developments of general hospital services, thereby helping to ensure the needs of people with learning disabilities are met more effectively.

The focus of the liaison models is on preadmission planning and assessments, thereby helping to ensure the appropriate care arrangements are in place. Alternatively there may be communication, consent or diagnosis concerns and the liaison nurse is well placed to help problem-solve and make referrals onto other specialists in learning disability health services. These models of practice present also an opportunity for research collaborations to determine their impact on health outcomes (Brown et al. 2005, Guidelines and Audit Implementation Network 2010, MacArthur et al. 2010).

The UK is fortunate to have specialists in learning disability healthcare; however, this is not the case across the world. Frequently these specialists work as part of community learning disability teams and comprise a range of professionals, including learning disability nurses, speech and language therapists, occupational therapists, physiotherapists, dieticians, clinical psychologists and psychiatrists. Collectively they are a resource available to nurses and others in emergency care to assist in the assessment and identification of health needs, as well as providing specialist interventions and treatments to people with learning disabilities with complex needs. Today links are being established between emergency care professionals and specialist learning disability teams, with liaison nurses acting as the central coordinating point, thereby ensuring that the most appropriate care and support is available to this vulnerable group.

Conclusion

The learning disability population is increasing and ageing, with more living into older age with more complex health needs. Healthcare professionals in emergency care need to become familiar with the distinct needs of this group. As the evidence base of the health needs of people with learning disabilities evolves and is better understood, it becomes apparent that their health needs when compared to the general population are different. Failure to recognize and respond to their distinct pattern of health needs contributes to and results in their health inequalities that in turn contribute to premature death.

Central to effective care is the need to recognize the patterns of communication used by people with learning disabilities and the important role that relatives and carers can play in facilitating and enabling an accurate assessment and identification of needs. Models of additional support are being developed and it is incumbent on nurses within the emergency care environment to be aware of and communicate with specialist learning disability teams in order to reduce challenges in assessing and providing care to this vulnerable group.

References

Alborz, A., Glendinning, C., McNally, R., 2005. Access to health care for people with learning disabilities: mapping the issues and reviewing the evidence. Journal of Health Services Research & Policy 10, 173–182.

Arnold, E., Boggs, K., 1999. Interpersonal Relationships: Professional Communication Skills for Nurses. WB Saunders Company, Philadelphia.

Balogh, R.S., Hunter, D., Ouellette-Kuntz, H., 2005. Hospital utilization among persons with an intellectual disability. Ontario, Canada, 1995–2001 Journal of Applied Research in Intellectual Disabilities 18, 181–190.

Barr, O., 2004. Promoting access: The experience of children and adults with learning disabilities and their families/carers who had contact with acute general hospitals in the WHSSB Area and the views of nurses in these hospitals. A Report to the Western Health and Social Services Board. WHSSB, Londonderry.

Blair, J., 2012. Caring for people who have intellectual disabilities Emergency Nurse 20 (6), 15–19.

Böhmer, C.J., Klinkenberg-Knol, E.C., Niezen-de Boer, M.C., et al., 2000. Gastroesophageal reflux disease in intellectually disabled individuals: how often, how serious, how manageable? American Journal of Gastroenterology 95 (8), 1868–1872.

Böhmer, C.J., Taminiau, J.A., Klinkenberg-Knol, E.C., et al., 2001. The prevalence of constipation in institutionalized people with intellectual disability. Journal of Intellectual Disability Research 45, 212–218.

Boore, J.R.P., 1978. Prescription for Recovery. Royal College of Nursing, London.

Brown, H., Stein, J., Turk, V., 1995. The sexual abuse of adults with learning disabilities. Report of a second two-year incidence survey. Mental Handicap Research 8, 3–24.

Brown, M., 2005. Emergency care for people with learning disabilities: what all nurses and midwives need to know. Accident and Emergency Nursing 13 (4), 224–231.

Brown, M., MacArthur, J., Gibbs, S., 2005. A New Research Agenda: Improving General Hospital Care for People with Learning Disabilities. NHS Lothian, Edinburgh.

Brown, M., MacArthur, J., McKechanie, A., et al., 2010. Equality and access to general health care for people with learning disabilities: reality or rhetoric? Journal of Research in Nursing 15 (4), 351–361.

Carling-Jenkins, R., Torr, J., Iacono, T., et al., 2012. Experiences of supporting people with Down Syndrome and Alzheimer's disease in aged care and family environments. Journal of Intellectual and Developmental Disability 37 (1), 54–60.

Center, J., Beange, H., McElduff, A., 1998. People with mental retardation have an increased prevalence of osteoporosis: a population study. American Journal of Mental Retardation 103 (1), 19–28.

Collacott, R.A., Cooper, S.A., 1998. Epidemiology of self-injurious behaviour in adults with learning disabilities. The British Journal of Psychiatry 173, 428–432.

Cumella, S., Martin, D., 2000. Secondary Healthcare for People with a Learning Disability. Department of Health, London.

Cumella, S., Ransford, N., Lyons, J., et al., 2000. Needs for oral care among people with intellectual disability not in contact with Community Dental Services. Journal of Intellectual Disability Research 44 (1), 45–52.

Cummings, S., 2012. How to tell whether patients can make decisions about their care. Emergency Nurse, 20 (5), 22–26.

Department of Health, 1992. Mansell Report on Services for People with Learning Disabilities or Challenging Behaviours or Mental Health Needs. Department of Health, London.

Department of Health, 2001a. Valuing People: A New Strategy for Learning Disability for the 21st Century. Department of Health, London.

Department of Health, 2001b. Seeking Consent. Working with People with Intellectual Disabilities. Department of Health, London.

Department of Health, 2001c. Reference Guide to Consent to Examination or Treatment. Department of Health, London.

Department of Health, 2008. Healthcare for All: Report of the independent inquiry into access to healthcare for people with learning disabilities (The Michael Report). Department of Health, London.

Department of Health, 2009. Valuing People Now. HMSO, London.

Department of Health, Social Services and Public Safety, 2004. Equal Lives: Review of Policy and Services for People with Learning Disabilities in Northern Ireland. DHSSPS, Belfast.

Disability Discrimination Act, 1995. London: HMSO.

Disability Rights Commission, 2006. Equal Treatment: Closing the gap: A formal investigation into physical health inequalities experienced by people with learning disabilities and mental health problems. Stratford Upon Avon, DRC.

Doody, G.A., Johnstone, E.C., Sanderson, T.L., et al., 1998. 'Pfropfschizophrenie' revisited. Schizophrenia in people with mild learning disability. The British Journal of Psychiatry 173, 145–153.

Dye, L., Hendry, S., Dougal, J., et al., 2004. Capacity to consent to participate in research: a reconceptualisation. British Journal of Intellectual Disabilities 32 (3), 144–149.

Emerson, E., Hatton, C., Roberston, J., et al., 2012. People with learning disabilities.

Lancaster University, Learning Disabilities Observatory. Equality Act, 2010. HMSO, London.

Evenhuis, H.M., Theunissen, M., Denkers, I., et al., 2001. Prevalence of visual and hearing impairment in a Dutch institutionalised population with intellectual disability. Journal of Intellectual Disability Research 45 (5), 457–464.

Gates, B., Barr, O., 2009. Oxford Handbook of Learning and Intellectual Disability. Oxford University Press, Oxford.

Gibbs, S.M., Brown, M.J., Muir, W.J., 2008. The experiences of adults with intellectual disabilities and their carers in general hospitals: a focus group study. Journal of Intellectual Disability Research 52 (12), 1061–1077.

Glasson, E.J., Sullivan, S.G., Hussain, R., et al., 2002. The changing survival profile of people with Down's Sydrome: Implications for genetic counseling. Clinical Genetics 62, 390–393.

Guidelines and Audit Implementation Network, 2010. Caring for People with a Learning Disability in General Hospital Settings. Department of Health and Social Services and Public Safety. DHSSPS, Belfast.

Hasle, H., Clemmensen, I., Mikkelsen, M., 2000. Risks of leukaemia and solid tumours in individuals with Down's syndrome. Lancet 355, 165–169.

Holland, A.J., 2000. Ageing and learning disability. The British Journal of Psychiatry 176 (1), 26–31.

Hollins, S., Perez, W., 2000. Looking After my Breasts. Gaskell Press, London.

Hollins, S., Attard, M.T., von Fraunhofer, N., et al., 1998. Mortality in people with learning disabilities: risks, causes and death certification findings in London. Developmental Medicine and Child Neurology 40, 50–56.

Houghton, B.M., 2001. Caring for people with Down's syndrome in A&E. Emergency Nurse 9 (2), 24–27.

House of Lords & House of Commons, 2008. A Life Like ANy Other? Human Rights and Adults with Learning Disabilities. HMSO, London.

Human Rights Act, 1998. HMSO, London.

Hutchinson, C., 2005. Addressing issues related to adult patients who lack the capacity to give consent. Nursing Standard 19 (23), 47–53.

Iacono, T., Davis, R., 2003. The experience of people with developmental disability in Emergency Departments and hospital wards. Research in Developmental Disability 24, 247–264.

Janicki, M., Davidson, P., Henderson, C., et al., 2002. Health characteristics and health service utilization in older adults with intellectual disability living in community residences. Journal of Intellectual Disability Research 46, 287–298.

Jansen, D., Krol, B., Groothoff, J., et al., 2005. People with intellectual disability and their health problems: a review of comparative studies. Journal of Intellectual Disability Research 48 (2), 93–102.

Jopp, D.A., Keys, C.B., 2001. Diagnostic overshadowing reviewed and reconsidered. American Journal on Mental Retardation 106, 416–433.

Kerr, D., Wilkinson, H., 2006. Responding to the pain needs of people with a learning disability/intellectual disability and dementia: what are the key lessons? Disability and Human Development 5, 69–75. Special Issue.

Kerr, D., Cunningham, C., Wilkinson, H., 2006. Responding to the Pain Experiences of People with a Learning Difficulty and Dementia. Joseph Rowntree Foundation, York.

Lund, J., 1985. The prevalence of psychiatric morbidity in mentally retarded adults. Acta Psychiatrica. Scandanavica 72 (6), 563–570.

MacArthur, J., Brown, M., Hayes, M., et al., 2010. Learning Disability Liaison Nursing Services in South East Scotland: A Mixed Methods Impact and Outcome Research Study. University of Edinburgh, CRFR.

McConkey, R., Truesdale, M., 2000. Reactions of nurses and therapists in mainstream health services to contact with people who have learning disabilities. Journal of Advanced Nursing 32, 158–163.

Medical Research Council, 2001. Review of Autism Research: Epidemiology and Causes. Medical Research Council, London.

Mencap, 2004. Trust Me Right! Better Healthcare for People with Intellectual Disabilities. Mencap, London.

Mencap, 2007. Death by Indifference. Mencap, London.

Mental Capacity Act, 2005. HMSO, London.

Merrifield, J., 2011. Meeting the needs of people with a learning disability in the emergency department. International Emergency Nursing 19, 146–151.

Moss, S., Emerson, E., Kiernan, C., Turner, S., Hatton, C., Iborz, A., 2000. Psychiatric symptoms in adults with learning disability and challenging behaviour. The British Journal of Psychiatry 177, 452–456.

National Patient Safety Agency, 2004. Understanding the Patient Safety Issues for People with Learning Disabilities. National Patient Safety Agency, London.

NHS Education for Scotland, 2004. Getting it Right Together: the Implementation of Recommendations 16, 17 and 20 from Promoting Health, Supporting Inclusion Report. NHS Education for Scotland, Edinburgh.

NHS Health Scotland, 2004. People with Learning Disabilities in Scotland: The Health Needs Assessment Report. NHS Health Scotland, Glasgow.

NHS Quality Improvement Scotland, 2006. Best Practice Statement. Promoting Access to Healthcare for People with a Learning Disability – A Guide for Frontline Staff. NHS Quality Improvement Scotland, Edinburgh.

NHS Quality Improvement Scotland, 2009. Tackling Indifference: Health Care Services People with Learning Disabilities National Overview Report. NHS Quality Improvement Scotland, Edinburgh.

Nursing and Midwifery Council, 2008. Code: Standards of Conduct, Performance and Ethics. Nursing and Midwifery Council, London.

PAMIS, 2001. The Views of Family Carers on the Contribution of Nurses to the Care and Support of People with Profound and Multiple Learning Disabilities (PMLD). University of Dundee, PAMIS.

Parliamentary and Health Services Ombudsman, 2009. Six Lives: The Provision of Public Services to People with Learning Disabilities. The Stationery Office, London.

Patel, P., Goldberg, D., Moss, S., 1993. Psychiatric morbidity in older people with moderate and severe learning disability. II: The prevalence study. The British Journal of Psychiatry 163, 481–491.

Patja, K., Eero, P., Livanainen, M., 2001. Cancer incidents among people with intellectual disability. Journal of Intellectual Disability Research 45, 300–307.

Public Health Institute of Scotland, 2001. Autistic Spectrum Disorders. Needs Assessment Report. Public Health Institute of Scotland, Glasgow.

Regnard, C., Reynolds, J., Watson, B., et al., 2007. Understanding distress in people with severe communication difficulties: developing and assessing the Disability Distress Assessment Tool (DisDAT). Journal of Intellectual Disability Research 51 (4), 277–292.

Reiss, S., Levitan, G.W., Szyszko, J., 1982. Emotional disturbance and mental retardation: diagnostic overshadowing. American Journal of Mental Deficiency 86, 567–574.

Richards, M., Maughan, B., Hardy, R., et al., 2001. Long-term affective disorder in people with mild learning disability. The British Journal of Psychiatry 179, 523–527.

Royal College of Nursing, 2011. Learning from the past - Setting out the future: Developing learning disability nursing in the United Kingdom. RCN, London.

Scottish Executive, 2000. The Same as You? A Review of Services for People with Learning Disabilities. The Stationery Office, Edinburgh.

Scottish Executive, 2002. Promoting Health, Supporting Inclusion: The National Review of the Contribution of all Nurses and Midwives to the Care and Support of People with Learning Disabilities. The Stationery Office, Edinburgh.

Scottish Executive, 2003. Home at Last? The Report on Hospital Closure Service Reprovision Sub Group – The Same As You? The Stationery Office, Edinburgh.

Scottish Executive, 2005. A Good Practice Guide on Consent for Health care Professionals in NHS Scotland: A Draft Consultation. Scottish Executive Health Department, Edinburgh.

Sillanpaa, M., Gram, L., Johannessen, S.I., Tomson, T. (Eds.), 1999. Epilepsy and Mental Retardation. Wrightson Biomedical, Stroud.

Sowney, M., Barr, O., 2006a. The perceived challenges encountered by nurses in accident and emergency caring for adults with intellectual disabilities. Journal of Advanced Nursing 55 (1), 36–45.

Sowney, M., Barr, O., 2006b. The challenges for nurses communicating with and gaining valid consent from adults with intellectual disabilities within the accident and emergency care service. Journal of Clinical Nursing 15 (1), 1–9.

Sowney, M., Brown, M., Barr, O., 2006. Caring for people with learning disabilities in emergency care. Emergency Nurse 14 (2), 23–30.

Tyler, F., Smith, L., McGrother, C., 2007. Mortality in adults with moderate to profound intellectual disability: A population-based study. Journal of Intellectual Disability Research 51 (7), 520–527.

United Kingdom Parliament, 2008. Joint Committee on Human Rights Written Evidence. Memorandum from the Royal College of Speech and Language Therapists. UK Parliament, London.

US Public Health Service, 2002. Closing the Gap: A National Blueprint to Improve the Health of Persons with Mental Retardation. Report of the Surgeon Generals Conference on Health Disparities and Mental Retardation. US PHS, Washington DC.

Van Schrojenstein Lantman-de Valk, H.M., Walsh, P., 2008. Managing health problems in people with intellectual disabilities. British Medical Journal 337, 1408–1412.

Walsh, M., Dolan, B., 1999. Emergency nurses and their perceptions of caring. Emergency Nurse 7 (4), 24–31.

Welsh Assembly, 2002a. Fulfilling the Promises: Proposals for a Framework for Services for People with Learning Disabilities. Welsh Assembly, Cardiff.

Welsh Assembly, 2002b. Reference Guide for Consent to Examination and Treatment. Welsh Assembly, Cardiff.

Wong, J.G., Clare, I.C.H., Gunn, M., et al., 1999. Capacity to make health care decisions: its importance in clinical practice. Psychological Medicine 29, 437–446.

Health promotion

34

Stewart Piper

CHAPTER CONTENTS

Introduction

It is interesting to note Beattie's (1991) observation that the major healthcare professions claim increasingly that health promotion underpins practice: interesting because while copious literature on health promotion and nursing is readily accessible in any nursing library, the emphasis tends towards practice and doing. Fundamental questions then about purpose, fit with practice and scrutiny of the different theoretical approaches and their pertinence for nursing, particularly in relation to specialist areas of practice, remain as much an underdeveloped area now as in 1991.

This debate was given fresh impetus in the UK by *The Health of the Nation* (HoN), the Government strategy for health in England (Department of Health 1992). This placed health promotion explicitly on the nursing agenda in general, and on the emergency care agenda in particular as accidents were one of the five key areas of the strategy with *The HoN* (Department of Health 1993a, p. 10) highlighting that:

> *'Tertiary prevention by Accident and Emergency departments … will contribute to the overall objective of reducing ill-health, disability and death from accidents.'*

Further to this, *Targeting Practice* (Department of Health 1993b) and *Saving Lives: Our Healthier Nation* (Department

of Health 1999), both of which include accident prevention, emphasize how health promotion has become more of a UK NHS priority. Likewise, *The NHS Plan* (Department of Health 2000), *Choosing Health* (Department of Health 2004a), *Better Information, Better Choices, Better Health* (Department of Health 2004b), *Benchmarks for Promoting Health* (Department of Health 2006) and, for example, from an international perspective the US *Healthy People 2010* (US Department of Health and Human Services 2000).

Given the health policy imperatives above, the intention of this chapter is not to provide an exhaustive account or the final word on health promotion in Emergency Departments (ED) per se, but to emphasize the benefits of a conceptual framework to explore the relationship between health promotion theory and ED nursing practice. Specifically, the mode and focus of intervention and the aims, methods, impact and outcomes of three models that can be operationalized and applied, to a greater or lesser extent, are discussed. The intention is to move the debate beyond any narrow or traditional view of health promotion as simply a form of information or advice giving, and highlight the need for a repertoire of approaches in the modern arena of healthcare and ED nursing.

Health promotion framework

To facilitate conceptual understanding, contextualize and map out the models of health promotion Piper's (2009) framework (Fig. 34.1), based on the work of Beattie (1991) and Piper & Brown (1998), is utilized. The framework comprises three models entitled The *Nurse as Behaviour Change Agent*, *The Nurse as Strategic Practitioner* and *The Nurse as Empowerment Facilitator* that derive from themes and deviant/paradigm cases generated in a qualitative study and constructive theorizing by the author to help illuminate the debate. As such, all require the tests of fit and transferability to be applied by the reader.

http://dx.doi.org/10.1016/B978-0-7020-4315-4.00034-6

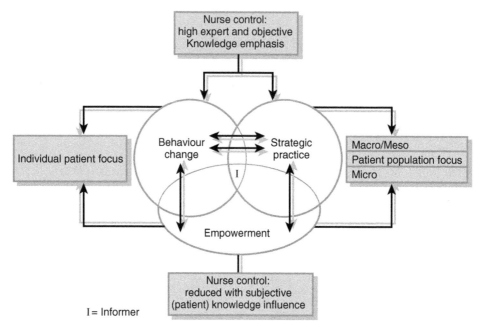

I = Informer

Fig. 34.1 ● Framework of health promotion models. I, Informer. ● (After Piper SM (2009) Health Promotion for Nurses: Theory and practice. Abingdon: Routledge.)

As can be seen, the combination of a nurse control axis (essentially a power continuum) and a patient focus axis creates three discrete but overlapping models of health promotion. The former unites *The Nurse as Behaviour Change Agent* and *The Nurse as Strategic Practitioner* models and reflects a 'top-down' nurse-led mode of intervention based on an objective assessment of need and nursing goals. However, they diverge on the individual/patient population axis as the former is concerned with individual action perspectives and outcomes and the latter with collective health gain.

Similarly, when concerned with individual patient health promotion needs, *The Nurse as Empowerment Facilitator* converges with *The Nurse as Behaviour Change Agent* but is polarized on the power continuum where the former is concerned with a more bottom-up mode of intervention from an individual patient and subjective perspective. It converges with *The Nurse as Strategic Practitioner* when the focus of intervention is at a population level while remaining divergent in terms of the locus of control. However, given the nature of ED practice, the wider micro-population aspect of *The Nurse as Empowerment Facilitator* that goes beyond individual and immediate ED patient problems is not explored herein, but can be found in Chapter 8 of Piper (2009). Its concern with community development and social capital and seeking to improve health by encouraging and supporting the development of social networks and 'social capital' (Cooper et al. 1999) is not explored herein as this is more the domain of public health practitioners.

Operational definitions

To avoid the debate surrounding the distinction between health education and health promotion (this is explored in Piper (2009)), for the purpose of this chapter the definition

of Tones (1990) is adopted. He states that health promotion: 'incorporates all measures deliberately designed to promote health and handle diseases' (Tones 1990, p. 3).

In addition, and consistent with Tones & Green (2004) and Piper (2009), primary, secondary and tertiary health promotion are defined as interventions that aim to:

- prevent new cases of disease or injury (primary)
- minimize the impact of disease or injury, prevent them from becoming chronic or irreversible and restore the patient to their former health status (secondary)
- maximize health experience within the context of chronic disease (e.g., diabetes, asthma, HIV), injury or disability, prevent further complications and assist rehabilitation (tertiary).

The nurse as behaviour change agent

The Nurse as Behaviour Change Agent reflects a 'medical model' approach to health promotion and is based on the assumption that individuals make rational, conscious decisions about their health-related behaviour. Primary interventions aim to prevent disease, illness and injury and promote optimum biological functioning by disseminating 'factual' information selectively derived from objective and medically based scientific research to the public. This takes the form of edicts from healthcare professionals, or the ever-present mass media awareness-raising campaigns such as the Clunk Click television car seatbelt campaigns of yesteryear, encouraging the use of cycle helmets, No Smoking Day and Drug Awareness Week, etc. It is suggested to the public that if they fail to follow a prescribed course of action their 'health' is at risk. The aim is to trigger a 'do-it-yourself' attitude and then behaviour/lifestyle changes consistent with the recommended advice given.

The Nurse as Behaviour Change Agent as a primary health promotion intervention engages ED nurses in an information-based approach. This includes themed displays in the waiting room on a variety of topics such as disease and accident prevention, first aid, the dangers of alcohol misuse, HIV and sexual health or healthy eating. These must be visually appealing, regularly changed and could reflect national initiatives such as Drinkwise Day or World AIDS Day. They should be supported by a wide range of leaflets in display racks, posters strategically placed around the ED and health promotion videos showing in the waiting room if it is suitably equipped. This approach also uses patient information to encourage people to use the healthcare services most appropriate to their needs i.e., right patient, right place, right time.

It is important to acknowledge that, while effective at raising awareness about particular health risks, the complexity of the relationship between social experience and health-related behaviour means that the outcomes are likely to be at best uncertain (Naidoo & Wills 2009). In emphasizing the personal controlling of risks and the correcting of individual inadequacies, it is assumed that free choice exists and that lifestyle is the primary cause of ill-health. In isolation such an approach denies that health is a social product, ignores and implicitly condones inequalities and minimal state intervention. For an excellent, albeit old and general (i.e., not related to nursing), critique of such a stance the reader is referred to Mitchell (1982); for a critique related to nursing, but not specific to ED, see Brown & Piper (1997) and Chapter 6 in Piper (2009).

The purpose of secondary health promotion for patients discharged home from the ED is patient compliance with prescribed treatment regimens. The goal is optimum management of injury and disease by patients to maximize the chances of full recovery and to minimize the risk of complications or relapse. The ED nurse determines the specific behaviour(s) required and supplies the appropriate information, discharge advice, reassurance and patient teaching to achieve this. Obvious examples of daily practice include, for example, advice and information on how to care for a fractured limb in a plaster cast, a sprained ligament or minor head injury, an outline of what potential problems to be alert to and what rehabilitative and preventive actions the patient can take. This is reinforced by an information sheet that the patient and their significant others can take away for reference and the ED contact telephone number should a problem arise. It is important to stress that the information sheet is not a substitute for nurse-patient health promotion interaction but a supplement to this process.

Tertiary health promotion essentially adopts the same methods as secondary but is applied to patients presenting to the ED with exacerbations of chronic problems. The issues for consideration are likely to be more complex and detailed health promotion input may be provided by specialist healthcare professionals from outside the department prior to discharge. The author concedes, however, that the severity of the presenting condition may warrant emergency admission and thus health promotion of the type described above may be problematic, ineffective and inappropriate.

At a simplistic level, elements of *The Nurse as Behaviour Change Agent* can be likened to an electrical system model (Hills 1979). This undermines the complexity of the nurse–patient interpersonal interaction by reducing it to a mechanistic relationship, but it serves a purpose and can be illustrated as follows:

Input > Coding > Channel > Decoding > Output

The nurse provides the input and the coding and the patient is the decoder. The method is concerned with the sender (ED nurse/expert) validating facts and transmitting knowledge to the receiver (patient), with the latter feeding back information on how the sender's messages have been received.

Ewles & Shipster (1984) take this one step further and refer to intervention of this nature as a three-stage process as follows:

- giving information or advice to a patient about his/her injury/disease
- ensuring that the patient understands and remembers that information or advice
- ensuring that the patient is able to act on the information or advice.

They stress the need to define the objectives and desired outcome for the intervention, to give the information in a structured way emphasizing and repeating the important aspects and the need to use short words and short sentences to avoid any misunderstanding. If there are any dangers with this important facet of ED nursing they are that the nurse tells rather than listens and adopts a didactic (Macleod Clark et al. 1991), top-down, one-way stance that reinforces their professional status and power base and engenders patient deference and dependence. In pursuing health promotion outcomes based on professionally determined needs there may also be a failure to consider the patient's perception of their problems and solutions, their social, economic or environmental context or to achieve their participation in care. Examples of the aims, methods, impact and outcomes of *The Nurse as Behaviour Change Agent* are summarized in Table 34.1.

Table 34.1 The ED nurse as behaviour change agent

Aims	Methods	Impact	Outcomes
Primary prevention	Posters/leaflets on disease prevention in line with national campaigns Patient information	Change in health-related behaviour	Reduction in: Accidents Disease Mortality Morbidity Complications Relapse Inappropriate service use
Secondary prevention	Verbal and written discharge advice/instructions on injury/disease management, complications, etc.	Compliance with treatment regimens/discharge advice	
Tertiary prevention		Self-management by patient	
Appropriate use of services	Patient teaching	Right patient, right place, right time	

The nurse as strategic practitioner

Part of this model of practice fits with what Beattie (1991) refers to as 'Legislative Action for Health'. Here, social factors and social conditions are seen as the major determinants of health status. Social class is considered to be beyond the control of individuals but instrumental in influencing their way of life and thus health status with poor health experiences and higher accident rates attributable to socio-economic inequalities (Townsend & Davidson 1990, Whitehead 1990, Acheson 1998, Department of Health 2002b, Marmot 2010).

Contributions to population (macro) health gain can be achieved by legislative and environmental interventions governing issues such as welfare provision, taxation, the distribution of resources and pollution. The action of industry and persuasive advertising can be monitored and controlled and laws can be enacted. With regard to the latter, and with a particular resonance for ED nurses, Tones & Tilford (2001) report that behaviour change based health promotion to encourage the wearing of front seatbelts was successful to a degree, but that legislation has been much more successful in enforcing their use and has changed the pattern of injury following a road traffic collision helping to reduce mortality and morbidity.

In line with this way of working, *The Nurse as Strategic Practitioner* approach could engage ED nurses in collecting data to construct a profile of the pattern of local accidents to use to campaign for traffic-calming measures in residential areas or improved street lighting. This would involve nurses lobbying local policy-makers by submitting written and verbal evidence to appropriate forums (within the boundaries of confidentiality and professional codes of conduct) and taking every opportunity to be involved in partnership and multi-agency working. Nationally, ED nurses can lobby power-holders through their professional organizations and specialist forums. Piper (2008) highlights that this is consistent with the UK Royal College of Nursing Emergency Nurses Association Conference (2008) encouraging Emergency Nurses to use their collective voice on issues beyond the confines of the ED.

Collectively then, ED nurses can align themselves with pressure groups to address such issues as poverty and welfare provision, car design, drinking and driving, health and safety laws governing the workplace and advertising bans, e.g., tobacco, or the emphasis placed on the high performance of cars, etc.

More closely related to patients, Piper (2008) has applied this model of health promotion at a meso level (Tones & Tilford 2001), i.e., from an organizational perspective specifically to ED nursing. This is a settings approach to health promotion and derives from the concept of Health Promoting Hospitals (World Health Organization 1991, 1997, Dooris & Hunter 2007). From an ED perspective the focus is on resource management, clinical governance, health promotion quality and standards such as customer care (Rushmere 2000) and patient information (Groene 2006), education and training issues and collaborative care planning, all of which are concerned with promoting ED patient population health gain.

In addition, resource management can enhance standards of care delivery by effective skill mix, e.g., numbers of nurses on a shift having undergone recognized post-registration training courses and the careful deployment of senior ED staff so that patients' needs are met by the most appropriate healthcare professional. Standard setting should state the quality levels expected within the department and be aligned with promoting evidence-based practice. Implementation of recognized processes such as trauma scoring, the use of nationally recognized protocols such as those for advanced life support, asthma, etc. and appropriate directives from the National Service Frameworks can also be closely monitored. These examples of how *The Nurse as Strategic Practitioner* might be adapted and applied by ED nurses are summarized in Table 34.2 in relation to the aims, methods, impact and outcomes of practice.

The nurse as empowerment facilitator

Of the previous strategies explored, *The Nurse as Behaviour Change Agent* and *The Nurse as Strategic Practitioner*

Table 34.2 The ED nurse as strategic practitioner

Aims	Methods	Impact	Outcomes
Health policy change (national/local) Organizational development, innovation and implementation at department level.	Lobbying: • national/local Service and resource management e.g. on: • Clinical governance • Service review • Staff rostering, skill mix and deployment • Timing of clinics • Use of protocols, pathways etc. • Trauma scoring • Risk registers • Inter-agency and multidisciplinary liaison and training • Collaborative care planning • Clinical audit	↓ Inequalities ↑ Safety Evidence-based practice Right staff, right place, right time; Inter-agency and multidisciplinary working Seamless service Support for the vulnerable ↑ service efficiency ↑ clinical outcomes.	Reduced: • Accidents • Mortality • Morbidity • Disability • Complications ↑ Clinical outcomes ↑ Patient satisfaction

involve professionally led direct and indirect health promotion, respectively, and a more traditional demeanour. Neither set out with the purpose of achieving health promotion outcomes in a patient-centred, non-hierarchical, non-coercive way aiming at active participation and thus pragmatic empowerment. *The Nurse as Empowerment Facilitator*, where the focus of intervention is the individual patient, seeks to achieve this by enabling patient reflection on and clarification of existing health-related behaviours and by facilitating informed choice.

While empowerment is a complex and contested concept (Lewin & Piper 2007, Piper 2009, 2010), this model of health promotion practice is flagged up because it fits with the developing consumer culture and moves to empower patients, for example, the UK Department of Health (2002a) policy 'Patient and public involvement in health'. Examples of developments in this direction also include moves to actively promote an expert patient persona in those with chronic illness (Department of Health 2001) and representation for patients via patient advice and liaison services (Department of Health 2002a).

Providing information about the cause and effect of disease may be an important facet of such health promotion, but fundamentally ED nurses would listen rather than just tell. They would strive towards individual patient empowerment through acknowledging and enabling their right to participate actively in decisions on clinical matters, ensuring they were aware of the options open to them and able to exercise informed choice at every opportunity. ED nurses would support patients during this process, act as advocates when required and assist them to acknowledge and draw on their personal resources and strengths to maximize their autonomy. As such, existing power relations between the nurse and the patient would be challenged and equalized and the distance between the two parties reduced.

A model currently popular and compatible with *The Nurse as Empowerment Facilitator* is the Stages of Change (Prochaska & Diclemente 1982). A detailed outline of this work is beyond the scope of this chapter and the reader is referred to the authors' original work for a clear exposition of this process and to Naidoo & Wills (2009). Briefly, however, the cycle has stages through which people who change successfully move whatever the variety of behaviour. 'Contemplation', the point at which people enter the cycle, represents a form of cognitive dissonance where people become aware of themselves, the nature of their behaviour and its negative consequences and think about the positive consequences of change. At this stage they continue the behaviour, e.g., smoking. 'Action' is when a person has decided to effect change, 'Maintenance' is the point at which there is a belief in the ability to maintain change and 'Relapse', an integral part of the cycle, is where the behaviour and contemplation or pre-contemplation stage is reverted to.

It is of course unrealistic to think that ED nurses would accompany a patient through the entire cycle of change. The process is referred to as it is desirable for ED nurses to have an understanding greater than that alluded to here to enable appropriate supportive intervention in relation to the stage the patient has reached. This would include, for example, referring people who want to stop smoking to smoking-cessation services during the 'contemplation' stage of the cycle.

Where there is a micro-population empowerment role for ED nurses it is in acknowledging the impact of social factors on health, having a knowledge of national and local self-help and support groups and being able to direct appropriate patients towards these. This would necessitate accident departments holding directories of local activity and key contacts. Such groups help reduce isolation, enable patients and/or their relatives and loved ones to use their collective resources to determine their common needs, shape their agenda for 'health' and build support networks. The group members can share experiences, offer coping strategies and draw strength from each other. They can also challenge the medical and nursing professions and lobby for change in both service provision and societal attitudes. Examples of the aims, methods, impact and outcomes of *The Nurse as Empowerment Facilitator* are summarized in Table 34.3.

Table 34.3 The ED nurse as empowerment facilitator

Aim	Methods	Impact	Outcomes
Empower-ment	Non-hierarchical patient-centred interaction and partnership working Neutral information provision Stages of change model Advocacy Peer support	Health agenda determined, directed and validated by patient with support from healthcare workers ↑ Informed patient decision-making ↑ Coping strategies Support group accessed	↑ Feelings of control Feeling supported ↑ Patient self-esteem

Conclusion

This chapter has endeavoured to combine a brief theoretical discussion on the nature of health promotion outlining a framework for practice and translating how the complementary and contradictory models within the framework, each with different aims, methods and outcomes, relate to ED nursing. It is the author's contention that health promotion is an intrinsic part of holistic ED nursing and that the three models outlined enable legitimate ED health promotion activity, but to varying degrees. Clearly *The Nurse as Behaviour Change Agent* has considerable and obvious application for individual patients while the collective patient agenda can be addressed by *The Nurse as Strategic Practitioner* for indirect health gain. The contribution of the individual and micropopulation *Empowerment Facilitation* model to ED nursing is perhaps more limited, but still has a place. In particular the former is important in terms of the absolute right of patients to have control over their own health and health-related decision making where possible and is in line with the developing consumer culture in healthcare. Finally, the author is aware that this chapter may re-label as health promotion, rather than re-shape, elements of existing practice.

References

Acheson, D., 1998. Independent Inquiry into Inequalities in Health Report. The Stationery Office, London.

Beattie, A., 1991. Knowledge and control in health promotion: a test case for social policy and social theory. In: Gabe, J., Calnan, M., Bury, M. (Eds.), The Sociology of the Health Service. Routledge, London.

Brown, P.A., Piper, S.M., 1997. Nursing and the health of the nation: schism or symbiosis? Journal of Advanced Nursing 25, 297–310.

Cooper, H., Arber, S., Fee, L., et al., 1999. The Influence of Social Support and Social Capital on Health: A Review and Analysis of British Data. Health Education Authority, London.

Department of Health, 1992. The Health of the Nation: A Strategy for Health in England. HMSO, London.

Department of Health, 1993a. The Health of the Nation: Key Area Handbook Accidents. HMSO, London.

Department of Health, 1993b. Targeting Practice: The Contribution of Nurses, Midwives and Health Visitors. The Health of the Nation. HMSO, London.

Department of Health, 1999. Saving Lives: Our Healthier Nation. HMSO, London.

Department of Health, 2000. The NHS Plan: A Plan for Investment, a Plan for Reform. HMSO, London.

Department of Health, 2001. The Expert Patient: A New Approach to Chronic Disease Management for the 21st Century. Department of Health, London.

Department of Health, 2002a. Patient Advice and Liaison Service. Department of Health, London.

Department of Health, 2002b. Tackling Health Inequalities: Summary of the Cross-cutting Review. Department of Health, London.

Department of Health, 2004a. Choosing Health: Making Healthy Choices Easier. TSO, London.

Department of Health, 2004b. Better Information, Better Choices, Better Health: Putting Information at the Centre of Health. Department of Health, London.

Department of Health, 2006. Benchmarks for Promoting Health. Department of Health, London.

Dooris, M., Hunter, D.J., 2007. Organisations and settings for promoting public health. In: Lloyd, C.E., Handsley, S., Douglas, J., Earle, S., Spurr, S. (Eds.), Policy and Practice in Promoting Public Health. Sage, London.

Ewles, L., Shipster, P., 1984. One to One Health Education. South East Thames Regional Health Authority, London.

Groene, O., 2006. Implementing Health and Promotion in Hospitals: Manual and Self-assessment Forms. WHO Europe, Copenhagen.

Hills, P., 1979. Teaching and Learning as a Communication Process. Croom Helm, London.

Lewin, D., Piper, S.M., 2007. Patient empowerment within a coronary care unit. Intensive and Critical Care Nursing 23, 81–90.

Lowthian, J.A., Curtis, A.J., Cameron, P.A., et al., 2011. Systematic review of trends in emergency department attendances: An Australian perspective. Emergency Medicine Journal 28 (5), 373–377.

Macleod Clark, J., Wilson-Barnett, J., Latter, S., 1991. Health Education in Nursing Project: Results of a National Survey on Senior Nurses' Perceptions of Health Education Practice in Acute Ward Settings. Department of Nursing Studies, King's College, University of London Education Authority, London.

Marmot, M., et al., 2010. Fair Society, Healthy Lives: Strategy Review of Health Inequalities in England Post 2010. The Marmot Review. Department of Health, London.

Mitchell, J., 1982. Looking after ourselves: an individual responsibility? Royal Society of Health Journal 4, 169–173.

Naidoo, J., Wills, J., 2009. Foundations for Health Promotion, third ed. Elsevier, London.

Piper, S.M., 2008. Promoting health. Emergency Nurse 16 (8), 12–14.

Piper, S.M., 2009. Health Promotion for Nurses: Theory and Practice. Routledge, Abingdon.

Piper, S.M., 2010. Patient empowerment: Emancipatory or technological practice? Patient Education and Counselling 79 (2), 173–177.

Piper, S.M., Brown, P.A., 1998. The theory and practice of health education applied to nursing: a bi-polar approach. Journal of Advanced Nursing 27, 383–389.

Prochaska, J.O., Diclemente, C.C., 1982. Transtheoretical therapy: towards a more integrated model of change. Psychotherapy: Theory, Research and Practice 19 (2), 276–288.

Rushmere, A., 2000. Health Promoting Hospitals and Trusts: Self Assessment and Peer Review Toolkit. The Wessex Institute for Health Research and Development, Southampton.

Tones, K., 1990. Why theorise? Ideology in Health Education. Health Education Journal 49 (1), 26.

Tones, K., Green, J., 2004. Health Promotion: Planning and Strategies. Sage, London.

Tones, K., Tilford, S., 2001. Health Education: Effectiveness, Efficiency and Equity, third ed. Nelson Thornes, Cheltenham.

Townsend, P., Davidson, N., 1990. Inequalities in Health. The Black Report. Penguin, London.

US Department of Health and Human Services, 2000. Healthy People 2010: Understanding and Improving Health. US Department of Health and Human Services, Washington.

Whitehead, M., 1990. Inequalities in Health: The Health Divide. Penguin, London.

WHO, 1991. The Budapest Declaration on Health Promoting Hospitals. WHO, Geneva Budapest, Hungary, 31 May–1 June.

WHO, 1997. Health Promoting Hospitals: Working for Health, The Vienna Recommendations. 3rd workshop of National/Regional Health Promoting Hospitals Network Coordinators The Hospital Unit, WHO Regional Office for Europe, Vienna.

Triage

35

Janet Marsden

CHAPTER CONTENTS

Introduction

Triage is a system of clinical risk management used in urgent care settings (Emergency Departments (EDs), walk-in centres, minor injury units, general practice) where an undifferentiated and unexpected caseload arrives at a point of care. It is used worldwide to manage the patient flow through these areas safely, when need exceeds the capacity of the service and its aim is to sort patients according to clinical urgency (van der Linden et al. 2012). This chapter will focus on the development of triage roles, types and systems.

The concept of triage

The word triage originates from the French verb 'trier', meaning 'to sort'. The origins of triage are well documented and it was originally used as a means of grading the quality of goods such as coffee beans and wool, and was first adopted for use in a medical context during the Napoleonic wars (Bracken 2003). For the first time, casualties were treated on the basis of medical need rather than rank or social status although at this time, those treated first were those who needed minimal attention in order that they could return to the battlefield. Triage, in the form we recognize now, where the most injured are dealt with first, emerged rather later in the Korean War. It has been used in every war since, as a means of managing mass casualties. While the term triage is used in both military/disaster triage and EDs, it must be recognized that the two processes fulfil very different functions.

Peacetime nursing triage emerged in the US in the early 1960s during the war in Korea. Highly trained paramedics moved across into civilian hospitals, taking their triage skills with them and adapting the process for use within EDs. It was not until the 1980s that the concept of nurse triage became popular in the UK. EDs began introducing schemes around this time, based largely on the experiences of American nursing colleagues.

Emergency department attenders

The unpredictability of workloads within emergency settings and the steadily increasing numbers of attenders are well recognized and documented (Mallet & Woolwich 1990, National

Audit Office 2004, Department of Health 2010). During a 24-hour period a wide spectrum of accidents and emergencies may be seen, sometimes stretching the resources of the department and staff to their limit. Walk-in centres and NHS Direct have not been demonstrated to reduce attendance in EDs (Cooke 2005).

Prior to nurse triage, the waiting room was an unknown quantity for the ED staff. It could be full of patients with a diverse range of illnesses and injuries, of varying degrees of severity and without any screening there was a risk of a patient's condition deteriorating while waiting to be seen. It is inevitable that with the ever-increasing demands on a finite service, longer waiting times develop and the most vulnerable group of patients, i.e., those who are seriously ill and in need of immediate emergency care and treatment, may not be identified and prioritized. Recognition of all these factors highlights the need for all patients to be assessed on arrival in the ED by a person skilled in triage.

The purpose of triage

The purpose of triage in the emergency care setting is not to reduce the overall waiting time for all patients. Mallet & Woolwich (1990) have shown, in line with other studies, that while the waiting times for the more seriously ill were reduced, overall departmental waiting times steadily increased. The purpose of triage is to 'make the best possible use of the available medical and nursing personnel and facilities' and it is there to assist in determining 'which patients need immediate care … and which patients can wait' (Potter 1985).

The role and aims of triage

In a joint statement, the College of Emergency Medicine, the Emergency Nurse Consultants Association, the Faculty of Emergency Nursing and the Royal College of Nursing Emergency Care Association (2011) defined triage as 'a complex decision making process to manage clinical risk'. Therefore, the primary aim of the triage nurse must be the early assessment of patients, in order to determine the priority of care according to the individual's clinical need. There are other aspects of care, however, that nurse triage can meet (Handyside 1996), for instance, more efficient use of the department facilities and resources as patients are allocated to the most appropriate clinical areas within the department and are seen and treated within an appropriate time. As triage should be a dynamic process, regular reassessment of patients ensures that the appropriateness of the care implemented can be modified as necessary.

The early and appropriate requesting of medical records or relevant previous X-rays will aid clinical assessment and diagnosis. Appropriate first-aid measures can be taken without delay and analgesia appropriate to the patient's level of pain can be given.

The waiting area is now a known quantity and patient flow can be controlled and organized. Patients and their relatives have an easily identifiable and reliable source of information for any enquiries. This helps to relieve anxiety and reduce aggression and can increase patient satisfaction with the service (Dolan 1998).

Types of triage

Non-professional triage

Patients arrive in the ED, register with the receptionist and then sit in the waiting area, without any form of assessment, until they are called to be seen by the clinician. The receptionist will only call a clinician if there appears to be some reason for concern.

In the UK, non-professional triage can still be found functioning in some departments and is more frequently used at certain times, e.g., at night when staff and resources are limited. Mallet & Woolwich (1990) identified this as an area of great concern in their study of nurse triage in an inner-city ED and recommended the provision of a nurse triage service during the night shift. Their concerns are echoed in the findings of a large study of the use of health care assistants (HCAs) in English EDs, which found that HCAs assessed patients on arrival in 28.7% of the 282 departments that responded to the survey (Boyes 1995).

Triage tends to have been recognized as a system which must be undertaken by a competent clinician; however, there are a number of emergency care settings where non-professional triage may be, while not the system of choice, the system which has to be lived with. Walk-in centres and minor injury units may not have levels of professional staff in which a qualified nurse can be allocated to a triage role. Nurses undertaking advanced practice roles are likely to be dealing with existing patients, away from the waiting area and therefore are not aware of the clinical need of those patients walking into the department.

Similarly, in general practice, the receptionist is always the first point of contact for the patient and there is little chance of a clinician being present when a patient who needs urgent care walks in. In these circumstances it is imperative that reception staff have a clear set of guidelines to work from to help them to identify those patients for whom urgent professional care must be obtained. Algorithms may be developed which reception staff are able to work through and appropriate training must be given to aid reception staff to undertake this crucial role.

Professional triage

Triage may be undertaken by a range of professionals in emergency care settings such as nurses, medical staff, ambulance paramedics and emergency care practitioners (ECPs). What needs to be common among these clinicians is experience and education. Because triage often uses algorithms to enable reproducible decisions in the care setting, it might be felt that it could be undertaken by anyone working in the setting. The level of decision-making which takes place within the rapid triage encounter requires sound clinical judgement which must be based on professional experience, knowledge and skill. The triage practitioner must be able to interpret, discriminate and evaluate the information he gathers from the patient, relative and carer and must be able to reflect on their decision-making and critically appraise it (Mackway-Jones et al. 2005).

Telephone triage

A major expansion of the triage process has been the recognition and development of telephone triage. As in the case of face-to-face triage, this strategy was first identified in the US (Simenson 2001).

Advice-giving over the telephone has always been a part of the clinician's role, although not one that has been recognized as having a particularly distinct identity. Formalized advice-giving by telephone has the potential to be a valuable tool in many settings – a fact that has been recognized in the development of NHS Direct in England and Wales and NHS 24 in Scotland. Some 5 million calls were made to NHS Direct in England in 2009/10 (NHS Direct 2010).

Telephone triage was first described as a useful emergency care strategy in the UK by Buckles & Carew-McColl in 1991. Various benefits have been attributed to it, including reduced attendance due to explanations and self-care advice, redirection of patients to more appropriate agencies, pre-identification of patient problems, cost-effectiveness, in terms of reduction in workload, and patient empowerment.

Telephone triage has many difficulties. The patient is not visible, so many of the cues that experienced clinicians take from the patient's appearance and behaviour are not available. The information may be gained from an intermediary such as a relative or neighbour or another health professional who may not know the patient well (Marsden 2000, Purc-Stephenson & Thrasher 2010).

Telephone triage must be approached as a distinct role and not undertaken by the member of staff who happens to be passing the telephone when it rings. Early studies of telephone triage suggested that patient assessment in telephone triage was, on the whole, subjective and required careful questioning which was often poor and carried out by unqualified personnel. A designated telephone triage clinician should be the first point of contact for telephone advice or triage in the emergency care setting. Decisions should be as reproducible as those made in face-to-face triage and, therefore, protocols or algorithms need to be developed. A key feature of these must be advice for the patient or carer – advice on self care if the decision is made that this is appropriate, but also advice for the patient or carer about what do to in the interim period between the call and the access to emergency care. This might include advice on basic life support while the ambulance service is directed to the caller.

The demarcation line between telephone advice and telephone triage is debatable. But it may be considered that triage occurs when a formalized process of decision-making takes place which allows identification of a clinical priority and allocation to predetermined categories of urgency of need for clinical evaluation and care. Many EDs and walk-in centres no longer offer telephone advice and have a direct transfer to NHS Direct or NHS 24 as appropriate.

What professional triage can become

As stated above, proponents of triage have never claimed that it reduced waiting times in the emergency care setting, merely that it acts as a risk-management tool, prioritizing services in a setting where demand often outstrips capacity. The triage encounter should be a rapid and reproducible assessment which accurately allocates a priority to each patient based on clinical need. A national triage system has been adopted in Portugal, using one of the systems most often used in the UK, the Manchester Triage System, and reports, nationally, that the triage encounter need take no more than 90 seconds (Lipley 2005).

At this initial assessment, opportunities have often been taken for clinicians to 'add in' other aspects of examination and investigation and the triage encounter includes much more than assessment, first aid and prioritization. It is used as a time to administer analgesia, to refer patients to X-ray or other investigations, to give advice about self-care and to initiate patient pathways to other specialties. This vastly increases the time taken to triage each patient and, whereas the triaged patients in the waiting room are a known quantity, the risk is transferred to the queue for triage. The triage assessment has become an 'MOT' rather than the 'pit stop'.

See and Treat

The premise at the beginning of this chapter is that triage is used to prioritize resources when supply does not meet demand. Where there is sufficient capacity in the emergency care setting, it is clear that prioritization is not required. One of the developments in emergency care in the UK has been the utilization of a 'See and Treat' model in the 'minor' areas of emergency care settings.

The challenge for EDs in the UK is to provide fast, fair and convenient access to health care in all sectors. There should be minimal wait for care with the right clinicians caring for the right patients at the right time (Windle 2005) and this had been a major challenge for emergency settings. A survey of patient experiences showed that patients prioritized waiting times, especially for less severe conditions, as their main issue of concern (Cooke et al. 2002).

See and Treat is a system of ED organization where patients with minor conditions are seen very quickly after they arrive in an ED by a senior clinician. Providing their problem is appropriate, such patients are examined, have definitive treatment and are then discharged (NHS Modernisation Agency 2004). This system of care emerged from the need to deal with long waiting times in EDs experienced particularly by those with the most minor presentations.

Key concepts in See and Treat

- on arrival, patients are seen, treated and referred or discharged by one practitioner
- the first person to see the patient, usually a nurse or doctor, is able to make autonomous clinical decisions about treatment, investigations and discharge

- other, more seriously ill patients or those requiring in-depth assessment or treatment should be streamed to, and dealt with in, the appropriate area
- triage of walk-in patients is unnecessary when See and Treat is in operation and patients are seen shortly after arrival
- dedicated staff allocated to separate areas and only withdrawn in exceptional circumstances.
- the system should operate with enough people to allow effective consultations without a queue developing; for instance, one doctor and one nurse has been shown to be effective for an arrival rate of up to 10 walk-in patients per hour
- staff development should be undertaken to ensure that all staff involved in See and Treat are able to make the system work effectively (NHS Modernisation Agency 2004).

There is no doubt that streaming in the ED and the use of See and Treat models has had a major effect on patient throughput (Shrimpling 2002) and has been endorsed by both the RCN Emergency Care Association and British Association for Emergency Medicine (BAEM). However, See and Treat is not without criticism, including the problems of the most senior clinicians dealing with the least serious presentations, thus potentially leaving the small number of seriously ill or injured patients being cared for by less experienced and less well supervised staff, the burn-out or boredom of senior clinicians dealing with interminable minor problems (Leaman 2003, Windle & Mackway Jones 2003) and the lack of adequate evaluation and evidence on which to roll out such programmes (Wardrope & Driscoll 2003). Literature search reveals little evaluation of See and Treat since this date with Maull et al. (2009) stating that although their fast-track strategy significantly improved service delivery to patients with minor conditions, service for patients with more acute conditions was not proportionately improved. Overall, however, department waiting times decreased.

It is clear though that where See and Treat services work optimally, where there is little or no queue and where there are always enough clinicians to manage the patient at the point of entry, triage is not necessary.

In many EDs though, while this may be a true picture on occasion, it is not likely to be the case all the time, with high patient attendance and sub-optimal staffing being the norm in most EDs. There is no doubt that waiting time is reduced using a See and Treat model in many cases but, while waiting times may be reduced, they still exist and where there is any wait at all to be seen by a clinician the waiting room becomes an unknown quantity and clinicians are back to the situation pre-triage where there was no knowledge of who was waiting and a major clinical risk-management issue. Just because a patient walks into the ED, it cannot be assumed that his problem is minor.

In any such situation, triage is essential in order to evaluate and prioritize waiting patients and manage the clinical risk. Many departments have implemented a policy of restarting triage when the queue for See and Treat reaches a critical point. The critical point should be determined centrally, after a careful analysis of case mix and workload predictions, and may be anything from 15 to perhaps 45 minutes and

beyond. The decision to take the risk of not assessing patients who walk into the department for this length of time is one of 'acceptable' risk and the validity of the acceptability of the risk will only be indicated by the lack of critical incidents associated with it over time. The issues around stopping and restarting triage are clear though – when the wait for See and Treat has increased, who will be made available to begin to triage patients when taking a clinician away from an area will inevitably lead to further delays? This must be balanced though against the clinical governance issues involved here, and flexibility needs to be built into streaming systems to allow them to function safely when their performance is sub-optimal due to problems with workload or staffing.

See and Treat is a strategy for use with those patients with minor conditions. For those patients who do not fall into this category, triage is an essential first part of the prioritization and risk management process.

Patient assessment

Triage, as stated earlier, should be a rapid, relatively superficial assessment taking no longer than a few minutes. Its purpose is to elicit information from the patient in order to determine their presenting problem. While in some cases this may be a quite straightforward process, e.g., a patient presenting with a clear history of simple uncomplicated trauma to an extremity, a significant proportion of attenders to the ED present with a more complex history involving various contributing factors which pre-empted their current illness or injury. It is the latter presentation that calls on the skills of the triage nurse. Diagnosis is not, and never should be, an aim or outcome of the triage encounter. Spot diagnosis, based on minimal information, may be correct when undertaken by an experienced clinician but it does not necessarily equate to priority and if incorrect, the potential for disaster is high, for both patient and clinician.

Various assessment tools have been developed which will aid the nurse in decision-making and encourage standardization of patients' assessments and subsequent collation of information. SOAP is an assessment tool devised in the US in 1969 (Lee & Fraser 1981). An 'I' for 'implementation' has been added after SOAP and an 'E' to emphasize the need for continual evaluation (Blythin 1988). Blythin's SOAPE became one of the first and most extensively used triage tools in the UK.

One of the potential problems with using this tool for the less experienced nurse is that by working systematically through the acronym, the nurse becomes caught up with the S – subjective assessment – and fails to reach the A, the actual assessment. Although S is the first letter, A and O are crucial elements of the tool. It is the objective assessment (O) which is often the best indicator of a patient's urgency for need of care. There is a rapid absorption of data which combines with a mental comparison with previous cases as the general appearance of the patient is assimilated by the triage nurse from the moment he comes into view. Along with a triage first impression (A), the objective assessment is often the critical factor when making a triage decision. It needs to be understood that the documentation of a triage decision, using any

Box 35.1

The SOAP model of triage

S Subjective assessment – The patient's evaluation of their illness or injury

O Objective assessment – An evaluation based on observable and measurable data

A Assessment – The clinical impression

P Plan of care

Box 35.2

PQRST model of triage assessment

P Provokes – What makes the pain better or worse?

Q Quality – What does it feel like? Suggestions may be offered to encourage a description, such as, 'burning, stabbing, crushing'

R Radiates – Where is the pain? Where does it go? Is it in one spot? Show me where it is

S Severity – Give the pain a score out of ten

T Time – How long have you had it? When did it start? When did it end?

Box 35.3

Systematic assessment model of triage

EYES List all the things that you can see

EARS What is the patient saying and not saying? Listen for breath sounds, audible wheeze

NOSE Smell for ketones, alcohol, incontinence, infection

HANDS Take the pulse, feel the skin temperature, assess capillary perfusion. Touch 'where it hurts'

BRAIN Use an assessment tool to aid your triage decision, e.g., SOAPE or PQRST

of the assessment tools devised, is secondary to the process of making that decision.

Other assessment tools have included the mnemonic P (provocation or palliation), Q (quality of pain), R (region and radiation), S (severity), T (time/history) to assess pain (Budassi & Barber 1981). They also suggest a tool involving the use of the five senses – looking, listening, smelling, touching and thinking – to evaluate a patient's chief complaint (see Boxes 35.1, 35.2 and 35.3).

Decision-making strategies

There are many theories of decision-making and a number of strategies used in the decision-making process. Unstructured triage methods may involve the triage clinician coming to a decision about a triage category with very little structure on which to base the decision.

Symptom clustering is a method used to assist in determining the clinical need of the patient. Using existing knowledge and experience, the nurse groups together symptoms and aims to identify the severity of the patient's condition. In this manner, 'chest pain' can be more easily associated with a cardiac condition if the symptom cluster includes nausea, shortness of breath on exertion, grey or clammy pallor, radiation of pain to the jaw or left arm, 'crushing' type pain or a 'tight band' across the chest. Conversely, a symptom cluster which includes increased pain on coughing and deep inspiration, shortness of breath on talking, and a productive cough would be more indicative of a respiratory or pulmonary condition.

'Clinical portraits' or pattern recognition is a strategy very commonly used by clinicians (Alfaro-LeFevre 2004). There are some illnesses and injuries that are so easily recognizable and that present so often in the ED that a very clear 'clinical

portrait' can be recognized. A symptom cluster narrows the options to a recognized injury or disease process in a particular system. Clinicians interpret the information they gain from the patient and compare it with previous cases. The very fast processing of information undertaken along with years of experience of different presentations and groups of symptoms is recognizable in expert practitioners. This is a technique which develops with experience and may appear to be intuitive.

Benner's (1984) model of skill acquisition looks at the way in which expertise in an area develops through an individual's experience. The novice, proficient or competent practitioner tends to use conscious decision-making where the expert is able to utilize pattern recognition.

Repetitive hypothesizing is a technique also employed by clinicians to test their diagnostic reasoning. By gathering data to prove or refute a particular hypothesis, a decision can be made.

It has been suggested that if the triage categories are clear and unequivocal, the role of the triage nurse can be carried out by any nurse, novice or expert, after the minimum training (Burgess 1992). The presence of a series of signs or symptoms will inherently warrant a particular priority, usually through the adherence to a written protocol in the form of flow charts, algorithms or simply lists of conditions in pre-designated priority categories.

Expertise is needed, however, as it is the experienced practitioner who is able to differentiate, for example, between cardiac and pleuritic chest pain; who understands that not all presentations of myocardial infarction are classical; who has an evidence base that tells them that women present with MI in different ways to men and is able to use all this knowledge to accurately allocate a triage category in a very rapid manner (Benner et al. 2009).

It should be recognized that the ability to ask the 'minimum of questions with the maximum of value' (Rund & Rausch 1981) comes with experience in the clinical area.

Priority setting

A reliable system of establishing priorities of care is the linchpin that determines the effectiveness of nurse triage. There may be circumstances whereby there are few data on which to determine a priority. Poor communication due to language difficulties is not uncommon, and the age or condition of the patient may also hinder the triage nurse in making an initial assessment.

Documentation

The accurate documentation of nurse triage findings cannot be overemphasized. Estrada (1979) argued that it is a 'professional judgment made by a professional nurse' deserving of careful documentation. It is a means of communication and becomes an integral part of the patient's permanent medical record. As such, it also becomes a legal document for which the triage nurse becomes accountable and responsible and Yu & Green (2009) note, the ED chart is the only lasting record of an ED visit, and attention must be paid to proper and accurate documentation. Indeed, the principle of personal accountability is fundamental to nursing practice. Documentation should be generated for all patients presenting to the emergency setting. If the patient leaves the department without waiting to see the doctor, it may be the only record of his attendance (Southard 1989).

When documenting the triage findings, a diagnosis should not be made. The purpose of nurse triage, as previously discussed, is not to establish a diagnosis. The initial assessment made by the triage nurse is no substitute for a full clinical examination, as diagnostic investigations may need to be carried out prior to any definitive diagnosis being made. In quieter departments, if the size of the caseload allows, other clinical information may be added: past medical history, allergies, medication, etc. These data may be used to initiate patient care plans and structured around the nursing model being used in the department. Duplications of information should be avoided, however, as the patient will be asked similar questions by the doctor or nurse practitioner.

It must be recognized that there is little point in a triage episode which delays the patient being examined by a clinician and it should be kept as short as possible.

Audit

As triage is a fundamental cornerstone of clinical risk management in the emergency care setting, inaccurate triage is as much of a problem for the department as no triage, as there is no guarantee of safe clinical priorities and this would soon become a governance issue.

Triage systems must be both reproducible, so that every clinician will come to the same triage decision about the same patient, and continuous audits should be carried out to ensure that the quality of triage is consistent and that practitioners who are less than accurate are identified so that support mechanisms can be put in place. Initial training of staff in triage methodology does not guarantee ongoing competence. Mentoring after initial training is required and an assessment of competence should be carried out. Audit ensures ongoing competence and underpins the quality agenda. Areas that need to be examined include completeness of the documentation and accuracy of the decisions made.

Without complete documentation, the decision made may still be accurate, but there is no way of proving how and on what basis the decision was made. It might then have been a random decision which just happens to be correct.

A simple method of audit is to take a number of randomly generated triage episodes for each practitioner and examine them:

- completeness of the episode can be expressed as a simple proportion
- accuracy can be expressed as a simple proportion
- feedback is given to the practitioner
- causes of inaccuracy are fed back to the practitioner.

The auditor should be an expert triage practitioner who is fully conversant with the triage method used in a particular department. Unless clinicians within the area are experienced triage practitioners and undertake triage regularly, it is not appropriate for them to audit the practice of those who do.

To ensure consistency of audit, a sample, perhaps 10% of episodes assessed, should be assessed independently by a second expert practitioner. Any differences in perception or decision would be moderated by discussion between the two.

Continuous audit can be time-consuming but is more effective than a set audit period where the triage practitioners know that their work is going to be scrutinized and may perform to a different standard than usual.

A national triage scale

The issue of uniformity and triage practice has been the subject of considerable discussion and debate. Following similar initiatives in Australia and Canada, a joint working party with members from both the Royal College of Nursing (RCN) ED Association and the British Association for ED Medicine (BAEM) led to the development of a standard five-point triage scale (Crouch & Marrow 1996). The scale was defined in terms of the maximum time the patient should wait before definitive clinical intervention.

Triage categories are linked to 'time to clinician' targets and, while the scale has been modified as reforms in emergency care and system redesign have led to 98% of patients being discharged from the ED within a window of four hours, in general, the categories still apply to all patients attending the emergency care setting.

The categories are colour-coded, in rainbow fashion, from red for the patient needing immediate attention to blue for those patients who have a non-urgent problem.

Triage systems

A number of triage systems are in place throughout the world and some of these are discussed here.

Emergency Triage – the Manchester Triage System

Emergency Triage, which has become known as the Manchester Triage System (MTS) was first published in 1996 and was the result of the recognition by clinicians in EDs around Manchester,

UK, that triage over the health economy was a muddle. A group of around 20 senior emergency physicians and nurses from each general and specialist ED spent a considerable amount of time formulating a solution that would be used in all EDs across the city. It was never envisaged that the system would extend outside the city; however, it seemed to appear at a time when triage was identified as an absolute necessity in most EDs and MTS became the triage system of choice in at least 90% of the UK's EDs. It appears that the system is generic enough and timely enough to have caught the imagination of EDs across the world (Martins et al. 2009, van der Linden et al. 2012). MTS has become the national triage system of Portugal and Brazil and is used extensively in a number of European countries and beyond. It is now used, translated into many languages, to triage tens of millions of ED attenders each year.

This triage method aims to give a clinical priority to each patient. It was recognized very early on in the group's deliberations that the length of the triage consultation means that any attempt to diagnose at triage is fraught with difficulty and doomed to fail. Even if diagnosis were possible, it is not necessarily linked to the patient's clinical priority, as other issues, such as the level of pain, will change the triage priority. It was also recognized by the group that the triage practitioner tends to look for a symptom and then hypothesize around a particular presentation or diagnosis, seeking symptoms and signs that give them permission to allocate the patient a higher triage priority, rather than assuming the worst and then eliminating signs and symptoms and moving down to a lower priority – a much safer way of working.

The key feature of the MTS is that it is reductive. The worst scenario and highest triage category is used until the patient can definitely be removed from that category (Mackway-Jones et al. 2005). Categories are time-based and this time is the time to clinical intervention rather than time to physician.

The triage practitioner is required to choose from a range of 50 presentational flow charts and seek a limited number of signs and symptoms at each level of priority. The signs and symptoms that discriminate between the different priorities are called discriminators and the assessment is carried out by finding the highest level at which the answer given to a discriminator question is positive.

Presentational flow charts are consistent in their approach so that whether the triage practitioner chooses the 'Unwell Adult' chart or the 'Diarrhoea and Vomiting' chart with which to assess a patient, the same priority will apply.

A number of general discriminators apply to every chart:

- life threat (vital ABC functions)
- haemorrhage
- pain
- conscious level
- temperature
- acuteness.

From the perspective of the patient, pain is a major factor in determining priority and the use of this as a general discriminator in every chart recognized the priority placed on pain by the patient. The MTS has been criticized for giving pain this level of priority, the concern being that patients will exaggerate their pain in order to achieve a higher priority for care; however, this is not borne out in practice. Pain should be part of every triage assessment as it is the most frequent symptom which prompts a patient to attend any emergency care setting (Fry et al. 2012). Ignoring pain is to ignore what is often most important to the patient. The use of a pain tool with behavioural characteristics such as that in the MTS allows the clinician to amend a pain score based on whether behaviour matches the patient's perceived pain matching the objective with the subjective pain scores, and this may be a move upwards as well as downwards. The use of appropriate analgesia at triage enables pain to be managed early in the patient encounter, and dynamic triage should ensure that a triage priority can be amended if required as pain is controlled. As Fry et al. (2012) also note, unnecessary suffering may be avoided if the public had a better understanding of pain and the benefits of pain management.

One of the key tenets of the MTS is that clinical priority should not be confused with management. Different patients will be managed differently in different emergency settings. It may be appropriate to manage, for example, children, quickly, but this decision should not effect a change in clinical priority. The priority is decided by their presentation and the management by the needs and particular circumstances of the department.

There has been some criticism of the MTS triage model since its inception, based on the lack of evidence for its claim to fitness for purpose and its lack of evaluation. While consensus may be the weakest form of evidence, where it is the only evidence it has credibility. Since its introduction, research has emerged to validate the system, in contrast to many other triage systems and a number of publications are available (Cooke & Jinks 1999, Roukema et al. 2006, Matias et al. 2008, Martins et al. 2009, van der Linden et al. 2012).

Each presentation is based on the best available evidence and has been updated in the second edition as clinical guidelines have changed. A national training strategy is in place for those units who use this method of triage.

Another use of MTS

MTS has now been validated by research and by its use throughout the world. Changes in emergency care practice have led to the recognition that it can be used as part of the streaming process in a concept known as the presentation priority matrix (Mackway-Jones et al. 2005). As the emergency care 'village' becomes more of a reality, the ED may not be the most appropriate place for the presenting patient to receive care.

Presentations and discriminators can be mapped against disposition for each emergency care setting: for example, chest pain priority 1 will always go to the resuscitation area.

An eye problem may always go to an Emergency Eye Centre where there is one, but may be seen in the general ED where there is no specialist eye provision. Torso injury at level 4 or 5 might be appropriately streamed to the minor injury unit.

Each emergency 'village' can create a matrix of presentations and dispositions for their local health economy in discussion with all those involved in emergency care provision, including the ambulance service, who can then also work to ensure that patients get the best care in the best place at an appropriate time.

Disposition will, of course, be influenced by what services are available at a particular time. For instance, the minor injury unit or primary care centre may be closed in the evenings, by the current pressures on these services and by the patient's choice.

The Australasian Triage Scale

The Australasian Triage Scale (ATS) was developed in Australia from a comprehensive review of the Australian National Triage Scale and was released in 2001 (Fitzgerald et al. 2011). The five categories are based on time to doctor, although this is being debated as nurse clinician roles are ever-developing. The category 1 patient is immediate and the category 5 should be seen within 2 hours.

All patients presenting to an ED should be triaged on arrival by a specifically trained and experienced registered nurse. The triage assessment and ATS code allocated must be recorded. The triage assessment involves a combination of the presenting problem and general appearance of the patient and may be combined with pertinent physiological observations. Vital signs are only measured at triage to estimate urgency or if time permits.

Clinical descriptors are listed for each triage category based on available research evidence and expert consensus. The list is not exhaustive or absolute and is considered to be indicative only. Physiological measurements should not be used as the only indicator for allocating to a triage category (Australasian College for Emergency Medicine 2005).

During revision of the National Triage Scale, it was recognized that there were many problems associated with inconsistency of application of the scale and also with education for the triage role and, in 2002, the Australian Commonwealth funded the development of a Triage Education Resource Book. The content of the book was developed with the assistance from professional organizations that represent ED nurses and the Australasian College for Emergency Medicine and this is used as the basis for triage training (Australasian College for Emergency Medicine 2005).

Canada Triage and Acuity scale

The Canada Triage and Acuity Scale was developed, based on the National Triage Scale in Australia. Its use became official policy in Canada in 1997 (Zimmermann 2006a). Categories are time-based and congruent with the ATS.

The Canadian ED triage and acuity scale is based on establishing a relationship between a group of sentinel events which are defined by the ICD9CM diagnosis at discharge from the ED, or from an in-patient database, and the 'usual' way patients with these conditions present. There are over 160 possible presentations with many additional modifiers which change priority.

Re-evaluation of patients is built into the system and nurses are encouraged to upgrade the triage level of patients with lower triage scores if the time objective has not been met. Reassessment is also recommended, at different intervals for different categories of patients; level 4 patients should be reassessed every hour and level 5 every 2 hours.

The Canadian Association of Emergency Physicians (CAEP) states that:

1. all patients should be assessed, at least visually, within 10 minutes of arrival
2. full patient assessments should not be done in the triage area unless there are no other patients waiting; only information required to assign a triage level should be recorded
3. a primary survey (rapid assessment) should be used when there are two or more patients waiting to be triaged, and only after all patients have had some assessment done should level 4 and 5 patients have a more complete assessment done by a triage or treatment nurse
4. priority for care may change following a more complete assessment or as patient's signs and symptoms change. There should be documentation of the initial triage as well as any changes. The initial triage level is still used for administrative purposes
5. level 1 and 2 patients should be in a treatment area and have the complete primary nursing assessment done immediately.

Lists of 'usual' presenting complaints and case scenarios are available to the triage nurse but are, again, not considered to be absolute. Triage personnel are encouraged to use their experience and instincts to 'up triage' priority, even if the patient does not seem to fit exactly with the facts or definitions on the triage scale, and the triage practitioner is asked to consider 'If they look sick then they probably are'. The CAEP strongly suggest that the triager's instinct should not be used to lower the triage level assignment when the facts suggest there may be a problem, but to take the more serious possibilities first and have someone find the proof that nothing is wrong (Canadian Association of Emergency Physicians 2006). Lee et al. (2011) found it to have high validity for elderly patients, and it is an especially useful tool for categorizing severity and for recognizing elderly patients who require immediate life-saving intervention.

The Emergency Severity Index Triage Scale

This was developed in the US in the late 1990s. Acuity and complexity are summarized on a 5-point scale where 1 is the highest acuity (Friedman Singer et al. 2012). Triage is based on acuity and on the likely resource consumption required to achieve a disposition and add what the patient needs on to when they need it (Zimmermann 2006b). Resources include radiography, medications and laboratory tests and resource determination is the triage nurse's best guess based on experience of what the patient is likely to need. After the most life-threatening presentations are dealt with, patients needing 2 or more resources are Emergency Severity Index (ESI) 3, one resource is ESI4 and none is ESI5. Vital signs are used to make a triage decision about patients at ESI level 3 and above.

Conclusion

Emergency care continues to develop and care settings and organizations continually strive to meet the needs of patients and the demands of purchasers of services and central government. What is clear is that emergency care is dealing with infinite demand in a context of finite resources. Strategies such as Streaming and See and Treat aim to address some of the problems of a demand-led service, and where the resources match the service needs, where every patient in a minor stream can be met at the door and treated immediately, triage in the minor areas of emergency

care settings is not required. The moment that definitive management is delayed and a queue develops, risk is generated where patients with unknown problems are waiting for assessment.

Triage in other areas of ED must follow the same pattern. Where each patient can be treated immediately, triage is not required; however, for almost all of the time, a robust triage system will be needed to discriminate between those patients who need immediate and life-saving intervention and those who have a lower clinical priority.

Triage, when undertaken correctly as a rapid assessment and prioritization strategy, is the gold-standard risk-management tool in emergency care throughout the world, however, as Kunz-Howard (2011) notes, triage is a process not a place. Experience and continuous education along with continuous audit lead to expert clinicians who can triage effectively and manage the work of the emergency care setting in the way that the patients deserve.

References

Alfaro-LeFevre, R., 2004. Critical Thinking and Clinical Judgment: A Practical Approach. Elsevier Science, Philadelphia.

Australasian College for Emergency Medicine, 2005. Guidelines on the Implementation of the Australasian Triage Scale in Emergency Departments. Australasian College for Emergency Medicine, Sydney.

Benner, P., 1984. From Novice to Expert: Excellence and Power in Clinical Nursing Practice. Addison-Wesley, Menlow Park, CA.

Benner, P., Tanner, C., Chesla, C., 2009. Expertise in Nursing Practice: Caring, Clinical Judgment, and Ethics, second ed. Springer Publishing Company, New York.

Blythin, P., 1988. Triage: A nursing care system. In: Wright, B. (Ed.), Managing and Practice in Emergency Nursing. Chapman and Hall, London.

Boyes, A., 1995. Health care assistants: delegation of tasks. Emergency Nurse 3 (2), 6–9.

Bracken, J., 2003. Triage. In: Newbery, L. (Ed.), Sheehy's Emergency Nursing: Principles and Practice, fifth ed. Mosby, St Louis.

Buckles, E., Carew-McColl, M., 1991. Triage by telephone. Nursing Times 87 (6), 26–28.

Budassi, S., Barber, J.M., 1981. Emergency Nursing Principles and Practice. CV Mosby, St Louis.

Burgess, K., 1992. A dynamic role that improves the service: Combining triage and nurse practitioner roles in A&E. Professional Nurse 7 (5), 301–303.

Canadian Association of Emergency Physicians, 2006. CTAS Implementation Guidelines. CTAS, Ottowa.

College of Emergency Medicine, the Emergency Nurse Consultant Association, the Faculty of Emergency Nursing and the Royal College of Nursing Emergency Care Association, 2011. Triage Position Statement. College of Emergency Medicine, London.

Cooke, M., 2005. Towards Faster Treatment: Reducing Attendance and Waits at Emergency Departments. Department of Health, London.

Cooke, M., Jinks, S., 1999. Does the Manchester triage system detect the critically ill? Journal of Accident & Emergency Medicine 16, 179–181.

Cooke, M.W., Wilson, S., Pearson, S., 2002. The effect of a separate stream for minor injuries on accident and emergency department waiting times. Emergency Medicine Journal 19 (1), 28–30.

Crouch, R., Marrow, J., 1996. Towards a UK triage scale. Emergency Nurse 4 (3), 4–5.

Department of Health, 2010. Hospital Activity Statistics. Department of Health, London.

Dolan, B., 1998. A dynamic process (Editorial). Emergency Nurse 6 (4), 1.

Estrada, E.G., 1979. Advanced triage by an RN. Journal of Emergency Nursing 5 (6), 15–18.

Fitzgerald, G., Jelinek, G.A., Scott, D., et al., 2011. Emergency department triage revisited. Emergency Medicine Journal 27, 86–92.

Friedman Singer, R., Infante, A., Oppenheimer, C.C., et al., 2012. The use of and satisfaction with the Emergency Severity Index. Journal of Emergency Nursing 38 (2), 120–126.

Fry, M., Hearn, J., McLaughlin, T., 2012. Prehospital pain management patterns and triage nurse documentation. International Emergency Nursing 77, 20–83.

Handyside, G., 1996. Triage in Emergency Practice. Mosby, St Louis.

Kunz-Howard, P., 2011. Do we need triage? Journal of Emergency Nursing 37 (6), 597.

Leaman, A.M., 2003. See and Treat: a management driven method of achieving targets or a tool for better patient care? One size does not fit all. Emergency Medicine Journal 20 (2), 118.

Lee, G., Fraser, S., 1981. ED Nursing SOAP Notes. Journal of Emergency Nursing 7 (5), 216–218.

Lee, J.Y., Oh, S.H., Peck, E.H., et al., 2011. The validity of the Canadian Triage and Acuity Scale in predicting resource utilization and the need for immediate life-saving interventions in elderly emergency department patients. Scandinavian Journal of Trauma, Resuscitation and Emergency Medicine 19 (1), 68–75.

Lipley, N., 2005. Foreign Exchange. Emergency Nurse 13 (7), 5.

Mackway-Jones, K., Marsden, J., Windle, J., 2005. Emergency Triage, second ed. Blackwell Publishing, Oxford.

Mallet, J., Woolwich, C., 1990. Triage in accident and emergency departments. Journal of Advanced Nursing 15, 1443–1451.

Marsden, J., 2000. Telephone Triage in an Ophthalmic A&E Department. Whurr Publishers Ltd, London.

Martins, H.M.G., De Castro Dominguez Cuña, L.M., Freitas, P., 2009. Is Manchester (MTS) more than a triage system? A study of its association with mortality and admission to a large Portuguese hospital. Emergency Medicine Journal 26, 183–186.

Matias, C., Oljveira, R., Duarte, R., et al., 2008. The Manchester triage System in Acute Coronary Syndromes. Portuguesa de Cardiologia 27 (2), 205–216.

Maull, R.S., Smart, P.A., Harris, A., et al., 2009. An evaluation of 'fast track' in A&E: a discrete event simulation approach. The Service Industries Journal 29, 923–941.

National Audit Office, 2004. Improving Emergency Care in England. NAO, London.

NHS Direct, 2010. NHS Direct Performance statistics. Department of Health, London.

NHS Modernisation Agency, 2004. Making See and Treat Work for Patients and Staff. NHS Modernisation Agency, London.

Potter, D. (Ed.), 1985. Emergencies Nurses Reference Library, Springhouse Corporation, Pennsylvania.

Purc-Stephenson, R.J., Thrasher, C., 2010. Nurse's experience with telephone triage and advice: a meta-ethnography. Journal of Advanced Nursing 66 (3), 482–494.

Roukema, J., Steyerberg, E.W., van Meurs, A.M., et al., 2006. Validity of the Manchester Triage System in paediatric emergency care. Emergency Medicine Journal 23, 906–910.

Rund, D.A., Rausch, T.S., 1981. Triage. CV Mosby, St Louis.

Shrimpling, M., 2002. Redesigning triage to reduce waiting times. Emergency Nurse 10 (2), 34–37.

Simenson, S.M., 2001. Telephone Health Assessment: Guidelines for Practice, second ed. Mosby, St Louis.

Southard, R., 1989. COBRA legislation: complying with ED provisions. Journal of Emergency Nursing 15 (1), 23–32.

van der Linden, C., Lindeboom, R., van der Linden, N., 2012. Managing patient flow with triage streaming to identify patients for Dutch emergency nurse practitioners. International Emergency Nursing 20, 52–57.

Wardrope, J., Driscoll, P., 2003. Turbulent times. Emergency Medicine Journal 20 (2), 116.

Windle, J., 2005. 'To triage or not to triage.' Emergency Nurse 13 (2), 11.

Windle, J., Mackway Jones, K., 2003. Don't throw triage out with the bathwater. Emergency Medicine Journal 20 (2), 119–120.

Yu, K.T., Green, R.A., 2009. Critical Aspects of Emergency Department Documentation and Communication. Emergency Medicine Clinics of North America 27 (4), 641–654.

Zimmermann, P., 2006a. Canada triage and acuity. In: Zimmermann, P., Herr, R. (Eds.), Triage Nursing Secrets. Mosby-Elsevier, St Louis.

Zimmermann, P., 2006b. The Emergency Severity Index Triage Scale. In: Zimmermann, P., Herr, R. (Eds.), Triage Nursing Secrets. Mosby-Elsevier, St Louis.

PART 8

Professional issues in the ED

Leadership

Lynda Holt

36

CHAPTER CONTENTS

Introduction

This chapter takes a broad look at leadership, a principle of organizational development that has been debated and studied for over 50 years. During this time the theories have changed considerably (Huczynski & Buchanan 2003, Bass & Bass 2008, Lang & Rybnikova 2012); however, one thing has remained consistent, human behaviour is a fundamental part of leadership. It is also clear that in an increasingly political healthcare environment strong clinical leadership is essential for effective patient care, and for nurses' well-being. This chapter will look at some aspects of leadership behaviour and identify the key components of effective clinical leadership as well as some of the principles of clinical supervision.

http://dx.doi.org/10.1016/B978-0-7020-4315-4.00036-X

What is leadership?

Leadership is a much debated term with many conflicting theories, definitions and qualities to describe successful leaders (Wade-Grimm 2010). Most people recognize a good leader, but it is often harder to identify why that individual is a good leader. It does, however, differ from management in that specific status or organizational position is not necessary for an individual to be a leader. So, if position is not the key factor, what is? Skills are important, but not necessarily the ones that may be expected. For example, management skills, attention to detail, organization, intelligence and planning are not consistent among great leaders (Owen 2005). The same inconsistencies exist when considering styles of leadership. Where consensus does exist it is around a collection of behaviours that together can create a leader; these include honesty and integrity, the ability to motivate others, vision, decisiveness, confidence and intuition. In short, leadership is the ability to influence others without threat or coercion (Huczynski & Buchanan 2003).

In healthcare, the profile and priority given to effective leadership has grown slowly, but its importance continues to increase, along with the evidence base showing how powerful effective leadership can be (Young-Ritchie et al. 2010). Effective leadership should not be confused with good management; the two often co-exist, but can also come from two different sources, as the behaviours demonstrated by leaders are not absolutely necessary for effective management.

Management can be seen as the organizational and technical tasks that have to be achieved in order to ensure the fluid delivery of services. Management is head-driven, rational and pragmatic. Leadership can be seen as the inspiration of others, the skills employed, often subtly, to galvanize a group of staff to commit to deliver a quality service. Leadership is heart-driven, emotive and enthusing. The most effective environments have both, and both leaders and managers are most effective when able to use a range of behaviours and skill from each domain, depending on circumstances.

Clinical leadership

Leadership skills are essential in any clinical environment, and the nature of Emergency Department (ED) work is such that priorities and pace can change dramatically over a very short period, with a potential for staff to feel threatened by the perceived chaos. To maintain a safe, effective service to patients the clinical leader needs to foster an environment where care delivery has some structure, staff have guidance and security, therefore trust can develop (Jonas et al. 2011). These rapidly changing high-pressured clinical areas are the environments where leadership and management are mostly likely to intertwine. It is not uncommon for the management role to become dominant, resulting in both perceived leaders and their clinical staff feeling disempowered and demoralized with their work. For clinical leadership to be successful, and not just clinical management, an overarching environment where individuals feel empowered and able to develop relies on access to information, power, opportunity and resources (Upenieks 2003). It is only when individuals feel empowered that they can truly lead change, take risks and create the innovation needed to develop clinical care.

The challenge for those leading care on a day-to-day basis in emergency care environments can seem daunting alongside the practical tasks of managing the workload, but often what is required is conscious application of principles used every day. Stanley (2006) discusses the value of congruent leadership as a basis for developing clinical care and describes clinical leaders as individuals who are experts in their field, positive clinical role models and good communicators. They are followed because they can translate what they believe about nursing into good clinical care. This is in fact a simple phenomenon; congruent leaders are successful because their values and beliefs and their actions match up; as a result they are credible.

Effective clinical leaders can adapt congruence theory to enhance their current practice. It creates a bridge between the necessary management role and the desired leadership role. The most important component in creating congruence is passion; this comes from trusting, valuing and believing in what you are doing (Thompson 2000).

Congruent leadership can be summed up as leading from the heart, trusting your instincts, and valuing your knowledge and beliefs (Box 36.1).

Step 1: how you feel It is no accident this is step one, and in the clinical environment nurses do this all the time; they get a feel for when a patient is 'going off' or when they should be wary or feel threatened by some patients and not others

displaying similar behaviour. This can be explained as intuition, sixth sense, or tacit or expert knowledge (Benner 1984, Benner et al. 2009). The key is to trust these feelings and act in congruence with them; they are based on both experience and intrinsic beliefs. Leadership behaviour will appear natural and confident, fostering trust and motivation to comply, as opposed to ignoring 'feelings', which can have the reverse effect on leadership behaviour, leaving the leader and the followers feeling anxious and lacking in confidence.

Step 2: walk the talk This is about personal congruence, the leader's values and purpose, but most of all their ability to take responsibility for their own thoughts, behaviours and actions, whatever the outcome. So when things do not go to plan, for example, blood results get lost, the leader takes responsibility for the appropriate delegation of that task, discusses the incident with those involved, and does not just pass on blame but follows through with any necessary action to prevent a repeat.

Step 3: constantly interact Most information in the clinical environment is gained through face-to-face interaction and observation; a leader remote from this cannot lead with passion and congruence. It is also worth remembering that individuals' experiences are different, and therefore their understanding and interpretation of situations may be different too. Interaction ensures the leader understands the reality for others in the clinical area they are leading.

Step 4: build trust This comes from demonstrated consistency in the leader's behaviour, from equity towards all staff and integrity. Being a role model in the clinical area helps to build trust.

Step 5: lead by example Again the leader's behaviour determines their success; the role should be carried out with passion, purpose and commitment, instilling confidence and enhancing motivation in followers.

Step 6: resolve conflict Conflict should not be left to fester, it grows and poisons. Most clinical teams rely heavily on each other to be effective, therefore the leader needs to step in and address conflict rapidly even when it is uncomfortable to do so.

Step 7: select followers A clinical team is no different to any other team, it needs complementary skills and differing personalities to work, so when selecting new members consideration should be given to what the team needs rather than selecting those in the leader's mould. People with genuine passion for their role usually have a natural energy which spills into the team. They are worth looking out for even if they do not yet have all the skills needed.

Garbett (1995) described leaders as people who have a vision; they make things happen, and at the same time they strengthen and support their followers, inspiring them to trust the leader. These appear to be the core qualities needed to lead the clinical team in ED.

Developing personal leadership behaviour

There are four key components to leadership behaviour:

1. self-awareness
2. positivity
3. focus
4. influence.

Box 36.1

Seven steps to congruent leadership

1. How you feel
2. Walk the talk
3. Constantly interact
4. Build trust
5. Lead by example
6. Resolve conflict
7. Select followers

Self-awareness

Personal effectiveness stems from self-awareness. It is only through true understanding of her/his strengths, likes and dislikes that a leader can find an authentic set of leadership behaviours. Through self-awareness the leader can understand what makes her/him feel strong or vulnerable, where she/he feels effective and where she/he is less sure, and what she/he is confident about. It is also through self-awareness that a leader can examine her/his expectations, and beliefs about herself/himself. Many individuals are far better at criticizing themselves than celebrating their strengths; this is probably the single most effective way of undermining self-confidence (Gonzalez 2012). Often this internal criticism is based on long-held beliefs and expectations that have no genuine validity. Once the leader becomes aware of this behaviour he/she is better placed to reverse it and replace negative internal dialogue with positive comments and praise for what is good. Box 36.2 offers some areas for self-examination to enhance self-awareness.

It is only with self-awareness that a leader can really understand the impact of her/his behaviour on others, as well as what expertise she/he needs from other team members to enhance the team. It is also worth remembering that behaviours individuals dislike in themselves they usually dislike in others, so a self-aware leader will be able to head off potential conflict by understanding where those feelings come from. An effective leader is someone who not only understands herself/himself well, but is also willing to challenge her/his make-up and change their viewpoint (Welford 2002). The dogmatic leader may appear strong and purposeful but will often close their minds to alternatives that may actually be better.

Box 36.2

Enhancing self-awareness

Know what you like
- Passion
- Experience
- Fun
- Talents
- Needs

Passion
- What gets you going?
- What do you really love?
- What makes you laugh?

What do you need?
- To show yourself affection
- To be happy
- To really get satisfied

Self-sabotage
- What you do to yourself
- Beliefs and values
- Fear
- Criticism
- Blame

Positivity

Leaders are positive in their attitudes, their direction and their responses. Being positive is not down to chance or personality, it is learned behaviour. Being positive is about creating solutions and learning to be lucky. Being lucky is an attitude, a way of behaving, and a way of seeing the world. Fundamentally, individuals create their own luck, and appearing lucky to others is often down to sheer hard work and creating enough opportunities (Box 36.3).

Effective leaders create opportunities, they take risks and they act. They believe outcomes will be positive, and convey a positive and passionate image to others. Positivity as described here is all about attitude and a personal belief system applied to life. It does not mean leaders should gloss over difficult issues, as this can equally alienate staff. Being able to recognize when a situation is genuinely challenging, and being prepared to acknowledge and discuss this with staff, makes the leader credible and 'in touch'. Being able to convey a way forward and potential resolution where staff feel involved, supported and engaged is genuine leadership.

Box 36.3

Being lucky

Perspective – how you look at situations
Choice – how you respond to situations
Responsibility – take responsibility for yourself
Persistence – sticking at something is often the only difference

Focus

Focus is an ability to look beyond what is immediately obvious, beyond personal need, and to focus on the overall aim, on what the individual is trying to achieve. This necessitates vision and the ability to create direction, not just provide effective crisis management or reactionary direction as is often seen in clinical environments. When truly focused a leader needs to be both decisive and proactive to ensure action.

This is the ability of the leader to see a finished product, which may be as simple as prioritizing and organizing the nursing work to ensure all demands are met. In terms of clinical leadership, however, focus is often the ability to take an external directive and find creative ways of achieving care standards while keeping the activity acceptable to the nurses delivering care.

Vision is the ability to see a way forward to the desired outcome. Selling that vision with enthusiasm, realism and commitment creates followers. It is important to remember that vision is a fluid concept and open to change. Opinions and ideas of followers can help to mould a vision to ensure success; the effective leader will set the destination and involve the team in planning the route.

Influence

This is perhaps the most fundamental skill of leaders; without the ability to influence others a leader may have no followers. All of the above components depend on the ability to influence others, but your ability to influence relies on understanding the impact you make (Box 36.4).

Box 36.4

Having influence

- Communication
- Empowering others
- Team building
- Political savvy

Having a vision that others want to be part of is important, but it is more important to have the ability to sell that vision to others. This is easier if the individual is seen as positive, credible and having integrity.

Communication

Becoming a clinical leader is a time of great personal vulnerability. The leader's knowledge, ability to organize and sustain direction, and skills in supporting others will all come under scrutiny before followers decide to adopt the leader's vision. Effective communication is fundamental to gaining acceptance as a leader. Most ED nurses have experienced a shift where the nurse in charge keeps information about patient progress to him- or herself and does not keep staff informed of activity. This results in a withdrawal from the situation; nurses continue to function under direction, but they have no ownership of the activity and offer little support to the leader. Conversely, where communication is good and ideas are welcomed from other nurses, staff work as a team, supporting each other and the leader. The success relies on the ability to communicate effectively with other staff members. This means the leader is able to give direction and feedback to staff, but also can receive feedback, air ideas and develop strategy (Box 36.5).

Box 36.5

Effective communication

Listening – not waiting to speak, really listening to what is being said and not said

Talking – conveying ideas, direction, discussing issues

Body language – these are perhaps the biggest communication cues

Confidence – a message delivered with confidence and conviction is much stronger and more motivating

Credibility – act with self-awareness, within personal values, and consistently

Time – be careful to allow enough time for important conversations, and not too much for corridor conversation. Remember the impact that urgency has on messages delivered and heard

Trust – this is fostered through communication action and credibility

Empowerment

Empowerment of individuals or a team can be a lengthy process; it is sometimes difficult to imagine this taking place in a busy ED when decision-making is necessarily rapid. The clinical leader needs to work periodically with nurses on an individual basis. She/he needs to understand and appreciate the nurse's contribution, give constructive feedback and invest in the nurse's individual development. This way when rapid decisions do need to be made, the followers are more likely to trust their leader and accept and support the action proposed.

Empowerment does not mean a lack of managerial control. The clinical leader must set boundaries on what are acceptable standards and behaviours and what are unacceptable. These must be communicated to others in the clinical environment and should remain constant. This way the team is free to participate in decision-making within a preset structure. For most people, boundaries provide a sense of stability and security. This can be particularly important when trying to maintain a departmental direction and vision. Leadership, however, is as much about risk-taking as it is about control. The effective leader will allow her team to make decisions that may be inappropriate or less than efficient (Bowles & Bowles 1999). The risk that should be considered, balanced and judged is whether the consequences of the staff making the wrong decision will be catastrophic. If this is likely then the leader would be foolish not to make a decision and pass it on; if it will not be then it may be worth allowing others to make the choice and let them glory in their success or learn from their lesson, depending on how things turn out. It might be easier as a leader to just take control and make the decisions; there is little risk of things going wrong, particularly in a busy ED. This fails, however, to empower the team. This lack of empowerment and overly controlling approach can lead to disenfranchisement of staff from the organizational process of their department, simply turning up at work to do their job; or worse the team become so disempowered that staff become unable to make even the most basic and simple of decisions. Every leader must remember that if there is constant downward management there will be constant upward referral. This does nothing to develop the skills of others and is exhausting for the leader. The challenge for the leader is one of balance; in order to empower and develop staff they must feel trusted, capable and supported. In order to achieve this, the leader must feel comfortable with the degree of risk he/she is taking.

Team-building

The ability to build and sustain a team is fundamental to being an effective leader. Part of the role of the leader is to draw people together, create common goals and encourage a sense of collaboration. This way a team can be formed that will face challenges together. This is best demonstrated by a well-run resuscitation – the team comes together, each member has a role, and a comprehensive package of care is given.

These teams last only for a short while. In building a team that is expected to work closely for a sustained period, such as a project group within a department, the leader must have an understanding of group dynamics. An effective team is one where there is diversity among the team members and the collective qualities those individuals bring offer a richness to the breadth of skills the team has at its disposal to achieve its goals. Effective leaders will look at their team and understand the differences between the individuals, celebrate these differences, and use them to the benefit of the service and the patients.

There are a number of systems available to analyse the personality profiles of individuals. It can be helpful to undertake such analysis in order to appreciate where the strengths lie within a team (Dolan 2011). By understanding this, the allocation of tasks can be made based upon people's strengths, so ensuring the best outcome. The effective leader, however, will also use such understanding to identify where an individual's weaknesses lie and sometimes allocate tasks to stretch and develop skills. This can be an uncomfortable experience for the individual that may result in resistance to the leader. The leader must, therefore, ensure that such development is backed up with support, reassurance and positive feedback.

A crucial factor in team-building is the function of the leader. To be successful, this person must remain part of the team, giving direction and support to the other team members. The leader must be secure enough in her/his own knowledge to encourage and utilize the abilities and knowledge of other team members without being threatened. It is important for leaders to recognize their own limitations, but recognition is not sufficient. Declaration of one's own limitations can often encourage loyalty and affiliation to the leader by the followers. This must be undertaken positively and with care and judgement. Listening effectively to the views and opinions of others, while acknowledging one's own short-comings, can lead to better decisions and a stronger team (Caplin-Davies 2000).

Political savvy

As a professional group, nurses are often less aware of how to manage organizational politics than other professional groups in healthcare (Nelson & Gordon 2006). This can have a detrimental effect on leadership ability. The principles of influence are the same regardless of the target audience, so whether the Chief Executive, Director of Nursing or Healthcare Assistant is the person to be influenced, the following principles apply.

Clinical leaders should use charm in the same way many medical colleagues do; it will engage others, make them want to talk, and more importantly listen to others' views (Box 36.6).

Box 36.6

How to charm

- Smile
- Make others feel comfortable
- Remember names or personal details
- Ask about people
- Involve others in conversation and activity
- Welcome others' views without agreeing
- Give praise
- Be consistent

As trust grows they will provide the clinical leader with information that increases their political intelligence, but also trust the leader's views and ideas, give the benefit of the doubt because that leader is a known and trusted entity,

and as credibility grows other professionals and Trust directors will want to work with the leader who has charmed them because they now know her, trust her/him and rate her/him. That alone makes the clinical leader's job a whole lot easier.

Clinical leaders should see organizational meetings as an opportunity, not an ordeal to be avoided with the slightest excuse. They are where issues are discussed and decisions are made and if the clinical leader is not there, her/his opinion is lost: worse, her/his power of influence is diminished. Instead clinical leaders should be political, plan for the meeting, read the agenda, and decide in advance what subject's impact on their clinical area. Prior to the meeting identify natural allies, and discuss issues beforehand, identify critics and have answers for their criticisms. On the day of the meeting arrive early, try to sit facing the chairperson as it is easier to get heard, and watch listeners as well as speakers, as they often give away much information about their stance on the discussion. The clinical leader should have prepared what she/he wants to say, and be clear and concise, avoiding any complex clinical analogies, which may lose the attention of non-clinicians. Finally the leader should stay on message responding, not reacting, to others comments. It is often worth practising this technique in meetings with little risk first, but it quickly becomes a habit. Other professional groups have practised in this way for a long while, and nurse leaders are disadvantaged if they do not engage in this process.

Leadership is fundamentally about influence; it is worth thinking about the impact clinical leaders make as individuals to ensure it is the impact they want to make (Armstrong 2012).

Clinical supervision

The importance of clinical supervision was emphasized in the light of serious concerns identified by the Allitt Inquiry (1991), named after Beverly Allitt, a paediatric nurse in England who assaulted 13 children in her care, murdering four during the early 1990s. The Health Service Ombudsman at that time repeatedly raised concerns about a number of flaws identified in the delivery of nursing care, including the quality of record-keeping. Clinical supervision offered a potential solution to some of the difficulties being encountered by the nursing profession on an individual and organizational basis. Some areas of nursing, such as psychiatry, have used supervision for many years; however, in acute nursing the concept has been underdeveloped.

The King's Fund (1994) has described clinical supervision as a formal arrangement in which nurses can discuss work with another professional colleague. It has been promoted as a support mechanism for nurses, a tool for professional development and a method of quality control.

Principles to support clinical supervision

The Nursing and Midwifery Council (2002) supports the concept of clinical supervision, however it has stopped short of identifying any particular model of delivery to allow for local adaptation. It does stipulate a set of guiding principles that should be used (Box 36.7).

Box 36.7

Nursing and Midwifery Council principles of clinical supervision

- Clinical supervision supports practice, enabling you to maintain and improve standards of care
- Clinical supervision is a practice-focused professional relationship, involving a practitioner reflecting on practice guided by a skilled supervisor
- The process of clinical supervision should be developed by practitioners and managers according to local circumstances. Ground rules should be agreed so that you and your supervisor approach clinical supervision openly, confidently and are both aware of what is involved
- Every practitioner should have access to clinical supervision. Each supervisor should supervise a realistic number of practitioners
- Preparation for supervisors should be flexible and sensitive to local circumstances. The principles and relevance of clinical supervision should be included in pre-registration and post-registration education programmes
- Evaluation of clinical supervision is needed to assess how it influences care and practice standards
- Evaluation systems should be determined locally

(Reproduced from Nursing and Midwifery Council (2002) Supporting Nurses and Midwives Through Life-long Learning. London: Nursing and Midwifery Council.)

For its introduction to be successful in any clinical environment, it is essential for participants to share a common understanding of their interpretation of clinical supervision. One approach to this is for emergency nurses to explore the many activities and skills in nursing work, including:

- caring
- curing
- supporting
- empowering
- teaching.

These activities all involve interaction with others, such as patients and their relatives or friends, and are not without personal risk. In emergency care, the patient's stay is relatively short and the onus is on the nurse to develop a therapeutic relationship quickly, but how do nurses maintain this relationship when someone is off sick, the shift is busy or the relative has complained about the ever-increasing waiting times?

Types of supervision

Clinical supervision must be clearly separated from issues relating to pay, promotion or discipline. Only then can a trusting relationship be fostered. Several ways of addressing supervision have emerged. These include:

- one-to-one supervision with an expert from a nursing or related background
- one-to-one supervision within a peer group
- group or network supervision
- action learning sets.

Peer supervision means the supervisor and supervisee are involved in similar clinical work, and possibly face similar challenges. The advantages are increased awareness, potentially greater trust and a relationship that is less threatening to the supervisee. The disadvantage is that without effort and commitment from both parties, the activity can become purely one of support and not development. Group and network supervision have been developed in some areas of healthcare, particularly in community settings. This involves a group of similar professionals sharing experiences and developing their practice using one another. For this to be successful, a large degree of trust and commitment is needed from participants. It does have disadvantages in that some members of the group can remain non-participative or dominate activity. It is perhaps organizationally easier to facilitate than one-to-one supervision. Whichever method of supervision is adopted, it is essential that the clinical supervisor remains clinically challenging. The success of clinical supervision relies on its perceived value to the department (Jones 2006); therefore agreeing the aims and process before implementation is imperative. Bishop (1994) identifies three overall aims that act as a bedrock for supervision activities:

- to facilitate professional expertise
- to improve patient care
- to safeguard standards of care.

To achieve these objectives, clinical supervision should be seen as a continuum along with mentorship and preceptorship. A mentor helps to develop clinical competence by guiding a nurse through learning a new skill, such as cannulation. A preceptor helps the nurse gain confidence in that role. A clinical supervisor aids professional development from acquisition of new skills. But for clinical supervision to be successful it is important to consider the impact of the nurse as a whole and not as a technician.

The philosophical approach to clinical supervision does not have to be complicated. Proctor (1986) suggested a simple tripartite approach to supervision (Fig. 36.1). The formative role is one of education, supplementing the supervisee's knowledge and facilitating growth. The restorative aspect relies on support, exploring anxieties or critical incidents and allowing the supervisee to resolve stress. The normative function is one of quality control, looking at actual practice and challenging methods to maintain high standards of patient care.

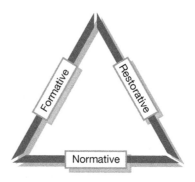

Figure 36.1 • Functions of clinical supervision.

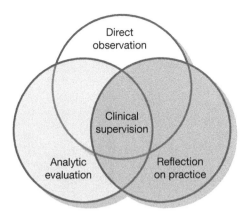

Figure 36.2 • Activities of a supervisor.

The success of clinical supervision relies on its perceived value to the department and staff commitment. The activities of clinical supervision revolve around the provision of regular space for reflection on the content and process of work (Fig. 36.2). Its functions are to develop the understanding and skills of the supervisee, to ensure quality nursing care and to provide space to explore and express distress about work. Done effectively this will result in the supervisee feeling valued and validated both as a person and as a nurse, as she/he is able to receive feedback and therefore gain new perspectives on her/his work. This empowers the nurse to plan and utilize personal resources and become proactive and innovative. Clinical supervision should not be a forum for self-congratulation or self-destruction, nor should it be personal therapy. The supervisor can facilitate this by observation of practice, encouraging retrospective reflection and participation in evaluating outcomes (RCN 2000).

Getting clinical supervision

Clinical supervision is not without personal risk, because the nurse is being asked to expose anxieties or perceived areas of weakness to a close colleague. Trust and confidentiality are therefore pivotal to a successful relationship. The nurse has a responsibility to seek supervision actively by going into a meeting with identified areas for support. She/he must ask for help in these areas and not rely on the supervisor to work it out. For supervision to succeed, the nurse needs to be able to share her/his feelings and be open to feedback, monitoring any tendencies to defend practice, but also monitoring what feedback is useful. Perhaps most important to the success of the relationship is the ability to be creative about clinical practice.

Self-awareness helps to minimize the impact of any blocks the nurse may have towards supervision, such as negative past experiences, inhibition, misunderstandings or relationship problems such as personality clashes. Much of this can be overcome if the nurse being supervised has a choice of who acts as supervisor. In making this choice it is important that the supervisee chooses a supervisor based on that person's ability to challenge and develop nursing practice and not because of popularity with the supervisee. This person is most

likely to be another nurse from the same or a similar specialty. The supervisor needs to apply clinical knowledge in a manner that promotes innovation, is constructive and creative, and facilitates the professional growth of the supervisee. It is not enough to be more senior or more experienced; the supervisor also needs advanced skills in listening, giving positive and negative feedback, facilitating reflection and defusing distress.

Before clinical supervision is established in a department, its ground rules should be identified and agreed by participants (Simms 1993); for example, it should be agreed that any unacceptable breach of the Code of Professional Conduct (Nursing and Midwifery Council 2008) may need to be taken outside the supervisory relationship (Box 36.8).

 Box 36.8

Ground rules and responsibilities for clinical supervision

- Commitment to confidentiality
- Open and honest learning
- Sharing best practice
- Seeking research for evidence-based practice
- Facilitating new learning opportunities
- Relevance to clinical practice

(Reproduced from Royal College of Nursing (2002) Ground Rules and Responsibilities for Clinical Supervision. London: RCN.)

In addition to these, some practical considerations such as the frequency and length of meetings, criteria for supervisors and termination routes if sessions become destructive should all be agreed. A robust audit tool is useful to measure quantitative data about activity such as the frequency and duration of supervision sessions. Evidence of its value to nurses is largely subjective, but potential benefits are outlined in Box 36.9.

There remains much debate about the real value of clinical supervision. Shanley & Stevenson (2006) argue that it is potentially hazardous in its current form, and models need to become more sophisticated if they are to be successful. Despite the ongoing concern in acute and primary care, clinical supervision has been successful in mental health nursing for many years.

Clinical supervision is a complex activity; it facilitates the development of clinical practice and supports the provision of quality patient care. Perhaps most importantly, clinical supervision provides a forum for innovation and creativity to flourish. Its implementation has been hampered by misunderstanding of its function, not aided by the inference of its title 'supervision'. It is, however, a real opportunity for nurses to develop their nursing practice further, challenge professional boundaries and celebrate the value of nursing.

360 degree feedback

In this chapter self-awareness has been discussed in relation to leadership skills. Becoming self-aware is something that most people have to constantly work at developing. Getting

Box 36.9

Potential benefits of clinical supervision

Benefits to the nurse

- Offers support and aids in confidence building
- Invests in staff and acknowledges the value of nurses and nursing
- Helps to develop nursing practice
- Allows nurse to review practice creatively and critically
- Can aid objective setting at individual performance reviews and reveal deficits
- Allows practice to change
- Promotes critical reflection on and in practice
- Develops individual accountability
- Aids personal and professional growth
- Helps link theory and practice
- Increases self-awareness

Benefits to the manager

- Helps monitor/maintain standards
- Promotes innovation
- Facilitates professionally accountable practitioners
- Links with organizational audit
- Challenges poor practice
- Strengthens collegiate relationships
- Maximizes training resources
- Creates a dynamic, changing environment
- Improves communication systems

Box 36.10

Benefits of 360 degree feedback

For the individual

- Increases self-awareness
- Gives a window to how he/she impacts on others
- Feedback is from people they know, work with and whose opinions matter to the appraisee, therefore it can be extremely powerful
- Offers feedback from a variety of work-based settings
- Motivating and focuses development

For the organization

- It measure skills and behaviours relevant to the appraisee's role
- Reinforces the organization's values and culture
- Can improve staff retention
- Identifies organizational strengths and weaknesses
- Focuses learning and development activity and resources to areas of genuine need
- Creates openness and trust amongst the team

feedback from other people is a critical part of this and giving feedback is an important part of being a leader. Very often this only happens when something has gone wrong, but feedback about strengths and things done well is equally as important and often leads to greater personal growth and performance improvement. The 360 degree feedback model is a good way of getting this type of information. It is popular for both clinicians and managers in the health sector. 360 degree feedback is where an individual (the appraisee) receives feedback from a selection of people, such as seniors, peers and juniors, in a range of predetermined competency areas (Holt 2011). While 360 degree feedback is predominantly a development tool, it can be used as part of a formal appraisal process, or in isolation. It is particularly valuable because it examines more than one work relationship and the impact the appraisee has in a number of different roles (Box 36.10).

Most people put a lot of time and emotional energy into their 360 degree feedback, and managed properly it is a motivating, powerful and positive experience. Managing 360 degree feedback properly takes time, effort and care, before, during and most of all afterwards. This way the organization, big or small, gets return on its 360 degree investment (Holt 2012).

Conclusion

This chapter has identified a range of clinical leadership and supervision issues which emergency nurses should consider when developing themselves and their practice. In an increasingly complex emergency service, support for and by those responsible for developing services is needed in order to recruit, retain and value that most precious commodity – the staff. The chapter highlights the importance of effective clinical leadership, both for those working within the ED environment and for their benefit within the organization. The chapter reinforces the need for clinical leaders to become more aware of professional and organizational politics, in order to get the best results for their clinical environment, those working in it and their patients. Finally, the chapter identifies that leaders exist at all levels within an organization, and because leadership is learned behaviour anyone can become a leader with a bit of self-awareness, willingness to stand out from the crowd, and the ability to influence others.

References

Allitt Inquiry, 1991. Independent Inquiry Relating to Deaths and Injuries on the Children's Ward at Grantham and Kesteven General Hospital During the Period February to April 1991. HMSO, London.

Armstrong, H., 2012. Spirited Leadership: Growing Leaders for the Future. In: Roffey, S. (Ed.), Positive Relationships: Evidence Based Practice Across the World. Springer, New York.

Bass, B.M., Bass, R., 2008. Handbook of Leadership: Theory, Research & Managerial Applications, fourth ed. Free Press, New York.

Benner, P., 1984. From Novice to Expert: Excellence and Power in Clinical Nursing Practice. Addison-Wesley, Menlo Park.

Benner, P., Tanner, C., Chesla, C., 2009. Expertise in Nursing Practice: Caring, Clinical Judgment, and Ethics, second ed. Springer Publishing Company, New York.

Bishop, V., 1994. Clinical supervision for an accountable profession. Nursing Times 90 (39), 35–37.

Bowles, N., Bowles, A., 1999. Transformational leadership. Nursing Times Learning Curve 3 (8), 2–4.

Caplin-Davies, P., 2000. Nurse manager: Change thyself. Nursing Management 6 (9), 16–20.

Dolan, B., 2011. How to work with people you'd rather kill! Nursing Review 12 (1), 11.

Garbett, R., 1995. Leading questions. Nursing Times 91 (27), 26–27.

Gonzalez, M., 2012. Mindful Leadership: The 9 Ways to Self-awareness, Transforming Yourself and Inspiring Others. John Wiley & Sons Canada Ltd, Ontario.

Holt, L., 2011. How to get the best ROI from 360 feeedback in your organization. The Grapevine 3, 18–19.

Holt, L., 2012. Get Out of Your Own Way: Stop Sabotaging Your Business and Learn to Stand Out in a Crowded Market. NABO (UK) Ltd, London.

Huczynski, A., Buchanan, D., 2003. Organisational Behaviour: An Introductory Text, fifth ed. Prentice Hall, London.

Jonas, S., McCay, L., Keogh, B., 2011. The importance of clinical leadership. In: Swanwick, T., McKimm, J. (Eds.), The ABC of Clinical Leadership. BMJ Publishing, London.

Jones, A., 2006. Clinical supervision: what do we know and what do we need to know? A review and commentary. Journal of Nursing Management 14 (8), 577–585.

King's Fund, 1994. Clinical Supervision: An Executive Summary. King's Fund Centre, London.

Lang, R., Rybnikova, I., 2012. Leadership is going global. In: Benscoter, G.M. (Ed.), The Encyclopaedia of Human Resource Management, vol. 3. Pfeiffer Books, San Francisco.

Nelson, S., Gordon, S., 2006. Moving beyond the virtue script in nursing. In: Nelson, S., Gordon, S. (Eds.), The Complexities of Care: Nursing Reconsidered. Cornell University Press, Ithaca, New York.

Nursing and Midwifery Council, 2002. Supporting Nurses and Midwives Through Life-long Learning. Nursing and Midwifery Council, London.

Nursing and Midwifery Council, 2008. Code: Standards of conduct, performance and ethics. Nursing and Midwifery Council, London.

Owen, J., 2005. How to Lead. Pearson Education Ltd, Edinburgh.

Proctor, B., 1986. Supervision: a co-operative exercise in accountability. In: Marken, M., Payne, M. (Eds.), Enabling and Ensuring.

Leicester Youth Bureau and Council for Education and Training in Youth and Community Work, Leicester.

Royal College of Nursing, 2002. Ground Rules and Responsibilities for Clinical Supervision. RCN, London.

Shanley, M.J., Stevenson, C., 2006. Clinical supervision revisited. Journal of Nursing Management 14 (8), 586–592.

Simms, J., 1993. Supervision. In: Wright, H., Giddey, M. (Eds.), Mental Health Nursing. Chapman & Hall, London.

Stanley, D., 2006. Recognizing and defining clinical leaders. British Journal of Nursing 15 (2), 108–111.

Thompson, C.M., 2000. A Congruent Life. Jossey Bass Publications, San Francisco.

Upenieks, V., 2003. Nurse leaders' perceptions of what compromises successful leadership in today's inpatient environment. Nursing Administration Quarterly 27 (2), 140–152.

Wade-Grimm, J., 2010. Effective leadership: Making the difference. Journal of Emergency Nursing 36 (1), 74–77.

Welford, C., 2002. Transformational leadership – matching theory to practice. Nursing Management 9 (4), 7–11.

Young-Ritchie, C., Spence Laschinger, H.K., Wong, C., 2010. The effects of emotionally intelligent leadership behavior on emergency staff nurses' workplace empowerment and organizational commitment. Nursing Research 22 (1), 171–194.

Clinical decision-making

37

Emma Tippins

CHAPTER CONTENTS

Introduction

Appropriate clinical decision-making is an intrinsic and frequently complex process at the heart of clinical practice (Hardy & Smith 2008) with some situations being more complex than others as they involve more unknowns and uncertainties (Cioffi & Markham 1997, Cioffi 1998). Decisions should be based on best practice and have an evidence base to them, this is essential to optimize outcomes for patients, improve clinical practice, achieve cost-effective nursing care and ensure accountability and transparency in decision-making (Canadian Nurses Association 2002). This process should not, therefore, be underestimated. The assessment, evaluation and subsequent changes made to a patient's care are intrinsically involved. The assessment process and the effective use of assessment information through appropriate decision-making are essential to improve outcomes of care (Aitken 2003). Within the patient assessment the nurse should, through a systematic approach, support clinical findings with hard scientific fact.

Requesting tests and the analysis of data completes this process. Simply put, if a nurse omits to request a relevant test there will be no scientific evidence to support the initial working diagnosis. Bochund & Calandra (2003) identified that requesting relevant tests during the initial assessment significantly reduced morbidity and mortality rates.

Within the modern protocol-driven emergency department (ED) a working diagnosis is essential to provide an efficient and structured patient experience through the department, concluding in their discharge or referral to a specialist service.

This chapter focuses on the importance of applying the key skills of critical thinking and clinical decision-making to everyday practice and the ways of facilitating nurses into the acquisition of these key skills. The chapter commences with an overview of emergency nursing and the importance of applying critical thinking to the assessment process. The focus will then be divided between the application of the nursing process within emergency nursing, how nurses construct their thought processes in relation to initial and continual patient assessments, and how the application of the key skills of critical thinking and clinical decision-making within their everyday practice will benefit both patient and nurse.

When assessing a patient the ED nurse must decide what data to collect; this is dependent on the nurse's initial clinical findings. In an age of clinical resource management and target-focused quantitative care it is essential that appropriate tests are ordered, to reduce an unnecessary workload resulting in wasted laboratory test time, to reduce false positives, and to facilitate a proficient cost-effective qualitative service. The importance of these initial data cannot be overemphasized, as analysis of these data will form the pathophysiological basis from which the medical diagnosis is made.

In order to understand the processes involved in clinical decision-making it is essential to consider the context in which decision-making activities are being performed. The ED was the portal for over 12.3 million annual visits in England in 2007–8, of which 20 % required hospital admission (Health and Social Care Information Centre 2009). These millions of patients attend with any number of clinical presentations and complaints requiring the assistance of every medical specialty. The role of the emergency nurse is unique in this respect, as in no other clinical setting is the nurse called upon to assess and identify the needs of such a wide range of potential patient conditions.

Initial assessment

The ED is the interface between patients and emergency care. Within this setting a patient's first contact with a healthcare professional will usually be with a nurse; the process of initial assessment. Nursing triage is a dynamic decision-making process that will prioritize an individual's need for treatment on arrival to an ED and is an essential skill in emergency nursing (Smith 2012). An efficient triage system aims to identify and expedite time-critical treatment for patients with life-threatening conditions, and ensure every patient requiring emergency treatment is prioritized according to their clinical need. The ethos of triage systems relates to the ability of a professional to detect critical illness, which has to be balanced with resource implications of 'over triage' i.e., a triage category of higher acuity is allocated. A decision that underestimates a person's level of clinical urgency may delay time-critical interventions; furthermore, prolonged triage processes may contribute to adverse patient outcomes (Travers 1999, Dahlen et al. 2012).

In this context, the triage nurse's ability to take an accurate patient history, conduct a brief physical assessment, and rapidly determine clinical urgency are crucial to the provision of safe and efficient emergency care (Travers 1999). These responsibilities require triage nurses to justify their clinical decisions with evidence from clinical research, and to be accountable for decisions they make within the clinical environment. The legal significance of undertaking an assessment relates to whether the nurse has sufficient knowledge to perform the assessment competently: if the patient care is compromised a tort of negligence could be issued (Dimond 2004).

It has been identified that many factors impact on the nurse's ability to make accurate decisions; for example, an unpredictable workload, poor professional continuity in relation to communication, and inexperience of the initial nursing assessor, or subsequent nursing staff (Tippins 2005). This has been exacerbated by demographic changes, such as an ageing population and the subsequent associated chronic pathologies, which have placed an enormous strain on primary care services (Dolan & Holt 2007), and secondly on the subjective clinical decision-making of the triage nurse (Cooke & Jinks 1999). If there is a failure to recognize deterioration in a patient's condition and intervention is delayed, the condition of these patients can potentially become critical. The care provided during the ED stay for critically ill patients has been shown to significantly impact on the progression of organ failure and mortality (Rivers et al. 2002, Church 2003). It is, therefore, essential that the care provided in the ED reflects the severity of the condition of the patient, the focal point being that accurate and dynamic patient assessment is imperative.

Continued assessment

The continued assessment and monitoring of patients is imperative in order that subtle changes in their condition can be recognized and intervention instigated and evaluated.

Physiological monitoring and the identification of deterioration in patients' conditions are an essential part of the role of the ED nurse; however, it remains uncertain whether this translates into the clinical setting. Patients who are critically ill are more likely to be recognized as such at initial assessment than if they deteriorate following that assessment (Cooke & Jinks 1999, Tippins 2005). For example, a patient who presents to the ED with a blood pressure of 89/38, pulse of 127 and respiratory rate of 31 is likely to be allocated a high clinical priority. In contrast, if the same patient presented an hour earlier with a blood pressure of 109/72, pulse of 98 and a respiratory rate of 24, they may not be allocated as high a priority on initial assessment, and their subsequent deterioration an hour later (after their first set of observations) will not necessarily result in a reallocation of priority (Cooke & Jinks 1999, Tippins 2005).

This phenomenon can be explained by a failure in the reassessment process and priority reallocation necessary to reflect the patient's changing physical condition. The introduction of education programmes, such as the Acute Life-threatening Events, Recognition and Treatment (ALERT) course, and tools such as the Modified Early Warning Score (MEWS), may be of benefit to assist staff in identifying patients who are deteriorating or are at risk of doing so. At the very least they ensure a structured approach to patient assessment and the regular and accurate recording of basic physiological observations, a crucial first step in recognizing patients at risk. Other possible explanations for the delay in recognizing patient deterioration could be external factors such as workload pressures, breakdown of communication, and lack of senior input (National Confidential Enquiry into Patient Outcome and Death 2009). The inexperience of staff in dealing with critically ill patients, the impact of teamwork and complacency when faced with certain conditions have also been shown to have an impact on clinical decision-making and, therefore, the care of critically ill patients (Bakalis & Watson 2005, Tippins 2005).

Clinical decision-making

In emergency care, nurses make multiple decisions rapidly in highly complex environments in order to deliver expert individualized care. Emergency care is different from other areas of nursing, as many patients are critically ill and frequently highly unstable. As a result their rapidly changing condition demands intelligent and decisive decision-making from nurses in short timeframes (Ryan & Tatumm 2012). Despite this there remains minimal research on the clinical decision-making skills of emergency nurses.

Decision-making can be divided into three categories: normative, descriptive and prescriptive approaches. Each of these categories has its own unique features, ideas and terminology. Normative decisions can be described as assuming the decision-maker is logical, rational and concentrates on how decisions are made in the ideal world. In comparison, descriptive theories attempt to describe how decisions are made and so are more concerned with the process of decision-making and how individuals reach that decision. Prescriptive theories try to improve the individual's decisions by looking at how decisions are made by understanding how a decision is formulated

(Thompson & Downing 2009). Of these different approaches to decision-making, prescriptive and descriptive approaches are the most common approaches used by practitioners (Cioffi & Markham 1997, Lurie 2012).

Clinical decision-making can be defined as the process nurses use to gather patient information, evaluate that information and make a judgement which results in the provision of patient care (White et al. 1992). This process involves collecting information with the use of both scientific and intuitive assessment skills. This information is then interpreted through the use of knowledge and past experiences (Cioffi 2000a, Evans 2005, Evans & Tippins 2007).

There are many theories on how to teach these essential and dynamic skills; however, learning or the acquisition of new knowledge does not necessarily guarantee the clinical application of expert practice (Tippett 2004) or critical thinking. Many theories of teaching and learning the art of critical thinking and expert clinical decision-making exist; behaviourist, cognitive, and humanistic being the commonly used three (Sheehy & McCarthy 1998). The behaviourist theory relates to reactionary learning whereby the learning occurs when an unmet need causes the learner to embrace the learning process; unfortunately the inclination to learn is often stimulated due to the learner feeling inadequate due to uncertainty and a lack of confidence. The cognitive theory relates to the interaction between the learner and their immediate environment, i.e., learning through experience and professional stimulation. The humanistic theory relates to adult-based learning where the focus is clearly on the learner to ascertain new knowledge through the process of self-discovery. A teacher who has understanding will present organized subject matter that is relevant to the learner's need and will, therefore, propagate learning. The expert practitioner perceives the situation as a whole, uses past concrete situations as paradigms and moves to the accurate region of the problem without wasteful consideration of a large number of irrelevant options.

Nursing process

The nursing process is a tool used by nurses to assist with decision-making and to predict and evaluate the results of nursing actions (Reeves & Paul 2002). The deliberate intellectual activity of the nursing process guides the professional practice of nursing in providing care in a systematic manner. The nursing process has evolved over recent years to incorporate five or six phases or stages (Box 37.1 and Fig. 37.1) (Reeves & Paul 2002, Ryan & Tatum 2012).

Movement between these phases is unusually linear; there is free movement among the phases during clinical practice. Once an assessment begins the nurse should begin to formulate diagnoses and eliminate others. As more information is gathered, through physical and technological findings, the practitioner should begin to narrow the possibilities. The worst possible diagnosis should be paramount in the practitioner's hypotheses, as this must be addressed and eliminated before moving on. By using a systematic approach patient problems can be identified and acted upon in the most effective way to ensure the best possible outcome for the patient. Examples of a systematic approach are those adopted by the

> ### Box 37.1
>
> **The nursing process**
>
> **Assessment** – collection of subjective and objective clinical data to provide a rationale for care
>
> **Nursing/working diagnosis** – analysis of physical presentation confirmed by scientific fact (data collection results)
>
> **Planning/outcome identification** – plan of care and realistic goals discussed with patient
>
> **Implementation** – performing interventions, reassess plan following each intervention to determine initial response
>
> **Evaluation** – have expected outcomes been achieved? Determine patient's level of clinical need and regularity of subsequent assessment

Resuscitation Council (2011) on the Advanced Life Support (ALS) course with the ABC mnemonic (airway, breathing and circulation) and ABCDE (airway, breathing, circulation, disability and environment), taught by the Royal College of Surgeons (2005) and American College of Surgeons (2008) in the Advanced Trauma Life Support (ATLS) course.

An obvious nursing diagnosis, such as difficulty in breathing in the patient with acute exacerbation of asthma, may be developed while data collection is still ongoing. In this situation implementation of life-saving actions, such as administration of oxygen therapy and bronchodilators, in which the desired outcome is obvious, may have begun before the assessment, diagnosis, outcome identification, and planning phases can occur. Throughout the phases, reassessment can lead to immediate changes in any of the previous phases. Reassessment and the further collection and analysis of data is a continuous, ongoing dynamic process and should not be confused with evaluation, which measures outcomes. Reassessment may lead to a change in the working diagnosis, which in turn could lead to a change in outcome identification, planning, implementation and evaluation as the process continues.

In order to demonstrate the nursing process a clinical scenario will be presented and discussed to demonstrate the practice from both a unilateral and a critical thinking perspective (Box 37.2 and Fig. 37.2).

> ### Box 37.2
>
> **Scenario 1**
>
> A 28-year-old female attends the ED at 08.30 via the ambulance service as a result of a collapse while on a bus. She is alert and oriented and able to recall the events prior to the collapse, and has not sustained any obvious injuries. The patient states that she has not eaten breakfast as she has been feeling nauseous and has been vomiting for the past 48 hours. The patient also adds that she is 13 weeks pregnant.

The nurse assessing the patient in a one-dimensional way will focus only on the patient's presenting complaint, and in this case attempt to establish a cause for the collapse. The nurse demonstrating critical thinking, however, will take into

Nursing process	One-dimensional nursing process	Dynamic nursing process utilized by a nurse demonstrating critical thinking
Assessment	Simplistic view of clinical presentation	Collection of objective and subjective data Construct care rationale
Working/nursing diagnosis	Linear view of one-dimensional hypothesis	Formulation of a working diagnosis/hypothesis confirmed by scientific fact
Planning/outcome identification	Goal identification	Holistic overview discussed with patient Specific realistic goals agreed
Implementation	Interventions performed	Appropriate interventions performed Plan reassessed Modifications as indicated
Evaluation	Established goal achievement	Have outcomes been achieved? Established subsequent care plan

Figure 37.1 • The nursing process illustrating a one-dimensional and a dynamic nursing process.

account all available information gained from the assessment and utilize it in order to establish a working diagnosis. In this example the one-dimensional process disregards the fact that the patient is pregnant. The dynamic model will take this information into account and process it along with all other available information, considering the bigger picture. With the use of critical thinking a working diagnosis/hypothesis will be formulated: hyperemesis; and appropriate scientific fact sought to either confirm or refute it. When the evaluation phase is reached, the nurse in the one-dimensional example may not have established a cause for the patient's collapse and, as a result, may have to go back to previous phases. In contrast, the critical thinker may have confirmed a working diagnosis, established a subsequent care plan and moved on.

The current demands placed on clinicians require the ED practitioner to be proactive and dynamic in their utilization of the nursing process. They need to know which stages can be safely omitted, combined or delayed, and also which situations warrant a rigorous, comprehensive approach (Alfaro-LeFevre 2004). There is, therefore, a clear need to implement a tool or structure to the diagnostic process directly aimed at ED nurses to facilitate the application of critical thinking. Novice practitioners frequently require a clear-cut approach to patient assessment; this can be achieved by applying the DEAD mnemonic as an aide-memoire or self-questioning

analytical tool. This approach is outlined in Box 37.3 (Evan & Tippins 2007).

By utilizing this structured framework, those less experienced in critical thinking will have a clear systematic outline to assist them in the organization of their thought process. This, in turn, could facilitate development of critical thinking and decision-making skills.

Critical thinking

The clinical scenarios outlined in Box 37.4 will be discussed to demonstrate the critical thinking and clinical decision-making involved in the initial and continuing assessment process.

Data The data the initial assessor will require are based on the patient's presenting complaint and medical history. The initial nursing or working diagnosis in this case would be an acute coronary syndrome (ACS). The nurse should be quick to ascertain the nature of the patient's pulse. A radial pulse can reflect the onset of physiological shock or the presence of life-threatening arrhythmias, including complete heart block, atrial fibrillation and tachycardias. The nursing diagnosis and need for immediate intervention can be either validated or negated by the recording of an ECG which would reflect the pathological changes associated with acute ST segment elevated myocardial infarction

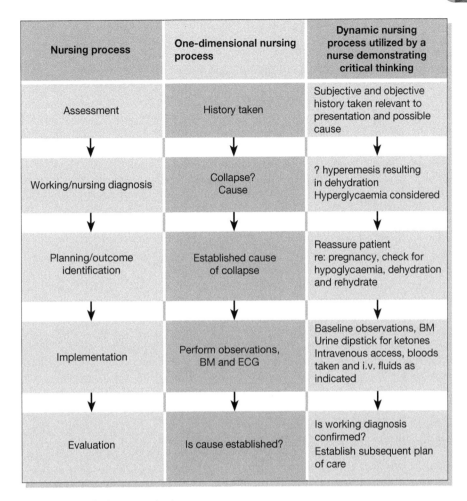

Figure 37.2 • The nursing process applied to scenario 1.

Box 37.3

The DEAD mnemonic

D: Data (scientific facts) – this should be based on what facts the nurse has and what other data the nurse can collect to validate or negate them.

E: Emotions – intuition or gut feelings/reactions, what are your instincts telling you, how can you consolidate or negate these.

A: Advantages – what advantage to others would result from actions the nurse takes, i.e., would an action instigated at the initial assessment improve the patient's prognosis, an example being the dispensing of an anti-platelet drug to a patient experiencing an acute coronary syndrome. The practitioner should also consider that a test requested when the patient presents may hasten their visit and result in an increasingly proficient service.

D: Disadvantages (differential diagnoses) – what could go wrong, in the worst case scenario what could this be, how I can rule this out?

Box 37.4

Scenario 2

A 76-year-old woman is admitted to the emergency department via the ambulance service complaining of a sudden onset of left-sided chest pain that commenced two hours previously. The pain radiates through to the centre of her chest; she also complains of a vague discomfort in her left arm. On examination, she has severe pain in her chest and back, she is pale and drowsy.

Vital signs reported: BP 110/60 mmHg, and a weak radial pulse.

(STEMI). The data recording at this point should include the requesting of blood tests, particularly as other co-existing pathologies may be exacerbating this presentation, such as anaemia.

Emotions The assessor's gut reaction in this case should be to consider the working diagnosis of STEMI. Comparing the current presentation with previously experienced situations

should alert the nurse to the potential severity of the condition, the process of pattern recognition and experiential learning (Cioffi 2001, Muir 2004, Tippins 2005).

Advantages The advantages involved in this situation would be an early door to treatment time, which has been shown to dramatically improve morbidity and mortality rates. The rapid diagnosis and treatment of life-threatening pathologies such as ACS is essential (Department of Health 2000a).

Disadvantages (differential diagnosis). The priority in this case is to confirm or dispel STEMI. The assessor also needs to consider other possible diagnoses, for example a dissecting aneurysm, which would be a contraindication to therapy. This possibility would result in the assessor returning to the data collection phase of the process in order to negate a potential aneurysm via further data collection.

Based on the clinical presentation the nurse will apply the DEAD mnemonic to aid critical thinking and decision-making.

Data What facts does the nurse have? This patient is presenting with the classical clinical signs of a respiratory infection. The fact that he smokes initially reinforces the nurse's first impression. The patient discussed having chest pain; the nurse should ascertain the nature of this pain, and ask whether it increases on inspiration, for example. The data needed to justify the nursing diagnosis will include the patient's respiratory rate, rhythm and depth. Oxygen saturation and a sample of the sputum should be requested. The nurse should look for clinical manifestations of chronic related pathophysiological changes associated with smoking; these include peripheral and potential central cyanosis and nail bed changes. Radial pulse and capillary refill time should be ascertained; the patient's blood pressure should be noted. An ECG should be recorded, as much respiratory-related pathology coincides with cardiac pathology. The patient's temperature should also be recorded. By recording and requesting data the nurse is validating the working diagnosis and negating other or coexisting pathologies.

Emotions Intuition and previous experience (experiential learning) have instigated this plan of care; the nurse is now applying critical thinking to the intuitive process to provide hard facts to justify gut reactions.

Advantages The nursing goal is to provide the patient with a quick efficient service. From the initial clinical signs and vital sign data collection the nurse has established this is not a life-threatening presentation. Within many departments the nurse will be able to request a chest X-ray, which will save time if requested early on.

Disadvantages The clinical decision-making process must include a quick analysis of the patient's presentation; this should include 'what is the worst case scenario?' Has the assessor negated immediate life-threatening pathologies? The ongoing process of excluding differential diagnoses now begins and the nurse may still think of other possible rule-out tests that could be requested.

Past experiences

In decision-making involving complexity, studies have shown that decision-making strategies are dependent on the individual's experiences (Cioffi 1998, Tippins 2005). Nurses use past experiences to assist in decision-making by comparing the current situation to previously experienced situations held in their memory (pattern recognition). This can manifest itself in a variety of forms, including recognizing a similarity between the present patient's condition/situation and a group of patients previously cared for with this presenting condition/situation, to describing quite specifically identified characteristics (Grossman & Wheeler 1997, Cioffi 1998, 2001). For example, a nurse who has previously cared for a patient with meningococcal meningitis may identify a future patient with the condition by recognizing a specific sign or symptom witnessed in the first instance, such as the petechial rash. Benner (1984) discusses the differences between a novice

and an expert and proposes that they can be attributed to the know-how that is acquired through experience.

Furthermore, past experiences with patients' symptoms and their probable outcomes is a factor that will determine the action a nurse will take in response to a patient's presentation (Radwin 1998). A recommendation for practice, therefore, must be to provide teaching to staff on conditions and situations common, but infrequently experienced, within the ED. This could facilitate the development of pattern-recognition skills, and improve response to critical care events. This could also address the retention of knowledge and skills gained in continuing professional development courses (Department of Health 2000b).

The use of reflection to assist in personal debriefing has an impact on the management of future practices when patients present with similar conditions (Evans 2005, Tippins 2005). By reflecting both on and in practice, with the use of critical thinking, best outcomes can be hypothetically discussed. This will result in modifications in an individual's clinical practice, and ultimately a positive impact on the care of future patients. Reflective practice has become an integral part of daily nursing life (Johns & Freshwater 1998). The need to reflect, critically analyse, develop and, where possible, improve is the constant aim of the nursing profession in the twenty-first century.

Intuition

Generally it is accepted that hard facts or science are the base from which nursing practice is delivered, and that intuition or logic do not directly influence clinical practice. In contrast the reality is very different, the rationalist paradigm of knowledge is logic, and the empiricist paradigm is science. Interestingly, empirical knowledge is less certain than logic; it is tentative, responsive to new evidence and better research, and always open to re-testing. The primary aim of applying theory in practice is to improve the patient's quality of care. Experts are able to generate better hypotheses due to a larger database of knowledge from which to pull ideas. This expert knowledge may also be assembled from intuition. Robinson (2000) identifies that clinical decision-making is the foundation of how an expert clinician can utilize their experientially based knowledge base to draw conclusions when assessing each new encounter.

Nurses' experience plays a major role in the development of critical observations, skills and subsequent intuition (Benner & Tanner 1987). When confronted with situations in which clinical judgements are characteristically uncertain, the nurse will rely upon the use of intuition to assist with their clinical decision-making (Benner & Tanner 1987). It has been argued that intuition actually accelerates the analytical process that leads to a nursing intervention (King & Appleton 1997). The use of intuition and systematic processes of decision-making has predominantly been believed to have occurred only in the more experienced and expert nurses (Benner & Tanner 1987, Watkins 1998, Rew 2000). Intuitive aspects of decision-making may, however, commence in nurses at an early point in their career and strengthen or lessen with time depending on their experiences and developing expertise (Sirkka et al. 1998, King & MacLeod Clark 2002).

Emergency nurses often have to deal with patients with life-threatening conditions, and sometimes reach a critical stage of perceiving a change in a patient's condition signifying that the patient may soon deteriorate. This use of intuitive judgement has been shown to be useful in the recognition of patient deterioration (Cioffi & Markham 1997, Cioffi 2000b, Tippins 2005, Harties et al. 2011). When used to identify deterioration this feeling is associated with knowing the patient (Cioffi 2000b), for which continuity of care is necessary (Grossman & Wheeler 1997).

Conclusion

The ultimate aim of emergency education is learning how to apply knowledge and understanding within the clinical setting. In order to achieve satisfactory outcomes the nurse must use elements from both the rationalist and empirical paradigms. The characteristics associated with advanced nursing practice centre on the practitioner utilizing the process of lateral thinking. Experts within the field of clinical decision-making suggest that in the absence of critical thinking, change and subsequent progress within the nursing profession would not have occurred. The ability of the nurse to reflect upon their role within the assessment process enables them to develop key analytical skills, which are essential within the role of emergency practitioners. Once the practitioner is able to demonstrate critical thinking they are able to construct more in-depth hypotheses. Emergency nurses play a pivotal role within the patient's journey by instigating the plan of care through the validation of the working diagnosis or hypothesis. Their role is, therefore, unique and paramount to the patient's subsequent care and clinical outcome.

References

Aitken, L.M., 2003. Critical care nurses' use of decision-making strategies. Journal of Clinical Nursing 12, 476–183.

Alfaro-LeFevre, R., 2004. Critical Thinking and Clinical Judgment: A practical approach. Elsevier Science, Philadelphia.

American College of Surgeons, 2008. Advanced Trauma Life Support, eighth ed. American College of Surgeons, Chicago.

Bakalis, N.A., Watson, R., 2005. Nurses' decision-making in clinical practice. Nursing Standard 19 (23), 33–39.

Benner, P., 1984. From novice to expert: Excellence and power in Clinical Nursing Practice. Addison-Wesley Publications, California.

Benner, P., Tanner, C., 1987. Clinical judgment: how expert nurses use intuition. American Journal of Nursing 87, 23–31.

Bochund, P.Y., Calandra, T., 2003. Science, medicine and the future: Pathogenesis of sepsis: new concepts and implications for future treatment. British Medical Journal 326, 262–266.

Canadian Nurses Association, 2002. Evidence-Based Decision-Making and Nursing Practice. Canadian Nurses Association, Ottawa.

Church, A., 2003. Critical care and emergency medicine. Critical Care Clinics 19 (2), 271–278.

Cioffi, J., 1998. Decision making by emergency nurses in triage assessment. Accident and Emergency Nursing 6, 184–191.

Cioffi, J., 2000a. Recognition of patients who require emergency assistance: a descriptive study. Heart and Lung 29 (4), 262–268.

Cioffi, J., 2000b. Nurses' experiences of making decisions to call emergency assistance to their patients. Journal of Advanced Nursing 32 (1), 108–114.

Cioffi, J., 2001. A study of the use of past experiences in clinical decision making in emergency situations. International Journal of Nursing Studies 38, 591–599.

Cioffi, J., Markham, R., 1997. Clinical decision making: managing case complexity. Journal of Advanced Nursing 25, 265–272.

Cooke, M.W., Jinks, S., 1999. Does the Manchester triage system detect the critically ill? Journal of Accident and Emergency Medicine 16, 179–181.

Dahlen, I., Westin, L., Adolfsson, A., 2012. Experience of being a low priority patient during waiting time at an emergency department. Psychology Research and Behaviour Management 5, 1–9.

Department of Health, 2000a. National Service Framework for Coronary Heart Disease. Department of Health, London.

Department of Health, 2000b. Comprehensive Critical Care – A Review of Adult Critical Care Services. Department of Health, London.

Dimond, B., 2004. Legal Aspects of Nursing, fourth ed. Longman, London.

Dolan, B., Holt, L., 2007. Preface. In: Dolan, B., Holt, L. (Eds.), Accident and Emergency Theory into Practice, second ed. Baillière Tindall, London.

Evans, C., 2005. Clinical decision making theories: patient assessment in A&E. Emergency Nurse 13 (5), 16–19.

Evans, C., Tippins, E., 2007. Foundations of Emergency Care. McGraw-Hill, Maidenhead.

Grossman, S.C., Wheeler, K., 1997. Predicting patients' deterioration and recovery. Clinical Nursing Research 6, 45–58.

Hardy, D., Smith, B., 2008. Decision Making in Clinical Practice. British Journal of Anaesthetic & Recovery Nursing 9 (1), 19–21.

Harties, C., Morgenthaler, B., Kugler, C., et al., 2011. Intuitive decision making in emergency medicine: An explorative study. In: Sinclair, M. (Ed.), Handbook of Intuition Research, Edward Elgar Publishing, London.

Health and Social Care Information Centre, 2009. Accident and Emergency Statistics in England. NHS Information Centre, Leeds.

Johns, C., Freshwater, D., 1998. Transforming Nursing Through Reflective Practice. Blackwell Science, Oxford.

King, L., Appleton, J., 1997. Intuition: a critical review of the research and rhetoric. Journal of Advanced Nursing 26, 194–202.

King, L., MacLeod Clark, J., 2002. Intuition and the development of expertise in surgical ward and intensive care nurses. Journal of Advanced Nursing 37 (4), 322–329.

Lurie, S.J., 2012. History and practice of competency based assessment. Medical Education 46 (1), 49–57.

Muir, N., 2004. Clinical decision-making: theory and practice. Nursing Standard 18 (36), 47–52.

National Confidential Enquiry into Patient Outcome and Death, 2009. Caring to the End? A review of the care of patients who died in hospital within four days of admission. NCEPOD, London.

Radwin, L.E., 1998. Empirically generated attributes of experience in nursing. Journal of Advanced Nursing 28, 590–595.

Reeves, J.S., Paul, C., 2002. Nursing theory in clinical practice. In: George, J.B. (Ed.), Nursing Theories: The Base for Professional Nursing Practice. Prentice Hall, New Jersey.

Resuscitation Council, 2011. Advanced Life Support Course Provider Manual, sixth ed. Resuscitation Council (UK), London.

Rew, L., 2000. Acknowledging intuition in clinical decision-making. Journal of Holistic Nursing 18, 94–108.

Rivers, E., Nguyen, H., Bryant, M.D., et al., 2002. Critical care and emergency medicine. Current Opinion in Critical Care 8 (6), 600–606.

Robinson, D., 2000. Clinical Decision-Making: A Case Study Approach, second ed. Lippincott, Philadelphia.

Royal College of Surgeons, 2005. Advanced Trauma Life Support. Royal College of Surgeons, London.

Ryan, C., Tatumm, K., 2012. Objective measurement of critical-thinking ability in registered nurse applicants. Journal of Nursing Administration 42 (2), 89–94.

Sheehy, C., McCarthy, M., 1998. Advanced Practice Nursing Emphasizing Common Roles. Davis Company, Philadelphia.

Sirkka, L., Salantera, S., Callister, L.C., et al., 1998. Decision-making of nurses practising in intensive care in Canada, Finland, Northern Ireland, Switzerland and the United States. Heart and Lung: The Journal of Acute and Critical Care 27, 133–142.

Smith, A., 2012. Using a theory to understand triage decision making. International Emergency Nursing 20.

Thompson, C., Downing, D., 2009. Essential Clinical Decision Making and Clinical Judgement for Nurses. Churchill Livingstone, London.

Tippett, J., 2004. Nurses acquisition and retention of knowledge after trauma training. Accident and Emergency Nursing 12, 39–46.

Tippins, E., 2005. How emergency department nurses identify and respond to critical illness. Emergency Nurse 13 (3), 24–33.

Travers, D., 1999. Triage: how long does it take? How long should it take? Journal of Emergency Nursing 25, 238–241.

Watkins, M.P., 1998. Decision-making phenomena described by expert nurses working in urban community health settings. Journal of Professional Nursing 14, 22–33.

White, J., Nativo, D.G., Kobert, S.N., et al., 1992. Content and process in clinical decision making by nurse practitioners. Image 24, 153–158.

Ethical issues

38

Karen Sanders

CHAPTER CONTENTS

Introduction

Perceptions of ethics are as varied as the mores that inform individual behaviour. Some people see ethics as an esoteric abstraction that belongs firmly in the ivory towers of academe; others see it as an ethereal subject that parliamentarians manipulate in matters of political controversy. There are elements of truth in both these perspectives. Ethics is, however, much more than this. Nurses and healthcare professionals are involved in decision-making every day and these decisions may have an ethical component to them. The practice of health care requires not only scientific and practical knowledge, but also the ability to make judgements regarding a course of action or plan of care. The ability to make these judgements requires reasoning skills from differing approaches.

Unlike many words, the nature and essence of ethics cannot be succinctly reflected in a single definition. Taking this further, Sparkes (1992) questioned the usefulness of dictionaries and argued that the best which can be offered for ethics is a semantic interpretation. This is given as 'the philosophical study of moral conduct and reasoning'. More simply put, ethics is that branch of philosophy that deals with matters of right and wrong. Knowledge of ethical principles may provide a framework for reasoned thought but cannot provide universal answers.

Sparkes' interpretation gives direction and focus to the essential themes of ethics. In essence, it is concerned with the way in which reason can clarify situations that have a moral dimension. This last point gives a prima facie rationale for placing ethics at the centre of the nursing equation, since the focus of that profession is steeped with issues that demand ethical enquiry and a moral response. Mirroring the vibrancy ethical analysis can offer nursing, Tschudin (1993) asserts that 'ethics is not only at the heart of nursing; it is the heart of nursing. Ethics is about what is right and good. Nursing and caring are synonymous, and the way in which care is carried out is ethically decisive. How a patient is addressed, cared for and treated must be right not only by ordinary standards of care, but also by ethical principles'. Jones (2000) describes ethics as 'the application of the processes and theories of moral philosophy to a real situation' and states that 'ethics is concerned with the basic principles and concepts that guide human beings in thought and action and which underline their values'.

Unlike many of the sciences, ethics is not a precise discipline. While it seeks to find answers, on one level, to questions such as 'What is right? What is good?' and at another level to resolve practical dilemmas such as whether to carry out a particular treatment or not, it can seldom provide a definitive answer. What it seeks to do is provide a framework, a means of formulating answers to questions/problems/dilemmas and so guide actions. However, as will be seen, in many situations different people might arrive at differing answers and so take different actions which are neither necessarily correct nor incorrect. The important thing is to justify the decisions and actions on the basis of sound ethical reasoning.

The purpose of this chapter is to use philosophical reasoning to examine some areas of moral concern that frequently confront practitioners not only in emergency departments but in all emergency care settings. These areas will provide

http://dx.doi.org/10.1016/B978-0-7020-4315-4.00038-3

a philosophical adjunct to the legal issues that are covered in Chapter 39, e.g., a duty of care and consent. The reason for this is to conduct an ethical examination of concepts central to healthcare law in this country. The lines between law and ethics have become blurred over the years and to consider ethics in isolation could potentially distort practice. In an increasing litigious society it is apparent that subjects such as informed consent, access to care, confidentiality, rights, best interests, autonomy/competence, withholding and withdrawing medical care are more open to public scrutiny and possible legal challenge.

This exercise will also usefully show that what may be legal may not be moral and what may be moral may not be legal. History abounds with examples that support this position; once (not so long ago) there was no right for women to vote in the UK or for gay men to give physical expression to their sexuality. A pressing example from the contemporary arena is assisted dying and voluntary euthanasia. Proponents argue it is both a moral and a humane concept that liberates an individual's self-governance about the manner and time of death – it has, however, no legal standing. Advanced decisions that give an indication of an individual's care wishes may, however, need to be heeded (Katsetos & Mirarchi 2011).

Given that nurses have a legally enforced duty of care towards patients within the emergency care setting, its seems fitting that a chapter dealing with ethics should begin by considering the notion of 'duty' as a central theme in the development of a school of ethical analysis called 'deontology'. During this process, strong parallels will be drawn between deontology, duty as a traditional motivational force in nursing and, also, the Nursing and Midwifery Council (2008) *The Code: Standards of Conduct, Performance and Ethics for Nurses and Midwives*.

Duty as a moral endeavour

The historical dimensions of nursing are engulfed by the notion of duty. This tradition is succinctly entwined in the most central of nursing edicts, 'a duty of care'. Within contemporary nursing there remains a strong allegiance to this theme. This approach is based upon the intrinsic and inalienable relationship that exists between 'rights' and 'duties'. Broadly speaking, once a duty of care has been established, the patient has a right to be cared for and the nurse must facilitate care giving – this is both a legal and moral theme.

The Nursing and Midwifery Council (2008) *Code* encourages high standards during professional endeavours and expects all practitioners to operate within its framework and guidelines. In the edition published in 2008 the *Code of Professional Conduct* underwent a name change and has become the Nursing and Midwifery Council (2008) *The Code: Standards of Conduct, Performance and Ethics for Nurses and Midwives*. The principle that nursing practice is inextricably linked with ethics cannot be ignored.

In the UK, the Nursing and Midwifery Council is the organization set up by Parliament to protect the public by ensuring that nurses and midwives provide high standards of care to their patients and clients. It is the regulatory body responsible

for identifying the standards of these professions and requiring members of the professions to practice and conduct themselves within the standards and framework provided by the *Code*. Honesty and ethics are included in the list of the Nursing and Midwifery's core values.

Statements made in the code of professional conduct serve to reinforce notions of duty and the statements made within the code provide motivational guidelines for nursing actions. Basing actions upon duties, rules or motives has a long history in ethics and is known as deontology. As Kendrick (1993) observes 'this school of ethical analysis maintains that being moral entails acting from a sense of moral duty, respecting others' rights and honouring one's obligations.'

This interpretation clearly aligns itself with the themes of the Nursing and Midwifery Council (2008) *Code* and the onus that it places upon registered practitioners. The person most closely associated with deontology is the philosopher Immanuel Kant. He was a prolific writer and fervently advocated that people had intrinsic worth and value. Furthermore, he argued that an essential part of being human was the ability to use reason in deliberating over the moral worth of an action. For Kant, this ability invariably found itself rooted in a sense of duty.

There are many attractive elements of Kantian ethics. In particular, it places a great deal of emphasis upon respect amongst persons and encourages a fervent sense of individual duty. Tschudin (1986) summarized these themes by stating 'a right action is only so if it is done out of a sense of duty, and the only good thing without qualification is a person's good will: the will to do what one knows is right'.

Kant devised a complex moral theory, consisting of three formulations, that he called the categorical imperative. Their precise interpretation and mutual relations are a matter of controversy. Kendrick (1993) simplified the different formulations as follows:

- an action is only moral if you are willing for it to be applied to everyone, yourself included, as a universal law; 'do as you would like to be done by'
- for an action to be moral it must never lead to people being seen just as 'means to an end' but always as 'ends' in their own right
- in wishing to be moral, individuals must act as members of a community where everybody is seen as having intrinsic worth (ends in their own right).

The essence of the categorical imperative can be readily applied to the duty-based nature of nursing; this will now be discussed with particular relevance to practice in emergency care.

Applying the imperative to practice

The first part of the imperative indicates that all people have intrinsic worth and should attribute respect to each other; for example, most societies would agree that it is intrinsically wrong to murder another person. The implications of Kant's theory are that persons wishing to undertake such acts should be willing to accept the same being done to themselves – as if they were governed by a universal law that related to that given activity. Expressed simply, the first principle is a moral edict that requires us to ask: 'Would I like this act to be done either to myself or to those close to me?' If the answer is 'no', then Kant would have serious reservations about the moral worth of the motives underpinning the action.

These themes are often introduced to the novice nurse who is asked to care from a basis of duty. While this may initially seem a little simplistic, it can act as a strong image for mental reinforcement and maintaining standards during the delivery of care throughout a nurse's career.

The second of Kant's principles further emphasizes the notion of equal respect amongst persons and resolutely argues that individuals should never be seen or treated solely as means to an end. This does not mean that people cannot work together or help each other – the key theme is that this should involve some degree of mutual reciprocity.

An example of this is the staff nurse who needs to attain the skills of suturing. Obviously, to be able to perform this task safely and competently requires the cooperation of a willing patient. While a patient may be used as a means to an end – the end being the nurse suturing competently – this does not echo the full essence of this part of the imperative. Suturing an open wound also offers some therapeutic worth to the patient; thus the process has benefited the nurse through the acquisition of a skill and the patient through the closure of a wound. Kant did not object to individuals being used as a means to an end as long as they are also valued as ends in their own right.

The essence of the second principle in the imperative does not just apply to the nurse/patient relationship but extends to all interaction within the professional milieu. Not only are nurses required to respect patients as being of equal worth, but this must also govern the professional ethos in dealing with colleagues. This duty to enact the principle of respect for persons is a cogent thread throughout the *Code* (Nursing and Midwifery Council 2008) and is alluded to under the following headings and themes:

- make the care of people your first concern, treating them as individuals and respecting their dignity
- work with others to protect and promote the health and wellbeing of those in your care, their families and carers, and the wider community
- provide a high standard of practice and care at all times
- be open and honest, act with integrity and uphold the reputation of your profession.

Such themes are vitally important given that recent years have seen the blurring of roles between doctors and nurses. If practitioners from both professions are to have shared working practices, it must be through mutual respect and the fervent desire to embellish the care that is offered to patients. Such notions offer the opportunity to embrace the themes of shared governance and create an organizational milieu where all concerned can achieve their potential. Such themes were given sharp focus for nursing by the introduction of the *Scope of Professional Practice* (United Kingdom Central Council for Nursing, Midwifery and Health Visiting 1992) and the associated concept of advanced practice (Kendrick 1997).

Respect is a central element in Kantian thinking and the word appears frequently throughout the Nursing and Midwifery Council *Code* (2008). A strong emphasis upon respect emerges from the third and final part of the imperative; its essential message is that persons form a community where each member has equal worth as a moral decision-maker. Nurses meet colleagues or patients who may have very different values or beliefs from their own. Sometimes these differences are informed by cultural or religious diversity. Kantian ethics suggests that the key issue is to respect the freedom of other individuals to hold moral perspectives and to act upon them – this is part of what it means to treat others as ends. If this is applied to the professional setting, it asks that all people have equal authority to express and defend their respective positions. Once again, it can be suggested that this theme runs throughout the *Code* (Nursing and Midwifery Council 2008).

To this point it has been seen that duty-based approaches to ethical thinking and analysis have a long history in moral theory. This has been supported with reference to deontology and the philosopher most closely associated with it, Immanuel Kant. Moreover, clear links have been drawn between the deontological approach and the duty-based themes that run throughout nursing.

The Nursing and Midwifery Council *Code* (2008) provides a series of guidelines and principles that inform a practitioner's professional obligations and preserve the traditional emphasis upon duty-based care-giving. However, while it may be suggested that principles of duty provide indications that can help give directions about professional conduct, there are problems with such approaches that demand clarification and analysis.

Duty as a moral problem

A glaring problem with duty-based approaches to morality and Kantian ethics in particular is that they tend to portray certain maxims as absolute, universal and all-encompassing. There are many examples from the real world that highlight an unquestioning bond to duty-based dictums; for example, certain religions require their members not to accept whole blood products during medical treatments. There is much room for debate about whether or not a principle/duty can ever be thought to be ubiquitous and applied as a categorical tenet.

Within nursing there are certain rules that are perceived, as has already been discussed, as absolute; principal among these is the duty of care. However, sometimes the maxims within a duty of care can be at variance with each other. Consider the following principles:

- a duty to do good (beneficence)
- a duty to do no harm (non-maleficence).

At first glance these principles seem closely related. However, further analysis does reveal distinct differences between the two themes. Nurses always try to ensure that their actions promote good and preserve the best interests of the patient. This leads nurses to an interesting and penetrating question: 'Can we say that nursing actions always promote good results for patients?' It is very doubtful that nurses can say 'yes' to this question; to a large extent this is because harm is an intrinsic part of some nursing actions.

The simplest example of this is when a nurse gives an intramuscular injection. Every time the syringe is introduced, it causes pain which, even to a very small degree, can be equated with harm. Many other nursing interventions carry the same ethos; antibiotics may cause an irritating rash; aspirin can cause gastric erosion; and diamorphine or other opiate derivatives can cause chronic constipation. Some of the more advanced nursing practices, e.g., intubation or cannulation, carry a host of risks that can, if realized, greatly harm the patient. Given the amount of harm that can result from some of our actions, the nurse needs to ask if the principle of non-maleficence is appropriate and applicable as a universal tenet in nursing.

Harris (1985) has argued that healthcare professionals do not have any special obligations, but are subject to the same sort of duties as any other person in society. All individuals have a duty to respect persons or to do no harm; however, it has been seen that the Nursing and Midwifery Council *Code* (2008) identifies certain obligations as part of the professional role.

Above all, do no harm

Believing the absolute notion that nursing actions will never do any harm is impractical because it can never be totally achieved within the professional role. Some of the 'harm' which can be induced by nursing actions has already been seen. This theme has been explored and analysed by Illich (1975), with particular reference to the medical profession, but may be applied with equal resonance to nursing, especially now that advanced practice involves nurses performing tasks that formerly fell under the sole auspices of doctors. Based on what is increasingly understood about patient safety (Johnstone 2007a,b, Gawande 2010), Illich's claims from the 1970s proved remarkably prescient.

Illich (1975) used the word 'iatrogenesis' to describe the harmful results and illnesses that can result from the intervention of doctors. For example, Illich (1975) claimed that 'it has been established that one out of every five patients admitted to a typical research hospital acquires an iatrogenic disease, sometimes trivial, usually requiring special treatment, and in one case in thirty leading to death. Half of these episodes resulted from complications of drug therapy; amazingly, one in ten comes from diagnostic procedures. Despite good intentions and claims to public service, with a similar record of performance a military officer would be relieved of his command and a restaurant or amusement centre would be closed by police'.

Illich (1975) has been criticized for not placing enough emphasis upon the amount of good that medicine achieves. This is a valid criticism and it leads to the centre of the debate about absolute duties as all-encompassing principles. It can be stated with a degree of certainty that the primary intention of practitioners is to promote beneficence and to strive to achieve non-maleficence. However, to place these two themes in the language of absolute duties is no more than an exercise in rhetoric and cannot be upheld in the 'real' world of delivering care.

The key issue is not to insist that health professionals abide unquestioningly by a duty to do good and a duty to do no harm – clearly the two duties are not always reconcilable as consummate themes. The essential worth of the two principles is found in balancing them both together, not viewing them as isolated absolutes. Returning to the example of the intramuscular injection, while the initial result may be pain or harm, this is usually outweighed by the amount of good that results from the therapeutic worth of the injected drug. This serves to highlight that the balance between beneficence and non-maleficence can help practitioners to reflect upon the worth of an action.

The essential problem with this is that the consequences of an action cannot always be forecast beforehand – crystal ball gazing is a poor basis for moral analysis. Despite this drawback, trying to weigh the moral worth of an action against the harm that it may produce at least asks for a degree of questioning, reflection and analysis; this is surely more acceptable than a passive acceptance of absolute, but conflicting, duties.

Practitioners at the 'cutting edge' of healthcare delivery have always had an intuitive awareness of the precarious balance between beneficence and non-maleficence. Unfortunately, the power relationship between doctors and nurses has usually resulted in the nurse handing issues of a moral nature over to the doctor, who then tries to deal with them through the value-free objectivity of a 'clinical decision'. Contemporary practice challenges such themes; 'teamwork' and parity in the decision-making process demand input from all interested parties; this is further supported by Kendrick (1997), who states 'in the UK, doctors need to stop seeing situations that are ethically relevant as something to be subsumed under the broad notion of a 'clinical decision'. In essence, this should mean shared governance with other practitioners – after all, ethics belongs to us all and is not the sole domain of doctors.

This section has presented an argument that highlights the inadequacies of duty-based principles as moral panaceas which can be applied and invoked for all ethical 'ills'. Emerging from this is a clear theme that moral duties can rarely stand as absolute and isolated 'ends'. Moral duties, whatever their nature, remain rhetorical unless they give clear and non-conflicting directions for the pathways of practice.

Chapter 39 gives a focused overview of the legal themes that inform a 'duty of care'. In comparison, this section has given an adjunct to the legal scenario and shown that using duty-based approaches to moral reasoning is often self-limiting. Taking this further, duty has been considered here in relation to such themes as: duty as a traditional force in nursing, the *Code of Professional Conduct* (Nursing and Midwifery Council 2008), the nurse/patient relationship, interprofessional relationships and, finally, the moral conflict that results when duties conflict. However, and this is vital, while nurses may liberally question the philosophical foundation of duty-based methods of ethical analysis, our legal requirement to fulfil a duty of care to patients, once established, remains absolute (Jones 1997).

It has been seen that the duties of beneficence and non-maleficence must have value as means to an end if they are to have meaning and essence for practitioners. This can be said with equal efficacy about the principles embodied in the *The Code: Standards of Conduct, Performance and Ethics for Nurses and Midwives* (Nursing and Midwifery Council 2008).

In essence, they provide the starting point for discussion, analysis and professional discernment but they are not categorical absolutes. Chadwick & Tadd (1992) pursue this line of enquiry and note 'a code of conduct or ethics should perhaps be seen, not as the last word on ethics, but as a stimulus to moral thinking'. Such themes are vital when considering the moral milieu of nursing practice in emergency care settings. What is also essential is an understanding of the ethical issues that engulf the notion of consent. In Chapter 39, consent is considered within a legal framework; the next part of this chapter will explore the moral dimensions of that concept.

Consent as an ethical process

Informed consent, by its very nature, demands that nurses give patients all the information needed to make an informed decision. This theme is reflected by Gillon (1985a), who argued that consent can be defined as 'a voluntary and uncoerced decision made by a sufficiently competent or autonomous person, on the basis of adequate information and deliberation, to accept rather than reject some proposed course of action that will affect him or her'.

However, a key issue is: how do nurses define 'adequate information'? For example, how many nurses would divulge to a male patient, brought into the ED with acute urinary retention, the remote possibility that catheterization may result in a perforated urethra? Intrinsic to this notion is a complex and controversial question: how much information should be given to patients before an informed consent can be given to the treatment or intervention offered? (Kendrick 1994).

Broadly speaking, there are two opposing perspectives towards this question. Kendrick (1991) argues that 'at one end of the spectrum there are those who believe that the patient should have access to every conceivable issue involved in their treatment or care. This is based on the understanding that a patient who is privy to both negative and positive aspects of their treatment or care will be able to make an informed and valid consent. In contrast to this perspective is the paternalistic view that a nurse has the necessary insight and professional knowledge to judge when the giving of certain information would be harmful to the patient'.

Both of these positions contain elements which make a valid argument and deserve further examination. This demands an exploration of the key ethical principles which support the notion of a full and informed consent.

The myth of self-governance

In its most basic form, autonomy is concerned with an individual's level of self-government. Gillon (1985b) broadened this to offer an interpretation that can be directly applied to nursing practice: 'Personal autonomy allows one to think, decide and act on the basis of such thought, making decision freely and independently, developing personal interests, setting and achieving personal goals, and giving meaning and coherence to such life'. However, the idea of absolute autonomy is something of a myth – nobody can be fully independent and self-governing. Consider the term 'autonomous nurse'; it is facile to think of an individual's practice as something that is free of constraints. Nurses have to work within a framework that is influenced by *The Code: Standards of Conduct, Performance and Ethics for Nurses and Midwives* (Nursing and Midwifery Council 2008), the organizational milieu and the needs of patients; thus, total autonomy is not reconcilable with the limitations of the real world. These themes are reflected by Henry & Pashley (1990), who state 'full autonomy is an ideal notion and we can only approximate to it. It is obvious that, in reality, some situations, states and circumstances will diminish a person's autonomy, such as the ability to control his or her actions, or both, through being restricted in some way, for example, illness, psychological impairment, physical or mental disability'. Ardagh (2004) offers the practical example of resuscitation where the patient's competence is impaired, as he or she is unable to receive information, undertake rational deliberation or express a decision free from coercion.

However, despite many practical difficulties, nurses must always strive to eliminate barriers which may hinder a patient's autonomy and freedom of choice.

Freedom to choose

There is a close relationship between autonomy and informed consent, the former being concerned with freedom and choice, the latter being the key which unlocks and enables their expression. Taking this further, it would be extremely difficult for patients to take an active part in decisions relating to care if they did not have the necessary information on which to make choices.

If autonomy is respected in practice, then patients should feel uninhibited about identifying their own needs and actively deciding how these should be met. However, a problem with discussing autonomy is that it can create an impression that all patients want to take part in such a full and dynamic role. A missing element here is that patients are, by definition, sick and often vulnerable. This may be particularly relevant to the patients you meet in emergency care – especially given the often shocking nature of sudden illness or trauma. This may conjure up different images for different people. Some patients may see it as a place of safety where their illness or trauma will be addressed, while others see it as a reflection of their own mortality and hear the ringing of the death knell.

For patients who see the ED as a symbol of fear, it may be inappropriate to expect them to take an active role in the decision-making process. This is not paternalism. If, after the choice has been offered, patients express no wish to take an active role in their care, then it should be accepted as an expression of autonomy. Kendrick (1991) supports this notion and states 'the patient should be given the freedom to say to the nurse that he wishes to surrender any role within the decision-making process. This agreement may be temporary or permanent in nature. What must be emphasized here is that when a patient gives the nurse responsibility for decisions he does not relinquish autonomy, but gives acknowledgement of it'.

Such approaches indicate the patient's right to freely decide what may or may not be done to his body. Indeed, irrespective of ethical considerations, performing an act without the patient's permission may, as is discussed in Chapter 39, constitute negligence in legal terms. All of this reflects an ethico-legal emphasis that is intended to protect the vulnerable status of patients. Such themes, however, frequently place practitioners in emergency care in very precarious positions; perhaps the most telling example of this is when an unconscious person is brought into the department after taking an overdose. Practitioners do not usually have the benefit of time and must act quickly if life is to be preserved. This is frequently when the maxim 'act first, ask questions later' comes into its own. What happens, however, when a patient is semi-conscious and gives the expressed desire to be left to die? There is no time to get a psychiatrist's opinion, little time to think about the patient's level of competence, establish whether a valid advance decision exists or what the patient's best interests are; just a real dilemma that needs an immediate decision. This is where ethics finds its most cutting edge.

The legal grounds for acting without the patient's consent could well be based on urgency and necessity and best interests (Mental Capacity Act 2005) – remembering also that failing to act holds the risk of being accused of negligence (see Chapter 39) and failure to act in the patient's best interest runs the risk of being accused of the wilful neglect and ill-treatment of a person who lacked capacity (Mental Capacity Act 2005) or assault and battery if the patient were competent. It is an unfortunate aspect of contemporary practice that practitioners may be 'damned if they do and damned if they don't'. Proponents of a literal and absolute interpretation of autonomy (self-governance) may argue that, irrespective of legal defences, health care professionals never have a sufficient moral mandate to override the expressed wish of a patient to be left to die; Brown et al. (1992) offered a brief and cogent comment on such themes: 'we cannot solve the dilemmas by saying that we should always do what the patient wishes'.

A further issue is whether a patient or groups of patients should be eligible for cardiopulmonary resuscitation. In an attempt to answer this question two related issues need to be addressed. Firstly, medical futility and secondly who should be involved in the decision-making process.

The medical futility debate involves two questions. Firstly, are there medical interventions administered to a specific patient with a particular disease that we can label *futile* or *useless*, because we are sufficiently confident that they will not be beneficial? Secondly, if so, are physicians entitled, or

indeed obligated, to refuse to provide those interventions to the patient in question even if the treatment is requested or demanded by the patient or appropriate surrogate? (Brody 1997).

The decision to resuscitate or not is generally made by the physician in collaboration with other health professionals if time allows. There is an assumption that people want to be resuscitated and therefore the only occasions when, if at all, the question is discussed with patients is when there are reasons for not resuscitating.

Yet, should not patients have the right to be involved in either decision if time allows? Bandman & Bandman (1990) argue that it should not be the health professional who decides but the patient: 'Playing God by deciding who has the required quality of life and who therefore lives or dies also reveals a serious moral pitfall of arbitrarily abrogating the equal rights of individuals to decide whether to live or die'. There may be patients who, although they meet the medical criteria for cardiopulmonary resuscitation would choose not to be resuscitated.

These are by no means easy questions to answer but health professions cannot escape them. Firstly, healthcare is an expensive enterprise dependent upon public funds so the justification for spending funds on interventions which have little or no medical benefit, has to be addressed. Secondly, we need to address the question as to what extent specific interventions are beneficial to the individual patient.

Such sober insights give buoyancy to the essential elements of moral reasoning in healthcare. Ethics is not about providing a panacea for all the moral ills of practice. It can, however, offer a focused means of reaching rational decisions about the issues that confront practitioners in emergency departments.

Conclusion

This chapter has critically explored two major ethical themes that continually challenge practitioners in emergency care: duty and consent. Within these broad concepts, a host of other issues have also been considered that often cause moral concern. It would be impossible, in a chapter of this size, to do justice to all the dilemmas that confront practitioners in emergency care; such an endeavour would command a book in its own right. However, it is hoped that this chapter has charged the reader with enough creative energy to read further and explore other areas that confront one's own practice.

References

Ardagh, M., 2004. Ethics of resuscitation. In: Cameron, P., Jelinek, G., Kelly, A.M., Murray, L., Brown, A.F.T., Heyworth, J. (Eds.), Textbook of Adult Emergency Medicine, second ed. Churchill Livingstone, Edinburgh.

Bandman, E.L., Bandman, B., 1990. Nursing Ethics Through the Life Span, second ed. Prentice Hall, Englewood Cliffs, NJ.

Brody, H., 1997. Medical futility: a useful concept? In: Zucker, M.B., Zucker, H.D. (Eds.), Medical Futility and the Evaluation of Life-sustaining Interventions. Cambridge University Press, Cambridge.

Brown, J.M., Kitson, A., McKnight, T.J., 1992. Challenges in Caring: Explorations in Nursing and Ethics. Chapman and Hall, London.

Chadwick, R.F., Tadd, W., 1992. Ethics and Nursing Practice: A Case Study Approach. Macmillan, Basingstoke.

Gawande, A., 2010. The Checklist Manifesto: How to Get Things Right. Profile Books, London.

Gillon, R., 1985a. Autonomy and consent. In: Lockwood, M. (Ed.), Moral Dilemmas in Modern Medicine. Oxford University Press, Oxford.

Gillon, R., 1985b. Autonomy and the principle of respect for autonomy. British Medical Journal 290, 1806–1808.

Harris, J., 1985. The Value of Life. Routledge, London.

Henry, C., Pashley, G., 1990. Health Ethics. Quay Books, Lancaster.

Illich, I., 1975. Medical Nemesis: The Expropriation of Health. Calder and Boyers, London.

Johnstone, M.J., 2007a. Patient safety ethics and human error management in ED contexts. Part I: Development of the global patient safety movement. Australasian Emergency Nursing 10 (1), 13–20.

Johnstone, M.J., 2007b. Patient safety ethics and human error management in ED contexts. Part II: Accountability and the challenge to change. Australasian Emergency Nursing 10 (2), 80–85.

Jones, G., 1997. Liability in A&E nursing. Emergency Nurse 5 (5), 18–20.

Jones, S.R., 2000. Ethics in Midwifery, second ed. Mosby, Edinburgh.

Katsetos, A.D., Mirarchi, F.L., 2011. A living will misinterpreted as a DNR order: confusion compromises patient care. Journal of Emergency Medicine 40 (6), 629–632.

Kendrick, K.D., 1991. Partners in passing: ethical aspects of nursing the dying person. International Journal of Advances in Health and Nursing Care 1 (1), 11–27.

Kendrick, K.D., 1993. Ethics and nursing practice. British Journal of Nursing 2 (18), 920–926.

Kendrick, K.D., 1994. Freedom to choose: the ethics of consent. Professional Nurse 9 (11), 739–742.

Kendrick, K.D., 1997. What is advanced nursing? (Editorial) Professional Nurse 12 (10), 689.

Mental Capacity Act, 2005. Code of Practice. TSO, London.

Nursing and Midwifery Council, 2008. The Code: Standards of Conduct, Performance and Ethics for Nurses and Midwives. NMC, London.

Sparkes, A.W., 1992. Talking Philosophy: A Workbook. Routledge, London.

Tschudin, V., 1986. Ethics in Nursing: The Caring Relationship. Heinemann Nursing, London.

Tschudin, V., 1993. Ethics: Aspects of Nursing Care. Scutari Press, London.

United Kingdom Central Council for Nursing, Midwifery and Health Visiting, 1992. Scope of Professional Practice. UKCC, London.

Law

39

Nicola Meeres

CHAPTER CONTENTS

Introduction

The society in which we live is an increasingly litigious one and as such it is in the best interests of those working in the emergency department (ED) to keep up to date with the relevant areas of law. This chapter highlights the key areas where knowledge of law is essential and discusses some of the legal dilemmas that may arise. Attendance, assessment, treatment and care, consent to treatment, detention of patients, confidentiality, the police, the press and staff health and safety are considered.

Law in the UK

The four countries of the UK have developed separate legal systems. England and Wales have identical legal systems and whilst the law in Northern Ireland has developed along similar lines, Scottish law has not. In this chapter, the law stated applies to England and Wales: where there are marked differences in Northern Ireland and Scotland, these will be noted. Otherwise, the reader can assume that the law is broadly applicable across the whole of the UK.

The two main sources of law are statute law and case law. Statute law is created either by Acts of Parliament or through a system of delegated legislation. Statutory Instruments, or Rules, form part of delegated legislation and they empower statutory bodies to expand or amend law for enactment by the Secretary of State. Delegated legislation has become increasingly important due to the pressures on parliamentary time.

Case law has developed through the judicial system as judges make decisions on the interpretation of law within the court setting. Once an outcome has been reached then a precedent is set for all other judges to follow in similar circumstances. Decisions made are binding on all courts below that where the precedent was set. For example, decisions made by the House of Lords are binding on all lower courts in the UK, but the House of Lords can overturn its own decisions and The European Court of Justice can set precedent for member states. Case law is of particular relevance to health care (Montgomery 2002).

Department of Health circulars and the Nursing and Midwifery Council (2008) *The Code: Standards of Conduct, Performance and Ethics for Nurses and Midwives* are not legally binding but they are recommended practice. The Nursing and Midwifery Council was established under the Nursing and Midwifery Order (2001), came into being on 1 April 2002 and has authority to prepare rules that carry the weight of law. *The Code* (Nursing and Midwifery Council 2008) is 'about being professional, about being accountable, and being able to justify your decisions', laying a moral responsibility rather than a statutory duty on members of the profession. A marked failure to abide by *The Code* could, in turn, lead to the Nursing and Midwifery Council using its disciplinary function, with legal implications of removal of the nurse's name from the register.

Classification of law

Law may be classified in various ways; one of the main divisions of law is civil and criminal law. Criminal law is concerned with the relationship between the state and individuals. Criminal offences are committed against the state and are punishable by the state, e.g., drug offences and theft. Civil law is concerned with the rights and duties of individuals towards each other. Legal action is taken by a private citizen rather than the state, and a successful outcome results in an award of monetary compensation only, e.g., a patient suing a hospital for damages following some harm that has resulted from treatment or the lack thereof. Some civil wrongs can also be crimes, e.g., assault and battery and gross negligence, which could become manslaughter.

Probably the two most relevant areas of civil law in the ED are firstly negligence, as this relates to the standard of care given to the patient. And secondly the law on assault and battery, as this is relevant to the patients' rights and encompasses where the giving of consent may act as a defence against a charge of assault and battery.

Negligence

For negligence of any kind to be proved, it must be shown that the following components exist (Mason & Laurie 2010, Cornock 2011a):

- that the defendant (nurse) owed a duty of care to the plaintiff (patient) (established in the case of *Donoghue* vs *Stevenson* [1932])
- that the defendant was in breach of that duty (*Bolam* vs *Friern Hospital Management Committee* [1957])
- harm to the plaintiff, which was reasonably foreseeable, resulted directly from the breach of duty of care (*Barnett* vs *Kensington & Chelsea Hospital Management Committee* [1969]).

The Bolam case (Pannett 1997) laid down the principle of how to judge the standard of care that must be given as that of the 'reasonably skilled and experienced doctor as accepted by a responsible body of medical men skilled in that particular art' (*Bolam* vs *Friern Hospital Management Committee* 1957). The Wilsher case (*Wilsher* vs *Essex* AHA 1988) made it clear that the standard of care required was that of the post held not of the post-holder (Tingle & Cribb 2002). These precedents are applicable to all health care workers (Box 39.1).

Clinical documentation can be pivotal in cases of negligence and the Nursing and Midwifery Council (2009) describes record-keeping as an integral part of nursing and midwifery. The approach that the law tends to take to

Box 39.1

Negligence checklist

1. Did the nurse have a duty of care? If 'yes', continue. If 'no', there can be no liability
2. Was there a breach in the appropriate standard of care? If 'yes' continue. If 'no', there can be no liability
3. Did the breach of the standard cause the losses? If 'yes' continue. If 'no', there can be no liability
4. Are the losses of a kind recognized by law? If 'yes' continue. If 'no', there can be no liability
5. Were the losses too remote? If 'no' continue. If 'yes', there can be no liability
6. Did the patient contribute to the happening or extent of his or her losses? If 'yes' there has been contributory negligence and the damages will be proportionately reduced.

(After Carson D, Montgomery J (1989) Nursing and the Law. Basingstoke: Macmillan.)

record-keeping is that if it has not been recorded, it has not been done. ED nurses should be scrupulous in the documentation of their actions to reduce the risk of legal difficulties should a case be brought against them or their colleagues.

The Nursing and Midwifery Council (2009) makes clear that for records to be effective they must:

- be factual, consistent and accurate
- be written as soon as possible after the event
- be clear and permanent and able to be photocopied
- be accurately dated, timed and signed, with the name printed by the first signature. A qualified nurse must countersign all records that a student completes
- be unambiguous, with any alterations crossed through, with the original still being legible. All alterations should be dated, timed and signed.

Assault and battery

Assault and battery is the civil wrong of trespass committed to the person. Assault is an attempt or threat to apply unlawful force to the person of another, whereby that other person is put in fear of immediate violence or at least bodily contact. Battery is the actual application of force, however slight, to the person of another against his or her will.

There are a number of important defences against a legal action for trespass to the body (Box 39.2). The success in suing for trespass is not high and a number of patients have a better outcome using the law on negligence that is in relation to inadequate information given in order to gain consent (Pattison 2009).

Attendance

There is a clear legal duty on the hospital running an emergency service to see and treat all those who attend. Purely by virtue of their coming within its doors, the hospital accepts

Legal defences to a civil action for assault and battery

- Consent
- Urgency and necessity
- Acting under a statutory power, e.g., the Mental Health Act
- Public health risks
- Patient's 'best interests'

responsibility, even without formally admitting them. A failure to treat those who present themselves could be negligence.

Many people who attend the ED are under the influence of alcohol and/or drugs and can be both difficult and disruptive. Healthcare professionals have an obligation to undertake clinical assessment before any decision not to treat is made, even in circumstances where a patient is uncooperative. For example, a hypoglycaemic patient will present as aggressive and uncooperative, often appearing drunk; left untreated hypoglycaemia is life-threatening. The onus is on the nurse to ensure sufficient history or investigation has taken place to determine whether there is a clinical cause for the behaviour. Once such assessment has taken place and the outcome been documented, removal or refusal to treat can be ordered with the support of security staff or the police when appropriate.

In such situations, security staff are allowed to use reasonable force to protect themselves, prevent injury or damage to property and to use reasonable force to contain uncooperative persons until the police arrive. Theoretically this situation could possibly give rise to a claim of assault and battery against security staff and/or the police; however, where reasonable force as opposed to excessive force can be identified, this is unlikely to happen or to be upheld.

The situation would be different if those causing these difficulties were not there as patients, but as friends or relatives, or if the patient had already been seen and treated. In this case, the individuals can be asked to leave; a failure to do so would mean they were then trespassing on hospital property and can be evicted.

It is imperative that all incidents of this nature should be accurately and thoroughly documented.

Assessment

Most EDs have a system of assessing the urgency of patients' conditions on arrival. The criteria used to allocate patients to certain treatment groups largely rely on some degree of diagnosis. For the nurse, the crucial issue of undertaking patient assessment is whether he has sufficient knowledge to make an assessment competently, act on this assessment and to know his own limitations. Assessing a patient as less critically ill than in fact is the case, with a subsequent delay in treatment, could result in negligence.

The Nursing and Miwifery Council's *Code* (2008) makes a nurse undertaking such roles personally accountable for his practice, that is, answerable for all acts and omissions and for the maintenance of his/her professional knowledge and competence. However, *The Code* also states that the nurse must 'recognize and work within the limits of his competence'.

If the nurse is required to carry out patient assessment, the manager must provide the necessary training and carry the legal responsibility of delegating appropriately, as there can be negligence in delegation (Cornock 2011b). In addition, where patient assessment is seen as part of the nurse's role, the employer will be vicariously liable for any negligence of the employee. This employer liability arises from the old law of master and servant relationship, where the employer has to carry this legal responsibility by reason of having a contract with the employee. This vicarious liability may also exist with agency staff, but its extent may depend on the exact nature of the contract.

Under Section 2 of the Limitation Act (1980), a case for negligence must be commenced within three years of the date of the cause of the action or when the effects become apparent to the plaintiff (Pannett 1997). It may be considerably longer before the case comes to court. Section 14 of the Act also requires that the injury is significant and relates this to the plaintiff's knowledge of the injury. The lengthy timescale underlines the importance of record-keeping for nursing and medical staff.

Treatment and care

A vitally important question is: what is the standard of care that is expected and must be reached in the ED in order to avoid potential legal repercussions? From a number of legal cases relating to medical care, it is clear that the standard must be safe care and one that is accepted as proper by a responsible body of medical opinion (Mason & McCall-Smith 2002). Reasonable, rather than excellent, skill is considered sufficient. The standard in the ED will be that considered acceptable and reasonable in the conditions and circumstances in which nursing care is given.

The standard must relate to the specialty to which it is applied. Thus, nurses new to emergency department work must be aware that inexperience can never be an excuse for negligence. This was stated very clearly in *Wilsher vs Essex AHA* (1988), when inexperience in the work of the neonatal intensive care unit was put forward as a reason for the doctor's mistake in taking the wrong blood reading from baby Wilsher and subsequently prescribing the wrong level of oxygen (Tingle & Cribb 2002). Both appeal judges were emphatic that the standard of care must be that of the post held, not of the post-holder. The lesson to be learned from this is that adequate training and supervision are vital until the nurse is competent in the skills required.

The legal significance of the above applies to both the varied nature of the work as well as the range of skills of the workforce. For example, a number of people present to an emergency department with mental health problems; ideally these people should be cared for by Community Psychiatric Nurses (CPNs), but in reality most EDs do not employ CPNs directly. The general/adult trained nurses therefore have to manage these patients to the best of their ability. In these circumstances, the standard is probably not that of the CPN, but of a nurse experienced in dealing with the range of circumstances presented by those with mental health problems in this particular setting.

The importance of multidisciplinary teamwork is recognized in most patient care settings and is particularly relevant to emergency departments where a number of different professionals work together. Traditionally, doctors had overall legal responsibility for the patient, but care roles have become blurred and this is no longer the case. Patients can now be solely managed by other health professionals, who take responsibility for their care. Nurses should ensure that they are adequately trained and are working within parameters agreed with the organization, which the organization would then be vicariously liable for. In order to safeguard the different members of the team, care must be taken in delegating tasks to members, whether it is across professional boundaries or from more senior members of the nursing team to those more junior.

Three checks can be made in order to avoid negligence:

- the extent of the nurse's knowledge
- the level of skill in the task delegated either through asking about past experience or through direct observation
- by teaching and supervision over a period.

With regard to the safeguarding of vulnerable adults in hospital, the Department of Health (England) issued a guidance document entitled 'No Secrets' (Department of Health 2000) and the Care Standards Act (2000) included a scheme to protect vulnerable adults. The Protection of Vulnerable Adults (POVA) scheme has been replaced by the Vetting and Barring Scheme regulated by the Independent Safeguarding Authority, although this is currently under review (Home Office 2011). The Safeguarding Vulnerable Groups Act (2006) contains a scheme for vetting and barring those unsuitable for working with vulnerable adults, including health and social care workers (British Medical Association 2012).

Nurses' prescribing powers

Many emergency nurses are either supplementary or independent prescribers. An independent prescriber takes responsibility for the clinical assessment of the patient, establishing a diagnosis and the clinical management required, as well as prescribing where necessary (Department of Health 2004). A supplementary prescriber works with an independent prescriber to implement an agreed patient-specific clinical management plan.

Legislation in the form of a Statutory Instrument has extended nurses' prescribing powers (Medicines for Human Use 2005). The changes, which came into force on the 1st May 2006 in England, allow qualified nurse independent prescribers to prescribe any licensed medicine for any medical condition within their competence, including some controlled drugs. This is a significant change, as independent prescribers can now prescribe from the British National Formulary based on their clinical competence rather than from the nurses' formulary. Both independent prescribers and supplementary prescribers are now able to prescribe opiates in some circumstances.

Death and organ donation

Laws and policies governing the use of organs for transplantation are evolving rapidly in response to sensitivity to ethical concerns and increasing shortages of transplantable organs (Price 2012). There are a number of legal issues surrounding death in the ED: the first is the legal definition of death. The determination of brainstem death requires confirmation of the 'irreversible loss of the capacity for consciousness combined with the irreversible loss of the capacity to breathe' and relies on the fact that key components of consciousness and respiratory control, the reticular activating system and nuclei for cardiorespiratory regulation, reside in the brainstem (Smith 2012). Although this still stands as the total stoppage of circulation of blood and cessation of animal and vital body functions, the concept of brain-stem death is now accepted by the courts. There will not, therefore, be a legal difficulty in turning off a life-support system once brainstem death has been diagnosed. In situations where death has not occurred but prognosis and quality of life are so poor that to continue with treatment seems to have no useful purpose, the law accepts decisions not to do so. Appropriately qualified healthcare professionals can verify that death has taken place; however, brain-stem death can only be certified by a doctor.

Organ donation can create legal as well as ethical dilemmas in an emergency department (Wilkinson 2000). The Human Tissue Act (2004) makes consent a fundamental principle. If the deceased has not given consent before death, then the consent of a nominated representative is required; in the absence of this, then it will be the consent of a 'qualifying relative' that is needed. These 'qualifying relatives' relationships are ranked in order when consent is being sought to use tissue or organs for scheduled purposes (Box 39.3).

Box 39.3

Qualifying relatives to give consent (in descending order)

1. Spouse or partner
2. Parent or child
3. Brother or sister
4. Grandparent or grandchild
5. Child of a brother or sister
6. Stepfather or stepmother
7. Half-brother or half-sister
8. Friend of longstanding

Patient property

The same rules apply for the care of property in the ED as in a ward, but the clinical condition of some patients demands the nurse to become a 'bailee' for the property of those unable to take this responsibility themselves; this may be involuntary bailment (Dimond 2008). The task of checking property soon after arrival in these cases is important, due to the open nature of the environment and the high risk of theft.

Preferably, two people should together check, list, sign and ensure valuables are locked away safely. When death occurs, valuables should not be given to relatives, but again the proper hospital procedures should be followed.

In an emergency, such as cardiac arrests, clothing may have to be cut off, but this should only be done as a last resort. If clothes are heavily contaminated by blood or parasites and need to be destroyed, the patient's permission should be sought where possible and documentation of items destroyed should be made. Additionally, where there is a possibility of legal action, for instance, following criminal activity, resulting in alleged stabbings, gunshot wounds or sexual assault, care must be taken to cut and bag clothing, in ways that will enable forensic examiners to undertake their role to the satisfaction of the courts. Where items may form part of a criminal investigation, it is important that these are bagged in paper rather than plastic bags due to risk of degradation of material evidence.

Consent to treatment

For treatment to be given, a patient's consent must be gained in order to avoid being sued for assault and battery. For this consent to be legally effective, the patient must be able to understand and come to a decision about what is involved. Under common law, the patient has the right to give or withdraw consent for treatment or a procedure at any time.

Consent can be given in writing, orally or be assumed from the patient's actions, e.g., from the fact that the patient voluntarily attends the ED. However, Cable et al. (2003) argue that the nurse must not assume that a patient is giving consent by virtue of his or her voluntary attendance. Listening to each patient's responses and observing his or her non-verbal behaviour is an essential part of the process of ensuring that legally valid consent is also informed consent. Dimond (2005) cautions that where there is a dispute, written consent is the preferred evidence that consent was given. However, the signature on the consent form should not be seen as the consent itself, but evidence that, following a process of communication between the health professional and the patient which was understood by the patient, consent was given to the proposed intervention. The Department of Health (2001b) has also been keen to promote best process in securing informed consent following recommendations that emerged from the Bristol Royal Infirmary Inquiry Report (Department of Health 2001a, Vincent 2010).

Written consent is usually reserved for those treatments or investigations carrying a marked risk and is usually obtained by the person undertaking the procedure or by the doctor. The nurse may be able to help clarify a patient's lack of understanding or assist the patient in finding out the information required, but the nurse must ensure that he or she is competent to undertake this role and that any information is accurate.

For most nursing actions, consent will be gained orally and this is better practice professionally than assuming consent. Oral consent should be recorded in the clinical record. It is not an unusual occurrence for patients to be brought into the department who are either unable or unwilling to give consent to treatment. As shown in Box 39.2, there are a number of legal 'defences' or reasons that treatment can be given, apart from consent, without there being a case for assault and battery.

When a patient cannot give a valid consent due to a lack of understanding, treatment that is urgent and necessary can still be given. Thus the unconscious, semiconscious or mentally confused patient can be treated on this basis.

Under the Mental Capacity Act (2005a), everything that is done for or on behalf of a person who lacks capacity must be in that person's best interests. The Mental Capacity Act Deprivation of Liberty Safeguards (formerly known as the Bournewood Safeguards) was introduced into the Mental Capacity Act (2005b) through the Mental Health Act 2007 and has been in operation since April 2009. The Deprivation of Liberty Safeguards gives special protection to those who are unable to make a decision about the way they are being treated or cared for in a hospital.

In law, the health professionals care for patients in the absence of consent as part of their duty to care for them out of necessity in an emergency, and they would have to defend any subsequent action for trespass to the person on that basis. Those suffering the effects of alcohol or drugs could also be included in this category.

Under the Police Reform Act (2002), where the police believe that for a medical reason a person is incapable of giving valid consent to having a blood specimen taken, following involvement in a road traffic accident, the police may now request that a blood specimen be taken by the medical practitioner and stored. However, if the medical practitioner in charge of the patient believes that this would be prejudicial to the proper care and treatment of the patient, then the request can be objected to and it will not be carried out.

With a child it is usual, if the child is under 16, for the consent of the parents or guardian to be sought. In the case of unmarried parents, only the mother's consent is legally binding unless the father has legal guardianship. If the situation is too urgent to await the arrival of a parent, the child can give consent if she has sufficient understanding, or the urgency and necessity rule can be used. The Children Act (1989) also makes it clear that the child's wishes are paramount and no court direction overrides the child's right of refusal to be examined provided she has sufficient understanding. A 'Gillick competent' minor is deemed to have sufficient understanding and intelligence to enable him to understand fully what is proposed (*Gillick vs W. Norfolk & Wisbech Area Health Authority* [1985]).

'Gillick competence' (also called Fraser Guidelines) relates to the particular child and the particular treatment: there have been cases where a 17-year-old has been found to be insufficiently competent to refuse medical treatment, while in other cases much younger children have been deemed sufficiently competent. Under the Sexual Offences Act 2003, it is a criminal offence to procure sexual intercourse with a child under 16 years. Thus contraceptive treatment should also be given on clinical grounds (Carvalho et al. 2011). In order to protect nurses from being accused of breaching the Sexual Offences Act 2003, the Fraser Guidelines have been extended and may mean not telling the child's parents about the treatment if it is deemed it is in the interest of the child's welfare not to do so.

Predicaments can arise in any of these situations when relatives either take a different view from the patient or claim that the patient, if mentally capable, would have refused consent. The often-quoted example is of the unconscious patient who is a Jehovah's Witness and requires a blood transfusion. The ED team can still proceed on the basis that, as this is an unforeseen emergency, it would be impossible to know the patient's wishes if faced with possible death.

Relatives may also expect to be in the position of giving consent on behalf of an adult patient unable to do so. There is no legal basis for asking relatives for their consent in these circumstances. They may be consulted about the patient's preferences, but the decision to proceed with treatment will be a medical one on the basis of urgency and necessity. The Nursing and Midwifery Council (2008) also supports the notion of proceeding if it is in the patient's 'best interests', stating 'You must be able to demonstrate that you have acted in someone's best interests if you have provided care in an emergency'. While this guidance creates an ethical dilemma for healthcare practitioners, in terms of the law, both a decision to treat and a decision not to treat based on evidence of the patient's beliefs would be acceptable.

Health carers also face a difficulty when caring for a patient who is still conscious but is refusing treatment following a drug overdose. The Mental Health Act (1983), as amended by the Mental Health Act (2007), may appear to provide a treatment pathway by placing the patient under the emergency section of the Act and then giving treatment against her will, but it would be wrong to assume that all those attempting suicide are mentally disordered under the terms of the Act. It is also unlikely the Act could be applied, as assessment of the patient's mental state could be impaired by the drugs taken. An apparently irrational refusal can still be a competent one and the decision whether to treat or not may then become an ethical one. Proceeding against the patient's will lays the carers open to an action for assault and battery; however, in reality, the likelihood of a patient's bringing and pursuing any such action through the courts is low. Abiding by the patient's wishes, on the other hand, whilst legally correct, places a responsibility on the healthcare practitioner to ensure that the patient understands the potential outcome of no treatment; the healthcare practitioner then has to make a professional decision based on what they perceive the patient's state of mind to be.

In many of these predicaments, the legal difficulty may be one of balancing patients' rights against a possible accusation of negligence in failing to act. Whatever is decided, both arguments should be considered and, if they are particularly contentious, a written record should be made of how the decision was reached.

Detention of patients

As well as times when it is legally acceptable to treat without the patient's consent, there are also occasions when individuals can be detained against their will (Dimond 2008). Of relevance to the healthcare worker in the ED are the following: patients may be detained under Section 4 of the Mental Health Act (1983), as amended by the Mental Health Act 2007. Admission to hospital for assessment in cases of emergency lasts for 72 hours. The grounds for using this order are an urgent necessity that the patient should be admitted and detained for assessment and that compliance with the normal procedure would involve undesirable delay. The recommendation of only one medical practitioner is required. There will be arrangements made for an on-call psychiatrist to attend the ED.

The only other section likely to be met is Section 136. This order can be invoked by the police on finding a person in a public place who appears to be suffering from a mental disorder and in immediate need of care or control. Such a person has to be taken to a designated place of safety; ideally this would be attached to a mental health unit, but in some localities this would be an emergency department. Some patients may be mentally confused due to physical illness, e.g., hypoxia following heart failure. The patient can be detained in the short term for emergency treatment, the law accepting the necessity for this. A failure to do so could be deemed negligence.

Much rarer is the situation of an individual with a certain infectious disease potentially dangerous to others who refuses to stay for treatment. An order made by a magistrate or sheriff can be issued to detain the person, who will then be rapidly transferred to an appropriate unit.

The police may detain a person in the ED. For example, the patient may have been injured at the time of arrest. In this case it is the police's responsibility to detain, never the nurse's. Even if the police request the nurse to assist them in preventing the patient leaving the department, he should refuse to become involved. The fact that someone is a detained prisoner does not lessen her right to treatment, confidentiality or refusal to consent to procedures.

Confidentiality, the police and the press

Patient information is generally held under legal and ethical obligations of confidentiality (Department of Health 2003). Professionally, nurses are required to treat information about patients as confidential and use it only for the purposes for which it was given and to protect information from improper disclosure at all times: Nursing and Midwifery Council *Standards of Conduct, Performance and Ethics* (2008). Both the Data Protection Act (1998) and the Human Rights Act (1998) seek to preserve and protect the privacy and confidentiality of the individual. The Freedom of Information Act (2000) gives a general right of access to all types of information held by public authorities. However, there are a number of situations where disclosure of information without the patient's consent can be made. These include the following:

- orders from the court before or during legal proceedings
- public interest
- statutory obligation such as
  - ○ infectious diseases regulations
  - ○ notification of registration of births and stillbirths
  - ○ Police and Criminal Evidence Act (1984)
  - ○ Health and Social Care Act (2008)
  - ○ Prevention of Terrorism Act (2005)
  - ○ Road Traffic Act (198).

If the nurse has to give evidence in court, privilege on the basis of professional position cannot be claimed and the nurse will have to give the information required. The courts can also order the release of medical and nursing notes prior to the court case. The public interest would cover situations where serious harm is feared to the patient or another person, or in a child protection situation (Dimond 2005). Most departments will have clearly laid down guidelines to follow if symptoms point to child protection concerns. The disastrous consequences of not taking action have been well publicized, as has the distress caused to both child and parents when action has been taken on grounds that are later found to be unsubstantiated. A team approach is usually seen as essential.

Under the Prevention of Terrorism Act (2005) it is an offence for any person having information that he or she believes may be of material assistance in preventing terrorism or apprehending terrorists to fail, without reasonable cause, to give that information to the police.

While nurses have an obligation to provide police with a statement regarding their own actions and observations, they do not have to provide a statement regarding the patient's medical condition. This can be referred on to the clinician in charge of the patient's care. While inter-agency cooperation is important, healthcare professionals should not feel pressurized into providing statements immediately. In most circumstances, it is quite acceptable to arrange a mutually agreeable time for statements. This enables the health professional to organize their thoughts and seek advice about confidentiality and disclosure if needed.

While there is a need for valid sharing of information between health professionals to ensure the safe care of patients, the Caldicott principles (NHS Executive 1997) should be followed (Box 39.4).

Box 39.4

Caldicott principles

- Justify the purpose
- Do not use patient-identifiable information unless it is absolutely necessary
- Use the minimum necessary patient-identifiable information
- Access to patient-identifiable information should be on a strict need-to-know basis
- Everyone should be aware of their responsibilities
- Understand and comply with the law

The healthcare worker in the ED is sure to have a certain amount of contact with the police and, possibly, the press. It is important to be aware of the respective rights of patients, hospital employees and police in these circumstances. The police have a number of powers regarding search and arrest and these will apply to a hospital in the same way as to a private dwelling because hospitals are Crown property, not public property. Police can enter premises without a search warrant if the person they wish to search for is suspected of an arrestable offence. An intimate search of body orifices can be authorized if the person concerned is likely to have concealed an item to injure herself or others, or for drugs. Police are entitled to use reasonable force in carrying out an intimate search.

In relation to arrest, police may arrest without a warrant if they suspect that an arrestable offence has been, is being or is about to be committed. Examples of an arrestable offence are unlawful possession of drugs, rape and most offences of violence (English & Card 2003). If the police suspect that an individual who is currently a patient in the ED has committed a serious offence, the staff should not hinder the police in their work, but should ensure the medical condition of the individual is not jeopardized.

A final situation where patient confidentiality may be put at risk is through press enquiries. Most hospitals will have strict rules on which staff are allowed to talk to the press. It is wise for staff always to refer these enquiries to the appropriate senior member of staff.

Staff health and safety

Both verbal abuse and physical violence against staff are not unusual occurrences in the ED. Police attendance at such incidents can be requested and the nurses involved will need to make statements to the police. However, quite often no charges will be brought against the individual.

The law can be relevant in a number of ways. First, violent actions could be the crime of assault, battery or causing grievous bodily harm. However, the police are often unable to charge a person on the basis of these crimes as there is often some doubt as to whether the person intended to commit the crime. Proving intention is necessary for a successful prosecution. If the patient is mentally ill, drunk or under the influence of drugs, they could claim that they could not form the necessary intention. Increasingly, however, courts take a poor view of acts of violence carried out under the influence of drink or drugs that offenders have taken to deprive themselves of their self-control or their knowledge of what they were doing. There are moves to try to bring nurses into line with the police, in as much as when a police officer is assaulted, it is automatically a criminal offence.

For most criminal charges, not only is self-induced intoxication no defence but, if the offender claims that she/he only did it because of intoxication, the prosecution are absolved from proving any mental element and need simply prove that the act was done. It is thus easier to obtain a conviction. It also underlines the need for clear, contemporaneous notes to be taken by staff and witnesses in case of legal action being taken. If injuries are sustained, the statement will provide evidence of the event and the nurse may be able to claim from the Criminal Injuries Compensation Authority even in the absence of a successful prosecution.

Assault and battery are also civil wrongs. This means the nurse could sue the individual through the civil courts for damages. In this context, intention does not have to be proved, so evidence of the incident would lead to a successful legal action. It is rare, however, for nurses to take this route. Finally, the nurse could complain to the employer that there has been a failure to provide a safe working environment, under common law, the Occupiers Liability Act (1957) and the Health and Safety at Work etc. Act (1974). However, the employer only has to take reasonable steps to ensure the health, safety and welfare of the employees. It is difficult for the employer to create a totally safe environment in EDs, because of the nature of the work undertaken and the open access of the department to the public. If the employee considers further measures should be taken, she should consult the health and safety representative of her trade union or professional body.

Other health and safety issues in the ED are very similar to those elsewhere, e.g., infection risks, moving and handling patients and fire hazards. European Union Directives, laid out in a number of UK Health and Safety (General Provisions) Regulations (1992), have resulted in the broadening of the requirements and improved protection of staff in the area of safety. The provision of training and adequate equipment are key elements of any statutory requirements. Health and Safety issues are examined in detail in Chapter 40.

Conclusion

In the medico-legal sense, the ED has been described as the most dangerous part of a hospital (Knight 1992). It is therefore important for all emergency nurses to have a working knowledge of the law if they are to try to prevent legal problems arising in the first place. This chapter has introduced the main areas of law relevant in emergency care and discussed the implications for emergency care practitioners. Like practice, however, the law is constantly evolving and it is in the nurse's best interest to maintain an up-to-date knowledge of the law.

References

Barnett vs Kensington & Chelsea Hospital Management Committee (1969) 1 QB 428.

Bolam vs Friern Hospital Management Committee (1957) 1WLR 582.

British Medical Association, 2012. Medical Ethics Today: The BMA's Handbook of Ethics and Law. BMA, London.

Cable, S., Lumsdaine, J., Semple, M., 2003. Informed consent. Nursing Standard 18 (12), 47–53.

Carson, D., Montgomery, J., 1989. Nursing and the Law. Macmillan, Basingstoke.

Care Standards Act. 2000. HMSO, London.

Carvalho, S., Reeves, M., Orford, J., 2011. Fundamental Aspects of Legal, Ethical and Professional Issues in Nursing, second ed. Quay Books, London.

Cornock, M., 2011a. A legal commentary on negligence. Paediatric Nursing 23 (1), 21–23.

Cornock, M., 2011b. Legal definitions of responsibility, accountability and liability. Paediatric Nursing 23 (3), 25–26.

Data Protection Act. 1998. HMSO, London.

Department of Health, 2000. No Secrets: Guidance on Developing and Implementing Multiagency policies and Procedures to Protect Vulnerable Adults from Abuse. Department of Health, London.

Department of Health, 2001a. Learning from Bristol: The Report of the Inquiry into Children's Heart Surgery at Bristol Royal Infirmary 1984–1995. Command Paper CM (5207) HMSO, London.

Department of Health, 2001. Reference Guide to Consent for Examination and Treatment. Department of Health, London.

Department of Health, 2003. NHS Code of Conduct. Department of Health, London.

Department of Health, 2004. Medicines Pharmacy and Industry Group. Department of Health, London.

Dimond, B., 2005. Legal aspects of trauma nursing. In: O'Shea, R.A. (Ed.), Principles and Practice of Trauma Nursing, Elsevier Churchill Livingstone, Edinburgh.

Dimond, B., 2008. Legal Aspects of Nursing. Pearson Education, Essex.

Donoghue vs Stevenson (1932) AC 562.

English, J., Card, R., 2003. Butterworth's Police Law. Lexis Nexis, London.

Freedom of Information Act. 2000. HMSO, London.

Gillick vs West Norfolk and Wisbech Area Health Authority [1985] 3 All ER 402

Health and Safety at Work etc. Act. 1974. HMSO, London.

Health and Social Care Act. 2008. HMSO, London.

Health and Safety (General Provisions) Regulations. 1992. HMSO, London.

Home Office, 2011. Vetting and Barring Scheme Remodelling Review: Report and Recommendations. Home Office, London.

Human Rights Act. 1998. The Stationery Office Limited, London.

Human Tissue Act. 2004. HMSO, London.

Knight, B., 1992. Legal Aspects of Medical Practice, fifth ed. Churchill Livingstone, Edinburgh.

Limitation Act. 1980. HMSO, London.

Mason, J., Laurie, G., 2010. Legal and Ethical Aspects of Healthcare. Medical Media, Greenwich.

Mason, J.K., McCall-Smith, R.A., 2002. Law and Medical Ethics, sixth ed. Lexis Nexis, London.

Medicines for Human Use (Prescribing) (Misc Amendments) Order (2005), Statutory Instrument 2005 No. (1507).

Mental Capacity Act. 2005a. The Stationery Office Limited, London.

Mental Capacity Act, 2005b. Deprivation of Liberty Safeguards introduced through the Mental Health Act 2007. HMSO, London.

Mental Health Act. 1983. HMSO, London.

Mental Health Act. 2007. HMSO, London.

Montgomery, J., 2002. Health Care Law, second ed. Oxford University Press, Oxford.

NHS Executive, 1997. Caldicott Committee: Report on the Review of Patient-identifiable Information. Department of Health, London.

Nursing and Midwifery Council, 2008. The Code: Standards of Conduct, Performance and Ethics for Nurses and Midwives. Nursing and Midwifery Council, London.

Nursing and Midwifery Council, 2009. Record Keeping: Guidance for Nurses and Midwives. Nursing and Midwifery Council, London.

Occupiers Liability Act. 1957. HMSO, London.

Pannett, A.J., 1997. Law of Torts, seventh ed. Prentice Hall, London.

Pattison, D., 2009. Medical Law and Ethics. Sweet and Maxwell, London.

Police and Criminal Evidence Act. 1984. HMSO, London.

Police Reform Act. 2002. The Stationery Office Limited, London.

Prevention of Terrorism Act. 2005. The Stationery Office Limited, London.

Road Traffic Act. 1988. HMSO, London.

Price, D.P.T., 2012. Legal framework governing deceased organ donation in the UK. British Journal of Anaesthesia 10 (Suppl 1), i68–i72.

Safeguarding Vulnerable Groups Act. 2006. HMSO, London.

Smith, M., 2012. Brain death: time for an international consensus. British Journal of Anaesthesia 108 (Suppl 1), i6–i9.

The Children Act. 1989. HMSO, London.

The Nursing and Midwifery Order, 2001. Statutory Instrument 2002 No. 253. The Stationery Office Ltd, London.

Tingle, J.H., Cribb, A. (Eds.), 2002. Nursing Law and Ethics. Blackwell Science, Oxford.

Vincent, C., 2010. Patient Safety, second ed. Wiley-Blackwell/BMJ Books, Oxford.

Wilkinson, R., 2000. Organ donation: the debate. Nursing Standard 14 (28), 41–42.

Wilsher vs Essex AHA (1988) 1 All ER 871.

Health and safety

40

Kim Sunley

CHAPTER CONTENTS

Introduction

It seems incongruous that a service set up to provide emergency care sometimes causes harm to the staff involved in delivering that care. In 2003, the National Audit Office carried out a survey on health and safety risks to staff in the NHS in England (National Audit Office 2003a). They reported that there were 135 172 staff accidents in 2001–2, with wide variations between similar Trusts in the number of accidents per 1000 staff. They also highlighted that there is significant under-reporting, so the true figure is likely to be much higher. In 2009 a comprehensive review into the health and well-being of the NHS workforce found that NHS staff have a greater propensity to work-related illness or accident than other comparative groups (Department of Health 2009). This is despite the complex set of statutes and regulations, some based on European legislation, designed to provide a safe environment for employees and others, such as patients, visitors, contractors' employees and agency staff. This chapter considers various aspects of accidents at work, describes the main legal responsibilities of employers and employees, and also how this legislation is applied to hazards found in emergency departments (EDs).

Preventing accidents

The Health and Safety Executive (1993) use the term 'accident' to refer to any unplanned event that results in injury or ill health of people, or damage or loss to property, plant, materials or the environment, or a loss of business opportunity. Before any action can be taken to prevent accidents, the causes must be identified. Causes can be divided into unsafe conditions (e.g., wet floors, trailing cables, insufficient manual handling aids, faulty equipment) or unsafe acts (e.g., nurses' failure to wear protective equipment or ignoring safety instructions). Unsafe acts arise from lack of training or nurses' attitudes towards their own safety (Lynch & Cole 2006). Workplaces should be regularly inspected to check that hazards do not exist and, although trade union safety representatives have this as part of their role, it should be a cooperative process between staff, managers and safety representatives. Local policies should encourage nurses to report hazards before accidents occur so that preventive action may be taken. In fact there is a specific duty contained within the *Management of Health and Safety at Work Regulations 1999* (Health & Safety Executive 2000) that requires employees

http://dx.doi.org/10.1016/B978-0-7020-4315-4.00040-1

to report to their employer details of any work situation that might represent a serious and imminent danger.

If an accident does occur, accurate records are needed. From the employer's point of view there is a duty to report certain types of accidents defined within the Reporting of Injury, Diseases and Dangerous Occurrence Regulations (RIDDOR) (1995) to the Health and Safety Executive. Failure to do so is a criminal offence. The employer needs information about an accident so the event can be investigated to prevent its recurrence and risk assessments can be reviewed. Employees are obliged to report accidents and it is in their interests to accurately complete accident forms and accident books to protect themselves in the event of future loss of income or long-term effects of injury or disease.

It has always been difficult to arrive at the true costs of accidents, and yet this information could provide an incentive to tackling the problem of workplace accidents by providing a measurement against which financial loss can be judged. The National Audit Office (2003a) survey of health and safety in hospitals estimated that accidents cost the NHS £173 million in England alone. This is a crude estimate and does not include staff replacement costs, medical treatment costs or court compensation, so the true costs are likely to be much higher. The cost of an accident is directly related to the outcome of that accident, but this can be difficult to predict, as, for example, a needlestick injury may or may not result in a nurse contracting a blood-borne virus such as hepatitis C. The total cost of accidents must include the cost of maintaining a safe environment. A relationship exists between underlying safety control and accident occurrence.

Implementing safety controls will involve some cost, such as staff communication and training, physical protection (alarm systems), publicity campaigns, time spent in risk assessment, inspecting the workplace for hazards and maintenance of equipment. These costs will be offset by the direct and indirect costs resulting from accidents and ill health, such as occupational sick pay, equipment damage, disruption in patient care, damage to the environment, costs of replacement staff and costs of litigation. The management responsibility is to reduce risks as far as is 'reasonably practicable', a term used in health and safety law that is a balance between the level of risk and the time, trouble and money needed to control it.

Legislation

The health service was not covered by any health and safety legislation until 1974 when the Health & Safety at Work etc. Act was passed. This is still the major legislative power and any new regulations come under its framework. The Health & Safety at Work etc. Act (1974) specifies the duties of the employer with the general requirement to 'ensure, so far as is reasonably practicable, the health, safety & welfare at work of all his Employees' (Section 2(1)). The Act then specifies the particular areas where this duty applies (Box 40.1).

Another section of the Health & Safety at Work etc. Act (1974) defines the duty of the employer to non-employees, including patients, visitors and contractors' employees, to

---

Box 40.1

Duties of employer in the Health & Safety at Work etc. Act 1974

- The provision of plant and systems of work that are without risk to health and safety. In addition, the equipment must be maintained so it remains safe. This could include systems of handling and moving patients, infection control procedures or extraction systems to remove hazardous fumes
- Making arrangements in the use, handling, storage and transport of articles and substances so that the risk is minimized. The safe disposal of clinical waste including sharps would be covered by this requirement
- Providing information, instruction, training and supervision so that employees are kept safe at work. General training on health and safety must be provided along with specific training on particular hazards of handling of loads and fire procedures
- Providing and maintaining a safe place of work so that there is adequate heating, lighting, ventilation and fire exits
- Provision of adequate welfare facilities. Welfare is a very broad area but could include access to occupational health services, vaccination against hepatitis B, facilities for changing, showers and toilets and a smoke-free working environment

---

ensure these people are also protected from harm whilst they are on the premises. Systems of work must be developed to protect these groups. Floor cleaning is an example of the need to ensure that staff and others are prevented from walking on wet, slippery floors by cleaning during quiet periods, temporarily rerouting pedestrian walkways or the use of cones and warning signs.

The approach to health and safety legislation is to involve both employers and employees. The Health & Safety at Work etc. Act (1974) specifies that all employees must take reasonable care for the health and safety of themselves and others who may be affected by their acts or omissions and cooperate with the employer to enable compliance with statutory requirements. If the employer provides any protective equipment, such as gloves, goggles or aprons, the employee must wear it. This presumes the employer has defined the need for the equipment, the equipment is suitable and the employer has trained staff in the correct use.

The Health & Safety at Work etc. Act (1974) is a wide-ranging piece of legislation and one that permits further regulations to be developed that refer to specific aspects of health and safety. In 1992, six new sets of regulations were enacted that were based on EC Directives (Health & Safety Executive 1992a–e), but during that period, 1974–1995, other regulations included:

- Safety Representatives & Safety Committees Regulations (1977), which define the rights and functions of trade-union-appointed safety representatives and the arrangements for safety committees
- Health & Safety (First-Aid) Regulations (1981), which provide a framework for the provision of first aid arrangements for employees. Even in emergency departments procedures need to be defined for staff who suffer an accident

- Reporting of Injuries, Diseases & Dangerous Occurrences Regulations (1995), which specify the duty on the employer to report to the Health & Safety Executive certain categories of injuries, dangerous occurrences and designated diseases.

In the case of disease, the nature of the work is specified. Hepatitis B infection is a reportable disease for anyone who comes into contact with blood, blood products or body secretions. The regulations specify the type of dangerous occurrences that must be reported, whether or not anyone has been injured. Similarly, the specific types of injury are defined along with a broad category of any injury that results in absence from work for seven days or more. The other reportable major injuries are outlined in Box 40.2. Any incidents where a staff member has a needlestick injury where the sharp was known to be contaminated with infected blood must be reported to the Health and Safety Executive under RIDDOR.

Box 40.2

Reportable major injuries under RIDDOR (1995)

- Fracture other than to fingers, thumbs or toes
- Amputation
- Dislocation of the shoulder, hip, knee or spine
- Loss of sight (temporary or permanent)
- Chemical or hot metal burn to the eye or any penetrating injury to the eye
- Injury resulting from an electric shock or electrical burn leading to unconsciousness or requiring resuscitation or admittance to hospital for more than 24 hours
- Any other injury leading to hypothermia, heat-induced illness or unconsciousness or requiring admittance to hospital for more than 24 hours
- Acute illness requiring medical treatment or loss of consciousness arising from absorption of any substance by inhalation, ingestion or through the skin
- Acute illness requiring medical treatment where there is reason to believe that this resulted from exposure to a biological agent or its toxins or infected material

Control of Substances Hazardous to Health Regulations (2002)

The Control of Substances Hazardous to Health (COSHH) Regulations (2002) was implemented in response to concerns about the effect on health of exposure to hazardous substances and replaced and revoked the earlier COSHH Regulations (1988). Dangerous substances must be categorized in terms of hazard and risk. A hazardous substance is one that has the potential to cause harm. The risk is the likelihood that it will cause harm in the actual circumstances where it is used. The regulations require the employer to carry out an assessment of the risk and subsequently to establish a safe system of work. The definition of a hazardous substance is any solid, liquid, gas, fume, vapour or microorganism that can endanger health

by being absorbed or injected through the skin or mucous membranes, inhaled or digested. One exclusion is substances administered as part of a medical treatment, although the impact on the healthcare worker would need to be assessed, for instance, during the preparation of cytotoxic drugs.

Once the assessment has been carried out, steps must be taken to prevent or at least control exposure. Elimination of the substance is the ideal solution to the problem, but there will be circumstances where this is not reasonably practicable. Glutaraldehyde, a potent cause of occupational asthma, used to be the most effective cold disinfectant available but has been substituted by less hazardous chemicals or even cold sterilization (Royal College of Nursing 2000). Examples of measures to control exposure include local exhaust ventilation, enclosing the process or, as a last resort, personal protective equipment such as goggles, masks and gloves. The regulations require the control measures to be properly used and maintained and for employees and non-employees to be informed, instructed and trained in what the risks are and how to control them.

Where nurses are exposed to risk there is a requirement to carry out health surveillance. Health surveillance is needed to protect the health of individuals by detecting adverse changes attributed to exposure to hazardous substances at the earliest possible stage. This will help in assessing the effectiveness of control measures. Where health surveillance is carried out, the employees' health records must be kept for 30 years.

Within EDs and fracture clinics there are three main areas of risk where COSHH assessments should be carried out. The first is chemical exposure, including drugs and plaster of Paris dust. The assessment and subsequent control measures should consider storage, local ventilation, waste disposal, need for personal protective equipment, training and air monitoring. Special attention should be paid to the type of environment and the potential for patients, accompanying relatives and children to gain unauthorized access to materials such as antiseptics.

The second group of substances comprises the disinfectants such as phenolics, hypochlorites, glutaraldehyde alcohol mixtures and idophors. Many of these can be an irritant to the skin and eyes.

The third group of hazards involves the microbiological hazards from contact with blood-borne infections such as human immunodeficiency virus (HIV), hepatitis B and hepatitis C that can be found in blood and body fluids of an infected patient. COSHH requires employers to assess the risks of infection and put measures in place to reduce the risks. Standard (universal) precautions such as hand washing, use of protective equipment such as gloves and goggles and decontamination of surfaces reduce the risks to both patients and staff (UK Health Departments 1998, Royal College of Nursing 2012).

However, care must be taken when decontaminating surfaces following spillages. Chlorine-releasing disinfecting agents used in spillages of urine can be used as an example of the application of COSHH. The indiscriminate use of powdered or granular products designed to disinfect and contain spills of body fluids can lead to ill effects in staff and patients through exposure to chlorine. The use of such a substance must be controlled so it does not become a greater danger than the risk of infection. A COSHH assessment in this instance would consider both biological and chemical hazards. It would take into account the urgency of any situation, the nature of the spillage, the quantities that might be spilt and the degree of ventilation. With this information a system of work may be defined to cover storage, handling and use of any disinfecting agent, the procedure for dissolving or diluting it before use and the need for any personal protection for the user.

Legislation since 1992

Health and safety is an issue that has featured prominently in European legislation. Article 118A of the Single European Act 1986 (European Union 1986) states that member states shall pay particular attention to encouraging improvements especially in the working environment as regards the health and safety of workers and shall set as their objective the harmonization of conditions in this area, whilst maintaining the improvements made.

Directly arising out of this article was a framework directive (EC Directive 89/391/EEC 1989) on health and safety, with a number of so-called 'daughter directives' covering manual handling, personal protective equipment, work equipment, the workplace, temporary workers and display-screen equipment. Once these directives were agreed, European Union member states were required to include the provisions of the directives into their own law by 1992. In the UK, this resulted in a set of regulations often referred to as 'the six pack', comprising:

- the Management of Health & Safety at Work Regulations 1999 (Health & Safety Executive 2000)
- the Manual Handling Operations Regulations 1992 (Health & Safety Executive 1992a)
- the Display Screen Equipment Regulations 1992 (Health & Safety Executive 1992b)
- the Personal Protective Equipment Regulations 1992 (Health & Safety Executive 1992c)
- the Work Equipment Regulations 1992 (Health & Safety Executive 1992d) (replaced by the Provision and Use of Work Equipment Regulations 1998 and the Lifting Equipment Regulations 1998)
- the Workplace Regulations 1992 (Health & Safety Executive 1992e).

Although all of these have relevance in emergency departments, the first two are considered in more detail.

The Management of Health & Safety at Work Regulations (1999)

These regulations build on and make more explicit the duties of employers and employees defined in the Health & Safety at Work etc. Act (1974). The regulations originally came into force in 1992 but were amended in 1999. The main requirement is the need to carry out a risk assessment for every hazard in the workplace (Box 40.3). All of the activities and processes carried out within the emergency service should be subjected to the process of risk assessment.

Box 40.3

Some possible hazards in the workplace

- Chemical hazards, e.g., glutaraldehyde and formaldehyde
- Biological hazards, e.g., blood-borne and airborne infections
- Electrical hazards
- Manual handling
- Physical hazards, e.g., violence
- Psychological hazards, e.g., stress
- Equipment, e.g., autoclaves, sharp instruments, computers
- Ionizing radiation, e.g., diagnostic X-rays
- Hot and cold working conditions
- Poor lighting
- Fire
- Workplace layout and design

Risk assessment

Employers are responsible for carrying out health and safety risk assessments; however, nursing staff should be involved in the process because they are familiar with the environment, the procedures and equipment used. Risk assessment is the starting point for total risk management. The aim is to identify where things could go wrong and what the effect would be. Risk may arise from physical hazards, e.g., unsafe flooring, poor lighting, no alarm systems, or working practices, e.g., failure to dispose of sharps safely, failure to wear gloves, failure to alter bed heights when moving patients. When carrying out risk assessments employers should:

- identify the hazards
- decide who may be harmed and how (including contractors, cleaning staff and visitors)
- evaluate the risks and decide on precautions
- record the findings and implement them
- review and update as necessary (e.g., following an accident or change to work environment) (Health and Safety Executive 2006).

Some risk assessment procedures apply numerical values to these items, which are multiplied together to produce an overall risk score, sometimes known as a risk matrix. This can be used to introduce greater objectivity and to look at relative risks from hazards, but in some cases it may be misleading. With manual handling, for example, an uncooperative patient will have an impact on the assessment. A skilled assessor, sensitive to all the variables, may produce a more useful assessment than the application of numerical values.

The process of risk assessment should result in a decision as to whether the risk is acceptable or not. If not, further work is required to control the risk. Elimination is the ideal solution but may not be always possible. Other methods of control are:

- to substitute a less hazardous process or substance
- to use engineering methods such as ventilation systems
- to redefine systems of work
- to provide personal protective equipment

- to immunize staff where possible
- to define emergency procedures.

The results of the risk assessment must be written and all staff affected must be informed about the risks and about the preventive measures or controls to be used (Clough 1998).

There are specific requirements relating to pregnant employees that were incorporated as a result of the *Pregnant Workers Directive* (EC Directive 92/85 EEC 1992). The risk assessment must cover any risks to the health and safety of a new or expectant mother from physical, biological or chemical agents. Where the risk cannot be avoided, the employer must alter the individual's working conditions or hours of work. If it is not reasonable to do so or if it would not avoid the risk, the employer must offer suitable alternative employment or suspend the employee from work. Furthermore, if the employee works nights and medical evidence states that this is a health risk, the employer must provide other employment or suspend her from work.

In addition to the requirement to carry out risk assessment, the Management of Health & Safety at Work Regulations (1999) (Health and Safety Executive 2000) contain other important duties. If the assessment identifies that nurses will be exposed to risk, it may be necessary to provide health surveillance. This is needed where there is an identifiable disease related to the work and where the techniques exist to detect indications of the disease. Under these regulations the employer must appoint one or more competent persons to provide health and safety assistance. This could be one person or a team depending on the size of the organization. They may be appointed from existing employees or brought in on a consultancy basis. In any event they must have adequate time and resources to carry out their functions.

The employer must take account of employees' capabilities, training and knowledge experience when allocating work. Training on health and safety must be given in working practices and systems introducing new equipment. The training must be repeated periodically and carried out during the employees' working hours. Specific reference is made to temporary staff. Where agency or bank staff are used, essential information must be provided about the workplace and about any particular risks to health and safety. These regulations clearly define what is needed to develop an organizational safety culture and provide the framework within which departmental approaches are developed.

Employees' duties

The duty of the employee to cooperate includes the use of equipment, dangerous substances, transport equipment, means of production or safety device and the need to operate these in accordance with training and instruction received. Additional duties are specified; each employee must inform the employer of any work situation which represents a serious and immediate danger to health and safety and any shortcoming in the protection arrangements for health and safety believed to exist by the employee.

This duty can be considered in the light of provisions within the Employment Rights Act (1996), which gives employment protection to employees in relation to health and safety. Employees and safety representatives have the right not to have action short of dismissal or be dismissed in the following circumstances:

- where they have been designated by the employer to carry out activities to prevent or reduce risks to health and safety and have done so or are proposing to do so
- where the employee is a safety representative and is acting in that capacity
- where the employee left the workplace because of serious and imminent danger
- where the employee took steps to, or proposed to take appropriate steps to, protect himself or others from the danger. The protection applies regardless of length of service.

Nurses are able to combine their responsibilities in *The NMC Code of Professional Conduct: Standards for Conduct, Performance and Ethics* (Nursing and Midwifery Council 2008) with health and safety regulations to take action to secure a safe working environment. For example, if a nurse believes staffing levels are insufficient to provide safe standards of practice, she has a responsibility to report this. It is also likely that such staffing levels would pose a risk to the health and safety of other staff and so the nurse would be required to report this under health and safety legislation.

Manual Handling Operations Regulations (1992)

The impact of manual handling on the health of nurses has long been recognized, but these are the first set of regulations to address the problem specifically. In the NHS sickness absence due to musculoskeletal disorders accounts for around 40 % of all sickness absence (NHS Employers 2009). Musculoskeletal disorders, including back injuries, are the main cause of ill health retirements in the health sector (Department of Health 2009).

The Manual Handling Operations Regulations 1992 (Health & Safety Executive 1992a) require the employer to avoid the need for employees to undertake any manual handling operations at work that involve a risk of injury. This is qualified by the phrase 'so far as is reasonably practicable' and where this applies the employer must carry out an assessment to reduce the risk to the lowest level reasonably practicable. The regulations cover both animate and inanimate objects. The approach in the risk assessment is based on ergonomic principles of optimizing the fit between the nurse and her work.

The guidance to the regulations identifies four factors for the assessment:

- the task
- the load
- the environment
- individual capability.

These factors are interrelated and may not be considered in isolation. No one working in a hospital should put their safety at risk when moving or handling patients. Risk assessments

Box 40.4

Risk factors in lifting patients

Patients

- Weight
- Cooperation
- Dependency
- Consciousness level
- Condition
- Pain
- Comprehension
- Behavioural problems

Task

- Frequency
- Repetition
- Job rotation
- Holding loads away from trunk, reaching upwards long distances
- Restrictions by uniform twisting/stooping
- Awkward posture
- Urgency of task

Environment

- Space to move freely
- Floor slippery, uneven, light inadequate
- Other tripping hazards, equipment available, equipment in good repair

Employee

- Training
- Danger to pregnant staff
- Danger to those with health problems, stress levels

Box 40.5

Control factors when lifting patients

Patient

- Use mechanical equipment
- Involve patient
- Explain to patient
- Consider patient's dignity
- Consider any attachments to patient

Task

- Sufficient number of staff
- Improved design of task
- Rest breaks for staff
- Decreased distances for moving patient, improved equipment
- Adjustable heights on equipment

Environment

- Use of ranges for easier movement
- Harmonize heights of work surfaces, location of equipment
- Improve lighting, temperature, noise levels
- Improve tidiness and cleanliness

Employee

- Improve individual technique
- Report unsafe systems
- Provide training
- Consider individual situations, e.g., pregnancy
- Increase level of supervision to eliminate poor practice

should identify what equipment, e.g., hoists or sliding aids, are needed to reduce the risk of injuries. Patients should be encouraged and allowed to move independently and contribute to the movement. A patient handling policy should be in place that commits to reduce the risk of injury as far as possible and to meet the needs of the patient and protect the staff from risk. Examples of the risk factors under the four headings are summarized in Box 40.4. Once the risk factors have been identified, the next stage is to take steps to eliminate or reduce the risk. Possible control measures are summarized in Box 40.5.

The assessment will take place at two levels. First, the workplace itself must be assessed by the department manager in conjunction with any specialist help. This assessment will take into account departmental accident and absence statistics, layout, availability of handling aids and training of staff. Once completed, the risk-reducing actions are likely to have been identified and action plans developed.

The particular needs of the nature of the work make a difference to the assessment. In emergency areas, it would be appropriate to develop generic assessments for many of the transfers that take place, e.g., trolley to bed, wheelchair to bed. In emergency situations, an on-the-spot assessment is needed by skilled staff to judge whether the generic

assessment is relevant. The risk assessment must be written and should be available to staff who need the information. If circumstances change so that the assessment is no longer valid, it must be updated.

The next level of assessment is in relation to individual patients. In wards or in the community, a manual handling assessment would be incorporated into the patient care plan. Within EDs a system should exist that would enable an initial manual handling assessment to be carried out; this would need updating as the patient's condition and treatment are known.

The duties of the employee under these regulations are to make full and proper use of the systems provided by the employer. Nursing staff have a responsibility for their own actions and their own competence. Where training on manual handling is available the nurse should attend. If the training is not provided, the nurse should be requesting that she has the opportunity to receive this training.

Infection prevention and control

Infection control is particularly important within EDs because the status of each patient arriving in the department will not be known and treatment may be necessary before there is any indication that the patient may present a risk. Specific local infection control policies are needed in relation to cleaning and decontamination of the workplace, use of disinfectants, hand washing, dealing with laundry, protective clothing, disposal of waste and transport of specimens.

Contact with patient's blood/body fluids carries with it the risk of occupational exposure to blood-borne infections such as HIV or hepatitis B or hepatitis C. Healthcare workers need to follow standard (universal) precautions to prevent contamination by blood/body fluids. These precautions include covering any abrasions to exposed skin, wearing gloves and plastic aprons, thorough hand-washing between procedures, and wearing eye protection if there is any risk of blood splashes or flying contaminated debris.

Accidental inoculation or splashes to the eyes or mucous membranes with infected blood present a real risk to the nurse although for most incidents there will be no harm to the nurse. However, sharps injury is a major cause of transmission of blood-borne viruses from patient to nurse. The Health Protection Agency (2008) reported that there had been 14 hepatitis C sero-conversions following significant exposure over a ten-year period and five HIV sero-conversions since 1999. Extreme care is needed with the use and disposal of sharps, and used sharps should never be recapped or re-sheathed. Risk assessment must be carried out and safer systems of work implemented. There are now technological solutions, with a wide range of safety-engineered devices that can significantly reduce the risk of a needlestick injury.

In the event of a needlestick injury, the immediate action is to make the puncture wound bleed by gentle squeezing of the area. Wash thoroughly with soap and water and apply a waterproof dressing. If the source patient is known, a record should be kept with the name of the patient. In any event, contact should be made with occupational health and an accident form completed. Procedures should be defined for spillages of blood and body fluids including COSHH assessments for the chemicals used to deal with spillages. A new European Directive (EC Directive 2010/32/EU 2010) on the prevention of sharps injuries to healthcare workers is due to be implemented by European member states by May 2013. The Directive places specific requirements on healthcare organizations to assess the risk of injuries to staff and put measures in place including safety engineered devices to reduce the risk of needestick injuries.

HIV

The most likely method of transmission of HIV to ED staff would be through inoculation of infected blood by a sharps injury or exposure of mucous membranes to blood. This reinforces the need for staff to adhere to the standard precautions. All patients attending an ED should be approached in the same way as far as infection control is concerned. If a nurse suffers a needlestick injury, blood samples for storage and possible testing for HIV antibodies must not be taken from the injured nurse or the source patient without informed consent and pre-test counselling. It is essential that the injured nurse follows local policies and seeks prompt expert advice following an injury so any

necessary post-exposure prophylaxis can be commenced without delay.

Hepatitis B

Hepatitis B has been known to be a problem to healthcare staff for over 20 years, and recently other strains of hepatitis have been identified. Hepatitis B is a stable virus, resistant to common antiseptics, and is therefore highly infectious. Hypochlorite, glutaraldehyde, chlorine and autoclaving at 134°C for a minimum of three minutes are known to destroy the virus (Royal College of Nursing 2000).

In EDs it is most unlikely that there will be any indication that a patient is infected with hepatitis B. It is advisable that all staff are vaccinated with the hepatitis B vaccine in accordance with Department of Health guidance (Department of Health 2007a).

The risk of transmission to a healthcare worker from an infected patient following such an injury has been shown to be around 1 in 3 when a source patient is infected with hepatitis B virus and is 'e' antigen positive, around 1 in 30 when the patient is infected with hepatitis C virus and around 1 in 300 when the patient is infected with HIV (Department of Health 2008).

Although risk of transmission of blood-borne infection from staff to patients is low, there are restrictions on working practice in place for staff that are infected with HIV, hepatitis C RNA-positive or hepatitis B e-antigen positive. Guidelines also require checks on viral loads to be made on healthcare workers who are e-antigen negative and perform exposure prone procedures. Exposure-prone working practices should be restricted, i.e., those where the worker's gloved hands may be in contact with sharp instruments, needle tips and sharp tissues, such as spicules of bone or teeth, inside a patient's open body cavity, wound or confined anatomical space where the hands or fingertips may not be completely visible at all times (Department of Health 2002, 2005, 2007b). It should be noted, however, that this policy is currently under review (Department of Health 2011).

Working Time Directive

It is clear that the organization of work in EDs, which normally provide a 24-hour service, is a factor that can have an impact on the health of staff. Working time had not been covered specifically by health and safety legislation until the European Directive on Working Time was agreed in 1993. The UK introduced regulations to implement the directive in 1998. The Working Time Regulations (1998) phased in the provisions for junior doctors. Since 2009 average working week for junior doctors has been reduced to 48 hours, which brings them in line with nurses. The basic provisions of the directive are outlined in Box 40.6.

All workers are entitled to four weeks paid annual leave. The implementation of the Working Time Directive (EC Directive 93/104/EC 1993) is likely to mean that working patterns and hours of work will be the subject of negotiation between employers and their employees, but the key purpose

Box 40.6

Basic provisions of Working Time Directive

- Entitlement to a rest break of 11 consecutive hours per 24-hour period
- Entitlement to an uninterrupted rest period of at least 24 hours per 7-day period. These provisions may be varied for healthcare workers provided that equivalent compensatory periods of rest are arranged
- Weekly working time including overtime must not exceed 48 hours. This can be averaged out over a period of 17 weeks or longer by agreement
- Normal hours of night work may not exceed an average of 8 hours in any 24-hour period. This can be averaged out over a period of time as agreed through collective bargaining
- Night workers are entitled to a free health assessment prior to starting night work and then at regular intervals
- Night workers suffering from health problems recognized as being connected with the fact that they perform night work are to be transferred to day work wherever possible
- Records of night workers are to be maintained and provided to competent authorities on request

is to ensure that the arrangements do not have a detrimental effect on the health of staff.

Framework for maintaining a safe environment

Health and safety is covered by extensive legislation aimed at producing working environments that are safe for both nurses and patients. The legislation must be translated into practical policies which are known and understood. The main employer must have an overall safety policy but particular areas should have departmental policies which address problems in those areas. In EDs, specific policies may be needed for manual handling, dealing with violence and aggressive behaviour, disposal of clinical waste and infection control. Each member of staff, whether clinical or not, should be clear about her responsibility for health and safety.

Procedures should be defined in the event of any accident taking place, from immediate first aid to the reporting procedures. The policy should specify the consultative arrangements that may exist. Normally this would be a safety committee with management and trade union safety representatives, along with specialist support such as occupational health and safety adviser, infection control and radiation protection adviser. Safety problems that cannot be resolved within the department should be addressed by the safety committee. Regular monitoring, such as health and safety audits, needs to be carried out to ensure that policies and risk assessments are effective.

Violence

In 2003, the National Audit Office carried out a survey examining the impact of violence and aggression in the NHS. This report demonstrated a rising incidence of violence and aggression and made wide-ranging recommendations (National Audit Office 2003b) (see also Chapter 12).

Following this survey, the NHS Security Management Service, now called NHS Protect, was established and given the operational and policy remit for security in the NHS (England) in 2003. It has developed a strategy which is being implemented. The key elements are:

- a national syllabus on conflict resolution. It is intended that all frontline NHS staff should have the opportunity to attend this training
- a national system for reporting physical assaults to the Security Management Service
- the appointment of local security management specialists in every trust with a programme of professional training
- the establishment of a Legal Protection Unit that will advise and support trusts in pursuing private prosecutions of offenders where the police and/or the Crown Prosecution Service take no action (Security Management Service 2003).

Across the UK there are a number of strategies in place to address the risk of violence against nurses and other healthcare workers including the Emergency Workers (Scotland) Act (2005) that makes it a specific offense to assault a nurse or other frontline staff who is delivering emergency care.

In a Royal College of Nursing Survey (2006) on nurses' working environment, nearly eight out of ten nurses working in emergency departments report having been assaulted in the previous 12 months and 95% reported experiencing verbal abuse at some time in their career. Violence is a complex problem with a range of causes, but clearly this is a significant risk in EDs with the potential for interaction with those whose behaviour is influenced by drugs or alcohol. The Management of Health and Safety at Work Regulations 1999 require the application of the risk-control approach to prevent as many incidents as possible by the use of technology such as CCTV, alarm systems, security staff and the design and layout of the environment. Medley et al. (2012) also found a correlation between ED crowding and higher rates of violence towards staff. It is unlikely that all incidents can be prevented, so systems are needed for supporting staff, reporting to the police and ensuring that there is a clear message to the public that violent and aggressive behaviour will not be tolerated.

Stress

The Health and Safety Executive (2005) reported that nurses, particularly in the public sector, are one of the occupation groups with the highest prevalence rates of work-related stress. The management of stress should be approached in the same way as any other health and safety hazard: identify the hazards, assess the risk, implement the control measures and review. The Health and Safety Executive has developed a set of six Stress Management Standards – called dimensions – to identify and tackle work-related stress. If the six dimensions are not properly managed they may become sources of workplace stress. These dimensions are:

- demands – such as workload, working patterns and the working environment
- control – the extent to which individuals can control the way they do their work
- support – level of support from the organization, line managers and colleagues in terms of encouragement, resources
- relationships – such as promoting positive working to avoid conflict and dealing with unacceptable behaviour
- roles – understanding roles within the organization and avoidance of role conflict
- change – management and communication of organizational changes.

The Royal College of Nursing (2006) incorporated these scales into a survey of nurses' working environment and found that nurses working in EDs scored most negatively compared with other groups, indicating that working in this specialty can result in workplace stress. The survey also used a measure of psychological wellbeing, and nurses working in emergency have poorer psychological health scores than those working in other areas of hospitals. Poor staffing levels leading to high workloads are a cause of stress in the nursing workforce (Royal College of Nursing 2010).

Conclusion

Professional competence must now include a positive attitude to health, safety and welfare. High standards of care can only be provided in an environment which is not going to cause harm to the nurse or the patient. Health and safety legislation is developing and is driven by European Directives. Nurses need a good basic knowledge of the statutory requirements and a thorough understanding of how these apply to their own workplace. This has been recognized within the Knowledge and Skills Framework (KSF) that supports Agenda for Change, as health, safety and security constitute one of the core dimensions to be included in every KSF job outline. Principles of health and safety should be incorporated in the culture of the department and not be considered as a separate issue. Managers should be regularly reviewing policies, setting performance standards and reviewing progress. All staff must take responsibility for identifying hazards and taking appropriate action. The majority of accidents are foreseeable and therefore preventable. Accident prevention will reduce costs, both direct and indirect, and will lead to a healthier, more productive workforce.

Acknowledgement

This chapter is dedicated to the memory of Sheelagh Brewer who authored this chapter in the first two editions of this textbook.

References

Clough, J., 1998. Assessing and controlling risk. Nursing Standard 12 (31), 49–54.

Control of Substances Hazardous to Health Regulations. 1988. HMSO, London.

Control of Substances Hazardous to Health Regulations. 2002. HMSO, London.

Department of Health, 2002. Hepatitis C Infected Healthcare Workers. Department of Health, London.

Department of Health, 2005. HIV Infected Healthcare Workers. Department of Health, London.

Department of Health, 2007a. Immunisation Against Infectious Disease. Department of Health, London.

Department of Health, 2007b. Hepatitis B Infected Healthcare Workers and Antiviral Therapy. Department of Health, London.

Department of Health, 2008. HIV Post Exposure Prophylaxis: Guidance from the UK Chief Medical Officers' Expert Advisory Group on AIDS. Department of Health, London.

Department of Health, 2009. NHS Health and Wellbeing Review – Final Report. Department of Health [Lead Reviewer: Dr. S. Boorman], London.

Department of Health, 2011. Management of HIV-infected healthcare workers: A consultation paper. Department of Health, London.

EC Directive 89/391/EEC Council Directive of the 12th June 1989 on the Introduction of Measures to Encourage Improvements in the Safety and Health of Workers at Work. 1989. EC, Luxembourg.

EC Directive 92/85 EEC Pregnant Workers Directive. 1992. EC, Luxembourg.

EC Directive 93/104/EC Concerning Certain Aspects of the Organisation of Working Time. 1993. EC, Luxembourg.

EC Directive 2010/32/EU Implementing the Framework Agreement on prevention from sharp injuries in the hospital and healthcare sector concluded by HOSPEEM and EPSU. 2010. EC, Luxemburg.

Emergency Workers (Scotland) Act, 2005. HMSO, London.

Employment Rights Act, 1996. HMSO, London.

European Union, 1986. Single European Act. EC, Luxembourg.

Health and Safety Executive, 1992a. Manual Handling Operations Regulations Guidance on Regulations L23. HMSO, London.

Health and Safety Executive, 1992b. Display Screen Equipment Work Guidance on Regulations L26. HMSO, London.

Health and Safety Executive, 1992c. Personal Protective Equipment at Work Guidance on Regulations L25. HMSO, London.

Health and Safety Executive, 1992d. Work Equipment Guidance on Regulations L22. HMSO, London.

Health and Safety Executive, 1992e. Workplace Guidance on Regulations. HMSO, London.

Health and Safety Executive, 1993. The Costs of Accidents at Work. Health & Safety series booklet HS(G) 96. HMSO, London.

Health and Safety Executive, 2000. Management of Health and Safety at Work Regulations 1999 Approved Code of Practice and Regulations Legal Series L21. HSE Books, Sudbury.

Health and Safety Executive, 2005. Working Together to Reduce Stress at Work. HSE Books, London.

Health and Safety Executive, 2006. Five Steps to Risk Assessment. HSE Books, London.

Health and Safety at Work etc. Act. 1974. HMSO, London.

Health and Safety (First Aid) Regulations, 1981. HMSO, London.

Health Protection Agency, 2008. Eye of the Needle – Surveillance of Significant Occupational Exposure to Blood Borne Viruses in Healthcare Workers. HPA, London.

Lynch, A., Cole, E., 2006. Human factors in emergency care: the need for team resource management. Emergency Nurse 14 (2), 32–35.

Medley, D.B., Morris, J.E., Stone, K., et al., 2012. An association between occupancy rates in the Emergency Department and rates of violence towards staff. Journal of Emergency Medicine 42 (4), 736–744.

National Audit Office, 2003a. A Safer Place to Work: Improving the Management of Health and Safety Risks to Staff in NHS Trusts. The Stationery Office, London.

National Audit Office, 2003b. A Safer Place to Work: Protecting NHS Hospital and Ambulance Staff from Violence and Aggression. The Stationery Office, London.

NHS Employers, 2009. Back In Work – Introduction and Key Messages. NHS Employers, London.

Nursing and Midwifery Council, 2008. The NMC Code of Professional Conduct: Standards for Conduct, Performance and Ethics. NMC, London.

Reporting of Injuries, Diseases and Dangerous Occurrences Regulations, 1995. HMSO, London.

Royal College of Nursing, 2000. Is There an Alternative to Gluteraldehyde? RCN, London.

Royal College of Nursing, 2006. At Breaking Point? A Survey of the Wellbeing and Working Lives of Nurses in 2005. RCN, London.

Royal College of Nursing, 2010. Guidance on safe nurse staffing levels in the UK. RCN, London.

Royal College of Nursing, 2012. Essential Practice for Infection Prevention and Control: Guidance for Nursing Staff. London, RCN.

Safety Representatives and Safety Committees Regulations (1977) London: HMSO.

Security Management Service, 2003. A Professional Approach to Managing Security. Department of Health, London.

UK Health Departments, 1998. Guidance for Clinical Health Care Workers: Protection Against Infection with Blood-borne Viruses. HMSO, London.

Working Time Regulations, 1998. (SI 1998 No. 1833). The Stationery Office, London.

Managing issues of culture and power in the ED

Sandra Richardson and Tracey Williams

41

CHAPTER CONTENTS

Introduction

This chapter looks at issues of power, diversity and the role of culture in the provision of nursing care in the Emergency Department (ED) environment. Emergency nurses are faced with a diverse population group; patients are representative of the wider multicultural society and there is no clearly defined 'best response' that will work in all situations. While the clinical expertise and practice of nurses continues to develop, there also needs to be an awareness of the importance of developing skills in assessing and managing socio-cultural contributors to patient presentations. This impacts on the ability to establish an effective nurse–patient relationship, and within healthcare the failure to acknowledge diversity and cultural needs can adversely impact on patient outcomes. Nurses have often been described as an 'oppressed group', yet nurses also hold considerable power, and the exercise of this power can potentially benefit or marginalize those directly affected (Dolan 2001, Dong & Temple 2011). Understanding culture, diversity and the use of nursing power is particularly relevant in the ED as patients and families are particularly vulnerable, often feeling anxious, fearful and uncertain. For many, there is no option or alternative for seeking care, and this alone creates a sense of 'power over' and loss of control for the patient (Malterud 2010). If care is not provided in a respectful and responsive way, this can ultimately lead to patient disengagement from the wider health system. The role of the emergency nurse has considerable significance and impact in assisting the patient to adapt to the hospital environment and to maintain their cultural integrity.

Defining culture and acknowledging diversity

Discussing culture, whether at an academic or clinical level is both challenging and potentially threatening. For many individuals, the specifics of cultural understanding are associated with emotional and social responses, and influenced by the individual's personal life experiences. Attempts to define culture have varied over time, between and within societies. While the concept of culture can be seen as an 'unstable metaphorical construct more or less open to differential analysis and transformation' (Leitch 1992), it also 'provides a recognisable symbol of the general and identifiable traits associated with particular sub groups in society' (Richardson 2004).

Culture is a broad term, and not limited to discussion of ethnicity. It includes elements such as individual and group values, social roles, taboos and beliefs. Clinicians therefore must understand the complexities of ethnicity and culture, its role in the life of each patient and its potential impact on one's understanding of and ability to treat patients effectively (Hickling 2012). One framework for recognizing the range of diversity is outlined in the cultural safety model's categories of difference (Box 41.1). Cultural diversity has been shown to impact on a patient's involvement with the health system, including their ability to access services and the type of diagnosis and treatment offered (Celik et al. 2008). Differences in patient presentations related to age, ethnicity and gender have been linked to particular conditions, one example being the variance in signs and symptoms associated with acute coronary

Box 41.1

Identifying aspects of cultural diversity

One framework for identifying areas of cultural diversity identifies the following eight categories, while noting that culture is not limited to these:

- Age or generation
- Sexuality
- Migrant status
- Ethnicity
- Occupational and socioeconomic status
- Religious or spiritual belief
- Gender

(After Nursing Council of New Zealand (2009) Guidelines for Cultural Safety, the Treaty of Waitangi, and Maori Health in Nursing Education and Practice. Wellington, New Zealand: Nursing Council of New Zealand.)

syndrome (Pezzin et al. 2007, Bosner et al. 2009). As well as variation in the type and range of patient-reported symptoms, differences have also been identified in the response of nursing and medical staff to individuals presenting with similar conditions (Takakuwa et al. 2006, Brown & Furyk 2009).

An individual, whether nurse or patient, may identify with more than one culture, and these can change in terms of priority and influence in response to internal and external forces. Nurses have traditionally sought to provide care 'regardless' of difference, assuming that the provision of a single standard of care, if set at an appropriate level, will result in 'best practice'. Similarly, the old adage often given is to provide the treatment that 'we would like to be given to our own relative/mother/child'. This assumes that the standard of care appropriate to one individual or within one culture is necessarily the best for all members of society. The presumption here is that, on one level, everyone is the same and that this sameness represents the ideal, which is usually the mainstream of society. For nurses, the assumption is often that the culture of healthcare is the most desirable, that patients should be compliant and responsive to directives, because they are presented in their best interests. When expressed bluntly like this, the paternalism is clear – the expert knowledge of healthcare is presumed to give the practitioner the ability to determine what is best for the patient, often overlooking the patient's expert knowledge of 'self'. The tendency is for nurses, and other health professionals, to integrate this approach at a subconscious level, rather than as a result of a deliberate decision-making process. Yet treating everyone the same does not guarantee an acceptable standard of practice. The care that one individual values may not be desirable or even acceptable within another culture. Rather than seeking to provide care 'regardless' of difference, it may be more appropriate to consider how to provide care 'regardful' of what makes people unique.

For emergency nurses, the benefits of recognizing and responding to cultural difference can be seen in improved ability to anticipate problems, recognize non-typical patient responses and become more responsive to individual needs. This has flow-on effects in terms of efficiency and effective use of time and the ability to defuse potential conflict. Patients who present to the ED do so for a variety of reasons,

and their attitudes and expectations towards care are similarly varied. Many of these patients appear agitated, aggressive, uncooperative or actively disruptive. While physiological responses can account for some behaviours, others appear socially inappropriate and can trigger negative responses from nurses and others attempting to care for them. Many emergency nurses thrive on the excitement and adrenaline rush associated with managing trauma and other life-threatening occurrences; dealing with non-urgent patient presentations can at times seem less worthy of time and resources. Whether this is an acknowledged response, often evident in the use of pejorative terms to describe certain groups of patients, or a more subconscious reaction, this can impact on patient care.

Nurses are expected to be non-judgmental, to uphold universal standards and to do so in a calm and conscientious manner. Yet nurses are also expected to make judgements, to prioritize care and to ration the use of resources in all aspects of clinical practice. Rather than simply labelling a patient as 'non-compliant' or 'difficult', nurses can seek to identify the areas of difference between their own expectations and those of the individual receiving care. The patient who sits sullen and unresponsive may not intend to be obstructive; without knowing what their previous experiences with hospitals, the health system and figures of authority has been, it is difficult to know how this may have impacted their behaviour. It may be that a physical impairment such as deafness or difficulty with language or understanding has led to a sense of isolation and frustration. It may be that the patient is simply so focused on other things, such as the circumstances that led them to present, concern about family and friends or fear of disclosing information related to their health and personal circumstances that this has resulted in the appearance of non-cooperation or aggression. While the potential causative factors are many, the risk remains the same. Nurses need to ensure that commonly encountered factors such as workload, patient acuity and other pressures do not impact their ability to assess a given situation. Failure to do so risks introducing assumptions and treatment based on misconceptions. An effective way to understand what is happening in a given situation is by asking the patient, and doing so in a manner that encourages the individual to feel safe in sharing relevant information. In an increasingly busy workplace it is important to find the time to reflect on practice and identify the unspoken moral judgements that are made.

Stereotyping, stigma and discrimination

The Oxford English Dictionary defines stereotype as 'a widely held but fixed and oversimplified image or idea of a particular type of person or thing' and cites as examples the stereotypes of women as carers and other racial and gender stereotypes. Stereotypes act like codes that give audiences a quick, common understanding of a person or group of people – usually relating to their class, ethnicity or race, gender, sexual orientation, social role or occupation. They are based on assumptions and generalizations about individuals and groups, and can be either positive or negative. There are certainly stereotypes present within the health system, and specific examples within the ED setting. These can have a positive impact, and at times are actively used to aid in recognition of conditions and to influence diagnoses. The constellation of signs and symptoms typically associated with myocardial infarction, support emergency nurses in the recognition of the patient with chest pain. However stereotypes can also perpetuate inaccurate and often damaging assumptions. They typically rely on reductionist, simplistic categorizations and can be used to exert power over marginalized groups. Use of stereotypes can result in expressions of social prejudice and tacit endorsement of inequalities in access to and availability of healthcare.

Whereas stereotypes can be either favourable or unfavourable, stigma relates to negative labelling that identifies some individuals as being less worthy than others (Feeg 2009). Common examples of stigmatization within healthcare include attitudes expressed towards people experiencing mental health issues, infectious and sexually transmitted diseases and self-inflicted injuries. Within the emergency care setting, typical patient groups for whom stigma can develop include those patients who are perceived as time-wasters, who exhibit drug-seeking or self-harm behaviours, present with non-urgent conditions or who are frequent attenders. Many of these patient groups are presumed to use a disproportionate or inappropriate amount of the limited resources available within the ED and to impact negatively on the acute care needs of others. Presumptions are also made around health and self-care behaviours that are seen as contributing to disease states, such as smoking, alcohol-related illnesses, and non-compliance with recommended treatments and medication regimens.

Discrimination occurs when one person is treated differently to another in the same or similar circumstances. Discrimination is not always illegal and at times is deliberately implemented in an effort to address issues of equity. Oppression, discrimination and marginalization have been associated with increased health risk amongst populations rendered vulnerable because of social deprivation, prejudice and violence. These vulnerable populations are also over-represented in the ED patient mix. Specific health-related conditions have been associated with marginalization and discrimination, such as obesity, mental illness and disability (Joachim & Acorn 2000, Latner et al. 2007, Verhaeghe et al. 2007, Bejciy-Spring 2008). Discrimination can result from prejudice that is triggered by personal responses to patient characteristics and imposed stereotypes. This has significance for the emergency nurse in that it can influence practice in conscious and unconscious ways, and affect the quality of care given.

A number of studies have linked variation in assessment and treatment of pain to presumptions and cultural stereotypes (Epps et al. 2008, Naryan, 2010). Rather than relying on generic expectations of pain behaviour linked to ethnicity or socio-cultural identification, it is important to acknowledge the significance of the pain experience to the individual. Chen et al. (2008) examined gender disparity in relation to the tendency to under analgise ED patients presenting with acute abdominal pain. This study identified that even when patients presented with similar symptoms and gave similar pain scores, women were consistently less likely to receive opioid analgesia and to wait longer for pain relief to be administered. Other examples include studies showing links to longer waiting times in EDs associated with ethnicity (Pines 2009) and health disparities associated with religious affiliation (Laird et al. 2007). Bias and assumption regarding some patient conditions and disease processes have been associated with the likelihood of receiving timely care. Dutch et al. (2008) found that descriptions of presenting complaints given at triage can lead to identification and avoidance of less desirable patients by emergency physicians. Emergency nurses have an ethical and professional duty of care and need to recognize and react to evidence of discrimination, and to reflect on aspects of their own practice that may involve unconscious expressions of marginalization.

Stereotypes are not only applied to patients; a number of assumptions are also made about the role and personal characteristics of nurses. These impact on the way in which patients, relatives and other health professionals view nursing as a profession and nurses as individuals. Misconceptions about the role of the nurse within the wider healthcare team can affect collegial relationships and expectations relating to authority, independence and autonomy in practice. Hierarchical structures remain in many health services and the nursing voice can at times be marginalized and the ability to act as a patient advocate impeded.

The culture of nursing

The profession of nursing has its own culture and associated cultural values and beliefs that guide practice. Nursing culture has been described as '…the learned and transmitted lifeways, values, symbols, patterns, and normative practices of members of the nursing profession of a particular society' (Leininger 1994). An understanding of nursing culture is important as it allows for the dissemination of core values, recognition of nursing assumptions and clarification of nursing ideologies and goals. Cultural values associated with nursing typically encompass concepts such as caring, respect for patient rights, autonomy and dignity alongside practice fundamentals such as quality improvement and use of an evidential base. More clinically orientated norms include beliefs around topics such as pain management and the patient role. Emergency nursing has its own specific values and clinical expectations. Personal and practice attributes that are valued include efficiency, flexibility, creativity and the ability to respond to rapidly changing and often stressful situations. Emergency nurses are expected to be leaders, to hold a range of knowledge, to show expert assessment and analytic skills and to act as a cohesive force in combining the input from a range of specialties. Cultural responses common in emergency nursing that might not be acceptable within wider society include the use of 'black humour' as a response to critical, traumatic or otherwise distressing incidents. While recognizing the value of this in debriefing and coping with stress, the ED nurse needs to reflect and recognize when this moves from being a defence mechanism to a genuine expression of bias or discrimination.

A number of different models of care seek to address issues of cultural and social difference. Many of these are influenced by understandings of power and draw on elements of Critical Social Theory, an approach that challenged the traditional assumptions around truth, power and knowledge. Recognition of the significance of knowledge formation and application is linked to notions of empowerment, enlightenment and emancipation. Applying these principles to emergency nursing encourages self-reflection and recognition of judgements based on unexamined beliefs, values and attitudes. There is emphasis on recognizing the significance of context and individual circumstances rather than relying on generic understandings of health and illness.

Models that address issues of culture in nursing include transcultural nursing, cultural sensitivity, cultural competence and cultural safety. Williamson (2010) suggests that these approaches follow two principal paths; the first of these focuses on learning about elements of culture such as values, beliefs, and traditions that are identified and categorized according to a specifically defined cultural group, often determined by language or location. However, assuming that a set of attributes apply to all members within a group risks perpetuating cultural stereotypes. These approaches are based on learning about other cultures, identifying key characteristics or preferred patterns of care associated with each specific, defined culture. This can result in a checklist approach to cultural knowledge that presumes that all members of a cultural group hold a similar intensity and range of beliefs and values. This presumes a degree of stasis within cultures and minimizes the ability to look for and respond to individual variation. In seeking to learn about the 'other', there is also a risk that the culture of the individual nurse becomes positioned as the norm, and those with different cultural identities by default are seen as deviating from the mainstream or social ideal.

A second approach looks to position cultural understanding within a wider framework, looking at issues such as the social construction of health, racism, power and oppression. These approaches are often linked to discussions around colonization, indigenous health needs and socio-political underpinnings. Criticisms of this approach focus on the difficulty of defining core features and evaluating its impact in practice (Johnstone & Kanitsaki 2007, Williamson & Harrison 2010).

Whichever type of approach is used, emergency nurses need to be consciously aware of the presumptions and judgements they and others are making. The use of techniques such as structured reflection, debriefing, case review and clinical supervision can all assist in identifying and where necessary altering patterns of response.

Expressions of power

The structure of nursing has been influenced by its historical origins that contributed to the development of formal role delineation and expression of status through use of uniforms and titles. Uniforms offer outward symbolism and are representative of the power underpinning nursing culture. The presence of uniforms can create an artificial barrier that has the potential to impact on personal, collegial and organizational relationships, whether this is acknowledged by the individual practitioner or not. The uniform can be seen as an intimidatory tool, sending a subconscious signal that has both positive and negative connotations in the healthcare setting. However, for many people, the uniform is easily identifiable, reassuring and recognizable. It signals authority, control and competence and as such can be seen as a clear representation of professionalism.

Emergency nurses hold considerable power, although this is often unrecognized and unacknowledged. Nurses have at times portrayed a victim mentality, describing themselves as an oppressed group. While stereotypes such as 'doctor's handmaiden' do tend to support this view, emergency nurses exercise considerable power and control over the patient environment, physical interactions and access to knowledge. Emergency nurses act as gatekeepers, mediating access to medical staff, resources and at times restricting family access and freedom of movement. By taking the time to reassure, explain and involve patients and their families, emergency nurses can share their power and reduce the sense of cultural distress that often follows entry to the health system.

Power and empowerment are concepts familiar to most nurses. There is an assumption that nurses actively seek to advocate for patients, and theories focusing on the role of the nurse-patient relationship and the goal of empowering patients to maximize their health status are well recorded (Chambers & Thompson 2009). The suggestion has been made that before being able to empower others, nurses need to empower themselves and their profession, with subsequent benefit in terms of improved clinical practice, patient and staff satisfaction and professional development. Donahue et al. (2008) identified a correlation between a nurse's own sense of empowerment in the work setting and patient satisfaction, suggesting that there are tangible benefits in terms of patient care from developing a context that values and empowers healthcare practitioners.

While patients can be seen as a potentially oppressed group, they can also be supported in gaining and expressing power (Dong & Temple 2011). This can be through acknowledgment of concepts such as the 'expert patient' that recognizes that while individuals may not have expertise in terms of nursing or medical knowledge they are often experts in their own right. This has been seen particularly in relation to the management of chronic conditions, with the expert patient defined as one who has 'the confidence, skills, information and knowledge to play a central role in the management of life with chronic diseases' (Department of Health 2001). While this may seem to embody the core concepts identified within healthcare, the practice reality can often see a less positive response. Despite the rhetoric of patient autonomy, it is often easier for nurses and other healthcare practitioners to act in a more directive, paternalistic manner and informed patients can be seen as less responsive and compliant. The reality of overcrowded EDs can see the emergence of a culture that values unquestioning acceptance of healthcare directives and the emergence of more limited interactions between nurses and patients. Power can be exerted as much through acts of omission as through concrete actions and nurses can generate and experience both active and passive expressions of power. Patients also express and utilize power in a number

Box 41.2

Skills toolbox for recognizing and responding to socio-cultural issues

- Critical thinking
- Clinical frameworks
- Reflective practice
- Case review
- Clinical supervision
- Debriefing activities

Box 41.3

Practice tips

- Care for patients regardful rather than regardless of difference
- Acknowledge the individual
- Do not assume all members of a particular culture hold the same beliefs or choose to express them in the same way

of ways. This can be passively through withdrawal of support, compliance or engagement with the healthcare process or actively through expressions of aggression, threats of complaint or demanding recognition of patient rights and care standards.

Implications for practice

The ED setting is one of constant change, with emergency nurses needing to be alert to potential complications, alterations in patient acuity and reactive to fluctuations in patient flow. Acknowledgement of the potential implications of culture and power in the ED can help maintain both nurse and patient safety. Techniques and skills that aid in this include use of clinical frameworks that provide 'trigger' questions around aspects of culture, the development of critical thinking skills, willingness to question one's own and others practice, and the application of critical reflection into clinical practice (Boxes 41.2 and 41.3).

Awareness of culture and power within the ED setting can be actively encouraged by senior staff, managers and institutional policy. Creating an environment within the ED that encourages questioning, participation in decision-making and which values the patient contributes to the ability of the individual nurse to practice in an effective professional manner. Recognition of unspoken concerns and potential issues can be

achieved by raising the index of suspicion, incorporating active strategies for identifying socio-cultural forces and anticipating their implications. This allows the nurse to be proactive and to minimize complication, defusing situations and supporting patients and their families/significant others.

Conclusion

It is necessary for emergency nurses to understand what is happening in terms of culture and power within the healthcare interaction, as this can impact on the range and scope of care provided. Direct implications include those that are primarily centred on the nurse, including risk of burnout, moral distress and horizontal violence (Rowe & Sherlock 2003, Hutchinson et al. 2008, Hughes & Clancy 2009). The practice implications in terms of nursing care include unconscious endorsement and support of racism, culturally based discrimination and variations in care based on value judgements rather than medical need. Aspects that are centred on the patient include recognition of the impact that societal discrimination, bias and stereotyping can have in terms of care standards, access and equity of healthcare. These can lead to patients disengaging from the health system, failing to seek care in a timely manner and receiving inadequate or unprofessional care.

Failure to recognize and reflect on the inherent power struggles in nursing practice places both the nurse and patient at risk. To maximize optimum patient outcomes and role satisfaction of nurses in their professional practice may require an adjustment between theoretical ideals and the realities of the ED setting.

References

Bejciy-Spring, S.M., 2008. R-E-S-P-E-C-T: A model for the sensitive treatment of the bariatric patient. Bariatric Nursing and Surgical Patient Care 3 (1), 47–56.

Bosner, S., Haasenritter, J., Hani, M., et al., 2009. Gender differences in presentation and diagnosis of chest pain in primary care. BMC Family Practice 10 (1), 79.

Brown, R., Furyk, J., 2009. Racial disparities in health care: Emergency department management of minor head injury. International Journal of Emergency Medicine 2 (3), 161–166.

Celik, H., Abma, T.A., Widdershoven, G.A., et al., 2008. Implementation of diversity in healthcare practices: Barriers and opportunities. Patient Education and Counselling 71 (1), 65–71.

Chambers, D., Thompson, S., 2009. Empowerment and its application in health promotion in acute care settings: nurses' perceptions. Journal of Advanced Nursing 65 (1), 130–138.

Chen, E.H., Shofer, F.S., Dean, A.J., et al., 2008. Gender disparity in analgesic treatment of emergency department patients with acute abdominal pain. Academic Emergency Medicine 15 (5), 414–418.

Department of Health, 2001. The Expert Patient: A New Approach to Chronic Disease Management in The 21st Century. Stationery Office, London.

Dolan, B., 2001. Diffusive attitudes in care. Emergency Nurse 9 (1), 1.

Donahue, M.O., Piazza, I.M., Griffin, M.Q., et al., 2008. The relationship between nurses' perceptions of empowerment and patient satisfaction. Applied Nursing Research 21 (1), 2–7.

Dong, D., Temple, B., 2011. Oppression: A concept analysis and implications for nurses and nursing. Nursing Forum 46 (3), 169–176.

Dutch, M.J., Taylor, D., Dent, A.W., 2008. Triage presenting complaint descriptors bias emergency department waiting times. Academic Emergency Medicine 15 (8), 731–735.

Epps, C.D., Ware, L.J., Packard, A., 2008. Ethnic wait time differences in analgesic administration in the emergency department. Pain Management Nursing 9 (1), 26–32.

Feeg, D., 2009. Stigma: Subtle poison with underestimated potency. Pediatric Nursing 35 (5), 267.

Hickling, F.W., 2012. Understanding patients in multicultural settings: a personal reflection on ethnicity and culture in clinical practice. Ethnicity & Health 17 (1-2), 203–216.

Hughes, R.G., Clancy, C.M., 2009. Complexity, bullying, and stress: Analyzing and mitigating a challenging work environment for nurses. Journal of Nursing Care Quality 24 (3), 180–183.

Hutchinson, M., Jackson, D., Wilkes, L., et al., 2008. A new model of bullying in the nursing workplace: Organizational characteristics as critical antecedents. Advances in Nursing Science 31 (2), E60–E71.

Joachim, G., Acorn, S., 2000. Stigma of visible and invisible chronic conditions. Journal of Advanced Nursing 32 (1), 243–248.

Johnstone, M.J., Kanitsaki, O., 2007. An exploration of the notion and nature of the construct of cultural safety and its applicability to the Australian health care context. Journal of Transcultural Nursing 18 (3), 247–256.

Laird, L.D., Amer, M.M., Barnett, E.D., 2007. Muslim patients and health disparities in the UK and the US. Archives of Disease in Childhood 92 (10), 922–926.

Latner, J.D., Rosewall, J.K., Simmonds, M.B., 2007. Childhood obesity stigma: Association with television, videogame, and magazine exposure. Body Image 4 (2), 147–155.

Leininger, M., 1994. The tribes of nursing in the USA culture of nursing. Journal of Transcultural Nursing 6 (1), 18–22.

Leitch, V.B., 1992. Cultural Criticism, Literary Theory, Poststructuralism. Columbia University Press, New York.

Malterud, K., 2010. Power inequalities in health care: Empowerment revisited. Patient Education & Counseling 79 (2), 139–140.

Narayan, M.C., 2010. Culture's effects on pain assessment and management. American Journal of Nursing 110 (4), 38–47.

Nursing Council of New Zealand, 2009. Guidelines for Cultural Safety, the Treaty of Waitangi, and Maori Health in Nursing Education and Practice. Nursing Council of New Zealand, Wellington, New Zealand.

Pezzin, L.E., Keyl, P.M., Green, G.B., 2007. Disparities in the emergency department evaluation of chest pain patients. Academic Emergency Medicine 14 (2), 149–156.

Pines, J.M., 2009. Racial disparities in emergency department length of stay for admitted patients in the United States. Academic Emergency Medicine 16 (5), 403–410.

Richardson, S., 2004. Aoteaoroa/New Zealand nursing: from eugenics to cultural safety. Nursing Inquiry 11 (1), 35–42.

Rowe, M.M., Sherlock, H., 2003. Stress and verbal abuse in nursing: do burned out nurses eat their young? Journal of Nursing Management 13 (3), 242–248.

Takakuwa, K.M., Shofer, F.S., Hollander, J.E., 2006. The influence of race and gender on time to initial electrocardiogram for patients with chest pain. Academic Emergency Medicine 13 (8), 867–872.

Verhaeghe, M., Bracke, P., Bruynooghe, K., 2007. Stigmatization in different mental health services: a comparison of psychiatric and general hospitals. The Journal of Behavioral Health Services and Research 34 (2), 186–197.

Williamson, M., Harrison, 2010. Providing culturally appropriate care: a literature review. International Journal of Nursing Studies 47 (6), 761–769.

Creating patient flow

42

Richard Hamilton, Brian Dolan and Michael Ardagh

This book is dedicated to the improvement of individuals' clinical and professional skills in emergency care. For some time now all the authors have been studying and working in wide-scale health system reforms and this work has exposed us to a wealth of knowledge that has enabled us to reconsider how we best serve communities of health need (Dolan & Hawes 2009, Ardagh et al. 2011). We realize now that in healthcare we have a responsibility as health practitioners beyond the patient in front of us right now; we have a responsibility to the patient in the waiting room, arriving in the ambulance, and to the patient who may not know they will shortly be on their way to the Emergency Department (ED). In other words, ensuring we are ready to handle the next patient that comes through the door in the same way we manage the patient in front of us right now, no matter how busy it gets.

This chapter introduces the key concepts of patient flow and how this impacts on both the immediate work environment and the journey of the patient seeking care. It introduces some of the techniques used in manufacturing and service industries and its application to health systems. This is by no means a comprehensive study of methods and tools, but an introduction to some key concepts and should act as a guide in the journey to making not just the patient but the health system better.

Health system environments

Health systems have not evolved significantly in the way they are organized in the last 100 years. New technology, bigger, brighter and more welcoming buildings and new clinical techniques mask what essentially is an industry that has kept its Victorian design into a new millennium. Just like craftsman-type industries prior to the 20th century industrial revolution in manufacturing techniques, health is a collection of inter-related cottage industries (Swensen et al. 2010). Every clinical service can be compared to a craft-based business of old, where highly specialized individuals within a particular clinical specialty deliver specialist knowledge and techniques. A hospital is often like a large mall full of specialist businesses to which a patient is sent for expert assessment. As a result the patient gets passed from service to service, from cottage industry to cottage industry, during the course of their care and treatment.

The organization and leadership of hospital resources further exposes this sense of passing the patient from one process area to another. Figure 42.1 highlights how a hospital setting is a matrix of services attempting to get patient outcomes via a series of functional business areas that are vertical silos. Traditionally, the management model of hospital systems has focused on managing the functional business units, or the vertical slices of the patient journey, often as discrete businesses. Each functional business unit is charged with being as efficient as possible with the resources they are given, where the resources are usually monetary based. In this way each independent business is seeking to maximize the use of its resources to achieve either more revenue, reduce costs or higher utilization of resources. These functional business units serve many different clinical specialities whose needs can be very different and competing; therefore, by default, they create their own rules and business practices that may not align with the other functional business units.

http://dx.doi.org/10.1016/B978-0-7020-4315-4.00042-5

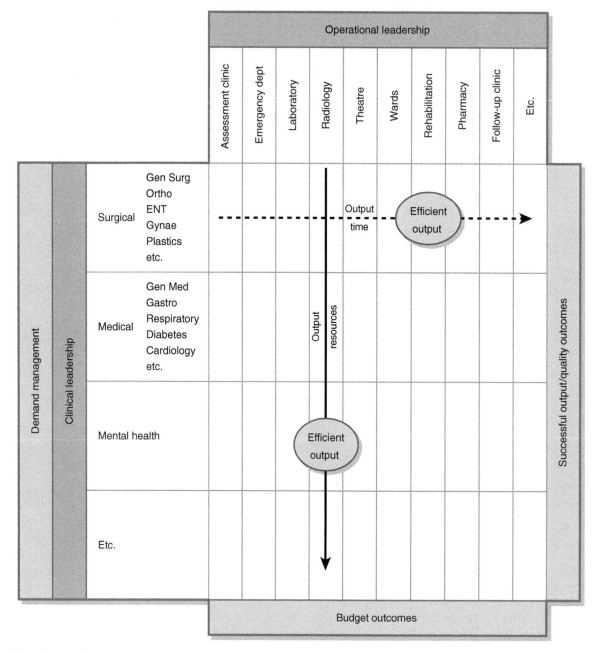

Figure 42.1 ● Matrix of healthcare.

In the clinical service context (the horizontal slice), they are looking to move patients through the functional areas at a regular rate. The clinical services must meet the patient demand on their service and navigate the patient through each of the functional business units to create the right patient outcome.

This process can be very frustrating and disempowering for the clinical teams. The response can be to shrug one's shoulders and say 'that's how it's done around here'. Again each clinical service creates its own way of responding to the pressures on its service. So, while surgeons may take a long time to appear in the ED and make prompt decisions about patient admissions, physicians may be prompt in arrival but take an apparently protracted time to make a decision to admit. From a patient perspective there is an equally large variation in response and service in this type of environment. No two clinical events will be the same from a patient perspective,

even when they attend regularly with the same presenting symptoms.

This traditional approach to hospital and specialist care creates a focus on episodic care rather than holistic care of the patient. How do we view this system with a fresh perspective?

Patient time

Health systems operate as complex supply chains where the goal is to achieve timely and appropriate outcomes for the population's needs. Where manufacturing systems are moving inventory and parts around the world to wholesalers and assembly plants; health systems are managing time – patients' time. Where Toyota is concerned about limiting its inventory to the next few hours of production as a way to reduce the time from paying suppliers to being paid by product buyers (Womack & Jones 1996), the health system has a focus on reducing the time a patient spends in the health system from the start of a health issue to the time the issue is resolved. In many respects, patient time is the health system equivalent of inventory.

Why is patient time so important?

Hospital systems can be likened to large warehouses of a supply chain where instead of storing parts and products like a manufacturing business, we are storing patients. Patients are stored in waiting rooms, cubicles, clinic rooms, beds, trollies, wards and discharge lounges; indeed, we even store them in their own home; with the home being the default waiting place for most patients on 'waiting' lists. A lot of the patient's time in the health system is spent waiting; waiting for appointments, assessment, diagnostics, the next decision, clinical intervention, admission/discharge, etc. Some of the patient's time in a health system is necessary such as waiting for a therapeutic response to treatment, but much of the patient's time is wasted. Practitioners see these waits and delays, but become inured to them as we are always busy and having to prioritize our time where it can best be spent.

As a result, the health system has been inadvertently designed around staff needs, where staff are considered a precious and scarce resource that needs to be optimized. In some health systems staff are seen as a high cost so resource time must be optimized.

But what about the patient's time, does that not have value as well? Imagine you are 81 years old and have just been advised that you need a hip replacement but cannot be seen for another six months, how would you feel knowing, on average, you probably only have another 24 months of life left. Time becomes very precious and the quality of time even more so. You do not want to be spending the latter years of your life in a hospital or at home on a waiting list, waiting for something to happen to you.

In the movie The Bucket List, Jack Nicolson and Morgan Freeman play two men, brought together in hospital, living on borrowed time, who are determined to live the last days as if they were the first. They remind the viewer of how precious time is, especially in the twilight years of life. So in a patient-focused health system, patient time and quality of life are guiding principles to system design. There are other reasons why patient time is such an important metric to the efficiency of any health system.

How Lean Thinking principles value time

Over 40 years, Toyota Motor Company has developed the Toyota Production System using techniques that are known more widely as Lean Thinking (Womack & Jones 1996, Stone 2012). Lean Thinking is a culture focused on delivering the most value with the least waste, for the end consumer (Liker & Convis 2011, Kaplan 2012). It has been designed to support complex supply chains, focusing on:

- 'just-in-time' (JIT) delivery of products thus minimizing storage space

- error-proofing processes, thereby minimizing waste and delays due to poor parts
- continuously eliminating excessive product movement/handling to create the fewest steps, therefore lessening the chance of errors (Westwood et al. 2007).

Staff in a Lean Thinking environment understand the importance of time and quality and the role they play in the supply chain. The goals of Lean Thinking are simple but intuitive and are based on a set of values where time is considered the most precious. The time it takes from paying suppliers and being paid by the consumer for the end product; or the time a patient spends in the health system.

The focus behind this philosophy is to keep inventory levels low, as the more parts sitting around in the supply chain the greater the cost of production and the longer the time it will take for the part to add value to an end product that the consumer will buy. The larger the number of parts in the system the bigger the warehouses we need to store them, therefore the more people needed to manage the warehouses and therefore the more money tied up earning no value for the shareholder; the risk of parts being scrapped goes up as well. This is the key driver of Lean Thinking; reducing the materials, effort and lead time required to produce a product that the customer is willing to pay for.

In patient terms, the longer patients wait, the more staff effort is involved, bigger waiting rooms are required, poorer quality of care can result. There is a direct correlation between waiting times in EDs and increased morbidity and mortality (Ardagh & Richardson 2004, Richardson 2006, Sprivulis et al. 2006, Richardson & Mountain 2009, Johnson et al. 2012, Mahler et al. 2012). Industry has much more to teach healthcare than we sometimes imagine, as it has addressed metaphorically similar issues many years ago. To achieve this focus Toyota recognized the contribution of staff, and in particular they recognized and valued frontline staff as long-term partners that learn, adapt and empower improvements. Managers and leaders in Toyota are driven to value frontline staff and their time; with particular emphasis on removing barriers to staff creating more value. Having staff spend time on producing a part that is not needed now, it may be needed but not now, is seen as disrespectful of the staff's time; the work has added no value (Liker & Franz 2011). Having staff skills and capabilities under-utilized is also considered disrespectful of staff time, i.e., the time they have invested in developing these skills.

Lean Thinking during the first decade of the new millennium has been adopted widely by health systems and is increasingly recognized for its potential to transform individual business processes (Baker & Taylor 2009, Millard 2011, Stone 2012). The true value and opportunity is where the tools of Lean Thinking are applied across the health system, across the patient's journey, where the patient is a substitute for inventory in a manufacturing environment, which must be moved through the health system in a timely manner. It is important to stress that in viewing the patient as metaphorical inventory is not about being disrespectful, rather the opposite, it is underlining that principles that apply in industry can readily be applied in healthcare. A true Lean Manufacturing culture seeks to have inventory valued in the same way we value people, with respect.

The concept of patient time being important in health systems and the reasons why it is so important can be hard to understand as it can be counter-intuitive to logic and professional training. The process for managing patients has its roots in Napoleonic warfare and is now pervasive in all clinical practice. The use of triaging and prioritization scores is viewed as a normal and necessary practice for determining who needs help now and who can wait, and who will never be seen (Allen & Jesus 2012). In war, where demand can rapidly outstrip supply of clinical resources, the use of battlefield triage makes sense; but why does this methodology continue in everyday practice? The underlying assumption of triage is there are not enough resources to treat everyone that seeks our help (see Chapter 35).

However, is this really true for normal population clinical needs? Most health systems are adept at treating the demand on the system; it's just a matter of when they are treated. With the exception of emergency care where critical care demand may impact on resources, most of healthcare demand is stable and predictable. The biggest variable is created by us, the health professionals. By prioritizing demand (triaging), patients are placed into queues based on urgency of need. Every time someone with a higher need enters the system, someone of a lower need is asked to wait longer. This reprioritization may not be transparent to the majority of patients and staff as it happens on waiting lists, where the patient is waiting at home; but what about the patient that comes to the ED who may be categorized as triage 3 and ultimately is assessed as needing surgery? Every time a patient with a higher need comes into the system this patient will be asked to wait longer. In extreme examples, these patients may have been 'nil by mouth' for three to four days, sitting in a hospital bed waiting for access to a treatment room or operating theatre. The patient's condition may have deteriorated and they pick up a hospital-borne infection. This patient initially needed a fifteen-minute surgical procedure, and would have gone home the same day. Instead they spent a week in hospital using up resources that could have been applied in other ways, as well as suffering needless pain, harm and distress. In patients with fractured neck of femur, the correlation between non-medical delays in surgery and increased morbidity and mortality is now well established (Bottle & Aylin 2006, Kalson et al. 2009).

This all too common story highlights how health professionals prioritize patients based on immediate medical need, with the underlying assumption being 'we do not have enough resources to treat everyone right now', so people have to wait. Health systems that are focused on valuing patient time understand this dynamic, and like Toyota realize the potential to release resources from tasks that add no value, such as storing patients that are waiting – waiting on waitlists, in waiting rooms, in ward beds, etc. The mindset of a Lean Thinking health system focuses on the way resources are used, before considering if there are enough resources.

EDs that use 'streaming', for example , split their capacity and resources into two separate patient streams, minors and majors, are focused on applying a key principle of Lean Thinking, First In First Out (FIFO). By streaming patients based on need, it is possible to prioritize patients based on time of arrival rather than just need. In this way patients with relatively minor conditions are processed faster (high turnover) with a focus on creating flow. This is also the theoretical basis of See and Treat (NHS Modernisation Agency 2004, King et al. 2006, Hoskins 2010).

Such an approach requires careful consideration of clinical capacity; understanding how much work is required in each stream, how frequent the work comes in, and having tools to predict future demand and potential changes in demand. Having event plans and buffer resources for those true emergency events that only occur occasionally and are outside normal variation of demand is another key design consideration. This chapter does not address the topic of capacity design in detail.

Creating goals of patient flow

Manufacturing companies create value for their shareholders by reducing the time inventory is in the supply chain; but health systems don't create money by reducing patient time. Or do they?

Average length of stay in hospitals is an important measure of ward capacity performance as the higher the number of days, or indeed hours, a patient spends in the system the more direct resources they consume, such as beds/chairs, rooms, food, laundry, etc. The more time people spend in hospital, the bigger the hospital space and staffing resources required to store and manage patients and their visitors; therefore, the more patient time in the system, the more resources we need to have, either directly managing patient treatment or indirectly managing the patient journey, such as waitlist, etc. The other risk for patients is that the more time they spend in hospital than is essential, the greater their risk of picking up healthcare-acquired infections (HCAI), which not only adds to their length of stay, but more importantly, adds needless harm and suffering. In Europe, HCAIs cause 16 million extra bed days and 37 000 attributable deaths and contribute to an additional 110 000 deaths every year (World Health Organization 2010).

For this and other reasons, access goals are expressed in patient time, e.g., no patient will spend longer than four hours in the ED, no patient will wait longer then 24 hours for an emergency operating theatre; no patient will wait longer than 2 hours for a radiology report.

By defining goals as stated outcomes, we intuitively seek information about why these goals are not achieved. Reasons patients breach the goal are analysed and we seek to modify the conditions that enabled the failure to occur. We seek out information and learning that will help us understand the cause and effect, and strive to find alternative methods that ultimately make it better for all patients.

Does your environment have clear goals? Are these goals based on patient time or quality of outcome; and do they encourage continuous improvement? Without these clear goals how do we know if we are making a difference. Beyond gut feeling, how do we know if we have had a good shift today or a difficult one? While EDs in most countries now have goals or more commonly 'targets', usually four or six hours from ED arrival to discharge or admission/transfer, staff frequently feel they are imposed. They remain an ED and not an organizational health system target, and in reality it's the nurses who make it happen. Even when the target is reached, too often it is with more a sense of relief than achievement. This is not what Lean Thinking and patient flow is about, which is to create sustainable and in many ways self-sustaining systems that continue to focus on improvement not plateauing and ultimately reversing earlier success. Lean Thinking is not about the tools, it's about the thinking that underpins it, and a relentless focus on eliminating everything that does not add value to the patient's experience and safety of care.

Identifying waste in the health system

As indicated above, waste is a significant problem in healthcare and indeed all service and manufacturing industries. As little as 10% of all activities provide value, which may be defined as adding 'value' to the customer, be they a patient or member of staff (Baker & Taylor 2009). Box 42.1 defines and provides numerous examples of waste using the mnemonic

TIMWOODS and underlines that, perhaps counter intuitively, the greatest challenge in healthcare is not necessarily the lack of resources, but the enormous levels of waste that exist.

Linked to waste, and usually masking inventory waste, is an opportunity to create a cleaner, calmer and more pleasant work environment using 5S. Decades old, 5S as translated from Japanese are seiri (sort), seiton (set in order), seiso (shine), seiketsu (standardize), and shitsukie (sustain). 5S is the starting point of any lean improvement process. Combined with the seven wastes it is often misunderstood as being the purpose of Lean Thinking rather than the start of understanding and practicing lean production principles. The reader is encouraged to view Lean Thinking as a series of inter-related tools and methods designed to support continuous patient flow with the least time and resource requirement whilst achieving the highest quality outcome.

Each stage of the 5S process is specifically designed to transform the workplace and set in motion a culture of waste elimination (Hodge & Prenovost 2011). Box 42.2 defines and describes 5S.

Box 42.1

Identifying waste

Waste may be defined as anything other than the minimum amount of equipment, people, materials, space and worker's time which are essential to add value to the product or service. Put in a different way, if it does not add value then it is waste. Waste is a symptom, and not a cause of a problem.

Waste may be described using the mnemonic TIM WOODS standing for:

Transport
Inventory
Motion
Waiting
Over production
Over processing
Defects
Staff under-utilization

Transportation

Moving patients or products that are not required to perform the process:
- Transporting patients to surgery prematurely
- Placing a ED trolley in the hall and constantly having to move it
- Staff looking for patients' notes
- Excessive movement of patients
- People not returning equipment to the correct place

Inventory

Too much work in progress (WIP), work piles, excessive supplies, signature requirements, information:
- Extra or outdated manuals, newsletters or magazines
- Excessive office supplies
- Obsolete supplies, charts, files, and equipment
- Duplicate medications
- Stockpiling supplies of any kind
- Waiting lists

Motion

Unnecessary movement of people, paper, and/or electronic exchanges (see Figure 42.2 spaghetti diagram for example of motion waste):
- Searching for paperwork, case notes, medication charts, and/or medications
- Searching for patients
- Searching for poorly located supplies, e.g., needles and syringes at opposite ends of a clinic room
- Walking to equipment that is not centrally located, e.g., printer
- Searching for files on your computer desktop

Waiting

For people, signatures, equipment and/or information. It is a waste that cannot be recovered as it relates to time:
- Waiting for admissions from ED, ICU, theatres, etc.
- Delays for lab/radiology test results
- Waiting for discharge letters/prescriptions
- Patient back-up due to equipment not working properly
- Delays to fit staff schedules
- Excessive signatures or approvals required

Over-production

Producing more than is needed, or earlier than needed by the next process:
- Putting a patient on a waiting list
- Keeping investigation slots, 'just in case'
- Delivery of samples, drugs, equipment too early or too late
- Entering repetitive information on charts or forms
- Repeating the same questions across multiple assessments
- Ordering more tests or services than what is required by the patient
- Producing reports that no one needs or reads

Continued

Box 42.1—cont'd

Over-processing

Putting more work or effort into the work required by internal or external customers:

- Retesting, for instance, doing same bloods and X-rays on patients who have had them done the day before by GPs
- Completing excessive paperwork
- Entering repetitive form information
- Repeated clerking before the patient is admitted to an inpatient bed
- Copying too many people into email distribution list

Defects or mistakes

Refers to all processing required creating a defect or mistake and the additional work required to correct it:

- Medication errors
- Adverse events, e.g., sentinel events/serious untoward incidents

- Wrong or missing information
- Adverse drug interactions
- Retesting due to inadequate sample, correct information not provided or wrong process earlier
- Out-of-date stock – often due to excess inventory
- Wrong patient, wrong site, wrong dosage, wrong time

Staff under-utilization

A result of not placing people where they can, and will, use their knowledge, skills and abilities to the fullest. It is, perhaps, one of the greatest wastes:

- Basing work on job title not competence
- Inadequate performance management system
- Rosters mismatched to patient workload
- Not using staff ideas

How many examples of waste can you identify where you work?

Box 42.2

Applying 5S in practice

Sort

To get rid of non-essential items, make sure most frequently used items are close by. Sort enables the elimination of clutter and unwanted items that so often make an area feel unsafe, disorganized and hard to work in. Sort is completed in five steps.

Step 1: Ask yourself the following questions

Systematically go around the room/area sorting the clutter and dispose of or quarantine for later recycling/disposal

At the same time red tag items by asking the following key questions:

Is it needed?

How many are needed? Are there too few/too many?

Where should it be located?

Step 2: Identify how often the item is used

Frequently: Items used constantly (once a day, every hour (green tag):

- Keep them at the workstation

Sometimes: Items used often (at least once a week) (yellow tag):

- Keep within easy reach

Occasionally: Items needed from time to time (every few months) (yellow tag):

- Store them at a distance from the workstation

Rarely: Items Never/Not used in the last 6 months (red tag):

- Discard or move to the quarantine area

In practice, most places simply red tag

Step 3: Team review of the red tags

All staff review red tags over a 7-10-day period. Staff add a sticky dot if they disagree along with a comment to explain why.

Step 4: Validate the amount needed

How many of each item is required?

- You may need to validate the amount with a tally chart/ inventory sheet

- Also obtain this information from stores
- Use the ward-based data to help inform your decisions

Set in order

'A place for everything and everything in its place.' It should take no longer than 30 seconds to locate any item. Whilst the red tags are being reviewed by staff, complete the following preparation to help clarify or answer their questions:

Step 1: Preparation

Collect background information related to the red tags as appropriate, e.g.:

- How many items or stock are needed? Relate this to number of patients or times the item will be used before it can be reordered rather than from existing stock levels
- Analyse the task that people use the items for and how people use them in the work area:
  - activity tally sheet
  - spaghetti diagrams (Fig. 42.2)
- Consider 'relationships' with other items, i.e., look at bringing equipment such as catheterization materials together if it is used in the one task and where is the best location for it in relation to its use
- Inform staff of findings to generate discussion and gain agreement

Step two (undertaken by the 5S Team)

Attend to every red tag in the work area:

- Discard those items which are no longer required, e.g., out-of-date stock. Capture cost of these items and/or photograph
- Quarantine those red tag items that are rarely/never used or while deciding on stock levels. Remove these items from the immediate area and store where items can be collected if required

Box 42.2—cont'd

- Establish locations of where things *should* be and reorganize the work area. Remember to arrange items to suit your processes and work flow

NB. Look with fresh eyes – challenge current practices.

Step 3: Establish visual controls with labelling
- Borders
- Home address – where does the item 'live'?
- Identification label on each item
- Shadows

NB. It should be easy to identify if something is missing or not placed back properly.

Shine

Inspecting, maintaining and keeping the work area clean.
- Undertake a basic 'spring clean'
- Create standards to keep it clean
- Create a 5S cleaning plan so everyone knows what needs to be cleaned and who is responsible for ongoing activities to keep the area clean
- Make it an *everyday* task so it becomes a natural part of the work, i.e., incorporate cleaning as part of completing the activity not something done at a later date

Shine ensures that broken equipment and clutter is identified and eliminated. Educate staff of the system to follow for broken equipment:
- Remove equipment from use and attach a label so others will not use it
- Note in detail the issues relating to the equipment failure
- Inform the relevant manager of broken equipment and/or

- Send requisition directly to Clinical Engineering/other department.

Standardize

Making different work areas with the same function the same, i.e., establishing 'standard workflows'

The advantage of this approach is that Units can jointly agree on the order and location of clinical forms, stock items and clinical equipment, etc. This reduces the amount of time spent by staff looking for items and is helpful for staff unfamiliar with that particular unit.
Standardizing is about:
- Agreeing a standard
- Communicating the standard
- Documenting the standard
- Following the standard

Standards can be presented in many forms:
- Photos
- Guidelines and checklists
- Visual aids
- Make standards visual, e.g., labelling, colour-coding, min/max levels, etc.

Without a standard you can slip back.

Sustain: Driving continuous improvement

The final step is to ensure the process is more than just a big clean up.
- The final step to ensure the process is more than just a big clean up and the hardest!
- Naturalizing the activity as part of everyday work
- Monitor the area to ensure compliance - audits
- Continuous improvement (improve the standards)

Moving to flow

Conceptually patient flow is about moving the patient through a series of process steps in a continuous manner with no waits and delays between process steps and within processes.

There are two methods of moving patients through a health system. The first is to create batches of like patients, and the second is to create single patient continuous flow. In the emergency setting continuous flow is the predominant method; while in elective care and acute medical environments, batch processing tends to be the main method, which often as a result impacts on the discharge end of ED activity. A batch is created when patients are grouped together for an event such as assessment clinics, theatre sessions, ward rounds, imaging clinics, etc.

Every time a batch is created we create greater variation for the next process step, which in turn means it is more likely that a queue will form. In this way, we have become immune and accept internal queues and consider a queue as necessary to the efficient management of any health system.

An understanding of Lean manufacturing techniques teaches the impact that batching has on achieving timely outcomes for patients. In the manufacturing environment, the goal is to create 'single piece flow' where product is moved from one process to another process one at a time. In this way the total time it takes to get a product through a series of processes is reduced to the minimum.

In most businesses, including health, batches of products or patients are created. The larger the number of products or patients in the batch the longer it takes to get through a series of processes, and therefore the more likely an expediting process is developed to ensure an outcome is delivered on time. When an expediting process is implemented then effectively we are creating a prioritization process, or another unique product that disrupts the use of resources and flow of activity. Removing batches is the ideal goal, reducing batch sizes is the practical focus. For example reducing the number of patients per ward round will decrease the time it takes to complete tasks from the ward round, which in turn will shrink the time it takes to make the next decision for the patient. The next step is to then increase the frequency at which ward rounds are undertaken to remove any delay for the next set of decisions being made. This concept is about moving to continuous flow by reducing batch sizes; which supports the goal of valuing the patient time.

The goal of continuous flow is impacted on by fluctuations or variation in demand and resources. Lean Thinking seeks to smooth out variation and create consistent flow, from which work can be balanced between resource functions. Workload

Figure 42.2 • Spaghetti diagram of drug round (15 minutes).

balancing concepts are not covered in this chapter, but need to be understood in conjunction with the following section on understanding variation.

Understanding variation in demand

For most patients their General/Primary Practice or ED team is their first contact when a health need arises. The quality of training and knowledge is very similar among these teams; but the knowledge of treatment options available within their health system varies significantly based on the relationships and exposure the teams have within the wider health community. This results in variation between clinicians as to how they refer patients between hospital and specialist care systems.

Variation in demand and capacity is the biggest cause of service failure. Having an understanding of demand variation is critical to developing strategies to eliminate queues such as waitlists for surgery. Many waitlist initiatives, such as cleaning up waitlists to remove demand that cannot be seen, or demand that exceeds capacity, fail because no change has been made to the causes for the waitlists developing in the first place. Waitlists or queues form because there is a mismatch between demand and capacity. Most queues form because there is significant variation in demand and variation in capacity which amplifies the gap between demand and capacity.

Silvester, Steyn and colleagues have studied the impact of variation on health services, and published a series of articles on the art of understanding and managing variation in the health system (Silverster et al. 2004, Walley et al. 2006,

Allder et al. 2011). Their work is based, among other things, on Queuing Theory first developed by Agner Erlang, a Danish engineer in 1909 who worked for the Copenhagen Telephone Exchange to help the telecommunication industry to assign sufficient switchboard capacity to meet the majority of demand (Erlang 1909). Too much capacity would mean money wasted, too little capacity and calls would not connect. Queuing theory is the mathematical study of waiting lines or queues and is widely used in telecommunication, traffic engineering, computing, manufacturing and service industries and health.

The two key messages of this work are: reduce the causes of variation in demand and capacity; and then set capacity to 70–85 % of the variation in demand (see Box 42.3). It is important to note that understanding when to use 70 % versus 85 % is based on how much variation occurs in demand, and is outside the intent of this chapter.

Any process that has allocated capacity based on the average volume, will create a queue. If the size of the ED has been based on average daily volumes, then in theory 50 % of the time demand will exceed capacity; but in reality it will be higher than this as variation of staff availability impacts as well as the variation in demand.

Pulling all the flow elements together

When clinicians lead service improvements, supported by managers, the level of change can be significant and, as important, sustained. One of the authors (Ardagh) co-led a major reform of emergency department's processes, plant and

Box 42.3

Establishing demand and setting capacity

If the number of patients being admitted to the ED daily for minors varies between 75 and 120 then the variation would be 45 a day. Using Erlang's theory:

    80% of the variation (45 x 80%) = 36
    add the minimum daily attendances = 75
    then the optimal patient volume to base capacity = 111

    This means that every day the ED will have capacity to see 111 patients. Note there is a different set of questions to determine when this demand comes in, what mix of patients makes up the 111 patients, and lastly what does capacity for 111 patients mean; i.e., if 12 of these patients are trauma-related then the resources required need will be different to the 54 minor, 15 surgical and 30 medical patients.

Box 42.4

Project RED: improving flow in ED

In 2007, the ED at Christchurch Hospital, New Zealand, was suffering severe overcrowding. In response, three senior ED clinicians conceived and implemented Project RED (Rejuvenating the Emergency Department). The overarching principles of the methodology were that the project was: patient-focused, clinician-led, management-supported, action-orientated, prioritized, transparent and accountable. Principles of Lean Thinking, Theory of Constraint and Six Sigma were well known to the leaders of the project and pervaded its methodology.

The methodology categorized the project into people (staff), plant (space and other physical resources) and processes (ways of doing things). Under these headings an 'Action Plan' was populated with a number of problems and/or actions required to resolve problems. Each of the specific problems/actions was graded according to two dimensions: urgency (U) (based on assessment of degree of risk already present because of the problem); and importance (I) (based on the contribution resolving the problem would make to resolving the risk, and achieving the objectives of the project).

Under these two headings (U and I) each specific action was graded as either high (H), moderate (M), or low (L) level of urgency or importance. Specific actions were further graded under the heading of Time (T), according to whether the intended solution was a 'Quick Fix' (Q), because of an urgent need for solutions, or whether it would take longer to see results – slower to achieve (S) (or somewhere in between – Q/S). Some problems were addressed by more than one action with one addressing an urgent need and the other addressing the longer-term need, and proceeding in parallel.

The first Action Plan was large, consisting of many pages of concentrated actions. Initially, with so many things needing to be done, the project concentrated almost exclusively on the 'HHQs' (High Urgency, High Importance, and Quick to Achieve).

All ED staff were involved in defining the problems, the solutions, and their priorities. As a sub-project a 'Lean Team' was established in the ED, consisting of doctors, nurses, clerical staff, allied health staff and radiographers, to review processes within the ED that might be improved without recourse to people outside the ED. Meanwhile the 'RED team', consisting of ED clinicians and representatives throughout the hospital, worked on wider system issues including access to hospital beds, processes for moving patients out of the ED and pathways for management of specific patient groups.

Waiting times to see a doctor and length of stay in the ED improved significantly (Ardagh et al. 2011), but the more subjective outcomes of reduced ED overcrowding, infrequent corridor placement of patients, and improved staff morale were most appreciated by ED staff. Christchurch ED is currently in the top 1% of hospitals in New Zealand and Australia for shortest ED length of stay.

people. The case study of Project RED (Rejuvenating ED) can be found in Box 42.4.

Conclusion

This chapter has outlined three key concepts:

1. **Identify the goal:** What is the service goal in your department? Is it related to time? And does it challenge us?

2. **Understand value:** what parts of the patient journey are value adding? Can we eliminate the non-value components to a patient's journey, such as the waits and delays or repeated steps? What staff work is necessary and what can be reassigned? Should a staff member be expected to do certain work, have they been trained sufficiently and will it benefit the patient outcome? Understanding value can be challenging as we need to analyse what *we* do and impartially assess is this necessary or is it waste. Identify the seven wastes in the patient's journey and in your work. Seek to eliminate as many wastes as possible.

3. **Create flow:** the ultimate goal is to create health outcomes at the rate the community needs them. Removing batches of patients from the system reduces variation and reduces the time to treatment and discharge. Any demand system will have natural variation, but most variation is created by us through poor understanding of demand and capacity, and poor process. Variation is the cause of most queues in health, and as such is the most misunderstood driver of health outcomes.

These are starting points to understanding how service design can best be improved. On their own they are not sufficient to achieving high performance; but should act as the guiding principles of any redesign of service.

A key concept of any redesign is to involve the whole health system in the design and improvement process; especially on creating flow. To improve ED service delivery requires a combination of partners from across the health system to ensure that the true system constraints are identified and fixed, which may involve the role of ED changing or the management of patient conditions changing (Holden 2011). Focusing the principles of this chapter on departments in isolation to the health system or patient journey across the health system, will limit the success and benefits of Lean methods.

Any process needs to understand demand and workload, and should seek to create standard workflow, or a common understanding of how work is done. Predicting demand has been well proven to work within health (Martin et al. 2010); translating this demand into capacity consumption or workload is a subject beyond the focus of this book. It is, however, a key consideration in designing patient flow, as the goal is to predict demand on the ED by shift and to translate this demand into resources such as beds, doctors, nursing, allied health, etc.

Patient safety, although not discussed in this chapter, is about two key concepts taken from Lean Thinking; error proofing and standard workflow. Creating work methods that minimize errors is the goal of error proofing. Standard workflow is about embedding this method into the work activity so it is the only acceptable way to perform any tasks.

Lastly, any patient journey study and improvement cannot be undertaken without the active involvement of the user of this system. Patient design sessions should be implemented to understand what the experience is like and consciously redesigning to maximize the value and minimize the non-value components of the patient's journey to an appropriate health outcome. The user is very aware of time and places a value on having their time respected. However, the user is very rarely given the opportunity to discuss this aspect of healthcare, as they are grateful to the staff for achieving an outcome, even if it came with long waits and little awareness of what was going to happen next.

The goal of any health system is to create health outcomes in the least possible time, for all. As health professionals we are good at creating clinical outcomes for people, we know how to respond and to treat those in need; but how do we achieve these outcomes and does it respect and value time? Have we created a system and process built around our needs or the patient's needs? Whose time do we value the most? Your time, your staff's time, or the patient's time?

Ultimately, it's a matter of reframing our thinking to a whole systems view, and recognizing that while our time is busy and important, our patients' time is scarce. Designing systems and patient flow around patient time will mean that access becomes less about 'targets' and more about delivering the access standards and quality care that we want for our patients.

References

Allder, S., Walley, P., Silvester, K., 2011. Is follow-up capacity the current NHS bottleneck. Clinical Medicine 11 (1), 31–34.

Allen, M.B., Jesus, J., 2012. Disaster Triage. In: Rosen, P., Adams, J., Derse, A.R., Grossman, S.A., Wolfe, R. (Eds.), Ethical Problems in Emergency Medicine: A Discussion-based Review. J Wiley & Sons, New York.

Ardagh, M., Richardson, S., 2004. Emergency department overcrowding. Can we fix it? The New Zealand Medical Journal 117 (1189), 774–779.

Ardagh, M., Pitchford, A., Esson, A., et al., 2011. Project RED – a succesful methodolgoy for improving emergency department performance. The New Zealand Medical Journal 124 (1344), 54–63.

Baker, M., Taylor, I., 2009. Making Hospitals Work: How to Improve Patient Care While Improving Saving Everyone's Time and Hospitals' Resources. Herefordshire, Lean Enterprise Institute, Ross-on-Wye.

Bottle, A., Aylin, P., 2006. Mortality associated with delay in operation after hip fracture: observational study. British Medical Journal 332, 947–951.

Dolan, B., Hawes, S., 2009. Lean Thinking & Leadership, third ed. NSW Health, Sydney.

Erlang, A.K., 1909. The Theory of Probabilities and Telephone Conversations. Nyt Tidsskrift for Matematik B vol. 20.

Hodge, C., Prenevost, D., 2011. 5S and demand flow: Making room for continuous improvement. In: Wellman, J., Hagan, P., Jeffries, H. (Eds.), Leading the Lean Healthcare Journey: Driving culture Change to Increase Value. Productivity Press, New York.

Holden, R.J., 2011. Lean thinking in emergency departments: a critical review. Annals of Emergency Medicine 57 (3), 265–278.

Hoskins, R., 2010. Is it time to 'Lean' in emergency care? International Emergency Nursing 18 (2), 57–58.

Johnson, E.J., Smith, A.L., Mastro, K.A., 2012. From Toyota to the bedside: Nurses can lead the lean way in health care reform. Nursing Administration Quarterly 36 (3), 234–242.

Kalson, N.S., Mulgrew, E., Cook, G., et al., 2009. Does the number of trauma lists provided affect care and outcome of patients with fractured neck of femur? Annals of the Royal College of Surgeons of Edinburgh 91 (4), 292–295.

Kaplan, G., 2012. Waste not: The management imperative for healthcare. Journal of Healthcare Management 57 (3), 160–166.

King, D.L., Ben-Tovim, B.I., Bassham, J., 2006. Redesigning emergency department patient flows: application of lean thinking to health care. Emergency Medicine Australasia 18, 391–397.

Liker, J., Convis, G.L., 2011. The Toyota Way to Lean Leadership: Achieving and Sustaining Excellence Through Leadership Development. McGraw-Hill, New York.

Liker, J., Franz, J.K., 2011. The Toyota Way to Continuous Improvement: Linking Strategic Excellence to Achieve Superior Performance. McGraw-Hill, New York.

Mahler, S.A., McCartney, J.R., Swoboda, T.K., et al., 2012. The impact of emergency department overcrowding on resident education. The Journal of Emergency Medicine 42 (1), 69–73.

Martin, M., Champion, R., Kinsmand, L., 2010. Mapping patient flow in a regional Australian emergency department: A model driven approach. International Emergency Nursing 19 (2), 75–85.

Millard, W.B., 2011. If Toyota ran ED: What lean management can and cannot do. Annals of Emergency Medicine 57 (6), 13A–17A.

NHS Modernisation Agency, 2004. See and Treat. Modernisation Agency, London.

Richardson, D.B., 2006. Increase in patient mortality at 10 days associated with emergency department overcrowding. Medical Journal of Australia 184 (5), 213–216.

Richardson, D.B., Mountain, D., 2009. Myths v facts in emergency department overcrowding and access block. Medical Journal of Australia 190 (7), 369–374.

Silvester, K., Lendon, R., Bevan, H., et al., 2004. Reducing waiting times in the NHS: is lack of capacity the problem? Clinician in Management 12 (3), 105–109.

Sprivulis, P.C., Da Silva, J.A., Jacobs, I.G., et al., 2006. The association between hospital overcrowding and mortality among patients admitted via Western Australian emergency departments. Medical Journal of Australia 184 (5), 208–212.

Stone, K.B., 2012. Four decades of lean: a systematic literature review. International Journal of Lean Six Sigma 3 (2), 112–132.

Swensen, S.J., Meyer, G.S., Nelson, E.C., et al., 2010. Cottage industry to postindustrial care – the revolution in health care delivery. The New England Journal of Medicine 362 (5) e12(1)–e12(4).

Walley, P., Silvester, K., Steyn, R., 2006. Managing variation in demand: Lessons from the UK National Health Service. Journal of Healthcare Management 51 (5), 309–322.

Westwood, N., James-Moore, N., Cooke, M., 2007. Going Lean in the NHS. NHS Institute for Innovation and Improvement, Warwick.

Womack, J.P., Jones, D.T., 1996. Lean Thinking: Banish waste and Create Wealth in your Organization. Simon & Schuster, New York.

World Health Organization, 2010. The Burden of Healthcare Acquired Infections: A Summary. WHO, Geneva.

Appendix

Normal values

Note: These values may vary. Please check with your local laboratory. Reproduced with permission from Kumar P., Clark M.L., Kumar and Clark's Clinical Medicine, 8th edition, 2012, Elsevier Saunders.

Haematology

Haemoglobin
Male	13.5–17.7 g/dL
Female	11.5–15.5 g/dL

Mean corpuscular haemoglobin (MCH)
27–32 pg

Mean corpuscular haemoglobin concentration (MCHC) 32–36 g/dL

Mean corpuscular volume (MCV) 80–96 fL

Packed cell volume (PCV) or haematocrit
Male	0.40–0.54 L/L
Female	0.37–0.47 L/L

White blood count (WBC) $4–11 \times 10^9$/L

Basophil granulocytes $<0.01–0.1 \times 10^9$/L
Eosinophil granulocytes $0.04–0.4 \times 10^9$/L
Lymphocytes $1.5–4.0 \times 10^9$/L
Monocytes $0.2–0.8 \times 10^9$/L
Neutrophil granulocytes $2.0–7.5 \times 10^9$/L

Platelet count $150–400 \times 10^9$/L

Serum B_{12} 160–925 ng/L (150–675 pmol/L)

Serum folate 4–18 µg/L (5–63 nmol/L)

Red cell folate 160–640 µg/L

Red cell mass
Male	25–35 mL/kg
Female	20–30 mL/kg

Reticulocyte count 0.5–2.5% of red cells
($50–100 \times 10^9$/L)

Erythrocyte sedimentation rate (ESR)
<20 mm in 1 hour

Plasma viscosity 1.5–1.72 mPa.s

Coagulation

Bleeding time (Ivy method) 3–10 min

Activated partial thromboplastin time (APTT)
26–37 s

Prothrombin time 12–16 s

International Normalized Ratio (INR) 1.0–1.3

D-dimer <500 ng/ml

Biochemistry

(serum/plasma in alphabetical order)

Alanine aminotransferase (ALT) <40 U/L

Albumin 35–50 g/L

Alkaline phosphatase 39–117 U/L

Amylase 25–125 U/L

Angiotensin-converting enzymes 10–70 U/L

α1-antitrypsin 2–4 g/L

Aspartate aminotransferase (AST) 12–40 U/L

Bicarbonate 22–30 mmol/L

Bilirubin <17 µmol/L (0.3–1.5 mg/dL)

BNP threshold 100 pg/ml

Caeruloplasmin 1.5–2.9 µmol/L

Calcium 2.20–2.67 mmol/L (8.5–10.5 mg/dL)

Chloride 98–106 mmol/L

Complement
C3 0.75–1.65 g/L
C4 0.20–0.60 g/L

Copper 11–20 µmol/L (100–200 mg/dL)

C-reactive protein <5 mg/L

Creatinine 79–118 µmol/L (0.6–1.5 mg/dL)

Creatine kinase (CPK)
Female	20–170 U/L
Male	30–200 U/L
CK-MB fraction	0–7 U/L (<6% of total activity)

Ferritin
Female	15–200 g/L
Post menopausal	4–230 µg/L
Male	30–300 g/L

α-fetoprotien <10 kU/L

Glucose (fasting) 4.5–5.6 mmol/L (70–110 mg/dL)

Fructosamine up to 285 µmol/L

γ-glutamyl transpeptidase (γ-GT)
Male	11–58 U/L
Female	7–32 U/L

Glycosylated (glycated) haemoglobin (HbA$_{1c}$)
3.7–5.1%

Hydroxybutyric dehydrogenase (HBD)
72–182 U/L

Immunoglobulins (11 years and over)
IgA	0.8–4 g/L
IgG	5.5–16.5 g/L
IgM	0.4–2.0 g/L

Iron 13–32 µmol/L (50–150 µg/dL)

Iron binding capacity (total) (TIBC)
42–80 µmol/L (250–410 µg/dL)

Lactate dehydrogenase 240–480 U/L

Magnesium 0.7–1.1 mmol/L

β2-microglobulin 1.0–3.0 mg/L

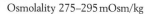

Osmolality 275–295 mOsm/kg

Phosphate 0.8–1.5 mmol/L

Potassium 3.5–5.0 mmol/L

Prostate-specifi c antigen (PSA) up to 4.0 µg/L

Protein (total) 62–77 g/L

Sodium 135–146 mmol/L

Urate 0.18–0.42 mmol/L (3.0–7.0 mg/dL)

Urea 2.5–6.7 mmol/L (8–25 mg/dL)

Vitamin A 0.5–2.01 µmol/L

Vitamin D (seasonal variation) 25-hydroxy
37–200 nmol/L (0.15–0.80 ng/L)
1,25-dihydroxy 60–108 pmol/L
(0.24–0.45 pg/L)

Zinc 11–24 µmol/L

Lipids and lipoproteins

Cholesterol 3.5–6.5 mmol/L
(ideal <5.2 mmol/L)

HDL cholesterol
Male   0.8–1. mol/L
Female   1.0–2.3 mmol/L

LDL cholesterol <4.0 mmol/L (ideal
<2 mmol/L)

Lipids (total) 4.0–10.0 g/L

Lipoproteins
VLDL   0.128–0.645 mmol/L
LDL   1.55–4.4 mmol/L
HDL
  Male   0.70–2.1 mmol/L
HDL
  Female   0.50–1.70 mmol/L

Phospholipid 2.9–5.2 mmol/L

Triglycerides
Male   0.70–2.1 mmol/L
Female   0.50–1.70 mmol/L
TSH   0.3–3.5 mu/L

Blood gases (arterial)

$PaCO_2$ 4.8–6. Pa (36–46 mmHg)

PaO_2 10–13.3 kPa (75–100 mmHg)

[H+] 35–45 nmol/L

pH 7.35–7.45

Bicarbonate 22–26 mmol/L

Urine values

Calcium 7.5 mmol per 24h or less
(<300 mg daily)

Copper 0.2–1.0 µmol per 24h (15–40 mg/24h)

Creatinine 0.13–0.22 mmol per kilogram body
weight, per day

5-hydroxyindole acetic acid (5HIAA)
<47 µmol daily; amounts lower in females
than males

Protein (quantitative) <0.15 g per 24 hours

Sodium 60–180 mmol per 24 hours

Serum/urine values

eGFR
Male   90–140 mL/min
Female   80–125 mL/min

Index

Page numbers followed by an *f* indicates figures; *t*, indicates tables; and *b*, indicates boxes.